Perspectives on Purposeful Activity: Foundation and Future of Occupational Therapy

Perspectives on Purposeful Activity: Foundation and Future of Occupational Therapy

Edited by
Rita P. Fleming Cottrell, MA, OTR

The American Occupational Therapy Association, Inc.
Bethesda, MD

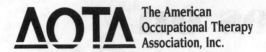

The American
Occupational Therapy
Association, Inc.

Preface

As some readers may know from my previous text (Cottrell, 1993), my entry into the profession of Occupational Therapy (OT) was deeply rooted in my personal life experiences. My life was forever changed and greatly enriched by my brother Kevin and his lifelong struggle with the degenerative neuromuscular disorder, Friederich's Ataxia. I would like to share our personal experience with the profession of OT with you, the reader, for it clearly highlights the meaningfulness of purposeful activity and is a major precipitant for this publication. When I finally discovered the field of OT and its emphasis on the use of purposeful activity to maximize a person's functioning and enhance the quality of life, I was literally thrilled. Here was a profession that finally offered what Kevin and others with disabilities and their families so desperately needed.

I began attending New York University (NYU) to obtain my OT degree and promptly had Kevin's physician refer him to an internationally known hospital for rehabilitation. The initial care he received seemed highly competent. He was given a custom wheelchair and scads of adaptive equipment. As an OT student, I was impressed with these obviously skilled practitioners and their thoughtful interventions.

It quickly became obvious, however, that Kevin's greatest needs were not being addressed by the rehabilitation team. Most striking was the total lack of interest in who Kevin was or what he wanted to achieve. As a 22-year-old living at home with no job or social network, Kevin clearly needed a complete OT evaluation. Unfortunately, his entire evaluation and treatment focused on his motor functioning, wheelchair mobility, and the self-care task of dressing. Increasing his strength and coordination were generally helpful to Kevin, but wheelchair mobility and dressing were difficult and extremely exhausting for him. Also, due to the nature of his illness, it was likely that these difficulties would increase as his disease progressed. Dressing in the morning took a frustrating 2 hours to complete and left him so fatigued that he could not even hold a book to read or put a record on his turntable. This was devastating to Kevin because he was extremely intelligent and craved the fine literature and music that still filled his life with meaningful activity. To be so weary that one can not enjoy life's pleasures is sad; to have this fatigue brought on by an ill-conceived treatment plan is tragic.

My brother's assertive nature fortunately remedied this unproductive situation. He quickly (and loudly!) refused to independently dress himself and threw out all the adaptive equipment. This act of self-preservation was viewed by his Occupational Therapist and rehabilitation team as a clear indication that he was a "difficult, unmotivated" client, and he was promptly discharged from the OT program! (He was "allowed" to continue in the wheelchair clinic, "as needed.") Not once during the time he was involved with this treatment program did anyone fully assess his values, interests, or goals; they assessed only his muscle strength, range of motion, coordination, and sensory awareness.

Fortunately, I was continuing in my OT studies and developing a strong appreciation for the holistic and therapeutic use of purposeful activity. After consulting with Kevin (and using him as a guinea pig for a number of my school assignments) we decided he would become a student at NYU during my senior OT year so that I would be available to assist him with his transition to independent living. His choice of a political science major, as he stated, was one of "pure selfish interest." It would have questionable use after graduation, but Kevin did not care because the progressive nature of his illness precluded employment at that time (this was pre-Americans with Disabilities Act).

Kevin's primary goals for attending college were to be intellectually stimulated, develop a social network, and live independently. He accomplished all of these goals with me serving as a novice Occupational Therapist and adapting his dorm and activities to meet his needs.

Kevin's success was truly a testament to his character, but I often found myself wondering what would have happened to him and his ability to attain his goals if his sister had not been an Occupational Therapist? Why was it so difficult for the Occupational Therapists working with him to see him as a whole person with interests, hopes, and dreams, not just a set of weak, uncoordinated muscles?

Years went by, and Kevin obtained his Bachelor's and Master's degrees from NYU. He accomplished many goals and found meaning in the pursuit of a number of purposeful activities. Yet, the question about the lack of holism in OT practice came back to haunt us many times. To preserve our sibling relationship, I tried not to be Kevin's "OT," and periodically we obtained physician's referrals for OT to meet his needs as his disease progressed.

Although I was always available as the family representative when a new therapist began working with Kevin, I never initially mentioned that I was an Occupational Therapist, for I was serving as a family member not as a professional colleague. Invariably, each Occupational Therapist would competently assess his physical status, prescribe built-up handled utensils, and begin a morning dressing program. Only one Occupational Therapist ever asked Kevin what he did for leisure, work, or meaningful occupation. This same Occupational Therapist was the only one to question if there were any psychosocial needs that were not being met for Kevin and our family. Unfortunately, this gifted Occupational Therapist did not stay in her position for long due to a lack of administrative support for her holistic approaches.

Kevin responded to all the other Occupational Therapists by discontinuing treatment after only a few sessions because, as Kevin said, "it's pointless." This served to perpetuate his reputation as a difficult, unmotivated client. Invariably, I resumed my dual role of "sister–OT," adapting activities and modifying Kevin's environment according to his interests and needs. Again, we asked ourselves in frustration, What if I wasn't an Occupational Therapist? How could our family help Kevin, manage a devastating illness, and maintain quality of life? My OT professional literature was replete with holistic views about the therapeutic use of purposeful activities, but why did we see it in so few of my brother's OT interventions?

Kevin passed away in 1989, but the lessons he taught me about life and the questions he raised about my profession continue to influence me and my teaching. In many respects, I cannot separate my personal self from my professional self because they were intertwined for so long. Therefore, I often use my brother and our life experiences as examples to underscore fundamental OT principles to my students. Thankfully, these examples are generally well-received, for I do not think I could teach OT any other way.

My experience as an OT educator has been rewarding, and many of my students seem to integrate these personal examples about the meaningfulness of purposeful activities into their own professional philosophies. Their work often reflects a strong, holistic view of clients, regardless of diagnosis. When they enter fieldwork, however, they are often told, "Forget everything you learned in school; this is the real world, and we don't have time for activities."

If OT doesn't have time for activities who will? Yes, today's health care system is demanding. Length of stays have decreased and treatment is reimbursement driven. If we meet these challenges by denying what is fundamentally OT and eliminate the use of purposeful activity, how will we survive as a unique profession? As Gail Fidler, OTR, FAOTA (personal communication, April 22, 1994) asks, do we become "pseudo–Physical Therapists" and "pseudo–Social Workers," or do we return to authentic OT with its emphasis on meaningful, purposeful, and productive activity? I strongly vote for the latter alternative, and I believe Kevin would have wholeheartedly agreed.

Recently, the American Occupational Therapy Association (AOTA) adopted a definition of OT practice to be used as a guide in state regulation laws (AOTA, 1994). (See Appendix A for the complete definition.) It is reassuring to note that this definition emphasizes the use of purposeful activity for health promotion, injury prevention, and improvement of function. Even more heartening are the current health care trends that emphasize functional outcomes, community-based treatment, and wellness and prevention programs. All of these trends—and the preference for a generalized, holistic approach to evaluation and treatment rather than a specialized, narrow approach—are highly congruent with OT's philosophical base and activity heritage (see Appendix B for the official AOTA statement on The Philosophical Base of Occupational Therapy). I truly believe that if we maintain our holistic philosophy and continue to use purposeful activity as our primary tool of practice, we will become leaders in the health care system of the next millennium. I was encouraged when my research for this text uncovered substantial literature supportive of this belief.

This text attempts to provide a philosophical, yet practical, link between OT's heritage, current clinical realities, and future practice. To complete this publication, I have conducted an extensive literature review to gather the "best of the best" in the OT professional literature. Original OT literary classics along with thought provoking recent works were selected to provide the reader with a solid theoretical foundation and basic tools of practice to meet the challenge of practicing authentic OT in a changing health care system. This compilation seeks to save OT educators, clinicians, and students from time-consuming literature searches and cumbersome copyright release procedures, thereby increasing the time and energy available for thoughtful study and dynamic discussion of these vital topics.

I would also encourage readers to join the American Occupational Therapy Association's (AOTA's) Special Interest Sections and to subscribe to *Activities, Adaptation and Aging, Physical and Occupational Therapy in Geriatrics, Physical and Occupational Therapy in Pediatrics* and/or *Occupational Therapy in Mental Health*. These resources are invaluable in increasing knowledge of current occupational therapy practice in today's health care system. Many of the chapters in this text are compiled from these superb resources and clearly reflect a proactive stance towards the use of purposeful activities in OT practice.

This text begins with a comprehensive review of the historical and philosophical foundations of purposeful activity and continues with an exploration of the environmental contexts of purposeful activities. Developmental aspects of purposeful activities and the impact of the therapeutic relationship on facilitating engagement in purposeful activities are then analyzed. Tools of practice, including media, methods, and strategies for using purposeful activities in clinical interventions, and research on the use of purposeful activity in practice are also presented. An analysis of current realities and future directions for purposeful activity in OT closes the text.

Appendixes include AOTA's definition of OT and position papers on the core values and attitudes of OT, OT and the Americans with Disabilities Act, purposeful activity, and physical agent modalities. Fidler's Lifestyle Performance Profile and an address in honor of Eleanor Clarke Slagle are also included. The 3rd edition of "Uniform Terminology for Occupational Therapy," activity analysis forms, a sample activity analysis, activity resource lists, and references complete the publication. Each section is preceded by an introduction that raises topical questions to challenge the reader's perceptions and to enhance integration of personal issues with professional knowledge, skills, and attitudes.

Although articles for the chapters were judiciously selected from quality professional juried publications to accurately reflect the depth and breadth of the use of purposeful activity in OT, there are realistic parameters to the text. Frames of reference and activity group process were intentionally omitted since there are a number of excellent comprehensive publications already available on these topics. Readers are urged to use the reference lists at the end of each chapter and in the appendix to further study topics of interest. Readers should also note that because all the chapters are reprinted from other sources covering a broad time period, they vary in style and some approaches may seem dated.

However, the overall content of these chapters still provides significant, relevant information worthy of the reader's thoughtful perusal. (Please see the Note to Readers on page *vi* and refer to references for more current information).

While some individuals may continue to question the applicability of purposeful activity to current and future clinical practice, it is my hope that the quality of the chapters in this text will foster an increased awareness and a renewed appreciation of the relevance, variety, and richness of the skilled use of purposeful activity in all areas of OT practice. This compilation strives to reaffirm our professional heritage and validate OT's unique contributions to persons with disabilities and their families. Employing the philosophies and practices described in this text will support the reader's development of a professional identity rooted in the art and science of using purposeful activity. This well-grounded professional identity will enable OT practitioners to clearly articulate their unique role in the health care system of the next millennium while using meaningful therapeutic activities to enhance the quality of life for clients and their families. Based upon my life experience, this is the true purpose of Occupational Therapy and the gift my brother and I embraced many years ago.

References

American Occupational Therapy Association. (1994). Definition of Occupational Therapy Practice for state regulation. *American Journal of Occupational Therapy, 48*, 1072–1073. (Reprinted as Appendix A).

Cottrell, R.P. (Ed). (1993). *Psychosocial occupational therapy. Proactive approaches.* Rockville, MD: American Occupational Therapy Association.

Dedication

To my brother, Kevin Michael Fleming. As my guardian angel, Kevin still guides me in my daily life and teachings, helping me remain focused on the vital need for a holistic therapeutic approach, regardless of diagnosis. His memory continually reaffirms my commitment to the use of meaningful occupation and purposeful activities in Occupational Therapy.

To all past, current, and future OT students, practitioners, and scholars who dare to withstand the pressure to treat just a part of a person, respectfully considering all aspects of the individual, physically, psychologically, socially, and spiritually by using meaningful occupation and purposeful activities to enhance the quality of life for persons with disablities, and their families.

Acknowledgments

I would like to thank my best friend and husband, Michael, who lovingly nurtures my soul and performed many additional purposeful activities while I completed this text, ensuring our home was still maintained, our family well-nourished, and time was available to sustain role balance; my son Christopher Michael, a budding actor, PR man, chef, goalie, storm tracker, skier, songwriter, woodsman, and joy of my life, who enlivens my spirit and adds laughter to my day as he pursues his many meaningful occupations; and Henry Zelin, who patiently compensated for my computer illiteracy to competently type this manuscript.

Table of Contents

Section II: The Environmental Contexts of Purposeful Activity: Physical, Sociocultural, and Temporal Influences on Activity

Section III: The Developmental Continuum: Purposeful Activities across the Lifespan

Section IV: The Therapeutic Relationship: Facilitating Engagement in Purposeful Activity

Section V: Tools of Practice: Media, Methods, and Strategies for Clinical Interventions

Section VI: Research: Applied Scientific Inquiry on Purposeful Activity and Occupational Therapy

Section VII: Current Realities and Future Directions for Purposeful Activity in Occupational Therapy

Note to Reader

Due to the need to comply with copyright laws, all of the chapters in this text were reprinted as originally published—while editorial efforts were made to ensure grammatical accuracy and gender-neutral language, readers will note some inconsistencies in several chapters. These chapters contain relevant content, but their formats do not always adhere to the American Occupational Therapy Association's (AOTA's) publication guidelines. Areas of concern include various styles of referencing and usage, non-gender-neutral language, and potentially dated (or nonexistent) author credentials. Readers are advised to review all chapters critically—recognizing the strengths of each while acknowledging their limitations according to current professional standards.

Section I

Occupational Therapy's Heritage: Historical and Philosophical Foundations of Purposeful Activity

Introduction

Purposeful activity has been firmly rooted in Occupational Therapy (OT) since the profession's inception in the early 1900s (Quiroga, 1995). The founders of OT emphasized the therapeutic value of activity throughout their writings and in their work, providing us with a rich heritage and a strong foundation for the use of purposeful activity in OT practice.

This section begins with five chapters that explore OT's philosophical base by presenting scholarly writings that examine the lives, times, values, and philosophies that influenced the development of our profession. Subsequent chapters by esteemed OT scholars build on this historical base, presenting solid philosophical and practical arguments that support the therapeutic application of purposeful activity. Many of these chapters are considered classics in the field, and it is an honor to include them in this text. It is hoped that thoughtful exploration of the richness of OT's heritage and a critical review of the dynamic, proactive thinking of our profession's past and current scholars will foster an appreciation for these timeless principles and develop an allegiance to the use of purposeful activity in current and evolving OT practice.

In Chapter 1, Peloquin begins this historical review by analyzing the writings of the founders of the National Society for the Promotion of Occupational Therapy. Her comprehensive literature review provides the reader with an insightful inquiry into the contemporary historical events and the shared beliefs that influenced the founders of OT and resulted in the development of our multifaceted profession. She discusses the founders' understanding of service with respect to three primary agents: the patient, the therapist, and the occupation. The interrelationships between these agents is emphasized throughout the chapter. The personal narratives, life stories, and unique perspectives of the founders are explored and supported by numerous quotes from their original writings, enabling the reader to share their vision for a profession rooted in care and function.

This personalization of the early years of OT is continued in Chapter 2, which presents Adolph Meyer's landmark speech to the attendees of the Fifth Annual Meeting of the National Society for the Promotion of Occupational Therapy, in 1921. Although the profession was very young at that time, and many years have since passed, the reader will be struck by the timelessness of Meyer's "Philosophy of Occupation Therapy." His call for the individuation of activity based on the personal interests and the natural capacities of the patient and the provision of opportunities for meaningful occupation, rather than the use of predetermined treatment prescriptions, has remained relevant despite the passage of many decades. Meyer's presentation traces the development of the therapeutic use of occupation from the 1890s to his time, and it looks toward a future in which all individuals will be able to engage in gratifying activity to productively use their time.

The next three chapters expand on this historical review by exploring two movements that began in the 18th century and greatly influenced the founders of OT in the early 19th century. The arts and crafts movement provided early occupational therapists with a theoretical base for the use of arts and crafts as treatment activities. In Chapter 3, Schemm explores the similarities and differences in the ideas and beliefs of the proponents of the arts and crafts movement and the founders of OT. She describes the historical, philosophical, political, and socioeconomic issues that lead to ideological conflicts within the field of OT, underscoring the overwhelming influence the environment has on the development of a profession.

The tremendous impact that historical contexts and societal trends have on a profession's development is further analyzed in Chapter 4 by Peloquin. Her presentation describes the moral treatment movement, its characteristics, and the course of its practice, detailing the successful therapeutic use of occupation within the asylums. The societal changes, ideological conflicts, and lack of leadership, which ultimately led to the demise of this movement, are clearly traced. The resulting inequity in treatment, the decrease in quality of care, and the often total lack of care are carefully considered, leading Peloquin to call for occupational therapists to reaffirm a humanistic view of practice that is committed to the effective use of occupation.

The exploration of the influence of moral treatment on the development of the profession of OT is continued by Bing in Chapter 5, who postulates that OT is a retitled form of moral treatment. He supports this viewpoint with a comprehensive analysis of the beginnings of moral treatment in Europe, its expansion in the United States, its disappearance in the last quarter of the 19th century, and its reemergence in the early 20th century as OT. The activity-based principles and definitions of OT identified by the founders of the profession are reviewed. This activity heritage is elaborated upon in Bing's presentation of the second generation of Occupational Therapists, as exemplified in the life and work of Beatrice Wade. This chapter is replete with personal vignettes and quotes from the founders of OT and Beatrice Wade, offering a unique perspective on the rich history of OT. Bing ends his historical analysis with a thoughtful summation of his views on the lessons current occupational therapists can learn from the first and second generation of our profession's leaders.

Chapter 6, written by a leader of the third generation of occupational therapists, Mary Reilly, is widely recognized in the field as a literary classic and contains perhaps the most widely quoted passage in OT literature. Her discourse seeking to answer the question, "Is occupational therapy a vital and unique service for medicine to support and for society to reward?" is answered with a resounding "yes" in the form of her hypothesis, "That man, through the use of his hands as they are energized by mind and will, can influence the state of his own health." Although over 35 years have passed since Reilly presented this lecture, her views on OT's unique body of knowledge and her concerns for future directions in the field remain relevant to this day.

Another classic in OT literature is presented in Chapter 7 by Fidler and Fidler, whose unique perspectives on OT remain pertinent today. Their exploration of sociological and psychological theoretical constructs provides a basis for a definition of "doing" and a foundation for the use of "doing" in OT. They define "doing" as purposeful action that enables one to become humanized. Prescribing interventions based on doing to develop performance skills, maintain health, and prevent

pathology is strongly advocated by Fidler and Fidler. Their discussion provides the reader with an understanding of the humanness of purposeful activity and its vital role in the development of adaptation.

The inherent value of doing and the impact of purposeful activity on adaptation is discussed further in Chapter 8 by King, who proposes adaptation as a unifying concept for OT. King recognizes the diverse areas of OT practice and the growth of specialization within the field. However, she also expresses concern that the lack of a shared theoretical framework for all OT practice will result in the increased fragmentation of our profession. Therefore, she offers adaptation as the foundation for a common theoretical structure for OT. She examines the characteristics of adaptation and analyzes developmental learning as an adaptive process. The maladaptive effects of sensory deprivation; the use of activity as an adaptive response to stress; and the role of OT in health maintenance, disease prevention, and health restoration are also explored. King acknowledges that other practice models can be developed for OT, and she calls on the reader to consider alternative models or to contribute to the construction of a science of adaptation.

The relevance of theory to OT practice is strongly emphasized in Chapter 9 by Williams, who begins with a clear discussion of the structure, development, and verification of theory. He defines terms and analyzes the nature of a profession's theoretical foundations. The means of relating theoretical systems to clinical practice, by use of the linking structures of practice theories and frames of reference, are explored. Several neurobehavioral frames of reference are specifically discussed, and concern is voiced that the application of these frames of reference in clinical practice is frequently incongruent with the philosophical base of OT. Williams calls for neurobehavioral frames of reference that reflect OT's heritage by actively engaging the individual in functional tasks and life roles through the use of purposeful activities. He clearly describes his clinic's critical review of their neurobehavioral treatment sessions and the year-long efforts they made to integrate the use of purposeful activity with neurobehavioral techniques. The success of this integrated approach clearly reflects the unique perspective of OT. Williams concludes with a realistic discussion of the relationship between theory and research in clinical practice and emphasizes the value of clarifying one's theoretical base to ensure meaningful, effective interventions.

Clear, well-developed practice models proposed by prominent OT scholars are presented in the next two chapters, providing the reader with two distinct theoretical frameworks useful in clarifying the link between theory and practice. Although these models differ in content, structure, and format, both emphasize the use of meaningful, purposeful activity or occupation in OT intervention. A complete presentation of practice models and frames of reference is beyond the scope of this text. Therefore, the reader is referred to Appendix L for a listing of several excellent references on frames of reference and models of practice.

In Chapter 10, Trombly's Model of Occupational Functioning conceptualizes occupational performance as a descending hierarchy of roles, tasks, activities, abilities, and capacities. Each component of her model is clearly defined and supported by pertinent examples and relevant research. Trombly distinguishes occupation as a treatment end goal from occupation as a means to remedial impairment, but she emphasizes that both are therapeutic if purposeful and meaningful. She hypothesizes that purposefulness organizes behavior, and meaningfulness motivates behavior; she then analyzes their relationships to both forms of therapeutic occupation. She recognizes that these aspects of occupation require exploration, clarification, and interpretation through research and proposes a number of highly relevant research questions. A comprehensive literature review of research related to the use of occupation in the motor domain is presented, however, it is apparent that more definitive research is needed. Trombly expresses her hope that her model will spark an explosion of research to further clarify and strengthen the link between occupation and therapeutic outcomes.

The relationships among meaningful interventions, goal attainment, and research are also explored in Chapter 11 by Fidler, who presents her Life Style Performance Model. This practice model offers an organized, holistic framework for knowing and understanding a person's lifestyle and activity repertoire within the context of his or her human and nonhuman environment. The functions, underlying principles, and major hypotheses of this model are reviewed, providing a basis for conceptualizing the interrelatedness of person, environment, activity profile, and quality of life. Fidler emphasizes the assessment of an individual's interests, capacities, patterns of daily living, and the analysis of potential activities and environmental contexts before defining and prioritizing intervention. This assessment ensures that the plan of OT treatment is motivating to the individual and pertinent to his or her lifestyle. She poses five fundamental questions on whose answers OT intervention can be planned and implemented. Four primary interrelated domains of performance that are relevant throughout the life span are also described. According to Fidler, the use of personally, socially, and culturally relevant activities that are designed to create and enhance the facilitative elements of the environment provides congruence among the person, activity, and environment, thereby increasing treatment efficacy and enhancing quality of life.

The inherent worth of purposeful activity and meaningful occupation is emphasized by all of the authors in this section, from our profession's founders to our contemporary scholars. The historical writings, philosophical foundations, and theoretical frameworks presented here provide a number of definitions of purposeful activity and occupation. This section concludes with Chapter 12 by Brienes, which attempts to define purposeful activity. Brienes acknowledges the ongoing debate in the field regarding the definition of purposeful activity as it relates to OT roles and tools of practice. Her definition is offered here as one way to view purposeful activity with the understanding that there are different definitions in the professional literature. The reader is referred to Appendix L for a listing of references that explore and contrast definitions of purposeful activity and occupation. Although some may argue strongly for one definition, others will appreciate a diversity of viewpoints. As evidenced by this section, there is a wealth of scholarly writings on the foundations of purposeful activity in our professional literature, with numerous definitions offered. A critical analysis of this professional literature will facilitate the reader's ability to develop a personal definition of purposeful activity that is congruent with the unique heritage of OT.

Questions to Consider

1. What were the historical trends, sociocultural issues, and sociopolitical forces influencing the development of the profession of OT? How did ideological conflicts influence this development? Do these trends, issues, forces, and conflicts continue to influence current OT practice?

2. What were the beliefs, values, and philosophies of the founders of OT? What are common views about the use of purposeful activity in OT that have stood the "test of time"?

3. Explain the relevance of theory to OT practice. How do frames of reference and practice models help link theory to practice? What key theoretical principles guide the use of purposeful activity in OT evaluation and intervention?

4. How would you define purposeful activity? How would you explain the therapeutic value of purposeful activity to consumers, families, and health care professionals?

Reference

Quiroga, V.A. (1995). *Occupational Therapy: The First 30 Years— 1900 to 1930.* Bethesda, MD: American Occupational Therapy Association.

Chapter 1

Occupational Therapy Service: Individual and Collective Understandings of the Founders

Suzanne M. Peloquin, PhD, OTR

This chapter was previously published as Looking back: Occupational Therapy Service: Individual and collective understandings of the founders, Part 1. *American Journal of Occupational Therapy, 45,* 352–360 and as Looking back: Individual and collective understandings of the founders, Part 2. *American Journal of Occupational Therapy, 45,* 733–744. Copyright © 1991, American Occupational Therapy Association.

Florence Stattel (1977) pleaded for a comprehensive history of occupational therapy, because such a history would provide perspective for contemporary understanding and future growth. Her rationale was also that occupational therapists might, in formulating a history, seize the awareness that occupational therapy has "extended an idea" in the universe (p. 649). The present paper is an attempt to explore those beliefs held by occupational therapists in the earliest years of our history and to examine the personal understandings of service found in the occupational therapy literature between 1917 and 1930. This seems an apt place to start. Any idea, including the idea of service, rarely exists in the abstract, but emerges instead from the larger context of the understandings and experiences of the person who holds it.

Sutton wrote in 1925 that "service is, or should be, one of the stellar ideals of occupational therapy" (p. 54). In 1972, a special task force of the American Occupational Therapy Association (AOTA) issued a comprehensive definition of occupational therapy that included the statement, "occupational therapy provides service" (AOTA, 1972, p. 204). An early characterization of the occupational therapist was that "she must have a deep desire to serve" (Northrup, 1928, p. 267). Because service is an idea articulated by most professions, some unique character of service must account for occupational therapy's emergence as a profession distinct from others. The ideas held individually and collectively by our founders reflect contemporary values and norms, forces that shaped their understanding of how they might serve others in a unique manner.

An Idea Extended

The service particular to occupational therapy involves three primary agents: patient, therapist, and occupation. These agents interrelate; forces across time shape both their nature and their relationships. The character and quality of service provided to any person thus exist within a particular context shaped by contemporary trends. Our current understanding of practice acknowledges distinct patient-therapist-occupation interrelationships as well as the trends that shape them. If, for example, one considers a hand therapist in private practice, the image of service in this context differs from that of a therapist treating patients in an acute psychiatric setting, even though both situations include the patient, the occupational therapist, and some form of occupation. The characteristics of a therapist that shape the type of service provided include his or her personal traits, education and experiences, frame of reference regarding occupation and patient rapport, understanding of professional roles, position and authority held within the treatment environment, and degree of commitment to standards within the particular agency. Similarly, the particular patient and his or her occupational performance strengths and problems, expectations for service, goals for treatment, attitude toward therapy, and environmental circumstances shape the service received. The particular occupations selected from self-care, work, or play-related arenas, whether targeting functional increases in cognitive, psychological, neuromuscular, sensory integrative, or social interactional performances, also characterize the service provided. There can be many pictures of occupational therapy practice. Although no single picture of service exists, invariant features enable us to identify a practice as occupational therapy. The existence today of many forms of occupational service reflects the multifaceted yet singular understanding of our founders in 1917.

Historical inquiry discloses the invariant features of a service that may persist while also assuming different forms across time. A seminal idea can be extended while also being shaped in time. My particular inquiry aims to identify the founders' characterizations of the relationships among patient, therapist, and occupation, in order to better grasp their understanding of service in the earliest decades of occupational therapy practice. My search has constituted an attempt to "search out those unusual roots carefully planted and nurtured by our forebears" (Bing, 1983, p. 800). These roots intertwine with major forces that shaped early service: hospital treatment, industry, and war. Additional societal trends toward science, education, sex stereotyping, and professionalization nourished the subsoil that shaped our growth.

I hope that this inquiry will help therapists to estimate the value of our current reflections about caring. Yerxa (1980), for example, said that "caring means being true to our humanistic and functional heritage with its concern for the quality of daily living of our patients" (p. 534). She appealed for our allegiance to that heritage. Johnson (1981) (see Chapter 63) later cautioned against current forces that shape occupational therapy service into a form that might embarrass our forebears: "Part of

the price we now pay is that our directions frequently seem to be predicated not upon the observations and concepts of our founders but upon external sources and influences" (p. 593). Many of us seem in this decade to regret the passing of a time in which we believe that it was somehow easier to care, to be humane, and to resist the forces that shape practice and service. The present inquiry aims to retrieve that time and to explore its influence in shaping the particular brand of caring that constituted occupational therapy.

Because the emphasis of this search is on the personal understandings that our founders had of the best way to serve in their time, a significant portion of the literature reviewed considers persons, personal stories, and personal philosophies. It seems apt to explore such narratives when researching a profession whose early aim was "not in the making of a product, but in the making of a MAN, of a man stronger physically, mentally, and spiritually than he was before" (Barton, 1920, p. 308). I also think it essential to consider, at least in broad strokes, what kind of world could want, shape, and nurture a service designed to reconstruct persons.

Crafting a New Service: Founders and Near Founders

In 1917, six persons gathered to found the National Society for the Promotion of Occupational Therapy: those attending the meeting at George Edward Barton and Dr. William Rush Dunton, Jr.'s, invitation were Thomas B. Kidner, Isabel G. Newton, Susan C. Johnson, and Eleanor Clarke Slagle. Because Susan Elizabeth Tracy was teaching a new course in occupation and could not attend, she was listed as an incorporator instead of a founder. Because Barton did not accept Dunton's nomination of Dr. Herbert Hall, Hall was not included as a member of the founding group, but became an early member and later president of the Society. Tracy and Hall might thus be called *near founders*. Johnson (1981) (see Chapter 63) described the group:

> Our founders were physicians, architects, social workers, secretaries, teachers of arts and crafts, nurses.... Each brought a different perspective and came from a unique background and orientation, yet each observed the effects of occupation in their individual environments and believed in its curative powers. (p. 592)

Johnson (1981) characterized the group as a gathering of specialists who supported the wide use of occupation as a curative service. Each founder shared life in the world of 1917, a world quite different from that which we experience today. Dr. Sidney Licht (1967) permitted a colorful glimpse of contemporary self-care, work, and play in that era when writing about the founding of occupational therapy.

In 1917 there was neither television nor radio. For the first time that year, color movies ran in commercial theaters in New York. Admission to local movie houses was a dime for an adult and a nickel for a child. Children were not admitted unless accompanied by an adult. A loaf of bread cost a nickel; the annual cost of living for a family of four was $1,843. Dollar bills were longer and wider and obviously stretched farther. Homogenized milk had not been invented, but milk was delivered to homes 7 days a week by horse-drawn wagons. Neither electric refrigeration nor supermarkets existed. Oranges were prized Christmas stocking fillers, rare treats in winter. It cost a penny to send a postcard, a penny more to mail a letter. Most people who had telephones had party lines. There were no commercial flights. Ford's touring car sold for $360. There were no traffic lights and no parking meters; 729 people were killed in automobile accidents during that year. Street lamps were turned on each night by persons called *lamplighters*. In that year, Binet developed the IQ test; Dewey endorsed new educational techniques that proposed learning by doing. Sanitation was not particularly good. Most cities had a hospital for contagious diseases, and because antibiotics were nonexistent, a large part of medical practice was concerned with infection. A man with a bilateral inguinal herniorrhaphy was immobilized for 20 days. Houses were heated with wood or coal. The United States would enter its first world war, known then as the Great War. Though perhaps simpler because of fewer inventions and options, occupational tasks in 1917 were not easy by today's standards.

Beyond these daily exigencies, other societal concerns and trends greatly influenced the ideas of the founders of the National Society for the Promotion of Occupational Therapy. The major forces that shaped their perceptions of the need for occupational therapy emerge from their respective narratives; these forces include industry, war, educational reforms, and the nature of hospital care. A brief overview may prove helpful.

A recently industrialized society was increasingly aware of the adverse psychological and physical effects of mechanization. Arts-and-crafts societies emerged in a number of cities to restore pride in individual and quality workmanship against the increasing monotony and vanishing autonomy of factory work. Powerful machines maimed bodies at an alarming rate. Social workers such as Jane Addams of Chicago's Hull House recognized the negative effects of both industrialization and city living among poor persons and offered educational, recreational, and community-enhancing activities in neighborhood settlement houses. Advocates for reform in education, industry, and treatment of the ill used settlement houses as centers for generating changes in living and working conditions. Efficiency engineers such as Frank and Lillian Gilbreth promoted techniques to make persons and machines more effective on the job and at home. The crippling effects of war on neighboring countries and the ways in which their governments reconstructed their war heroes prompted a readiness in the United States to do the same. Hospital care was scrutinized. Inhumane conditions in state hospitals for "the insane" received public exposure, and the National Committee for Mental Hygiene sought to promote better treatment for institutionalized patients. Doctors, nurses, and patients increasingly criticized the failure of general hospitals to prepare patients for a society that valued effectiveness and productivity. Nurses and social workers strove for professional respect and credibility, often using contemporary pleas for reform as catalysts for changes in their practices. Each of our founder's conclusions about the kind of service that would be most helpful connects back to personal experiences with and personal understanding of these broader issues.

Changes occurring within medical settings during these early years seem particularly important, because much of the expressed need for occupation as therapy came from hospital workers:

This was a time of significant medical advance. Medicine moved from a discipline concerned solely with treatment to one involved with preventing the occurrence and the recurrence of disease. However, as such infectious and epidemic illnesses as typhoid and small pox were being eliminated, new medical problems, which were to result in an increased number of chronic patients, became apparent. These included heart disease, arteriosclerosis, and diabetes. The number of the institutionalized mentally ill increased five times.... As more people were able to survive illness and accident due to rapid medical advances, more were left with lasting impairments. The war, a severe polio epidemic in 1916, industrial accidents, and the widening use of the automobile all contributed to the need for new methods of treating residual disabilities. (Woodside, 1971, p. 226)

Each founder of the Society drew a common understanding from this larger context of 1917: the right occupation might in some way help. Exploration of each founder's unique view of patients, therapists, and occupations clarifies the manner in which occupational therapy became multifaceted yet rooted in one basic idea.

George Edward Barton

George Edward Barton was a successful architect who originated the idea of founding a society to promote occupation as therapy. Because his background included a year's work in nursing and some studies in medicine, he had a working knowledge of medical matters (Staff, 1923). He was also knowledgeable of the patient's point of view. He spent a year in a sanitarium for treatment of tuberculosis and had recurrent attacks of the disease.

Two of his toes, which had frozen and become gangrenous, were amputated after a trip during which he was investigating famine among farmers for the governor of Colorado. After his surgery he developed a hysterical paralysis on the left side of his body. He was sent to Clifton Springs Sanitarium in New York, where he counseled with the Reverend Dr. Elwood Worcester and developed an interest in occupation as therapy. Aware that he could not return to architecture, he determined to spend the rest of his life "devoted to the subject of reclamation of the sick and crippled" (Barton, 1968, p. 340). He bought a small old house and barn and named them Consolation House, where in 1914 he opened a school, a workshop, and a vocational bureau for convalescents (Barton, 1914; Licht, 1967). Barton hired a secretary, Isabel G. Newton, who helped him in his work and whom he later married. She described his early efforts: "Paralyzed in his left side, he could scarcely do more than stand. With no motion possible in his left hand and arm, he used his own body as a clinic to work out the problem of rehabilitation himself" (Barton, 1968, p. 342). She remembered that his medical friends, appreciating his results, sent patients to him for help. These referrals launched his "first experimental practice of occupational therapy" (p. 342). In 1917, Barton invited Newton to become one of the founders of the Society. She agreed and became its first secretary. She worked alongside her husband, teaching occupation to convalescents until his death in 1923.

Barton's early views on the subject of occupational therapy are of considerable interest. In his earliest writings he called the therapy "occupational nursing" (Barton, 1915a, p. 335). He regretted that the work was "unfortunately called Occupational Therapy ... because the subject has so very many different sides that most people ... have such difficulty in making out what it is all about anyhow" (Barton, 1920, p. 304). He viewed occupational therapy's goal as the making of a person, that is, a productive individual. He was critical of the hospital's restricted role in treatment:

> To get the patient well has been the aim and the end of it all.... But if the hospital world expands, as the public is demanding that it shall expand, so that to merely get the patient well is not the whole thing, but to get him well for something. (Barton, 1920, p. 305)

Barton (1920) argued that a man "is not a normal man just because his temperature is 98.6. A man is not a *normal* man until he is able to provide for himself" (p. 306). He believed that the hospital had lost a vital opportunity by becoming focused on the X ray and laboratory, thereby turning out "paupers instead of producers" (Barton, 1920, p. 307). He maintained that a patient fared better during the convalescent period with something to do (Barton, 1920). Occupying his or her

mind with something worthwhile enabled that patient to sleep and heal at night. Barton thought that worthwhile activity meant activity with earning power. He reminded his audiences that concern over the inability to earn often impelled a patient to seize a nurse and say, "In God's Name, tell me what I'm going to do!" (Barton, 1915a, p. 335).

Barton (1920) believed that a "proper occupation" promoted physical improvement, "clarified and strengthened the mind," and could become "the basis or the corollary of a new life upon recovery" (p. 307). He believed that a person's spirit could resurrect in "greater strength and purity" to triumph over disability and despair (Barton, 1920, p. 308). He therefore chose a phoenix rising from the flames as the emblem for Consolation House. Barton recommended an extensive occupational diagnosis to include consideration of the patient's education and inclinations; present status, habits, and ambitions; and expectations. The diagnosis would suggest the prescription: the proper occupation in the proportion necessary to produce the desired physical, mental, and spiritual results. Barton believed that any prescription from *materia medica* (as cited by Barton, 1915b) could be translated into occupational terms. He explained that if medicine prescribed benzol to a patient as a leukotoxin for leukemia, occupational therapy would put the same patient to work in a canning factory where the fumes of hot benzine would "keep her in good health" while she supported herself (Barton, 1915b, p. 139). Each human activity could be associated with a physical effect. Barton's unique belief that every occupation had an effect analogous to that of a drug distanced some physicians and resulted in his being considered an extremist (Licht, 1948).

Barton thought that the teacher of the occupation must monitor its therapeutic effects. He called for scientific reeducation with an argument from Frank Gilbreth: "The teaching element is more important in this new phase of adequate placement than it has ever been before, because in every case a new or changed worker must be made useful, self-supporting, and interested" (as cited by Barton, 1920, p. 306). Gilbreth was himself elected to honorary membership in the Society at its founding meeting (Dunton, 1967).

Barton believed strongly that the teacher of occupation should be a nurse. He saw occupational work as an opportunity for the nursing profession to develop, expand, and become more important and useful (Barton, 1920). He exhorted nurses not to sit idly by while others took up this new line of work, leaving them to handle the "crescent basin" (Barton, 1915a, p. 338). Barton's commitment to occupational therapy's alliance with medicine is clear. He suggested that when Adam was cast from the Garden of Eden he was given a divine prescription to earn his bread by the sweat of his brow (Barton,

1915b). Barton used numerous medical analogies. One finds a now humorous medical reference in the paper entitled "Preparation of Patients for Inoculation [sic] of 'Bacillus of Work'" (as cited by Dunton, 1967, p. 287), which Barton read at the Society's founding meeting.

Barton was also the first secretary of the Boston Society of Arts and Crafts, a group allied with the arts-and-crafts movement against industrialization. He supported quality work crafted by conscientious persons. He was particularly fond of our Society's, if not our therapy's, name, including in his rationale a trait of the nonindustrialized worker:

> I am strongly in favor of the National Society for the Promotion of Occupational Therapy as a title. I know that it is long but it does tell the story and the S.P.O.T. suggests the ever alert "Johnnie." (as cited by Licht, 1967, p. 272)

Barton's understanding of occupational therapy was that the person providing occupation would be an advanced nurse who would be teaching scientifically from a medical and occupational knowledge base. This nurse-therapist would ensure harmony between occupational and medical treatments and use a frame of reference for treatment broader but parallel to that of medicine. The therapist would regard the patient as a mental, physical, and spiritual being and consider the patient's individual strengths, goals, and ambitions in these three realms when planning treatment. The addition of occupational therapy to hospital treatment would enable staff to remake a whole person who could lead a useful life.

Susan Elizabeth Tracy

Because Barton encouraged nurses to engage in occupational therapy, it seems fitting to next consider the legacy of one nurse who did: Susan Elizabeth Tracy. I refer to Tracy as a *near founder* because although not one of the founders, she was invited to the Society's founding session. Licht (1967) believed that "no one did more in this country to resurrect and establish occupational therapy than did Miss Tracy" (p. 275). Moodie (1919), herself a nurse, argued that "Occupational Therapy, in other words, the application of various forms of handicraft to meet the individual limitations of invalids and the physically handicapped was first brought into being by Miss Susan E. Tracy" (p. 313). During her training, Tracy had noticed that those patients on surgical wards who kept occupied seemed happier than those who remained idle (Licht, 1967). After completing her course work she became director of the nurses' training school at the Adams Nervine Asylum, Boston, where she initiated a program of manual arts. Her program was the first course in the United States designed to prepare instructors for patients' activities (Licht, 1948). Tracy also taught nurses in practice in the Boston area, including those at the city's Massachusetts General Hospital. One indica-

tion of her positive relationships with others and her ability to share her convictions is that an early surgical patient published her *Studies in Invalid Occupations* (Licht, 1967).

Tracy's (1913) book communicates her values and her ideas about service. She valued the support of physicians. In the chapter that introduces Tracy's ideas, Dr. Daniel H. Fuller of the Adams Nervine Asylum noted that "suitable occupation is a valuable agent in the treatment of the sick ... as an important adjunct to other forms of treatment, and sometimes it is quite all the treatment necessary" (Tracy, 1913, p. 1). Tracy no doubt perceived it important to include a physician's endorsement. She must have thought it also meritorious to include Fuller's characterizations of the quality of personal care required:

> Nurses are constantly being impressed with the fact that the technical and mechanical part of their work is but one aspect of their professional duty, that a broader conception must be attained—a sense of obligation to minister to the individual as well as to the disease. The value of wise human sympathy, of cheerfulness in work and mien, of tactful dealing with unreasonableness and irritability, of skillful diversion of thought from pessimistic channels ... are essential parts of the trained nurse's equipment to do her work. (Tracy, 1913, pp. 9–10)

Although Fuller saw occupation as helpful in meeting a physician's goals, he did not believe that a nurse had to be the provider. He believed instead in possession of the proper character:

> Without the constant cooperation of the teacher or nurse, without the daily expression of interest and the stimulus of example, the work is either never begun, or if begun, is thrown aside. The personality of the teacher and nurse therefore becomes an important factor. Her real enthusiasm and love for the work react most powerfully on the patient. (Tracy, 1913, p. 3)

In subtitling her book A *Manual for Nurses and Attendants*, Tracy also extended the role of providing occupation to those competent persons who had not been trained to nurse.

Tracy (1913) believed that a physician could prescribe work for the patient "whose physical, nervous, mental and moral characteristics he had made the object of keen observation and study" (p. 5). The result of such broad prescription was "cure in the broadest sense, in that the mental attitude toward life has been changed" (Tracy, 1913, p. 3).

Tracy (1913) used Dewey's definition of occupation as it related to education: "A mode of activity on the part of the child which runs parallel to some form of work carried on in the social life" (p. 13). She felt challenged to identify parallel occupations for hospitalized patients:

The real problem of the nurse is to find means whereby she may initiate and actually lead and cooperate in forms of occupation suited to every invalid condition and any natural temperament. (Tracy, 1913, p. 18)

Tracy (1913) pleaded for a certain dignity and quality to the work, for employment of time on worthy materials and purposeful productions. She believed that although a handicraft teacher was perhaps suited to the hospital shop or workroom, sicker patients required special care: "When the shop is a sick-room, and the bed the bench, it is almost a necessity that the nurse be the teacher" (Tracy, 1913, p. 10). Whatever their background or training, Tracy (1913) believed that teachers of occupation in hospitals must have similar traits:

They must possess resourcefulness, unfailing patience, quick perception of capacities and limitations, an enthusiasm which can anticipate for the patient the attractiveness of the finished product and the insight which substitutes a new piece of work or a new phase of the old before the patient is conscious of weariness or distaste.... The first requirement then in a teacher for this work is that she be able to understand abnormal conditions. (p. 18)

Tracy (1913) then proceeded to a chapter-by-chapter consideration of methods for the teaching of occupations to children and to patients in restricted positions, in quarantine, able to use only one hand, possessed of waning powers, without sight, and with clouded minds. Regardless of the patient's condition, Tracy believed that the teacher must be "thoughtful of the deeper needs of her patient" (Tracy, 1913, p. 10). She supported empathy because "in a large majority of the cases the trouble is local and the patient is like an animal caught in a trap" (as cited by Licht, 1948). Consideration of deeper needs would benefit patient and nurse alike:

If a nurse can prove to the patient who chafes against his limitations that there is really a broad highway of usefulness opening before him of which he knew not, the mental friction is diminished and satisfaction steals in, while the whole physical organism prepares to respond by improved conditions. In this connection the effect upon the nurse herself must not be overlooked. She too will forget the tiresome routine. (Tracy, 1913, p. 171)

Almost a decade later, Tracy (1921) was calling occupational therapy a "healing force which should be used whenever possible" (p. 399). She personified occupational therapy:

Suppose the door (to the hospital) is suddenly opened and Occupational Therapy is permitted to walk swiftly down the corridors to the wards. What is she looking for? If she is wise she is endeavoring to discover the human impulse for activity. It is certainly there. Here is a crowd of loafing, foot-

swathed men on the veranda; no impulse to work visible. If work is proposed it may be, and often is, scouted. This is no signal for discouragement.

Of what is this crowd composed? A young house-painter who has fallen hurt from a staging and is pretty badly hurt.... Next a psychopathic patient in bed held in a restraining jacket.... Third a man who repairs furniture. Only one of his hands are [sic] available at present.... Then, a three-year-old baby with a new arm in place of the one crushed by an automobile.... Occupational Therapy sets down her basket.—There is always something interesting for each person. (Tracy, 1921, p. 398)

Tracy served as a nurse under the supervision of doctors and psychiatrists in hospital environments, and she was an instructor of other nurses. She had been exposed to multiple disabilities, she used occupation as a service provider rather than as a patient, and her training in occupations had been in the manual arts. These circumstances no doubt shaped her distinct perspective. She supported the use of occupation on wards with the more acutely ill and bedridden patients as a treatment well suited to a medical setting even in the earliest stages. She saw occupational treatment as a continuum along which the patient might move from bed to shop. She supported the physician's claim to authority in matters of the prescription for occupation, perhaps because the subordinate role in prescription writing was familiar or because the patients whom she wanted to treat were acutely ill. She must have recognized the slim chance of success for a hospital treatment that was not medically prescribed. Possibly, she also believed that her acknowledgment of their authority over occupation would enable physicians to admit, as did Fuller, that it was sometimes the only treatment required.

Tracy supported the employment of crafts teachers and attendants in hospital workshops. She valued occupation for the happiness and changed attitude that it produced and for that attitude's curative effect on disabilities. To Tracy, the *worthwhileness* of handicrafts referred to the quality and purposefulness of the end product, not to its earning power. She saw occupation as a means for the nursing profession to help and care for the whole patient. She emphasized interpersonal traits without which a nurse-teacher could not engage the patient successfully.

Barton and Tracy differed slightly in their understanding of how to provide occupations to patients; the differences relate largely to their respective life experiences. The narratives of other founders and near founders explain the additional facets of our heritage as reflections of their personal perspectives about how occupation might help.

William Rush Dunton, Jr.

Also concerned with the care of hospitalized patients, particularly with patients with mental illness, was William Rush Dunton, Jr., a psychiatrist whose contributions to the early Society can scarcely be enumerated. Dunton responded readily to Barton's suggestion that a national society be established. He was an organizer by nature, having himself founded both the Maryland Psychiatric Society and the Baltimore Physicians Orchestra (Licht, 1967). He was convinced of the merit of occupation in the treatment of persons with mental illness. Early in his 30-year career at Sheppard and Enoch Pratt Hospital, Towson, Maryland, he had discussed the value of occupation with its director, Dr. Edward Brush. In 1912, Brush appointed Dunton in charge of occupation; by 1915 Dunton had published a book on the subject.

Dunton described his early encounter with patients and occupation while he was an assistant physician. At that time, he organized dramatic performances for the patients, thus earning the "sobriquet of Charles Frohman Dunton" (Dunton, 1943, p. 245). He remembered an interaction with one patient:

> At this period we had a scene painter as a patient and I was able by much bossing to make him paint some attractive sets. Each morning he would say: "Won't you let me off today?" And I would harden my heart and refuse.... It is probable that in later years I would not have been so brutal in my treatment of my scene-painter patient and I would have drawn him back to his vocation by easy stages, but experientia docet and I wanted new scenery. (Dunton, 1943, p. 245)

Dunton described his concurrent activities: "In order to interest patients I sought various craftsmen, such as bookbinders, leather toolers, and others who were kind enough to show me the rudiments of their craft so that I could by a little practice start a patient on a craft which attracted his interest and helped him on the way to recovery" (Dunton, 1943, p. 246). Dunton's personal experience with occupation deepened his commitment to moral treatment, a treatment practice used by psychiatrists many years before.

Of all the founders, Dunton articulated more than most the belief that his use of occupation constituted an earlier form of treatment that he was simply extending into a new period of history. His practice in a psychiatric hospital enabled his ready access to articles in the *American Journal of Insanity* about moral treatment in the 19th century. As a psychiatrist, he was perhaps eager to claim occupational therapy's roots among his forebears. Much of Dunton's (1919) writing included references to moral treatment. He regretted the passing of moral treatment toward the end of the 19th century:

> It is a strange thing that the physician is so often willing, even anxious, to discard remedies which have proved efficacious in his practice and in that of others, for something new to him and perhaps hitherto untried, so that we have fashions in therapeutics, some of which seem quite as bizarre to us in after years as do those of costume. (p. 17)

Although Dunton accurately identified one factor that contributed to its discontinuance, there were multiple societal, professional, and institutional circumstances that contributed to the demise of moral treatment (Peloquin, 1989) (see Chapter 4). Because moral treatment's particular form is not so much at issue here as is the core of its service, my discussion will be broad and brief.

Dunton (1919) cited Sir James Connolly, who in 1813 caught the essence of moral treatment when speaking of the York Retreat in Pennsylvania:

> The substitution of sympathy for gross unkindness, severity, and stripes; the diversion of the mind from its excitements and griefs by various occupations, and a wise confidence in the patients when they promised to control themselves led to the prevalence of order and neatness, and nearly banished furious mania from this wisely devised place of recovery. (p. 21)

Stories of interactions among therapist, patient, and occupation contribute to an understanding of moral treatment. Leuret (1948) shared one:

> I had one patient, an old fiddler, whom I had not been able to draw out. He believed that he was being trailed by the police and consequently did not dare or care to budge. In order to make him rise, walk, or feed himself, entreaty and even compulsion were necessary. I was unable to make further progress with him until I thought of the violin. I led the patient into the bathing-room, turned on the shower, and at the same time gave him a violin. He had to choose between them. I greatly feared that he would choose the shower. He hesitated for quite some time but finally the memory of his calling returned; he took the violin and played a tune of his choice.... Two months after resuming his instrument he was discharged cured, to continue the practice of his calling and for his entire treatment I had used only music. (p. 30)

A more contemporary description of moral treatment is that it was "a grand scheme for activities of daily living, which placed the patient in a total program with the goal of arranging healthy living" (Kielhofner & Burke, 1977, p. 678). Bockoven (1971) indicated that the significant attitudinal features of moral treatment were "respect for human individuality and the rights of individuals... and respect for the need of every individual to be engaged in creative and recreational activity with his fellow citizens" (p. 223). Most recently, King (1980) argued that in moral treatment "caring for and caring about the patient was as implicit as occupation" (p. 523).

One must not unduly romanticize the practice of moral treatment. Asylum reports did verify that patients benefitted from individual attention, engagement in a wide variety of occupations, small patient–staff ratios, a family atmosphere, and a system that classified and treated patients according to severity of illness. But the patients' benefit was not the exclusive motivation for the practice. Moral treatment brought prestige to asylums and physicians alike. Systems for the classification of patients and for the involvement of patients in occupations reflected a class and sex bias: wealthy patients had carriage rides while poorer patients labored in the fields. Conceptualizations of the good life were those held by upper-middle-class physicians who managed the asylums. Patient occupation was also a form of patient labor that helped to maintain the asylum. The particular form that moral treatment took lent itself to some distortions and to its eventual demise (Peloquin, 1989 [see Chapter 4]). Licht (1948) believed that "the disturbing element of this diminution is that it was world-wide, which points to a basic error in its conduct during that period" (p. 455).

Dunton warned always against repeating late-19th-century distortions of the use of occupation and in an issue of the *American Journal of Occupational Therapy* cited a cautionary segment written in 1892 by his former supervisor, Dr. Brush:

> Occupation is undoubtedly of very great importance in the treatment of the insane, but the idea of occupation which is satisfied by putting a row of twenty dements to picking hair or making fiber matts is as far short of the true aim of occupation as is the attempt to get labor out of cases of acute mania or melancholia already subject to exhaustive changes and waste ... a misconception of its true value. (as cited by Dunton, 1955, p. 17)

The ideal of moral treatment was that occupations of all kinds be used for the benefit of persons with mental illness. Shaw (1929) reflected early-20th-century thinking about this ideal: "By a new name, an old idea has had rebirth, and is called occupational therapy" (p. 199). The structural invariants of patient, therapist, and occupation mutually acting to improve the patient's condition constitute those strands of the 19th-century idea that Dunton believed the Society had extended into the 20th century.

The extension was timely. Clifford Beers, himself a patient in three mental institutions in Connecticut between 1900 and 1905, had framed a plea for the reform of contemporary abuses. Inhumane conditions after the demise of moral treatment had led Beers to organize the National Committee for Mental Hygiene. Through this organization, Beers (1917) advocated numerous hospital reforms, including individualized care of patients, occupations, recreation, and a more homelike atmosphere.

In the personal chronicle of his experiences, Beers maintained that he had contributed to his own cure through his initiative in engaging himself in reading, writing, and drawing. He often struggled against the system to procure materials with which to occupy himself. When reflecting about the origins of the use of occupation in treatment, Dunton (1921) admitted that "possibly the credit belongs to a number of patients, each one of whom found a tranquilizing influence in work casually undertaken and so continued it in the form originally begun, or in other ways" (p. 11). Dunton thus credited persons such as Beers with having influenced the development of occupational therapy.

The appendix to the 1917 edition of Beers's book details his organizational efforts for institutional reform. He included a letter from Julia Lathrop of Hull House, who had agreed to become an honorary trustee. Lathrop wrote that she had "felt for some time that a national society for the study of insanity and its treatment, from the social as well as the merely medical standpoint, should be formed" (Beers, 1917, p. 326). Lathrop's name is significant in the history of occupational therapy also because of her association with another founder, Eleanor Clarke Slagle. Another letter supporting Beers came from Dr. Adolph Meyer, Director of the Phipps Clinic at Johns Hopkins Hospital in Baltimore. Beers (1917) thanked Meyer, "who, because of his profound knowledge of the scientific, medical and social problems involved, helped more than anyone else" (p. 322). Meyer also worked to support the growth of occupational therapy in substantial ways. He presented a paper entitled "The Philosophy of Occupational Therapy" at the Fifth Annual Meeting of the Society, in which he said:

> A pleasure in achievement, a real pleasure in the use and activity of one's hands and muscles, and a happy appreciation of time began to be used as incentives in the management of our patients, instead of abstract exhortations to cheer up and to behave according to rules. The main advance of the new scheme was the blending of work and pleasure. (Meyer, 1922, pp. 2–3) (See Chapter 2.)

One passage from Beers's (1917) book resembles other passages in which he decried the lack of activity, even in the better institutions:

> For one year no further was paid to me than to see that I had three meals a day, the requisite number of baths, and a sufficient amount of exercise.... As I shall have many hard things to say about attendants in general, I take pleasure in testifying that, so long as I remained in a passive condition, those at this institution were kind, and at times even thoughtful. (p. 68)

When Dunton read his paper at the founding meeting of the Society for the Promotion of Occupational Therapy, it consisted of a history filled with references to the use of occupation in antiquity and to the practice of moral treatment. He encouraged the use of work, recreation, and exercise among persons with mental illness by invoking the success of an earlier time (Licht, 1967). Dunton thus responded to the need and push for hospital reform from persons such as Beers by proposing occupational therapy as a viable solution.

The Shaping Force of World War I

William Rush Dunton, Jr., became president at the Second Annual Meeting of the Society in 1918. At that meeting, he outlined the effectiveness of occupational therapy in treating shell shock, and he addressed the need for occupational workers in the war effort. He thought it important to articulate fundamental therapeutic principles, because many persons entering military service erroneously equated skill in handicrafts with occupational therapy (Dunton, 1919). Dunton's contemporaries were divided on the type of training required to teach occupations. Some considered craftsmen suited for the job; others believed that some form of medical training was necessary and that those most qualified were nurses (Licht, 1948). Dunton expressed his personal preference by establishing the first occupational training course for nurses.

Before discussing principles, Dunton (1919) classified occupational work into three types: invalid occupation, occupational therapy, and vocational training. *Invalid occupation*, primarily diversional, was the simplest form of occupational work. It helped recovery by promoting cheerfulness, rest, and freedom from worry. *Occupational therapy* described occupation whose primary object was to restore the patient's mental or physical function. *Vocational training*, although not occupational therapy per se, became so when used to restore function to persons with disabilities (Dunton, 1919). In all cases, Dunton argued that "the primary purpose of occupational therapy [is] cure" (p. 317). He enumerated nine curative principles that he believed essential to each type of occupational work:

1. The work should be carried on with cure as the main object.
2. The work must be interesting.
3. The patient should be carefully studied.
4. One form of occupation should not be carried to the point of fatigue.
5. It should have some useful end.
6. It preferably should lead to an increase in the patient's knowledge.
7. It should be carried on with others.
8. All possible encouragement should be given the worker.
9. Work resulting in a poor or useless product is better than idleness. (p. 320)

Dunton continued to propose that there were different types of occupational work, saying "there are many facets to the gem of occupational therapy and one of them has been humorously expressed" (Dunton, 1930, p. 349). He then recited a poem titled "Decorative Therapeutics," which linked medicine with occupation while also identifying occupational work as a primary therapeutic agent:

Do you wish to lead a healthy, happy life?
Be particular what furnishings you choose.

For there isn't any question
That these things affect digestion
And have much to do with biliousness and blues.

Old candlesticks are excellent for colds,
And pewter is a panacea for pain;
While a pretty taste in china
Has been known to undermine a
Settled tendency to water on the brain.

A highboy is invaluable for hives,
Or a lowboy if you're feeling rather low.
Colonial reproductions
Will allay internal ructions
And are splendid for a case of vertigo.

Old Chippendale is warranted for coughs.
And Heppelwhite is very good for nerves.
If your stomach is unstable
There is nothing like a table,
If it have the proper therapeutic curves.

Decorative therapeutics are the thing
If you happen to be feeling out of whack
We are happy to assure you
That these things are bound to cure you,
For there's virtue in the smallest bric-a-brac.
(Dunton, 1930, p. 350)

Dunton communicated his belief in the power of occupation with a creed that introduced his book on wartime reconstruction therapy:

That occupation is as necessary to life as food and drink. That every human being should have both physical and mental occupation. That all should have occupations which they enjoy. These are more necessary when the vocation is dull or distasteful. Every individual should have at least two hobbies, one outdoor and one indoor. A greater number will create wider interests, a broader intelligence. That sick minds, sick bodies, sick souls, may be healed through occupation. (Dunton, 1919, p. 17)

The philosophical grounding of this creed supports the use of occupation with persons who are well. The concept of health maintenance through occupation constitutes yet another facet of the early legacy.

Dunton (1921a) identified war as a catalyst for clarifying the principles of occupational therapy. Within months of the Society's founding, the United States entered World War 1. This event was important in that (a) the wartime need for occupational workers prompted the founders to more clearly articulate the service that they were promoting, (b) the war actively engaged three of the founders (Dunton, Slagle, and Kidner), and (c) the war validated the successes of occupational therapy. Dunton described the effect: "I can well remember the thrill experienced at the second annual meeting of the

National Society for the Promotion of Occupational Therapy, in September, 1918, when it was announced that General Pershing had cabled to send over two thousand more aides as soon as possible" (p. 17).

The war also influenced an early understanding of what type of person was best suited to provide occupation. The first few wartime aides to go overseas had achieved much success. The circumstances of their recruitment and early engagement are fascinating. Dr. Frankwood Williams, then Associate Director of the National Committee for Mental Hygiene, wanted to include occupational workers on his staff for Base Hospital 117. He had gathered a group of women who were ready to serve, but he could not get Washington officials to appoint them. He then noticed openings for civilian aides—scrubwomen with no official connection to the army. He proposed that he get the recruits overseas by identifying them as scrubwomen, and they agreed (Myers, 1948). One of the original aides wrote the following:

> The Aides were small in number, but large in optimistic plans for the work ahead—of which we knew practically nothing. Our unit did attend two or three lectures at the Academy of Medicine.... There were only four of us to teach handicrafts. (Myers, 1948, p. 209)

Myers (1948) also confirmed the aides' scrubbing tasks on Ellis Island. The nature of the task is important in light of the aides' backgrounds. Cordelia Myers had graduated from Columbia University in New York and was working in the occupational therapy department at Bloomingdale Hospital. Her "scrubwoman" companions were Eleanor Johnson, a psychologist; Amy Drevenstedt, a history teacher at Hunter College; Corrine Dezeller, a Columbia graduate; and Laura LaForce, a graduate nurse (Myers, 1948). Spackman (1968) described these women as skilled teachers of crafts or commercial subjects with no medical background. The aides who followed these pioneers were required to obtain a general education from a secondary school; normal school and college graduates were preferred. The age preference was between 25 and 40 years. Personal qualifications sought were those held by good teachers: knowledge and skill in the particular occupation; attractive, forceful personalities; sympathy; tact; judgment; and industry (Spackman, 1968).

Many schools opened to meet the war emergency and gave basic medical instruction. A sample course of studies lasted 4 months and included lectures on psychology, blindness, hearing problems, orthopedics, subnormal mental conditions, disorders of the central nervous system, and hospital etiquette (Spackman, 1968). Hospital practice was required for half a day per week. Spackman (1968) observed that "the occupational therapists so trained were equipped as teachers of arts and crafts, and not as therapists" (p. 68). Although she did not elaborate, she seemed to regret, as did Dunton, the

aides' lack of understanding of curative principles and the superficiality of their medical training. Some courses were more accelerated than the one that Spackman criticized. The Chicago chapter of the Red Cross, for example, gave a 6-week course directed by Eleanor Clarke Slagle at the Henry B. Favill School of Occupations, Illinois Society for Mental Hygiene, Chicago. Twenty young women, most with training in social services or special work in sociology, attended (Dunton, 1919).

A comment from Dunton (1921a), made 3 years after his cautionary note about wartime training, clarified his initial concern:

> There not being enough cafeterias to accommodate all the silly society girls who wanted to do war work, and there being a call for occupational therapists, a number of them took emergency training courses and proved their earnestness by sticking through and getting certificates. Those of us concerned with the training of this group found that as a rule they were not silly society girls at all, but were fine, earnest women despite their veneering of silly society girlism. (p. 18)

This comment identifies another force that shaped the determination of who should be occupational therapists at the time: The feeling that occupational therapy was women's work. Aides recruited for the war effort were women. Dunton (1921a) attributed a measure of their success in the war to their sex: "It had been found that the presence of energetic women who went through the wards of hospitals stimulating the patients to occupy themselves making things had had a wonderful effect in keeping up the morale of the patients" (p. 17).

Dunton was not alone in this belief. A writer for *Carry On*, a war journal reporting reconstruction efforts, argued that women alone could have a powerful effect on the recovery of injured soldiers:

> To prevent his losing hope, to keep his sense of responsibility is in the power of his womankind.... In every step the help of women is essential; not only in cheering him during the first stages, but in encouraging him to follow patiently and exactly the detail of his training....The recovery of our disabled soldiers—their return to a useful life—is in the control of the women of this country. (Miller, 1918, pp. 17–18)

The rationale for this endorsement of women was the belief that a man's state of mind reflected that of his wife or his mother. The writer was a woman expressing a common view that women created a moral refuge for their men, sustaining their spirits so that they could return refreshed to the world of men. These female reconstruction aides returned to the United States to join the ranks of other occupational therapists.

Few studies in the literature that I reviewed for this inquiry suggested that nurses complained that this advanced form of nursing had been snatched from them. Reverby (1987) noted that the scarcity of nurses during the war "brought nursing more damnation than blessings" (p. 163). Her reference, however, was not to a loss of the use of occupation, but to the war's having contributed to an increase in the number of country girls training as "subnurses" (p. 163).

The wartime shift away from a conviction that nurses made the best occupational workers may well have strengthened the belief that a physician should prescribe occupation; someone had to know medical conditions in depth. Dunton (1919) offered another reason for medical supervision:

> If the [occupation] director has not had medical training it has been found that there will be a lack of sympathy between the medical staff and the occupational department so that this valuable therapeutic agent is not used so well as it should be.... For this reason alone, if for no other, it is believed that the director should be one of the senior physicians, who should at rounds, conferences, and elsewhere, instruct the juniors as to the value of occupation. (p. 55)

Dunton's argument for a physician's use and support of occupation reflected his role as the president of a society founded to promote occupation. His argument that the physician-director should train the staff and the teachers, arrange for the purchase of supplies, and supervise the shops seems consistent with a desire to replicate the managerial control held by physicians in the Moral Treatment era.

Dunton's (1919) estimation of the personal qualities required of the occupational director included tact, the "precious gift of inspiring others," knowledge of the psychology of everyday life, interest in occupation as therapy, "fertility of invention," and an artistic sense of form (pp. 43–45). These traits paralleled those thought necessary for occupational nurses and craft teachers. Physician-directors would provide a service centered on occupation and similar to that provided by nonphysicians.

The war also nurtured an idea of the kind of patient-therapist relationship that worked in occupational therapy. A soldier revealed the quality of the service that he as a patient experienced:

> I got a new vision of life.... I saw that men made unfit for the work of the past must be equipped for work in the future ... saw the dignity of labor made new and interesting, and even more powerful because of the handicap. (Cooper, 1918, p. 24)

The biography of Ora Ruggles, a reconstruction aide, chronicled this kind of service. Ruggles, a school teacher who had graduated from San Diego Normal School and had taken additional courses in the manual arts, responded to the war call for crafts experts. She quickly integrated the importance of engaging the interest and the heart of each patient. Physicians and administrators acknowledged her accomplishments. Ruggles's competence, warmth, and concern inspired awe, loyalty, and gratitude in her patients. She creatively adapted activities that allowed even patients with the most severe disabilities to succeed. Without having been trained to apply them, she understood many of the principles of occupational therapy:

> By now, Ora and the other reconstruction aides were keenly attuned to the word useful. It was a vital key to what they were trying to do. Whenever possible, they thought up projects that the patients could see had tangible use, particularly for the outside world, the world of the well. In this way they could literally work themselves to the level of the normal world. (Carlova & Ruggles, 1946, p. 81)

Ruggles summed up the essence of her view of service: "It is not enough to give a patient something to do with his hands. You must reach for the heart as well as the hands. It's the heart that really does the healing" (Carlova & Ruggles, 1946, pp. 249–250).

If the war shaped conceptualizations of the patient–therapist relationship, it acted similarly on the meaning of occupation. The founders' idea of prewar services was that occupation could be an effective treatment that would enable occupation after recovery. Occupation could serve both as the means and the goal of treatment. The wartime experience of occupational work affirmed this assumption while also emphasizing "the physical side of occupational therapy" (Dunton, 1919, p. 56). Wartime occupational therapy, often called *curative work*, was prescribed to "restore usefulness, overcome deformities or teach to the remaining portion of a limb or another member new functions" (Mock, 1919, p. 12). War injuries focused attention on the use of occupation to restore the patient to a functional condition.

During the war years, Frank Gilbreth had operationalized the efficiency principle of "fitting the machine to the man"; he designed numerous work adaptations that occupational therapists readily implemented as part of the goal of returning the patient to useful occupation (Dunton, 1919, p. 107). Dunton's (1919) book entitled *Reconstruction Therapy* contained several of Gilbreth's photographs of men wearing prostheses (e.g., the Amar claw, the Carnes artificial arm, and the Hanger leg). The book also included photographs of men using self-help devices for dressing, doing farm work, and driving a car. If the disabled person could be equipped with some adaptive device that would facilitate accomplishing the task, the occupational therapist would modify the instructions accordingly. The idea seemed a logical extension of the founders' views. If the prosthetic device were considered part of the person, and occupational therapy taught the whole person, then teaching its use became part of teaching the person. Conversely, if the device were considered a tool required to get the job done, then teaching its use would be inherent in teaching the occupation. One is struck by photographs of men wearing hooks and gadgets, crude by today's standards. The devices permitted a restorative role for the machine that otherwise excelled at maiming, wounding, or dehumanizing. The machine advanced into treatment to touch the patient.

The language of science peppered the occupational therapy literature during the war years. It had been there before, both in the group's plea that occupations be taught with the best scientific methods and in the scientific aims articulated by the original Society. The war experience operationalized this philosophy with methods that appeared to be scientific. Dunton (1919) mused about the many terms describing occupational therapy at the time and thought the term *ergotherapy* the best and the most scientific. He thought it "a very simple matter to trace the development of occupational therapy from simple tasks and amusements to the more scientific occupational therapy or re-education applied to all forms of mental and physical disability" (p. 29). Dunton believed that a scientific evolution was evident in the growing number of studies on occupation, such as the one conducted by Kent at the Government Hospital in Washington, DC. Kent's study suggested that "definite practice effects can be obtained, by means of a short series of tests, from advanced cases of dementia praecox" among female patients (pp. 30–32).

The belief that occupational therapy's problems needed to be framed in a scientific manner appeared early in the literature. Dunton (1919) argued that much remained to be done before occupational therapy could be considered an exact science. He hoped that the task would attract the attention of the research worker:

> There are many difficulties to be encountered, chiefly centered about the emotional reaction of the patient. Why does one form of work, say carpentry, appeal to one man and not to another, when they are apparently of similar mental caliber and from the same social level?... In all probability the answer lies somewhere in the associative activities, but how can we most quickly stimulate the association which will give us the best co-operation of the patient? (pp. 30–31)

Occupational therapists were interested in answers to questions about how people learned; they were teachers of occupations. They were also concerned with human motivation because so much of their service consisted of interesting the patient in occupation (Mock, 1919, p. 13). Not surprisingly, much of the early literature about occupational therapy included discussions of recent developments in education and psychology. The war experience directed the application of occupations within the context of the growing body of knowledge in arenas related to teaching occupations and in the increasing use of technology designed to enhance individual functioning. The war challenged the founders to examine their service within this context in terms of both immediate applications and unanswered questions.

Eleanor Clarke Slagle

Eleanor Clarke Slagle completed a course given by Julia Lathrop at the Chicago School of Civics and Philanthropy. Lathrop had pursued Beers's (1917) cause for reform in treating persons with mental illness by designing a course in curative occupations and recreations for attendants and nurses in institutions and by resigning from the State Board of Control in Illinois in 1908 to protest poor conditions in that state. Most patients in Illinois state hospitals at that time sat idly through each day, with an able few engaging in hospital industries that consisted of monotonous work designed to help the hospital (American Occupational Therapy Association, 1940). After completing Lathrop's course in 1911, Slagle taught a similar course in Michigan. She then went to the Phipps Psychiatric Clinic of the Johns Hopkins Hospital, Baltimore, to direct the occupational therapy department under the supervision of Dr. Adolph Meyer.

Meyer had experienced occupational conditions similar to those seen by Slagle and had also supported Beers in his reform efforts. He described "industrial shops and work in the laundry and kitchen and on the wards...very largely planned to relieve the employees" (Meyer, 1922, p. 2). At the Phipps Clinic, he "secured the services of Mrs. Slagle," whose efforts he acknowledged as having positively contributed "to the level [then] represented at the Phipps Clinic" (Meyer, 1922, p. 4). While at the Phipps Clinic, Slagle gave 3-week courses on occupation to groups of nurses in training at the Johns Hopkins Hospital. The instructions included both occupations and the principles underlying their use (Dunton, 1921b). She discussed with Dunton her ideas about their new form of therapy (Licht, 1967).

Slagle returned to Chicago in 1915 to establish the Henry B. Favill School of Occupations and directed the school from 1918 to 1922. She had taken courses in social work and had worked with Meyer, who advocated "the creation of an orderly rhythm in the atmosphere" of the hospital. (Meyer, 1922, p. 6). These influences shaped Slagle's perspective: She taught habit training through occupation. She selected severely regressed and chronically ill patients for her training program. It is not surprising that she started habit training with this group, because Meyer had characterized the patient with dementia praecox as "suffering from disorganized habits" (Wilson, 1929, p. 189). An original principle of occupational therapy permeates the concept of habit training: Occupations could be useful and curative by fostering their habitual use among patients with mental illness.

In habit training, small groups of patients were given close supervision throughout the day. They followed a carefully designed schedule that included self-care and personal hygiene, occupational class, walks, meals in small groups, recreational activities, and physical exercise. Each patient was encouraged to get into a routine and then to assume responsibility for that routine. Excerpts from one care report on a patient convey a sense of the personal service that Slagle initiated:

May 3, 1926—Admitted to habit training. Will not dress or undress self. Clothing untidy and unbuttoned. Mute. Will not wash self. Wets and soils the bed. Eats excessively. Masturbation frequent.

June 1 to June 30, 1926—Washes and dresses self. Wets and soils less frequently. Polishes floor when continuously supervised. Does low-grade occupation.

July 10 to September 22, 1926—Speaks occasionally. Told superintendent that he was "slightly improved." Works on braid-weave rug. Helps attendant with cleaning and cleans dishes from table at meals. Appetite more normal. (Wilson, 1929, pp. 196–197)

Physicians like Charles Vaux (1929) believed that habit training caused a "turning point that started [patients] on the road to recovery" (p. 329). He regretted that other physicians found it difficult to accept this "new viewpoint" and "work of reclamation" (p. 328). Slagle's reclamation work with occupation extended to those patients considered beyond the reach of contemporary treatments.

Slagle did not believe that the director of occupation had to be a physician, having herself assumed that role. She indicated that the "capability of such a person involved not only arts and crafts training, but, and most chiefly, personality and character" (Slagle, 1927, p. 126). Although she insisted on solid knowledge of materials and processes, she emphasized the personal element:

For, if lacking in this—in understanding, in give and take, in spiritual vision of the "end problem" of all too many of the cases, the craftsman may make some initial showing, but the work will eventually flag and be largely a failure. (Slagle, 1927, p. 126)

Given her early training in social work, Slagle's belief in the therapist's personal influence made sense. An early conceptualization in social work held that the social worker's (or friendly visitor's) character and his or her relationship with the patient together constituted the agent of change.

Although she did not believe that the director of occupations should be a physician, Slagle sought medical authority in occupational prescriptions. She believed that the physician should prescribe at least the kind of occupation needed, "such as stimulating, sedative, mechanical, intellectual, academic or varied" (Slagle, 1927, p. 128). She argued that all therapeutic measures were the responsibility of the physician in charge. Her definition of occupational therapy included a medical metaphor: "It is directed activity and differs from all other forms of treatment in that it is given in increasing doses as the patient's condition improves" (Slagle as cited by Hull, 1931, p. 219).

Slagle regarded her 3-week training courses as an orientation to nurses about the merits of occupation rather than training in what they might themselves do. She believed that although some nurses completed a period of service in an occupational therapy department, "this did not mean that the nurse would become a specialist...but that she would become acquainted with the nature and possibilities" of the therapy (Slagle, 1927, p. 129). Slagle included attendants in habit training, much as Tracy (1913) had endorsed their direct involvement in invalid occupation with medically stable patients.

Slagle was a leader. She was described as "a woman whose presence was felt by all who were in her company. She was regally tall and there were those who found that some of her pronouncements were in keeping with her appearance and bearing" (Licht, 1967, p. 271). Ruggles remembered Slagle's inspiring words during a personally difficult time. Slagle had told Ruggles that the occupational therapy movement needed her to "get behind it and push!" (Carlova & Ruggles, 1946, p. 113). This urging prompted Ruggles to return to service. Elected vice-president at the first Society meeting, Slagle eventually held every office in the Association and did so for a longer period than anyone else (Licht, 1967). She also agreed to direct occupational therapy for the Illinois Department of Mental Hygiene (Smith, 1929).

Slagle's leadership was exceptional. Men held the highest positions of authority in those early years. In treatment, occupational therapists deferred to physicians, who were predominantly men; in promotional and organizational efforts, men were most often elected to the highest position. The view that women were most effective with patients shaped a leadership pattern that placed men in administrative and supervisory roles and made Slagle's leadership remarkable. (Editor's note: See Appendix E for Adolf Meyers' address in honor of Eleanor Clarke Slagle.)

Herbert J. Hall

Licht (1967) reported that although Dunton had nominated Dr. Herbert J. Hall for inclusion at the founding meeting, Barton rejected his nomination. Because Hall was nearly selected, because his involvement with occupation was widely cited by the other founders, and because he assumed leadership roles early in the Society's history, Hall's views can be considered, like Tracy's, to be those of a near founder.

As early as 1904, Hall was prescribing occupation as a means of regulating his patients' lives (Hopkins, 1978). In 1906, Harvard University awarded him a grant to study the use of occupation in the treatment of neurasthenia. As a part of this grant project, Hall established an experimental workshop in Marblehead, Massachusetts. In a presidential address to the Society in 1921, he characterized the workshop as an experimental laboratory that addressed the technical problems of occupational therapy. The Society officially accepted his project as the Medical Workshop.

Hall's vision of service provided yet another understanding of the helping potential of occupation:

> The writer of these chapters undertook ten years ago to meet in a small way the needs of a class of people who were not in actual want but who from illness or the overstrain of modern life had been obliged to give up their usual occupations. (Hall & Buck, 1915)

Hall reached out to single young people, "nervous invalids" who had "gone to pieces" from a lack of "depth and substance in their lives" (p. 57). Hall believed that these persons learned something of the dignity and satisfaction of "work with the hands" when engaged in occupation (Hall & Buck, 1915, p. 58). His goal was to simplify life through occupations that could rest the mind. One recognizes Hall's concurrence with contemporary criticisms of the "strain of modern life" (Upham, 1917, p. 409). One can also recognize Hall's support of a popular view of "women's work." He believed that the absence of home-like occupations and nurturing functions caused problems among single women; these could be remedied with occupations that substituted one means of creative satisfaction for another.

Another of Hall's unique views was that industries should be established specifically for persons with disabilities. Although he urged the development of workshops within hospitals, he believed that a further step was necessary. Because "the regular industries could not change their rules and systems for the sake of giving him employment ... the way out seems to lie in the establishing of special industries where the handicapped may be favored" (Hall & Buck, 1915, pp. xiii, xiv). Hall predicted a time when hospitals and sanatoriums would recognize the value of remunerative occupation for their patients and would conduct industries as adjunctive treatments (Hall & Buck, 1915). Hospital workshops and industries would help the patient take a first step toward later employment in special industries for disabled persons; there would be a continuum of restorative occupation. He described with deep feeling the patient who would otherwise face a life of idleness and dependence: "Put yourself in that man's place—imagine the despair and the final degeneration that must sap at last all that is brave and good in life" (Hall & Buck, 1915, p. viii).

Barton (1914) thought well of Hall's views because he thought that they represented a nonmedical orientation. Hall argued, however, for medical involvement in the use of occupations. He recommended the use of a prescription for occupation, providing illustrative models:

> May 1, 1914
> Occupation Work
> Mrs. X—Room 50
> Light occupation in bed
> Basketry or knitting
> Not more than 1 hour daily
> [Physician's name], MD (Hall & Buck, 1915, p. 76)

Hall (1921) called occupational therapy the "science of prescribed work" (p. 245). He believed that there had previously been a "fatal gap" in medicine that had released the patient cured but "totally unfit because of weakness or discouragement, to take his place immediately among competitive labor" (p. 245). He believed that nurses and social workers needed training in the use of work as treatment and in 1908 provided such training at the Devereaux Mansion, Marblehead, Massachusetts (Hopkins, 1978).

Hall differed from other founders in his belief that the medical diagnosis and the patient's problems should remain unknown to the teacher of occupations. He argued that "work was one of the few normal habits left to the patient, and the nearer he could approach to health in his relations with the teacher the better" (Hall & Buck, 1915, p. 77). Only an unbiased teacher could relate normally with the patient. He further believed that medical information might be easily misunderstood and misapplied by nonmedical personnel. He argued that the ideal teacher would be a nurse serving under a craftsman, because the doctor could then share information necessary for dealing with the "whole problem" (Hall & Buck, 1915, p. 55).

Hall sought teachers with traits that enabled a low-conflict interpersonal approach. He thought that individualized teaching was important (Hall & Buck, 1915). He reasoned that "praise for effort should be given ungrudgingly; but praise of results should not be too lavish" (Hall & Buck, 1915, p. 87). He thought it wise to allow the patient a "liberty of choice" (Hall & Buck, 1915, p. 88). He believed that special effort was the hallmark of caring. As an example, he discussed the case of a choreic boy, aged 11 years, who had at first been dull and discouraged in occupation. The boy had eventually recovered the use of his hands. Hall associated his recovery with the fact that "the teacher took pains to show him exactly how to use his hands, and he gradually became quite expert in fretsawing and other crafts" (Hall & Buck, 1915, pp. 138–139). Special, individualized effort had made the difference. If a teacher had to address a patient's symptoms directly, as in the case of a neurasthenic patient, Hall (Hall & Buck, 1915) hoped that she would "use tact as well as skill" (pp. 138–139). She should also be flexible, using "common sense in the application of all rules" (Hall & Buck, 1915, pp. 168–169). Hall (1921) believed that this profile created a new field for women:

> We are at the beginning of a new profession for educated women. The actual work must be done for the most part by women. Feminine tact and perseverance alone can be depended upon to break down the barriers of prejudice, and to secure the cooperation of difficult patients. (p. 246)

Hall (1921) elaborated on his meaning, while also qualifying the nature of the prejudice he described:

> The theory is so divertingly simple that we may fall easily into error, and fail to realize that we are concerned with the very sources of human power.... Occupational therapy is a means to an end. Some of its proceedings may seem trivial, but they gain in importance through the opportuneness of their application. Practice in this field is not so simple as it looks. All the ingenuity in the world may not be sufficient to overcome the shiftlessness, the hopelessness, the lack of ambition, the evasion, the prejudice which stands in the way. (p. 245)

Hall joined the other founders in recognizing occupation as one of the sources of human power.

Susan Cox Johnson

Susan Cox Johnson studied and taught high school arts and crafts in Berkeley, California. In 1912, she travelled in the Orient, eventually residing in the Philippines to teach crafts for 2 years. On her return, she accepted a position in the Hospital of New York City on Blackwell's Island and also agreed to direct the occupations committee for the Department of Public Charities of New York State. In this capacity, she aimed to prove that occupations could improve the mental and physical condition of patients and inmates in public hospitals and almshouses, that these persons could contribute to their self-support, and that occupation could be morally uplifting (Licht, 1967, p. 276). Her aim embodied her belief in the curative and restorative potential of occupation, a belief that was invariant among all the founders.

Johnson's work impressed Barton, who believed that she had "by all odds the most important job in the world, together with a very level head, a keen insight, good experience and a tremendous interest in the therapeutic side" (Reed & Sanderson, 1983, p. 196). Dunton had submitted Johnson's name for inclusion in the Society after Barton's rejection of Hall; Barton had readily agreed to her inclusion (Licht, 1967, p. 271). Shortly after the establishment of the Society and the United State's entrance into war, Columbia University in New York invited Johnson to teach occupational therapy in their nursing department. She accepted the position and soon directed

the course (Licht, 1967). She simultaneously organized and directed an occupational therapy department at Montefiore Home and Hospitals, New York.

Five of Johnson's articles published in *Modern Hospital* addressed the training of personnel and the function of occupational therapy in the hospital (Reed & Sanderson, 1983). Her continued emphasis on the reeducational aspect of work and on the educational requirements for practitioners reflected her teaching background. Johnson shared the concerns of her cofounders about educational prerequisites. She regretted a "difference of opinion among those who are working with the same end in view" (Johnson, 1919, p. 221). She wrote:

> What seems to be a difference ... is often not a real difference at all, but is a misunderstanding due to our failure to keep always before us the several natural divisions of our work and the different purposes of each, as well as the fact that each must overlap and merge one into the other instead of being separate and aloof. No standards for training teachers can be set without the recognition of these different elements. (Johnson, 1919, p. 221)

Johnson (1919) believed that teaching occupations to invalids differed from other teaching; there was need to "plan with much greater consideration for the individual than is done in any system of instruction under normal conditions" (p. 221) . She outlined various training programs suitable for working with specific populations. She reasoned that persons teaching invalid occupations in a hospital needed more understanding and training in handling sick people, whereas those teaching in curative workshops or outpatient shops needed more educational courses, because their teaching would "fall into more nearly normal lines" (p. 222).

Johnson's arguments resembled Tracy's. She believed strongly that the educational curriculum mattered; the "great field of occupation would never bear full fruit until the dignity and importance of the position of the teacher in this field is recognized" (Johnson, 1919, p. 223). She thought it "dangerous" that the pendulum might swing toward "losing sight of the nursing aspect of the work of the teacher" (Johnson, 1919, p. 223). She predicted that there would "always be a problem keeping a definite middle path between the nursing and teaching aspects of this work" (Johnson, 1919, p. 223).

Johnson (1919) recognized that the debate over suitable therapists' qualifications had escalated during the war:

> The idea that it was desirable to have teachers specially trained for this work and that they could well be nonmedical people was just coming to be accepted when the avalanche of war necessity descended upon us. The great demand for nurses and the need for numbers of teachers in this field swept occupations out of the hands of the nurse without further discussion and made necessary either the

absorption of a foreign group into the hospital regime or the discard of the whole idea of using occupation for a therapeutic purpose. (p. 221)

Johnson (1919) urged occupational workers to resolve the conundrum of suitable training, and in so doing to balance the need for specialized skills against the need for skills required across all settings. She believed that all teachers of occupation needed "an understanding of the psychology of both normal and abnormal minds" and a grounding "in the principles and methods of teaching the sick," regardless of their practice settings (p. 222).

Johnson argued that the product of the patient's work should be of high quality. Her emphasis on "maintaining high standards in the products of occupation" seems reasonable after so many years teaching and learning crafts (Johnson, 1919, p. 223). Recognizing that the field was in a "formative period," she cautioned against any hasty standardization, but encouraged the Society to instead provide "practical aid to the teacher in maintaining the best standards in products" (Johnson, 1919, p. 223). She perhaps supported the Society's establishment in 1920 of an occupational therapy bureau in Boston to investigate the market and the wholesale purchase of staples to sell at a low price to occupational therapy departments everywhere (Hall, 1921).

Johnson's background distinguished her from many other founders. Her views and questions, born of her personal competencies, pushed for a balanced view of occupational therapy as a part-medical, part-teaching function.

Thomas Bessell Kidner

Barton invited Thomas Bessell Kidner to the founding meeting because Kidner resided in Canada and thus would give the Society an international flavor (Reed & Sanderson, 1983). Kidner's foreign status was not the exclusive criterion for his selection, however. In 1915, he had been appointed Vocational Secretary to the Canadian Military Hospitals to develop a vocational rehabilitation system. Before that, Kidner had established a number of technical educational programs in various Canadian provinces. Dunton described Kidner's chief aims in life as being "to prevent the convalescent soldier from falling into habits of idleness and self-indulgence, to educate the crippled soldier in some vocation by which he can support himself " (Dunton, 1967, p. 288).

Like Barton, Kidner had been trained as an architect. He included several architectural drawings in his journal articles that detailed the planning of occupational therapy departments. Kidner served as president of the Society for six terms (Licht, 1967). Barton (1968) described Kidner as "outgoing in expressing his enthusiasm about the use of occupation, a fascinating personality, so very British, even the tailoring of his morning

coat, striped trousers, winged collar and tie" (p. 345). During Kidner's presidency in 1923, the American Occupational Therapy Association (formerly known as the Society for the Promotion of Occupational Therapy) adopted an official insignia, which included a caduceus, and made this insignia available for use by Association members (Kidner, 1923; "Occupational Therapists Meet Again With A.H.A.," 1923). The pin symbolically fixed the affiliation of this new service to that of medicine.

Kidner (1923) spoke often about the progress of occupational therapy and the growing valuation of "curative work in practically every kind of disability" (p. 55). He reminded therapists that the Industrial Rehabilitation Act of 1920 had extended the use of occupation to many hospitals:

Indeed, I think it is fair to say that many hospitals have had their attention drawn to the value of occupational therapy by the federal and state industrial rehabilitation authorities who are doing their best to place persons disabled by accident or disease in industry. (p. 500)

Kidner also credited the Act with introducing curative work into many new non-hospital-based service arenas. One new arena was the world of homebound persons, whom Kidner (1924) described as "the product of industrial accidents" (p. 500). Kidner (1923) estimated that the number of persons disabled by industrial and other accidents annually equaled the number of those who might be disabled in an army of 1.5 million men active in the field. He believed that the great number of disabled persons and the consequent "growth and development of occupational therapy naturally led to the evolution of standards" (Kidner, 1929b, p. 243).

In 1923, the year in which the standards were developed, the officers of the Association were mostly men; one of the three was a physician. Slagle was the only woman, reelected secretary–treasurer. Of the eight persons elected to the Board of Managers of the Association, five were physicians ("Occupational Therapists Meet Again With A.H.A.," 1923). In response to a growing interest in securing occupational therapists, "several doctors called the attention of the American Occupational Therapy Association" to the hurried wartime educational programs that gave "practically nothing more than instruction in simple manual arts" (Kidner, 1929b, p. 244). A committee that included physicians studied the problem of occupational therapy education; the membership then adopted a statement of minimum standards at their annual meeting (Kidner, 1930). These first educational standards for training in occupational therapy further shaped the early characterization of the occupational therapist.

The standards outlined prerequisites for candidates and curriculum content. Admission to a training course required at least a high school education or its equivalent. A year's special training in some related field such as applied art, crafts, social service, or advanced academic work was desirable. Successful employment or experience could replace time spent in training school or some other educational institution (Kidner, 1924). The training course had to last a minimum of 12 months, with no less than 6 hr of work and lectures daily. The year's course had to include no less than 8 months of theoretical and practical work and no less than 3 months of hospital practice training and supervision. The official statement required that adequate instruction be given in (a) psychology, normal and abnormal; (b) anatomy, kinesiology, and orthopedics; (c) mental diseases; (d) tuberculosis; and (e) general medical cases, including cardiac diseases. At least 1,080 hr were required in practical handiwork such as "woodworking, weaving, basketry, metal work and jewelry, drawing and applied design" (Kidner, 1924, p. 55). The standards also required lectures on work in several types of hospitals, the principles of hospital management, hospital ethics, the history and development of curative occupations, arts and crafts in relation to the development of civilization, modern industry and the factory system, and the relation of occupational therapy to vocational rehabilitation (Kidner, 1929b).

Course titles and recommended lectures did not specifically include the principles for use of occupation that had been endorsed by Dunton, then serving on the Board of Managers. Neither did the listing include occupations such as habit training or recreational activities. These omissions are of interest because Kidner (1923) mentioned that "the original group of incorporators of the association [except Barton, who was deceased] continued active in its affairs" ("Occupational Therapists Meet Again With A.H.A.," 1923, p. 500). Among those persons with the greatest investment in the inclusion of their own perspectives, none disputed the minimum standards. Kidner (1924) did mention the existence of various views (p. 55) and suggested that the standards would warrant upcoming revisions, probably to increase their rigor. His summative statement that the standards "provided a fair and workable basis for the training of occupational therapists, and...represented the consensus of opinion on the subject of the great majority of those interested" (p. 55) suggests comfort with the standards. Kidner (1924) explained that "the board of managers endeavored to avoid the Scylla of placing the requirements so high that too few students would undertake the training, and, on the other hand, the Charybdis of lowering the standards of the work" (p. 55). Comprehensive requirements, although ideal, might stymie the development of a new group of therapists.

Whatever the rationale for the minimal curriculum, the standards purported to train the early therapist as both a medical worker and a crafts instructor, thereby resolving the question of which function, that of nurse or teacher, was more important. The occupational therapist had to be a bit of both. The therapist would understand the hospital world and the authority that the physician held in that world, and he or she would perform his or her service within that context. The therapist would be an instructor in crafts whose real end product would be a restored person.

Kidner (1924) detailed the end product of occupational therapy. He cautioned against misconstruing the value of occupation as the "making of a more or less useful and attractive object" for sale (p. 57). He reminded the membership that the "real value of curative work lay in the result obtained in the patient" (p. 57). He believed that to construe the "incidental products of occupational therapy to be the end and aim of treatment" was to not appreciate "the real meaning and significance of work" (Kidner, 1929b, p. 243). Although not acknowledged as such in the literature, Kidner's reminder might have constituted a redirection of members, trained primarily in handiwork, toward a valuation of the work process.

Kidner (1929a) spoke often of rehabilitation. When addressing graduating students, he shared his conception of the quality of service that they ought to provide:

In your chosen field, a part of the noblest work of man—the care and relief of weak and suffering humanity—may you realize in increasing measure the value of certain spiritual things which are the real making of life, but which we call by many common names. Kindness, humanity, decency, honor, good faith—to give these up under any circumstances whatever would be a loss greater than any defeat, or even death itself. (p. 385)

Concern for the patient and for the quality of his or her personal relationship with the therapist wove through Kidner's statements on standards, medical affiliation, and the curative goal of occupation. Kidner contributed much to legacy. In a memorial tribute, Dunton (1932) characterized Kidner's connection with occupational therapy as a "bond of interest in advancing a body of knowledge of occupational therapy" that "grew into a firm friendship which death has ended" (p. 195).

The National Society for the Promotion of Occupational Therapy

Each of the founders contributed a unique perspective to the multifaceted service that constituted occupational therapy. The founders also shaped the early service when acting collectively as the Society. Early signs of this collective shaping appeared at the first meeting. The certificate of incorporation of the National Society for the Promotion of Occupational Therapy identified its objectives for "the advancement of occupation as a therapeutic measure; for the study of the effect of occupation upon the human being; and for the scientific dispensation of this knowledge" (Reed & Sanderson, 1983, p. 272). Concerns for science, for humanity, and for the advancement of this new therapy were clear. To operationalize their objectives and to recruit additional members to the Society, the founders appointed each other to chair six district committees: Barton, the Committee on Research and Efficiency; Slagle, the Committee on Installations and Advice; Dunton, the Committee on Finance, Publicity, and Publication; Johnson, the Committee on Admissions and Positions; Tracy, the Committee on Teaching Methods; and Kidner, the International Committee (Dunton, 1967). Barton outlined the plan:

> Let each member, that is, each chairman of a standing committee select from his own acquaintances four others who will become members of the committee and of the society at the next meeting.... Then for the next step—let special subjects be assigned to each member of the society, or rather to the 20 new members, according to the strength, interest, and ability of the individual member. Then let each of these members secure from his personal friends four others to be members of his subcommittee.... Thus the work will "pyramid." (Barton as cited by Licht, 1967, p. 272)

The plan virtually assured the perpetuation of the varied perspectives of the founders as well as the common objectives of the Society. It enabled the growth of special interest groups with a central interest in promoting occupation as therapy.

In 1921, Hall, then president, had suggested that the name of the Society be replaced by the "crisper and more descriptive" American Occupational Therapy Association (Reed & Sanderson, 1983, p. 182). Simultaneously, the larger membership generated by the pyramid plan adopted a new constitution that established two governing bodies—a Board of Managers and a House of Delegates. The House of Delegates voted in 1922 to hold the meetings of the American Occupational Therapy Association in conjunction with those of the American Hospital Association so that hospital executives might better understand occupational therapy (Reed & Sanderson, 1983). These joint meetings promoted occupational therapy while also sealing its affiliation with physicians and its practice in hospitals. The lectures on hospital management and ethics required by the 1923 standards affirmed this liaison.

In 1922, Hall articulated the goals of the Association and the service that it promoted:

> The association is a responsible, incorporated body with officers of large experience, and active committees encouraging research, collecting data and recommending standards. It seems reasonable to assert that here is a work of national importance, a human reclamation service touching vitally on matters of vast social and economic consequence. Mere encouragement, even placement in industry cannot restore men and women who have not learned through careful bedside training how to use their disabled bodies. The association is literally helping the helpless to help themselves. (pp. 164–165)

Much of the spirit and vitality of the individual founders permeates the statement.

When the official insignia was accepted in 1923, the House of Delegates also voted to establish a national registry, a measure that Kidner had promoted during his presidency. Numerous physicians had sought to secure the registration of occupational workers before 1921. The opinion of Dr. Salmon, a psychiatrist, is representative:

> We badly need a list of qualified workers in this field to which a hospital superintendent could refer with as much assurance in finding correct information with regard to an applicant for a position in an occupational therapy department as he could refer to the directory of the American Medical Association for the information regarding a doctor. (Salmon as cited by Kidner, 1929b, p. 245)

The Society's cooperation with physicians parallels that found in personal narratives of the founders. The early Association strived to cooperate with a number of groups. It endorsed a service that extended not only to the disabled patient and his or her family, but also to physicians, hospital managers, employers, and members of the scientific community. This accountability to many persons structured the Pledge and Creed for Occupational Therapists submitted by the Boston School and adopted by the Association in 1926:

> Reverently and earnestly do I pledge my wholehearted service in aiding those crippled in mind and body.
> To this end that my work for the sick may be successful, I will strive for greater knowledge, skill and understanding in the discharge of my duties in whatsoever position I may find myself.
> I solemnly declare that I will hold and keep whatever I may learn of the lives of the sick.
> I acknowledge the dignity of the cure of disease and the safeguarding of health in which no act is menial or inglorious.
> I will walk in upright faithfulness and obedience to those under whose guidance I am to work, and I pray for patience, kindliness and strength in the holy ministry to broken minds and bodies. (as cited by Welles, 1976, p. 45)

After an exploration of their personal understandings and stories, we can almost hear the voices of Barton, Tracy, Dunton, Slagle, Hall, Johnson, and Kidner reciting this creed.

Other than the writings of Barton, who was himself disabled, there was little written by patients about the early years of occupational therapy service. One article, "A Patient Looks at Occupational Therapy," written anonymously in 1930, is noteworthy. It coincides with what I consider the end of the early years. The patient wrote:

> It is hard when the rudiments of many crafts must be mastered ... to keep the fuller vision of all that occupational therapy does and must mean if we are to be really helpful to those who need us.... The broader and more inclusive our outlook as to the wholesome interest in real things the more helpful and effective our work. (p. 277)

Conclusion

This inquiry has supported a broad view of the nature of occupational therapy's early service: that the right occupation could resolve many problems, and that the patient, therapist, and occupation could interrelate therapeutically. These understandings of the founders reflect their sensitivity to the problems and issues of their times, that is, hospital care, industrialization, and war. Also reflected are the founders' responses to contemporary trends toward science, education, sexual stereotyping, and professionalization. Both individual narratives and the collective activities of the Society support Yerxa's (1980) claim that the heritage of occupational therapy includes a focus on care and function. To use occupation as a way of helping persons live their lives in a way that is meaningful to them is to care about persons and about function.

The heritage of occupational therapy was shaped by numerous societal forces and historical events that enabled each founder to visualize occupation as helpful. Events in the early years affirmed the merits of the vision. Had there not been a need created by war; discomfort with the depersonalization and machine-maiming of industry; a push for hospital and other societal reforms; growing knowledge about teaching, psychology, and efficiency; and advances in medicine sufficient to permit a focus on chronic illness, one wonders whether the outcome might have been the same.

To regret the passing of the early 20th century as a time during which the founders resisted forces that threatened to undermine their essential idea constitutes a misreading of the time and a romanticizing of the founders. The founders, visionary and caring people with varied backgrounds and life experiences, shaped the unique, multifaceted character of occupational therapy. Although the idea of the use of occupation was not new, having been used before by psychiatrists, attendants, nurses, and social workers, the founding of a Society to name and promote occupational therapy extended that idea in time and into many places. The multifaceted character of occupational therapy practice today, when centered on occupation and relationships, rooted in a concern for care and function, and sensitive to broader societal issues and problems, extends the legacy into the 21st century.

References

American Occupational Therapy Association. (1940). History. *Occupational Therapy and Rehabilitation, 19,* 30.

American Occupational Therapy Association. (1972). Occupational therapy: Its definition and functions. *American Journal of Occupational Therapy, 26,* 204–205.

Barton, G. E. (1914). A view of invalid occupation. *Trained Nurse and Hospital Review, 52,* 327–330.

Barton, G. E. (1915a). Occupational nursing. *Trained Nurse and Hospital Review, 54,* 335–338.

Barton, G. E. (1915b). Occupational therapy. *Trained Nurse and Hospital Review, 54,* 138–140.

Barton, G, E. (1920). What occupational therapy may mean to nursing. *Trained Nurse and Hospital Review, 64,* 304–310.

Barton, I. G. (1968). Consolation house, fifty years ago. *American Journal of Occupational Therapy, 22,* 340–345.

Beers, C. W. (1917). *A mind that found itself.* New York: Longmans, Green.

Bing, R.K. (1983). Nationally Speaking—The industry, the art, and the philosophy of history. *American Journal of Occupational Therapy, 37,* 800–801.

Bockoven, J. S. (1971). Occupational therapy—A historical perspective: Legacy of moral treatment—1800's to 1910. *American Journal of Occupational Therapy, 25,* 223–225.

Carlova, J., & Ruggles, O. (1946). *The healing heart.* New York: Julian Messner.

Cooper, G. (1918). Re-weaving the web: A soldier tells what it means to begin all over again. *Carry On, 1*(4), 23–26.

Dunton, W. R. (1919). *Reconstruction therapy.* Philadelphia: Saunders.

Dunton, W. R. (1921a). The development of reconstruction therapy. *Trained Nurse and Hospital Review, 67,* 16–21.

Dunton, W. R. (1921b). *Occupational therapy: A manual for nurses.* Philadelphia: Saunders.

Dunton, W. R. (1930). Occupational therapy. *Occupational Therapy and Rehabilitation, 9,* 343–350.

Dunton, W. R. (1932). Thomas Bessell Kidner. *American Journal of Psychiatry, 89,* 194–196.

Dunton, W. R. (1943). How I got that way. *Occupational Therapy and Rehabilitation, 22,* 244–246.

Dunton, W. R. Jr. (1955). Today's principles reflected in early literature. *American Journal of Occupational Therapy, 9,* 17–18.

Dunton, W. R. Jr. (1967). Occupations and amusements: Organization of the National Society for Promotion of Occupational Therapy. *American Journal of Occupational Therapy, 21,* 287–289.

Hall, H. J. (1921). Forward steps in occupational therapy during 1920. *Modern Hospital, 16*, 245–247.

Hall, H. J. (1922). Editorial—American Occupational Therapy Association. *Archives of Occupational Therapy, 1*, 163–165.

Hall, H. J., & Buck, M. M. (1915). *The work of our hands*. New York: Moffat, Yard.

Hopkins, H. L. (1978). An historical perspective on occupational therapy. In H. L. Hopkins & H. D. Smith (Eds.), *Willard and Spackman's occupational therapy* (5th ed., pp. 3–23.) Philadelphia: Lippincott.

Hull, H. H. (1931). A survey of occupational therapy. *Occupational Therapy and Rehabilitation, 10*, 217–234.

Johnson, J. (1981). Old values—New directions: Competence, adaptation, integration. *American Journal of Occupational Therapy, 35*, 589–598. (Reprinted as Chapter 63.)

Johnson, S. C. (1919). Occupational therapy, vocational re-education and industrial rehabilitation. *Modern Hospital, 12*, 221–223.

Kidner, T. B. (1923). Planning for occupational therapy. *Modern Hospital, 21*, 414–428.

Kidner, T. B. (1924). Occupational therapy in 1923. *Modern Hospital, 22*, 55–57.

Kidner, T. B. (1929a). Address to graduates. *Occupational Therapy and Rehabilitation, 8*, 379–385.

Kidner, T. B. (1929b). Standards of occupational therapy. *Occupational Therapy and Rehabilitation, 8*, 243–247.

Kidner, T. B. (1930). The progress of occupational therapy. *Occupational Therapy and Rehabilitation, 9*, 221–223.

Kielhofner, G., & Burke, J. P. (1977). Occupational therapy after 60 years: An account of changing identity and knowledge. *American Journal of Occupational Therapy, 31*, 675–689.

King, L. J. (1980). Creative caring. *American Journal of Occupational Therapy, 34*, 522–528.

Leuret, J. (1948). On the moral treatment of insanity. *Occupational Therapy and Rehabilitation, 27*, 27–33.

Licht, S. (1967). The founding and founders of the American Occupational Therapy Association. *American Journal of Occupational Therapy, 21*, 269–277.

Licht, S. L. (Ed.). (1948). *Occupational therapy source-book*. Baltimore: Williams & Wilkins.

Meyer, A. (1922). The philosophy of occupational therapy. *Archives of Occupational Therapy, 1*, 2–3. (Reprinted as Chapter 2.)

Miller, A. D. (1918). How can a woman best help? *Carry On, 1*, 17–18.

Mock, H. E. (1919). Curative work. *Carry On, 1*(9), 12–17.

Moodie, C. S. (1919). The value of occupational therapy to the nursing profession. *Hospital Social Service Quarterly, 1*, 313–315.

Myers, C. M. (1948). Pioneer occupational therapists in World War I. *American Journal of Occupational Therapy, 2*, 208–215.

Northrup, F. M. (1928). Work on wards: Methods, crafts and equipment. *Occupational Therapy and Rehabilitation, 7*, 267.

Occupational therapists meet again with A.H.A. (1923). *Modern Hospital, 21*, 499–502.

A patient looks at occupational therapy. (1930). *Occupational Therapy and Rehabilitation, 9*, 277–280.

Peloquin, S. M. (1989). Looking Back—Moral treatment: Contexts considered. *American Journal of Occupational Therapy, 43*, 537–544. (Reprinted as Chapter 4.)

Reed, K. L., & Sanderson, S. R. (1983). *Concepts of occupational therapy* (2nd ed.). Baltimore: Williams & Wilkins.

Reverby, S. M. (1987). *Ordered to care: The dilemma of American nursing, 1850–1945*. Cambridge, England; Cambridge University Press.

Shaw, C. N. (1929). Occupation as an aid to recovery. *Occupational Therapy and Rehabilitation, 8*, 199–206.

Slagle, E. C. (1927). To organize an "O.T." department. *Occupational Therapy and Rehabilitation, 6*, 125–130.

Smith, P. (1929). The value of occupational therapy from a medical inspector's standpoint. *Occupational Therapy and Rehabilitation, 8*, 331–334.

Spackman, C. S. (1968). A history of the practice of occupational therapy for restoration of physical function: 1917–1967. *American Journal of Occupational Therapy, 22*, 67–71.

Staff. (1923). Nurse's appreciation of George Edward Barton. *Modern Hospital, 21*, 658.

Stattel, F. M. (1977). Occupational therapy: Sense of the past—Focus on the present. *American Journal of Occupational Therapy, 31*, 649–650.

Sutton, B. (1925). Enthusiasm in occupational therapy. *Modern Hospital, 24*, 54.

Tracy, S. E. (1913). *Studies in invalid occupation: A manual for nurses and attendants*. Boston: Whitcomb & Barrows.

Tracy, S. E. (1921). Getting started in occupational therapy. *Trained Nurse and Hospital Review, 67*, 397–399.

Upham, E. G. (1917). Some principles of occupational therapy. *Modern Hospital, 8*, 409–413.

Vaux, C. L. (1929). Habit training. *Occupational Therapy and Rehabilitation, 8*, 327–329.

Welles, C. (1976). Ethics in conflict: Yesterday's standards—Outdated guide for tomorrow? *American Journal of Occupational Therapy, 30*, 44–47.

Wilson, S. C. (1929). Habit training for mental cases. *Occupational Therapy and Rehabilitation, 8*, 189–197.

Woodside, H. H. (1971). Occupational therapy—A historical perspective: The development of occupational therapy—1910–1929. *American Journal of Occupational Therapy, 25,* 226–230.

Yerxa, E.J. (1980). Occupational therapy's role in creating a future climate of caring. *American Journal of Occupational Therapy, 34,* 529–534.

Related Readings

Aims of the American Occupational Therapy Association. (1922). *Modern Hospital, 18,* 54.

Billings, F. (1919). Leaving too soon: The disabled soldier should remain in the hospital for full restoration, physical and mental. *Carry On, 1,* 8–10.

Boltz, 0. H. (1927). The rationale of occupational therapy from the psychological standpoint. *Occupational Therapy and Rehabilitation, 6,* 277–282.

Bonner, C. A. (1929). Occupational therapy: Its contribution to the modern mental institution. *Occupational Therapy and Rehabilitation, 8,* 387–391.

Bowman, E. (1922). Psychology of occupational therapy. *Archives of Occupational Therapy, 1,* 171–178.

Brannan, J. W. (1922). Occupational therapy. *American Journal of Public Health, 12,* 367–376.

Carroll, R. S. (1910). The therapy of work. *Journal of the American Medical Association, 54,* 2032–2035.

Crane, B. T. (1919). Occupational therapy. *Boston Medical and Surgical Journal, 181,* 63–65.

Cromwell, F. S. (1977). Eleanor Clarke Slagle, the leader, the woman. *American Journal of Occupational Therapy, 31,* 645–648.

Cullimore, A. R. (1921). Objectives and motivation in occupational therapy. *Modern Hospital, 17,* 537–538.

Dunton, W. R. (1944). Some older occupational therapy literature. *Occupational Therapy and Rehabilitation, 23,* 138–141.

Dunton, W. R. Jr. (1913). Occupation as a therapeutic measure. *Medical Record, 83,* 388–389.

Durgin, D. D. (1923). The value of occupational therapy. *State Hospital Quarterly, 8,* 382.

Elton, F. G. (1924). Relationship of occupational therapy to rehabilitation. *Archives of Occupational Therapy, 3,* 101–108.

Gilfoyle, E. M. (1980). Caring: A philosophy of practice. *American Journal of Occupational Therapy, 34,* 517–521.

Gilligan, M. B. K. (1976). Developmental stages of occupational therapy and the feminist movement. *American Journal of Occupational Therapy, 30,* 560–567.

Grant, I. (1920). Practical side of occupational therapy. *Modern Hospital, 15,* 504–505.

Grant, I. (1928). Bedside, ward, porch and shop methods. *Occupational Therapy and Rehabilitation, 7,* 95–98.

Gundersen, P. G. (1927). Dynamic occupational therapy. *Occupational Therapy and Rehabilitation, 6,* 131–135.

Haas, L. J. (1925). *Occupational therapy for the mentally and nervously ill.* Milwaukee: Bruce.

Hills, F. L. (1909). Work as an immediate and ultimate therapeutic factor. *Journal of the American Medical Association, 53,* 892.

Houston, I. B. (1928). Occupational therapy submerged. *Occupational Therapy and Rehabilitation, 7,* 413–415.

Kahmann, W. C. (1967). Fifty years in occupational therapy. *American Journal of Occupational Therapy, 21,* 281–283.

Kenna, W. M. (1927). Occupational therapy and hospital industries. *Occupational Therapy and Rehabilitation, 6,* 453–461.

Kielhofner, G., & Burke, J. P. (1983). The evolution of knowledge and practice in occupational therapy: Past, present and future. In G. Kielhofner (Ed.), *Health through occupation: Theory and practice in occupational therapy* (pp. 3–54). Philadelphia: F. A. Davis.

Livingston, W. H. (1923). Useful occupational therapy vs. useless occupational therapy. *Modern Hospital, 21,* 51–52.

Mabie, H. R. (1919). A plea for occupational therapy. *Woman Citizen, 4,* 344.

Matthews, W. H. (1923). Work—The cure. *American Journal of Nursing, 24,* 164–167.

McNew, B. B. (1923). "Useless" versus useful occupational therapy. *Modern Hospital, 21,* 62–64.

Occupational therapy, vocational re-education and industrial rehabilitation. (1919). *Modern Hospital, 12,* 221–223.

Occupational therapy. (1921). *Hospital Progress, 2,* 265.

Patients make attractive toys. (1921). *Modern Hospital, 16,* 42.

Patients to be trained. (1920). *Modern Hospital, 15,* 465.

Pennington, L. E. (1925). O.T. known for nearly 2,000 years. *Hospital Management, 19,* 37–38.

Reilly, M. (1962). Eleanor Clarke Slagle Lecture—Occupational therapy can be one of the great ideas of 20th century medicine. *American Journal of Occupational Therapy, 16,* 1–9. (Reprinted as Chapter 6.)

Robinson, G. C. (1919). Occupational therapy in civilian hospitals. *Modern Medicine, 1,* 159–162.

Sands, I. F. (1928). When is occupation curative? *Occupational Therapy and Rehabilitation, 7,* 115–122.

Second annual meeting of the National Society for the Promotion of Occupational Therapy. (1918). *Modern Hospital, 11,* 298.

Six "musts" for occupational therapy. (1921). *Modern Hospital, 16,* 169.

Slagle, E. C. (1921). To organize an "O.T." department. *Hospital Management, 12,* 43–45.

Spear, M. R. (1927). The value and limitations of attendants in occupational therapy departments in mental hospitals. *Occupational Therapy and Rehabilitation, 6,* 225–227.

Thayer, A. S. (1908). Work cure. *Journal of the American Medical Association, 51,* 1485–1487.

True occupational therapy. (1924). *Modern Hospital, 22,* 66.

Value of occupational therapy. (1921). *Hospital Progress, 2,* 316.

War brought wider recognition to O.T. (1923). *Modern Hospital, 20*(1).

What is occupational therapy? (1921). *Modern Hospital, 17,* 234.

Zamir, L. J. (1966). Editorial—Whither occupational therapy. *American Journal of Occupational Therapy, 20,* 195.

Chapter 2

The Philosophy of Occupation Therapy

Adolph Meyer

This chapter was previously published in the *Archives of Occupational Therapy, 1,* 1–10.

This paper was originally "Read at Fifth Annual Meeting of the National Society for the Promotion of Occupational Therapy (now the American Occupational Therapy Association), held in Baltimore, Md., October 20–22, 1921."

There was a time when physicians and the public thought the art of medicine consisted mainly in diagnosing more or less mysterious diseases and "prescribing" for them. Each disease was supposed to have its program of treatment, and to this day the patient and the family expect a set of medicines and a diet, and a change of climate if necessary, or at least a rest-cure so as to fight and conquer "the disease." No branch of medicine has learned as clearly as psychiatry that after all many of these formidable diseases are largely problems of adaptation and not some mysterious devil in disguise to be exorcised by asfetida and other usually bitter and, if possible, alcoholic stuffs; and psychiatry has been among the first to recognize the need of adaptation and the value of work as a sovereign help in the problems of adaptation.

It so happened that in the first medical paper I ever presented, about December, 1892, or January, 1893—curiously enough before the Chicago Pathological Society, where one would least expect discussions of occupation—I asked my new neighbors and colleagues for suggestions as to the tastes and best lines of occupation of American patients. The proper use of time in some helpful and gratifying activity appeared to me a fundamental issue in the treatment of any neuropsychiatric patient. Soon after that, May 1, 1893, I went to Kankakee and found in that institution some ward work and shop work, and later, under the inspiration of Isabel Davenport, some gardening for the women in her convalescent cottages. But I also found there a little of a feeling which pervaded quite conspicuously much of the contemporary attitude toward this question.

Among a most interesting collection of abstracts from the history of American institutions put at my disposal by Dr. Wm. R. Dunton, I find a report on the employment of the insane by a committee from the Michigan institutions, dated 1822 and signed by Dr.

Henry M. Hurd. The committee had visited European institutions and had been especially impressed by the use of occupation as a substitute for restraint. But they have a fear that the presence of *private* patients would interfere with the introduction of occupation. The conclusions contain the following statements:

> Employment of some sort should be made obligatory for all able-bodied patients ... (But) it would be feared that such measures would meet with much opposition from all quarters .... It might, consequently, be best to arrange at first for the employment of state patients and to procure legislative sanction of the step. If this works advantageously it will be comparatively easy to extend the system to other patients.

This represents the attitude of many hospital men of the time. Industrial shops and work in laundry and kitchen and on the wards were the achievements of that problem—very largely planned to relieve the employees.

A new step was to arise from a freer conception of work, from a concept of free and pleasant and profitable *occupation—including recreation and any form of helpful enjoyment as the leading principle.*

When in 1895 I was transplanted to Worcester, Mass., there was little in the atmosphere to foster interest in occupation: ward-work and a few shops managed merely from the point of view of utility. Only the McLean hospital had the beginnings of some organized recreative occupations. From 1902 it was my good fortune to have to work on Ward's Island in a division which then was under the immediate direction of an unusually active and enterprising man, Dr. Emmett C. Dent, always eager for therapeutic results and untiring in his development of hospital principles in the face of very cramped opportunities. In this new atmosphere I was greatly assisted by the wholesome human understanding of my helpmate, Mrs. Meyer, who under these conditions may have been one of the first, if not the first, to introduce a new systematized type of activity into the wards of a state institution.

She had become a great help to my patients in visiting them in my ward and had started the visiting of the homes, as probably the first social worker with a systematic program of help to patient, family and physician, just before Miss Louise Schuyler urged the introduction of a very eleemosynary type of aftercare in November, 1906. When in 1907 a real social worker, Miss Horton, was appointed, Mrs. Meyer turned her attention to the occupation and organized recreations of the patients on the ward, not only in the shops and amusement hall, but in the employment of the available time on the ward.

Shortly after that, in 1909, Miss Lathrop and the Chicago School of Civics and Philanthropy undertook a course of training in play and occupation for nurses, and Miss Wright was chosen to attend it and she returned to organize the work throughout the institution—with a wise balance between organized shopwork and more individual work on the wards.

It had long been interesting to see how groups of a few excited patients can be seated in a corner in a small circle of two or three settees and kept wonderfully contented picking the hair of mattresses, or doing simple tasks not too readily arousing the desire for big movements and uncontrollable excitement and yet not too taxing to their patience. Groups of patients with raffia and basket work, or with various kinds of handwork and weaving and bookbinding and metal and leather work, took the place of the bored wall flowers and of mischief-makers. A pleasure in achievement, a real pleasure in the use and activity of one's hands and muscles and a happy *appreciation of time* began to be used as incentives in the management of our patients, instead of abstract exhortations to cheer up and to behave according to abstract or repressive rules. The main advance of the new scheme was the blending of work and pleasure—all made possible by a wise supplementing of centralization by individualization and a kind of redecentralization.

When the Phipps Clinic was opened, we were able to secure the services of Mrs. Slagle, who, with her successors—Mrs. Price and Miss DeHoff, and Mrs. Marion, Mr. Russell, and Mr. Cass—brought us to the level you find now represented at the Phipps Clinic.

This contact with the evolution of occupation therapy gave a good opportunity to see this movement grow to a position which we now want to consider more closely.

Somehow it represents to me a very important manifestation of a very general gain in human philosophy. There is in all this a development of the *valuation of time and work* which is not accidental. It is part of the great espousal of the *values of reality and actuality* rather than of mere thinking and reasoning and fancy as characteristic of the nineteenth century and the present day.

As I said in my brief abstract, we feel today that the culminating feature of evolution is man's capacity of imagination and *the use of time with foresight* based on a corresponding appreciation of the past and of the *present*. We know more definitely than ever that the twenty-four hours of the day are the problem of nursing and immediate therapy, and not the medicines taken *t. i. d.* Somehow something apparently *self-evident* has taken its *proper position* in our attention. Just as in the medical aspects we have come to value an appreciation of the exceedingly *simple* facts of basal metabolism (that is, the simple measure of the amount of CO_2 we produce), so the simple fact of employment of *time* has become an important measure and problem for physician and nurse. The most important factor in the progress lay *undoubtedly* in the newer conceptions of *mental problems* as *problems of living*, and not merely diseases of a structural and toxic nature on the one hand or of a final lasting constitutional disorder on the other. The formulation in terms of habit-deterioration of even those grave mental disorders presently the serious problem of *terminal dementia* made *systematic engagement of interest, and concern about the actual use of* TIME *and work an obligation and necessity.*

It is very interesting that the progress of all the fundamental sciences has shown the same trend during the last thirty years. The nineties of the nineteenth and the first decade of the twentieth century marked the rise of *energetics* (so effectively brought home to all scientists by Professor Ostwald in his lectures in this country some fifteen years ago)—a determination to replace the interest in *inert matter* by a broad conception of the world of physics and chemistry in terms of *energies*, which means literally "applications of *work*." Similarly, during this same period of study of human and of animal life gave birth to the concept of *behaviorism* with its emphasis on performance as the fundamental formulation of what had figured up to that time on the throne of an abstract timeless psychology, curiously enough, first invaded by science in the form of studies in reaction-*time*. Direct *experience* and performance were everywhere acknowledged as the fullest type of life. Thought, reason and fancy were more and more recognized as merely a *step* to *action*, and mental life in general as the integrator of *time*, giving us the fullest sense of past, present and future, but after all the best type of reality and actuality only in real *performance*. We all know how fancy and abstract thought can go far afield—undisciplined and uncensured and uncorrected; while *performance* is its own judge and regulator and therefore the most dependable and influential part of life. Our body is not merely so many pounds of flesh and bone figuring as a machine, with an abstract mind or soul added to it. It is throughout a live organism pulsating with its rhythm of rest and activity, beating time (as we might say) in ever so many ways, most readily intelligible and in the full bloom of its nature when it feels itself as one of those great self-guiding *energy-transformers* which constitute the real world of living beings. Our conception of man is that of an organism that maintains and balances itself in the world of reality and actuality by being in active life and active use, i.e., using and living and acting its *time* in harmony with its own nature and the nature about it. It is the use that we make of ourselves that gives the ultimate stamp to our every organ.

This growing conviction that personality is fundamentally determined by *performance* rather than by mere good-will and good intention rapidly became the backbone of our psychology and psychopathology. It became a fair task for our ingenuity to *obtain* performance wherever it had failed to come *spontaneously* and thereby to serve the organism in the task of keeping itself in good form.

This philosophy of reality, of work and time, seen in all the sciences appeals to me because it expresses, with respect for fact, the simple and yet most valuable experiences of real life.

The whole of human organization has its shape in a kind of rhythm. It is not enough that our hearts should beat in a useful rhythm, always kept up to a standard at which it can meet rest as well as wholesome *strain* without upset. There are many other rhythms which we must be attuned to: the *larger rhythms* of night and day, of sleep and waking hours, of hunger and its gratification, and finally the big four—work and play and rest and sleep, which our organism must be able to balance even under difficulty. The only way to attain balance in all this is *actual doing*, *actual practice*, a program of wholesome living as the *basis* of wholesome feeling and thinking and fancy and interests.

Thus, with our *patients*, we naturally begin with a natural simple regime of *pleasurable* ease, the creation of an orderly *rhythm* in the atmosphere (a wise rule of using all our natural rhythms), the sense of a day simply and naturally spent, perhaps with some music and restful dance and play, and with some glimpses of activities which any one can hope to achieve and derive satisfaction from.

In this frame of rhythm and order of time, we naturally heed also the other factors—the personal interests and personal fitness. A large proportion of our patients present inferiority feelings, often over a sense of awkwardness and inability to use the hands to produce things worth while, i.e., respected by themselves or others. To get the pleasure and pride of achievement and use of one's hands and muscles, the feeling of worthwhileness of a little effort and of a well fitted use of time, is the basic remedy for the blasé tedium that characterizes the indifference or the hopeless depression (that stands in the way of rallying thwarted personalities). I am convinced that a premium should be put on the production of things that are finished in one or a few sittings and yet have an independent emotional value. They must give the satisfaction of completion and achievement, and that in the eye of the maker and of those for whom he has tried to work. Performance and completion form also the backbone and essence of what Pierre Janet has so well described as the "fonction du real"—the *realization* of reality, bringing the very soul of man out of dreams of eternity to the full sense and appreciation of actuality.

Our role consists in giving *opportunities* rather than prescriptions. There must be opportunities to work, opportunities to do and to plan and create, and to learn to use material. There are bound to be valuable opportunities for timely and actually deserved approval and encouragement. It is not a question of specific *prescriptions*, but of opportunities, except perhaps where suggestions can be derived from the history of the patient and a minute study of the trends of fancy and even delusions reveals the lines of predilections and native longings—yet even here the physician would only exert his ingenuity to adapt *opportunities*.

In a meeting like this, the personal contact of many practical inspirers brings out an interchange of experiences and resources from the side of the instructors and helpers.

It takes rare gifts and talents and rare personalities to be real pathfinders in this work. There are no royal roads; it is all a problem of being true to one's nature and opportunities and of teaching others to do the same with themselves. I went through the occupation departments of a large institution the other day and was profoundly impressed by the wide differences of the personnel and the manifold ways of approach leading to success with the work. It takes, above all, resourcefulness and ability to respect at the same time the native *capacities and interests* of the patient. Freedom from premature meddling, and tact in avoiding false comparisons or undue expectations fostering disappointment, orderliness without pedantry, cheer and praise without sloppiness and without surrender of standard-these may be the rewards of a good use of personal gifts and of good training.

Somehow I see in all this profound importance extending far beyond our special field. Our efforts seem to me destined to be the soil for helps of much wider applicability. Present day humanity seems to suffer from a deluded craze for finding substitutes for actual work. It seems more difficult than ever to guide with the traditional preachments.

Our industrialism has created the false, because onesided, idea of success in *production* to the point of overproduction, bringing with it a kind of nausea to the worker and a delirium of the trader living on advertisement and salesmanship, instead of sound economics of a fair and sane distribution of the goods of this world according to need, and an education of the public as to where and how to find the best and worthiest.

The man of today has lost the capacity and pride of workmanship and has substituted for it a measure in terms of money; and now his money proves to be of uncertain value. A great deal of activity, to be individually and socially acceptable and exciting enough and mentionable for social exhibition of one's worth, has to be of the nature of conspicuous waste, a class performance like athletics and golf and racing about the country, and a display of rapidly changing fashions. Work and play, ambition and satisfaction, are apt to lose their natural contact with the natural rhythms of appetite and gratification, vision and performance, and finishable cycles of completion—of work and play and rest and sleep.

Our special work, which tries to do justice to special human needs, I feel is destined to serve again as the center of a great gain for the normal as well. It will work like the Montessori system of education. Grown out of the needs of defective children, it has become the source of inspiration and methods for a freer education for *all* children.

What satisfactions you may develop in the guidance in difficult conditions may bring out the best principles and philosophy for the ordinary walks of life.

We are often told, and I suppose it is largely true, that the world cannot and will not move back. A new sense of *uses of time*, new satisfactions from that inexhaustible fountain, that one thing, time, that will come and come, and only waits to become an opportunity used—that seems to me the gospel and salvation of the day. Human ideals have unfortunately and usually been steeped in dreams of timeless *eternity*, and they have never included an equally religious valuation of *actual time* and its meaning in wholesome rhythms. The awakening to a full meaning of time as the biggest wonder and asset of our lives and the valuation of opportunity and performance as the greatest *measure* of time; those are the beaconlights of the philosophy of the occupation worker. I have often felt that Dr. Herbert James Hall represents the true *religion* of work, leading us to a new sense of the sacredness of the moment—when fitted rightly into the rhythms of individual and social and cosmic nature. Another apostle of the Gospel is announced by Prof. Cassimir J. Keyser in his Phi Beta Kappa address in Science (September 9, 1921)—Count Alfred Korzybski's "Manhood of Humanity,"—the science and art of human engineering.

We might well sum up our philosophy in this way:

In the great process of evolution there is a great law of unfolding which shows in every new and higher step what we call the *integration* of the simpler phases into new entities. Thus the inorganic world continues itself into the plant and animal world. The laws of physics and chemistry expand into laws of growth and laws of function, still physical and chemical, but physical and chemical in terms of plans and in terms of the active animal, and finally in terms of more or less highly gifted man, with all that capacity to enjoy and to suffer, to succeed and to fail, to fulfill the life-cycle of the human individual happily and effectively or more or less falteringly. The great feature of man is his new sense of time, with foresight built on a sound view of the past and present. Man learns to organize time and he does it in terms of *doing* things, and one of the many good things he does between eating, drinking and wholesome nutrition generally and the flights of fancy and aspiration, we call *work and occupation*—we might call it the ingestion and digestion and proper use, and we may say a religious *conscience*, of *time* with its successions of *opportunities*.

With this type of background, we may well be able to shape for ourselves and our patients an outlook of sound idealism, furnishing a setting in which many otherwise apparently insurmountable difficulties will be conquered—and in which our new generations will find a world full of ever new opportunity and achievement in healthy harmony with human nature.

Chapter 3

The Influence of the Arts-and-Crafts Movement on the Professional Status of Occupational Therapy

Ruth Levine Schemm, EdD, OTR/L, FAOTA

This chapter was previously published in the *American Journal of Occupational Therapy, 41,* 248–253, under the name of Ruth Ellen Levine. Copyright © 1987, American Occupational Therapy Association.

The arts-and-crafts movement ultimately came to be regarded as an oddity; yet in its beginnings, it was widespread and deeply influential. Its origins can be traced to the work of John Ruskin, a mid-nineteenth-century British university professor.

Ruskin (1884b) maintained that machines and factory work limited human happiness. He urged a return to simpler ways of life where experience was "more authentic" because less complicated by modern bureaucratic and industrial structures. Ruskin was a romantic, looking back to similar ages when humankind purportedly was healthier because more connected with its environment, its work, and its religious values.

He found the Middle Ages especially attractive and lectured on facets of medieval life. Architecture especially interested him, and he pointed to the construction of Gothic churches as an example of how values were incorporated into people's lives: Workmen completed uplifting projects which gave a central meaning to their lives (Ruskin, 1884a). He also maintained that humans, not machines, completed objects; therefore, work was not abstracted from life but had a place at its very core. The manufactured goods of his own time he found to be both aesthetically and morally unsatisfying because the worker was treated like an extension of the machine, completing only a part of the finished product.

Ruskin's ideas were further refined by William Morris who criticized machine "gimcrackery" as threatening the foundation of civilized life (Rodgers, 1974, p. 77). These ideas struck a responsive chord in the United States as well as in Britain. They were most warmly received by the socially advantaged—not because of any widespread disaffection with the capitalist economic system, but because of a discomfort in some circles with excessive materialism and the shoddiness of mass production.

By the turn of the 20th century, the arts-and-crafts movement's advocates formed a network which reached across America. Proponents were eager reformers celebrating nature, authentic experience, and honest design. Like their British contemporaries, they displayed a patrician contempt for the system of mass production, which was keyed to lower class tastes. They advocated the use of natural materials and processes and the purchase and use of handmade items that were straightforward and simple in design. Indeed, for some advocates, the arts-and-crafts movement meant quality of design as much as quality of life.

In the United States, 25 arts-and-crafts societies appeared from 1895 to 1907 (Rodgers, 1974, p. 78). These handicraft clubs where filled with middle- and upper-middle-class Americans striving for self-improvement as well as social stability (Lears, 1981). Reverence for authentic objects and simple but substantial designs for homes and furnishings testified to the good taste of arts-and-crafts proponents while at the same time conveying a comforting and traditional set of moral values (Wright, 1980). This was helpful in a world where strong ambitions threatened permanence and rapid social change heightened the need for stability.

Wiebe (1967) described late nineteenth century America as a "society without a core" (p. 12). Rapid social, economic, technological, civic, and cultural changes had created a "distended" society; yet people were still trying to understand the expanding American society in terms of their familiar, small-town environment. This simplistic orientation created even more problems since a larger vision of the future was required to deal with destabilizing forces such as westward expansion; millions of Eastern European immigrants; rising impersonal, industrialized work; technological advances that linked the country together; declining birth and death rates; changing roles of women; and economic instability.

The smug security of small-town America was ending and local community members felt as if they were losing control over their lives although the "enemy" was not always clear. People yearned for a slower paced life, governed by the old and authentic values. Thus, the arts-and-crafts movement rose in popularity, offering the promise of a more meaningful life-style.

The Transformation of Medicine

Medicine was in part responsible for the initial direction taken by occupational therapy. By the turn of the twentieth century, American physicians were shifting to a scientific foundation. Disease was understood in terms of physiological processes rather than in terms of suffering or personal disorientation; specialists concerned themselves with organs and tissues rather than the whole patient; hospitals removed the sick from their environments and treated them as abstractions; and vital signs collected through such new instruments as the X-ray machine and interpreted by the laboratory obviated the need for the physician to listen to patients' complaints or win the patient's active partnership in treatment planning.

Yet some physicians, often those connected with the most prestigious institutions, believed that science, by itself, did not offer a complete answer to illness. They argued that earlier notions of mind-body unity were being overlooked in the new high-technology medicine. Dr. Herbert J. Hall was one such dissenter. He was interested in neurasthenia, a medical problem that did not reduce itself easily to the limitations of the new medicine. This disease was not obviously physiological, its symptoms were diverse and could be linked to the strain of American life. The malady was identified in middle- and upper-class persons who complained of "morbid anxiety, unaccountable fatigue, irrational fears, and compulsive or inadequate sexual behavior" (Beard, 1881, pp. 7–8; also Lears, 1981, p. 50).

Hall (1910) developed a work cure to take the place of the commonly prescribed bed rest. He based his therapeutics squarely on the philosophy espoused by the arts-and-crafts enthusiasts. After securing financial backing from the prestigious Proctor Fund, he developed a sanatorium in Marblehead, Massachusetts, and began to validate the success of his work cure. Hall joined a network of likeminded physicians.

Two other physician dissenters who also became interested in curative occupations were Adolf Meyer and William Rush Dunton. Both searched for ways to humanize the care of chronically ill patients. Meyer was impressed with the results he saw at Worcester Massachusetts State Hospital where his wife, Mary Potter Brooks Meyer, a social worker, developed an occupations program for ward patients. Adolf Meyer, as a researcher, was usually removed from direct patient care. Mrs. Meyer, therefore, operationalized his ideas on adaptation and the therapeutic prescription of activities (Hopkins, 1979).

In Chicago, the collaboration between Meyer, a medical leader, and Julia Lathrop, a social worker and civic activist, resulted in the application of arts-and-crafts ideology to chronically ill mental patients. Lathrop studied bookbinding at Kelmscott Press under Morris. She wanted to improve the lives of the less fortunate by applying the principles of the arts-and-crafts movement to patient programs. She fulfilled this goal by using her influence as a member of the Illinois State Board of Charities and Correction. She and another Board member, Rabbi Emil Hirsch, in 1906 organized one of the earliest occupations training courses (Addams, 1935).

Dunton, who also came to believe in the curative effect of goal-directed activity, applied the occupations cure to his patients at the Sheppard and Enoch Pratt Asylum in Towson, Maryland, as early as 1895. By 1908, his observations of patients' undirected efforts led him to search for an arts-and-crafts teacher. Using *Studies in Invalid Occupations: A Manual for Nurses and Attendants* by Susan E. Tracy (1912), a nurse, Dunton established his own training program.

In her book, Tracy described an occupations training course she designed in 1906 for nurses working at Adams Nervine Hospital in Boston. The text, which is basically a craft book, offered teaching strategies, supply lists, and treatment rationales for a variety of settings, including the homes of advantaged and disadvantaged patients. These progressive physicians, Meyer, Hall, and Dunton, worked with social caretakers Lathrop and Tracy to link the holistic treatment of the past with modern, scientific approaches (Burnham, 1972). Combining ideas that were once important in medical practice with ideas from the arts-and-crafts movement, these individuals founded a new profession, which was later named occupational therapy.

The Arts-and-Crafts Origins in Occupational Therapy

Early occupational therapy practice combined the therapeutic and medical with the diversional and recreational use of activities. One of the earliest sources of overlap between these applications was the sheltered workshop. Hall and other physicians championed the development of sheltered workshops where patients produced carefully designed, well-made objects such as hand towels, ceramic vases, and cement pots. The craft objects were sold in shops that had three purposes—to employ talented people who could earn a living by making authentic objects, to give spiritual support to craftspeople who pursued crafts as an avocation, and to help employ the mentally and physically handicapped ("Craftsmanship," 1906; Evans, 1974; Roorbach, 1913; Simkhovitch, 1906). These purposes frequently overlapped, and it soon became difficult to separate rehabilitation goals from the aesthetic ideology of the arts-and-crafts movement.

Following Hall's lead, George Barton, an architect familiar with Morris, joined the Boston Society of Arts and Crafts in 1901. Barton was not a healthy man, and after a long struggle with tuberculosis he decided to move to Denver where he lost his left foot to frostbite in 1912. Depressed and ill, he returned to the East and sought the advice and counsel of both a physician and a minister who urged him to direct his energies toward a productive mission. Barton decided to help others instead of focusing on his own health problems and opened Consolation House in Clifton Springs, New York, in 1914. He received referrals from physicians and applied the principles of therapeutic arts and crafts to disabled individuals such as himself (Reed and Sanderson, 1983).

Barton joined a group of workshop managers who had to balance conflicting personnel and production goals. Goods had to be appealing, well made, and relatively cheap. Thus, the arts-and-crafts workshop proved a difficult venture even for nondisabled craftsmen because of the competition from mass-produced goods (Boris, 1984). The successful therapeutic workshop also had to address the additional factor of varied and inconsistent client needs. Above all, the goal of the therapeutic workshop was to move successful performers back into the workforce.

Solvent workshop endeavors were rare even if workers were nondisabled, skilled, and efficient. Machine-made goods proved to be stiff competition in the marketplace, lowering prices on workshop-produced goods and squeezing profits (Boris, 1984). To survive, workshops shifted their focus from therapeutics to cost-conscious ventures that would reap profits. The individualistic thrust of early occupational therapy was lost in this shift to economic considerations.

The early occupational therapy link to the arts-and-crafts movement did not end with the demise of the therapeutic workshop. This influence was still evident in the 1930s and 1940s, long after the ideas and beliefs of the proponents of the arts-and-crafts movement disappeared from the American culture. Evidence is plentiful: Black (1935) discussed the employment of sheep herders in the Arts and Crafts League of New Hampshire, Ash (1940) presented the use of handicrafts with blind and retarded patients, annual conferences included craft instructions, and the 1932 Annual Institute of Chief Occupational Therapists devoted 25% of its conference to a folk dance, a lecture, and a demonstration (Annual Institute for Chief OT's, 1932).

Glaser (1930) noted that the eye, hand, mind, and creative imagination are stimulated by arts and crafts. In line with this thinking, occupational therapy schools offered courses in needlework, weaving, metalwork, bookbinding, and leatherwork. The missions and philosophies of occupational therapy and the arts-and-crafts movement were so intertwined that few therapists would have disagreed with Will Levington Comfort when he remarked that "there is something holy in the crafts and the arts" (as cited by Glaser, 1930, p. 131).

Healthy individuals were drawn to the arts-and-crafts movement because involvement with arts and crafts promised to settle nervous lives. The occupational therapy founders creatively applied these ideas to a neglected group of chronically disabled patients. These applications were varied and creative and included the management of pain during recuperation, the redirection of the wandering minds of elders, and the diversion of self-indulgent thoughts of depressives. Therapists were slow to depart from the prescriptions of the founders who had argued that the "scientific" prescription of arts and crafts could cure a variety of chronic problems generally considered outside of the domain of medicine (Tracy, 1912; Hall & Buck, 1916; Dunton, 1918).

Changes in Social Values Create Conflicting Philosophies

Only a thin line divided the arts-and-crafts philosophy from occupational therapy. Arts-and-crafts persons were diversionists using an activity to achieve a cure; yet to them the craft product was as valued as the process. Therapists differed slightly, they focused more on the concept of function and were less concerned with the product, but they still used crafts.

Trained in specific modalities, many diversionists neglected the patient's interest in the activity at hand. Consistent with their crafts training, they searched for information about specific crafts rather than exploring why the occupation cure succeeded. Diversionists fervently believed that craftwork alone was curative. This belief was based on the work ethic. The differences between therapists and diversionists grew more and more obvious in the 1930s and 1940s.

The overlap between personal interests and professional roles and responsibilities was also confusing. Even Dunton demonstrated a mixture of personal and professional interests, displaying his quilt collection at an occupational therapy meeting held at the Baltimore Handicraft Club ("OT Notes," 1930). This mixture of values proved difficult for early therapists who were trained in fine arts and specific crafts. To abandon their commitment to craftsmanship, to embrace the process over the end product was a violation of their cherished belief in the arts-and-crafts movement. Diversionists were so tied to the arts-and-crafts ideology that they overlooked the process by which the therapist elicits the patient's goals, values, and interest in the activity process (Dunton, 1928).

Furthermore, the professional occupational therapist was under severe strains. Health care's focus on the individual further eroded as the status of physicians rose and medicine was transformed into a specialty practice based on scientific principles. In this milieu, the holistic philosophy of early occupational therapy practice was increasingly compromised as diversionists continued to focus on specific craft concerns (Hall, 1922).

The Depression contributed to the changes in health care delivery. In some states, over 40% of the population subsisted on relief. The national income plummeted to less than half of what it had been in 1929 (Stevens, 1971). The bleak industrial situation created shortages in health services and providers. Physicians' incomes fell, nurses were unemployed, and hospitals developed insurance to guarantee payment. For many Americans, medical care became a luxury (Starr, 1982).

Occupational therapy survived using strategies such as "classes" to provide treatment to large numbers of patients. At the same time, leaders pushed therapists away from the values of the arts-and-crafts mission and toward the medical model (Mock, 1930; Munger, 1935). Occupational therapy leaders embraced functional concerns; arts-and-crafts values were subordinated to the functional orientation. Occupational therapy, like medicine, assumed responsibility for making decisions for the patient's welfare. Unlike the developing science of medicine, however, therapists had no technology to measure the accuracy of their prescriptions.

Occupational therapy was caught in a web of conflicting ideas. The scientific goals of medicine pulled against the holistic goals of the arts-and-crafts movement. Change did not come smoothly. In 1930, Eleanor Clarke Slagle, a prominent occupational therapy leader, felt obligated to warn new graduates of Sheppard and Enoch Pratt Hospital that "handiwork alone was insufficient" (p. 271).

Joseph Doane (1931), a physician and president of the American Occupational Therapy Association, was equally emphatic when he differentiated between two groups of occupational therapists: "There are those who believe that the occupationalist who diverts and amuses and who as a by-product perhaps spiritually improves the sick, contributes the greatest good to the community" (p. 365). Doane maintained that the "occupationalist" is likely to possess less vision and training than the therapist who uses supplies as a means to the performance end. Doane rejected the arts-and-crafts movement and promoted the science of occupational therapy. He noted that "Occupational therapy is not a fad which like many others seizes the imagination of a community or country and then suddenly relinquishes its hold" (p. 364).

Dr. Horatio M. Pollock (1934) traced occupational therapy back to Galen in the second century but noted that occupational therapy "has not yet won a place in the consciousness of a large part of the medical profession" (p. 362). In the same vein, Oscar M. Sullivan (1935), also a physician, predicted the future thrust of occupational therapy when he explained that although "craftwork constitutes the bulk of what is known as occupational therapy," there was no reason that "another kind of practical work should not develop quite as much" (p. 107). It was merely a matter of opportunity and facilities.

Thus, the profession struggled during the 1930s and 1940s and ultimately lost the momentum enjoyed during the initial years of organizing. Pulled by internal tensions regarding the focus of the occupation process, therapists were also influenced by shrinking health resources, the rising status of physicians, the limited roles of professional women, and most distressing, the doubts raised by patients who questioned the merit of craft therapy. In short, few therapists, physicians, or patients remembered the lofty mission of the forgotten arts-and-crafts movement.

Dr. Harry Steckel (1934) noted "it is quite possible that patients do not fully realize or recognize the true value of occupational therapy, even if they are not particularly interested in the project worked on by them" (p. 494). Steckel believed that occupational therapy could be improved by using a variety of projects with "more opportunity for personal choice, with a closer check upon the reaction of the patient to the type of work offered" (p. 498).

Thus occupational therapy survived the 1930s but was moored to the values of a forgotten social movement. Meanwhile, the medical profession had shifted from a holistic to a reductionist focus. During World War II, the occupational therapy profession struggled with the same unresolved tension between craft proponents and therapists, but the context had changed. Younger physicians no longer understood or valued the arts-and-crafts philosophy. Since occupational therapy practice did not seem scientific or theory based, they tended not to take it seriously. The example of a specific hospital offered below demonstrates that therapists changed little in their philosophy, theory, and therapeutic modalities during the first 35 years of practice. Few acknowledged that the context for health services had changed.

The Example of Norristown State Hospital

In 1884, Norristown State Hospital used occupations to control patients or as a "conspicuous feature of the management" ("Official Report," 1884, p. 35). A physician reported that it was not necessary to restrain patients because "employment and varied diversions of the mind" (p. 60) were prescribed. Overcrowding compromised this idealistic beginning. Only such production-oriented activities as farming; sewing dresses, shirts, and sheets; and housekeeping chores survived. Overcrowding continued, and only a few patients were given occupations ("Sixth Annual Report," 1885).

In response to the arts-and-crafts influence, a craftsperson, Nancy Cresson, was hired in 1904 to teach Indian basket making. The focus on occupations was minimal until 1920 when the department for men's occupational therapy was used as a supplement to medical treatment, a means to get the mentally afflicted back into the work force ("41st Annual Report," 1920). That year, 52 men were so engaged. Yet at the same time, a nursing staff shortage caused the closing of the women's arts-and-crafts workroom. Activities were moved to the wards.

The male occupational therapy department was formally organized in 1924. Four therapists were assigned to over 4,000 patients. The department's year end report contained the following facts for 1925: Activities included basketry, art, weaving, and sewing. The patients completed 245 rugs, 257 reed baskets, 324 raffia baskets, 27 leather items, 74 wood items, 92 embroidered objects, 97 lace objects, and 20 fiber mats (Norristown State Hospital, 1925). The arts and crafts focus is clear.

The hospital plant was in disrepair by 1930, and a drought also affected the farm. Yet occupational therapy thrived with four therapists and a supply and material budget. Physician turnover was problematic, but occupational therapy was even mentioned in the hospital mission although the main emphasis was on returning patients to the community. This was a time of opportunity when occupational therapists could have chosen to increase their influence because of the shortage of physicians and the limited status of other professionals. Therapists, nevertheless, were not prepared to take advantage of this opportunity.

Instead, the occupational therapists treated 600 patients during the year, producing 1,662 arts-and-crafts products. The occupational therapy department was described thus:

> Among the diversional methods of treating the mentally sick and hastening recovery is Occupational Therapy-the scheme of scientifically arranged activities which tend to improve the mental and physical health of patients. ("Fifty-Second Annual Report," 1931, p. 27)

The department organized two pageants and other forms of hospital entertainment. By 1934, occupational therapists used small ward groups to "prevent further deterioration in patients" ("Fifty-Fifth Annual Report," 1934, p. 30). Music, movies, bridge, French classes, and dance activities were also part of the department's responsibilities. An elaborate May Day pageant involved over 100 patients. Photos depict patients proudly posing in elaborate costumes and staging activities for patients functioning at a high level. Annual reports and occupational therapy department reports mention only craft and diversional activities.

In the 1937 annual report ("Fifty-Eighth Annual Report"), nursing and occupational therapy were combined. The occupational therapy chief worked with six aides (therapists), and together they offered classes on nine wards. An average of 438 patients participated in occupational therapy programs, and the products were sold for a total of $1,178.23. Program changes in the department were minimal through the 1930s; the occupational therapy department basically continued the same work it had done in the 1920s.

On the other hand, psychologists, nurses, and other health professionals were paralleling the specialization of medicine in their own fields (Burnham, 1974). Occupational therapy was ill prepared to explain the activity process except in the idealistic language of the art-and-crafts movement. The resulting criticism from physicians and other professionals indicates that occupational therapists failed to explain the value of the activity process except in terms of a long forgotten social movement.

The Unresolved Conflict of Values

As the profession matured, confusion regarding our therapeutic mission, goals, and treatment techniques still remained. The use of arts and crafts boosted professional visibility during the early years of development, but the profession paid a price for capitalizing on a therapeutic form that was part of a lay health movement. In fact, occupational therapy became locked into treatment modalities that reflected the social values of a forgotten era. Arts-and-crafts proponents and therapists did not always have similar goals. Surprising evidence of these differences can be found in a telling exchange that took place in 1935.

In a letter to William Rush Dunton, the editor of *Occupational Therapy and Rehabilitation*, Susan Colson Wilson suggested that occupational therapists needed a patron saint. She selected St. Birgetta for the role of patroness. This seemed to upset Dunton, an occupational therapy founder and leader. In a 1935 editorial, Dunton responded sarcastically that

> St. Birgetta might be an admirable patron for the Needlework Guild of America, but her selection as a patron of occupational therapy seems to unduly emphasize a particular craft rather than the special object to be gained by use of any occupation. (p. 223)

Wilson, the chief occupational therapist at Brooklyn State Hospital, was an experienced therapist and an active member of the association. Her suggestion and Dunton's subsequent reply symbolize the conflicting philosophies that continued to surface between the arts-and-crafts proponents and the medically oriented therapists.

Summary

This paper traced the effects of changing health care demands on occupational therapy founders and arts-and-crafts proponents. The Founders were responding to the emerging needs of patients whereas the proponents of the arts-and-crafts movement continued to focus on their original ideas. A study of past events underscores the overwhelming influence of the environment on professional practice. This influence must be recognized so that newly emerging public needs can be addressed.

Acknowledgments

I thank Morris Vogel, PhD, Professor of History at Temple University, Philadelphia, for his helpful comments on an earlier draft of this article and Doris Kaplan, OTR/L, Director of Occupational Therapy, Norristown State Hospital, Norristown, Pennsylvania, for lending supporting documents and artifacts.

References

Addams, J. (1935) *My friend Julia Lathrop*. New York: MacMillan.

Annual institute for chief OT's. (1932). *The Psychiatric Quarterly, 6*, 384–387.

Ash, F. (1940). The value of handicraft for the retarded blind. *Occupational Therapy and Rehabilitation, 19*, 339–343.

Beard, G. M. (1972). *American nervousness, its causes and consequences* [Reprint of 1881 ed.]. New York: Arno Press.

Black, W. D. (1935). League of arts and crafts of New Hampshire. *Occupational Therapy and Rehabilitation, 14*, 29–37.

Boris, E. (1984). *Art and labor: John Ruskin, William Morris, and the craftsman ideal in America 1876–1915*. Philadelphia: Temple University Press.

Burnham, J. C. (1972). Medical specialists and movements toward social control in the progressive era: Three examples. In J. Israel (Ed.), *Building the organizational society* (pp. 19–30). New York: Free Press.

Burnham, J. C. (1974). The struggle between physicians and paramedical personnel in American psychiatry, 1917–41. *Journal of the History of Medicine and Allied Science, 29*, 93–106.

Craftsmanship for crippled children. (1906). *The Craftsman, 9*, 667–677.

Doane, J. C. (1931). Presidential address. *Occupational Therapy and Rehabilitation, 10*, 363–368.

Dunton, W. R. (1918). The principles of occupational therapy. *Public Health Nursing, 10*, 316–321.

Dunton, W. R. (1928). *Prescribing occupational therapy*. Springfield, IL: Charles C Thomas.

Dunton, W. R. (1935). Editorial. *Occupational Therapy and Rehabilitation, 14*, 223.

Evans, P. (1974). *Art pottery of the United States: An encyclopedia of producers and their marks*. New York: Charles Scribner's Sons.

Fifty-eighth annual report of the Norristown State Hospital at Norristown, Pa., S. E. District of Pennsylvania for year ending May 31, 1937. (1937). Norristown, PA: Hospital Printing Office and Bindery.

Fifty-fifth annual report of the Norristown State Hospital at Norristown, Pa., for the year ending May 31, 1934. (1934). Norristown, PA: Hospital Printing Office and Bindery.

Fifty-second annual report of the Norristown State Hospital at Norristown, Pa., for the year ending May 31, 1931. (1931) Norristown, PA: Hospital Printing Office and Bindery.

41st annual report of the State Hospital for the Insane, S. E. District of Pennsylvania, Norristown, Pa., for the year ending May 31, 1920. (1920). Norristown, PA: Hospital Printing Office and Bindery.

Glaser, L. (1930). Some notes on a St. Louis weaving shop. *Occupational Therapy and Rehabilitation, 9*, 127–131.

Hall, H. J. (1910). Work-cure. *JAMA, 54*, 12–14.

Hall, H. J. (1922). President's address. *Archives of Occupational Therapy, 1*, 435–442.

Hall, H. J., & Buck, M. M. C. (1916). *Handicrafts for the handicapped*. New York: Moffat, Yard, and Co.

Hopkins, H. L. (1979). *The status of occupational therapy: Implications for program development*. Unpublished doctoral dissertation, Temple University, Philadelphia.

Lears, J. T. (1981). *No place of grace: Antimodernism and the transformation of American culture*. New York: Pantheon.

Mock, H.E. (1930). The rehabilitation of the disabled. *JAMA, 95,* 31–34.

Munger, C.W. (1935). Fitting OT into the institutional scheme. *Occupational Therapy and Rehabilitation, 14,* 111–119.

Norristown State Hospital. (1925). *Report of occupational therapy for year ending June 1, 1925.* Norristown, PA: Author.

Official report of the trustees and officers of the State Hospital for the Insane for the S.E. District of Pennsylvania at Norristown, Pa., for the Year ending September 30, 1884. (1884). Allentown, PA: Allen W. Haines.

OT Notes. (1930). *Occupational Therapy and Rehabilitation, 9,* 253–258.

Pollock, H.M. (1934). The relation of occupational therapy to medicine. *Occupational Therapy and Rehabilitation, 13,* 361–366.

Reed, K.L. & Sanderson, S.R. (1983). *Concepts in occupational therapy.* Baltimore: Williams & Wilkins.

Rogers, D.T. (1974). *The work ethic in industrial America, 1850–1920.* Chicago: University of Chicago Press.

Roorbach, E. (1913). Making pottery in the California hills. *The Craftsman, 24,* 342–346.

Ruskin, J. (1894a). *Lectures on architecture and painting delivered at Edinburgh in November, 1853.* New York: John Wiley & Sons.

Ruskin, J. (1884b). *Pre-Raphaelitism.* New York: John Wiley & Sons.

Simkhovitch, M.K. (1906). Handicrafts in the city—What their commercial significance is under metropolitan conditions. *The Craftsman, 11,* 363–365.

Sixth annual report of the State Hospital for the Insane for the S.E. District of Pennsylvania at Norristown, Pa., for the year ending September 30, 1885. (1885). Norristown, PA: Hospital Printing Office.

Slagle, E.C. (1930). Address to graduates. *Occupational Therapy and Rehabilitation, 9,* 271–276.

Starr, P. (1982). *The transformation of American medicine.* New York: Basic Books.

Steckel, H. (1934). Retrospective evaluation of therapy. *Psychiatric Quarterly, 8,* 489–498.

Stevens, R. (1971). *American medicine and the public interest.* New Haven: Yale University Press.

Sullivan, O.M. (1935). Relation of occupational therapy to state and federal rehabilitation service. *Occupational Therapy and Rehabilitation, 14,* 105–110.

Tracy, S.E. (1912). *Studies in invalid occupations: A manual for nurses and attendants.* Boston: Whitcomb & Barrows.

Wiebe, R.H. (1967). *The search for order, 1877–1920.* New York: Hill & Wang.

Wright, G. (1980). *Moralism and the model home, domestic architecture and cultural conflict in Chicago. 1873–1913.* Chicago: University of Chicago Press.

Chapter 4

Moral Treatment: Contexts Considered

Suzanne M. Peloquin, PhD, OTR

Moral treatment is intriguing in its emergence, its essence, and its decline. The fascination with moral treatment deepens when one encounters the 20th-century term *occupational therapy* used in historical commentaries about the 19th-century practice. Digby (1985), in discussing moral treatment, noted that "occupational therapy took a variety of forms" (p. 63). Bell (1980) and Grob (1973) both identified occupational therapy as a component of moral treatment. Although this identification is incorrect in the strict historical sense, it is perhaps apt in other ways.

Three views provide different representations of the nature of the relationship between moral treatment and occupational therapy. Bing (1981) (see Chapter 5), an occupational therapist, described the relationship as evolutionary: "Occupational therapy's roots are in the subsoil of the moral treatment developed in Europe during the Age of Enlightenment .... Moral treatment came to the U.S. as part of the Quaker's religious and intellectual luggage .... During the last quarter of the 19th century moral treatment disappeared. It re-emerged in the early decades of the 20th century as Occupational Therapy" (p. 499). In contrast, Bockoven (1971), a psychiatrist, insisted that "the history of moral treatment in America is not only synonymous with, but *is* the history of occupational therapy before it acquired its 20th century name of 'occupational therapy'" (p. 225). Engelhardt (1977), a philosopher familiar with Bockoven's work, suggested a similarity between moral treatment and occupational therapy in the attempt to "effect more successful adaptation to society through organizing certain activities for patients in special environments" (p. 668). These divergent views suggest that a clearer understanding of the nature of moral treatment is relevant for occupational therapy professionals. Such an understanding seems particularly valuable in light of the continued desire within the profession to clarify its identity and its lineage.

A Definition of Moral Treatment

Dr. Thomas Kirkbride (1880/1973), a physician and the superintendent of the Pennsylvania Hospital for the Insane from 1841 to 1883, described moral treatment in terms of daily efforts to provide "system, active movements, and diversity of occupation" to the patients (referred to then as "inmates") (p. 275). Dr. Amariah Brigham (1847), a contemporary of Kirkbride, interpreted moral treatment as "the removal of the insane from home and former associations, with respect and kind treatment upon all circumstances, and in most cases manual labor, attendance on religious worship on Sunday, the establishment of regular habits of self control, [and] diversion of the mind from morbid trains of thought" (p. 1).

More than 150 years later, Dain and Carlson (1960) characterized the theory and practice of moral treatment as the psychological medicine that constituted milieu therapy in the 19th century. Tomes (1984) believed that moral treatment was based on the assumption that one could appeal to the patient's innate capacity to live an ordered and rational existence. To allay any concern that moral treatment meant the enforcement of moral standards, Bockoven (1963) argued that early psychiatrists used the word *moral* to mean *psychological* or *emotional*. He viewed moral treatment as "the first practical effort made to provide systematic and responsible care for an appreciable number of the mentally ill" (p. 12).

Other interpretations articulate various goals and principles underlying moral treatment. Several of these suggest that moral standards were, in fact, guiding principles. Grob (1973) described the goal of moral treatment as the "inculcation, through habit and understanding, of desirable moral traits and values" (p. 12). Rothman (1971) viewed the process of moral treatment as the arrangement of a disciplined routine that provided stability for a person suffering from environmentally generated ills. Bell (1980) considered moral treatment to be a distinct method of therapy that enabled the patient to understand right from wrong within a total therapeutic community. Through moral treatment, the physician manipulated both the environment and the patient to help the patient overcome past associations and to create an atmosphere in which natural restorative elements could assert themselves (Grob, 1983). The image of moral treatment emerging from these interpretations is one of a treatment of the mentally ill that occurred in virtually all institutions; it included humane treatment, a routine of work and recreation, an appeal to reason, and the development of desirable moral traits.

Moral Treatment within Its Various Contexts

An understanding of certain 19th-century conditions is crucial to an appreciation of the significance of moral treatment's emergence. Two environments—the medical community and 19th-century society as a whole—did much to influence the characteristics of moral treatment and its emergence in institutions.

The medical community's perception of insanity greatly influenced the development of moral treatment. A shift in 19th-century thinking revolutionized medical thought: persons with mental disorders, then labeled "the insane," were capable of reason. Before this awareness, insane persons had been considered subhuman because they were believed to be devoid of reason (Deutsch, 1949). Torturous methods were used to treat insane persons. These methods were used not to inflict pain, but to frighten the irrational beast. Methods congruent with contemporary theory included chaining the patients, placing them in cold showers, and lowering them into water-filled wells. The physician's goal was to dominate patients to cure them (Carlson & Dain, 1960). Only when it was acknowledged in the early 19th century that insane persons retained intellectual and rational capacities could treatment methodologies change.

The new philosophy of insanity generated the first humane systems for treatment in Europe. Philippe Pinel, a physician in France, and William Tuke, a Quaker in England, established the specific regimen of moral treatment. Pinel first used the term *moral treatment* (*traitement morale*) in 1801, but it was not until 1817 that a hospital was founded in the United States expressly for the purpose of providing moral treatment. This hospital, built by Pennsylvania Quakers for members of their Society and patterned after Tuke's York Retreat in England, was named the Friend's Asylum. Within 7 years, three more privately endorsed mental asylums (called *corporate asylums*) were built: McLean Hospital in Massachusetts, Bloomingdale Hospital in New York, and the Hartford Retreat in Connecticut. All of these corporate asylums practiced moral treatment (Bockoven, 1963).

This humane system of moral treatment became identified with institutional care. Its character was shaped by the medical men of these early institutions. Scull (1981) called the first four asylums the "earlier generation of asylums" (p. 151). Many developments among this earlier generation significantly influenced later institutions. The first influence related to lines of authority for providing treatment. The Bloomingdale Hospital and the Friend's Asylum, which were patterned after the York Retreat in England, were initially managed by lay superintendents, a custom prevalent in Europe. These superintendents oversaw the provision of moral treatment, and resident physicians provided mild medical treatments for physical conditions. At the Hartford Retreat, a physician named Eli Todd was superintendent. Todd endorsed and supervised traditional therapeutics as well as an increasing use of opium and morphine to complement moral treatment. He campaigned for medical treatment at the other three asylums. As a result of his efforts, medical treatment came to figure more prominently at all of these institutions. Over time, an uneasy relationship developed between the medical leadership and the moral leadership. In 1850, the tension culminated in a codification: An asylum superintendent would be a well-qualified physician. This new role that combined moral and medical functions became the leadership model adopted by the second generation of asylums (Scull, 1981).

A second early asylum influence was the adoption of public relations measures in the community. Superintendents realized that the negative image of European "madhouses" was powerful. They made a point of using annual reports to communicate the advantages of asylum treatment. The widespread communication of these messages was continued by later superintendents.

A final measure through which early superintendents ensured their influence on second-generation asylums was their personal involvement in the establishment of the first state asylums: Worcester State Hospital and Utica Asylum. These two facilities, though designed more for public than for private use, were patterned after the early asylums. These second-generation asylums, in turn, became models for later state facilities. The consolidated physician–superintendent role, the public relations efforts, and the tutelage of second-generation superintendents solidified the manner in which moral treatment would be practiced. The setting would continue to be institutional, the overseers would be physicians, and the public would remain convinced of the utmost practicality of this arrangement.

Changing social patterns during the 19th century helped to place the practice of moral treatment in institutions. America was industrializing, and many people moved from farms to urban centers. The urban family clustered into smaller units and became less able to deal effectively with its ill members. Not surprisingly, the new view of insanity was linked to these changing social patterns of industrialization and urbanization. Dr. Isaac Ray (1861), superintendent of the Butler Hospital, noted that many of his patients displayed deranged moral faculties of the will and of the emotions, although their intellectual faculties remained apparently intact. Deranged moral faculties could be attributed to societal tensions and chaos in the community, which social observances and institutions of the time were unable to handle. The result, for some, was moral insanity (Rothman, 1971).

Given the environmental causes of insanity and the family unit's growing inability to keep a family member with insanity at home, upper- and middle-class members of the community saw the asylum as a new, less chaotic, and more effective environment that could first halt and then reverse the process of insanity. The acceptance of institutions was not a desperate measure. With physician–superintendents and asylum supporters ad-vertising their effectiveness in curing insanity, families admitted the insane with a sense of optimism (Rothman, 1971). The community supported physicians in this new movement toward institutionalization of a class of the population heretofore treated at home. Poor persons, commonly housed in local jails and poorhouses, were minimally affected during the early years of moral treatment (Dain, 1964; Deutsch, 1949; Galt, 1846/1973).

American superintendents shaped the practice of moral treatment. In Europe, the prevalent belief was that moral treatment alone cured insanity; in the United States, some form of medical treatment accompanied moral treatment (Scull, 1981). Tomes (1984) claimed that American superintendents reworked Pinel's original concept of moral treatment to justify treatment by medical doctors. This reworking is evident in Brigham's (1844) writings. He believed that deranged moral and intellectual faculties were generally the result of a diseased brain, although he thought that emotions and great trials of affection could derange brain function and cause insanity. Treatment of insanity stayed within the province of medical practice because physicians continued to link insanity to a disease process. Additionally, moral treatment in the United States was considered most appropriate for recent cases of insanity; more chronic cases (often the long-standing cases among the poor) were considered less likely to be reversed. The chronicity of disease among the poor made them less suitable candidates for moral treatment. For the most part, the asylum community consisted mainly of upper-middle-class doctors treating upper- and middle-class patients.

The Asylum: Structuring a New Environment

American physicians became involved in the design of the new therapeutic environments. As asylum superintendents, they were responsible for individual patient care, management of daily operations, and supervision of asylum personnel. Largely from the upper middle class, they were said to prefer treating patients from their own social stratum (Bell, 1980). They enforced the admission policies specific to their asylums, although they sometimes made concessions to local authorities and accepted a few poor people. Admission policies varied widely. Many corporate institutions totally excluded the poor; others, such as the Quaker asylums, admitted them more freely.

The standards set by the private asylums also set the example for state institutions eager to attract curable patients (Tomes, 1984). The Pennsylvania Hospital for the Insane, a public institution that began receiving patients in 1841, has been called by much of the literature one of the best American mental institutions of that era. Superintendents of corporate asylums welcomed public institutions as an alternative for poor inmates. The previous two-tier treatment system of the asylum versus the poorhouse or jail was evolving into one of the private versus the state institution.

Appropriate construction was a critical factor. Kirkbride thought "a properly constructed building . . . indispensable for such an effect [cure]" (Dain, 1964, p. 76). The building design was also important because it had to appeal to the public. The typical state hospital of the 19th century was constructed according to the Kirkbride Plan, which was officially endorsed by the Association of Medical Superintendents of American Institutions for the Insane. The Kirkbride Plan called for a large central administration building, from which extended several long, straight wings for housing patients. The design of the wings, with windows spaced evenly, embodied the belief that insanity could be cured by an ordered and rational environment (Rothman, 1971).

The internal structure of the asylum was considered as important to the ability to effect a cure as was the external structure. Classification of patients was an essential component of moral treatment and was incorporated into the building's internal structure. In the 19th century, physicians classified insane patients as manic, melancholic, or demented. These categories continued to form one basis for their classification in the asylum. Inmates were also separated according to sex, behaviors, and degree of illness (Tomes, 1984). At the private Friend's Asylum, for example, quiet convalescent inmates were separated from more acutely ill, violent, and noisy patients. Asylums that admitted more heterogeneous populations housed and grouped their inmates according to classes as well. Tomes described the rationale: "Since, in a non-institutional setting, patients would have expected to see class distinctions in housing and employment, the asylum replicated these features of everyday life" (p. 126).

Classification dictated various levels of care. Private asylums usually gave paying patients better treatment than they gave poor patients; this meant better accommodations and more attention. Moral treatment methods for individual patients, then, varied according to their socioeconomic status, sex, degree of illness, and ability to gain admission to an asylum.

Occupations within the Asylum Context

Pinel (1806/1962) said that silence and tranquility prevailed in the Asylum de Bicetre when the Parisian tradesmen supplied the patients with employment that held their attention. He noted that even "the natural indolence and stupidity of ideots [sic] might in some degree be obviated, by engaging them in manual occupations, suitable to their respective capacities" (p. 203).

American superintendents made daily routine and occupation a central component of moral treatment. They claimed that the ultimate results of these two components outweighed the considerable initial cost of the arrangements necessary for their implementation. Labor, or occupation, judiciously used, contributed not only to patient comfort but also to health and recovery (Kirkbride, 1880/1973). Asylum staff went to exceptional lengths to engage patients in manual tasks. Kirkbride encouraged his patients to do any task; the critical thing was to keep busy. The therapeutic rationale was that occupation inculcated the regular habits necessary for recovery (Rothman, 1971). Throughout each carefully structured day, men engaged in agricultural pursuits, carpentry, painting, and general maintenance. Women performed domestic chores and manual crafts. The superintendents agreed that productive labor was the most important element in moral treatment (Grob, 1973). A precise schedule and regular work characterized the best private and public institutions.

The superintendents assigned occupations according to a patient's classification. Not all occupations were considered suitable at all stages of illness; superintendents were cautious about overtaxing patients or exposing them to potentially hazardous situations. Brigham felt that the members of the curable class benefitted most from the rational engagement of the mind through reading, writing, drawing, music, and various studies and recreational pursuits. Patients viewed as incurable benefitted more from manual labor to preserve whatever mind they still possessed (Brigham, 1847). In some cases, hardworking patients could reduce their board payments or earn placement on the free list (Tomes, 1984). Cooperative and industrious behaviors could also result in the acquisition of special privileges or "advancement to a better gallery" (Galt, 1846/1973, p. 497). In most asylums, occupation was supplemented by religious exercises, regular physical exercise, and group amusements organized by the staff. The use of occupations reflected an awareness of individual differences, of comfort level, and of degree of illness, but it also revealed a class and sex bias.

Dr. Lee, the superintendent at McLean Hospital, described the results of occupation: "Give a man constant employment, treat him with uniform kindness and respect, and, however insane he may be, very little may be feared from him, either of mischief or indolence" (Galt, 1846/1973, p. 50). He said that bodily labor proved immeasurably superior to all other aspects of treatment with a large class of male patients. The asylum staff encouraged patients to engage in energetic labor as a way to work off irritability. Perseverance and ceaseless efforts resulted in a patient's return to industrious habits, even with chronic cases. In these cases, attendants often helped patients initially with the motion required for a task until it was mastered. Asylum reports touted the successes at length and in great detail. Labor helped to inculcate moral habits in the patients; as a secondary benefit, labor often helped maintain the asylum.

Besides occupation, other treatment operatives were used in the early asylum. The superintendents in all institutions invoked the use of kindness. The patient population was kept low to facilitate individual care, and doctors met with individual patients daily. The Hartford Retreat, for example, housed only 40 patients (Deutsch, 1949). The staff used restraints minimally, appealing instead to patients' rationality. A system of rewards and privileges replaced a system of punishments. Cooperative patients could be promoted in classification, which encouraged self-control (Galt, 1846/1973). Radical medical treatments such as bleeding and the use of purgatives and emetics were replaced by the use of tonics and narcotics such as opium (Galt, 1846/1973). Family members were discouraged, but not forbidden, from visiting, because new associations were essential. The attendants became the patients' constant companions, and each attendant cared for one to six patients. The superintendents were diligent in obtaining attendants and nurses of the best character (Galt, 1846/1973). Families were encouraged to commit patients for a minimum of 3 to 6 months, time enough to demonstrate some progress. Confinement in a new environment and isolation from previous associations marked the beginning of a cure for environmentally caused insanity (Rothman, 1971).

Early Successes

In the small early asylum, success meant a cure. Statistics from the Worcester State Hospital between 1833 and 1842 show recoveries in 70% to 75% of the patients admitted, and improvements in 3% to 8% of the patients. Dr. Eli Todd of the Hartford Retreat reported recovery in 90% of the patients admitted with mental illness of less than 1 year's duration (Bockoven, 1963). Kirkbride (1880/1973) described his clinical observations of patients' behaviors both before and after the introduction of evening amusements. He said that a comparison of results "leaves no room to question the importance and great superiority of the last" (p. 273). Countless case histories validated moral treatment's success. Many of these case histories appeared in Galt's *The Treatment of Insanity* (1846/1973) and in the asylum's annual reports. One man, for example, reportedly suffered violent fits at least once a month. After he took up gardening and became involved, he was subsequently free of attacks (Rothman, 1971).

Grob (1973) thought that the success of the early asylum rested on a series of circumstances: (a) the small number and homogeneous nature of patients, (b) the internal therapeutic atmosphere arising from the enthusiasm of the superintendent's personality, and (c) close interpersonal relationships. All this success resulted in a wild optimism that Deutsch called "the cult of curability" (Dain, 1964, p. 78).

The Demise of Moral Treatment

Moral treatment can perhaps be called a system. The systematization of moral treatment contributed in part to its own demise. Certain aspects of the practice and principles characterizing moral treatment made its survival incompatible with later 19th-century conditions.

Changes that led to the demise of moral treatment occurred first in 19th-century society, and second, in the medical community. While the providers of asylum care were touting its curative effects, a social reform movement was pushing to extend humane care to all insane persons. The push was successful; thousands of persons were crowded into existing asylums. A Civil War-taxed economy could not provide the rapid institutional growth that was needed to house this influx of patients. Asylum conditions deteriorated both from overcrowding and from a radical change in the types of patients treated. Because it was almost impossible to provide moral treatment, custodial care prevailed. Curative moral treatment was eliminated. Meanwhile, medicine was committing itself to more scientific inquiry and somatic treatments of all illnesses. A shift in thinking had occurred: insanity was caused by lesions in the brain. Therefore, consideration of environmental causes or treatments for what was essentially a physiological problem was unnecessary.

This course of events contributed to the demise of moral treatment partly because of certain characteristics inherent in the moral treatment system. For all its successes, moral treatment had its problems from the outset. One significant problem was the early superintendents' reluctance to deal with the poor, whether because of class bias or because of a genuine belief that the advanced condition of their disease precluded a cure. The early asylum experience tended to validate the assumption that poor persons presented hopeless cases. This validation occurred in the following manner. Superintendents sometimes labored under financial limitations. Public officials capable of providing funds were less concerned with effectiveness of treatment than with convenience of placement. These officials pressured superintendents to accept less curable cases to the asylum in greater proportions than had been recommended (Rothman, 1971). Additionally, it had been assumed that a therapeutic asylum would have a transient population because of a constant turnover of cured patients. In practice, a percentage of more chronic cases stayed at the asylum. This situation created a different type of institution from that originally envisioned (Grob, 1973). The poor and the chronically ill, because they stayed, validated physicians' assumptions about their hopelessness. This would create a major obstacle when larger numbers of poor persons were later admitted.

Given their original expectations, physicians embraced middle-class behaviors and values as the norm; their emphasis was on the order, moderation, and self-control inherent in a middle-class life-style (Rothman, 1971). The initial theoretical and practical groundwork of moral treatment (that insanity was curable and that moral treatment was the cure) could have inspired a vigorous progressive movement across all classes. Instead, asylums were small-scale experiments that reached only a select group. Moral treatment was isolated amid a scene of widespread stagnation begging for reform (Rothman, 1971). At the time, public provision for poor persons consisted of sending the "dangerous and violent" to prison; the harmless and mild "paupers" went to auction or the almshouse (Deutsch, 1949, p. 115). The asylum superintendents showed little desire to treat the very patients who were to dominate asylum populations after the reform movement.

Michel Foucault (1965), a harsh critic of institutions in any form, for any reason, described moral treatment of mentally ill patients as a gigantic moral imprisonment: a "structure that formed a kind of microcosm in which were symbolized the massive structure of bourgeois society and its values ... centered on the theme of social and moral order" (p. 274). Digby (1985) countered that any experience of moral imprisonment in the subjective estimation of patients would "turn on the extent to which they shared the moral values of the establishment" (p. 54). Real treatment successes would come from inducing self-control in patients sharing the values, assumptions, and objectives of their therapists. Those not sharing institutional values would only conform superficially; problems would surface with discrepancies in values (Digby, 1985). In fact, as Bell (1980) wrote, "When poor people having different values formed the majority of the patient population, moral treatment ran into difficulties" (p. 14).

Another problem of the moral treatment system was its administration by physicians. The patients might have fared better had asylums been under the direction of lay superintendents (Bockoven, 1963). Physician-superintendents focused on the cure. When scientific theory was to later challenge moral treatment's curative potential, physicians rejected their recovery statistics and early successes. Eager to join the mainstream of scientific medicine, they increasingly distanced themselves from the moral care of the institutionalized mentally ill patients (Grob, 1983). Bockoven described the situation as one in which psychiatry did not have the courage to pursue its original course.

Moral Treatment in Crisis

Moral treatment in the asylum meant cure. Social reformers thought that all insane persons should have access to asylum cure. A widespread reform movement in the 1830s and 1840s worked to improve the lot of persons who were blind, deaf, slaves, alcoholics, convicts, or insane. Dorothea Dix, using superintendents' annual reports as testimony, led state after state to construct asylums. Her dream, however, soon turned into a nightmare (Bell, 1980). New state laws mandated that dangerously insane persons be sent to asylums. Those insane persons previously housed in jails and almshouses also went to asylums. This rapid admission of large numbers of patients taxed superintendents and facilities prepared for small homogeneous patient groups. Psychiatrist-superintendents were largely unsuccessful in their protest against the influx and their suggestion that violent or chronic patients be segregated (Bockoven, 1963).

Overcrowding restricted the practice of moral treatment. Rooms used for leisure activities and workshops became sleeping quarters. Individualized patient care was no longer possible in the congested asylum maze. Overcrowding stressed the sewage, ventilation, and water systems; the health of the patients was compromised. Epidemics struck at numerous institutions (Bell, 1980). The superintendents became increasingly concerned with order, regularity, and control among growing numbers of patients. They reinstituted the use of restraints among patients who were noisy or violent. The attendants assumed responsibility for larger groups of 8 to 15 patients each. Inmates were often appointed as temporary nurses and attendants because of the staff shortage. The most critical personal quality sought in an attendant shifted from kindness to obedience (Grob, 1973). Overtaxed institutional facilities provided fewer patients with meaningful work; idleness further complicated behavioral problems. The superintendents recognized a growing gap between their original theory and their practices; their powers to close the gap were diminishing.

The wide range of persons admitted to the asylum jeopardized adequate care. Older patients with dementia accounted for 10% of the number of admissions from 1830 to 1875, thereby complicating hospital management considerably (Grob, 1973). Insane criminals often required maximum security. Alcoholic patients, mentally retarded patients, and patients suffering from general paresis (resulting from the advanced stage of a syphilitic infection) or other organic diseases often required individual care at a time when none was possible. Under these conditions, chronic patients failed to respond to treatment. They became troublesome, engaging in disruptive behaviors, escapes, and physical violence that perpetuated the need for restraint (Tomes, 1984).

Poverty-stricken immigrants joined this influx in the post-Civil War years. American physicians had difficulty empathizing with "foreign insane paupers" (Bockoven, 1963, p. 25). Admitted to already deteriorating institutions, foreign patients quickly became apathetic, leading physicians to believe them less capable, less motivated, and less curable. A vicious cycle developed, with predictable consequences. Because they were thought to be incurable, poor patients received less care. Without care, these patients showed little improvement—This confirmed their incurability.

New theories about mental illness dealt moral treatment yet another incapacitating blow. One school of thought linked mental illness with heredity; another linked mental illness with a somatic, mechanical defect. Both views led to a decline in optimism about a cure and to a total disillusionment about moral treatment in the 1850s. By the 1870s, pessimism was the trend; by 1900, moral treatment was reduced to a minor form of therapy even in the most affluent of corporate asylums (Dain, 1964).

Emphasis on hereditary predisposition began to fill the psychiatric literature. Heredity was thought to predispose the poor person to poverty and insanity (Bockoven, 1963). Inferior biological stock was thought to produce conditions leading to insanity. Some physicians debated the logic of heredity as an explanation for insanity; they argued against the heredity explanation in defense of a somatic view (Bell, 1980). Although earlier in the century it had been understood that a weakening of the body's vital forces could damage the brain, microscopic lesions now found in the central nervous system of mentally ill patients upset previous environmental theories and confirmed the somatic cause of insanity (Bockoven, 1963).

The early successes of moral treatment were challenged. In 1877, Dr. Pliny Earle published a critique of pre-Civil War curability statistics and accused early superintendents of having exaggerated their figures (Bockoven, 1963). Earle questioned the validity of the high cure rates cited because in the 1870s corporate asylums could no longer replicate these cure rates. Some physicians argued in response that insanity was becoming less curable because society was becoming more chaotic. Others claimed that insanity had become more complex in the late 19th century; it was less curable because the categories of insanity, such as general paralysis, senile dementia, and hereditary insanity, had multiplied. Many thought that the physiological causes of insanity were intensifying: Organic alterations in the nervous system were more involved in producing insanity than before (Bockoven 1963).

Conversion toward a more somatic view seemed inevitable. From 1840 to 1860, three men had been responsible for most of the psychiatric research in the United States: Luther Bell, Amariah Brigham, and Isaac Ray. Their work had largely involved data gathering, certainly not serious research by 20th-century standards. Even the curability statistics gathered between 1833 and 1842 by superintendent Samuel Woodward at Worcester State Hospital had failed to delineate criteria used to determine the recovery or improvement of patients. Those succeeding the early superintendents were deeply discouraged by the apparent failure of moral treatment and by their inability to validate its effectiveness scientifically. Articles in the *American Journal of Insanity* supporting the mechanical defect theory exhorted a move toward somaticism. Scientific medicine was gaining respect and credibility; any psychological approach to the treatment of insanity seemed outdated, illogical, and irrelevant. In 1894, Dr. Weir Mitchell, a neurologist, castigated physicians for having ever believed in some mysterious therapeutic influence (Bockoven, 1963).

Therapeutic regimens differed among asylums, depending on the superintendent's viewpoint. Moral treatment suffered in this respect as well. Bockoven (1963) attributed the demise of moral treatment to the lack of inspired and committed leadership after the death of its innovators. Only 4 of the original 13 founders of moral treatment survived the 1870s, and 2 of these founders had returned to private practice. Leaders seemed to have lacked foresight. They had failed to train moral therapists who might have been able to articulate or redefine moral treatment's efficacy in the face of social changes and scientific inquiry. This seemed a major failure.

The asylum, diverted from its original mission of treatment, and pressured into merely containing insane persons, sank into a mire of apathy and indifference (Bell, 1980). Moral treatment, once considered vital to the cure of persons with mental disorders, disappeared from psychiatric practice.

Conclusion

The complexity of moral treatment precludes the opposing views that it was a short-lived triumph of humanitarian zeal or that it was a rationalization of middle-class morality (Tomes, 1984). Moral treatment was neither of these stereotypes. One thing is clear: Moral treatment cannot be understood outside of the framework within which it developed and disappeared.

One can hope that occupational therapy practice today is free of the limitations that precluded the survival of moral treatment. One would hope to find, in this century, a freedom from class and economic bias, a freedom from a push for professional credibility that is blind to patient need, and a leadership committed to defend those humane aspects of practice only empirically validated.

One can also hope that occupational therapy practitioners understand the powerful forces that often define the character of occupational therapy practice. During the 19th century, the medical community and the society as a whole shaped several guiding principles and treatment concepts into the practice of moral treatment. These two communities cannot be underestimated in the 20th century; their demands shape the duration, direction, location, and quality of occupational therapy. Preventive care, accountability, and documentation of measurable progress are but a few of the trends grounded in challenges from these two sectors.

Moral treatment's decline relates closely to a lack of inspired and committed leadership willing to articulate and redefine the efficacy of occupation in the face of medical and societal challenges. The desire to embrace the most current trend of scientific thought led to the abandonment of moral treatment in spite of its established efficacy. The failure to identify and address the social and institutional changes that had gradually made the practice and success of moral treatment virtually impossible led to the erroneous conclusion that occupation was not an effective intervention. The responsivity to trends supplanted any reaffirmation of basic assumptions.

Occupational therapists need to recommit, in this century and in the next, to the assumptions about man and occupation that inform the practice of occupational therapy. In the face of changing trends, therapists must continually redefine and rearticulate the value of a humane practice that transcends scientific validation and bureaucratic understanding.

Acknowledgments

Special thanks to Ellen More, PhD, whose flexibility and encouragement enabled the integration of course material with occupational therapy issues. Thanks also to Lillian H. Parent, MA, OTR, FAOTA, for her supportive suggestions.

References

Bell, L. V. (1980). *Treating the mentally ill*. New York: Praeger.

Bing, R. K. (1981). Occupational therapy revisited: A paraphrastic journey. *American Journal of Occupational Therapy, 35,* 499–518. (Reprinted as Chapter 5.)

Bockoven, J. S. (1963). *Moral treatment in American psychiatry*. New York: Springs Publishing.

Bockoven, J. S. (1971). Legacy of moral treatment—1800's to 1910. *American Journal of Occupational Therapy, 25,* 223–225.

Brigham, A. (1844). Definition of insanity—Nature of the disease. *American Journal of Insanity, 1,* 107–108.

Brigham, A. (1847). The moral treatment of insanity. *American Journal of Insanity, 4,* 1.

Carlson, E. T., & Dain, N. (1960). The psychotherapy that was Moral Treatment. *American Journal of Psychiatry, 117,* 519–524.

Dain, N. (1964). *Concepts of insanity in the United States: 1789–1865*. New Brunswick, NJ: Rutgers University Press.

Dain, N., & Carlson, E. T. (1960). Milieu therapy in the nineteenth century: Patient care at the Friend's Asylum, Frankford, Pennsylvania, 1817–1861. *Journal of Nervous and Mental Disease, 131,* 277–290.

Deutsch, A. (1949). *The mentally ill in America: A history of their care and treatment from colonial times*. New York: Columbia University Press.

Digby, A. (1985). Moral treatment at the Retreat, 1796–1846. In W. F. Bynum, R. Porter, & M. Shepherd (Eds.), *The anatomy of madness. Essays in the history of psychiatry* (pp. 52–72). New York: Tavistock.

Engelhardt, H. T. Jr. (1977). Defining occupational therapy: The meaning of therapy and the virtues of occupation. *American Journal of Occupational Therapy, 31,* 666–672.

Foucault, M. (1965). *Madness and civilization: A history of insanity in the Age of Reason*. New York: Vintage Books.

Galt, J. M. (1973). *The treatment of insanity*. New York: Arno Press. (Original work published 1846).

Grob, G. N. (1973). *Mental institutions in America: Social policy to 1875*. New York: Free Press.

Grob, G. N. (1983). *Mental illness and American society, 1875–1940*. Princeton, NJ: Princeton University Press.

Kirkbride, T. S. (1973). *On the construction, organization, and general arrangements of hospitals for the insane*. New York: Arno Press. (Original work published 1880).

Pinel, P. H. (1962). *A treatise on insanity*. New York: Harper Publishing. (Original work published 1806).

Ray, I. (1861). An examination of the objections to the doctrine of moral insanity. *American Journal of Insanity, 18,* 112–139.

Rothman, D. J. (1971). *The discovery of the asylum*. Boston: Little, Brown.

Scull, A. (Ed.). (1981). *Madhouses, mad-doctors, and madmen*. Philadelphia: University of Pennsylvania Press.

Tomes, N. (1984). *A generous confidence: Thomas Story Kirkbride and the art of asylum keeping*. New York: Cambridge University Press.

Related Readings

Beers, C. W. (1917). *A mind that found itself*. New York: Longmans, Green, & Co.

Chapter 5

Occupational Therapy Revisited: A Paraphrastic Journey

1981 Eleanor Clarke Slagle Lecture

Robert K. Bing, EdD, OTR, FAOTA

Try as one might, it is impossible to recount the evolution of occupational therapy so that it resembles the cliff-hanging biographies of Butch Cassidy and the Sundance Kid. Masters and Johnson, as well as Kinsey, who took years to amass their stories, had something going for them that does not exist for us. Somewhat puckishly I was tempted to entitle this paper, *Everything You've Ever Wanted to Know About Occupational Therapy, But Were Afraid to Ask*. That would not have been altogether misleading. Because of my part German heritage, and true to that cultural bias and tendency, I thought I should take us back to the Thirty Years' War and bring everyone up to date. After all, it is important territory occupational therapy has won and lost.

The title, *Occupational Therapy Revisited: A Paraphrastic Journey*, prevailed because this paper is a tour to what should be familiar historical landmarks and progenitors. For some of us, it will renew old friendships and acquaintances. For others, it will be a second-hand account of certain ancestors, not unlike those stories that emanate from grandmothers. For some, it will only be like an endurance of those pictures that inevitably get projected on the screen by vacationers returning home.

Because of the relative youthfulness of those of us in practice (most have entered within the past decade), now seems the time to critically examine our ancestral roots and subsequent grafts to determine the nature of the present and to offer some speculations about why we (and the profession) developed as we did through several generations. This is not *the* history of occupational therapy nor of the Association that supports our endeavors. Nor is it *a* history like someone else might well find it. It is *not* a detailed, definitive account of how we multiplied, divided, and invaded several areas of medicine and health care. It is *one person's* way of telling the story of who we are and citing some lessons to be learned. That is important! After several months of submergence just off the coast of Texas (as my colleagues in Galveston will attest), I have at long last come up for air and am ready to declare my findings.

This is a statement of how an idea, born in a philosophical movement, became activated through *the good works of men and women* who inalterably believed in the ideal that those who are sick and handicapped can regain, retain, and attain some semblance of function within the fundamental limitations of the human organism and the expectations of the society in which all must exist: that this may occur through the most obvious means of all—*one's reorganization through occupation, through activity, through leisure, and through rest.*

This journey about occupational therapy, its evolution and development, presents vexation: one must accept a fair number of ambiguities, something some today consider a fundamental problem in occupational therapy; a more than reasonable amount of astonishment; and a certain degree of messiness, closely akin to what is created by the beginner in fingerpainting. What can it all mean? What was taking place at the time? Will the patient recover? Most significantly, does it make any difference? To answer these and related questions I wanted to conduct some scholarly research that could be equally interesting, helpful, and valuable to students, occupational therapists, and others who are interested in our profession. This is how I interpret the intent of the originators of the Eleanor Clarke Slagle Lectureship.

Such an historical presentation should be long enough to say something, yet short enough to be tolerated.

To give you some idea of the continuing dilemma I encountered these past several months in preparing the lecture and in limiting its scope and length, I wrote:

> There once was an historian named Dan,
> Whose prose no one could scan,
> When, once asked about it,
> He said, "I don't doubt it,
> Because I try to cram as many facts and dates into each sentence as I possibly can."

Significant Landmarks

Let us start this paraphrastic journey and take note of some significant landmarks along the way—those recurring patterns and themes of the past 200 years that give us today's relevance:

1. There is an inextricable union of the mind and the body; the employment of activity or occupation must be based on this precept, which is unique to occupational therapy.
2. Activity, inherently, contains modes the patient may employ to gain understanding of and ascendancy over one's feelings, actions, and thoughts: these modes include the habits of attention and interest; the perceived usefulness of occupation; creative expression; the processes of learning; the acquisition of skill; and evidence of accomplishment.

3. Activity provides a balance between the practical and intellectual components of experience; therefore, a wide variety of activities must be accessible to meet human objectives for work, leisure, and rest.
4. One's approach to the patient is as significant to treatment and rehabilitation as is the selection and utilization of an activity.
5. Essential elements of occupational therapy practice are continuous observation, experimentation, empiricism, and analysis.
6. An appreciation of the pain that accompanies any illness or disability; a strong desire to reduce or remove it; a gentle firmness; and a knowledge of the patient's needs are fundamental characteristics of the provider of therapeutic occupations.
7. Therapeutic processes and modes of treatment are synonymous with the processes of learning and methods of education.
8. The patient is the product of his or her own efforts, not the article made nor the activity accomplished.

A Theory of Experience

We could go back to the Garden of Eden to begin this story, if time permitted, since occupational therapy could well have started in that idyllic spot. Dr. Dunton, one of the founders of the 20th century movement, insisted that those fig leaves had to have been crocheted by Eve, who was trying to get over her troubles. They had something to do with her being beholden to Adam and his rib. We will unfortunately pass over all that and begin the modern epoch with a brief description of what was taking place in Europe approximately 200 years ago.

It was the *Age of Enlightenment*, or, as some prefer, the *Age of Reason*. The roots of 20th century occupational therapy are visible in the empiricism of John Locke, an English philosopher and physician, who fostered confidence in human reason and freedom; in Etienne de Condillac, a French philosopher, who advanced the dualism of body and mind; and Pierre Cabanis, a French physician and theorist, who offered an explanation of the importance of the moral and social sciences in perfecting the art of medicine. These three, together with others, popularized the new ideas. Indeed, it was the *best of times*, a clear demarcation in the emergence of the modern world.

If one were to combine the thoughts of these three, one would arrive at a *theory of experience*. John Locke, in his famous *Essay Concerning Human Understanding*, published in 1690,[1] examines the nature of the human mind and the processes by which it learns about and comes to know the world. When born, the human is a blank tablet (tabula rasa). Because of an innate ability to receive sensations from the outside world, the human can assimilate and organize impressions. As contact with the environment stimulates the senses and causes impressions, the mind receives and organizes these into ideas and concepts. Since the human mind does not already contain innate ideas, all must come from without.[2(p287)]

There is a second source for the accumulation of experience, according to Locke. It is the mind itself: "… the perception of the operations of our own mind … (such as) thinking, doubting, believing, reasoning, knowing … this source of ideas every man has wholly within himself."[3(p74)] Locke strongly held that the body and mind exist as real entities and they interact. He spent a great deal of time developing his perspective. He spoke of the aim of education as the process of knowing and learning through experience and in striving toward happiness. Ideally, he contended, one should work toward a sound mind in a healthy body. To achieve this ideal, Locke advocated physical exercise as a hardening process, and an exposure to a wide variety of sensations from the physical and social worlds.

Condillac was Locke's apologist. He tried to simplify Locke's fundamental theory by arguing that all conscious experiences are the result of passive sensations: these sensations are the raw materials from which one forms complex and interrelated ideas. Learning is the noting of incomplete ideas, considering each separately, combining them into relationships, and ordering them. This process results in retaining the strongest degrees of association. Condillac asserted: "Then we shall grasp (ideas) easily and clearly and shall understand their origins entirely."[3(p7)]

Elsewhere in his writings Condillac presented his thoughts on analysis. One cannot have the proper conception of a thing until one is in a position to analyze it. "To analyze," claimed Condillac, "is nothing more than to observe in successive order the qualities of an object … the simultaneous order in which they exist."[4(p17)]

The third philosopher, Pierre Cabanis, tended to apply medicine to philosophy and philosophy to medicine. Cabanis considered illness and its impact upon the formulation of values and ideas. Through the social sciences, which emerged in the *Age of Enlightenment*, he explained *moral* as a psychological phenomenon on a physiological base. He concluded that moral impressions can have both physiological and pathological results. At last, there was a rational explanation for the psychological production of disease in which the so-called moral (emotional) passions play a significant part.[5(p37-38)] Cabanis contributed a socially based theoretical explanation of human experience that became the cornerstone for the moral management of the insane.

Age of Enlightenment and Moral Treatment

Moral treatment of the insane was one result of the *Age of Enlightenment*. It sprang from the fundamental atti-

tudes of the day: a set of principles that govern humanity and society; faith in the ability of the human to reason; and the supreme belief in the individual. The rapid changes caused by this new philosophy advanced the disappearance of the notion that the insane were possessed of the devil. Mental diseases became legitimate concerns of humanitarians and physicians. The discontinuance of the idea that crime, sin, and vice were at the core of insanity brought forth humane treatment. Up to this time the insane had been housed and handled no differently than were criminals or paupers—often in chains.

Two men of the 18th century working in different countries, and unknown to each other, initiated the moral treatment movement. "No two men could possibly have been chosen out of all Europe at that time of whom it could be said more truly that they were cradled, and nursed, and educated among widely differing social, political, religious influences …"[6(p24-25)] Philippe Pinel was a child of the French Revolution, a physician, a scholar, and a philosopher. He is described as "…far exceeding the bounds of pure humanitarianism … to encompass the goals of a naturalist, … a reformer, a clinician, … and, above all, a philosopher."[7(Intro)] William Tuke was a devout member of the Society of Friends (Quakers).

Philippe Pinel: Physician-Reformer

Whenever Philippe Pinel's name comes up in a conversation among health professionals, he is immediately mentioned as the striker of the chains at two French hospitals. His efforts and contributions go way beyond that reformational act. As a physician, he began his most serious work in 1792 as superintendent of Bicêtre, the asylum for incurable males in Paris.

As a natural scientist, Pinel achieved exceptional skill in the observation of human behavior and the bringing of "…some order into the chaos of … treatment methods by means of critical and objective investigations."[5(p42)] Pinel says this about himself: Desirous of better information, I resolved for myself the facts that were presented to my attention; and forgetting the empty honours of my titular distinction as a physician, I viewed the scene that was opened to me with the eye of common sense and unprejudiced observation.[8(p109)] From his own experience, he urged that observations "…be the basis upon which (one) should decide what opinions to believe."[9(p74-75)] Throughout his work, he held constantly before him his own motto of independent thought: "Chercher à èviter toute illusion, toute prèvention, toute opinion adoptèe sur parole" (to seek to avoid all illusion, all prejudice, all opinion taken on authority)[10(p8-9)]

Pinel's descriptions of the mentally deranged provide insight into his own compassionate nature. For him, the loss of reason was the most calamitous of human afflictions. The ability to reason principally separates the human from other living forms. Because of mental illness, the human's "…character is always perverted, sometimes annihilated. His thoughts and actions are diverted.... His personal liberty is at length taken from him.... To this melancholy train of symptoms, if not early and judiciously treated ... a state of the most abject degradation sooner or later succeeds." [8(p xv–xvii)]

What Pinel entitled *revolution morale*, or moral revolution, is the ultimate insight of the insane into the delusional and absurd nature of their experiences.[7(p256)] This, to him, was the basis for treatment. Some historians believe that he was stating that moral treatment is synonymous with the humane approach. His own writings do not bear this out. Pinel believed that each patient must be critically observed and analyzed; then treatment should commence. "To apply the principles of moral treatment, with undiscriminating uniformity, would be ... ridiculous and unadvisable." [8(p66)] The moral method is well reasoned and carefully planned for the individual patient.

According to Pinel, moral management is a maintained continuity of approach; a predictable routine, infused with vigor by personnel who inspire confidence. Moreover, moral treatment calls for a constant, observed study of patient behavior and performance. It included a gentle, but firm approach. Each patient is given as much liberty within the institution as he or she can tolerate. The approach is designed to give the patient a feeling of security as well as a respect for authority. Pinel asserted: "The atmosphere should be the same as in a family where the parents are quite strict. To establish this relationship, the doctor must convince the patient that he wishes to help him and that recovery is a real possibility." [9(p76)]

Occupations figured prominently in Pinel's conception of moral treatment. He used activities to take the patients' thoughts away from their emotional problems and to develop their abilities. He considered literature and music as effective in altering patients' emotions. Physical exercise and work should be part of every institution's fundamental program and be employed in accord with individual tastes. He concluded: "The (occupations) method is primarily designed and intended to reach man at his best which...means human understanding, intelligence, and insight." [3(p63–64)]

The concept of *moral treatment* belongs solely to Philippe Pinel. His fundamental belief was that its purpose is to restore the patient to himself, "...to use the patient's own emotions to balance his emotional excesses." [9(p76)] Truly, Pinel and his efforts, rooted in the *Age of Enlightenment*, mark the beginning of the modern epoch in the care of the mentally ill.

William Tuke: Philanthropist-Humanitarian

Across the channel, in England, things were astir at the same time. King George III, who was giving the American colonies fits, was himself in similar trouble. In 1788 it became public knowledge that the King was seized with mania. Questions arose about his fitness to continue ruling. Nevertheless, public sentiment was on his side. For the first time, insanity and its treatment formed a topic of public discussion: "The subject had been brought out of concealment in a way which defeated the conspiracy of silence."[11(p42)] This being the *Age of Enlightenment*, the public openly sympathized with the sufferer; there was no condemnation. No one suggested that the King was being visited by the Devil, or that he was being punished for his sins.

The Society of Friends, derisively called *Quakers*, originated in 17th century England and became one of the most distinctive movements of Puritanism: "They arose out of the religious unrest of England ... and stood for a radical kind of reform within Christendom which contrasted sharply with Protestant, Anglican and Roman patterns alike."[12(p118)] George Fox, founder of the Society, discovered "...the spirit of the living Christ and knew that it was an experience open to all men. 'This was the true light that lighteth every man that cometh into the world!'" [13(p1)]

William Tuke, a devout Quaker, wealthy merchant, and renowned philanthropist, was made aware of the deplorable conditions in the insane asylum in York, England. There were tales of extreme neglect and possible cruelty. He was an unusual man, not given to listening to sensational reports and acting rashly.[14(p12)] In true Quaker fashion Tuke presented a concern at a Friend's Quarterly Meeting in the spring of 1792—that an institution for the insane be established in York under the direction of the Society. At first, he was met with considerable resistance by those who believed that there were too few mentally ill Quakers, and that no one would want them concentrated in such a lovely, quiet locale.[15(p58)]

The York Retreat

Initially, Tuke was disheartened; yet, he pressed on, and within 6 months *The Retreat for Persons* afflicted with *Disorders of the Mind*, or simply, *The Retreat* came into being. Up until then the term *Retreat* had never been applied to an asylum. Tuke's daughter-in-law suggested the term to convey the Quaker belief that such an institution may be "...a place in which the unhappy might obtain refuge; a quiet haven in which (one) ... might find a means of reparation or of safety."[16(p20)] The cornerstone simply stated the purpose of the institution: "The charity or love of friends executed this work in the cause of humanity." [15(p19)]

William Tuke became the superintendent. Thomas Fowler, an unusually open-minded man, was appointed visiting physician. After a trial-and-error period, they came to believe that moral treatment methods were preferable to those involving restraint and use of harsh drugs. The new approach was a product of Tuke's humanitarianism and Fowler's empiricism.

Several fundamental principles became evident within a short time. The approach was primarily one of kindness and consideration. The patients were not thought to be devoid of reason, feeling, and honor. The social environment was to be as nearly like that of a family as possible, with an atmosphere of religious sentiment and moral feeling.[16(p35)]

Tuke and Fowler strongly believed that most insane people retain a considerable amount of self-command. Upon admission, the patient was informed that treatment depended largely upon one's own conduct. Employment in various occupations was expected as a way for the patient to maintain control over his or her disorder. As Tuke reported: "…regular employment is perhaps the most efficacious; and those kinds of employment … to be preferred … are accompanied by considerable bodily action."[16(p156)] The staff endeavored to gain the patient's confidence and esteem, to arrest the attention and fix it upon objects opposite to any illusion the patient might have. The fundamental purpose of employment and recreation was to facilitate the regaining of the *habit of attention*, as Tuke called it. Various learning exercises were used, such as mathematical problems, to help the patient gain ascendancy over faulty habits of attention.

Tuke and Fowler determined that "indolence has a natural tendency to weaken the mind, and to induce ennui and discontent…"[16(p180–181)] A wide range of occupations and amusements was available. Patients not engaged in useful occupations were allowed to read, draw, or play various games. Tea parties, walks, and visitations away from the institution were planned regularly in preparation for the patients' returning home. All activities were closely analyzed through observation in order to individualize patients' needs.

The pioneer work of William Tuke and his son, Samuel, who wrote the definitive treatise on *The Retreat*, opened a new chapter in the history of the care of the insane in England. Mild management methods, infused with kindness, and building self-esteem through the judicious use of occupations, resulted in the excitation and elicitation of superior, human motives. Patients recovered, left *The Retreat*, and rarely needed to return for further care. The entire regimen was carefully patterned "…to accord (patients) the dignity and status of sick human beings."[17(p687)]

Moral Treatment Expansion

As soon as Pinel's major work on moral treatment (1801) and Samuel Tuke's description of *The Retreat* were published (1813), there was a rush toward implementing many reforms in other hospitals, particularly in England and the United States. In both countries occupations were introduced as an integral part of moral treatment.[18(p83–84)] Some unusual experiments were undertaken by Sir William Charles Ellis, a physician, who became the superintendent of a pauper lunatic asylum. The mainstay of his asylum management was useful occupations. He moved well ahead of mere amusements

and "introduced a gainful employment of patients on a large scale and even had them taught a trade."[19(p62)] Ellis and his wife undertook other reforms. She organized the women patients into groups under the supervision of a *workwoman* to make useful and fancy articles.

Another Ellis innovation was the development of what would eventually be called *halfway houses*. Keenly aware of environmental and social influences on insanity, Ellis suggested "…after-care houses and night hospitals as a stepping stone from the asylum to the world by which … the length of patients' stay would be reduced and in many cases the cure completed…"[17(p871)] He insisted that convalescing patients should go out and mix with the world before discharge. His proposals were made in the 1830s!

In the United States, few public and private asylums existed in the post-Revolutionary era; however, institutional reforms were needed. Any recounting of this period must include two very important individuals and their work: Benjamin Rush and Dorothea Lynde Dix. Their efforts did not overlap; they did not know one another; nor was one influenced by the other. Just as in the cases of Pinel and Tuke, no two individuals this side of the Atlantic could have been more unlike one another in background, education, or experience. Nevertheless, each recognized the hapless plights of the institutionalized insane and set out to alleviate dire conditions and the inauguration of moral treatment, including occupations and exercise.

Benjamin Rush: Father of American Psychiatry

Benjamin Rush, often referred to as the *father of American psychiatry*, was a Philadelphia physician in the latter half of the 1700s. Through his training in Europe and several visits there, he adopted many of Pinel's practices; however, Rush did not adopt moral principles until later. As a member of the staff of Pennsylvania Hospital, he was placed in charge of a separate section set aside for the insane, the first hospital in America to reserve such a section. He was appalled by the conditions and he appealed to the staff and the public for change. Change did come and humane treatment was instituted. Rush saw to it that "certain employments be devised for such of the deranged people as are capable of working…"[20(p257)] This approach was based upon his philosophical stance that man, by his very nature, is meant to be active; "Even in paradise (Garden of Eden) he was employed in the health and pleasant exercises of cultivating a garden. Happiness, consisting in folded arms, and in pensive contemplation…by the side of brooks, never had any existence, except in the brains of mad poets, and love-sick girls and boys."[21(p115–116)]

In his major writing, *Medical Inquiries and Observations Upon the Diseases of the Mind*, Rush clearly differentiates between goal-directed activity and aimless exercise:

"Labour has several advantages over exercise, in being not only more stimulating, but more endurable in its effects;...it is calculated to arrest wrong habits of action, and to restore such as regular and natural..."[21(p224–225)]

Dorothea Lynde Dix: Humanitarian-Reformer

Dorothea Lynde Dix, a reform-minded humanitarian during the middle 1800s, vehemently pressed for improved conditions of the insane who were incarcerated in jails and almshouses. She presented a number of *Memorials* to state legislatures, believing that the public had an obligation to care for such individuals. By 1848 numerous states had responded to her efforts, and she decided to tackle a more formidable object— the Federal government. Dix envisioned the sale of public lands to finance the building of a federal system of hospitals for the indigent blind, deaf and mute, as well as the insane. For 6 years she wheedled and cajoled members of the Congress. Finally, in 1854, the bill was ready for President Franklin Pierce's signature. He was a close friend of Miss Dix and she felt highly confident of the outcome. The President vetoed the bill claiming unconstitutionality: "...every human weakness or sorrow would take advantage of this bill if it became law.... It endangers states' rights."[22(p20)] Through her contacts with physicians in several states, Miss Dix embraced moral treatment as the most humane method. She strongly advocated "...decent care, quiet, affection and normal activity (as) the only medicine for the insane."[22(p11)]

United States: Individual Treatment, Occupations, Education

The Quakers brought moral treatment to the United States as part of their intellectual and religious luggage. Through published accounts about *The Retreat* in York, some private asylums were established in which moral principles were practiced. A number of public institutions altered their programs to include individualized treatment, occupations, and education. Those patients who had remained for years unimproved and listless, even on the verge of apathy "...are seen in encouraging instances, when transferred to attendants who have more disposition to attend to them,...to waken (them) from their torpor, to become animated, active and even industrious...."[23(p487–488)]

Moral management also was taking on a new facet: the influence of a sane mind upon the insane mind. Those who daily attended the sick were to impress upon the insane the influences of their own character, designed to specifically improve the patients' behavior. Personnel must possess a number of traits: observational skills to see the "...actual condition of the patient's mind...and a faculty of clear insight...."[23(p489)] Other traits: "...seeing that which is passing in the minds of (patients)....Add to

this a firm will, the faculty of self-control, a sympathizing distress at moral pain, a strong desire to remove it...."[23(p489)]

Arguments appeared in the literature relative to the moral use of firmness and gentleness. Strong cases were made for both extremes; however, it took two alienists (the precursor to psychiatrist), John Bucknill and D. Hack Tuke, grandson of Samuel Tuke, in 1858 to settle the dispute: "The truth, as usual, lies between; and the (individual) who aims at success in the moral treatment of the insane must be ready to be all things to all men, if by any means he might save some."[23(p500)] They elaborate on their thesis by stating: "With self-reliance ... it requires widely different manifestations, to repress excitement, to stimulate inertia, to check the vicious, to comfort the depressed, to direct the erring, to support the weak, to supplant every variety of erroneous opinion, to resist every kind of perverted feeling, and to check every form of pernicious conduct."[23(p500)]

Bucknill and Tuke also wrote that moral treatment included the gaining of the patient's confidence, fixing his or her attention on interesting and wholesome objects of thought, diverting the mind from introspection, and loosening the hold on concentrated emotion. They explain: "For (these) purposes useful occupation is far superior to any form of amusement. The higher the purpose, and the more appellant the nature of the occupation ... the more likely it is to draw him from the contemplation of self-wretchedness, and effect the triumph of moral influences."[23(p493)]

The next step in institutional occupations emphasized education. Those occupations that require a process of learning and thought were determined far preferable, from a curative point of view, than those that require none. "Moral treatment is as wide as that of education; ... it is education applied to the field of mental phenomena..."[23(p501)] Therefore, it was not unusual to find specific mental activities included with occupations. The purpose was to educate the individual in order to provide him or her with "the power of controlling his feelings, and his thoughts, and his actions.[24(p166–167)]

With continued experience, a number of alienists decided that occupations and amusements also could serve as a prophylactic against insanity. One interesting prescription for the return and maintenance of sanity was: "...rest in bed, occupation, exercise and amusements."[25(p14)] D. Hack Tuke declared: "If idleness is a curse to the sane, it is the parent of mischief and ennui to the insane, especially to the pubescent and adolescent."[26(p315)] He urges that the same approach be taken with the sane and the insane: "Employment, Nature's universal law of health, alike for body and mind, is specially beneficial, ... seeing that it displaces ideas by new and healthy thoughts, revives familiar habits of daily activity, restores (and maintains) self-respect while it promotes the general bodily health."[26(p315)]

Decline of Moral Treatment

Moral management and treatment by occupations reached its zenith in the United States just before the outbreak of the War Between the States (Civil War). Corporate, private asylums continued to expand their efforts. State- and public-supported institutions withdrew their programs, so that by the last quarter of the 19th century, virtually no moral treatment was taking place.

Several reasons for this decline and eventual disappearance can be identified, including a nation at war with itself. Bockhoven cites others: 1. the founders of the U.S. movement retired and died, leaving no disciples or successors; 2. the rapidly increasing influx of foreign-born and poor patients greatly overtaxed existing facilities and required more institutions to be built with diminished tax support; 3. racial and religious prejudices on the part of the alienists, beginning to be called psychiatrists, reduced interest in treatment and cure; and 4. state legislatures became increasingly more interested in less costly custodial care.[27(p20–25)]

Essentially, there was no place in the public institutions for moral treatment. "The inferior physical plants and facilities, poorly trained and insufficient staff, ... and, worst of all, overcrowding, prohibited any attempts to practice moral management."[28(p128)] A belief emerged that many insane were incurable. One eminent psychiatrist stated: "I have come to the conclusion that when a man becomes insane, he is about used up for this world."[29(p155)] Such pessimism was predominant for a century in this country. Custodial care had come to stay for a very long time.

As we shall see next, moral principles and practices emerged in the early years of the 20th century through the efforts of individuals, then by a group who founded an organization dedicated to those principles. This group, in collaboration with others, established a definition and fundamental principles that have carried over through several generations of specifically educated practitioners of occupational therapy.

Once again, as with Pinel and Tuke, Rush and Dix, the individuals who founded and pioneered the 20th century occupational therapy movement could not have been more diverse in their backgrounds, experience, and education. They included a nurse, two architects, a physician, a social worker, and a teacher.

Susan Tracy: Occupational Nurse

Susan Tracy was this country's first proponent of occupations for invalids. A trained nurse, she initiated instruction in activities to student nurses as early as 1905 as part of their expanding responsibilities. She also developed the term *occupational nurses* to signify specialization.[30(p401)] By 1912 she decided to devote all her energies to patient activities and she distinguished herself by applying moral treatment principles to acute conditions. As Tracy stated, "The application of this most rational remedy to ordinary, everyday sick people, as found in the general hospital, is almost unknown."[31(p386)] She strongly claimed that remedial treatments "are classified according to their physiological effects as stimulants, sedatives, anesthetics ..., etc. Certain occupations possess like properties."[31(p386)] The physician may select stimulating occupations, such as watercoloring and paper folding; or sedative occupations such as knitting, weaving, basketry.

Throughout Tracy's many years of work she employed experimentation and observation to enhance her practice. Her carefully worded writings provide ample evidence of her intense desire to bring scientific principles to the application of invalid occupations. In 1918 she published a remarkable research paper on 25 mental tests derived from occupations; for example, by instructing the patient in using a piece of leather and a pencil, "require him to make a line of dots at equal distances around the margin and at uniform distances from the edge. This constitutes a test of *Judgement* in estimating distances."[32(p15)] Continuing with the same piece of leather, the patient is instructed to punch a hole at each dot. "In order to do this he must consider the two sides of leather, the two parts of his tool and bring these together thus making a *Simple Coordination* test."[32(p16)] Other tests in the fabrication of the leather purse include *Aesthetic Coordination and Rhythm, Differentiation of Form and Size, Purposeful Relation*. In all 25 tests, she stressed a completed, useful and "not unbeautiful" object.

Tracy's other writings state the value and usefulness of discarded materials to successful ward work.[33(p62)] She also emphasized high quality workmanship: "It is now believed that what is worth doing at all is worth doing well, and that practical, well-made articles have a greater therapeutic value than a useless, poorly made article."[34(p198)] A premium is placed upon originality and the "... adoption of the occupation to the condition and natural tastes of the patient."[35(p63)] Further, she believes that "... the patient is the product, not the article that he makes."[33(p59)]

Tracy's major work, *Studies in Invalid Occupation*, published in 1918,[36] is a revealing compendium of her observations and experiences with different kinds of patients, for instance: "the child of poverty and the child of wealth, the impatient boy, grandmother, the business man."

By 1921, Susan Tracy had adopted the term *occupation therapy* originally coined by William Rush Dunton, Jr., and defined it and differentiated it from vocational training. She felt this was necessary because of the arising confusion between the two concepts following World War I. She wrote: "What is occupation? The treatment of disease by occupation.... The aim of occupation is to get the man well; that of vocational training is to provide him with a job. Any well man will look for a job, but the sick man is looking for health."[37(p120)]

Throughout all of her writings she stated that nothing is "...too small to be pressed into the service of resourceful mind and trained hands toward ... the establishment of a healthy mind in a healthy body."[33(p57)]

George Barton: Re-education of Convalescents

George Edward Barton, by profession an architect, contracted tuberculosis in his adult life. This plagued him for the remainder of his years. His constant struggle led him into a life of service to the physically handicapped. Out of his own personal concerns came the establishment of Consolation House, an early prototype of a rehabilitation center. He was an effective speaker and writer, often given to hyperbole; he gained his point with the listening or reading public.

Barton's central themes were hospitals and their responsibility to the discharged patient; the conditions the discharged patient faces; the need to return to employment; occupations and re-education of convalescents. These were intense concerns to him because of his own health problems.

His first published article, derived from a speech given to a group of nurses, points out a weakness he perceived in hospitals: "We discharge from them not efficients, but inefficients. An individual leaves almost any of our institutions only to become a burden upon his family, his friends, the associated charities, or upon another institution."[38(p328)] In the same article, he warms to his subject: "I say to discharge a patient from the hospital, with his fracture healed, to be sure, but to a devastated home, to an empty desk and to no obvious sustaining employment, is to send him out to a world cold and bleak...."[38(p329)] His solution: "...occupation would shorten convalescence and improve the condition of many patients."[38(p329)] He ended his oration with a rallying cry: "...it is time for humanity to cease regarding the hospital as a door closing upon a life which is past and to regard it henceforth as a door opening upon a life which is to come."[38(p330)]

Barton established Consolation House in Clifton Springs, New York. Those referred to his institution underwent a thorough review, including a social and medical history, and a consideration of one's education, training, experience, successes, and failures. Barton believed that "By considering these in relation to the condition (the patient) must presumably or inevitably be in for the remainder of his life, we can find some form of occupation for which he will be fitted...."[39(p336)] He claimed that Consolation House was "getting down to our social difficulties."[39(p337)]

By 1915, Barton had adopted Dunton's term, *occupation* therapy, but preferred the adjectival form: occupational therapy. He declared: "If there is an occupational disease, why not an occupational therapy?"[40(p139)] He expansively stated: "The first thing to be done ... is for occupational therapy to provide an occupation which will produce *a similar therapeutic effect to that of every drug in materia medica*. An exercise for each separate organ, joint, and muscle of the human body. An exercise? An occupation! An occupation? A useful occupation! Then (occupational therapy) can fill the doctor's prescriptions... written in the terms of materia medica."[40(p139)] He even advocated a laxative by *occupation*.

Re-education entered Barton's terminology with the aftermath of World War I. He viewed hospitals as taking on a mission different from that previously adopted. A hospital should become "...a re-educational institution through which to put the waste products of society *back and into the right place*."[40(p139)] Using alliteration, he declared: "...by a catalystic concatenation of contiguous circumstances we were forced to realize that when all is said and done, what the sick man really needed and wanted most was the restoration of his ability to work, to live independently and to make money."[41(p320)]

Barton's major contribution to the re-emergence of moral treatment was the awakening of physical re-construction and re-education through the employment of occupations. Convalescence, to him, was a critical time for the inclusion of something to do. Activity "...clarifies and strengthens the mind by increasing and maintaining interest in wholesome thought to the exclusion of morbid thought ... and a proper occupation...during convalescence may be made the basis of the corollary of a new life upon recovery.... I mean *a job, a better job, or a job done better* than it was before."[42(p309)] With Susan Tracy, Barton held that the major consideration of occupations "...should be devoted to the therapeutic and education effects, not to the value of the possible product."[43(p36)]

William Rush Dunton, Jr.: Judicious Regimen of Activity

Of the founders of the 20th century movement, William Rush Dunton, Jr., was the most prolific writer and the most influential. He published in excess of 120 books and articles related to occupational therapy and rehabilitation; served as president of the National Society for the Promotion of Occupation Therapy; and, for 21 years, was editor of the official journal. As a physician, he spent his professional career treating psychiatric patients in an institutional setting. Key to his treatment methods is occupational therapy, a term he coined to differentiate aimless amusements from those occupations definitely prescribed for their therapeutic benefits. Before embarking on what he called *a judicious regimen of activity*, he read the works of Tuke and Pinel, as well as the efforts of significant alienists of the 19th century.

From his readings and from observations of patients in Sheppard Asylum, a Quaker institution in Towson, Maryland, Dunton concluded that the acutely ill are generally not amenable to occupations or recreation. The acutely ill exhibit a weakened power of attention. Occupations at this time would be fatiguing and harmful. The prevailing prescription is "…to let the patient alone, meanwhile improve (his) condition, restore and revivify exhausted mental and physical forces…."[44(p19)] Later, activities should be selected that use energies not needed for physical restoration. Stimulating attention and directing the thoughts of the patient in regular and healthful paths would ensure an early release from the hospital. Dunton developed a wide variety of activities from knitting and crocheting to printing and the repair of dynamos, in order to gain the attention and interest, as well as to meet the needs, of all patients.

Dunton's proclivities for history and research led him to extensive readings and experimentations—all related to the human, his need for work, leisure, rest, and sleep; the causal factors of mental aberrations; various cures of mental illness. Each excursion brought him back to *a judicious regimen of activity* as the treatment of choice, regardless of whether the patient was mentally or physically ill. He became more and more convinced that attention and interest in one's work and play are as efficacious, if not more so, than the many and varied other medications available. He stated it this way: "It has been found that a patient makes more rapid progress if his attention is concentrated upon what he is making and he derives stimulating pleasure in its performance."[45(p19)]

At the second annual meeting of the National Society for the Promotion of Occupational Therapy (AOTA) in 1918, Dunton unveiled his nine cardinal rules to guide the emerging practice of occupational therapy, and to ensure that the new discipline would gain acceptance as a medical entity: 1. Any activity in which the patient engages should have as its objective a cure. 2. It should be interesting; 3. have a useful purpose other than merely to gain the patient's attention and interest; and 4. preferably lead to an increase in knowledge on the patient's part. 5. Curative activity should preferably be carried on with others, such as in a group. 6. The occupational therapist should make a careful study of the patient in order to know his or her needs and attempt to meet as many as possible through activity. 7. The therapist should stop the patient in his or her work before reaching a point of fatigue; and 8. encouragement should be genuinely given whenever indicated. Finally, 9. work is much to be preferred over idleness, even when the end product of the patient's labor is of a poor quality or is useless.[46(p26-27)]

The major purposes of occupation in the case of the mentally ill were outlined in Dunton's first book.[47(p24-26)] The primary objective is to divert the attention either from unpleasant subjects, as is true with the depressed patient; or from day-dreaming or mental ruminations, as in the case of the patient suffering from dementia praecox (schizophrenia)—that is, to divert the attention to one main subject.

Another purpose of occupation is to re-educate—to train the patient in developing mental processes through "…educating the hands, eyes, muscles, just as is done in the developing child."[47(p25)] Fostering an interest in hobbies is a third purpose. Hobbies serve as present, as well as future, safety valves and render a recurrence of mental illness less likely. A final purpose may be to instruct the patient in a craft until he or she has enough proficiency to take pride in his or her work. However, Dunton did note that "While this is proper, I fear … specialism is apt to cause a narrowing of one's mental outlook…. The individual with a knowledge of many things has more interest in the world in general."[47(p26)]

Dunton continued to write and publish his observations, each one elaborating on a previous one. His texts became required reading for students preparing for practice. Even in his 90s, well beyond retirement from practice, he maintained an interest in our profession and continued to offer counsel.

Eleanor Clarke Slagle: Founder-Pioneer

Eleanor Clarke Slagle qualifies as both a founder and a pioneer. She was at the birth of the Association in 1917. Before that time she had received part of her education in social work and had completed one of the early Special Courses in Curative Occupations and Recreation at the Chicago School of Civics and Philanthropy. Following this, she taught in two courses for attendants of the insane; directed the occupations program at Henry Phipps Clinic, Johns Hopkins Hospital, Baltimore, under Dr. Adolf Meyer; returned to Chicago to become the Superintendent of Occupational Therapy at Hull House. Later, Mrs. Slagle moved to New York where she pioneered in developing occupational therapy in the State Department of Mental Hygiene. In addition, she served with high distinction in every elective office of the American Occupational Therapy Association, including President (1919–1920) and as a paid Executive Secretary for 14 years.[48(p122-125); 49(p473-474); 50(p18); 51]

She found occupational therapy to be "…an awkward term…" but felt "… it has been well defined as a form of remedial treatment consisting of various types of activities … which either contribute to or hasten recovery from disease or injury … carried on under medical supervision and that it be *consciously* motivated." Further, she emphasized that occupational therapy must be "a *consciously* planned progressive program of *rest, play, occupation and exercise*…."[52(p289)] In addition, she explained it is "…an effort toward normalizing the lives of countless thousands who are mentally ill, … the normal mechanism of a fairly well balanced day."[53(p14)] She enjoyed quoting C. Charles Burlingame, a prominent psychiatrist of her day: "What is an occupational therapist? She is that newer medical specialist who takes the joy out of invalidism. She is the medical specialist who carries us over the dangerous period between acute illness and return to the world of men and women as a useful member of society.'"[52(p290-291)]

Slagle placed considerable emphasis upon the personality factor of the therapist: "...the proper balance of qualities, proper physical expression, a kindly voice, gentleness, patience, ability and seeming vision, adaptability ... to meet the particular needs of the individual patient in all things.... Personality plus character also covers an ability to be honest and firm, with infinite kindness...."[54(p13)]

The issue would constantly arise about the use of handicrafts as a therapeutic measure in the machine age. Her response is a classic: "...handicrafts are so generally used, not only because they are so diverse, covering a field from the most elementary to the highest grade of ability; but also, and greatly to the point, because their development is based on primitive impulses. They offer the means of contact with the patient that no other medium does or can offer. Encouragement of creative impulses also may lead to the development of large interests outside oneself and certainly leads to social contact, an important consideration with any sick or convalescent patient."[52(p292–293)]

Habit training was first attempted at Rochester (New York) State Hospital in 1901. Slagle adopted the basic principles and developed a far greater perspective and use among mental patients who had been hospitalized from 5 to 20 years and who had steadily regressed. The fundamental plan was "...to arrange a twenty-four hour schedule ... in which physicians, nurses, attendants, and occupational therapists play a part...."[54(p13)] It was a re-education program designed to overcome some disorganized habits, to modify others and construct new ones, with the goal that habit reaction will lead toward the restoration and maintenance of health. "In habit training, we show clearly an academic philosophy factor...that is, the necessity of requiring attention, of building on the habit of attention—attention thus becomes application, voluntary and, in time, agreeable."[54(p14)]

The purposes of habit training were two-fold: the reclamation and rehabilitation of the patient, with the eventual goal of discharge or parole; and, if this was not reasonable, to assist the patient in becoming less of an institutional problem, that is, less destructive and untidy.

A typical habit training schedule called for the patient to arise in the morning at 6:00, wash, toilet, brush teeth, and air beds; then breakfast; return to ward and make beds, sweep; then classwork for 2 hours, which consisted of a variety of simple crafts and marching exercises. After lunch, there was a rest period; continued classwork and outdoor exercises, folk dancing, and lawn games. Following supper, there was music and dancing on the ward, followed by toileting, washing, brushing the teeth, and preparing for bed.[55(p29)]

Once the patient had received maximum benefit from habit training, he or she was ready to progress through three phases of occupational therapy. The first was what Slagle called *the kindergarten group.* "We must show the ways and means of stimulating the special senses. The employment of color, music, simple exercises, games and storytelling along with occupations, the gentle ways and means ... (used) in educating the child are equally important in re-educating the adult...."[54(p14)] Occupations were graded from the simple to the complex.

The next phase was *ward classes in occupational therapy.* "...graded to the limit of accomplishment of individual patients."[56(p100)] When able to tolerate it, the patient joined in group activities. The third and final phase was the *occupational center.* "This promotes opportunities for the more advanced projects ... (a) complete change in environment; ... comparative freedom; ... actual responsibilities placed upon patients; the stimulation of seeing work produced; ... all these carry forward the readjustment of patients."[56(p102)]

This founder, this pioneer, this distinguished member of our profession provided a summary of her own accomplishments and philosophy by stating: "Of the highest value to patients is the psychological fact that the patient is working for himself.... Occupational Therapy recognizes the significance of the mental attitude which the sick person takes toward his illness and attempts to make that attitude more wholesome by providing activities adapted to the capacity of the individual patient and calculated to divert his attention from his own problems."[54(p290)] Further, she declared: "It is directed activity, and differs from all other forms of treatment in that it is given in increasing doses as the patient improves."[57(p3)]

Adolf Meyer: Philosophy of Occupation Therapy

Dr. Adolf Meyer is cited in this account of the evolution of occupational therapy because of his outstanding support and because his approach to clinical psychiatry was entirely consistent with the emerging occupational therapy movement.

Adolf Meyer, a Swiss physician, immigrated to the United States in 1892 and accepted a position initially as pathologist at the Eastern Illinois Hospital for the Insane in Kankakee. Over the next 14 years he held various positions in the United States and became professor of psychiatry at Johns Hopkins University in 1910. Throughout this period he developed the fundamentals of what was to become the psychobiological approach to psychiatry, a term he coined to indicate that the human is an indivisible unit of study, rather than a composite of symptoms. "Psychobiology starts not from a mind and a body or from elements, but from the fact that we deal with biologically organized units and groups and their functioning ... the 'he's' and 'she's' of our experience—the bodies we find in action...."[58(p263)] Meyer took strong issue with those in medicine: "...who wish to reduce everything to physics and chemistry, or to anatomy, or to physiology, and within that to neurology...."[58(p262)] His enlightened point of view is that one can only be studied as a total being in action and that this "...whole person represents an integrate of hierarchically arranged functions."[59(p1317)]

His common sense approach to the problems of psychiatry was his keynote: "The main thing is that your point of reference should always be life itself.... I put my emphasis upon specificity.... As long as there is life there are positive assets—action, choice, hope, not in the imagination but in a clear understanding of the situation, goals and possibilities.... To see life as it is, to tend toward objectivity is one of the fundamentals of my philosophy, my attitude, my preference. It is something that I would recommend if it can be kept free of making itself a pest to self and to others."[60(p vi–xi)]

From the very beginning of his work in Illinois, he was concerned with meaningful activity. In time, it became the fundamental issue in treatment. "I thought primarily of occupation therapy," he stated, "of getting the patient to do things and getting things going which did not work but which could work with proper straightening out."[60(p45)] In a report to the Governor of the State of Illinois in 1895, Meyer wrote: "Occupation is, with good right, the most essential side of hygienic treatment of most insane patients."[60(p 59)]

By 1921, Meyer had become Professor of Psychiatry at Johns Hopkins University in Baltimore, and had extensive experiences with others, such as William Rush Dunton, Jr., Eleanor Clarke Slagle, and Henrietta Price, leaders in the occupational therapy movement. At the Fifth Annual Meeting of the National Society for the Promotion of Occupational Therapy in Baltimore, October 1921, Meyer brought together his fundamental concepts of psychobiology to produce his paper, *The Philosophy of Occupation Therapy* (see Chapter 2). Through time, this has become a classic in the occupational therapy literature. It bears study by all of us.

Psychobiology is clearly visible in his statement that "...the newer conceptions of *mental problems* (are) *problems of living*, and not merely diseases of a structural and toxic nature...."[61(p4)] The indivisibility and integration of the human are cited in this manner: "Our conception of man is that of an organism that maintains and balances itself in the world of reality and actuality by being in active life and active use...."[61(p5)]

Because of the nature of his paper, *The Philosophy of Occupational Therapy*, Meyer emphasized occupation, time, and the productive use of energy. Interwoven are the elements of psychobiology. He stated: "The whole of human organization has its shape in a kind of rhythm.... There are many ... rhythms which we must be attuned to: the larger rhythms of night and day, of sleep and waking hours...and finally the big four—work and play and rest and sleep, which our organism must be able to balance even under difficulty. The only way to attain balance in all this is actual doing, actual practice, a program of wholesome living is the basis of wholesome feeling and thinking and fancy and interests."[61(p6)]

According to Meyer, a fundamental issue in the treatment of the mentally ill is "...the proper use of time in some helpful and gratifying activity...."[61(p1)] He expands on this precept by stating: "There is in all this a development of the *valuation of time and work*, which is not accidental. It is part of the great espousal of the *values of reality and actuality* rather than of mere thinking and reasoning...."[61(p4)] The introduction of activity is "... in giving opportunities rather than prescriptions. There must be opportunities to work, opportunities to do and to plan and create, and to learn to use material.... It is not a question of specific prescriptions, but of opportunities ... to adapt opportunities."[61(p7)] He concluded his philosophic essay by returning once again to time and occupations: "The great feature of man is his new sense of time, with foresight built on a sound view of the past and present. Man learns to organize time and he does it in terms of doing things, and one of the many things he does between eating, drinking and ... the flights fancy and aspiration, we call work and occupation."[61(p9–10)]

Near the end of his working life, Meyer summed up his major efforts. He wrote of dealing with individuals and groups from the viewpoints of *good sense*; of *science*, "...with the smallest numbers of assumptions for search and research..."; of *philosophy*; and of *religion*, "... as a way of trust and dependabilities in life." [62, p100]

Occupational Therapy Definitions and Principles

As the founders and pioneers were experimenting with and writing their concepts, a definition of occupational therapy was emerging. It is remarkable that so early in the formation of the 20th century movement, a definition could be developed and stand for several decades and several generations of occupational therapists. Many of us were required in school to immortalize it through needlepoint, embroidery, and even printing.

H.A. Pattison, M.D., medical officer of the National Tuberculous Association, advanced his view at the annual conference of the National Society for the Promotion of Occupational Therapy in Chicago, September 1919. It was also adopted by the Federal Board of Vocational Education: "Occupational Therapy may be defined as any activity, mental or physical, definitely prescribed and guided for the distinct purpose of contributing to and hastening recovery from disease or injury."[63(p21)] Twenty-one years later, in 1931, John S. Coulter, M.D., and Henrietta McNary, OTR, added one phrase: "...and assisting the social and institutional adjustment of individuals requiring long and indefinite periods of hospitalization."[64(p19)] This was inserted in order to recognize occupational therapy's involvement in chronicity.

By 1925, a committee, made up of four physicians including William Rush Dunton, compiled an outline for lectures to medical students and physicians.[65(p277–292)] Though their document never received the official imprimatur of the AOTA, it nevertheless served for several years as a guide for practice.[66(p347)] Fifteen principles were enunciated: "Occupational therapy is a method of training the sick or injured by means of instruction and employment in productive occupation; ... to arouse interest, courage, confidence; to exercise mind and body in...activity; to overcome disability; and to re-establish capacity for industrial and social usefulness."[65(p280)] Application called for as much system and precision as other forms of treatment; activity was to be prescribed, administered, and supervised under constant medical advice. Individual patient needs were paramount.

The outline stressed that "employment in groups is ... advisable because it provides exercise in social adaptation and stimulating influence of example and comment...."[65(p280)] In selecting an activity, the patient's interests and capabilities were to be considered and as strength and capability increased, the occupation was to be altered, regulated, and graded accordingly because "The only reliable measure of the treatment is the effect on the patient."[65(p280)]

Inferior workmanship could be tolerated, depending upon the patient's condition, but there should be consideration of "...standards worthy of entirely normal persons ... for proper mental stimulation."[65(p281)] Articles made were to be useful and attractive, and meaningful tasks requiring healthful exercise of mind and body provided the greatest satisfaction. "Novelty, variety, individuality, and utility of the products enhance the value of an occupation as a treatment measure."[65(p281)] While quality, quantity, and the salability of articles made could be of benefit, these should not take precedence over the treatment objectives. As adjuncts to occupations, physical exercise, games, and music were considered beneficial and fell into two main categories: gymnastics and calisthenics, recreation and play.

One last principle spoke of the qualities of the occupational therapist: "...good craftsmanship, and ability to instruct are essential qualifications; ... understanding, sincere interest in the patient, and an optimistic, cheerful outlook and manner are equally essential."[65(p281)]

Occupational Therapy's Second Generation

The die was cast. Practice rapidly expanded in a phenomenal number of settings following the establishment of the founders' principles and definition. A *second generation* of therapists emerged during the late 1920s and the 1930s. They were the practitioners and educators who elaborated, codified, and applied the initial theory upon which present-day practice is based. A chronicle of their efforts would offer a highly valuable and valued study in itself. The names of Louis Haas, Mary Alice Coombs, Winifred Kahmann, Henrietta McNary, Harriet Robeson, Marjorie Taylor, and Helen Willard would figure prominently in such an account.

For the purpose of *this history*, a composite of these and others is drawn into one individual who exemplifies the spirit and deeds of the *second generation* of occupational therapists—those whose efforts are lasting and ensure our present and future education and practice.

Understandably, it would be a woman. She would devote her professional career to either teaching, practicing, or administering. Quite possibly she would combine two or more of these. She would acquire an expertise in one area of practice, such as the mentally ill.

Her belief in the treatment of the total patient would guide her thoughts and actions. Occupational therapy, she would declare, "since its founding has concerned itself with the basic tenet—the treatment of the total patient. This approach is unique to occupational therapy among the ... health disciplines.... There has always existed a strong component concerned with the behavior of the physically ill or disabled, as well as the mentally sick; with the entirety of man and his functioning as a patient. This occupational therapy concept," she would continue, "prevented (as has occurred in medical practice) an undesired separation of the psychiatric therapist from those who develop knowledge and skills centered in the treatment of the physically disabled."[67(p1)] Stated another way, "The major emphasis in occupational therapy is not the body *as such* but the individual *as such*. The therapist's background is strongly weighted in an understanding of personality adjustment and reactions to social situations; ... and in the patients' attitudes toward an adjustment to acute and chronic disabilities."[68(p9)]

At some point in her work, she would be asked to serve as a consultant to one or more medical facilities, possibly a state hospital system. In time, she would produce a report and re-state her definition of occupational therapy. It might well go this way: "The goal of all treatment in a modern mental hospital is the physical, social and economic rehabilitation of the patient.... The accepted function (of occupational therapy) ... is the scientific utilization of mental and physical activities for the purpose of raising the patient to the highest level of integration; to assist him in making his initial adjustment to the hospital; to sustain him while his body responds to physical treatment and his mind to psychotherapy; or to assist him in making a satisfactory adjustment to chronic illness."[69(p24)]

In the report she would also call for an atmosphere as normal as possible, where a patient could be encouraged to respond in as normal a manner as possible: a balanced program of work and play, with flexibility to meet individual needs: "There must be organized a succession of steps through which the patient will be gradually led to his highest level of integration.... At each level ... the patient experiences a feeling of success and self-respect. One cannot overemphasize the importance of careful planning ... in order that there be a systematic progression up this ladder of integration."[69(p24)]

In another context, supportive care, as a vital concern to the therapist, would also be described, particularly in the care of the physically disabled: "To name only a few of its treatment objectives, occupational therapy may function as a diagnostic evaluative instrument; as corrective treatment; ... or a design for effecting prevocational evaluation. Incorporated in each ... is a treatment phase referred to as supportive care. This is a most fundamental and yet less definitive and indeed the least spectacular element of the total rehabilatory program. In supportive care, the occupational therapist (is concerned) with the behavioural factors which have and will affect the patient's response to the rehabilitation program...." Convincingly, she would say: "...it can be said with conviction that successful rehabilitation can be effected only when the patient has attained a true state of rehabilitation 'readiness.'"[70]

Not just a woman of words, she would find one or more ways to activate her philosophy. She might well become active with a group of former patients and assist in organizing an association of and for individuals who have been hospitalized—for instance, the mentally ill. Such an endeavor would be the first of a kind. Through such an experience, she would conclude: "One difficulty which presented itself again and again was the need to instill in these (former) patients a philosophy toward their own rehabilitation: ... an organized effort beyond the hospital which would offer special training, guidance and professional evaluation of their potentials."[71(p3)]

This would lead her to even greater endeavors on behalf of a whole category of patients. As an example, she would find that the 1920 Federal Vocational Rehabilitation Act excluded former psychiatric patients. In the manner of Dorothea Lynde Dix, whom she probably emulated, she would wage a relentless battle to right such a wrong. By enlisting the assistance of physicians' associations and veterans' groups she would see the legislation change. As part of her campaign she would write: "The former mental patient, in his struggle for economic rehabilitation, incurs the burden imposed on the physically handicapped 'plus' the stigmatization based on the popular misconception of mental disease. He must cast aside self-pity or the idea that the world owes him a living. The world does owe him understanding and guidance."[72(p114)] Finally, amendments to **Public Law 113** were passed and signed by President Franklin Roosevelt. Psychiatric patients could now qualify for the benefits of the vocational rehabilitation act.

With such efforts the therapist's personal beliefs about emotional illness become even more strongly felt: "The majority of mentally ill are (sick) through no fault of their own ... any more than one who has contracted a physical illness. Persons suffering from mental disease are generally ill as a result of an accumulation of unsuccessful efforts...to adjust to his environment."[72(p83)]

Two continuing concerns of all occupational therapists would be commented upon: the qualifications of the therapist and the use of media. One is as significant as the other. "The personality of the therapist," she would say, "must command respect, admiration, hope and confidence, ... for no therapy is better than the therapist who directs it."[72(p83)] Therapeutic media have a number of inherent qualities, such as providing a vehicle for objectively recording patient performance, and, for the patient, affording opportunities for "...creative expression and evidence of accomplishment. The therapist should have a wide variety of activities (available) in accordance with the interests, aptitudes, and mental state of the patient. A craft track mind had no place in preparing such a program," she would state.[72(p103)]

The accumulation of experiences as a clinician, and educator, or an administrator, or possibly a combination of these, would lead this *therapist of the second generation* to arrive at a new definition of occupational therapy. It would precede by several years an altered definition by the national organization. It would incorporate the social and behavioral sciences, with a diminished emphasis upon medicine. Human development would appear for the first time as a focus for the treatment of physical and psychosocial dysfunction. She would declare: "Occupational therapy's function is to provide skilled assistance in influencing human objectives; its approach is inextricably conjoined with the behavioral factors involved. It is interested in how the process of growth and development is modified by hospitalization, chronic illness or a permanent handicap."[73(p2)]

This re-focus was quite explainable and understandable to her since occupational therapy, and its ancestral emphasis, has always been the totality of the human organism. She would say, "It was inevitable, therefore, that there evolve an ever increasing emphasis in occupational therapy ... a greater understanding of the part that the developmental process plays in the preventive and therapeutic factors of this form of treatment."[74(p3)]

The foregoing has been a descriptive composite of a whole generation of therapists and assistants. The composite is actually the story of one individual; her observations alone have been cited. That individual is *Miss Beatrice D. Wade*, OTR, FAOTA.

The story is far from finished. Without a doubt, someone sometime will chronicle the lives and works of those who are still making contributions from that era to the present generation. Among them are Marjorie Fish, Virginia Kilburn, Mary Reilly, Ruth Robinson, Clare Spackman, Ruth Brunyate Wiemer, Carlotta Welles, and Wilma West. Each one, together with many others, continues to serve us well as clarifiers and definers of reasonable and reasoned alternatives. As counselors, they confirm old values and clearly point out *new directions* as well as our faithfulness or infidelity to those timeless principles established by our professional ancestors.

Lessons From Our History

The history of occupational therapy is the most neglected aspect of our professional endeavors. Seemingly, *old values* are least considered when charting *new directions*. On occasion we have been accused of taking leave of our historical senses. More to the point is that we have no historical sense. The problem primarily lies in not taking the time to assiduously locate our profession's diggings, to excavate what is relevant, and, then, to learn from what has been unearthed.

Archival materials from the past 200 years have been abundantly used in the development of this paper. Location and excavation has been difficult at times; however, it is reassuring to note that records and accounts still exist that are extremely relevant to today's endeavors. Lessons can be learned and they must. May I encourage each of you to determine for yourself what you have learned from this paraphrastic journey to our profession's diggings. To assist in this endeavor, may I cite a few lessons I have gained.

Mind and Body Inextricably Conjoined. No less than our professional ancestors, we must refuse to accept any alternative to the belief in the wholeness of the human—that the mind and body are inextricably conjoined. Illness, treatment, and the return to a healthful state simultaneously affect the physiological and emotional processes. Indeed, should these processes ever become separated, then occupational therapy would be of no value. The patient has died!

The Natural Science of the Human. The inextricable union of the human leads to another lesson. The science fundamental to our practice is the natural science of the human. No amount of neurophysiology, psychology, sociology, or child development alone can determine the differential diagnosis, treatment, or prognosis of the patient undergoing occupational therapy. The current trend toward specialization, with its varying emphases upon one or another science, to the neglect of other human sciences, and indeed to the neglect of other nonscientific aspects of occupational therapy, borders on superstition and mythology. It is the continuous acquisition and scientific synthesis of the ingredients of the human organism and its surround that guarantees authentic occupational therapy.

The Human Organism's Involvement in Tasks. Occupational therapy is the only major health profession whose focus centers upon the *total* human organism's involvement in tasks—a making or doing. In spite of the many grafts we have effected, our roots remain in the subsoil of the *art*, the *craft*: a paradigm of the total activity of the human. Just as those who have come before us, we think of ourselves and others fundamentally as makers, as users, as doers, as tools. We look at: "...craft as a way in which man may create and cross a bridge within himself and center himself in his own essential unity."[75(p vii)] The procedures one goes through in rearranging and reassembling the basic elements in art or craft operate upon and within the doer: "... his material modifies him as he modifies it, in proportion to his openness, his awareness of the exchange that is taking place."[75 (px)]

The Differentiation of Occupational Therapy. Any definition, any description, any differentiation between ourselves and other health providers must have as its major theme occupation and leisure. Without it, we become a blurred copy, a xerography of a host of others.

Without the dynamics of human motion inherent in purposeful activity, we become quasi-physical therapists. Without the interaction between human objects and the objects of work and leisure, we become quasi-social workers, psychologists, or nurses. Without the demonstrated and proven interrelationships between healthful, normal growth and development, activity, and the pathology of illness and disabling conditions, we become quasi-physicians and psychiatrists.

The more we intermingle our fundamental philosophy and our treatment techniques with others, the more likely we will become enfeebled, the more likely we will degenerate, the more likely we will eventually disappear.

A Refusal to Accept the Common Verdict. As Hugh Sidey has noted, "History is a marvelous collection of stories about men and women who refuse to accept the common verdict that certain achievements (are) impossible."[77(p18)] The history of occupational therapy is the story of the ideals, deeds, hopes, and works of *individuals*. Changes and advancements came from those who eliminated inhumaneness, which prevented or discouraged the sick and disabled from achieving their potential. These same individuals were willing to assume the care and responsibility for those *who were not highly valued by the society*: the mentally ill and retarded, the severely disabled—all those defined as "non-producing, ... an economic burden."[65(p277)]

In numerous places and on countless occasions these same individuals were derided, hated, or, at best, ignored, because they pressed for change in the human condition. Yet, they persevered, knowing there was nothing innately unusual about themselves or what they wished to achieve. Few ever saw their names inscribed on monuments.

They were a *cast* quite diverse in character, and largely obscure because of the immensity of the saga being enacted. A few received *speaking parts*, primarily through reporting their own clinical findings. Only very few were singled out to be stars. None ever became members of the *audience*, passively observing events. All were *actors*.

The very same can be said of the present occupational therapy generation. We are actors, not observers. We continue to willingly strive on behalf of those who are not highly valued by the society. We refuse to see this as a burden. Rather, we perceive it as an obligation, as an opportunity, as a way of life.

Legacy of Experience. Too often we are disposed to think that those lessons another generation learned do not apply to the present generation. We should be remindful that there are two ways to learn: by our own experience and from those who have made discoveries, regardless of how long ago they were made. The experience of others is a magnificent heritage, and the more we learn from them, the less time we waste in the present, proving what already has been proved.

Those of us who are teachers and clinicians have a special obligation to pass on the legacy of experience, the knowledge of timeless principles and practices that do not change merely because times change.

Who They Were, What They Did. The legacy of experience suggests one more lesson. So often we are caught up in our daily activities we tend to forget what it is we owe those who came before us. All probably agree that each occupational therapy generation seemingly acquires a sense of self-sufficiency. It is true that we of the present occupy the positions that once were filled by others.

It is, however, of great import that we realize we are influenced by those who came before us more than we can truly know. Who they were and what they did has immeasurable bearing upon what we are and what we do. No generation is capable of isolating itself from its past. The past, plus what we are and what we do, greatly assists in fashioning our future.

The archives, the portraits and photographs, the published accounts, the personal memorabilia and scrapbooks are records of considerable moment. At the least, they are a profound reminder of the possibility that someday, someone may be looking back and may be wondering who we were and what we did.

Conclusion

It is altogether fitting and proper to conclude this lecture with the observations of two former Presidents of the Association, Mr. Thomas B. Kidner and Mrs. Eleanor Clarke Slagle. In 1930, Mr. Kidner offered a personal impression of the state of occupational therapy at the annual meeting of the Connecticut Occupational Therapy Society. In part, he said: "May we, therefore, look on occupational therapy—with the increased faith as the years go by—as a natural means of aiding in the restoration of the sick and disabled to health and working capacity (which means happiness) because it appeals to all our human attributes."[57(p11)]

Mrs. Slagle, a year after she retired in 1937, made this observation: "The story of the profession of occupational therapy will never be fully told, nor will that of the patients who have so abundantly appreciated the opportunities of the service. There has been no fanciful crusad-ing 'for the cause'; it has meant that a few have perhaps borne many burdens, but in the slow process that make permanent things of great value, it can be said that there is a fine body of professional workers, experienced and well trained, coming forward and being welcomed to a really great human service, that of helping to show the way to the person with large disabilities to make the best of his incomplete self."[78(p382)] Finally, in an editorial "From the Heart," she concluded: "The integrity of your profession is in your hands. I bid you all Godspeed in your work."[79(p345)]

Acknowledgments

A study of this nature and scope is not possible without the valuable and valued assistance of numerous individuals and sources. I wish to recognize the incomparable services provided by the staffs of the Moody Medical Library, The University of Texas Medical Branch at Galveston; the Quine Library, University of Illinois at the Medical Center, Chicago; the McGoogan Library of Medicine, University of Nebraska Medical Center, Omaha; and the Archives, Shapiro Developmental Center (Eastern Illinois State Hospital), Kankakee.

Finally, I wish to recognize Frances Sawyer, COTA, and the Board of Directors, The Texas Occupational Therapy Association, Inc., who placed my name in nomination for this exalted honor. My gratitude to them is immeasurable.

Dedication

I wish to dedicate the 1981 Eleanor Clarke Slagle Lectureship:

to my parents, who provided me with those cumulative experiences and values that inevitably led me to the decision to become an occupational therapist;

to a very great woman, Beatrice D. Wade, OTR, FOATA, who has been my valued teacher and beloved mentor for more than 30 years;

to my cherished colleagues, Lillian Hoyle Parent and Jay Cantwell, both occupational therapists, who constantly stimulate me and insist on a high level of constructive activity;

to Charles H. Christiansen, OTR, FOATA, whose personal and professional qualities and insistence on excellence from himself and others assure me of the future of occupational therapy.

Without the examples, teachings, guidance, counseling, and friendship of these individuals, I could never have achieved this exalted opportunity.

References

1. Locke J: *An Essay Concerning Human Understanding* (Two Volumes). New York: Dover Press, 1894F

2. Frost SE: *Basic Teachings of the Great Philosophers,* New York: Barnes and Noble, Inc., 1942

3. Riese W: *The Legacy of Philippe Pinel: An Inquiry into Thought on Mental Alienation,* New York: Springer Publishing Co., 1969

4. Condillac EB de: *Oeuvres Philosophiques de Condillac,* Paris: Presse Universataires de France, 1947

5. Ackerknecht EH: *A Short History of Psychiatry,* New York: Hafner Publishing Co., 1968

6. Tuke DH: *A Dictionary of Psychological Medicine* (Vol One). Philadelphia: P Blakinston, Son & Co., 1892

7. Pinel P: *Traité Médico-Philosophique sur 'Alienation Mentale,* Paris: Richard, Caille & Rover, 1801

8. Pinel P: *A Treatise on Insanity In Which Are Contained the Principles of a New and More Practical Nosology of Maniacal Disorders,* Translated by DD Davis. London: Cadell & Davis, 1806 (Facsimile published by Hafner Publishing Co., New York, 1962)

9. Mackler B: Philippe Pinel: *Unchainer of the Insane,* New York: Franklin Watts, Inc., 1968

10. Folsome CF: *Diseases of the Mind: Notes on the Early Management, European and American Progress,* Boston: A. Williams & Co., Publishers, 1877

11. Jones K: *Lunacy, Law, and Conscience: 1744–1845: The Social History of Care of the Insane,* London: Routledge & Kegan Paul, Ltd., 1955

12. Dillenberger J, Welch D: *Protestant Christianity: Interpreted Through Its Development,* New York: Charles Scribner's Sons, 1954

13. Philadelphia Yearly Meeting of the Religious Society of Friends: *Faith and Practice,* Philadelphia: Philadelphia Yearly Meeting, 1972

14. Tuke DH: *Reform in the Treatment of the Insane. Early History of the Retreat, York; Its Objects and Influence,* London: J & A Churchill, 1872

15. Tuke DH: *Reform in the Treatment of the Insane: An Early History of the Retreat, York: Its Objects and Influence,* London: J & A Churchill, 1892

16. Tuke S: *Description of The Retreat, An Institution Near York for Insane Persons of the Society of Friends: Containing an Account of Its Origins and Progress, The Modes of Treatment, and a Statement of Cases,* York, England: Alexander, 1813

17. Hunter R, Macalpine I: *Three Hundred Years of Psychiatry, 1535–1860: A History Presented in Selected English Texts,* London: Oxford University Press, 1963

18. Connolly J: *The Treatment of the Insane Without Mechanical Restraints,* London: Smith, Elder & Co., 1856 (Facsimile copy published by Dawson's of Pall Mall, London, 1973, with introduction by R Hunter and I Macalpine)

19. Ellis WC: *A Treatise on the Nature, Symptoms, Causes, and Treatment of Insanity,* London: Holdsworth, 1838

20. Goodman N: *Benjamin Rush: Physician and Citizen, 1746-1813,* Philadelphia: University of Pennsylvania Press, 1934

21. Rush B: *Medical Inquiries and Observations Upon the Diseases of the Mind* (4th Edition). Philadelphia: J Grigg, 1830

22. Buckmaster H: *Women Who Shaped History,* New York: Macmillian Pub. C., 1966

23. Bucknill JC, Tuke, DH: *A Manual of Psychological Medicine,* New York: Hafner Pub. Co., 1968 (Facsimile of 1858 Edition)

24. Barlow J: *Man's Power Over Himself to Prevent or Control Insanity,* London: William Pickering, 1843

25. Skultans V: *Madness and Morals: Ideas on Insanity in the Nineteenth Century,* London: Routledge & Kegan Paul, 1975

26. Tuke DH: *A Dictionary of Psychological Medicine: Volume Two,* Philadelphia: P Blakiston, Son & Co., 1892

27. Bockhoven JS: *Moral Treatment in American Psychiatry,* New York: Springer Publishing Co., Inc. 1963

28. Dain N: *Concepts of Insanity in the United States, 1789–1865,* New Brunswick, NJ: Rutgers University Press, 1964

29. Deutsch A: *The Mentally Ill in America: A History of Their Care and Treatment from Colonial Times* (2nd Edition). New York: Columbia University Press, 1949

30. Tracy SE: The development of occupational therapy in the Grace Hospital, Detroit, Michigan. *Trained Nurse Hosp Rev 66:* 5, May 1921

31. Tracy SE: The place of invalid occupations in the general hospital. *Modern Hosp 2:* 5, June 1914

32. Tracy SE: Twenty-five suggested mental tests derived from invalid occupations. *Maryland Psychiatr Q 8:* 1918

33. Barrows M: Susan E. Tracy, RN. *Maryland Psychiatric 1 6:* 1916–1917

34. Tracy SE: Treatment of disease by employment at St. Elizabeth's Hospital. *Modern Hosp 20:* 2, February 1923

35. Parsons SE: Miss Tracy's work in general hospitals. *Maryland Psychiatr Q 6:* 1916–1917

36. Tracy SE: *Studies in Invalid Occupation,* Boston: Witcomb and Barrows, 1918

37. Tracy SE: Power versus money in occupation therapy. *Trained Nurse Hosp Rev 66:*2, February 1921

38. Barton GE: A view of invalid occupation. *Trained Nurse Hosp Rev 52:*6, June 1914

39. Barton GE: Occupational nursing. *Trained Nurse Hosp Rev 54:*6, June 1915

40. Barton GE: Occupational therapy. *Trained Nurse Hosp Rev 54:*3, March 1915

41. Barton GE: The existing hospital system and reconstruction. *Trained Nurse Hosp Rev 69:*4, October 1922

42. Barton GE: What occupational therapy may mean to nursing. *Trained Nurse Hosp Rev 64:*4, April 1920

43. Barton GE: *Re-education: An Analysis of the Institutional System of the United States.* Boston: Houghton Mifflin Co., 1917

44. Sheppard Asylum: *Third Annual Report of the Sheppard Asylum,* Towson, MD: 1895

45. Dunton WR: The relationship of occupational therapy and physical therapy. *Arch Phys Ther 16:* January 1935

46. Dunton WR: *The Principles of Occupational Therapy. Proceedings of the National Society for the Promotion of Occupational Therapy: Second Annual Meeting,* Catonsville, MD: Spring Grove State Hospital, 1918

47. Dunton WR: *Occupational Therapy: A Manual for Nurses,* Philadelphia: WB Saunders, 1915

48. Komora PO: Eleanor Clarke Slagle. *Ment Hyg 27:*1, January 1943

49. Pollock HM: In memoriam: Eleanor Clarke Slagle, 1876–1942. *Am J Psychiatr 99:*3, November 1942

50. American Occupational Therapy Association: *Then and Now, 1917–1967,* New York: American Occupational Therapy Association, 1967

51. Loomis B, Wade BD: *Chicago...Occupational Therapy Beginnings: Hull House, The Henry B. Favill School of Occupations and Eleanor Clarke Slagle.*

52. Slagle EC: Occupational therapy: Recent methods and advances in the United States. *Occup Ther Rehab 13:*5, October 1934

53. Slagle EC: History of the development of occupation for the insane. *Maryland Psychiatr Q 4:* May 1914

54. Slagle EC: Training aids for mental patients. *Arch Occup There 1:*1, February 1922

55. Slagle EC, Robeson HA: *Syllabus for Training of Nurses in Occupational Therapy,* Utica, NY: State Hospital Press, date unknown

56. Slagle EC: A year's development of occupational therapy in New York State Hospitals. *Modern Hosp 22:*1, January 1924

57. Kidner TB: Occupational therapy, its development, scope and possibilities. *Occup Ther Rehab 10:*1, February 1931

58. Meyer A: The psychological point of view. In *Classics in American Psychiatry,* JP Brady, Editor. St. Louis: Warren H Green, Inc., 1975 (Also, In *The Problems of Mental Health,* M Bentley, EV Cowdey, Editors. New York: McGraw-Hill, 1934)

59. Arieti S: *American Handbook of Psychiatry* (Vol Two), New York: Basic Books, Inc., Publishers, 1959

60. Lief A: *The Commonsense Psychiatry of Dr. Adolf Meyer: Fifty-two Selected Papers, Edited with Biographical Narrative.* New York: McGraw-Hill Book Co., 1948

61. Meyer A: The philosophy of occupation therapy. *Arch Occup Ther 1:*1, February 1922 Also in *Am J Occup Ther 31* (10): 639–642, 1977 (Reprinted as Chapter 2.)

62. Meyer A: The rise to the person and the concept of wholes or integrates. *Am J Psychiatr 100:* April 1944

63. Pattison HA: The trend of occupational therapy for the tuberculous. *Arch Occup Ther 1* (1): February 1922

64. Coulter JS, McNarry H: Necessity of medical supervision in occupational therapy. *Occup Ther Rehab 10* (1): February 1931

65. An outline of lectures on occupational therapy to medical students and physicians. *Occup Ther Rehab 4* (4): August 1925

66. Elwood, ES: The National Board of Medical Examiners and medical education, and the possible effect of the Board's program on the spread of occupational therapy. *Occup Ther Rehab 6* (5): October 1927

67. Wade BD: *Occupational Therapy: A History of Its Practice in the Psychiatric Field.* Unpublished paper presented at 51st Annual Conference, American Occupational Therapy Association, Boston, October 19, 1967

68. Advisory Committee in Occupational Therapy: The Basic Philosophy and Function of Occupational Therapy. *University of Illinois Faculty—Alumni Newsletter of the Chicago Professional Colleges. 6* :4, January 1951

69. Wade BD: A survey of occupational and industrial therapy in the Illinois state hospitals. *Illinois Psychiatr 2* (1): March 1942

70. Wade BD: Supportive care, *Bull Rehab Inst Chicago,* date unknown

71. Wade BD: Supportive care. *Bull Rehab Rehabilitation of the Mentally Ill.* Unpublished paper presented to the Department of Public Welfare, State of Minnesota, June 26, 1958

72. Willard HS, Spackman CS: *Principles of Occupational Therapy* (First Edition). Philadelphia: JB Lippincott Co., 1947

73. Wade BD: *The Development of Clinically Oriented Education in Occupational Therapy: The Illinois Plan.* Unpublished paper presented at 49th Annual Conference, American Occupational Therapy Association, Miami, November 2, 1965

74. Wade BD: Introduction. *The Preparation of Occupational Therapy Students for Functioning with Aging Persons and in Comprehensive Health Care Programs: A Manual for Educators,* Chicago: University of Illinois at the Medical Center, 1969

75. Dooling EM: *A Way of Working,* Garden City, NY: Anchor Press/Doubleday, 1979

76. Sidey H: The presidency. *Time 116* (22):December 1, 1980

77. Slagle EC: Occupational therapy. *Trained Nurse Hosp Rev 100* (4): April 1938

78. Slagle EC: Editorial: From the heart. *Occup Ther Rehab 16* (5): October 1937

Chapter 6

Occupational Therapy Can Be One of the Great Ideas of 20th Century Medicine

1962 Eleanor Clarke Slagle Lecture

Mary Reilly, EdD, OTR

This chapter was previously published in the *American Journal of Occupational Therapy, 16,* 2–9. Copyright © 1962, American Occupational Therapy Association.

Specifying the Theme

As an occupational therapist honored by her peers, I join my Eleanor Clarke Slagle predecessors in feeling the awesome responsibility of the award. The occasion, it seems to me, makes it obligatory for an awardee to objectify a lifetime experience and then speak of an issue of concern to all. With this in mind, I have elected to present an issue which impinges upon the very root meaning of our existence. In developing the idea I have sought to reflect it against the changing background of the world in which we live. My hope is that its exploration will add to an understanding of the profession which we practice.

The question I would like to speak to is one which each one of us has asked at some time or other in our professional lives. Some of us have asked it many times. It has been raised in different ways and expressed in different words, both within and outside our field. In all probability, it will continue to be asked by those who follow us. I am referring to an anxiety about our value as a service to sick people. This theme I have identified by the question: Is *occupational therapy a sufficiently vital and unique service for medicine to support and society to reward*?

The anxiety begins in a primitive form when we stand before our first patient and sense the enormous demands that a treatment problem makes upon the occupational therapy brush, hammer or needle. The wide and gaping chasm which exists between the complexity of illness and the commonplaceness of our treatment tools is, and always will be, both the pride and the anguish of our profession. Anxiety accumulates as we become increasingly involved in treatment, teaching and research, and even more sophisticated questions tend to arise from that same source to plague us.

The theme of today's presentation is focused, therefore, on the critical appraisal of the essential worth of occupational therapy. I say critical because the technique of criticism will be the method by which the issue will be explored. The subject was selected because I found from my experience that the value of occupational therapy exists in a controversial state. Among any group of my colleagues who have practiced long and well, I found that this question of value constituted a continuous and almost lifelong dialogue.

The Theme Converted to an Hypothesis Test

Where and how does one begin to make dependable and hence usable judgments about value? Taking full advantage of the freedom inherent in the Slagle lectureship, I reasoned that the idea most basic to our practice ought to be searched out and then converted into a kind of a question which might be answerable to some degree. This search, I further reasoned, should begin in the time of our earliest days. I began there and found that there was a single root idea embedded deep in our foundation and this deeply imbedded belief is what we call occupational therapy. In the stormy years between then and now, I found that there were few opportunities given to examine the roots of our foundation and to consider the growth which sprang from it.

My re-examination of our early history revealed that our profession emerged from a common belief held by a small group of people. This common belief is the hypothesis upon which our profession was founded. It was, and indeed still is, one of the truly great and even magnificent hypothesis of medicine today. I have dared to state this hypothesis as: *That man, through the use of his hands as they are energized by mind and will, can influence the state of his own health.* This is the inherited occupational therapy hypothesis passed on for proof by the early founders.

The splendor of its vision goes far beyond rating it as an idea conceived once in a lifetime or even once in a century. Rather, it falls in the class of one of those great beliefs which has advanced civilization. Its magnificence lies in the optimistic vote of confidence it gives to human nature. It implies that there is a reservoir of sensitivity and skill in the hands of man which can be tapped for his health. It implies the rich adaptability and durability of the central nervous system which can be influenced by experiences. And more than all this, it implies that man, through the use of his hands, can creatively deploy his thinking, feelings and purposes to make himself at home in the world and to make the world his home.

For a profession organized around this hypothesis it sets few limits to its growth. It merely endows a group with the obligation to acquire reliable knowledge leading to a competency to serve the belief. Because this is an hypothesis about health, it requires that this knowledge be made available for the guidance of physicians and that it be made applicable to a wide range of medical problems.

The Role of Criticism

Before preparing a brief for its validation I would like to make a detour into a description of the method whereby the issue will be explored. The method is in harmony with my temperament because, by choice, I am neither a conservative nor am I a conformist. I am a devout and practicing, card-carrying critic. Since criticism as a technique of public discussion has yet to emerge in our association affairs, I feel a need to define and describe it. Its philosophy, techniques and tactics will constitute the point of view from which I will speak.

The public use of criticism by a profession has been spelled out best by Merton[1] who sees it as a prevailing spirit within a group necessary to maintain a group's progress. Its greatest usefulness is that it acts to repudiate a smugness which assures that everything possible has already been attained. Its presence commits an association to keeping its members from resting easily on their oars when they are so inclined. In general, Merton finds that criticism stings a profession into a new and more demanding formulation of purpose and maintains a policy position of divine discontent with the state of affairs as they are.

A disciplined person in either the sciences or the professions uses critical thinking as a personal tool of reality testing and problem solving. When a professional organization as a whole accepts criticism as the dominating mode of thought, then indeed, theorizing flourishes and the intellectual atmosphere of their gatherings is characterized by sweeping controversies. In this atmosphere of controversy, progress becomes somewhat assured.

But a card-carrying critic must do more than merely engage in critical thinking. Judgments made by a critic must emerge from a discreet use of techniques which are difficult to master and dangerous to apply. Basically, the skill is dependent upon an ability to analyze, interpret and synthesize. A critic must have a sharply developed capacity to see deficiencies in data and fallacies in interpretation. The best stock in trade that any critic has is a discerning eye for trends and an ability to pattern and verbalize them. Whether a critic is worth listening to is usually decided by an ability to use language well, by a creativeness in synthesizing new relations and by courage to propose provocative hypotheses. Ultimately, however, a good critic rests his case upon how well he has been able to restructure the issue so that the necessary powers for its resolution can be freed. These idealistic but difficult standards are the ones I hope to follow in restructuring the issue of how valuable is occupational therapy.

Design of the Presentation

Having discussed the point of view from which I will speak, it is now necessary to describe the plan of attack which will be made on this global theme. For the sake of this presentation let us suppose that the hypothesis I have proposed is the wellspring of our profession and that it is worth proving. It would not follow necessarily from this that it is provable. A large part of the power to act on the hypothesis, of course, resides with us, the members of the American Occupational Therapy Association. But the society in which our profession lives holds power too and can rule on its growth. Even before we begin the validation, we must look at the probability that this idea may not be capable of proof in this century. I plan to ask first whether the American culture can tolerate such an hypothesis. Next I shall question whether the 20th Century is the right time for the test. The most crucial aspect of the presentation will be an attempt to identify the point at which the process of proof ought to begin. This will be followed by an attempt to identify the basic pattern of our service by which the hypothesis will be proven. Finally, I shall comment on some ongoing crises which the hypothesis is undergoing and then leave for history its continuing proof.

Is America the Place to Test the Hypothesis?

Let us first consider the tolerance in America for the occupational therapy idea. In his social history, Max Lerner[2] identified certain dynamic forces which impelled the greatness of this country. He cited in the American mind two crucial images present since the beginning. One was the self-reliant craftsman, whether pioneer, farmer or mechanic. He was the man who could make something of the American resources, apply his strength and skill to nature's abundance, fashion new tools and machines, imagine and carry through new constructions. Without taking himself over-seriously, Max Lerner's American has generally regarded the great engineering, business, government and medical tasks as jobs to be done. Progress in technology was seen simply as agenda for the craftsman.

The second image Lerner drew was from the American environment. It was that of a vast continent on earth, as in space, waiting to be discovered, explored, cleared, built-up, populated and energized. Lerner contends that our culture is dominated by an American spirit which hates to be confined. A drive toward action, he postulated, is a part of the American character.

This drive towards action seems to me to make reasonable the American idea of a patient. Our cultural concept of the man of action suffers little change when an American moves into a hospital community. It has been supported by a series of principles which merged and fused into what we now call rehabilitation. Early in this century, there emerged the principle in medical management that patients were easier to handle when they were occupied with mild tasks. Later when it was found that an active patient tended to recover faster, early ambulation became an acceptable principle of physiology and blended well with the principal of patient occupation. Concern for the psychological nature of patients brought forth the widespread acceptance of craft, recreation and work programs in hospitals. The need to train patients in self-care became almost a crusade to insure the rights of patients to be independent. Within the community, laymen cooperated in ventures to assure the handicapped's right to return to work. Now we are implementing in full swing the socio-economic principle that it is good business for society to support such programs with public monies.

There are some obvious things which can be concluded about America's tolerance for the occupational therapy hypothesis. It would seem almost axiomatic that the American society in general, and medicine in particular,

has need of a profession which has as its unique concern the nurturing of the spirit in man for action. In every way it knows how, America has said that this spirit must be served and served in a special kind of way when it has been blocked by physical or emotional ills. That this need will be persistent in American culture seems fairly certain. That occupational therapy will persist is not quite so certain. It is true, however, that if we fail to serve society's need for action, we will most assuredly die out as a health profession. It is also most assuredly true that if we did dissolve from the scene, in a decade or so, another group similarly purposed and similarly organized and prepared would have to be invented. I believe, therefore, that the occupational therapy hypothesis is a natural one to be advanced in America.

Is the 20th Century the Time?

The timeliness of the hypothesis is the next question I should like to raise. Are we the people and these the times for the test? We are all deeply entangled in the forces and events of the century in which we live. But if this entanglement commits our energies to the endless treadmill of survival, then the hypothesis cannot get off the ground. The social scientists tell us that the world we live in is in a state of indigestion from too much change. We have yet to absorb the disorganizations brought on by a depression, two wars and an ongoing massive technological revolution. This change is being reflected by society into all its component institutions. It follows naturally that we feel its reflection in our professional lives.

But our state of turmoil was not always so, because occupational therapy was born in the quieter times of this century. In the first several decades of our existence, medicine offered us a tranquil and supportive setting. Our literature reveals that physicians tended to nurture the development of our schools and clinics. In these earlier times we were helped to meet the challenges of contributing to the ongoing medical scene. The last several decades, however, have put excessive stress for expansion upon a profession whose role had been barely defined. We have seen our practice organized into specialty fields by the demands of World War II. Our clinicians have only recently been systematized into team behavior by the pressures of rehabilitation. Now in the sixties we are confessing to a mounting sense of confusion and voicing a need for direction. We are keenly aware of the conflicting demands being made upon our practice. The problems that our schools face in digesting the accumulating technical knowledge which practice demands, is a matter of growing distress. Caught up in these forces how free can we be to control our growth?

If we are anxious today, the social scientist offers the explanation that it is because we are now aware that the hopes we had cultivated in gentler times of the past are being threatened by the pace of the world around us. Historians, however, are quick to counter that when times of great change appear, they are forecasting a death to the old and a birth to a new way of life. It is inconceivable that we or any other group with organized intelligence would stand idly by and permit the random destruction of the old and encourage blind birth to the new. Fortunately, most institutions have centralized their action for controlling change through planning groups variously called the Task Force, Master Plan Committee or the Role Definition Study. Our national association has not remained aloof from such efforts and is currently involved in three change controlling studies. As many of us know well, the studies involve professional curriculum and clinical practice, the functions of the organization and the future development of the profession.

We may conclude that we have shown by our action that we have felt the buffeting of great change and are attempting to control it. But how can we know whether the efforts we are making are sufficient and are of the right kind? This difficult question has some partial answers. One common sense answer is that we must recognize the fact that we have grown and have changed as we grew. In our forty years of existence our sense of purpose, our anchorage points have shifted. It is only logical to reason that we will not rediscover a sense of purpose by merely reflecting within our professions the problems of the larger society in which we exist. Few rewards are granted to those who are content to reflect problems. Society demands that its problems be answered. Therefore, to any group which aspires to be a profession, there is placed before it a clear-cut mandate. This mandate says that if we wish to exist as a profession we must identify the vital need of man which we serve and the manner in which we serve it.

I contend that this is the point at which the proof of the occupational therapy hypothesis begins. The reality of our profession depends upon an identification of the vital need of mankind that we serve. How free we are in these troubled times to reconstruct our thinking at this basic level I do not know. But I do know that the crucial nature of our service cannot be spelled out in the loosely constructed way that it is today. I personally have little trust that we can continue to exist as an arts and crafts group which serves muscle dysfunction or as an activity group which serves the emotionally disabled. Society requires of us a much sharper focus on its needs. As the next step in the development of the theme it becomes necessary to make a critical examination of what, if any, vital need we serve.

What Vital Need Is Served?

As the first order of the business at hand we ought to have it clearly in mind what constitutes a vital need. Of all the descriptions of the need states of man which I

have heard I like Eric Fromm's[3] the best. He says that needs are an indispensable part of human nature and imperatively demand satisfaction. The need we serve must fall within this category. He says further that they are rooted in the physiological organization of man and consist of hunger, thirst and sleep and that in general they all belong to self-preservation. He proposes a simple, forthright formula of self-preservation which is directly applicable to occupational therapy. According to Fromm, when man is born the stage is set for him. He has to eat, drink, sleep and protect himself from his enemies. Therefore, for his self-preservation he must work and produce. Work, in the Eric Fromm sense, is a physiologically conditioned need and therefore a need to work is postulated as an imperative part of man's nature.

In our forty years of practice we have accumulated some fascinating odds and ends of understanding about the need to work. For example, early in my training I was taught that work was good for people. All people needed to work and sick people even more so. This kind of justification of service reminds me of the old story about the man who died and woke up surrounded by all kinds of delights which were his for the mere bend of the finger. After he had satiated himself well, he called for the headman, expressed his appreciation for the manner in which he was treated and then said, "Now that I have pleasured myself well, it is my wish to do something. My good man, what is there for me to do in this paradise?" The answer given to him was, "You are doing it now." "But," replied our man, "I must do something or else my stay in heaven will be intolerable." "Who" replied the headman firmly, "said that you were in heaven?" In the past I have been guilty of believing and having my patients persuaded that work was good and heaven would prove me right. The rationale that man works because it is good for him, regardless of comfort to us, makes little contribution to our understanding of work as a basic need.

During the thirties, the economic depression gave us an unparalleled opportunity to learn that when able people could not find work, certain psychological disorganization occurred. These changes were deemed to be over and above the changes which could reasonably result from economic loss. We are able to generalize from the depression that human nature does not thrive in idleness. In the last several decades we have accumulated a few more broad generalizations. One is that the stress of work produces psychosomatic conditions in modern businessmen. Another generalization which is now being formulated is that when people retire from their work, they retire from life itself.

A vital need to be occupied however, is not to be inferred from such global generalizations. It is being left to the more rigorously controlled experimentations to do this. Now under laboratory conditions man's need-state for action is being rigorously investigated. In the United States and Canada basic research is going on in an area called sensory deprivation. The work began in reaction to the Russian brainwashing attempts. The research was designed on the principle of restricting man's interaction with the ongoing world of reality. Under controlled conditions of isolation man was found to suffer profound disturbances of his thought processes. In isolation men regressed to unrealistic and prelogical modes of behavior. The sensory deprivation findings suggest strongly that the concepts of man's response to his environment must be sharply revised. The behavioral aberrations which were observed in the idleness of depression and retirement, and the stress of overwork, appear to have been confirmed by the laboratory induced sensory deprivations. The data were checked out by neurologists, psychiatrists, biochemists, pharmacologists, mathematicians and engineers.

The final sensory deprivation report sums up to a concept that the mind cannot continue to function efficiently without constant stimuli from the external world. The central nervous system is now seen as a complex guessing machine oriented outward for the testing of ideas. The experimenters postulate that each individual constructs a different development pattern with respect to strategies for dealing with reality. Jerome Brauner[4], as one of the researchers, concluded that early sensory deprivation prevents the formation of adequate models and strategies for dealing with the environment. Later sensory deprivation in normal adults, he suggests, disrupts the vital evaluation process by which one constantly monitors and corrects the strategies one has learned to employ in dealing with the environment.

To summarize at this point, it seems to me that the American drive toward action as identified by Max Lerner and the human drive toward work as identified by Fromm have been verified in the laboratories. I believe that we are on safe ground right now to say that man has a vital need for occupation and that his central nervous system demands the rich and varied stimuli that solving life problems provides him and that this is the basic need that occupational therapy ought to be serving.

What Is the Unique Service?

A profession, however, must do more than identify the need it serves. There is a twin obligation to spell out its unique pattern of service. The next gigantic task which this presentation faces and with some trepidation, because of the limitation of time, is an attempt to identify the basic pattern of our service by which the hypothesis may be proven. The charge is gigantic because it makes it obligatory to define the occupational therapy body of knowledge, its treatment process and techniques.

A search for valid content, process and methods has been my preoccupation in the past ten years of reading,

study and practice. If I had the ability to do all this with any degree of clarity, I would not be here talking about it. I would be in a clinic doing it. However, I am now admitting to a rising sense of satisfaction in the project and a receding sense of frustration. At no time in technological history have the behavioral scientists been producing so much knowledge directly applicable to our field as they are now. The material is emerging from sources as divergent as neurological theory, animal psychology, developmental and personality theory and from psychologists as diverse as Allport, Murphy, Harlow, Hebb, Goldstein, Piaget and Schlachtel.

In order to plunge directly into this material I am going to have to make use of a device in logic known as a First Principle. For if we were to have a First Principle in occupational therapy it would provide us with a way to specify our knowledge. To those who may not be familiar with the meaning of First Principle, it is a device in reasoning to account for all that follows. For instance, the idea of God is a First Principle which accounts for the Universe. There has been a First Principle postulated to explain the nature of man. We are told that the first duty of an organism is to be alive. Medical science derives its premise from this first law of life. If it were not desirable to cure disease and prolong life, the rules of science and the skills and practice of medicine would be irrelevant. The second duty of an organism is to grow and be productive. Occupational therapy ought to derive its premise from the second law of life. If it were not desirable to be productive, the skills and practices of occupational therapy would be irrelevant.

These two laws merge into a concept of function which asserts that both the existence and the unfolding of the specific powers of an organism are one and the same thing. This concept of function is expressed as: the power to act creates a need to use the power, and the failure to use power results in dysfunction and unhappiness. The validity of the First Principle is easily recognizable in the physiological functions of man. Man has the power to talk and move, therefore, if he were prevented from using the power, severe physical discomfort would result. Freud utilized this First Principle to build a powerful theoretical position from which emotional illness was so successfully attacked. He accepted man's biological necessity to produce and generalized that when sexual energy was blocked, neurotic disturbances resulted. He endowed sexual satisfaction with all-encompassing significance. He developed his theory of sexual satisfaction into a profound symbolic expression of the fact that man's failure to use and spend what he has is the cause of sickness and unhappiness. The Freudian theory that human action is primarily sexually based has thrown a strong but restrictive shadow over other behavioral fields. It has been only lately that attention has been given to human productivity in non-sexual areas. Oc-

---

cupational therapy's focus, it is asserted here, lies in the non-sexual area of human productivity and creativity.

In Gardner Murphy's[5] brilliant defense of human productivity he makes us aware that there is a distinct path which leads to becoming human. This path is not seen as being sexually directed. The direction lies largely in the enrichment and elaboration of the sensory and motor experience and the life of symbolism which depends upon them. He maintains that the sheer fact that we have a nervous system, the sheer fact that we can learn, means that we can prolong and complicate sensory and motor satisfactions, can make them richer, can give them more connections, can avoid boredom, can recombine them, can feed upon them, can become immersed in them and make them a part of ourselves. In all these respects, Murphy says man is most completely human. His primary thesis is that man achieves satisfaction in using what he has, in using the equipment that makes him human; and this entails not only the sensory and motor equipment but that central nervous system upon which the learning and thinking processes depend.

Murphy's spirited description of the conditions necessary for being human can provide the basis for an occupational therapy First Principle. This logic constitutes our mandate to discover and organize our body of knowledge; to develop a treatment process; and to devise techniques for its application to the health of man. The logic of occupational therapy rests upon the principle that man has a need to master his environment, to alter and improve it. When this need is blocked by disease or injury, severe dysfunction and unhappiness results. Man must develop and exercise the powers of his central nervous system through open encounter with life around him. Failure to spend and to use what he has in the performance of the tasks that belong to his role in life makes him less human than he could be. With this principle in mind I would like to summarize my thoughts of the last several years of work on our body of knowledge, our treatment process and techniques.

Regarding the body of knowledge. Because our profession is focused on influencing the health of people there will always be a need to include in our body of knowledge the fundamental material of anatomy, neurophysiology, personality theory, social processes and the pathological states to which these functional areas are subject. However, I do not feel this is our unique content. We should have as a special contribution a profound understanding of the nature of work.

Knowledge of work capacity lies scattered over many behavioral fields. We do know, for instance, that man's ability to work has been developed in the long evolutionary process. It began when man hunted and fished for his food and continued as he grew his food and fabricated objects for his comfort. The lot of man was considerably improved when he freed himself from arduous labor through tools and machinery. His comfort was immeasurably assured by the social institutions he built and operated with increasing skill over the centuries. It is my contention that this evolutionary process, plus a bit more, is present, symbolically expressed in today's culture. The concept of work capacity as being an outgrowth of an evolutionary process I call the phylogenesis of work. I believe that cultural history of work ought to be deeply embedded in the occupational therapy body of knowledge and its phylogenetic nature considered particularly in program building.

We know that as a child grows, he recapitulates the history of his race in the stages through which he himself must pass enroute to maturity. The need to pass through phylogenetic experiences in work is necessary for mature work capacity to be developed. There is historical evidence that a child's ability to play, to explore his environment, to exercise his motor skills are the foundation for his later school experiences. The problem-solving processes and the creativity exercised in school work, craft and hobby experiences are the necessary preparations for the later demands of the work world. Because we know that the random movements of the infant progress in developmental sequence toward the job competencies of the mature adult, I postulate an ontogenesis of work. I believe that the ontogenetic nature of work ought to be considered in the case study approach to each treatment problem.

The occupational therapy body of knowledge should include therefore, an understanding of the developmental nature of the sensory-motor systems, the patterning of aptitudes, abilities and interests, the nature of the learning process involved in the acquisition of skills. It should include also an understanding of the developmental nature of the problem-solving process and process of creativity. My epistemological conclusion is that the biological, psychological or social knowledge we select as part of our thinking content must be intermeshed deliberately with the knowledge of work–phylogenesis and work–ontogenesis.

Regarding the treatment process. The capacity to work develops in the long socialization process through which a child becomes an adult. It proceeds along the path of growth as man learns to intermesh his motor with his intellectual functions and adapt this integration to the tasks of his life which satisfy his need to control his environment. Work capacity, in this sense, can be said to develop out of the struggle with gravity for motor control, the struggle with learning for manual and mental skills and the struggle with people and people purpose for economic and social control. When the struggle is great, the personal involvement is high; although conflict and frustration are high, so, too, is work satisfaction high. It follows, too, that when involvement is low, work satisfaction is low. The occupational therapy process becomes primarily concerned with that special aspect of the socialization process called work satisfaction. Its approach in treatment is biographical because work satisfaction is, by its nature, the result of past experiences expressed in the present ability to cope with the environment. Its focus is on the meaningful involvement in problem solving tasks or creative performances. The parameters of its concern are the ability to experience pleasure in achievement, to tolerate the frustrations of struggle, to sustain the burden of routine tasks and to maintain the level of aspiration within the reality level of work skills. The goal of the process is to encourage active, open encounter with the tasks which would reasonably belong to his role in life. The process is paced and guided by the supervision of the prescribing physician.

Regarding treatment techniques. Techniques which would emerge from the body of knowledge and the professional process as just described would be concerned with program and treatment execution. Methods would include all those administrative techniques of program building which would provide a laboratory setting for human productivity. The treatment technique would be all those procedures associated with modifying sensory-motor dysfunctions, perceptual difficulties and the difficulties inherent in coping with the world of play, work and school. It is suggested in terms of today's thesis that in the merging of our content, process and methods, the unique pattern of our function will be spelled out. If this pattern is focused strongly on man's need to be occupied productively and creatively, the hypothesis will grow stronger.

Major Tests of the Hypothesis

Of all the ongoing tests of the occupational therapy hypotheses, I have selected a few major ones upon which to comment. The first and obvious one is whether a need to accumulate substantial knowledge about human productivity and creativity will be recognized and acted upon in our schools and clinics. The problem of balancing our knowledge has been with us for some time. Until now our attention has been preoccupied with the medical science which supports the application of our craft knowledge to medical conditions. But medical science knowledge is a means for the application of our service and not an end in itself. A profound knowledge of human dynamics of productivity and creativity is the end to which our knowledge ought to be designed. As far as our practice today is concerned, we have more medical science knowledge than we know how to apply and we are applying more knowledge about human productivity than we actually have on hand.

The second, and not so obvious test, is the delimiting effect that psychoanalytical practice has on the promotion of a non-sexual concept of human productivity. The fundamental doctrine of the Freudian pleasure principle

is that the essential movement of a living organism is to return to a state of quiescence and that primary pleasure is sought in sensual gratification. A fundamental principal of work is that primary pleasure can be sought through efficient use of the central nervous system for the performance of those ego integrating tasks which enables man to alter and control his environment. In this sense psychoanalytical theory is seen to focus on subjective reality while work theory becomes largely concerned with objective problem-solving reality. It is not that these points of view run counter to each other. They simply do not meet or interact except under very special conditions of intimate supervision by a psychoanalyst.

In 1943 Hendrick[6] raised this issue in the *Psychoanalytic Quarterly*. He argued that the psychosocial activities of the total organism are not adequately accounted for by the pleasure and reality principles when these are defined, in accordance with Freudian tradition, as immediate or delayed response, respectively, to the need for sensual gratification. He suggests that work is not primarily motivated by sexual need or associated aggressions, but by the need for efficient use of the muscular and intellectual tools, regardless of what secondary needs (self-preservation, aggressive or sexual) a work performance may also satisfy. Hendrick postulated a need for a work principle which asserts that primary pleasure is sought by efficient use of the central nervous system for the performance of well integrated ego functions which enable the individual to control or alter his environment.

In psychoanalytic practice today sexual satisfaction is seen as being influenced by ontogenetic, phylogenetic and biographical considerations while no such considerations are seen needed for work satisfaction. Although many analysts have agreed that sexual capacity correlates highly with work capacity, the idea has not been developed much beyond the statement. Work is seen as a kind of experience a patient ought to have and whatever satisfaction he derives from it will be dependent upon his subjective state. As a result, extensive activity programs have grown up around psychiatric treatment which have been designed for participation, but not specifically for ego involvement. These programs are now being called activity programs and those implementing them are called activity therapists.

Such activity programs encourage the participation of large groups and usually appeal to the automatic, learned patterns of behavior. However, activity programs so designed, deny the dignity of a human being to struggle, to control his environment as witness the fact that they tend to make man quiescent within the hospital community. They tend to depersonalize, institutionalize and, in general, debase human nature. The occupational therapy hypothesis makes the assumption that the mind and will of man are occupied through central nervous system action and that man can and should be involved consciously in problem solving and creative activity. It is believed that psychoanalytical theory and the occupational therapy hypothesis can profitably co-exist if a work principle is postulated and executed. This will be even more true if occupational therapy deepens its understanding of the phylogenetic and ontogenetic nature of work and make a case study approach to ego involvement of patients. It is not so possible, however, that activity therapy and occupational therapy can co-exist. It is believed that the major crisis in the proof of our hypothesis will not be how to co-exist with psychoanalytical theory but to know the difference between activity and occupation and to act on the knowledge of this difference.

The last major test which I will discuss has to do with the physical disability field. In this specialty we have been placing heavy emphasis upon muscle efficiency and enabling devices. There is a long, perilous and complex ladder to be scaled between neuro-muscular efficiency and work satisfaction. The ontogenetic reconstitution of motor behavior is a tedious process and must be done step by step. It begins at the reflex muscle action stage and proceeds to the development of complex patterns of motor skills which are utilized in a rich variety of work skills. These, in turn, must be disciplined to a sustaining level of tolerance for routine labors. It is upon this broad pattern that human tolerance for working with people in people affairs is built. If any of these steps are missing, they must be re-fashioned and the whole pattern re-shaped accordingly. The proof of the occupational therapy hypothesis in the physical disability field will depend upon how much we know about the process of restoring work capacity. It cannot be done from prescriptions based upon a narrow understanding of human productivity. It cannot be done in cramped clinics dependent upon scrap material. Nor can it be done from our present ignorance of the world of industry for which we believe we are preparing patients. The challenge to the hypothesis in this area is severe, yet provocative. The technical literature of our profession is indicating that this challenge is not being ignored.

Summary and Conclusion

In summarizing the many ideas I have touched or expanded upon in this thesis, I once again return to my original question: *Is occupational therapy a service vital and unique enough for medicine to support and society to reward?* In answering it, I have said that we have had a magnificent hypothesis to prove and if it could be proven, even to some degree, the answer would be that we are valuable to medicine and to society. The hypothesis that I presented for evidence of proof was that *man, through the use of his hands, as they are energized by mind and will, can influence the state of his own health.* I asked if this were a kind of idea that America could subscribe to and to that I replied with

a resounding yes. I wondered about the stress that the terrible 20th Century was putting on this idea and worried some about the energy left to us to advance it. I suggested the hypothesis would begin its proof when we identified the drive in man for occupation and would continue as we shaped our services to fill that need. I speculated on some of the crises the hypothesis was now undergoing and left the decision not in the lap of the gods but in our own laps for us to think and act upon in our daily practice.

I have said that our profession has a magnificent medical purpose. Whether we shall fulfill it or whether it shall ever be fulfilled I have not said because I do not know. But this I can say from personal experience, that we belong to a profession that requires the mind to look at the history of man's achievements throughout civilization. It requires the spirit to respond to the wonders of what man has accomplished with his hands. It gives us a mandate to apply this knowledge and more to help man influence the state of his own health.

Bibliography

1. Merton, Robert K. "The Search for Professional Status." *American Journal of Nursing,* March, 1959.

2. Lerner, Max. *America as a Civilization.* New York: Simon and Schuster, 1957.

3. Fromm, Eric. *The Fear of Freedom.* London, England: Routledge and Kegan Paul Ltd., 1960.

4. Solomon, Philip, & etc. *Sensory Deprivation.* Cambridge, Massachusetts: Harvard University Press, 1961.

5. Murphy, Gardner. *Human Potentialities.* New York: Basic Books, 1958.

6. Hendrick, Ives. "Work and the Pleasure Principle." *Psychoanalytic Quarterly,* Vol. VII, No. 3, 1943.

BIBLIOGRAPHICAL NOTES

Work has been studied from the viewpoint of economics, philosophy, sociology and psychology, and although the literature is considerable, and is being added to constantly it is a comparatively recent focus for scholars. So far no general study of work has been written, but to some extent a student in this field need not be left entirely without guidance. He needs to remember, however, that the literature is too extensive for one individual to investigate thoroughly. This bibliography noting is designed to serve as an introductory guide. Many of the recommended writings also include full bibliographies of the topic with which they are concerned.

Anyone who seeks to be a student of human occupation should attempt first to build a historical perspective of the field. A *History of Technology,* edited by Charles Singer, E. J. Holmyard and A. R. Hall, is a massive five volume series published by Clarendon Press in Oxford from 1954 to 1958 and provides a general historical background as far as science, economics and technology is concerned. An account of the effect of labor and technology on the culture of the west is set forth at another series titled *The History of Civilization*, edited by C. K. Ogden and published in New York by Alfred A. Knopf, 1926 to 1929.

The sociological nature of work may be approached through a study of the socialization process and the field of industrial social psychology. This aspect of study is excellently covered in *The Handbook of Social Psychology*, edited by Gardner Murphy and published in two volumes by Addison-Wesley Company in 1952. A recent perceptive and illuminating view of the social and economic nature of work and the worker is presented by *Theories of Society* Vol. I and II, edited by Parsons, Stills, Naegele and Pitts published by the Free Press of Glencoe, Inc., in 1961.

The specific classics regarding human occupations are exemplified by: Theodore Caplow's *The Sociology of Work*, (Minneapolis: The University of Minnesota Press, 1954); Eli Ginzberg's *Occupational Choice: An Approach to a General Theory* (New York: Columbia University Press, 1951); Anne Roe's *The Psychology of Occupations* (New York: John Wiley and Sons, 1956); Donald Super's *The Psychology of Careers: An Introduction to*

Vocational Development (New York: Harper and Brothers, 1957) and John Darley and Theda Hagenah's *Vocational Interest and Measurement: Theory and Practice* (Minneapolis: The University of Minnesota Press, 1955).

The classics concerned with human creativity are: Vikor Lowenfeld's *Creative and Mental Growth*, revised edition, (New York: The Macmillan Company, 1952); Edwin Ziegfeld's *Education and Art: A Symposium* (Paris: 19 Avenue Kleber, United Nation's Educational, Scientific and Cultural Organization, 1953) and Harold Anderson's *Creativity and its Cultivation* (New York: Harper and Brothers, 1958).

The author further recommends: Robert Gagne and Edwin Fleishman's *Psychology and Human Performance* (New York: Henry Holt and Company, 1959); Ernest Schachtel's *Metamorphosis* (New York: Basic Books, 1959); Gordon Allport's *Personality and Social Encounter* (Boston: Beacon Press 1960); Hannah Arendt's *The Human Condition* (New York: Doubleday Anchor Books, 1959); Erich Fromm's *Man for Himself*; (New York: Rinehart and Company, 1945); Gerald Gurin, Joseph Veroff and Sheila Feld's *Americans View Their Mental Health: Number Four* (New York: Basic Books, 1960); and Frederick Herzberg, Bernard Mausner and Barbara Snyderman's *The Motivation to Work* (New York: John Wiley and Sons, 1959).

Chapter 7

Doing and Becoming: Purposeful Action and Self-Actualization

Gail S. Fidler, OTR, FAOTA

Jay W. Fidler, MD

This chapter was previously published in the *American Journal of Occupational Therapy, 32,* 305–310. Copyright © 1978, American Occupational Therapy Association.

A ristotle made the following observations: "Now we realize our being in action (for we exist by living and acting) and the man who has made something may be said to exist in a manner through his activity.—So he loves his handiwork because he loves existence. It is part of the nature of things. What is potential becomes actual in the work which gives it expression."

During the intervening centuries the behavioral sciences have contributed little to the elaboration of the relationship between handiwork and individual development. Belief in the value of activity for the mentally ill has nevertheless been sustained for many years and is reflected in the universal use of activity programs in community mental health and psychiatric hospital services. However, despite the historical use of activity experiences for patients, understanding it has remained limited. Human action and doing continue to be viewed as peripheral components of intervention. Motivation for such programming seems to be to avoid immobility, rather than for providing positive help. When aftercare programs emphasize medication, psychotherapy, and social service as having priority over the development and improvement of those functional skills that make it possible to achieve a sense of mastery of self and the environment, services remain tangential to mental health or human needs. Also, when services consist of activity programs characterized by single techniques such as art, dance, music, or poetry, a comprehensive perspective on human productivity is sacrificed.

If health professionals are to assume a major responsibility for designing environments and experiences for the prevention of illness, for the maintenance and restoration of health, they need to achieve a more sophisticated understanding of *doing*. The word *doing* is selected to convey the sense of performing, producing, or causing. It is purposeful action in contrast to random activity in that the action is directed toward the intrapersonal (testing a skill), the interpersonal (clarifying a relationship), or the nonhuman (creating an end product). *Doing* is viewed as enabling the development and integration of the sensory, motor, cognitive, and psychological systems; serving as a socializing agent, and verifying one's efficacy as a competent, contributing member of one's society.

All organisms are born to act. Although lower forms of animals come equipped with behavioral patterns enabling them to cope with the external world, humans are dependent upon their social and cultural environments for learning and developing the action patterns necessary for both survival and satisfaction. That action is essential to human existence has been known and pursued by philosophers for many years, although the fields of medicine and psychiatry, with few exceptions, have viewed action (in the sense of doing) as peripheral to the human condition. Today, developments in social psychiatry, ethology, brain research, and developmental psychology reflect a growing sophistication in understanding the relationship of mental activity to motor behavior. There is an accumulation of significant data to support the thesis that the drive to action, transformed into the ability to "do," is fundamental to ego development and adaptation.

Becoming—"I"

The ability to adapt, to cope with the problems of everyday living, and to fulfill age-specific life roles requires a rich reservoir of experiences gathered from direct engagement with both human and nonhuman objects in one's environment. *Doing* is a process of investigating, trying out, and gaining evidence of one's capacities for experiencing, responding, managing, creating, and controlling. It is through such action with feed-back from both nonhuman and human objects that an individual comes to know the potential and limitations of self and the environment and achieves a sense of competence and intrinsic worth.

The play of childhood is a striking manifestation of the natural drive to action in the service of learning—of exploration and discovery about the body, the self, and the external world. Bruner's studies of perception and learning emphasize the need for on-going engagement with the world of reality as the means by which behavioral patterns and strategies for dealing with the environment are learned. His recent explorations into the meaning and uses of play (1) provide impressive evidence of the critical value of all aspects of play in individual development and evolution. Piaget's (2) observations about play and other exploratory behaviors led him to define these as the processes by which the child assimilates experiences while accommodating to the world. His remarkable studies continue to expand the body of knowledge regarding adaptive human action in a world of objects. Reilly (3) views play as a "connectivity" phenomenon leading to competence and adult "workmanship." She makes some valuable observations about the development of adaptive function and productivity. Erickson continues to emphasize the value of *doing* in achieving a sense of mastery, personal integrity, and in successfully participating in one's external world. His psychoanalytic background and ego psychology orientation are reflected in his focus on the expressive aspects of play (4) and on *doing* in the process of self-actualization and acculturation. (5)

In his study of the nonhuman environment, Searles (6) convincingly argues that relatedness to nonhuman objects is a significant force in the development of the sense of self as human, as differentiated from the nonhuman. He describes how involvement with one's nonhuman environment is a means for learning about self and others, and for both symbolically and realistically dealing with one's affective states, needs, and ideations.

In another work, the authors (7) hypothesize that when an activity relates both realistically and symbolically to an individual's needs and personal characteristics, it is an agent for learning and growth. *Doing* within this context is seen as a means for communicating feelings and ideas, expressing and clarifying individuality, and achieving gratification. The authors and Edelson (8) emphasize that *doing* in this sense can mediate between one's inner and outer world, nurture the capacity to invest, teach realistic responses to success and failure, provide concrete evidence of one's capacities and limitations, test the reality base of fantasy and perceptions, and validate the ability to achieve and influence one's environment.

The writings of John Dewey articulate the criticality of *doing* for developing a sense of "I" and in accumulating a store of action experiences essential for human functioning. Becker (9) explores how the sense of self is developed by and sustained in action. He adds dimension to Dewey's earlier hypothesis, emphasizing the significance of the inherent feedback loop process in *doing*. He views such action an essential for coming to know the realities of self and the world and for testing out the truth of one's perceptions and mental images. Becker's thesis considers schizophrenia and other psychiatric disorders as occurring when internal and external factors limit or preclude an individual's acting on—trying out—an idea or thought.

In defining "objective orientation," Black (10) states that the process of acting enables knowing or "taking account of" the presence of independent, material objects, and emphasizes that it is such action processes that make possible the distinction between reality and illusion.

Neurophysiologic theory seems to be converging on a similar description of behavior. In Karl Pribram's (11) intriguing use of the holographic paradigm, an organism perceives a reality, conceives an intended reality or goal, and learns what motor activity is needed to achieve the goal through a constant series of "tests" to define each increment of change in perceived reality.

A counterpoint to *doing* as the means for defining reality is made by Don Juan as he explains *not-doing* to Castaneda. The sorcerer discovers a separate or nonordinary reality by freeing himself from consensual reality. Don Juan explains, "that a rock is a rock because of all the things you know how to do to it—I call that "doing."—A man of knowledge—knows the rock is a rock only because of "doing," so if he doesn't want the rock to be a rock, all he has to do is—"not-doing." (12, p 227)

In another context, each individual has personal evidence of the sense of well-being, the excitement of challenge, the satisfaction of achievement that comes, for example, from a particular job success: mastering the calculator, planting the garden, repairing the carburetor, "teeing off" in form, or painting a landscape. Whatever limitations there may be in the "artistry" of the end product from the viewpoint of the "expert," there is a keen satisfaction and sense of competence in having accomplished it from one's own resources. Such gratification, the joy of being a cause, can be understood within the context of the human being's innate drive to master the environment.

Robert W. White (13) for a number of years has articulated the thesis that there is an innate human drive to explore and master the environment and that this drive can best be understood as motivation toward competence. White views a sense of competence and efficacy as emerging from direct encounters with and mastery of the environment. He further suggests that gratification from such mastery is intrinsic "in the sense that strictly speaking it requires no social reward or ratification from others. The child acts on the intention, for instance, to climb a stone wall; the outcome of the ensuing struggle between his muscles, hard surfaces, and the law of gravity is brilliantly clear to him even if no one is around to pronounce upon it." (14, p 273)

White urges that the "helping" professionals become more knowledgeable about the phenomenon of competence and more alert to the patient's sense of competence. He suggests that to become "as sensitive to the client's feeling of competence as we are to anxiety, defensiveness, love and hate, would open a wide additional channel to being of help." (14, p 274)

When one's accomplishments, one's sense of competence is verified and given value by others, one's efficacy and value as a human being is confirmed. If, for example, climbing the stone wall has no relevance to the child's social group, the intrinsic gratification may be short lived, or limited as an exploratory learning experience. The meaning and worth of one's doing or mastery is appreciably determined by the views and values of significant others. Humans are inextricably dependent upon others for learning and thus for the feedback that verifies that something has been learned and that the new function has value to others. Self-esteem can therefore be understood as evolving from the intrinsic gratification of accomplishment and the feedback from others regarding the achievement.

The significance of doing and feedback from others in developing a realistic sense of competence and efficacy was illustrated in one of the author's experience with a patient group. The group was composed of patients who persistently refused any aspect of occupational therapy programming. With few exceptions, they acted out provocatively in the community and in the hospital. Their actions were random. A decision was made to see them in a talking group and to move cautiously toward action with a purpose. It became evident that action planned toward productivity and achievement generated tremendous anxiety. Their nonverbal behavior in this setting and the groups' reflections on the experiences, strongly suggested that, "to do" was to risk verification of their incompetence, lack of control over self and the environment, inability to master the environment, and of their "nonhumanness." Subsequently, several members of the group were able to describe that. Their expectations were that what they produced, the "fruits" of their actions, would replicate what they were. Their appallingly limited "action-learning" experiences and the negative or nonexistent feedback from the environment had left them with few action alternatives.

Action leading to achievement is in contrast to random activity. Action is both the *product* of a mental image that sets the objective and the *creator* of a mental image. The mental image that is created includes the refinement of strategies for achieving the objective and an affective evaluation of the achievement. The actor builds a self-image as a competent actor, confronts the realities of the results of the action, finds the boundaries for reasonable objectives, and learns the social relevance of competent actions. When the motivation or ability to act on mental images or ideation is blocked or inhibited by forces in the environment or by sensorimotor deficits, coping behaviors and adaptive skills are not learned.

Becoming—"A Social Being"

Humanization, becoming part of human society, may be defined as the process whereby the individual, beginning life as a biologic organism, becomes a person whose primitive actions are gradually transformed into behavior that concomitantly satisfies individual needs as well as contributes to societal development. In this sense humanization can be viewed as the process of learning about self and one's world, of developing those perspectives and related performance skills essential to a functional society and a functional individual with satisfaction to both.

Mead (15) suggests that social roles are learned through the activity of play and games. Game playing teaches a perspective about the significant other and begins the process of internalization of social roles and values. Let us return again to White's child and the stone wall. As the child struggles to master the hard surface, the pull of gravity, the child is exploring, testing, and developing age-appropriate motor planning, physical skills, and agility. If peers share in the climbing experience, there is additional exploration and learning about "the significant other." If the activity becomes a game, it is reasonable to assume that the rules for playing the game will be defined according to the cognitive, psychologic, and social learning needs appropriate to the developmental level of those participating and congruent with their culture. If significant adults applaud the achievement, then the efficacy of the action is reinforced and verified as socially significant.

The task-oriented groups described by one of the authors (16) are based on such hypotheses regarding *doing*, with the group providing consensual validation of the efficacy of action and interpreting social/cultural norms: the choices of tasks and the action process per se both reflect and meet the individual's developmental and learning needs.

Moore and Anderson (17) hypothesize that all societies have created "folk models" for dealing with the most critical features of their relationship with the environment. These models can be understood as games, the rules of which teach the necessary perspectives and skills. The authors identify first the nonrandom aspects of nature; second, the random or chance elements; third, interactional relations with others; and fourth, the normative aspects of group living. These are correlated with four types of games: puzzles, which teach a sense of agency, the joy of being a cause; games of chance, which teach a relationship to events over which one has no control; games of strategy, which teach the individual to attend to the behavior and motivation of significant others; and aesthetic entities, or art forms, which teach people to make normative judgments and evaluations of their experiences. Learning experiences planned from this folk model are thus structured to include activities that incorporate varying aspects and characteristics of these models, and are matched with the developmental level and personal characteristics of the learner.

As reviewed here, such perspectives about *doing* bring into focus two critical dimensions for determining the value of any activity for a given individual. First, the activity or *doing* must match the individual's sensory, motor, cognitive, psychologic, and social maturation, as well as their developmental needs and skill readiness. Second, it must be recognized by the social, cultural group as relevant to their values and needs.

The information that is available from the various social sciences for research is impressive. However, what is not known about *doing* and human productivity and what is not being investigated is even more impressive.

Constraints on Doing

Middle class values place great significance on verbal skills. Professionals frequently reinforce the priority of this value in both their educational and treatment orientations and practices regardless of what they know about learning and human functioning.

In mental health practice, there is the familiar problem posed by those patients who, with impressive verbal skill, can describe the psychodynamics of their difficulties and articulate the psychotherapeutic process, but are much less able to act on such cognitive awareness. These are most frequently the clients who disdain activity programs and view action and doing as irrelevant to their needs, problems, or life style. As community mental health programs have broadened the base of psychiatric services, practice has come to include those persons whose culture and learning experiences place a priority on action. These persons most frequently view talking as oblique to their needs, problems, and life style.

There is a need to pursue investigation into the neurological, perceptual, and social components of action in relation to mental health. Simultaneously, conscious efforts need to be made toward breaking down the stereotypes regarding priorities on introspection and talking in isolation of *doing*. Both the quality and variety of *doing* is critical for ego development and adaptation.

Social change and technological development have altered the interaction of the person and the world. Direct life-supporting and life-threatening contacts with flora and fauna are almost eliminated. Communication and information are dramatically extended. People hear of events immediately but do not interact with them. The accuracy of reality testing is always dependent upon one's neurological idiosyncrasies, perceptual distortions, the results of prior actions, and social responses. Contemporary psychopathology is fashioned by the current demands on all neurologic functions, on perceptual accuracy, on reduced opportunity for learning through action, and by the enlarged input of information and language.

One can, for instance, easily visualize the different possibilities in the world of John who lives on a farm near a wooded hillside with his parents, grandparents, three siblings, and an uncle. He is expected to be responsible for a number of chores to maintain the household. He is free to endlessly explore nature with all manner of physical skills. He gets direct and consistent response from several generations while also observing them in their work roles. He receives indirect response from family members reacting with value judgments to each other. Finally, he has the direct and indirect responses available to all children at school.

Compare John to Peter who lives in an apartment in a city with two working parents, a cat, and a neighborhood that holds personal threat during much of the 24 hours. He may have some chores but they may not be viewed as critical to the maintenance of family life. He is given very limited freedom to explore. He receives some direct response from two people whose work he does not observe except in the housework about which they complain. He gets vestigial, indirect response from his parents and many hours of passively received indirect response from television or radio. Finally, he has the direct and indirect responses available to all children at school. Once Peter has learned to manipulate his predictable toys he is limited to exploring the behavior of his cat, which is limited in its own behavioral possibilities. A sense of mastery, especially for the new and unexpected, is difficult to achieve. A sense of value and social role identity is even more difficult. Feelings, actions, and meanings do not become integrated.

It can be hypothesized that the prevalence of senseless, purposeless violence by children and adolescents who show no remorse can be generated by hours of viewing television violence that has no relation to their behavior and that is not accompanied by action on their own part. When action does not follow thought, perception is distorted and the critical learning that comes from confronting the consequences of an act is precluded. This dissociation of thought, affect, and action so characteristic of schizophrenia can follow this process of "learning without action." Schizophrenic dissociation can occur when neurologic and perceptual deficits preclude action and when the nature of one's environment inhibits doing or does not support doing in a variety of contexts. The limited learning of functional, adaptive skills that occur when there is a paucity of opportunity for doing is emphasized by Winn (18). She discusses the faulty reality testing, loose distinction between illusion and reality, and the passivity of response evident in children whose daily hours are filled with TV viewing as opposed to psychomotor activity.

There is increasing evidence that limited action experiences are no less significant for the adult. Speaking to the role of activity in maintaining normal human functioning and the consequences of sensory deprivation, Bruner points out that "an immobilized human being in a sensorially impoverished environment soon loses control of his mental functions." (19, p 7) Greenberg quotes Stainbrook commenting on thrill seeking as reflecting a search for individual mastery, "So much of our life has become sedentary, inhibitive action. There has been an over-emphasis on cerebration—thrill seeking behavior is expressing an almost desperate need for active, assertive mastery at something. We are programmed for action,—but where there is so much less adaptive behavior which requires physical action, there is an insidious anxiety about the concept of mastery. We need to restore a sense of physical mastery and assertion; a sense of control, of self doing rather than merely thinking." (20, p 21)

Prescribing Intervention

The complexities of a rapidly expanding, industrialized society make it imperative for the health professions to attend to those factors that preclude or inhibit *doing*. A reduction in *doing* generates pathology. When pathology is identified, *doing* must be used in the service of personality integration. If treatment is heavily biased toward verbal communication, and if treatment responds to symptoms rather than to performance skill development and reinforcement, then it will have a limited effect. Likewise, when activity programs fail to relate to the specific development of performance skills, their impact is more like random activity and much of their potential benefit is lost. The extent of carry over of learning and changes from the treatment setting to the *home* environment is frequently determined by the degree to which treatment modalities are relevant to the adaptive and performance skill demands and expectations of the *home* setting.

Programming for the prevention of ill health or for the remedy of dysfunction must reflect an appreciation for and understanding of the internal relationship among internal and external systems in the generation and shaping of human behavior. Selective attention to one system, one skill area or component of coping, fragments the totality of the human being.

The question then is how to elaborate concepts about *doing* to create plans or prescriptions to enhance critical human functions? Different periods in the life cycle demand different configurations of skills, both those relating to the internal realities and those relating to the external realities. Performance can be understood as the ability, throughout the life cycle, to care for and maintain the self in a more independent manner, satisfy one's personal needs for intrinsic gratification, and contribute to the needs and welfare of others. The balance among these performance skill clusters, that is, the proportion of time, attention, and energy allocated to each, is critical in achieving and maintaining a way of life that is satisfying to self and others and is health sustaining.

The level and kind of skills and the balance among them at any one point are determined by age, developmental level, unique biology, and culture. For example, what is an adequate level of independent self care and what are appropriate self-care activities will vary in accordance with age as well as with cultural norms. Likewise, what is considered a healthy balance among caring for self, pursuing personal need gratification, and caring for others, changes with the different stages of life and varies according to one's culture.

Planning for intervention requires an initial assessment of the nature and level of the individual's intact skills, skill limitations, and balance among performance skill clusters. Once such assessments have been made, it is necessary to identify those components or sub-systems of performance that inhibit or prevent skill development. This description includes evaluations of the sensory, motor, psychologic, and social deficits as well as identification and assessment of those human and nonhuman factors in the environment that impact on being able *to do*.

Concepts regarding the components of *doing* make it possible to analyze activities or doing experiences in relation to skill acquisition. Planning therefore requires that activities be understood and analyzed in terms of the level and kind of motor skill requirements, sensory integrative components, psychologic meaning, cognitive requisites, interpersonal and social elements, and cultural relevance and significance. Such knowledge then makes it possible to match activity experiences to the individual's deficits, learning readiness, intact functions, and values. On the basis of such data and planning, *doing* can be designed to provide the action-learning experiences necessary for the development of the critical components of performance and for skill acquisition.

Each human action calls on some neurologic function. It is done within some social context and has various potential values and meaning. Understanding the nature and relevance of *doing* to human adaptation should make it possible to plan intervention programs to facilitate learning and change, increase the chances of helping others maintain a state of health, contribute to a better understanding of the basis of pathology or dysfunction and, thus, hopefully develop more effective prevention strategies.

Acknowledgment

This article is adapted from a paper presented to the Sixth International Congress of Social Psychiatry, Opatjia, Yugoslavia, October 1976.

References

1. Bruner JS, Jolly A, Sylva K (Editors): *Play, Its role in Development and Evolution,* New York: Basic Books, 1976.

2. Piaget J: *Play, Dreams, and Imitation in Childhood,* New York: W.W. Norton, 1962.

3. Reilly M (Editor): *Play as Exploratory Learning,* Beverly Hills, CA: Sage Publications, 1974.

4. Erickson EH: Play and actuality. In *Play, Its Role in Development and Evolution,* JS Bruner, A Jolly, K Sylva, Editors. New York: Basic Books, 1976.

5. Erickson EH: *Childhood and Society,* New York: W.W. Norton, 1963.

6. Searles HF: *The Nonhuman Environment,* New York: International University Press, 1960.

7. Fidler GS, Fidler JW: *Occupational Therapy: Communication Process in Psychiatry,* New York: MacMillan, 1964.

8. Edelson M: *Ego Psychology, Group Dynamics and the Therapeutic Community,* New York: Grune and Stratton, 1964.

9. Becker E: *The Revolution in Psychiatry,* New York: The Free Press, 1964.

10. Black M. The objectivity of science. *Bull Atomic Scientist 33:* 55–60, 1977.

11. Pribam KH: *Languages of the Brain,* Englewood Cliffs, NJ: Prentice Hall, 1971.

12. Castaneda C: *Journey to IXTLAN,* New York: Simon and Schuster, 1972.

13. White RW: Motivation reconsidered: the concept of competence. *Psychol Rev 66:* 297–333, 1959.

14. White RW: The urge toward competence. *Am J Occup Ther 25:* 271–274, 1971.

15. Mead GH: *Mind, Self and Society,* Chicago: University of Chicago Press, 1934.

16. Fidler GS: The task oriented group as a context for treatment. *Am J Occup Ther 23:* 43–48, 1969.

17. Moore OK, Anderson AR: Some principles for the design of clarifying educational environments. In *Handbook of Socialization Theory and Research,* D Goslin, Editor. Chicago: Rand McNally, 1968.

18. Winn M: *The Plug-in Drug,* New York: Viking Press, 1977.

19. Bruner JS: *On-Knowing—Essays for the Left Hand,* Cambridge, MA: The Belknap Press of Harvard University Press, 1962.

20. Greenberg PF: The thrill seekers. *Human Behav 6:* 17–21, 1977.

Chapter 8

Toward a Science of Adaptive Responses

Lorna Jean King, OTR/L, FAOTA

This chapter was previously published in the *American Journal of Occupational Therapy, 32,* 14–22. Copyright ©1978, American Occupational Therapy Association.

An "asset almost peculiar to occupational therapists is their high tolerance for puzzlement, confusion and frustration." (1) Ten years ago this was the opinion of Dr. J. S. Bockoven, one of our profession's most vocal admirers. Today one might argue about the tolerance, but who could dispute the puzzlement, confusion and frustration as we look back on a good many years of effort to define practice, to structure theory, and to build philosophies of occupational therapy.

Need for a Comprehensive Theory

And, as we look toward an era of increasing specialization, we are soberly aware that, without a unifying theory to insure cohesiveness, specialization could easily become fragmentation. In fact, back at the time when the profession's definition began "Occupational therapy is any activity, mental or physical, ... ," (2) recreation, art, music, and dance all fell under the rubric of occupational therapy. The responsibility for the fact that these modality-based specialties have become separate professions can be assigned in large measure to the lack of unifying theory.

It seems readily apparent that splintering into small professions results in watering-down of job development effectiveness, the scattering of progressively scarcer financial resources for education, and the loss of political "clout." The economics of the health care delivery system will not indefinitely support professional proliferation and duplication of effort. To allow future specialization to result in further fragmentation might well be suicidal. Therefore, we need a framework that will give specialists the bond of a common structure.

We must also cope with the fact that today's consumers, far more sophisticated than in the past, expect to understand what they are paying for. They will no longer accept "on faith" what they are told. This underscores the need for a coherent theoretical model understandable, not just to the professional initiate, but also to the consumer. We may develop complex theories, but, in order to be really useful, they will need to be based on a straightforward structure that can be widely understood, and is clearly related to the client's life functions.

Difficulties in Constructing a Science of Occupation

As a prelude to an attempt to identify a usable theoretical framework, let us look at the roots of some of our difficulties in achieving a science of occupation. One of the difficulties is related to the fact that occupational therapy was born of common sense; and common sense is, by definition, "what everyone knows." Everyone knows that it is a good thing to keep busy. There is the old proverb, "The devil finds mischief for idle hands." Carlyle said it with great-feeling, "An endless significance lies in work; in idleness alone is there perpetual despair." (3) One must reach far down on the evolutionary ladder to find organisms that are not active, that simply exist. Occupation, or employment, or activity, is quite literally bred in our bones. Occupational therapy, then, deals with purposeful behavior—with people *doing*. But isn't this what people are engaged in during most of their waking hours? It is hard to see what is significant about such a commonplace fact of life, and that is precisely the problem, or one of them—something so ever present is hard to grasp conceptually. Whitehead is credited with saying that the, more familiar something is to us, the more difficult it is to subject it to scientific inquiry (4). As a commonplace example, consider how many eons must have gone by before Man even thought to wonder about the nothingness that surrounded him. A great many more eons probably passed before Man realized that it was *not* nothingness, and named it atmosphere. I am suggesting, then, that the very universality of the filling or occupying of time with purposeful behavior has made it difficult to form concepts that would help us to construct a theory or science of occupation.

Who has not had the experience of trying to explain occupational therapy to someone, only to realize that people think they know all about it because, of course, they have *experienced* occupation and activity. They are thinking about it in everyday terms, and the therapist is, hopefully, thinking about it scientifically and analytically. So, although words are exchanged, frequently no communication takes place.

Another problem in constructing models is the difficulty that therapists sometimes have in communicating with each other because of the many levels on which purposeful behavior can be organized. One can talk about the effects of activity on the biochemistry of cells, or about its place as an essential component of neurodevelopment. Purposeful behavior is also basic to cognitive processes; and on the still broader scale of cultural anthropology, an individual's role in the cultural milieu can be thought of as determining purposeful behavior. Conversely, behavior may determine cultural roles. So, whether one looks at biochemical Man, psychological Man, social, economic or ecological Man, purposeful behavior is inextricably woven into the total fabric of human function. However, if one therapist looks at occupation solely in terms of its psychological implications, while another looks only at the cognitive issues, and a third describes chiefly the neurophysiological consequences, a situation results much like that of the blind men examining the elephant. One described the leg, another the ear, and another the trunk. Finally, they were convinced that they could not possibly be talking about the same creature. Certainly an outsider would be hard-pressed to find a principle unifying work simplification, sensory integration, hand splints, and acceptable outlets for aggression, to name just a few of the topics with which therapists may be concerned.

Naturally, attempts have been made to deal with this disparity of viewpoints. Development frameworks are appropriate for many clients, but are not particularly helpful with the normally developed adult who is suddenly faced with trauma or disabling disease. Other models deal with occupation in terms of chronic conditions or the sequelae of disease—a rehabilitative context. These are not readily applicable to developmental problems or acute, as contrasted with chronic, conditions. Few models that I am aware of have spelled out what it is that is peculiar to occupational therapy as contrasted with physical therapy or vocational counseling, for example. What *is* that factor which makes occupational therapy so uniquely valuable that, as Dr. Reilly says, if the profession were to disappear tomorrow, it would have to be quickly reinvented? (5)

General systems theory teaches that systems share common features, that large inclusive systems tend to recapitulate the features found in more specific units. As Laszlo says, "A system in one perspective is a subsystem in another." (6) It seems, then, that our task in finding a theoretical frame for occupational therapy is to identify a level of system that is not so specific as to shut out some of our areas of specialization, nor yet so general as to include a great many more areas than are applicable.

In short, in order to satisfy the profession's current needs, a theory or science of occupational therapy should provide:

1. a unifying concept that will apply to all areas of specialization;
2. a framework that will clearly distinguish occupational therapy theory and techniques from those of other disciplines;
3. a model that is readily explainable to other professionals and to consumers; and
4. a theory that is adequate for scientific elaboration and refinement.

Adaptation as a Unifying Concept

While mulling over some of these considerations, I read Konrad Lorenz's recent book, *Behind the Mirror*, A

Search for a Natural History of Human Knowledge (7). Lorenz deals essentially with the evolutionary and individual processes of adaptation that are involved in Man's active acquisition of knowledge and techniques. I was struck with the implications of his work for occupational therapy. Then Kielhofner and Burke's recent review of the ideological history of occupational therapy (8) drew my attention to Dr. Ayres' phrase, "eliciting an adaptive response," (9) which seemed a succinct and accurate description of what an occupational therapist does. I was at this time going over the occupational therapy literature, and suddenly the words *adaptation* and *adaptive* seemed to leap out from almost every page. In fact, few of our professional articles fail to mention adaptation, regardless of the author's specialty or point of view. I was struck, like Cortez, with "a wild surmise" (10); could the *adaptive process* be an adequate synthesizing principle for our profession? Is it too nebulous a concept to be useful? Surely it is too simple an idea—or is it? Has its very familiarity, like that of the word *occupation* blinded us to its true significance?

Certainly the words *adaptation* and *adaptive* are well known to us. We advertise on bumper stickers that occupational therapists are adaptive; we have large investments in adaptive equipment; and assumptions about adaptation are implicit in our literature. Adolph Meyer began his treatise on "The Philosophy of Occupation Therapy," in 1922, by defining disease and health in terms of adaptation (11) (see Chapter 2). But I have not found evidence that we have rigorously analyzed the concept or used it consciously to explain our functions in any broad sense. Perhaps it is time that some of our implicit assumptions about adaptation be made explicit. Only when these assumptions are articulated can their validity be examined through research.

At the outset we must distinguish between adaptation as an evolutionary concept and the process of individual adaptation. Evolutionary adaptation refers to changes in the structure or function of an organism or any of its parts that result from the process of natural selection (12). Natural selection, in turn, is the process by which a differential survival advantage is transmitted to successive generations. The process of evolutionary adaptation is very slow, requiring at the minimum hundreds of thousands of years for significant changes in form or function to occur.

Individual adaptation refers to adjustments made by the individual that primarily enhance personal rather than species survival, and secondarily contribute to actualization of personal potential. Tinbergen says, "Adaptedness is a certain relationship between the environment and what the organism must do to meet it." (13)

The idea of using adaptation as a model in a health-related profession is reinforced by Dr. Rene Dubos in his book, *Man Adapting* (14). He says "states of health or disease are the expressions of the success or failure experienced by the organism in its efforts to respond adaptively to environmental challenges."

Rappaport, the general systems theorist, says "Science is clearly a systematized search for simplicity." He adds, "Seek simplicity, and distrust it." (15) I would invite you, then, to keep a healthy skepticism as we explore the concept, a relatively simple one, that the adaptive process constitutes the core of occupational therapy theory, and that specific attributes of adaptation are also the significant and characteristic attributes of occupational therapy. This will make explicit and specific and testable some of our heretofore unexamined assumptions.

Characteristics of the Adaptive Process

Initially, let us discuss four specific features of individual, as opposed to evolutionary, adaptation. The first characteristic of adaptation is that it demands of the individual a positive role. The adapting person is defined as "adjusting himself to different conditions or environments." (12) In doing this he is acting not being acted upon. An adaptive response cannot be imposed, it must be actively created. To quote Nobel prize-winning ethologist Tinbergen again, "Living things do not move passively through the physical processes of the environment; they do something against it." (13) Active participation of the client in the treatment process has long been recognized as characteristic of occupational therapy.

Alexei Leontiev, Chairman of the Psychology Faculty of the University of Moscow, reminds us that "Even seemingly simple human functions develop as an interaction between sensory stimulation from the environment and the *person's own activity*." (16) (Italics by this author [King])

Even unprofitable or maladaptive adjustments to change are actively entered into. Withdrawal, for example, which is often considered a negative condition, is actually an active response, sometimes appropriate, sometimes maladaptive.

Secondly, adaptation is called forth by the demands of the environment. The challenge of something the individual needs or wants to do—obstructed by change or deficit in the self or the environment—calls forth a specific adaptive response. We could say that occupational therapy consists of structuring the surroundings, materials, and especially the demands, of the environment in such a way as to call forth a specific adaptive response. Another way of saying this is that occupational therapy uses the demands of tasks or other goal-oriented activities in a specially structured environment to trigger the unfolding of a needed adaptation.

Among the healing sciences, occupational therapy is unique in its utilization of the demands of the real-life environment. An adaptive response cannot truly be said to have occurred until the individual consistently carries it out in the course of ordinary activities. Thus an amputee may practice opening the hook of the prosthesis over and over, but has not truly adapted to it until the prosthesis is used habitually in a daily routine. The occupational therapist uses this knowledge by providing the amputee with many real-life activities in which to use the prosthesis. The therapist knows that pure exercise, no matter how repetitive, often does not generalize into daily activities, and therefore fails to be adaptive.

This brings us to the *third* characteristic of the adaptive response, namely that it is usually most efficiently organized subcortically, and, in fact, often can *only* be organized below the conscious level. Conscious attention to a task or an object permits the subconscious centers to integrate and organize a response. Dr. Yerxa, in her 1966 Slagle Lecture (17), gave an example that can hardly be improved upon. She said, "A year ago I helped evaluate a brain damaged client's function. She was asked to open her hand. No response occurred, except that she was obviously trying. Next she was moved passively into finger extension while the therapist demonstrated the desired movement. This time the client responded with increased finger flexion. In frustration she cried, 'I know, I know.' Finally she was offered a cup of water. As the cup was perceived, her fingers opened almost miraculously to grasp it." It would be hard to overemphasize the importance of the therapist's using his or her cognitive powers to structure situations that will elicit a subcortical adaptive response from the client. We tend to rely too much on the client's cognitive processes.

Another example of the importance of subcortical adaptive learning is less familiar to the therapist, but popular with the sports enthusiast. It is to be found in such concepts as "inner tennis." Gallweg, author of *The Inner Game of Tennis* (18), says, "There is a far more natural and effective process for learning and doing almost anything than most of us realize. It is similar to the process we all used but soon forgot as we learned to walk and talk. It uses the so-called unconscious mind more than the deliberate "self-conscious" mind, the spinal and mid-brain areas of the nervous system more than the cerebral cortex. This process doesn't have to be learned, we already know it. All that is needed is to unlearn those habits which interfere with it, and then to just *let it happen.*" This approach recognizes the frequently *disorganizing* effects of analyzing consciously what should be automatic sequences of movement.

I stress this point because it is another essential reason why occupational therapists use purposeful activity instead of exercise: namely, that tasks, including crafts, or other goal-directed activities, such as play (where the goal is fun), focus attention on the object or outcome, and leave the organizing of the sensory input and motor output to the subcortical centers where it is

handled most efficiently and adaptively. I am suggesting, then, that the distinguishing characteristic of occupational therapy, derived from a similar truth about adaptation, is that *there is always a double motivation*: first, the motivation of the activity itself—catching the ball, creating the vase, making the bed; and the second motivation, recovering from illness, maintaining health, preventing disability—in short, adapting. Now no *animal* recognizes the need to "adapt." It sets out to do something specific—escape a pursuer, or find food. The immediate objective provides the motivation. Adaptation is a secondary and unrecognized goal. But in dealing with humans we need to recognize that the double motivation of therapeutic activity may or may not need to be brought to the client's awareness, depending on age, cognitive function, and so forth. The therapist should see to it, however, that other professionals and the client's family are made aware of *both* motivations, and of how the direct motivation of the activity subserves the indirect, but *primary* motive of therapy.

The implications of the foregoing definitions of the nature of occupational therapy practice are important in light of certain current problems. As mentioned earlier, the profession has been concerned with role definition—how to delimit the boundaries that separate our practice from that of physical therapy or other professions. In a recent report of an American Occupational Therapy Foundation board meeting, to which Washington area therapists were invited, concern was expressed about occupational therapists "infringing on" exercise, the territory of physical therapy (19). And well may we be concerned, for it is *our* professional identity that will be diluted by this infringement, not theirs. Obviously all disciplines that are working with a client should work together cooperatively, but it seems equally obvious that it is uneconomic if there is duplication of function. Exercise has its important place, so also does purposeful activity as a producer of adaptive responses, and this latter is the realm of the occupational therapist. We need to be able to explain in terms of the principles outlined above why purposeful behavior can elicit adaptive responses that exercise alone cannot. Defining our role in this way will be much more satisfactory than the old way of dividing the patient in the middle and giving the top half to the occupational therapist and the bottom half to the physical therapist.

The *fourth* characteristic of the adaptive response is that it is self-reinforcing. In animal behavior the reward for successful mastery of environmental demand is survival, and the penalty for failure is death. In humans the results are seldom so immediate and stark. Nevertheless, mastery of environmental demand is a powerful reinforcer and Maslow lists the drive to master the surroundings as one of Man's innate needs (20). Mastery of one demand is rewarding and serves as a stimulus for attention to the next necessary response at a higher level of challenge. This is the genius of occupational therapy—that, as the old adage has it, "nothing succeeds like success." As the occupational therapist plans and structures successful efforts, each success serves as a spur to a greater effort. Exercise, psychotherapy, behavior modification are all means to an end. But with purposeful activity, the activity itself is an end, as well as being a means to a larger end, therapy or adaptation, hence the double motivation mentioned before.

To summarize the thesis thus far, I am implying that the essential purpose of occupational therapy is to stimulate and guide the adaptive processes through which an individual may best survive and develop. I have suggested that the basic characteristics of occupational therapy derive from the corresponding elements of adaptation; *first*, that it is an active response; *second*, that it is evoked by the specific environmental demands of needs, tasks and goals; *third*, that it is most efficiently organized below the level of consciousness, with conscious attention being directed to objects or tasks, and *fourth*, that it is self reinforcing, with each successful adaptation serving as a stimulus for tackling the next more complex environmental challenge.

Having tried to identify the basic characteristics of the adaptive process from which the significant features of occupational therapy derive, let us look at some familiar aspects or categories of practice in the light of adaptation, and also at the adaptive process as an organizing principle in two newer or less familiar areas of practice.

In broad general terms we can divide individual adaptation, on the one hand, into the phase that is synonymous with developmental learning, and, on the other hand, the process of adjusting to change or stress.

Developmental Learning as an Adaptive Process

The organizing of sensory input into information, and the subsequent integration of an appropriate motor response, is a continuous adaptive process. As mentioned earlier, Leontiev suggests that human functions consist of the interaction of sensory input and individual activity. For example, we learn to see by seeing. The visual figure-ground skills of a child raised in the green leafy lights and shadows of the jungle will be different from those of the child raised in the clear light and great vistas of the Navajo reservation. Each child begins with similar, basic visual equipment, but the process of learning to see in each environment is a process of adaptation in which available stimuli, combined with active sorting and filing, produce patterned vision.

There are a number of theoretical frames for considering the adaptive processes of early childhood, and the occupational therapy profession can be proud of the several outstanding developmental theorists among its

ranks. It is not the intention here to recapitulate developmental theories, but to emphasize the fact that "eliciting an adaptive response," in Dr. Ayres' apt phrase, is, in essence, eliciting goal-directed or purposeful behavior. This may be as basic as enticing an infant to lift its head to look at a toy, or more complex, such as suggesting to a child that he shovel sand into a wheelbarrow to trundle across the playground to a sand box. The child's goal is playing with the sand; the therapist's goal is stimulating co-contraction, heavy work patterns, and so forth, in the service of integrating and organizing sensory input and motor behavior.

The role of the occupational therapist in stimulating this sequence of integration and response appears deceptively simple to the consumer who cannot be expected to understand, without explanation, that it takes considerable knowledge and professional finesse to know which adaptive response is needed and to provide the proper setting and stimuli for a given action at the opportune moment when the individual's development makes it possible for him to make a successful response.

We have been considering the well-known field of developmental learning in children. However, it is not only in childhood that one must organize sensory data and respond appropriately. This process goes on throughout life. Afferent, or incoming impulses, particularly those characterized as proprioceptive feedback, play a crucial role in sensory integrative processes in adults as well as in children. The key concept is that sensory input is the raw material for adaptation at *any* age. If developmental adaptation does not take place normally in childhood, the adult will show various disabilities ranging, as an example, from mild motor planning problems to severe disabilities such as process schizophrenia. Recent studies, suggesting that the adult brain is relatively plastic, give some hope that even in adulthood developmental adaptations can be facilitated.

The role of sensory data in the adult has been strikingly illuminated in the last 25 years by a large number of sensory deprivation studies, which have, as a matter of fact, strengthened the theoretical base for sensory integration theory. However, the critical relationship between these studies and the health of the average citizen is just beginning to be appreciated. As an example, consider the scenario for an all too familiar tragedy that goes something like this. An elderly man, in somewhat precarious health, must undergo major surgery. As a precaution, he is kept somewhat longer than usual in the intensive care unit. When he is moved to a room, he is kept very quiet, sedated, curtains drawn, and visitors restricted. Somewhere between the third and fifth day, post-surgery, the nurse's notes show that the patient appears to be confused and disoriented. The following day he is hallucinating and has to be restrained because he is trying to get out of bed. There are no family members who are willing to care for him in his apparently deranged state, so he is transferred to a nursing home where he continues in a state of relative sensory deprivation, and his mental and physical condition deteriorates rapidly.

The tragedy is that this kind of occurrence is often preventable. And in the instances where confusion or disorientation occur in spite of precautions, it is important to note that it is often reversible if suitable sensory input is provided. Lipowski, whose studies (21) suggest the reversibility of deprivation-caused psychiatric symptoms, also warns that around age 55 vulnerability to the effects of sensory deprivation increases quite sharply. Thus it is apparent that it is not just the very old who are at risk.

It is also important to note that the effects of deprivation are cumulative, and that the more sensory modes that are understimulated, the faster confusion and disorientation result. One of Lipowski's most significant findings appears to be that immobilization is the most disabling form of deprivation, and that, if added to other sensory losses, is very likely to produce psychiatric symptoms in the vulnerable.

In terms of the emphasis of this discussion on adaptation, we may think of confusion and disorientation as *dis*-adaptation—failure of organization and response. Hallucinatory and delusional phenomena, on the other hand, represent *mal*-adaptation; the sensory data is organized, but incorrectly, and therefore, of course, the response seems inappropriate. So-called unpatterned stimuli are as bad or worse than complete absence of stimuli. "White noise," such as the constant hum of a motor, is an auditory example, while the test pattern on a television set is an instance from the visual domain. Kornfeld, Zimberg, and Malm, in a paper on psychiatric complications of open heart surgery (22), report that "The patient might first experience an illusion involving, for example, sounds arising from the air conditioning vent or the reflection of light from the plastic oxygen tent. Many experience a rocking or floating sensation. These phenomena were often not reported to the staff and could then develop into hallucinatory phenomena and associated paranoid ideation." Kornfeld and his group confirm the harmful effects of immobilization, noting that many patients interviewed after recovery remembered as one of their chief discomforts not being able to move. Let us emphasize again that *sensory input is the raw material for adaptation*. Without adequate sensory data, the individual's adaptive capacity is greatly curtailed.

Motivational loss is another aspect of hospital-induced sensory deprivation that is of critical importance in rehabilitation or therapy. Zubek, in a report on electroencephalographic correlates of sensory deprivation (23), reports that not only were alpha frequencies progressively decreased during 14-day deprivation experiments, but this was also accompanied by severe motivational losses. The abnormal encephalograms persisted for a week after the subjects returned to normal living conditions, *but the motivational losses lasted even longer*. These findings have profound implications for all medical personnel who are trying to motivate patients toward independence. Perhaps the cart has been ahead of the horse! Perhaps the first thing to do is to provide sensory stimulation, particularly of the proprioceptors, through whatever degree of mobility is possible. Then motivation for independent behavior might follow more quickly and spontaneously.

I am indebted to Lillian Hoyle Parent for discussing with me some of the material on sensory deprivation, and, as she points out in her recent helpful summary of the deprivation studies (24), occupational therapists are better prepared than any other health care professionals to make use of this information. A dozen exciting research projects come readily to mind in reference to hospital-induced deprivation. For example, a control group receiving the usual post-operative care could be compared with an experimental group receiving systematic meaningful sensory stimulation under an occupational therapist's supervision. Comparisons could be made of number of hospital days post-surgery, incidence of complications, and amounts of pain and sleep medications.

We have suggested that sensory input and motor output are the essentials of individual adaptation as seen in the familiar field of developmental learning, and we have looked at the less familiar concept of sensory deprivation as a prime factor in *dis*-adaptation or *mal*-adaptation.

Therapeutic Adaptation to Change or Stress

The *second* general category of adaptive response is adaptation to change or stress. One aspect of response to change is represented by a very active current field of specialization in occupational therapy, namely the field of physical disabilities. This field concerns itself with the individual's adaptation to physical change.

Changes within the person can be of many kinds; what they have in common is the demand that the individual alter habitual responses. Arthritis, heart disease, amputations, spinal cord injuries, stroke, blindness are a few examples. The use of adaptive equipment, work simplification, splinting, development of strength and skill in residual body segments are among the adaptive considerations in this area of practice. Sometimes the acquiring of appropriate adaptive responses may actually be a matter of survival, as with the cardiac client. More often adaptation means the possibility of actualizing potential that would otherwise be wasted.

While the concepts of adapting to physical change are very familiar to us as therapists, we have had less direct experience with the relatively new field of adaptation as it relates to stress medicine. The role of activity in adapting to or coping with stress is an old idea whose scientific time has come. Dr. Hans Selye, who is considered the "father" of stress medicine, comments, "The existence of physical and mental strain, the manifold interactions between somatic and psychic reactions, as well as the importance of defensive-adaptive responses, had all been more or less clearly recognized since time immemorial. But stress did not become meaningful to me until I found that it could be dissected by modern research methods and that individual tangible components of the stress response could be identified in chemical and physical terms." (25) Dr. Selye called this stress response the "general adaptation syndrome." Today few literate people are unaware of the fact he demonstrated: that any stimulus which appears to pose a threat to survival elicits a response that includes the secretion of the cortico-steroids which prepare the body for a fight or flight reaction. The heightened blood pressure, pulse, and respiration that follow a danger signal had a distinct survival value when the appropriate reaction was running, or climbing, or hand-to-hand combat. In our present cultures, running, climbing, or fighting are seldom considered appropriate responses, and threats are often perceived as long continued, like the danger of losing one's job, or the daily stress of driving through rush-hour traffic. There are well-known stress diseases such as ulcers, high blood pressure, and heart disease, to mention the most common, that follow chronic stimulation of cortico-steroid secretion. The current vogue for jogging, marathon running, and other strenuous sports owes part of its very real usefulness as a health maintenance measure to the fact that exercise metabolizes and renders harmless the stress hormones that otherwise might accumulate and cause permanent damage to the body.

What is not so often considered is the effect of either subtle or overt stress on an already over-taxed system. A person who is already feeling ill is told he must enter the hospital. Whether it is for surgery or for tests, or for nursing care, everything about the experience spells danger: the strangeness, the uncertainty, the painful or uncomfortable procedures, but most of all the feeling of helplessness. Stress hormones are poured into a system that not only is already reacting to the stress of illness, but also has few opportunities for activity that might help to metabolize and dissipate the cortico-steroids. Stress hormones can make the sick person sicker and can retard recovery.

It is often assumed that *rest* is what is needed in the hospital, but, as Dr. Selye points out, unless the organism is completely exhausted, activity of some sort is much more appropriate to stress dissipation than too much rest. Many years ago an occupational therapist frequently stepped into a hospital room and made available purposeful, goal-directed activities that allowed the patient an adaptive response to stress. If we had known then what we know now, we might have called it *stress management* or *stress reduction therapy*. Instead, someone used the word *diversional*, with the result that the whole

area of human needs has been virtually abandoned, and the word *diversional* has become the equivalent of profanity. In fairness we must point out that few third-party reimbursement agents are willing to pay for something labeled *diversional*.

To turn to another aspect of this subject, before the stress hormones and their physiological effects had been identified by Dr. Selye, we often spoke of *tension*, and in the mental health field were able to recognize the usefulness of activity, even though the reasons were vague. Dr. Roy Grinker writes of the treatment of *battle fatigue* or *war neuroses* (26) and says, "In their free time physical activities are encouraged in order to dissipate accumulated tensions. Enforced idleness and rest are bad therapy for these states." Later he comments, "The patients are busy the whole day with physical and mental activities and various aspects of occupational therapy."

The high hopes held for the usefulness of the psychotropic drugs led to the serious curtailment of other forms of treatment such as those described by Grinker. Now that there is widespread disillusionment with the major tranquilizers, which seem to cause almost as many problems as they solve, perhaps the efficacy of what might be called *adaptational therapy* will be rediscovered.

The psychiatric disorders provide excellent examples of the interrelatedness of the various aspects of the adaptive process. In some instances, as in autism or in process schizophrenia, we are probably dealing with inadequate developmental adaptive learning and the attendant severe problems in perception and communication. These problems inevitably produce stress and the concomitant physical changes produced by the stress hormones. These, in turn, probably further derange the sensory-integrative processes. Many of the symptoms seen in the psychoses represent either disadaptations or maladaptive behavior. As the therapist is able to facilitate adaptive development, that is, sensory integration, coping behaviors improve. Activity also helps to metabolize stress hormones and thus increases the client's feeling of well-being. Though basic biochemical causes may ultimately be found for some of the major psychoses, there will probably always be a need for facilitating adaptive or coping skills in a society that seems increasingly stressful.

Psychologists Gal and Lazarus, it seems to me, have made the strongest case for activity as an adaptive response to stress. Their article, "The Role of Activity in Anticipating and Confronting Stressful Situations" (27), spells out the physiological correlation of activity with the reduction, or metabolism, of the stress hormones. They point out that while activity which is related to the cause of the stress is best, yet activity of any kind is better than none. Their useful analysis of the literature concludes with these words: "Regardless of the interpretation, it seems quite evident that activity during stressful periods plays a significant role in regulating emotional states. We are inclined to interpret activity as being a principal factor in coping with stress. As has been repeatedly argued by Lazarus a person may alter his/her psychological and physiological stress reactions in a given situation simply by taking action. In turn this will affect, his/her appraisal of the situation, thereby ultimately altering the stress reaction."

To summarize, we may divide adaptation in response to change or stress into three major components of concern to the occupational therapist:

1. adaptation to physical change (which includes a component of adaptation to stress because the physical changes are in themselves stressors);
2. adaptation to the stress of hospitalization or acute illness;
3. adaptation to reduce stress reactions in psychiatric conditions.

We have engaged in a lengthy exploration of stress and adaptation because it seems that in the foreseeable future coping with or adapting to stress is going to be one of the major health challenges facing humanity. Toffler, in his book *Future Shock*, (28) makes a good case for the thesis that the extremely rapid rate of change in almost all of our cultural institutions is a significant cause of stress for large segments of humanity, certainly including our own. Ethologist Tinbergen warns, "The amounts of strain now imposed on the individual may well overstretch man's capabilities to adjust." (13) If it is true that stress is a major health problem for modern man, and if, as Gal and Lazarus propose, activity is of major importance in stress adaptation, then occupational therapy has a major role to play in health maintenance and disease prevention as well as in health restoration.

One of my colleagues (Roene Shortsleeve) once drew a cartoon that expressed this rather well. She drew a bearded figure in the white robes of a prophet. In his hand was a placard which read, "The world is NOT coming to an end; therefore, you had better come to occupational therapy and learn to cope."

Conclusion

I have attempted to demonstrate in this paper that the adaptive process can provide a theoretical framework for occupational therapy that meets the criteria suggested at the outset: that it can be applied to all the specialty areas as a unifying concept; that it will differentiate occupational therapy from other professions; that it is readily explainable to other professionals and to consumers; and that it is adequate in depth to allow for scientific elaboration and refinement.

The adaptive process is probably not the only tenable model for occupational therapy. If this paper spurs others to articulate a more suitable theory, it will have served its purpose.

Toffler, in concluding *Future Shock*, comments that, as yet, there is no science of adaptation. Is it too ambitious to suggest that occupational therapists are uniquely prepared to begin constructing *a science of adaptive responses*? It is a challenge worthy of our best.

References

1. Bockoven JS: Challenge of the new clinical approaches. *Am J Occup Ther 22:*24, 1968.

2. Dunton WR: *Prescribing Occupational Therapy*, Springfield, IL: Charles C Thomas, 1947.

3. Carlyle T: *Past and Present*, Boston: Houghton Mifflin, 1965, p 196.

4. Thayer L: Communications systems. In *The Relevance of General Systems Theory*, E Laszlo, Editor. New York: Braziller, 1972, p 96.

5. Reilly M: The educational process. *Am J Occup Ther 23:*300, 1969.

6. Laszlo E: *The Systems View of the World*, New York: Braziller, 1972, p 14.

7. Lorenz K: *Behind the Mirror: A Search for a Natural History of Human Knowledge*, New York: Harcourt Brace Jovanovich, 1977.

8. Kielhofner G, Burke JP: Occupational therapy after 60 years; An account of changing identity and knowledge. *Am J Occup Ther 31:*657–689, 1977.

9. Ayres AJ: *Southern California Sensory Integration Tests Manual*, Los Angeles: Western Psychological Services, 1972.

10. Keats J: On first looking into Chapman's Homer. In *Century Readings in English Literature*, JW Cunliffe, Editor. New York: The Century Company, 1920, p 639.

11. Meyer A: The philosophy of occupation therapy. *Arch Occup Ther 1:*1–10, 1922 (Reprinted as Chapter 2).

12. Stein J (Editor): *Random House Dictionary of the English Language*, Unabridged. New York: Random House, 1966.

13. Tinbergen N, Hall E: A conversation with Nobel prize winner Niko Tinbergen. *Psychol Today*, March 1974, pp 66, 74.

14. Dubos R: *Man Adapting*, New Haven: Yale University Press, 1965, p xvii.

15. Rappaport A: The search for simplicity. In *The Relevance of General Systems Theory*, E Laszlo, Editor. New York: Braziller, 1972, pp 18, 30.

16. Leontiev AN, cited by Cole M, Cole S: Three giants of Soviet psychology, conversations and sketches. *Psychol Today 10:*94, 1971.

17. Yerxa E: Authentic occupational therapy. *Am J Occup Ther* *21:*2, 1967.

18. Gallweg WT: *The inner Game of Tennis,* New York: Random House, 1974, p 13.

19. The Foundation. *Am J Occup Ther 31:*114, 1978.

20. Maslow AH, Murphy G (Editors): *Maturation and Personality,* New York: Harpers, 1954.

21. Lipowski ZJ: Delirium, clouding of consciousness and confusion. *J Nerv Ment Dis 145:*227–255, 1967.

22. Kornfeld DS, Zimberg S, Malm JR: Psychiatric complications of open-heart surgery. *New Engl J Med 273:*287–292,1965.

23. Zubek JP: Electroencephalographic changes during and after 14 days of perceptual deprivation. *Science 139:*490–492,1963.

24. Parent LH: Effects of a low-stimulus environment on behavior. *Am J Occup Ther 32:*19–25,1978.

25. Selye H: *The Stress of Life,* New York: McGraw-Hill, 1956, p 263.

26. Grinker R: *Men Under Stress,* 2nd edition. New York: McGraw-Hill. 1962, pp 30, 218.

27. Gal R, Lazarus RS: The role of activity in anticipating and confronting stressful situations. *J Human Stress 4:*4–20, 1975.

28. Toffler A: *Future Shock,* New York Random House, 1970.

Chapter 9

A Heritage of Activity: Development of Theory

G. Gordon Williamson

To achieve a professional level of competence, an occupational therapist must be able to translate a body of knowledge into a plan of action that facilitates change in a predicted direction. Clinical practice is grounded on a theoretical base. The aim of this presentation is to increase understanding of theory and the ways it can be linked to practice. To accomplish this task, theory is initially viewed from a broad perspective before attention is focused on its specific relation to intervention.

The discussion first examines the structure and function of theory, its development and verification, and the nature of a profession's theoretical foundation. Next, two common methods for relating theoretical systems to clinical application are presented—practice theory and frame of reference. To illustrate this link between theory and practice, neurobehavioral treatment approaches are analyzed as frames of reference within occupational therapy. Last, the connection of research to theory and practice is described with an emphasis on interpretation of research findings.

Theory: Nature, Development, and Verification

The term *theory* evolves from the Greek word "theoria," signifying a "vision" or "a look at." The most basic definition of theory comes from the philosophy of science in which theory is considered a set of sentences whose purpose is to explain (1). Theory offers a systematic method for organizing and thinking about data. It provides a coherent view of phenomena by specifying relationships among concepts in order to describe, explain, and predict the phenomena (2).

A theory comprises well-defined concepts and the propositions that relate the concepts to each other (3, 4). Concepts are words or phrases that classify seemingly disparate phenomena according to common characteristics. They are symbolic ways of describing objects, properties, events, and relations among them, and are expressed at varying levels of abstraction and complexity. The concepts pertinent to occupational therapy range from concrete ones such as joint range and muscle strength to more abstract ones such as health, adaptation, and temperament.

Concepts are the basic units of a theory and delineate its subject matter. Precise definitions are essential for understanding since many concepts depend on what can only be indirectly observed or are defined in terms of their relationship to other concepts. Concepts such as intelligence, social roles, and pain are considered constructs because they are inferred from other concepts and are not directly observable. In the development of theory, concepts should be mutually exclusive, discriminating, parsimonious, appropriately abstract, and eventually operational (1, 5).

Propositions, the other structural component of a theory, are statements of a relationship between two or more concepts. Propositions can describe different types of relationships (6): for example, a causal proposition indicates an invariant stimulus-response link between two concepts. More common in the behavioral sciences is the correlational proposition that designates the degree to which events or objects are associated with each other. A temporal proposition states the sequence of events in time. Like concepts, propositions can be expressed in degrees of abstraction. Propositions are theoretical statements also identified in the literature as postulates, suppositions, assumptions, or premises.

A mass of isolated facts and propositions do not constitute a theory. Zetterberg (7) cites more than 1,000 propositions documented as research findings on human behavior. He emphasizes that only when empirical data are systematically arranged and interrelated within a theoretical system can they be interpreted and unified. In general, theories in the physical and biological sciences are more capable of explaining and predicting phenomena than theories in the younger social science disciplines and applied professional fields (8).

Verification of theory is achieved through scientific research (9). Concepts and their connecting statements are reduced to operational definitions stated in measurable, observable terms. In this redefining process concepts become variables, and propositions become hypotheses that can be tested. A theory is validated indirectly by accepting or rejecting hypotheses derived from the theory's propositions.

Accurate prediction of events is the major criterion for the relative merit of a theory (10). A particular theory is favored when its predictive power is greater than other theories describing the same phenomena. Theories, therefore, are considered tentative and provisional. The history of science is in large part a chronicle of the refutation of established theories: for example, the basic elements of the universe were once considered earth, fire, air, and water. This premise was later replaced by the theory of the atom as the smallest irreducible element with its electron, neutron, and proton composition. Beyond this level, a whole new universe of even smaller subatomic particles is now being exposed.

Theory and research are the cornerstones of scientific inquiry leading to the acquisition of knowledge. These activities necessitate use of both deductive and inductive reasoning. Reynolds (11) terms the deductive method as the "theory-then-research" approach. Through deduction, theory can be developed by a process of logical thinking before empirical investigation. In the inductive process, specifics of empirical situations lead to generalizations about the data that are interrelated to become theory. There is no best approach to building and evaluating theory. In reality these modes of theory construction are complementary, and both methods contain parts of the other (12).

The scope of a theory may range along a continuum of generality from concern for all the empirical events of a phenomenon or science to an isolated occurrence in the real world. A theory that addresses the entire field under consideration is described by Mills (13) as a "grand theory." These theories, which are global in nature and tend to be very abstract, have been criticized as explaining everything while explaining nothing (14). A collection of all-inclusive concepts and propositions is offered with often limited direct relevance. In contrast, a theory may deal with a specific event in the present with no attempt to generalize beyond. Mills terms this restricted theoretical scope "abstracted empiricism." For example, a theory with little capacity for generalization could conceivably be constructed about a clinical problem of a given client.

Merton (15) proposes the development of middle-range theories that avoid the extremes of both grand theory and abstracted empiricism. This range of theory is characterized by an intermediate level of generality and its ability to be tested. Theories of middle range focus on a selected aspect of reality and a limited number of concepts and propositions. This level of theory building seems particularly suitable for occupational therapy. No profession or academic discipline has successfully developed a grand theory that addresses its entire domain of concern (8). As an illustration, the field of psychiatry experienced a period of stagnation during the 1950s when it adopted psychoanalysis as its grand theory and consequently lost relevance to many patient populations. Occupational therapy needs to generate varying middle-range theories related to its interests in the nature of human occupation and the use of activities to achieve functional well being.

The theoretical systems that comprise the body of knowledge of occupational therapy are generated within the profession as well as drawn from the academic disciplines (e.g., the social and biological sciences) and other professional fields (e.g., medicine). Theories are selected, formulated, and adapted to have specific meaning to the profession's practice. So constituted, they form the body of knowledge or theoretical foundation of the profession. The body of knowledge is unique in its entirety but not in its component parts (16). The challenge to occupational therapy is to identify a body of knowledge that reflects its scientific base and philosophical assumptions in order to organize this knowledge in ways that serve clinical practice.

From a sociological perspective, all professions have a model that delineates their internal structure and content (17). Mosey (18) proposes that this model include the philosophical assumptions of the profession, its ethical code, theoretical foundation, domain of concern, legitimate tools for practice, and principles for identifying and solving client-related problems. In this context a model provides identity and unity to the profession and describes its relationship to other professions and society. Although the theoretical foundation forms an essential component of a profession's model, it is not the sole criterion for defining the profession's service or parameters.

The discussion so far has focused on the structure, development, and verification of theory as well as the nature of a profession's theoretical foundation. In theory building, concepts are formulated and defined, relationships between concepts are expressed as propositions, and hypotheses are tested for validation. Theories are refined or refuted depending on their degree of congruence with observed events. The theoretical foundation of a profession is in a state of continual alteration as knowledge expands through scientific investigation within and outside of the profession (9). The next issue to be explored is the means for relating theoretical systems to clinical application.

Relation of Theory to Practice

Traditionally, the function of theory is to explain, describe, and predict phenomena. Control of events is not a primary aim of scientific knowledge, although it may be a desirable outcome (1). For example, theories of motor organization describe the integrative processes of the neuromuscular system but do not address concrete methods of improving coordination. Any training procedures derived from theories are examples of their application and not the function of the theories per se.

In the applied professional fields one is concerned with the nature of the change process and the means to influence it. Two approaches are commonly used to relate theoretical systems to intervention—practice theories and frames of reference. They are two systematic ways of organizing and applying knowledge to effect change. Both models are similar since they share a common goal and use components of a theory. Practice theories and frames of reference serve as linking structures between theory and practice.

A practice theory provides a guide for specific actions to be taken to produce a desired change (19–22). Practice theories represent a departure from the standard view of theory since they offer ways of controlling phenomena. A practice theory uses concepts and propositions to develop a rationale for a coherent approach to assessment and intervention. From this rationale are derived principles that govern the treatment process.

A practice theory addresses the following issues (19-21):

1. Ideal state of the human organism (health or function),
2. Factors adversely influencing the attainment of this state (ill health or dysfunction),
3. Kind and extent of behavioral change deemed possible,
4. Predicted rate and duration of change,
5. Mechanisms or techniques for effecting change, and
6. Identification and role of change agents.

To focus the discussion, the remainder of this paper explores the model of a frame of reference as an approach for linking theory to practice. Frames of reference are produced from the body of knowledge of the profession and address a specific aspect of the profession's domain of concern. A frame of reference is a "set of interrelated internally consistent concepts, definitions, and postulates derived from or compatible with empirical data that provide a systematic description of or prescription for particular designs of the environment for the purpose of facilitating evaluation and change." (Mosey, personal communication, 1982)

A frame of reference is concerned with a specific practice area. It may address one or more performance components (e.g., sensory integration. motor skill, cognition) or an aspect of occupational performance (e.g., activities of daily living, leisure, work). Similar to a practice theory, it describes the change process and provides principles for assisting a client to move from a level of dysfunction to a level of function. It is prescriptive in nature. A practitioner may draw on several frames of reference at one time when interacting with a client: in a therapy session with a developmentally disabled child, one may simultaneously employ frames of reference from neurodevelopmental treatment, Piaget, and learning theory. Or the frames of reference may be used sequentially over time as the focus of intervention changes with a client.

According to Mosey (18, 23), a frame of reference has four components: 1. a statement of the theoretical base, 2. delineation of function-dysfunction continuums, 3. a listing of behaviors indicative of function and dysfunction, and 4. postulates regarding change.

The theoretical base of a frame of reference contains the structural elements of a theory—that is, well-defined concepts and propositions deduced from one theory or from a number of compatible theoretical systems. The theoretical base establishes the boundaries of the frame of reference by describing the nature of one or more human functions, the influence of the human and non-human environment upon that function, and interactions that facilitate more competent performance in the particular area of concern.

From this base one can derive continua that grade skills from the level of total deficiency to complete mastery in addition to the observable behaviors indicative of adequate or inadequate performance in each continuum. The postulates regarding change identify the type of environmental interactions that effect change in the direction of function. They are prescriptive statements that guide the selection of short- and long-term goals and govern the design of appropriate activities for intervention.

The link between theory and practice is now further examined using neurobehavioral treatment approaches as an illustration of frames of reference. Since these approaches have many commonalities, the discussion addresses them collectively. This section includes a description of their focus and use, an analysis of the theories upon which they are based, an examination of their status as frames of reference within the profession, and last, a personal account of ways to make them more relevant to occupational therapy.

Neurobehavioral Frames of Reference

Over the past 30 years Brunnstrom, Bobath, Knott, Voss, Rood, and their associates have evolved systems of intervention that have successively been referred to as neuromuscular facilitation and inhibition, neurophysiological approaches, sensorimotor treatment, neurodevelopmental therapy, and more recently, neurobehavioral approaches. Neufeld (24) suggests use of the last term since the ultimate focus in intervention is on human behavior and not simply on developmental or physiological processes.

The neurobehavioral approaches are primarily concerned with motor performance. The other performance components of sensory integration, cognition, and psychosocial skills are related to the neurobehavioral frames of reference but are not their focus. In the neurodevelopmental treatment approach of Bobath, function or health is viewed as an intact postural reflex mechanism that provides normal muscle tone, reciprocal innervation of opposing muscle groups, and automatic movement patterns such as righting and equilibrium reactions (25). Dysfunction or ill health is considered a derangement in the postural reflex mechanism caused by lesions in the central nervous system. Inadequate control by higher neurological centers results in abnormal postural tone and the release of tonic reflex activity.

In the proprioceptive neuromuscular facilitation approach advocated by Knott and Voss, health is viewed as a normal neuromuscular mechanism "capable of a wide range of motor activities within the limits of the anatomic structure, the developmental level, and inherent and previously learned neuromuscular responses." (26. p 4) Dysfunction or ill-health is considered a deficient neuromuscular mechanism that results in limitations of movement as evidenced by weakness, incoordination, and spasticity.

Neurobehavioral treatment within the context of occupational therapy can be employed in four primary modes: 1. direct therapeutic handling as preparation for functional performance, 2. the use of treatment procedure while teaching a specific life skill, 3. the provision of selected activities that elicit neurophysiological mechanisms to facilitate psychomotor competence, and 4. the use of adapted positioning and equipment. Neurobehavioral frames of reference are used for restorative purposes as well as to compensate for lost or impaired abilities.

The theoretical base of neurobehavioral treatment draws on numerous theories from neuroanatomy, neurophysiology, kinesiology, and the psychology of learning and development. The theories range on a continuum from the microscopic level such as concepts of neurotransmission and the law of reciprocal innervation to the macroscopic level of theories of motor learning and motivation. The strength of the neurobehavioral approaches is the breadth of their knowledge base within the biological, social, and medical sciences.

However, many theories within these fields are at an early stage of development. There is much controversy over such fundamental issues as the nature of motor control and recovery of function after brain damage. Frequently, definitions for neurobiological concepts are not mutually exclusive, discriminating, and readily reducible to operational terms for testing. For example, confusion exists regarding definitions for such concepts as mobility/stability, normal muscle tone, and spasticity. Propositions do not link together all the concepts within each theory in a coherent manner. Instead, the concepts are often haphazardly related, and at times the theories are a mere collection of isolated facts and propositions. All of these limitations in theory development in the neurosciences influence the clarity of neurobehavioral frames of reference that rely upon them for their scientific rationale.

The propositions in these theories are frequently correlational in nature; however, they are commonly viewed as causal propositions when integrated into the theoretical base of neurobehavioral frames of reference. The therapeutic approaches typically explain the effectiveness of specific treatment techniques on neurophysiological principles. Yet few controlled experiments relate the techniques to therapeutic manipulation of discrete neural mechanisms. For example, the PNF technique of "reversal of antagonists" is founded on the neural concept of successive induction. Its effectiveness, however, could also be explained in reference to the client's increased motivation and interest when interacting with the therapist.

With Mosey's criteria for a frame of reference, continued attention is required to refine and organize neurobehavioral treatment approaches into a more cohesive structure. Function–dysfunction continua and behaviors indicative of function and dysfunction are not well delineated in many neurobehavioral approaches. Consequently, some confusion exists relative to identifying specific continuums (i.e., what one treats) and behaviors indicative of dysfunction (i.e., the signs of a problem that will disappear as the problem resolves). General treatment principles are usually stated but are not expressed in the form of postulates for change. For instance, what does it *really* mean when one says that activities foster integration on a subcortical level?

Of primary importance is the degree to which neurobehavioral frames of reference are adapted to occupational therapy practice to be congruent with the profession's philosophical assumptions. Neurobehavioral approaches are legitimately concerned with one performance component. However, in normal development and the acquisition of skill, motor control is achieved through involvement in occupational performance—that is, tasks of daily living, play, leisure, and work. Therefore, these frames of reference should explicitly address the role of the individual in influencing his or her own state of health through engagement in goal-directed activities or occupation.

In our profession, movement per se is not an end product that defines health. Motor performance is viewed as *one* contributing component to satisfactory accomplishment of life tasks and roles. It is the purposeful application of movement within an environmental context that is important. Movement is only relevant in a field of action (27).

Function or health "is manifested in the ability of the individual to participate in socioculturally delineated and prescribed activities with satisfaction and comfort. ... As beacons of health, activities are the *ends* to which occupational therapy directs its energies." (27, p 33) Since activities also have therapeutic potential when applied in a systematic manner, they serve as the *means* to achieve those ends. The terms *activities* and *occupation* have this process-product ambiguity in that they refer both to a sequence of actions (process) and to an outcome (product).

Neurobehavioral frames of reference must reflect occupational therapy's heritage of activity and view of the individual as an active agent engaged in life tasks.

They may be employed concurrently, in clinical practice with frames of reference that address other performance components and occupational behaviors. Two positive trends are noted within the profession: 1. there is greater attention to the functional application of these neurobehavioral approaches in the context of the client's daily life, and 2. commonalities among the approaches are being synthesized as a basis for evolving new, better integrated frames of reference (28–31).

A personal account regarding strategies for relating neurobehavioral treatment to occupational therapy is relevant to this discussion. A few years ago the author shared with colleagues a concern that our clinic had lost its appreciation for activities-based therapy. Intervention was too frequently artificial and unreal, such as stacking cones in PNF patterns and cutting Theraplast with a rocker knife. Simulated activities are only therapeutic if they are familiar, promote positive associations, and resemble as closely as possible the activities pattern the individual will experience in the community.

For a week the activities patterns of our professional practice with neurologically impaired clients were documented. It was a simple procedure of recording on a time chart goals of treatment during the sessions and the means for achieving the goals. The results of this analysis indicated that therapy was splintered into discrete segments with a large percentage of time devoted to direct handling procedures, teaching self-care skills, and repetitive table-top activities presented as perceptual training.

In our occupational therapy clinic the *ends* had become independence in self-care tasks and achievement of perceptual-motor skills. The *means* were primarily therapeutic handling procedures and repetitive exercises. To broaden our perspective of activities as the process and product of intervention, numerous strategies were initiated.

We first reviewed and discussed the professional literature describing the nature and meaning of activity and occupation. We constructed activities histories with ourselves and learned to conduct an activities-based interview with clients. We divided into small groups to create ways to incorporate neurobehavioral therapy into independent living skills. The emphasis was on activity analysis and synthesis. To expand our repertoire of activities, therapists went to shopping centers to analyze what therapeutically relevant activities could be discovered in hardware, sporting goods, and toy stores. Last, we banned for periods of time certain over-used treatment modalities to force us to generate alternatives. Prohibited media included pulleys, bilateral sanders, mat tables, pegs, cones, and the ubiquitous Developmental Learning Materials.

The result of the inservice education program was appraised a year later when activities patterns of our professional practice were re-evaluated. It was difficult on this occasion to allocate therapy time according to segregated performance components. Neurobehavioral treatment was directed toward functional application in the environment, and activities served to integrate performance subskills into purposeful action. Thus, we found that neurobehavioral approaches had much to contribute to occupational therapy practice when modified to reflect the unique perspective of the profession.

Connection of Research to Practice

In order to refine our body of knowledge and develop more precise and utilitarian frames of reference, the relationship between research and practice needs clarification. The current knowledge explosion in the biological and behavioral sciences creates a dilemma for the clinician regarding ways to select and apply new concepts to therapy. Three common approaches are used to translate findings into practice (32). In the "popularization method" technical studies are reinterpreted into an easy, intellectually accessible form. Without caution, this approach can degenerate into isolated techniques segregated from their theoretical underpinnings. An example of this occurrence is the unrestricted use of bilateral sanding for hemiplegic clients out of context of Brunnstrom's frame of reference, which originally advocated the activity under carefully prescribed conditions (33, 34).

A variation on this theme is the voguish emphasis over the years in particular neurological structures. In need of a label, this trend is referred to as "the quest for the sacred homunculus." In reviewing my professional career, I first became enamored with the muscle spindle, expanded to the alpha-gamma coactivation system, moved to the reticular activating system, relocated to the limbic lobe, and later left half of my colleagues in the vestibular system while I raced across the corpus callosum between the right and left hemispheres. Although the popularization method can increase use of research data, precision is often lost in the interpretation.

A second approach is termed the "empirical method," in which the therapist reads research reports and case histories and applies their conclusions directly in practice. This strategy is severely limited by the lack of exact fit between a clinical condition described in the literature and the needs of a particular client. In addition, specific treatment procedures are seldom reported in a manner that allows for precise duplication of the intervention. It is hazardous to adopt therapeutic practices based on the results of one or two clinical research studies. Such findings may be particular to the research sample and the experimental design. A need exists for replication of studies to establish the generality of results to various clinical settings and populations.

The third and most effective approach is the process of relating research to an appropriate theory rather than attempting immediate application of the studies. In this method the research findings are taken into the body of knowledge of the profession to be studied, and they are tentatively included in the theoretical base of frames of reference. With further experimental investigation the theoretical statements can be confirmed, rejected, or modified. This approach demonstrates the manner in which research shapes the development of theory and theory directs research. As Krueger and associates have noted, "Without data theories are empty and without theory data are blind." (12, p 188)

All therapists have some system or viewpoint that monitors their practice (21). Actions are grounded on some expectation of behavioral outcome. What differentiates therapists is the degree to which their system has become elaborated and made explicit. Therapists vary in their level of awareness regarding the philosophical assumptions and theoretical foundations of their practice and their ability to communicate them to others. A professional is distinguished from a technician by knowledge of the propositions that guide his or her actions and the conscious selection of those propositions to influence change. In a practice based on theory, the therapist is able to ascertain the relationship between a client's need and a theoretical principle, and apply intervention procedures on the basis of accurate prediction of outcome (35).

The theories relevant to occupational therapy vary in their degree of verification through research. It should not be disheartening that many questions remain unanswered regarding the psychological and physiological processes of adaptive behavior. An old Gaelic maxim suggests that knowledge does not proceed from understanding but rather from questioning.

Acknowledgments

The author gratefully acknowledges contributions to his understanding of theory and practice by Simme Cynkin, M.S., OTR, FAOTA; Anne Cronin Mosey, Ph.D., OTR, FAOTA; and Barbara E. Neuhaus, Ed.D., OTR, FAOTA.

References

1. Roy C, Roberts SL: *Theory Construction in Nursing: An Adaptation Model,* Englewood Cliffs, NJ: Prentice-Hall, 1981.

2. Kerlinger FN: *Foundations of Behavioral Research: Educational, Psychological & Sociological Inquiry* (2nd Edition). New York: Holt, Rinehart & Winston, 1973.

3. Burr WR: *Theory Construction and the Sociology of the Family,* New York: Wiley, 1973.

4. Fawcett J: A declaration of nursing independence: The relation of theory and research to nursing practice. *J Nurs Adm* 10: 36–39, 1980.

5. Hage J: *Techniques and Problems of Theory Construction in Sociology,* New York: Wiley, 1972.

6. Hardy ME: Theories: Components, development, evaluation. *Nurs Res 23:*100–107, 1974.

7. Zetterberg HL: *On Theory and Verification in Sociology,* Totoux, NJ: Bedminster Press, 1954.

8. Jacox A: Theory construction in nursing: An overview. In *Readings on the Research Process in Nursing,* DJ Fox, IR Leeser, Editors. New York: Appleton-Century-Crofts, 1981, 24–35.

9. Payton OD: *Research: The Validation of Clinical Practice,* Philadelphia: FA Davis, 1979.

10. Gibbs JP: *Sociological Theory Construction,* Hinsdale, IL: Dryden Press, 1972.

11. Reynolds PD: *A Primer in Theory Construction,* New York: Bobbs-Merrill, 1971.

12. Krueger JC, Nelson AH, Wolanin MO: *Nursing Research: Development, Collaboration and Utilization,* Germantown, MD: Aspen Systems Corporation, 1978.

13. Mills CW: *The Sociological Imagination,* New York: Oxford University Press, 1967.

14. Hardy ME: Perspective on nursing theory. *ANS 1:*37–48,1978.

15. Merton RK: *Social Theory and Social Structure,* New York: Free Press, 1968.

16. Mosey AC: Involvement in the rehabilitation movement—1942 to 1960. *Am J Occup Ther 25:*234–236, 1971.

17. Hughes EC (Editor): *Education for the Professions of Medicine, Law, Theology and Social Work,* New York: McGraw-Hill, 1973.

18. Mosey AC: *Occupational Therapy—Configuration of a Profession,* New York: Raven Press, 1981.

19. Argyris, C, Schon D: *Theory in Practice: Increasing Professional Effectiveness,* San Francisco: Jossey-Bass, 1974.

20. Dickoff J, James P, Wiedenbach E: Theory in a practice discipline. *Nurs Res 17:*415–435,1968.

21. Ford DH, Urban HB: *Systems of Psychotherapy: A Comparative Study,* New York: J Wiley, 1963.

22. Wallace WL: *The Logic of Science in Sociology,* Chicago: Aldine-Atherton, 1971.

23. Mosey AC: *Three Frames of Reference for Mental Health,* New York: Charles B. Slack, 1970.

24. Neufeld PS: Neurobehavioral evaluation and management. In *Physical Disabilities Manual,* BC Abreu, Editor. New York: Raven Press, 1981, 117–140.

25. Bobath B: *Adult Hemiplegia: Evaluation and Treatment* (2nd Edition), London: W Heinemann, 1978.

26. Knott M, Voss DE: *Proprioceptive Neuromuscular Facilitation* (2nd Edition), New York: Hoeber Medical Division, Harper & Row, 1968.

27. Cynkin S: *Occupational Therapy: Toward Health Through Activities,* Boston: Little, Brown, 1979.

28. Farber S. *Neurorehabilitation: A Multisensory Approach,* Philadelphia: WB Saunders, 1982.

29. Gilfoyle EM, Grady AP, Moore JC: *Children Adapt,* Thorofare, NJ: Charles B Slack, 1981.

30. Heiniger MC, Randolph SL: *Neurophysiological Concepts in Human Behavior: The Tree of Learning,* St. Louis: CV Mosby, 1981.

31. Price A: Neurotherapy and specialization. *Am J Occup Ther 34:*809–815, 1980.

32. Burr WR, Mead DE, Rollins BC: A model for the application of research findings by the educator and counselor: Research to theory to practice. *Fam Coord 22:*285–290, 1973.

33. Brunnstrom S: Motor behavior of adult hemiplegic patients. *Am J Occup Ther 25:*6–12, 1961.

34. Brunnstrom S: *Movement Therapy in Hemiplegia: A Neurophysiological Approach,* New York: Harper & Row, 1970.

35. Shapiro D, Shanahan PM: Methodology for teaching theory in occupational therapy basic professional education. *Am J Occup Ther 30:*217–224,1976.

Chapter 10

Occupation: Purposefulness and Meaningfulness as Therapeutic Mechanisms

1995 Eleanor Clarke Slagle Lecture

Catherine A. Trombly, ScD, OTR/L, FAOTA

I chose the topic of therapeutic occupation because that was what attracted me to the profession and it is the concept about which I have thought most. I became an occupational therapist because I liked arts and crafts and "medical things." When I was about 11 years old, my friend's sister came home with paintings and jewelry and other things she had made at college. She was enrolled in the occupational therapy program at the University of New Hampshire and told me she was preparing to work in a hospital using arts and crafts to help people get better. I decided then and there that that was the profession for me. Eventually, I went to the university and enjoyed learning all those activities. Those were the days when a large proportion of the curriculum was devoted to developing knowledge and skill in crafts.

We learned technique from artists and theory in our occupational therapy classes. We learned that activities were therapeutic because they were purposeful, that is, they demanded certain responses that might be deficient in people who had a disease or injury and, that by doing activities, people improved their skills and abilities. We learned how to adapt activities to change the demands as the person changed. We also learned that because the person got to choose from several activities that demanded similar responses, the chosen activity was meaningful and kept the person interested and working. These beliefs were based on anecdotal observations passed down from early occupational therapists.

These beliefs are still taught, but have hardly been researched. Current economic and scientific forces in our society require us to provide support for the hypothesis that engagement in purposeful and meaningful occupation improves impaired abilities or produces occupational functioning. It would be to our advantage also to discover *how* therapeutic occupation brings about those changes so that we can treat more effectively.

Because I have always felt the need to know more about what made occupation therapeutic, I took the opportunity of this lecture to attempt to sort out some concepts concerning therapeutic occupation for myself and to pull together evidence for whether and how occupation is therapeutic. My goal is to spark an explosion of research concerning therapeutic occupation.

If there is novelty in this lecture, to paraphrase White (1959), it lies in examining pieces that already lie before us, in seeing how to fit those pieces into a larger conceptual picture, and in determining what new pieces are needed to complete the picture.

Occupation

In the early days of occupational therapy, crafts were used as diversions, as general methods of recovery from disease and injury (Llorens, 1993; Slagle, 1914), and for their utilitarian value because products were produced that could be sold (Haas, 1922). The purpose of the craft was to keep the patient occupied so that manic or depressive thoughts would be replaced (Dunton, 1914). Replacement happened because one cannot think about two things at once and occupation compelled attention. Believed prerequisite to the therapeutic value of the craft were the patient's feelings of interest and personal pride, which the instructor needed to instill if not evoked by the activity itself (Purdum, 1911). It was Susan Tracy who moved occupational therapy into the general hospital (Barrows, 1917; Editorial, 1929). She emphasized that the product was the patient, not the article he or she makes, and thereby changed the focus of occupation from a money-making enterprise to a specific therapeutic one (Barrows, 1917; Parsons, 1917). Occupation was primarily prescribed to remediate impairment (Barrows, 1917; Swaim, 1928), although there is a report that Tracy developed what we now call a *universal cuff* to enable persons to feed themselves (Cameron, 1917). By 1930, therapists were being invited to move beyond remediation to join the rehabilitation effort. The philosophy of rehabilitation is to focus not on what is lost, but on what capabilities remain, to prepare the person for return to the fullness of life's activities (Lowney, 1930). Occupation came to include activities of daily living (ADL) and prevocational training.

In the past several years papers have been written and several conferences held to discuss occupation, but consensus about what occupation is and is not continues to elude us. Nelson (1988) (see Chapter 41) presented a detailed conceptualization of occupation in which he defined occupation as the relationship between occupational form and occupational performance. By *occupational form* he meant the task demands and environmental context. By *occupational performance* he meant the act of doing. According to his view, *therapeutic occupation* is the synthesis of an occupational form by the occupational therapist that either enables the patient to compensate to achieve a goal activity or produces an adaptive change in what Nelson called the person's developmental structure (1990). In this conceptualization, any voluntary activity a person does of *whatever complexity* is considered occupation as long as the occupational form of the activity has meaning from the person's point of view and the performance is based on a sense of purpose. According to this conceptualization, reaching for something of interest and preparing one's lunch are both occupations.

Occupation is limited to complex activity sequences by others. Clark and her colleagues (1991) defined occupation as "chunks of culturally and personally meaningful activity in which humans engage that can be named in the lexicon of the culture" (p. 301). By that they meant such things as doing one's job, dressing, cooking, and gardening. Christiansen and Baum, as reported by Christiansen (1991), defined *occupation* as all goal-oriented behavior related to daily living, including spiritual and sexual activities. In their view, the basic unit of occupation is activity. They defined *activity* as specific goal-oriented behavior directed toward the performance of a task. Bathing is an example of a task; filling the bathtub and washing one's self are examples of activities. They acknowledged that abilities are required to engage in activities and tasks, but did not seem to include this level in their characterization of occupation. *Occupation*, as defined by Clark and her colleagues and by Christiansen and Baum, seems to assume ability to perform. For those who treat patients with physical impairments, occupation thus defined is problematic because most of our patients cannot perform.

A Model of Practice for Physical Dysfunction

I want to suggest a different way of considering therapeutic occupation, but first I need to tell you how I view the practice of occupational therapy for adults with physical dysfunction and define some terms. I am limiting my examples to physical dysfunction because that is what I know best, although the ideas apply to many areas of practice. The model I am presenting is not my original idea. I think it has been used since the inception of the application of occupational therapy to this population, but I have named it the model of occupational functioning (Trombly, 1993). This model of practice parallels a certain conceptualization of occupational performance. This conceptualization of occupational performance is a descending hierarchy of roles, tasks, activities, abilities, and capacities (see Figure 1).

In the model of occupational functioning, the goal of occupational therapy is to develop a sense of competency and self-esteem. A competent person has sufficient resources to interact effectively with the physical or social environments and to meet the demands of a situation (White, 1959). A sense of competency is highly associated with feelings of self-efficacy (Abler & Fretz, 1988; Bandura, 1977), a belief that one is capable of accomplishing a goal. To be competent means to be able to satisfactorily engage in one's life roles (or to voluntarily reassign a role to another). The American Occupational Therapy Association (AOTA) (1994) (see Appendix I) categorized roles into the three performance areas of work, play and leisure, and activities of daily living. However, I prefer to categorize roles from the point of view of the person (Trombly, 1993)—for example, roles that relate to self-achievement or productivity; roles that are essentially self-enhancing or that add pleasure or joy to one's life; and roles that maintain the self, which in my view includes family preservation and home maintenance.

Any categorization, however, is deceptive in that it implies that particular roles can be unequivocally classified into one category or another. They cannot. A particular person may categorize one role as an achievement–productivity role, whereas someone else may classify the same role as an enhancement–recreational role. The example that comes quickest to mind is the role of shopper. For some persons, shopping is recreation and adds joy to their lives; for others, shopping is a chore done simply to acquire the raw materials needed for living. The category depends upon the meaning that the role has for the person. This fact becomes readily apparent when we note the results of a study by Yerxa and Locker (1990) (See Chapter 19). They examined how 15 subjects with spinal cord injury categorized their daily activities. They found that the same activity was often placed into different categories. For example, eating was categorized by different subjects as self-maintenance, rest, play, and "other."

In order to engage satisfactorily in a life role, a person must be able to do the tasks and activities that make up that role within the natural context. Some tasks are essential to the role and must be mastered by whomever chooses the role. For example, the role of bus driver requires that the person be able to do the activity of steering the bus on a city street. Other roles are defined by the person so that the same role may be constituted in terms of different tasks by different persons. For example, one woman might consider the task of helping with homework an essential aspect of her mother role, whereas another, like the patient with chronic back pain interviewed by Nelson and Payton (1991), might consider roughhousing with her children as very important to that role. The patient, or a significant other, decides which roles the patient should work toward resuming. Furthermore, the person decides which tasks and activities constitute particular roles according to his or her values as well as sociocultural mores and expectations.

To go on with the description of the occupational functioning model, tasks are composed of *activities*, which are smaller units of behavior. For example, peeling a potato is an activity within the task of meal preparation. To continue further down the hierarchy, in order to be able to do a given activity, one has to have certain sensorimotor, cognitive, perceptual, emotional, and social abilities. A*bilities* are skills that one has developed through practice and that underlie many different activities—for example, eye–hand coordination. Abilities emanate from developed capacities that the person has gained through learning or maturation. D*eveloped capacities* are refinements, gained through maturation and learning, of biologically based capacities. Graded grasp to accommodate the size and shape of an object is an example of a developed capacity. Developed capacities depend upon first-level capacities. *First-level capacities* are reflex-based responses or subroutines that underlie voluntary movement and derive from a person's genetic endowment or spared organic substrate. For example, reflexive grasp and reflexive release, which underlie the higher capacity of graded grasp, are first-level capacities.

In this conceptualization, complex occupations, such as maintenance of one's clothes, have progressively simpler occupations nested within them (see Figure 2) (e.g., doing the laundry, hanging clothes on a clothesline, fastening the clothespin, grasping the clothespin). This nesting contributes to our quandary in characterizing what is, and what is not, occupation and in building

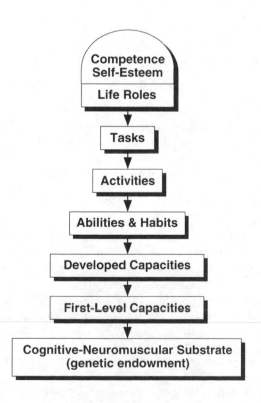

Figure 1. Conceptualization of occupational performance.

a theory of therapeutic occupation. A second dimension that makes occupation difficult to define is time: occupations comprise a range of time from brief moments to the entire lifespan (Nelson, 1988 [see Chapter 41]; Yerxa et al., 1990 [see Chapter 19]). So not only does occupation have a vertical dimension, complexity, as I have just described, but it also has a horizontal dimension, time.

Another Look at Occupation

For me, one way to begin the characterization of occupation was to notice, in the process of thinking about the occupational functioning model, that in some situations we consider occupation as the goal to be learned and in other situations we consider occupation as the change agent. I have termed these *occupation-as-end* and *occupation-as-means*. I suggest this distinction because I think the goals and therapeutic processes of these two forms of occupation are different. Furthermore, there is historical basis for this separation because these two uses of occupation came into occupational therapy practice at different times. I equate the idea of occupation-as-end to the levels of activities, tasks, and roles in the occupational functioning model. At each of these levels, the person has a functional goal and tries to accomplish it by using what abilities and capacities he or she has. I think this is close to how Clark and others (1991) and Christiansen and Baum (Christiansen, 1991) defined occupation. Occupation-as-means, on the other hand, is *the therapy* used to bring about changes in impaired performance components. Occupation at this level often is limited to simple behaviors. Both occupation-as-end and occupation-as-means garner their therapeutic impact from the qualities of purposefulness and meaningfulness.

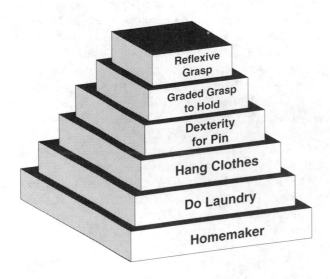

Figure 2. Nesting of levels of occupation.

Purposefulness in Occupation-as-End

Occupation-as-end is purposeful by definition. According to many occupational therapy writers, purposeful occupation-as-end organizes a person's behavior, day, and life (Kielhofner, 1985, 1992; Meyer, 1922/1977 [see Chapter 2]; Slagle, 1914; Yerxa & Baum, 1986; Yerxa & Locker, 1990 [see Chapter 19]; Yerxa et al., 1990). Early occupational "workers" imposed purposeful occupation on persons who could not choose it for themselves; they were then able to act in more healthy ways (Slagle, 1914). Time-use studies indicate that people who are mentally able to envision goals distribute their awake time among occupational tasks and activities. The studies also indicate that this distribution is affected by age (McKinnon, 1992) or disability (Yerxa & Baum, 1986; Yerxa & Locker, 1990 [see Chapter 19]). For example, Yerxa and Baum found that the number of hours that community-living subjects with spinal cord injury devoted to particular occupations differed significantly from the number of hours their friends without disabilities devoted to those occupations. The subjects with spinal cord injury worked fewer hours and devoted more hours to occupations categorized as "other," which for some subjects included shopping, going to church, eating, or watching television. The problem with this study, for our purposes, is that subject-designated categories were used as the data. Subjects categorized the same occupation (e.g., eating) differently. Further research is needed concerning purposefulness in occupation-as-end. Time-use studies inform us that persons fill their time with activities and tasks that they can name and categorize. However, I found no studies in our literature on how occupation-as-end organizes persons' lives. One paradigm that might be fruitful is to examine how persons without mental illness, who are recently retired, in extreme circumstances such as in prison or lost in the wilderness, or even on extended lazy vacations try to impose organization on their lives by planning and carrying out purposeful occupations of various complexities.

Meaningfulness in Occupation-as-End

Occupation-as-end is not only purposeful but also meaningful because it is the performance of activities or tasks that a person sees as important. Only meaningful occupation remains in a person's life repertoire. Meaningfulness as a therapeutic aspect of occupation derives from our belief in the mind–body connection. The actions of the body are guided by the meaning ascribed to them by the mind (Bruner, 1990). Meaningfulness of occupation-as-end is based on a person's values that derive from family and cultural experiences. Meaningfulness also derives from a person's sense of the importance of participating in certain occupations or performing in a particular manner; or from the person's estimate of reward in terms of success or pleasure; or perhaps from a threat of bad consequences if the occupation is not engaged in.

Meaning is individual (Bruner, 1990) and although the occupational therapist can guess what may be meaningful based on a person's life history, he or she must verify with each patient that the particular occupation is meaningful to that person *now* and verify that the person sees a value in relearning it. The therapist cannot substitute his or her own values in selecting appropriate occupational goals for the patient. Two studies concerning differences in valuing between therapist and patient come to mind. In 1974, Taylor reported that the values attached to goals by 19 occupational therapists differed significantly from those of 44 patients with spinal cord injuries. The patients valued development of work tolerance most, followed by bladder and bowel control. They did not value ADL skills highly. The therapists valued development of adapted devices and ADL skills most and bowel and bladder control least. Chiou and Burnett (1985) surveyed 26 patients living at home after stroke to determine the relative importance of 15 ADL tasks to each of them. Then the researchers paired each patient with one or more of 10 visiting occupational therapists and physical therapists who were treating these patients, to form 29 pairs. Patients and therapists, independently, ranked the 15 items from not at all important to very important for the particular patient. Scores for each patient and therapist pair were correlated. Only one of the 29 pairs yielded a significant correlation, and that was only of moderate strength [.57]. These results seem to indicate that therapists were not good judges of the value ascribed by patients to particular ADL tasks.

The meaningfulness of occupation-as-end is so profound that people at least partially define life satisfaction in terms of competent role performance. For example, in the study by Yerxa and Baum (1986) of 15 subjects with spinal cord injuries and their 12 friends without disabilities, a significant, moderate correlation of $r = .44$ was found between satisfaction with performance in home management and overall life satisfaction. A slightly higher correlation of $r = .62$ was found between satisfaction with performance of community skills and overall life satisfaction. Bränholm and Fugl-Meyer (1992) surveyed 201 randomly selected 25- to 55-year old northern Swedish persons without disabilities to determine what value they attached to certain roles in relation to their perceived level of life satisfaction. Roles associated with vocation, family life, leisure, and home maintenance correctly classified 62% to 78% of the subjects in terms of satisfaction with life. Smith, Kielhofner, and Watts (1986) (see Chapter 31) studied 60 persons with a mean age of 78 years, half of whom were institutionalized, to determine the relationship between engagement in daily occupations and life satisfaction. They found that those subjects who were classified into the high satisfaction category engaged in recreation and work significantly more and in ADL and rest significantly less than those classified in the low satisfaction category.

Therapeutic Achievement of Occupation-as-End

I think that occupation-as-end is brought about by teaching the activity or task directly, using whatever abilities the patient has at his or her disposal or providing whatever adaptations are necessary. It is the Rehabilitative Approach (Trombly, 1995a) or skills training approach (Rogers, 1982). In this approach, occupations are analyzed to ensure that they are within the capabilities of the patient, but are not used to bring about change in those capabilities, per se. The patient learns, with the help of the therapist as teacher and as adaptor of the task demands and context. In the therapeutic encounter, the therapist organizes the subtasks to be learned so that the person will succeed, provides the feedback to ensure successful outcome, and structures the practice to promote improved performance and learning. The purpose of the activity or task is readily apparent to the patient and, if the therapist has allowed patient goals to guide treatment, it is meaningful. Therapeutic principles for this approach derive from cognitive information processing and learning theories.

Occupation-as-Means

Occupation-as-means refers to occupation acting as the therapeutic change agent to remediate impaired abilities or capacities. Various arts, crafts, games, sports, exercise routines, and daily activities that are systematically selected and tailored to each person (Cynkin & Robinson, 1990) are examples of occupations-as-means. Occupation in this sense is equivalent to what is called *purposeful activity* (AOTA, 1993) (see Appendix C). Purposeful activity demands particular, more circumscribed responses than occupation-as-end.

The therapist analyzes the occupation to determine that it demands particular responses from the person and that the responses demanded are slightly more challenging than what the person can currently easily produce. The therapist provides the opportunity to engage in the potentially therapeutic occupation (Meyer, 1922/1977 [see Chapter 2]), and as the person makes the effort and succeeds, the particular impairment that the occupation-as-means was chosen to remediate is reduced.

Although occupation is provided, therapy may be absent. What makes occupation-as-means therapeutic? First, the activity must have a purpose or goal that makes a challenging demand, yet has a prospect for success. Second, it must have meaning and relevance to the person who is to change so that it motivates the will to learn and improve (Cynkin & Robinson, 1990). The therapeutic aspects of occupation used as a means to change impairments, then, are purposefulness and meaningfulness.

Purposefulness in Occupation-as-Means

Occupation-as-means is based on the assumption that the activity holds within itself a healing property that will change organic or behavioral impairments. We have further assumed that those inherent therapeutic aspects can be reliably identified through the activity analysis process (Llorens, 1986, 1993). However if that assumption were true, therapists should fairly unanimously identify the inherent characteristic components of particular activities. But Tsai (1994), who surveyed 120 therapists experienced in the treatment of stroke, found poor consensus on the sensorimotor, cognitive-perceptual, or psychosocial components demanded by five particular activities that are commonly used in the treatment of patients who have had a stroke, such as stacking cones, putting on a shirt, and making a sandwich. Neistadt, McAuley, Zecha, and Shannon (1993) also reported discrepancies among therapists in identifying components required to do common activities.

Research Related to Purposefulness of Occupation-as-Means in the Motor Domain

When analyzing activities to remediate motor impairments, we have assumed that there are inherent aspects of an activity that elicit particular muscular responses. However, this assumption is not supported by electromyographic evidence. If the therapeutic benefit were inherent in the activity, then whenever any person did that activity, the effects should be similar from trial to trial and similar from person to person, especially in those with normal biomechanical and neuromuscular systems. However, a colleague and I completed an electromyographical study some years ago that examined the responses of hand muscles of 15 persons without disabilities when they were doing 16 different occupational therapy hand activities (Trombly & Cole, 1979). I had assumed in designing this study that if the goal was the same (e.g., "open this lock with this key"), and placement of objects was the same from subject to subject, and if each subject was positioned the same in relation to the objects (i.e., if the task demands were the same), then the same muscles would be used at similar levels by the various subjects. However, the results indicated that each subject used his or her own muscle activation pattern and amount of muscle activity. This finding was contrary to my expectations, but fully in agreement with predictions of Bernstein (1967).

Bernstein theorized that neuromuscular variability between trials is due to the redundancies in the musculoskeletal systems. Such redundancies allow the same goal to be accomplished effectively by a wide variety of muscle combinations and movement patterns (Horak, 1991; Morasso & Zaccaria, 1986; Newell & Corcos, 1993). Bernstein's ideas, and the evidence that supports them, contributed to the paradigm shift to the dynamical systems theory of motor control. The term *dynamical systems* refers to any area of concern in which order and pattern emerge from the interaction and cooperation of many systems (Hawking, 1988). Applied to motor behavior, dynamical systems refers to movement patterns that emerge from the interaction of multiple systems of the person and performance contexts to achieve a functional goal (see Figure 3) (Mathiowetz & Haugen, 1994, 1995; Haugen & Mathiowetz, 1995).

According to Bernstein's hypothesis, the central nervous system temporarily yokes muscles together to constrain the number of degrees of freedom to within its capability of control at the moment, given the current resources of the person and the particular demands of the context. This synergic coupling, or coordinative structure, forms as needed at the moment and then dissolves. The next time the person does the same thing, his or her muscles may be more warmed up, or there may be a slight difference in placement of task object in relation to the active limb, so a new coordinative structure evolves. That is, different muscles may be recruited, or the same muscles used before may be more or less active in order

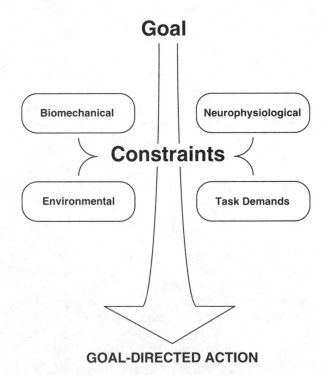

Figure 3. Dynamical systems theory of motor control hypothesizes that goal-directed action emerges from a synthesis of goal or purpose and personal and contextual constraints.

to accomplish the movement goal in the most efficient way. The motor goal is constant or invariant and requires a constant, invariant response, but this response can be fulfilled by a varying set of muscular contractions (Luria, 1973). The goal or purpose seems to organize the most efficient movement, given the constraints of person and context (see Figure 3).

What evidence is there that purpose organizes behavior? Motor commands issued to moving segments are not accessible to an experimenter and must be inferred from study of the limb trajectories that they ultimately produce (Jeannerod, 1988). Limb trajectories are recorded with instruments designed to track the spatial-temporal aspects of movement. Different spatial-temporal patterns, which are indicative of differences in movement organization, emerge for particular goals (Jeannerod, 1988). Movement organization can be detected from the shape of the velocity profile (Georgopoulos, 1986; Kamm, Thelen, & Jensen, 1990) that changes depending on goal (Nelson, 1983). The goal of reaching to a large target that does not demand accuracy produces a unimodal and bell-shaped velocity profile. The goal of reaching precisely to a target, which requires accurate, guided movement, on the other hand, has a left-shifted velocity profile because more time is spent in deceleration than in acceleration.

In 1987, Marteniuk, MacKenzie, Jeannerod, Athenes, and Dugas demonstrated for the first time the impact of goal on the organization of movement. They found that five university student subjects used a different movement organization when they reached for the same object for two different purposes. One goal was to pick up a 4-cm disk and place it in a slot; the other goal was to pick up the same disk and throw it into a basket. The task demands and the context were exactly the same. Only intent after the reach was different. The different purposes produced two different velocity profiles, indicating different movement organizations, for the reaches to the disk. Reaches before placing the disk into a slot produced a left shift of velocity profile in which a significantly greater percentage of total reach time was spent in the deceleration phase and the acceleration phase was significantly shortened as compared to reaches before the throwing condition.

Mathiowetz (1991) tested whether the same motor organization was elicited when 20 subjects with multiple sclerosis performed functional tasks in natural, impoverished, partial, and simulated conditions. In one of the experiments, the subjects actually ate applesauce with a spoon in the natural condition; pretended to eat applesauce, with no applesauce, spoon, or dish present in the impoverished condition; pretended to eat applesauce with a dish and spoon, but no applesauce present in the partial condition; or did, in the simulated condition, the feeding subtest of the Jebsen-Taylor Hand Function Test

(Jebsen, Taylor, Trieschmann, Trotter, & Howard, 1969) that requires the subject to pick up kidney beans with a spoon and transfer them to a can placed in front of him or her. The outcomes of each trial were described qualitatively in phase plane diagrams in which velocity is graphed against displacement. These should be replicable from trial to trial if the subject is using the same movement organization. However, the phase planes were judged, by experienced judges, to be different among the four conditions. Because subjects produced unique phase planes for each condition, Mathiowetz concluded that subjects perceived each condition as an unique activity, having a different goal.

In another test of differences in goal situation, Van der Weel, van der Meer, and Lee (1991) tested nine children of average intelligence, aged 3 to 7 years, who had right hemiparesis. They measured the children's range of supination and pronation movement when moving a drumstick back and forth in the frontal plane with the instruction 'to move as far as you can' (the abstract condition). The children had previously experienced the full range of movement passively. Range was also measured when the children were told to use the same drumstick to 'bang the drums' which were placed to require full range of motion (the concrete condition). Movement range was significantly greater ($t_8 = 6.75$, $p < .0001$) for the concrete task of banging the drums than for the abstract task, which had a vague goal.

Wu (Wu, 1993; Wu, Trombly, & Lin, 1994) investigated whether actually reaching for a pencil to write one's name, reaching the same distance for an imagined pencil, or reaching forward in a biomechanically similar way would produce different outcomes in terms of the organization of movement. In the sample of 37 college-aged subjects without disabilities, the materials-based occupation of reaching for an actual pencil elicited significantly different and more efficient organization of movement than imagery-based occupation of reaching for a pretend pencil or exercise. The reach was faster ($F_{2,62} = 20.44$, $p < .001$) and straighter ($F_{2,62} = 23.25$, $p < .001$), was more preplanned ($F_{2,62} = 22.13$, $p < .001$), and used less force ($F_{2,62} = 6.13$, $p < .005$). The imagery-based occupation, on the other hand, produced a more guided, longer, and more convoluted path than did the exercise condition, probably because the goal was more vague in that condition.

Sietsema, Nelson, Mulder, Mervau-Scheidel, and White (1993) tested the effect of goal on overall active range of shoulder motion of 20 adults with brain injury. Each subject reached to a point 3 in. above the center of a table placed to require full forward reach. Each also reached the same distance to play a computer controlled game of flashing lights and sounds. Overall active range of motion was significantly greater as a result of the game than simply reaching to the more vague target ($t_{19} = 5.77$, $p < .001$).

At least in terms of motor responses, then, purpose does appear to organize behavior. Of course, much more study is required to verify this finding.

Meaningfulness in Occupation-as-Means

Whereas a meaningful occupation has purposefulness, strictly speaking, a purposeful activity may or may not be meaningful. Sharrott (1983) stated that the purpose of an action gives that action meaning. He may have been using *purpose* to denote the reason that a person does something, or the motive, rather than the goal of the action. I think that confounding these terms will impede research. The purpose is the goal, the expected end result. The meaning is the value that accomplishment of that goal has for the person. I have an anecdotal example of the separation between the two concepts. Some years back, my father had a right cerebrovascular accident with resultant hemiinattention. The occupational therapist gave him parquetry blocks to do. There were two purposes. One was the goal of the activity—to place all the blocks on the diagram. He understood the goal and tried to do what he was told. However, it had no meaning to him; he viewed this activity as a children's game and found it degrading. The therapeutic purpose, of course, was to improve his hemiinattention. That purpose had no meaning to him either; he did not think he had hemiinattention and did not get the connection between the child's game and the therapeutic goal.

What do we mean by *meaningful* and how does that quality of occupation-as-means affect behavioral responses? Meaning related to occupation-as-means may relate to basic values held by the person—similar to the way meaning is derived for occupation-as-end. However, meaning is probably generated from a less profound source when it applies to particular, circumscribed, time-limited activities used to promote some performance component. The meaningful aspect of occupation-as-means may be the emotional value that an interesting and creative experience offers the patient (Ayres, 1958). Or meaningfulness may stem from familiarity with the occupation, or its power to arouse positive associations, or the likelihood that completion of it will elicit approval from others who are respected and admired (Cynkin & Robinson, 1990), or its potential to contribute to recovery.

Although we often count on meaningfulness to emanate from the activity, there is no inherent meaningfulness quality in a particular occupation. Meaningfulness is individual. Bruner (1990) said that "action is interpretable only by reference to what the actor says he or she is up to" (p. 20). In therapy, meaningfulness is developed through an exchange between the therapist and the person to construct the meaning of the activity within the context of culture, life experiences, disability (Fleming, 1990; Kielhofner, 1992), and present needs.

Table 1.
Mean Number of Repetitions as a Result of Preference and Purpose in Assigned Tasks

Purpose	Tasks Assigned	
	Preferred	Nonpreferred
Yes	63	63
No	83	84

Note. Based on Bakshi, R., Bhambhani, Y., & Madill, H. (1991). The effects of task preference on performance during purposeful and nonpurposeful activities. *American Journal of Occupational Therapy, 45,* 912–916.

Research Related to Meaningfulness of Occupation-as-Means

The importance of meaningfulness to us as therapists is that we believe that it motivates. What evidence is there that meaning motivates behavior?

Meaningfulness has been operationalized in occupational therapy studies in one of three ways. One is to offer a choice, another is to provide a product, and the third is to enhance the context. The response, motivation, has been operationalized as the number of repetitions or length of time engaged in the occupation or as the effort expended.

Choice. Bakshi, Bhambhani, and Madill (1991) studied 20 female college students who chose their most preferred and least preferred activity from eight offered activities. They completed each under conditions of purpose and nonpurpose, defined respectively as working on a product or not. There were no differences in number of repetitions performed between the preferred and nonpreferred occupation. Differences between product and no-product conditions were not significant due to high variability (see Table 1). On the other hand, LaMore and Nelson (1993), in a more controlled study, did find a significant increase in repetitions ($Z = 2.9, p < .01$) when 22

Table 2.
Effects of Product-Oriented and Non–Product-Oriented Activities

Measures	Product	
	Yes (Cutting Board)	No (Wood)
Preference	4.8	3.4*
Increased heart rate	13	17
Performance time	172	148

Note. Based on Thibodeaux, C. S., & Ludwig, F. M. (1988). Intrinsic motivation in product-oriented and non–product-oriented activities. *American Journal of Occupational Therapy, 42,* 169–175.
*$p=.001$

adult subjects with mental disabilities were given a limited choice of which ceramic object to paint as compared with when they were told to paint a particular one.

Product. Thibodeaux and Ludwig (1988) tested whether performance time and heart rate (effort) would be significantly different when 15 occupational therapy students sanded a cutting board that they could keep as compared with when they sanded wood for no reason. Although the subjects reported enjoying the product-oriented activity significantly more and they worked longer at it, there was too much intersubject variability to detect significant differences between conditions (see Table 2).

Enhanced context. Riccio, Nelson, and Bush (1990) (see Chapter 55) studied the effects of enhanced context. They tested the effect of imagery-based activity and exercise on the number of repetitions of 27 elderly nursing home residents when they reached up to pretend to pick apples and reached down to pretend to pick up coins versus when they simply reached up or down for exercise. There was a significant difference between the two conditions for the up direction ($Z = 2.25$, $p = .012$), indicating that pretending to pick apples was more motivating than exercise. The outcome for reaching down was in the same direction, but nonsignificant ($Z = 1.60$, $p = .055$), possibly because of a confounding effect of fatigue.

Lang, Nelson, and Bush (1992) tested the responses of 15 elderly nursing home residents under three conditions: materials-based activity, imagery-based activity, and exercise. In the materials-based condition, subjects actually kicked a red balloon. In the imagery-based condition, they pretended to kick a described balloon. In the exercise condition, they kicked as demonstrated. The number of repetitions associated with really kicking the balloon (54) was significantly greater ($F_{2,28} = 6.62$, $p = .004$) than those associated with imagining kicking the balloon (26) or kicking for exercise (18). This study was later replicated by DeKuiper, Nelson, and White (1993)

Table 3.

Average Effects of Materials-Based Occupation, Imagery-Based Occupation, and Role Exercise

Measures	Type of Occupation and Exercise		
	Materials-Based	Imagery-Based	Rote
Repetitions to fatigue	127*	51	75
Distance foot lifted (cm)	29	31	26
Speed (cm/sec)	71	71	67

Note. Based on DeKuiper, W. P., Nelson, D. L., & White, B. E. (1993). Materials-based occupation versus imagery-based occupation versus rote exercise: A replication and extension. *Occupational Therapy Journal of Research, 13,* 183–197.

*$p<.001$

on 28 elderly nursing home residents. Materials-based occupation produced significantly more repetitions than imagery-based occupation or rote exercise ($F_{2,54} = 12.1$, $p < .001$). In this study they also measured effort in terms of distance the foot was raised and speed of kick. There were no significant differences among the various contextual conditions for these variables (see Table 3).

A number of other researchers (Bloch, Smith, & Nelson, 1989; Kircher, 1984; Miller & Nelson, 1987 [see Chapter 54]; Steinbeck, 1986 [see Chapter 53]; Yoder, Nelson, & Smith, 1989) all demonstrated significantly greater numbers of repetitions or duration for what they termed purposeful versus nonpurposeful activity. The differences in the activities were actually differences in meaning in terms of context, not differences in purpose—the motoric purpose was the same: jump up and down or jump rope, stir dough for exercise or stir dough that will be made into cookies that the subjects could smell baking, squeeze a bulb to keep a ping-pong ball suspended in air or squeeze the same bulb for exercise. Some demonstrated significantly greater effort (heart rate) expended for the enhanced condition, but this was not a consistent finding (Bloch, Smith, & Nelson, 1989; Kircher, 1984; Steinbeck, 1986 [see Chapter 53]).

Meaningfulness, as operationalized by enhanced context, and possibly by choice, appears to motivate continued performance. However, more definitive research is needed. Additionally, basic research on what makes occupation-as-means meaningful and how best to operationalize this in both research and practice is needed.

Practice and Research

As occupational therapists we want our patients to achieve role competence. We use occupation-as-end and occupation-as-means now to achieve that. We need to document the successes of our current practices, but we also need to reconsider some of our practices. For example, practice based on an ascending hierarchical model has emphasized remediation of occupational components because it is assumed that lower level skills and abilities are prerequisite to higher level functioning. Although this assumption makes logical sense—persons who cannot lift their arms certainly cannot comb their hair in the usual way—practice has sometimes emphasized treatment to increase strength and other capacities and abilities to the exclusion of teaching functional skills. However, a thorough review of the literature on stroke rehabilitation (Wagenaar & Meijer, 1991a, 1991b) indicated that gains in component functions are small and do not automatically result in improved functional performance. When the results of several correlational studies were averaged together, the average correlation between motor impairment and ADL was .56 and between perceptual impairment and ADL was .58 (Trombly, 1995b). By squaring the *r*, the amount of variance of ADL accounted for by

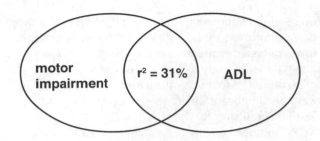

Figure 4. Pictorial description of r^2.

motor impairment was 31% (see Figure 4). Therefore, 69% of variance associated with ADL derives from other factors. Even if motor impairment were 100% remediated, would the patient be able to do ADL without specific training and adaptation? Studies are needed that compare skills training at the level of occupation-as-end with subskills training using occupation-as-means to effectively and efficiently achieve occupational functioning (Rogers, 1982).

How the purposefulness and meaningfulness aspects of both levels of occupation contribute to the therapeutic effect need explication to guide practice. We need to study in more detail how purposefulness organizes behavior and meaningfulness motivates performance. The literature reviewed here is a beginning in this regard. Some of the studies reviewed indicated that the organization of motor behavior is different when the purposes or contexts are different, even if they are similar. This finding suggests that treatment in simulated contexts using simulated objects and simulated goals may not help a patient learn occupational performance for real life. Studies are needed to compare effectiveness of treatment with actual objects in natural contexts versus treatment with simulated objects in clinical settings. Follow-up studies of carryover of occupational performance from treatment center to home are also needed.

Those golden moments that we have all experienced as therapists probably came about when the patient succeeded in doing something that had great meaning to him or her. Sometimes we get complacent, though, and offer activities and occupations that we think ought to be meaningful to the person but are not really, or we offer a choice of activities from a selection in which none of the choices are meaningful. Much more attention needs to be applied to discovering the meaning of, or creating meaning for, therapeutic occupation. Methods to evaluate meaningfulness are needed both for research and practice. We need more well-controlled studies that test the effect of meaningfulness on perseverance and effort during therapy.

Conclusion

Occupational therapy was founded on the belief that engaging in occupation brought about mental and phys-

ical health. Over the years we have redefined health, for our purposes, as occupational performance having many levels of organization. In this context, occupation can be seen both as end and as means. In both dimensions, meaningfulness and purposefulness are key qualities. Purposefulness organizes and meaningfulness motivates. Purposeful occupation-as-end seems to organize time and a person's description of his life. Meaningful occupation-as-end motivates the person's participation in life. Purposeful occupation-as-means organizes behavioral responses, at least as far as motor responses are concerned. Meaningful occupation-as-means seems to motivate the person to persevere in his efforts long enough to achieve a therapeutic benefit. Research is needed to verify each of these hypotheses. I hope each occupational therapist will join me in taking responsibility to contribute to that effort.

Acknowledgments

Figures 1, 2, and 4, as well as all the slides in the original presentation, were prepared by Elizabeth (Boo) Murray, ScD, OTR, FAOTA, to whom I am very grateful. I further want to acknowledge the support and constructive critique of my colleagues in the Neurobehavioral Rehabilitation Research Center (NRRC), which is the American Occupational Therapy Association and American Occupational Therapy Foundation Center for Scholarship and Research at Boston University: Sharon Cermak, EdD, OTR, FAOTA; Wendy Coster, PhD, OTR, FAOTA; Anne Henderson, PhD, OTR, FAOTA; Karen Jacobs, EdD, OTR, FAOTA; Noomi Katz, PhD, OTR; Boo Murray, ScD, OTR, FAOTA; and Elsie Vergara, ScD, OTR, FAOTA.

References

Abler, R. R., & Fretz, B. R. (1988). Self-efficacy and competence in independent living among oldest old persons. *Journal of Gerontology: Social Sciences, 43,* S138–143.

American Occupational Therapy Association. (1993). Position Paper—Purposeful activity. *American Journal of Occupational Therapy, 47,* 1081–1082. Reprinted as Appendix C.

American Occupational Therapy Association. (1994). Uniform terminology for occupational therapy—third edition. *American Journal of Occupational Therapy, 48,* 1047–1054. Reprinted as Appendix I.

Ayres, A. J. (1958). Basic concepts of clinical practice in physical disabilities. *American Journal of Occupational Therapy, 12,* 300–311.

Bakshi, R., Bhambhani, Y., & Madill, H. (1991). The effects of task preference on performance during purposeful and nonpurposeful activities. *American Journal of Occupational Therapy, 45,* 912–916.

Bandura, A. (1977). Self-efficacy: Toward a unifying theory of behavior change. *Psychological Review, 84,* 191–215.

Barrows, M. (1917). Susan E. Tracy, R. N. *Maryland Psychiatric Quarterly, 6,* 57–62.

Bernstein, N. (1967). *The coordination and regulation of movements.* Elmsford, NY: Pergamon.

Bloch, M. W., Smith, D. A., & Nelson, D. L. (1989). Heart rate, activity, duration, and affect in added-purpose versus single-purpose jumping activities. *American Journal of Occupational Therapy, 43,* 25–30.

Bränholm, I-B., & Fugl-Meyer, A. R. (1992). Occupational role preferences and life satisfaction. *Occupational Therapy Journal of Research, 12,* 159–171.

Bruner, J. (1990). *Acts of Meaning.* Cambridge, MA: Harvard University Press.

Cameron, R. G. (1917). An interview with Miss Susan Tracy. *Maryland Psychiatric Quarterly, 4,* 65–66.

Chiou, I-I. L., & Burnett, C. N. (1985). Values of activities of daily living. A survey of stroke patients and their home therapists. *Physical Therapy, 05,* 901–900.

Christiansen, C. (1991). Occupational therapy intervention for life performance (pp. 1–43). In C. Christiansen & C. Baum (Eds.), *Occupational therapy: Overcoming human performance deficits.* Thorofare, NJ: Slack.

Clark, F., Parham, D., Carlson, M. E., Frank, G., Jackson, J., Pierce, D., Wolfe, R. J., & Zemke, R. (1991). Occupational science: Academic innovation in the service of occupational therapy's future. *American Journal of Occupational Therapy, 45,* 300–310.

Cynkin, S., & Robinson, J. M. (1990). *Occupational therapy and activities health: Toward health through activities.* Boston: Little, Brown.

DeKuiper, W. P., Nelson, D. L., & White, B. E. (1993). Materials-based occupation versus imagery-based occupation versus rote exercise: A replication and extension. *Occupational Therapy Journal of Research, 13,* 183–197.

Dunton, W. R., Jr. (1914). Roundtable. *Maryland Psychiatric Quarterly, 4,* 20–32.

Editorial. (1929). Susan E. Tracy. *Occupational Therapy and Rehabilitation, 8,* 63–66.

Fleming, M. (1990). Untitled invited paper presented at the American Occupational Therapy Foundation planning meeting for the Occupation Symposium, Boston, MA.

Georgopoulos, A. P. (1986). On reaching. *Annual Review of Neurosciences, 9,* 147–170.

Haas, L. J. (1922). Crafts adaptable to occupational needs: Their relative importance. *Archives of Occupational Therapy, 1,* 443–455.

Haugen, J. B., & Mathiowetz, V. (1995). Contemporary task-oriented approach (pp. 510–528). In C. A. Trombly (Ed.), *Occupational therapy for physical dysfunction* (4th ed.). Baltimore: Williams & Wilkins.

Hawking, S. W. (1988). *A brief history of time: From the big bang to black holes.* New York: Bantam.

Horak, F. B. (1991). Assumptions underlying motor control for neurologic rehabilitation (pp. 11–27). In M. Lister (Ed.), *Contemporary management of motor control problems. Proceedings of the II STEP Conference.* Alexandria, VA: The Foundation for Physical Therapy.

Jeannerod, M. (1988). *The neural and behavioral organization of goal-directed movements.* Oxford: Clarendon.

Jebsen, R. H., Taylor, N., Trieschmann, R. B., Trotter, M., & Howard, L. A. (1969). An objective and standardized test of hand function. *Archives of Physical Medicine and Rehabilitation, 50,* 311–319.

Kamm, K., Thelen, E., & Jensen, J. L. (1990). A dynamical systems approach to motor development. *Physical Therapy, 70,* 763–775.

Kielhofner, G. (Ed.). (1985). *A Model of Human Occupation.* Baltimore: Williams & Wilkins.

Kielhofner, G. (1992). *Conceptual foundations of occupational therapy.* Philadelphia: F. A. Davis.

Kircher, M. A. (1984). Motivation as a factor of perceived exertion in purposeful versus nonpurposeful activity. *American Journal of Occupational Therapy, 38,* 165–170.

Lang, E. M., Nelson, D. L., & Bush, M. A. (1992). Comparison of performance in materials-based occupation, imagery-based occupation, and rote exercise in nursing home residents. *American Journal of Occupational Therapy, 46,* 607–611.

LaMore, K. L., & Nelson, D. L. (1993). The effects of options on performance of an art project in adults with mental disabilities. *American Journal of Occupational Therapy, 47,* 397–401.

Llorens, L. A. (1986). Activity analysis: Agreement among factors in a sensory processing model. *American Journal of Occupational Therapy, 40,* 103–110.

Llorens, L. A. (1993). Activity analysis: Agreement between participants and observers on perceived factors in occupation components. *Occupational Therapy Journal of Research, 13,* 198–211.

Lowney, M. E. P. (1930). The relationship between occupational therapy and rehabilitation. *Massachusetts Association for Occupational Therapy Bulletin, 4*(2), no pages.

Luria, A. R. (1973). *The working brain: An introduction to neuropsychology.* New York: Basic.

Mathiowetz, V. G. (1991). *Informational support and functional motor performance.* Unpublished doctoral dissertation, University of Minnesota.

Mathiowetz, V., & Haugen, J. B. (1994). Motor behavior research: Implications for therapeutic approaches to central nervous system dysfunction. *American Journal of Occupational Therapy, 48,* 733–745.

Mathiowetz, V., & Haugen, J. B. (1995). Evaluation of motor behavior: Traditional and contemporary views (pp. 157–186). In C. A. Trombly (Ed.), *Occupational therapy for physical dysfunction* (4th ed.). Baltimore: Williams & Wilkins.

Marteniuk, R. G., MacKenzie, C. L., Jeannerod, M., Athenes, S., & Dugas, C. (1987). Constraints on human arm movement trajectories. *Canadian Journal of Psychology, 41,* 365–378.

McKinnon, A. L. (1992). Time use for self care, productivity, and leisure among elderly Canadians. *Canadian Journal of Occupational Therapy, 59,* 102–110.

Meyer, A. (1977). The philosophy of occupation therapy. *American Journal of Occupational Therapy, 31,* 639–642. (Reprinted from *Archives of Occupational Therapy, 1,* 1–10, 1922) (Reprinted as Chapter 2.)

Miller, L., & Nelson, D. L. (1987). Dual-purpose activity versus single-purpose activity in terms of duration of task, exertion level, and affect. *Occupational Therapy in Mental Health, 1,* 55–67. (Reprinted as Chapter 54.)

Morasso, P., & Zaccaria, R. (1986). Understanding human movement. *Experimental Brain Research, 15,* 145-157.

Neistadt, M. E., McAuley, D., Zecha, D., & Shannon, R. (1993). An analysis of a board game as a treatment activity. *American Journal of Occupational Therapy, 47,* 154–160.

Nelson, C. E., & Payton, O. D. (1991). A system for involving patients in program planning. *American Journal of Occupational Therapy, 45,* 753–755. (Reprinted as Chapter 41.)

Nelson, D. L. (1988). Occupation: Form and performance. *American Journal of Occupational Therapy, 42,* 633–641.

Nelson, D. L. (1990). Untitled invited paper presented at the American Occupational Therapy Foundation planning meeting for the Occupation Symposium, Boston, MA.

Nelson, W. L. (1983). Physical principles for economies of skilled movements. *Biological Cybernetics, 46,* 135–147.

Newell, K. M., & Corcos, D. M. (1993). Issues in variability and motor control (pp. 1–12). In K. M. Newell & D. M. Corcos (Eds.), *Variability and motor control.* Champaign, IL: Human Kinetics.

Parsons, S. E. (1917). Miss Tracy's work in general hospitals. *Maryland Psychiatric Quarterly, 6,* 63–64.

Purdum, H. D. (1911). The psycho-therapeutic value of occupation. *Maryland Psychiatric Quarterly, 1,* 35–36.

Riccio, C. M., Nelson, D. L., & Bush, M. A. (1990). Adding purpose to the repetitive exercise of elderly women through imagery. *American Journal of Occupational Therapy, 44,* 714–719. (Reprinted as Chapter 55.)

Rogers, J. C. (1982). The spirit of independence: The evolution of a philosophy. *American Journal of Occupational Therapy, 36,* 709–715.

Sharrott, G. W. (1983). Occupational therapy's role in the client's creation and affirmation of meaning. In G. Kielhofner (Ed.), *Health through occupation: Theory and practice in occupational therapy.* Philadelphia: F. A. Davis.

Sietsema, J. M., Nelson, D. L., Mulder, R. M., Mervau-Scheidel, D., & White, B.E. (1993). The use of a game to promote arm reach in persons with traumatic brain injury. *American Journal of Occupational Therapy, 47,* 19–24.

Slagle, E. C. (1914). History of the development of occupation for the insane. *Maryland Psychiatric Quarterly, 4,* 14–20.

Smith, N. R., Kielhofner, G., & Watts, J. H. (1986). The relationships between volition, activity pattern, and life satisfaction in the elderly. *American Journal of Occupational Therapy, 40,* 278–283. (Reprinted as Chapter 31.)

Steinbeck, T. M. (1986). Purposeful activity and performance. *American Journal of Occupational Therapy, 40,* 529–534. (Reprinted as Chapter 53.)

Swaim, L. T. (1928). Does occupational work hasten recovery of the crippled? *Massachusetts Association of Occupational Therapy Bulletin, 2*(3), no pages.

Taylor, D. P. (1974). Treatment goals for quadriplegic and paraplegic patients. *American Journal of Occupational Therapy, 28,* 22–29.

Thibodeaux, C. S., & Ludwig, F. M. (1988). Intrinsic motivation in product-oriented and non-product oriented activities. *American Journal of Occupational Therapy, 42,* 169–175.

Trombly, C. (1993). Anticipating the future: Assessment of occupational function. *American Journal of Occupational Therapy, 47,* 253–257.

Trombly, C. (Ed.). (1995a). *Occupational therapy for physical dysfunction* (4th ed.). Baltimore: Williams & Wilkins.

Trombly, C. A. (1995b). *Relationships between motor and perceptual performance components and activities of daily living.* Unpublished paper, Boston University.

Trombly, C. A., & Cole, J. M. (1979). Electromyographic study of four hand muscles during selected activities. *American Journal of Occupational Therapy, 33,* 440–449.

Tsai, P-L. (1994). *Activity analysis and activity selection among occupational therapists: A survey.* Unpublished master's thesis, Boston University, Boston.

Van der Weel, F. R., van der Meer, A. L. H., & Lee, D. N. (1991). Effect of task on movement control in cerebral palsy: Implications for assessment and therapy. *Developmental Medicine and Child Neurology, 33,* 419–426.

Wagenaar, R. C., & Meijer, O. G. (1991a). Effects of stroke rehabilitation (1): A critical review of the literature. *Journal of Rehabilitation Sciences, 4,* 61–73.

Wagenaar, R. C., & Meijer, O. G. (1991b). Effects of stroke rehabilitation (2): A critical review of the literature. *Journal of Rehabilitation Sciences, 4,* 97–109.

White, R. W. (1959). Motivation reconsidered: The concept of competence. *Psychological Review, 66,* 297–333.

Wu, C-Y. (1993). *The relationship between occupational form and occupational performance: A kinematic perspective.* Unpublished master's thesis, Boston University.

Wu, C-Y., Trombly, C. A., & Lin, K-C. (1994). The relationship between occupational form and occupational performance: A kinematic perspective. *American Journal of Occupational Therapy, 48,* 679–687.

Yerxa, E. J., & Baum, S. (1986). Engagement in daily occupations and life satisfaction among people with spinal cord injuries. *Occupational Therapy Journal of Research, 6,* 271–283.

Yerxa, E., & Locker, S. (1990). Quality of time use by adults with spinal cord injuries. *American Journal of Occupational Therapy, 44,* 318–326. (Reprinted as Chapter 19.)

Yerxa, E. J., Clark, F., Frank, G., Jackson, J., Parham, D., Pierce, D., Stein, C., & Zemke, R. (1990). An introduction to occupational science, A foundation for occupational therapy in the 21st century. *Occupational Therapy in Health Care, 6,* 1–32.

Yoder, R. M., Nelson, D. L., & Smith, D. A. (1989). Added-purpose versus rote exercise in female nursing home residents. *American Journal of Occupational Therapy, 43,* 581–586.

Chapter 11

Life-Style Performance: From Profile to Conceptual Model

Gail S. Fidler, OTR, FAOTA

This chapter was previously published in the *American Journal of Occupational Therapy, 50,* 139–147. Copyright © 1996, American Occupational Therapy Association.

The Life Style Performance Model evolved from the Life Style Performance Profile originally conceptualized in the mid 1970s (Fidler, 1982, 1988b). The purpose of the profile was to identify and then relate the activity-focused aspects of daily living to the fundamental biopsychosocial needs of the human being. The profile represented an effort to discern the personal and interpersonal dimensions of daily living activities, articulate more clearly the relevance of such activities to each person's quality of living, and, thus, avoid the ambiguities and stereotypes inherent in the generalized terms of work, play, leisure, and self-care.

The profile proposed that a life-style that sustains health and enables life satisfaction includes a culturally relevant, age-specific harmony among four activity domains. These domains were identified as those occupations or activities concerned with self-care and self-maintenance, personally referenced pleasure and intrinsic gratification, societal contribution, and interpersonal engagement. The term *daily living activities*, within the context of the profile, refers to all of the activities that compose a person's daily life, not simply self-care. The Life Style Performance Profile provided the format for obtaining and organizing information that reflected a patient's personal and socially determined interests, skills, and limitations in each domain (see Appendix F for the Profile). The profile was expected to provide both the patient and therapist with a view of the patient's characteristic activity patterns of daily living and the harmony–disharmony or balance among them and then serve as a guide in defining occupational therapy interventions (Fidler, 1982, 1988b).

Exploration of the viability of these tenets, first in mental health practice and then in geriatrics and physical disabilities, led to the development of the model presented in this chapter. The questions that guided this development included

- Can activity patterns of daily living be explained in more personally meaningful terms than is possible in the traditional general categories of self-care, leisure, play, and work?

- Is it possible to explicitly describe and evaluate the relationship between a person's patterns of daily living and his or her quality of living?
- Can a format be designed that would facilitate arriving at more personally relevant treatment goals or interventions?
- What are the environmental elements that notably affect patterns of activity?
- Are such themes applicable to occupational therapy practice?

During maturation and socialization, each person develops a configuration of activity patterns that can be characterized as a life-style. These patterns of doing— these ways of engaging and being engaged in doing— emerge through the interplay of the person's intrinsic needs, desires, capacities, and unique expectations of the environmental context of living (Fidler & Fidler, 1978 [see Chapter 7], 1983). An overall sense of satisfaction and well-being depends on the sum of positive benefits derived from such interplay. A resulting sense of harmony, or life-style balance, then emerges from the congregate experiences of active engagement, gratifying emotional expression, evidence of personal achievement, societal contribution, positive response from significant others, and membership in a chosen group or groups. Development and maintenance of a repertoire of activity patterns that enable and support such experiences are essential to the quality of a person's life.

The existing strengths and limitations of a person's sensory processing, motor patterns, cognition, psychologic structure, and interpersonal perceptions are important variables in the development of activity patterns. Any impediment to these systems causes a temporary or long-lasting disruption of a person's physical integrity, psychologic structure, or interpersonal orientation. Likewise, achievement of a state of harmony or a sense of well-being is frequently disrupted or made unlikely when the external world presents barriers or limitations on either the development or the maintenance of positive activity configurations.

Occupational therapy practitioners are called upon to intervene when one or more domains of a person's lifestyle performance are deemed to be deficient to a degree that produces distress in that person or in those who are part of that person's social matrix. Thus, in addition to addressing a specific disability or dysfunction, establishing outcome objectives for occupational therapy requires working with a person to develop, or redevelop, a life-style pattern of activities that will enhance the quality of his or her way of living. In some instances, this process means establishing a more satisfactory life-style. In others, it is restoring a previously achieved life-style.

Function of the Model

Thus, building on the descriptive outline of the Life Style Performance Profile (see Appendix F), a practice model has evolved that offers a framework for defining individually relevant, wellness-generating, as well as remedial goals of occupational therapy interventions. The Life Style Performance Model provides a way of describing and examining the interacting, multiple dimensions of doing and living from an organized, holistic framework applicable to all ages, cultures, and persons. The configuration of the model makes it possible to identify the relationship of activity patterns to the pursuit of a person's unique needs to achieve a personal identity, to know self as a contributing member of society, and, thus, to confirm self as acceptably human. It provides a focus for study and practice of occupational therapy as a many faceted process of enabling a way of living that is intrinsically gratifying as well as socially contributory. The model extends the parameters of occupational therapy beyond reducing disability, shifts the focus of practice beyond the realm of our traditional daily living activities, and establishes as a top priority the development of an individualized life-style profile as both a first step in defining intervention goals and an outcome focus of practice.

A fundamental concept on which the model is based is that dysfunction and remedial interventions are definable only from the perspective of what constitutes a given person's state of health and well-being. The model therefore stresses an initial focus on individual interests, capacities, and customary patterns of daily living as the basis for defining and prioritizing any intervention. An inherent belief underlying the model is that quality of life is the single most important theme in human performance. Wellness and a sense of well-being are understood as a state of being that is optimally satisfying to self and to significant others. It is hypothesized that such satisfaction is gleaned from personally and socially relevant activities that focus on and maximize individual strengths, capacities, and interests. Most important is the concept that intrinsic motivation is elicited and sustained when there is congruence between the characteristics of an activity and the biopsychosocial characteristics of the person. An important function of the model is to facilitate such a match.

Although themes related to the holistic perspective of occupational therapy have repeatedly appeared in the literature, they are frequently an elusive goal for practice. There is a marked gap in efforts to specifically connect intervention activities with the quality of a person's way of living and, thus, with what holds personal meaning and is intrinsically gratifying for that person. Current practice environments, issues of reimbursement, and reduced lengths of stay all exert pressures that most often result in reductionistic practices. The need for a model or format that encourages and readily fosters a broader, more holistic perspective for our study and practice is evident.

Christiansen (1993) cautioned that we need to understand and consider the meaning of disability and the intervention process from the patient's point of view. Addressing the focus of assessments, he called for approaches that "better [reflect] the context (including the environment) of the patient's everyday life" (p. 258). "Without this context," Christiansen asserted, "interpretations of the meaning of assessment data will have limited validity and may lead to irrelevant goals for intervention" (p. 258).

Likewise, Trombly (1993) suggested that an initial "inquiry into role competency and meaningfulness would clarify the purpose of occupational therapy" (p. 253). She advised that "those roles that are important to the person, especially those that he or she engaged in prior to illness or trauma, become the focus of inquiry" (p. 253). Trombly conjectured that if a discrepancy among the past, present, and future role performance becomes evident, it serves to clarify the purpose and relevance of an occupational therapy intervention. More recently, Trombly (1995) (see Chapter 10) has expressed the need to find more personally relevant terms to describe what we have traditionally generalized as work, play, and leisure occupations. She has cited studies that ranked the importance given to daily living activities by patients and therapists. Such studies, she reported, indicated that occupational therapists were not always good judges of what is important to the patient.

Although the importance of the environment has become an increasing focus in occupational therapy literature, there are marked lags in the application of such perspectives to practice. Addressing issues of person–environment interactions, Kielhofner (1993) cautioned that the evaluation criteria we traditionally have used may "unwittingly rob individuals of both voice and power to determine the direction of their own lives" (p. 249). He stated that too frequently we assume that the problem resides in the person, and, thus, "issues [such as] environment or workplace conditions and incentives are largely ignored" (p. 249). In a similar context, Law (1993) emphasized the critical importance of understanding and relating a person to the environmental context. She stated that most occupational therapy assessments, for example, do not consider the patient's culture and roles or the environment in which he or she lives. Furthermore, she contended that occupational therapists "do not routinely consider balance in occupational performance over a day or across a person's life-style" (p. 235).

Underlying Principles of the Model

The Life Style Performance Model facilitates the practitioner's address of these concerns, bridging the gaps among current practice, our philosophic constructs of holism, personal relevance, and quality of life. Traditionally, the goal of occupational therapy is to improve function and enhance the ability of a person to perform. The question now is: To what end? The Life Style Performance Model proposes that the outcome of occupational therapy intervention is to enable a way of living that allows persons to develop and bring into harmony a configuration of daily living activities that have personal, social, and cultural relevance for them and their significant others.

The frames of reference underlying the Life Style Performance Model incorporate the basic principles and philosophic constructs of the occupational therapy profession. The relationship of a sense of well-being, self-fulfillment, and adaptation to active participation in one's world is one principle that has been explored throughout the history of occupational therapy as well as within other disciplines. The innate drive to explore and cope with one's environment is viewed as essential to human existence and adaptation not only as a means of survival, but most importantly as enabling personal and social development (Erickson, 1950; Fidler & Fidler, 1978 [see Chapter 7], 1983; White, 1971).

In occupational therapy, this perspective has led to the construct that the drive toward action, when channeled into personally and socially relevant occupational behavior, is fundamental to the development of a positive self-regard, coping, adaptation, and health (Fidler & Fidler, 1978 [see Chapter 7], 1983; White, 1971). Additionally, the profession has embraced the concept that the sense of competence and self-agency gained through occupational performance carried out in relation to others encompasses social role learning and societal contribution (Fidler, 1988a; Fidler & Fidler [see Chapter 7], 1978, 1983; Kielhofner, 1985; Reilly, 1971). From these perspectives, purposeful activity, as used in the Life Style Performance Model, means a personally referenced action that is concerned with testing a skill, ability, or level of competence or an activity that is focused on clarifying a relationship and discerning the nature of one's relatedness to another person (or persons) or to one's nonhuman world (Fidler & Fidler [see Chapter 7], 1978). In a related sense, an *activity* is understood to reference any act or series of interconnected acts requiring the active engagement of a person's mind and body in the pursuit of a discernible outcome. In the current construction of this model, *purposeful activity* and *occupation* are viewed as interchangeable terms.

I have offered several hypotheses regarding the motivational, developmental, sociocultural, and restorative potential of occupations and activities (Fidler, 1981). I suggested that

- mastery and competence in those activities that are valued and given priority in one's society or social group have greater meaning in defining one's social efficacy than competence in activities that carry less social significance
- a total activity and each of its elements have symbolic as well as reality-based meanings that notably affect individual experience and motivation

- mastery and competence are more readily achieved and the sense of personal pleasure and intrinsic gratification is more intense in those activities that are most closely matched to one's neurobiologic and psychologic structure
- competence and achievement are most readily seen and verified in the end-product or outcome of an activity, thus, the ability to do, to overcome, and to achieve becomes obvious to self and others.

These factors all play a major role in eliciting motivation and engagement and in defining personal meaning to the person.

Becoming part of human society has been described as the process that transforms primitive actions into behaviors that both satisfy personal needs and contribute to the development of society (Fidler & Fidler, 1978 [see Chapter 7], 1983; Moore & Anderson, 1968). The importance of doing—of occupational performance—in this transformation and in the consequent configuration of an individual pattern of daily living activities is a fundamental focus of occupational therapy and of the Life Style Performance Model. Understanding the relevance of occupational performance—of purposeful activity—to human development, health restoration, and the quality of life involves complex mixes of anthropologic, historic, physical, psychologic, sociocultural, political, and economic variables. It is from these multidimensional dynamics that the scientific base of occupational therapy must seek to explain how doing or being occupied relates to the dimensions of physical integrity, psychologic structure, and social relatedness. The scientific base, furthermore, must seek to explain how such relationships then generate a person's ability to fulfill personally relevant activities and roles of everyday living in ways that are mutually satisfying to self and significant others. The Life Style Performance Model offers a framework for the study, practice, and testing of such undertakings.

Because the model is concerned with identifying and describing a contextual configuration of daily living activities that optimize individual wellness and quality of life, and from which idiosyncratic dysfunction can be defined, two major components are addressed. First, the model seeks to identify and describe the nature and critical doing elements of an environment that supports and fosters achievement of a satisfying, productive lifestyle. Second, it proposes a way of looking at and categorizing those activity clusters, their contextual dynamics, and interrelationships that compose the critical activities of everyday living.

The Environmental Context of the Model

The importance of the interaction between persons and environment has been studied in many professions.

Literature in the fields of anthropology, psychology, sociology, psychiatry, and, more recently, occupational therapy provide a rich resource for conceptualizing the impact of both the human and nonhuman environment on human behavior. The era of Moral Treatment, for example, demonstrated the importance of the environment in shaping the behavior of persons with mental illness (e.g., Stanton & Schwartz, 1934). During the period of renewed interest in this philosophy, numerous studies were undertaken to define and create a treatment environment that would maximize the therapeutic potential of the mental hospital (Greenblatt, York, & Brown, 1955; Jones, 1953; Stanton & Schwartz, 1934). Moos's (1974) evaluation of treatment environments further influenced the design of institutions; Goffman's (1963) work contributed considerably to understanding the influence of institutions on behavior; Searles' (1960) offered impressive evidence of the role of the nonhuman environment both in health and in mental illness; and Wolfensberger's (1972) initiatives in describing the normalizing aspects of an environment transformed institutions and homes for persons with developmental disabilities. Anthropologic studies added dimension to the growing awareness of the dynamics of an environmental context in shaping patterns of behavior and, in turn, communicating values, customs, and beliefs (Benedict, 1934; Geertz, 1973; Langor, 1942; Mead, 1964; Schwedor & LeVine, 1986).

Environmental psychology has complemented the people focus of studies through research on the impact of the physical environment on behavior (Holohan, 1986; Prohansky, Ittleson, & Rivlin, 1970). Building on the seminal work of Dewey (1916), numerous studies evaluated the impact of the environmental context on learning (Bruner, 1962, 1989; Jarvis, 1992; Moos, 1979). Moore and Anderson (1968) identified environmental elements that they considered essential for maximizing individual potential for social role learning and personal development. More recently, Fidler and Bristow (1992) described the structure and process of creating a total institutional environment that maximized the competence of both staff members and patients. Similarly, in the field of management, there is a plethora of studies attesting to the influence of environmental factors on workers' performance and productivity (Bennis, 1989; Bolman & Deal, 1984; Hersey & Blanchard, 1982; Kantor, 1983; Senge, 1990).

Looking at the phenomenon of environmental congruence, Murray (1938) explored the relationship between persons and environment, coining the phrase *environmental press*. Kahana (1975) offered an intriguing perspective in her study of the necessary fit between environmental settings and individual preferences of older persons. Yarrow, Rubinstein, and Pederson (1975) explored the congruence of environment and infant cognitive and motivational development. Fidler and Bristow's (1992) Community-Family-Individual Resource Format addressed the issue of synergy between persons and environment by looking at a number of factors and characteristics of the family or family surrogate, the community, and the person. In this context, the relationship between a person's skills, limitations, and expectations and the characteristics, values, and expectations of the family and community is seen as defining the dimensions of congruence between the person and the environment.

The influence of the environment on performance has been a consideration in occupational therapy for some time (Barris, 1982; Dunning, 1972; Kiernet, 1990; Law, 1991; Llorenz, 1984; Parent, 1978). Further evidence of the extent to which the profession considers the environment to be a critical dynamic can be found in Christiansen and Baum (1991). In this publication, several authors explore the influence of public policy and the social, cultural, and physical environments on performance. Most recently, the challenging work of Dunn, Brown, and McGuigan (1994) (see Chapter 13) offered a framework for investigating the relationship between environment and performance. These authors considered such study essential to the development of a broadened perspective and studied approach to occupational therapy intervention.

Relationship of Self, Doing, and the Environment

The Life Style Performance Model presents a view of a person's environment as comprising the interactive dimensions of interpersonal, societal, cultural, physical, and temporal elements in which that person lives and acts. It contends that an environment can maximize individual performance to the extent that it includes, emphasizes, and ensures, by the nature of its structure, its operations, and interpersonal practices, those doing experiences that optimize the following:

- *Autonomy*—to be self-determining, gain a sense of being in control of one's life, and be as self-dependent as personal needs and capacities define.
- *Individuality*—to be self-differentiating, see and know one's uniqueness, verify the existence and identity of oneself, distinguish self from others, and confirm the entitlement of one's interests, skills, and differences.
- *Affiliation*—to have evidence of belonging; be part of a dyad, group, or cluster; have associations with others; and know interdependence.
- *Volition*—to have alternatives, access to sufficient information, and latitude to make and act on one's choice.

- *Consensual validation*—to have feedback from one's activity and from other persons that verify one's perceptions and reality and to be part of reciprocal exchanges that clarify and acknowledge one's contributions and actions.
- *Predictability*—to discern and evaluate cause and effect, be able to predict, limit ambiguity and chanciness, give order to one's world, and experience the comfort of predictables.
- *Self-efficacy*—to have evidence of one's competence, of being able to cope and manage one's everyday life, of being a cause, and of making things happen.
- *Adventure*—to seek and try out the new, the unknown; to explore; to look beyond the here and now; and to discover, experiment, and dare to risk.
- *Accommodation*—to be free from physical and mental harm and to function in an environment that is responsive to individual capabilities while compensating for individual limitations.
- *Reflection*—to have respite from activity, ponder on the meaning of things, and review and contemplate recent and past events.

These elements have relevance to hospitals, institutions, and residential settings as well as to living arrangements within the home and community. They provide a base from which guidelines can be developed for evaluating, creating, adapting, or managing a living or treatment environment. For example, although the positive impact of a hospital or nursing home environment on recovery is theoretically acknowledged, many institutional environments fail in this regard. Too frequently, the occupational therapist's singular focus on the patient's functional deficit precludes attention to the context in which services are being provided. The efficacy of intervention strategies is maximized when the occupational therapy process includes activity designed to create and enhance the elements of the environment as described in the previous paragraph. The life-style of any one person is a multidimensional, dynamic phenomenon created by the inner self shaping and being shaped by the unique characteristics and dynamics of that person's human and nonhuman external world.

Structure of the Model: Four Domains

As stated earlier, achievement of social efficacy, personal satisfaction, and a way of living that is more satisfying than not to self and significant others relates directly to achieving and maintaining an age-specific, culturally relevant synergy among four primary domains of performance:

- Taking care of one's self and maintaining one's self in as self-dependent a manner as personal needs and capacities determine

- Pursuing personally referenced pleasure, enjoyment, and intrinsic gratification
- Contributing to the need fulfillment and welfare of others
- Developing and sustaining reciprocal interpersonal relationships.

These domains form the structure of a Life Style Performance Profile (Fidler, 1982) (see Appendix F) and are seen as composing an occupational or activity repertoire that encompasses the patterns of daily living activity.

Because these domains represent the principal focus of daily living activities, they are viewed as relevant throughout the life span. What may be described for any one person, at any point in time, as an adequate, relevant, and balanced life-style depends on the age, cultural orientation, and neurobiologic endowment of that person as well as the values and resources of that person's social matrix. Performance skills and life-style expectations change with different stages of life and vary in accordance with cultural and social norms.

Although each of the activity domains is characterized as having a distinct purpose, the domains are not independent entities. Rather, they are interrelated parts of a life-style, a way of living that has meaning in defining and expressing a personal and social identity and a self-regard.

The Domain of Self-Care and Self-Maintenance

Self-care is both an expression of self and a self–other link. Our commercial world and its advertising offer ample testimony to the importance of dressing, grooming, and related activities as both social and personal statements. The unique dress codes that regularly emerge among each new generation of adolescents, ethnic dress and grooming styles, the arrangement and decoration of living spaces, food choices, and cooking methods are only a few examples of how such activities are part of one's theme of personal identity as weil as a link with others. Christiansen (1994) stated that self-care activity has importance as a "foundation for enabling a shared existence with others and as part of the continuing search to understand who we are and to make meaning of our existence" (p. i).

The care and maintenance of self in as self-reliant a manner as possible also addresses the universal human need to achieve and sustain a sense of autonomy. For example, the child's need to experience self as increasingly independent frequently is first manifested in dressing and other personal care activities. The need to express one's uniqueness, one's differentiation from others, is a strong force that is expressed during these early years in many self-care and self-maintenance activities. Only later is there a beginning discovery that the auton-omously unique self is not lost in affiliation, but rather strengthened by it. Thus, one's ways and manner of caring for and maintaining the self play out the paradox of the need for individuality and affiliation with others. "Self care is part of an intimate, ego invested portrait, a powerful narrative of one's self and one's relationship with others" (Fidler, 1994, p. v).

The Domain of Intrinsic Gratification

Engagement in an activity for the sheer joy of the experience is an essential part of defining self and one's personal worth. Developing an activity repertoire with no strings attached except for the fun and enjoyment in the doing is one important dimension of getting to know self, developing an awareness of one's skills, capacities, ability to commit; caring about self; and discerning one's capacity for joy and pleasure. Csikszentmihalyi (1990) observed that "when we act for the sake of action rather than for ulterior motives, we learn to become more than what we are" (p. 42). Fidler and Fidler (1978 [see Chapter 7], 1983) called attention to the importance of the sense of pleasure, the joy of doing, and being a cause. To acknowledge and legitimize one's uniquely personal interests and needs is an important theme in shaping the quality of one's way of living. Only as we know the dimensions of self can we come to know another; only as we are able to freely care about and treasure self can we care for and value another. We are reminded by Devereaux (1984) that "the ability to develop caring relationships with others is in direct proportion to the ability to care for self" (p. 795). Searles (1960) pointed out that it is "through engagement with one's non-human world that we become more deeply human, more committed to our status as a human being" (p. 89). This domain is therefore concerned with exploring patterns of activity related to the pursuit of one's personal interests, pleasure, and joy.

The Domain of Social Contribution

Contributing to the need fulfillment and welfare of others is another critical dimension in the evolution of a mutually satisfying way of living. The identity of self as a productive member of society is molded through social and economic contributions to one's society. Engagement in those activities that are necessary for the survival and well-being of a group in society enables a sense of self as essential and verifies such contribution. The child's delight in helping with household tasks and assisting with adult chores and the stature of volunteerism or community service in American society are testimony to the importance of activities that embody social contributions and adult responsibility (Fidler & Fidler, 1978 [see Chapter 7]; Kelly & Godbey, 1992; Mosey, 1986). The dimensions of a person's social roles, such as wage earner, homemaker, student, family member, and volunteer, are themes to be explored within this domain.

The Domain of Interpersonal Relatedness

Perhaps one of the most simple and fundamental constructs about human behavior is that one becomes human through association with humans. A sense of personal acceptability, of human and interpersonal worthiness, emerges through encounters and relationships with other human beings. The importance of mutually satisfying interpersonal relationships in all aspects of living has been studied and verified well beyond question. It is axiomatic to acknowledge that a repertoire of activity patterns focused on development and maintenance of reciprocal human relationships is essential to achieving a life-style that is mutually satisfying to self and to those with whom one shares living. Verifying one's humanness and connectedness with others is a critical theme of daily living, and engagement in reciprocal human relationships is a principal dynamic in that process. Jarvis (1992) stated that "only in reciprocal relationships can being and becoming be maximized" (p. 112). The description of the nature and extent of a person's activity repertoire that enables and sustains reciprocal patterns of relating, enabling friendships, intimacy, family relationships, and peer and group affiliations are all important components of the focus of this domain.

Application of the Model

A first priority in application is coming to know and understand what is or has been a person's characteristic way of living and how that way reflects or does not reflect personal and social needs and expectations. It must again be emphasized that any deficit or dysfunction can be defined, understood, and allocated meaning only within the context of a person's life-style needs and expectations. An occupational therapy plan for either prevention or remediation therefore includes

- the development of a Life Style Performance Profile that reflects what is and has been the person's typical life-style activity pattern
- a description of current performance skill strengths and limitations relative to each of the four activity domains
- the performance expectations and preferences in each of these domains in relation to self-interest and the needs of significant others
- the balance or imbalance of harmony among the domains within the context of age and social and cultural norms and interests
- the dimensions of the family and community's social and cultural values, performance expectations, interests, economic resources and limitations, and environmental resources and constraints
- evaluation of those components of performance that notably affect performance
- individual characteristics, interests, values, and attitudes that shape performance

- the design of a recommended Life Style Performance Profile that reflects current capacities, interests, and needs relative to each activity domain.

An occupational therapy intervention plan for either prevention or remediation is designed in response to five fundamental questions. First, what does the person need to be able to do—that is, what performance skills are essential and at what level? Second, what is the person able to do—that is, what are the strengths, capacities, and interests of the person and of the external environment that can be used to enable successful intervention? Third, what is the person unable to do—which internal and external factors interfere, and how should these be addressed? Fourth, what interventions must be undertaken and in what order of priority so that the person will be able to move toward fulfilling relevant life-style performance needs and expectations? Finally, what are the characteristics and patterns of activity and the environment that will enhance the quality of this person's living?

Summary

The use of personally relevant activity, of occupation, in the development and restoration of performance skills has been the hallmark of occupational therapy since its inception. It is this focus that distinguishes the profession from other disciplines in the health or behavioral sciences. Questions surrounding the relationship of occupation to performance in daily living, coping and adaptation, and the meaning and quality of life have consistently been a principal concern of practice and inquiry in occupational therapy. More recently, society's interest in wellness and in defining health as more than the absence of disease has far-reaching importance for occupational therapy. Thus, the questions for occupational therapy have broadened and become more complex. Further exploration and critique of the Life Style Performance Model should lead to our ability to raise increasingly sophisticated questions and pursue such inquiry.

Acknowledgment

This article was developed during the author's tenure as Scholar-in-Residence, Occupational Therapy Program, College Misericordia, Dallas, Pennsylvania.

References

Barris, R. (1982). Environmental interactions: An extension of the model of occupation. *American Journal of Occupational Therapy, 36*, 637–644.

Benedict, R. (1934). *Patterns of culture.* Boston: Houghton Mifflin.

Bennis, W. (1989). *Why leaders can't lead.* San Francisco: Jossey-Bass.

Bolman, L. G., & Deal, T. E. (1984). *Modern approaches to understanding and managing organizations.* San Francisco: Jossey-Bass.

Bruner, J. S. (1962). *On knowing: Essays for the left hand.* Cambridge, MA: Harvard University Press.

Bruner, J. S. (1989). *Acts of meaning.* Cambridge, MA: Harvard University Press.

Christiansen, C. (1993). The Issue Is—Continuing challenges of functional assessment in rehabilitation: Recommended changes. *American Journal of Occupational Therapy, 47,* 258–259.

Christiansen, C. (Ed.). (1994). *Ways of living: Self care strategies for special needs.* Rockville, MD: American Occupational Therapy Association.

Christiansen, C., & Baum, C. (Eds.). (1991). *Occupational therapy: Overcoming human performance deficits.* Thorofare, NJ: Slack.

Csikszentmihalyi, M. (1990). Flow: *The psychology of optimal experience.* New York: Harper & Row.

Devereaux, E. B. (1984). Occupational therapy's challenge: The caring relationship. *American Journal of Occupational Therapy, 38,* 791–798.

Dewey, J. (1916). *Democracy and education.* New York: Free Press of Glencoe.

Dunn, W., Brown, C., & McGuigan, A. (1994). The ecology of human performance: A framework for considering the effect of context. *American Journal of Occupational Therapy, 48,* 595–607. (Reprinted as Chapter 13.)

Dunning, H. (1972). Environmental occupational therapy. *American Journal of Occupational Therapy, 26,* 292–298.

Erickson, E. (1950). *Childhood and society.* New York: Norton.

Fidler, G. S. (1981). From crafts to competence. *American Journal of Occupational Therapy, 35,* 567–573.

Fidler, G. S. (1982). The life style performance profile: An organizing frame. In B. Hemphill (Ed.), *The evaluation process in occupational therapy.* Thorofare, NJ: Slack.

Fidler, G. S. (1988a). *Examining the knowledge base of occupational therapy.* Unpublished manuscript, American Occupational Therapy Foundation.

Fidler, G. S. (1988b). *The life style performance profile. In focus: Skills of assessment and treatment.* Rockville, MD: American Occupational Therapy Association.

Fidler, G. S. (1994). Foreword. In C. Christiansen (Ed.), *Ways of living: Self-care strategies for special needs* (pp. v–vi). Bethesda, MD: American Occupational Therapy Association.

Fidler, G. S., & Bristow, B. (1992). *Recapturing competence: A systems change for geropsychiatric care.* New York: Springer.

Fidler, G. S., & Fidler, J. W. (1978). Doing and becoming: Purposeful action and self-actualization. *American Journal of Occupational Therapy, 32,* 305–310. (Reprinted as Chapter 7.)

Fidler, G. S., & Fidler, J. W. (1983). Doing and becoming: The occupational experience. In G. Kielhofner (Ed.), *Health through occupation: Theory and practice in occupational therapy.* Philadelphia: F. A. Davis.

Geertz, C. (1973). *Interpretation of culture.* New York: Basic.

Goffman, E. (1963). *Asylums.* New York: Doubleday.

Greenblatt, H. M., York, R. H., & Brown, E. I. (1955). *From custodial to therapeutic care in mental hospitals.* New York: Russell Sage Foundation.

Hersey, P., & Blanchard, K. (1982). *Management of organizational behavior.* Englewood Cliffs, NJ: Prentice Hall.

Holohan, C. J. (1986). Environmental psychology. *Annual Review of Psychology, 37,* 381–407.

Jarvis, P. (1992). *Paradoxes of learning.* San Francisco: Jossey-Bass.

Jones, M. (1953). *The therapeutic community.* New York: Basic.

Kahana, E. (1975). Matching environment to the needs of the aged—A conceptual schema. In J. F. Gubrium (Ed.), *Communities and environmental policy.* Springfield, IL: Charles C Thomas.

Kantor, R. (1983). *The change masters.* New York: Simon & Schuster.

Kelly, J. K., & Godbey, G. (1992). *Sociology of leisure.* State College, PA: Venture.

Kielhofner, G. (1985). *A model of human occupation: Theory and application.* Baltimore: Williams & Wilkins.

Kielhofner, G. (1993). The Issue Is—Functional assessment: Toward a dialectical view of person–environment relations. *American Journal of Occupational Therapy, 47,* 248–251.

Kiernet, J. M. (1990). Considering the environment. In C. B. Royeen (Ed.), *AOTA Self Study Series: Assessing Function* (Lesson 6). Rockville, MD: American Occupational Therapy Association.

Langor, S. (1942). *Philosophy in a new key.* Cambridge, MA: Harvard University Press.

Law, M. (1991). The Muriel Driver Lecture: The environment: A focus for occupational therapy. *Canadian Journal of Occupational Therapy, 58,* 171–180.

Law, M. (1993). Evaluating activities of daily living: Directions for the future. *American Journal of Occupational Therapy, 47,* 233–237.

Llorenz, L. A. (1984). Changing balance: environment and individual. *American Journal of Occupational Therapy, 38,* 29–34.

Mead, M. (1964). *Continuities in cultural evolution.* New Haven, CT: Yale University Press.

Moore, O. K., & Anderson, A. R. (1968). *Some principles for the design of clarifying educational environments.* Pittsburgh: University of Pittsburgh, Research and Development Center.

Moos, R. H. (1974). *Evaluating treatment environments: A social ecological approach.* New York: Wiley.

Moos, R. H. (1979). *Evaluating educational environments: Procedures, methods, findings and policy implications.* San Francisco: Jossey-Bass.

Mosey, A. (1986). *Psychosocial components of occupational therapy.* New York: Raven.

Murray, H. R. (1938). *Explorations in personality.* New York: Oxford University Press.

Parent, L. H. (1978). Effects of a low-stimulus environment on behavior. *American Journal of Occupational Therapy, 32,* 19–25.

Prohansky, H. M., Ittleson, W. H., & Rivlin, L. G. (Eds.). (1970). *Man and his physical settings.* New York: Holt, Rinehart & Winston.

Reilly, M. (1971). The modernization of occupational therapy. *American Journal of Occupational Therapy, 25,* 243–246.

Searles, H. (1960). *The non-human environment.* New York: International Universities Press.

Senge, P. (1990). *The fifth discipline.* New York: Doubleday.

Schwedor, R. A., & LeVine, R. A. (Eds.). (1986). *Culture theory and essays on mind, self and emotion.* New York: Cambridge University Press.

Stanton, A. H., & Schwartz, M. S. (1934). *The mental hospital.* New York: Basic.

Trombly, C. (1993). The Issue Is—Anticipating the future: Assessment of occupational function. *American Journal of Occupational Therapy, 47,* 253–257.

Trombly, C. (1995). Occupation: Purposefulness and meaningfulness as therapeutic mechanisms—1995 Eleanor Clarke Slagle Lecture. *American Journal of Occupational Therapy, 49,* 960–972. (Reprinted as Chapter 10.)

White, R. W. (1971). The urge towards competence. *American Journal of Occupational Therapy, 25,* 271–274.

Wolfensberger, W. (1972). *The principles of normalization in human services.* Toronto: National Institute of Mental Retardation.

Yarrow, L. G., Rubinstein, J. L., & Pedersen, F. A. (1975). *Infant environment: Early cognitive and motivational development.* New York: Wiley.

Chapter 12

An Attempt to Define Purposeful Activity

Estelle B. Breines, PhD, OTR, FAOTA

An initial look at the term *purposeful activity* suggests it would be difficult to define except in terms of the individual. Because purposeful activities are unique constructions for individuals, the term eludes definition as a conceptual whole.

Elude, however, does not mean defy. To elude is to hide, to evade exposure. That the profession of occupational therapy has only recently attempted to synthesize a consistent and official definition for purposeful activity (1) despite a history of repeated use of the term, is evidence of this elusiveness.

In the past, the use of purposeful activity in treatment has been debated. This discussion often centered on the meaning of the term, with therapists taking opposing positions as to those modalities and activities that they considered appropriate to practice. I, too, shall enter the debate and attempt to examine the term *purposeful activity* by addressing issues that underlie the problem of achieving its definition.

A first step in definition is to analyze each word in the term. The dictionary defines purpose as "an end to be obtained, intention, determination" (2, p 736). Activity is defined as "vigorous or energetic action, liveliness, a process that an organism participates in or carries on by virtue of being alive, a similar process actually or potentially involving mental function" (2, p 10). These definitions, when seen in light of one another, reveal that personal will is integral to the understanding of each word. Further, individual intention and choice are inherently related concepts, both to each other and to the concepts of personal will. Finally, purposeful activity suggests both mental and physical involvement. Thus, the mind/body unity to which occupational therapy subscribes correlates with the term that has long been associated with its practice.

Philosophical Origins

The education philosopher, John Dewey, expressed the concept of purposeful activity before the occupational therapy literature. In 1916, Dewey proposed that occupation is conceptually allied with purposive action inherent in play and work (3). He believed that development was structured by independently constructed striving, relevant to the individual's personal explorations. Dewey also proposed that the elements of personal choice and self-direction are enabled by active occupation. This concept is among Dewey's principles that appear to have been adopted and adapted by occupational therapy's founders toward application in health care, which is not inconceivable considering their historical relatedness (4, 5). Although the occupational therapy literature does not refer to pragmatism, it does demonstrate it. Therefore, Dewey may represent the basic philosophy upon which occupational therapy is based.

Discussion

Arguments within the profession about defining the role and tools of occupational therapy have centered around the use of purposeful activities by occupational therapists. Because there had been no official definition of the term, the need for definition increased as the profession moved from its conceptual origins toward wider health applications. As these practice vistas have expanded, it has become less clear to therapists how to deliver practice and retain their unity and identity as occupational therapists.

Several authors represent various positions around which the argument has been drawn. Fidler (6) addresses the value of tangible creations and interaction toward increasing the patient's self-image. Similarly, Huss (7) asserts that action upon environment defines occupational therapy. Yet her view includes associated neurodevelopmental principles and techniques, a dimension absent from Fidler's view of practice. Huss goes on to address the use of mechanistic modalities and rejects their use for occupational therapy. In response, English et al. (8) refute this position, defending the use of such modalities in practice. Certainly it is common knowledge that therapists in all dimensions of practice differ widely in their use of tools. Those just mentioned represent some of the variety of views occupational therapists have expressed in practice.

In analyzing these positions, it seems evident that occupational therapists define their practice by the tools they use (9) rather than by the process in which patients engage. Therefore, the arguments about definition may reflect therapist role identity conflicts rather than conceptual foundation criteria. A profession that adopts a concept of mind/body synthesis must reach beyond the tools of the therapist to reflect on the motivation or intent of patients as they engage in living.

Occupational therapy is not what therapists do to their patients. It is a collaborative effect of therapist and patient directed toward eliciting cognitive/perceptual capacities of patients through development of skill in all levels of performance (10). Therefore, purpose or purposeful action cannot be defined in terms of the tools with which, or activities in which, therapists engage their patients. Purposeful activity must be defined in terms of the unique directions of individual patients and the enabling of patients toward enhanced growth and development, and by involvement and organization of self and environment, both structural and personal.

Using these parameters for definition, all activities requiring both mental and physical involvement in which occupational therapists and their patients engage collaboratively can be assumed to be purposeful activities, if they elicit choice and provoke development. It is the occupational therapist's role to identify and ameliorate or circumvent barriers to that development. The goals must be those of the patient. Goal-directed activities assume intention and purpose on the part of the individual. It is also the therapist's role to identify will and barriers to will, assuming that with all life there is will, although perhaps not the will idealized by the therapist.

Choice, intention, or purpose are not always in conscious awareness (11). The occupational therapist can serve two roles regarding choice or purpose. One role is to bring patients' intentions beyond choice and into automaticity. Automaticity is defined as behavior that occurs without conscious awareness. For example, proprioceptive neuromuscular facilitation and neurodevelopmental training can be interpreted as a means of solving praxis disorders through clarification of antigravity discontinuity. Praxis or motor *planning* reveals an element of choice or intention in its expression. Conscious attention, or planning, is an indication that skills are being attempted, but automaticity in performance is a sign that skills have been achieved. To be able to perform skillfully requires the ability to disregard, and disregard is enabled by automaticity. Sensory integration is directed at increasing spontaneous responses as a means of eliminating barriers created by the necessity to choose among behaviors. Moving behavior from conscious to below conscious awareness and into automaticity is viewed as enabling.

On the other hand, in the second role, the therapist may be directed toward bringing patients' automaticity to conscious awareness. Group tasks that highlight interactional patterns and the use of media to elicit symbolic representations are such examples.

Issues of personal intention, occupation, and relationships associated with development were of concern to early twentieth century philosophers outside occupational therapy (3, 12). Occupational therapy appears to have adopted these principles and applied them to health care.

Much attention in the education and practice of occupational therapists has been directed toward the technology of practice and away from these early principles. This attention to tools has clouded our understanding of the pragmatic principles of personal choice upon which our profession was founded. The dispute in our profession about tools is founded on an illusion, perhaps facilitated by the medical model by which we have been directed, which is leading us away from the educational and philosophical principles upon which I suggest we were founded.

Conclusion

I conclude that purposeful activity cannot be defined by one individual for any other individual, other than that it requires both mental and physical involvement. It is a personal construction, which is solely dependent on individual choice and subject to the influence of the structural and personal environment of the individual; this position is consistent with the philosophical principles upon which the profession probably was founded. Further, it may not be valuable to stress the tools of occupational therapists; rather, the developmental process in which our patients are engaged should be emphasized. With this emphasis, the tools must follow, as I believe has been demonstrated by our current admirable level of practice, which is founded on a sound philosophical heritage.

Acknowledgment

Ann C. Mosey, PhD, OTR, FAOTA, is acknowledged for having stimulated the discussion cited here in her course in Advanced Occupational Therapy Theory at New York University.

References

1. Hinojosa J, Sabari J, Rosenfeld MS: *Purposeful Activities.* AOTA Representative Assembly, April 1983.

2. *The New Britannica/Webster Dictionary and Reference Guide.* Chicago: Encyclopedia Britannica, Inc., 1981.

3. Dewey J: *Democracy and Education.* Toronto: Collier-MacMillan, 1916.

4. Cromwell FS: Eleanor Clarke Slagle, the leader, the woman. *Am J Occup Ther 31:* 645–648, 1977.

5. Dykhuizen G: *The Life and Mind of John Dewey.* Carbondale IL: Southern Illinois University Press, 1973.

6. Fidler G: From crafts to competency. *Am J Occup Ther 35:* 567–573, 1981.

7. Huss AJ: From kinesiology to adaptation. *Am J Occup Ther 35:* 574–580, 1981.

8. English C, Kasch M, Silverman P, Walker S: On the role of occupational therapists in physical disabilities. *Am J Occup Ther 36:* 199–202, 1982.

9. Mosey AC: *Configuration of a Profession.* New York: Raven Press, 1981.

10. Breines E: *Perception: Its Development and Recapitulation.* Lebanon, NJ: Geri-Rehab, 1981.

11. Hofstadter D: *Godel, Escher and Bach: The Eternal Golden Braid.* New York: Basic Books, 1979.

12. Mead GH: *The Philosophy of the Present.* Chicago: Open Court, 1932.

Section II

The Environmental Contexts of Purposeful Activity: Physical, Sociocultural, and Temporal Influences on Activity

Introduction

A basic philosophical premise of occupational therapy (OT) is that purposeful activity cannot be understood or used therapeutically without consideration of its environmental contexts. This premise was clearly evident in Section I in which the environmental aspects of OT were strongly emphasized by the founders of our profession and by later generations of OT scholars. These environmental contexts include the physical, social, cultural, and temporal aspects of performance (AOTA, 1994; see Appendix I). Some, if not all, of these factors will influence an individual's performance of purposeful activity; therefore, the occupational therapist must assess the individual's current and expected environment to ensure a comprehensive evaluation and a relevant plan of intervention (Mosey, 1986).

Although purposeful activity is an integral part of our entire life, the meaningfulness or value of this activity performance cannot be understood without considering the context of that performance (Dunn and Brown, 1994). Assessing a client's ability to prepare a meal in a large, well-equipped OT activities of daily living kitchen and providing intervention to teach meal preparation skills in this setting are totally irrelevant and virtually useless to the client whose only kitchen is a one burner hotplate in a single-room occupancy hotel. As Cynkin (1994) stated, "The nature of everyday activities emerges only from the context in which they are embedded" (p. 13).

Environmental contexts are critical variables in understanding, evaluating, and interpreting purposeful activity (Dunn and Brown, 1994). This section has, therefore, gathered literature that will provide the reader with the knowledge and skills needed to effectively assess the environmental contexts of everyday activities and to plan interventions that are pertinent to the environment of each individual client.

Chapter 13 begins this section with a presentation of a comprehensive framework for considering the effect of environmental contexts on human performance. The authors, Dunn, Brown, and McGuigan, provide a broad, encompassing definition of environmental contexts, emphasizing the importance of analyzing contextual features in OT evaluations and interventions. They review relevant literature from social science and OT to identify pertinent environmental concepts and definitions, establishing a foundation for their Ecology of Human Performance (EHP) framework. This EHP framework provides an organized structure for systematically considering the complexities of temporal, physical, social, and cultural contexts in OT practice. The authors describe context as a lens through which the individual views the world, with the interrelationships between the person and the contexts determining the tasks that are within the person's performance range. They propose and define five alternatives for therapeutic intervention that enable the occupational therapist to collaborate with the consumer and the family to meet performance needs within the person's environmental contexts. Numerous case examples, illustrated schemata, and clear practical suggestions complete their discussion. The use of the EHP framework to thoroughly consider context can be invaluable to a therapist for it removes the limitations and potential dangers of evaluating performance and planning intervention out of context.

This process of environmental analysis will facilitate congruence between the person and the environment, allowing for optimal functioning. However, this environmental analysis may also uncover deficits which make attaining this congruence challenging, especially when one considers the multitude of disabilities clients may have that can hinder occupational performance. As occupational therapists, we help develop adaptive environments that enable individuals to fulfill their roles and meet environmental demands for occupational performance. Therefore, guidelines and principles for designing environments supportive of maximum independent functioning for persons with disabilities are presented in Chapter 14 by Watzke and Kemp. Although this chapter specifically addresses the needs of elderly individuals, the principles and guidelines provided are highly relevant to individuals of all ages with functional limitations.

Watzke's and Kemp's discussion provides environmental design guidelines for older adults, emphasizing the attainment and maintenance of safety within the home. Their major focus is on safe mobility and environmental control. Selected environmental features, technological aids, and adaptive equipment that have the potential to enhance the in-home safety of an individual with a disability are presented. Practical suggestions for environmental modifications along the low- to high-technology continuum and resources for environmental design and technology are provided. (Additional resources and references are located in Appendix L of this text.) The authors conclude this chapter with a discussion of future needs for environmental design, product development, and empirical research.

Although Chapter 14 focussed specifically on physical environment contexts, the next two chapters study an equally important environmental context: culture. Culture influences all aspects of purposeful activity, i.e., "what we do, how, when, where, for how long, and with whom we do it" (Cynkin, 1994, p. 15). If activities are to be meaningful in clinical situations, they must meet the cultural and personal standards of the individual (Brienes, 1994). Therefore, occupational therapists must have a thorough understanding of a client's sociocultural background and environment to ensure the appropriateness of his or her evaluation and intervention.

In Chapter 15, Schemm provides a comprehensive discussion of how culture influences the OT process and the outcome of treatment. A historical analysis of views about culture held by OT founders and theorists is presented. Levine defines culture and identifies components of culture, examining how they pertain to and affect OT clinical practice. The influence of culture on a person's perception of illness, health, and therapy and a person's belief in the meaning of his or her own life and activities is explored. Guidelines for considering cultural factors during evaluation and treatment are provided along with a case study, highlighting the relevance of these factors to the ultimate outcome of OT.

Krefting, in Chapter 16 expands on Levine's exploration of culture, providing an in-depth analysis of the practical implications of culturally sensitive and culturally insensitive practice. She presents a multidimensional definition of culture, with emphasis placed on the individual level of culture and its effects on assessment and treatment. The importance of increasing awareness of one's own cultural orientation, values, and beliefs is highlighted. The costs of culturally insensitive therapy are analyzed, and strategies for enhancing cultural sensitivity are provided. Clinical examples from pediatric practice support these culturally sensitive principles, which are clearly relevant to all areas of OT practice.

One inherent component of culture that cannot be ignored in any OT practice is time. As Hall clearly explained in his landmark work on culture, "time is an element of culture which communicates as powerfully as language" (1959, p. 140). The temporal contexts of activity have a rich historical base in OT literature and practice, as evident in the founders' emphasis on the need for a temporal balance among work, self-care, play, and rest. Temporal contexts are still vitally important to OT evaluation and treatment, so the next three chapters are presented to explore the temporal aspects of activity and the nature of temporal adaptation.

In Chapter 17, Kielhofner begins this exploration with a comprehensive presentation of a conceptual framework for considering this concept in OT evaluation and intervention. Recognizing the value OT founders consistently placed on the temporal aspects of performance, Kielhofner calls for a renewed appreciation of this concept's influence on adaptation and dysfunction. He presents a review of the literature, describing characteristics of temporal adaptation and temporal dysfunction. A series of propositions about temporal adaptation are presented that can be used to develop strategies to evaluate temporal adaptation and treat temporal dysfunction in a socioculturally relevant manner. Two case examples demonstrate the application of this temporal adaptation framework to OT clinical practice.

The relevance of temporal contexts to OT practice is further explored in Chapters 18 and 19, which study the temporal patterns of two major patient populations with which occupational therapists traditionally and commonly work. Both schizophrenia and spinal cord injury (SCI) can have a devastating impact on the meaningfulness and quality of a person's use of time. Weeder presents a study that compared the temporal patterns and meaningfulness of daily activities of persons with schizophrenia and persons with no disability; Yerxa and Locker present a study contrasting the quality of time use for adults with SCI and adults with no disabilities. Weeder reviews literature relevant to temporal adaptation in general and diagnosis-related issues specific to schizophrenia, whereas Yerxa and Locker briefly describe occupational science. Both chapters identify their research questions, methods, and results. Analysis of the data reveals several significant differences and noteworthy trends in temporal patterns, meaningfulness of daily activity, and quality of time use between disabled and nondisabled populations in both studies. Implications for OT clinical practice are explored with recommendations for evaluation and treatment provided by Weeder, Yerxa, and Locker. The authors challenge occupational therapists to review their interventions to ensure that they are assisting clients with disabilities in finding alternative purposeful activities that give meaning to their lives. Although these two research studies have clear limitations and are not generalizable, their findings, discussions, and conclusions warrant thoughtful consideration and further study.

Chapter 20 by Rowles also presents a research study with significant implications for OT practice. This study explores clients' immersion into culturally defined spatiotemporal environments. Rowles' analysis integrates concepts of physical space, time, and culture with the human processes of knowing, doing, and being. An emphasis on the understanding of the nature of "being in place" and methods for researching this vital process are provided through the discussion of the extensive enthnographic study conducted by Rowles. This study clearly substantiates the relevance of understanding clients' immersion into their highly individualized life world, i.e., their "being in place." The way in which environment can become part of oneself is a significant theme with major implications for enhancing OT practice and improving clients' quality of life. Occupational therapists who are sensitive to the significance of the environment can identify interventions that are attuned to the client's lifeworld, whether that environment is a home of many years or a recent relocation. Rowles argues that increased attention and sensitivity to and concern for a persons' "being in place" is a vital part of OT practice that is highly relevant to all clients, whether they are living in a home environment or in a residential, institutional setting.

This call for an increased sensitivity to individual responses to the environment is continued in Chapter 21 by Kari and Michaels. Their presentation explores the effects of institutionalization and loss on elderly residents and the powerlessness of staff within long-term care facilities. The authors present a model project that aimed to create an empowering environment for residents, family members, volunteers, and those who work within a nursing home. Current hierarchical models for institutional governance are compared with a proposed alternative community model for residential living based on social support theory and democratic principles. The authors outline strategies for implementing this model to facilitate change within the existing power structure of an institution and to foster collaborative decision making and shared power among residents, staff, and administration. Kari and Michaels challenge occupational therapists to create environments that empower individuals with disabilities, thus enabling them to have control over their lives and to engage in meaningful life roles and purposeful activities. These empowering environments also support OT practice as a reflection of the broad holistic philosophy of our profession, rather than practice as narrowly defined by third party reimbursers and state and federal regulators.

Chapters 22 and 23 in this section expand on this concept of creating empowering environments. Crist and Stoffel discuss the impact of the Americans with Disabilities Act (ADA) on the evaluation and enhancement of work environments for persons with mental illness. Their comprehensive analysis integrates OT principles with literature on personal self-efficacy, employment readiness, and the ADA, and they provide a clear link between performance accomplishments and OT's focus on using purposeful activities and the "doing" process in intervention. ADA criteria for determining essential job functions, marginal job functions, and reasonable accommodations are clearly identified. Implications for OT practice are discussed, including the development of advocacy and attitude training programs to reduce stigma and the provision of concrete assistance to employers seeking to provide reasonable accommodation and to persons with mental illness seeking preparation for successful employment. Although Crist's and Stoffel's main focus is on clients with mental illness, the issues identified (particularly those regarding personal self-efficacy) are highly relevant to all persons with disabilities in a work setting. They challenge occupational therapists to assume leadership positions and act as agents of change to assist persons with disabilities in achieving efficacy and independence within their work environments.

In Chapter 23 Anne Grady amplifies this challenge to create enabling environments in her 1994 Eleanor Clarke Slagle Lecture on building inclusive communities. She analyzes the nature and meaning of community and examines the relationships among individuals, their families, their culture, environmental contexts, and community. Foundations for building personal communities of choice are identified. The interaction among a person's past experience, present situation, future aspirations, and ability to choose are explored as they affect the relationship between the occupational therapist and the consumer of OT services. Grady discusses the challenge for occupational therapists in understanding each person's unique community and its culture, context, and foundation. She calls for occupational therapists to develop skill in analyzing environments and environmental interaction. Current ideas about the philosophy of inclusion, societal mandates, and legislative initiatives for inclusion, along with contrasting views about disability are presented. Grady emphasizes the need to recognize disability as a dimension of diversity, not a limiting handicap. She proposes four key values for OT reflective of an interactive model of disability and supportive on inclusion and choice. She also entreats occupational therapists to create opportunities for persons with disabilities to develop their capacities within their chosen community environments. To achieve this goal, environmental barriers must be removed and supports and adaptations must be provided. Grady cautions that attitudinal and emotional barriers, supports, and adaptations must be considered along with the physical aspects of the environment. The removal of attitudinal barriers, the provision of emotional supports, and the development of physical adaptations will foster the person's ability to engage in meaningful activity within his or her natural environments. Grady also presents the spatiotemporal adaptation theory, which views development in children and ongoing functioning in adults as a transactional process between the individual and the environment. She describes a spiraling continuum of environments that promote inclusion, independence, interdependence, and successful adaptation. Interactive strategies for occupational therapists to use to build collaborative models of consumer-driven, community-based practice are presented with an emphasis on the therapeutic communication process.

Grady's call to occupational therapists to promote choice and inclusion by creating inclusive communities that welcome the gifts of diversity and by influencing sociopolitical systems and established institutions is certainly a timely one. Her advocacy for the development of proactive practice venues within the community—the environment in which engagement in "real occupation" takes place—is critical in today's evolving health care system that is emphasizing community-based care, yet limiting resources. As hospital lengths of stay decrease, clients are being discharged with a multitude of limitations affecting their ability to interact with their environment in a need-satisfying manner. Therefore, hospital-based occupational therapists must immediately evaluate the home and community environment to ensure OT intervention is relevant to the client's discharge goals. Home-care and community-practice occupational therapists must develop the necessary supports and provide the required adaptations and modifications to ensure the client's safe, active participation in his or her environment. School-based occupational therapists must expand their vision beyond the classroom to view the broader environmental contexts of children with disabilities. This view is particularly critical as students "age out" of educational systems and sadly find few opportunities to interact fully with their community environment. All occupational therapists have an ethical responsibility to advocate for sociopolitical change supportive of full inclusion and for the allocation of adequate resources to meet the needs of persons with disabilities. Our evaluations and interventions are rendered meaningless if persons with disabilities are not welcome members in their communities. A sociopolitical system that devalues persons with disabilities by providing insufficient resources will force full inclusion to remain an elusive goal, rather than becoming an achievable reality. I urge all occupational therapists to use their knowledge and skills to fight for inclusive communities that enable persons with disabilities to share their perspectives, abilities, and gifts with all of us, thereby enriching our environments and our lives.

Questions to Consider

1. Analyze your current living environment (i.e., your home and community). What are the physical, sociocultural, and temporal contexts of your occupational performance? What are environmental characteristics supportive of your performance of purposeful activities? What are environmental barriers or constraints that limit your occupational performance?

2. Imagine you acquired a serious, long-term disability. Describe your environment of choice. What environmental supports, adaptations, and modifications would be needed to maximize your occupational performance and ensure an acceptable quality of life? How would your use of time change? What purposeful activities would be essential for you to engage in to maintain temporal adaptation?

3. Pair up with a peer from a different cultural background. Discuss each culture's view of health, illness, treatment, and therapeutic relationships. Identify your culture's values, beliefs, and norms. How will these affect your role as an occupational therapist? What are potential biases within your cultural background that may affect your professional roles and tasks?

4. Visit several communities with different physical characteristics and a diversity of cultures. Identify existing supports and barriers for persons with disabilities. Be certain to consider attitudinal supports and barriers, along with the physical characteristics. What recommendations would you make for additional supports, adaptations, and modifications to create communities of inclusion? What are resources available to support your recommendations?

References

American Occupational Therapy Association (1994). Definition of occupational therapy practice for state regulation. *American Journal of Occupational Therapy, 48,* 1072–1073. (Reprinted as Appendix I).

Cynkin, S. (1995). Activities. In C. B. Royeen (Ed.). *The Practice of the Future. Putting Occupation Back into Therapy (Lesson 7).* Bethesda, MD: American Occupational Therapy Association.

Dunn, W., Brown, C., McClain, C. and Westman, K. (1995). The ecology of human performance: A contextual perspective on human performance. In C. B. Royeen (Ed.). *The Practice of the Future. Putting Occupation Back into Therapy (Lesson 1).* Bethesda, MD: American Occupational Therapy Association.

Hall, E. (1959). *The Silent Language.* New York, NY: Doubleday.

Mosey, A. (1986). *Psychosocial Components of Occupational Therapy.* New York, NY: Raven Press.

Chapter 13

The Ecology of Human Performance: A Framework for Considering the Effect of Context

Winnie Dunn, PhD, OTR, FAOTA
Catana Brown
Ann McGuigan

This chapter was previously published in the *American Journal of Occupational Therapy, 48,* 595–607. Copyright © 1994, American Therapy Occupational Association.

A person does not exist in a vacuum; the physical environment as well as social, cultural, and temporal factors all influence behavior. Taken together, those factors that operate external to the person are identified as *context* for the purposes of this article. Each person's contextual experience is unique, although many elements are shared among persons.

Consider the unique way that adults talk to young children. They may change the tone of their voices, carefully select their words, bend down to make themselves smaller, or use gestures that animate the conversation. Adults make these adaptations because they recognize the importance of context when talking to young children, such as the level of the child's communication skills or how the child might feel about talking to a big person. Use of these adaptive strategies by an adult speaking at a work meeting would be considered inappropriate because the context of a work meeting dictates other communication methods. The same need for contextually selected behavior exists in many realms of daily life. A Catholic who attends services at a synagogue derives different meaning from the experience than does her Jewish friend. When a family eats at a fast-food restaurant, a different repertoire of behaviors may be sanctioned than if that same family went to a restaurant with menus at the table. Context influences behavior and performance in many ways; disciplines that address human behavior must consider the effect of these contextual features on target behaviors.

A recurring theme in the occupational therapy literature is the concept that environment (i.e., context) is a critical factor in human performance. Despite this emphasis, the potential contribution of contextual features in evaluation and intervention relative to performance components and performance areas has received little attention. For example, occupational therapy has many assessments that examine muscle strength, social skills, vestibular function, dressing, or use of leisure time. However, contextual features such as the physical qualities of an environment, the cultural background of the person, or the effect of friendships on performance are often missing from assessment tools typically used in occupational therapy. The Ecology of Human Performance (EHP) framework has been developed by the occupational therapy faculty members at the University of Kansas in response to the lack of consideration for the complexities of context. The framework provides a structure for thinking of context as a key variable in assessment and intervention planning, while elucidating the inherent dangers in examining performance out of context.

Ecology is concerned with the interrelationships of organisms and their environments. Occupational therapy is interested in the interrelationship of humans and their contexts and the effect of these relationships on performance; hence this framework is entitled the Ecology of Human Performance.

The EHP framework provides guidelines directed at including contextual features in occupational therapy research and practice (Mosey 1992). It draws from occupational therapy and social science knowledge to contribute a complementary perspective of ecological principles. As a framework, it delineates and defines the relevant concepts and describes relationships among variables. It provides direction for the development of specific frames of reference concerned with context or the reexamination of existing frames of reference and their attention to context. The following literature review acknowledges the major contribution of others in the development of this framework and provides the groundwork for understanding the EHP.

Relevant Literature from Social Science

The EHP framework is founded on and synthesizes the work of scholars in several disciplines who have considered the interaction between person and environment. Much of the original work was conducted by environmental psychologists who examined the interrelationship of the physical environment and human behavior or experience. In environmental psychology, persons are considered to be interdependent with their immediate environment; the focus of research is on the interaction of the physical elements of a person's immediate environment with behavior (Holahan, 1986; Wicker, 1979).

Although the EHP framework shares this emphasis on examining the interdependent relationship between the person and the physical environment, it expands the concept of context–environment to include physical, temporal, social, and cultural elements. Employing a broader definition of environment allows researchers to make explicit those elements that have frequently been left implicit by the environmental psychologists. For example, Wicker (1979) described the effect of settings on behavior and detailed how behavior might be modified to be appropriate for a particular environment. Implicit in his analysis is the assumption of a shared concept of the external environment. The use of context in the EHP framework balances the emphasis on the external environment presented in environmental psychology and suggests that the researcher–practitioner consider what the environment means to the person.

Hart (1979) conceptualized the environment as an instrument of socialization. He presented the concept of environmental competence as the "knowledge, skill and confidence to use the environment to carry out one's own goals and to enrich one's experience" (p. 343). Like other environmental psychologists, he emphasized that the process of learning about self and the environment is interactional and he limited the concept of environment to the physical environment.

The idea that context and person are interactional is fundamental to the EHP. It is assumed that persons both affect and are affected by their context. Although the interactional relationship between person and environment is of primary importance to environmental psychologists, none has described this process as completely as Bruner (1989). He developed the concept of transactional contextualism as a process in which the person constructs the self in the context of the environment. For example, a child who grows up in a large family develops a different construction of self than a child who grows up without siblings.

Lawton's conceptualization of environment more closely resembles that of the EHP than do those of other environmental psychologists. He presented a broader concept of environment that includes the personal, suprapersonal, and social as well as the physical (Lawton, 1982). Applying Murray's (1938) concept of environmental press to the physical environment, Lawton (1982) developed an ecological model of aging that describes the dynamics of ecological change, competence, and environmental press in which a person's environment affects perceptions of competence. In this model, behavior is thought to be "a function of the competence of the individual and the environmental press of the situation" (p. 43).

Hall (1983) and Zerubavel (1981) have examined the concept of time as an aspect of environment. Both considered time as context. Hall portrayed time as a factor that is different when persons live it and when they consider it. He argued for a contextually bound, culturally idiosyncratic, realistic concept of time. Zerubavel asserted that time is a major parameter of environment and that the two must mesh to produce a meaningful gestalt. Csikszentmihalyi (1990) described "flow" experiences in which persons are so immersed in a selected task that they are unaware of the passage of time. These authors' discussions of time as context provide excellent examples of the importance of considering time to be a component of context.

Several issues have been raised by those who have considered the relationship of environment to behavior. Many authors have distinguished between the phenomenological and physical nature of the environment. The EHP recognizes the role played by both. Gibson (1986) discussed both these aspects in his consideration of the relation between ecological context and visual perception. He suggested that the environment is both physical and phenomenological in that persons perceive objects in the environment by the affordances they offer. The environment–context is meaningful to the person by what it offers or allows the person. The EHP framework incorporates this interpretive phenomenological perspective in its consideration of the relationship between the person and context.

Developmental psychologists have also examined the effect of environment on behavior. For the most part, they have emphasized social aspects of environment. Bronfenbrenner's (1979) ecological model for human development applied an ecological systems model to human development. It presented a system of social relationships that provided the context for child development. Bronfenbrenner also developed the concept of ecological validity, in which he argued that research was not valid unless it was grounded in context. The EHP framework might enable professionals to consider whether therapeutic intervention could be valid if it were not grounded in context.

Vygotsky (1978) also examined the contribution that social environment makes to development. Wertsch (1985) summarized Vygotsky's principles by describing how context could affect development in the theory of the zone of proximal development. For Vygotsky, the zone of proximal development was the distance between a child's actual development and a higher level of potential development. Vygotsky argued that intervention during periods of sensitivity might allow the child to develop to a higher level than might have otherwise occurred, that is, an alteration of the child's regular context could affect development.

The importance that the EHP framework places on context is consistent with the emphasis placed on ecology and context by Auerswald (1971). Auerswald's work on ecological epistemology was among the earliest applications of an ecological perspective to therapeutic intervention. He argued that the processing of information from a holistic ecological perspective should replace simpler linear cause-and-effect thinking in therapeutic intervention. He identified a keynote of this kind of ecological thought as the "concern with the context in which a phenomenon occurs" (1971, p. 263). His position was that contextual issues should be considered before any therapeutic intervention began.

Relevant Occupational Therapy Literature

The environmental psychologists have contributed to the thinking of many occupational therapists. Kiernat (1992) applied the Lawton-Nehamow ecological model in her discussion of the environment as a modality. Barris (1982) drew from the work of Wicker and Hall in her conceptualization of environmental interactions. Howe and Briggs (1982) described an ecological systems model for occupational therapy that included the theories of Auerswald, Bronfenbrenner, and Wicker, whereas Spencer (1991b) used the ideas of Hall and Lawton in her discussion of physical environment and performance.

The terms *environment* and *context* are used interchangeably in the present review, dependent on the word contained in the original work. Although the occupational therapy literature has most commonly used the term *environment*, more recent authors have used the term *context*. The latter term was chosen for the EHP framework because context encompasses more of the person's physical, social, and phenomenological experience.

The concept of environment in theoretical occupational therapy literature is typically explained from two positions. In one, the environment is described primarily as a tool employed by the therapist in the intervention process. For example, Llorens (1970) defined occupational therapy intervention as the provision of environments that assist persons whose developmental cycle has been disrupted. Fidler and Fidler (1978) (see Chapter 7) explained that persons develop skills and mastery through interaction with the human and nonhuman environment. She appreciated the individuality of this interaction and recognized the influence of social and cultural norms. King (1978) (see Chapter 8) described intervention as the use of the environment to elicit adaptive responses.

In the other position, the relationship of the environment and the person is characterized from the perspective of general systems theory. The application of general systems theory to occupational therapy has facilitated the understanding of person and environment interaction. Reilly (1962) (see Chapter 6) was the first to apply the constructs of general systems theory and to include the rules of hierarchy as organizing principles. The person and environment are therefore viewed as interdependent, interacting through a system of input, output, and feedback.

General systems theory and hierarchical structures provide a framework for the Model of Human Occupation (Kielhofner & Burke, 1980). The components of the environment are identified as objects, persons, and events that again interact with the person in an open system. Kielhofner and Burke included throughput as an element of the system that is made up of three hierarchically arranged subsystems: volition, habituation, and performance. Barris (1982) used the framework of the Model of Human Occupation to clarify environmental properties and their influence on the person.

Occupation science organizes the study of humans as occupational beings through the Model of Human Subsystems That Influence Occupation (Clark et al., 1991). This model, based on general systems theory, represents the person as six hierarchically arranged subsystems that interact with the environment in an open system.

Howe and Briggs (1982) developed the Ecological Systems Model, which uses general systems theory to portray interconnections of the person and the environment as concentric circles with the person at the center surrounded by environmental layers. They detailed the model's view of function and dysfunction, which considers both the person and the environmental context.

In defining occupation, Nelson (1988) (see Chapter 41) described the dynamics of occupational form and occupational performance within the framework of a system. Occupational form was defined as "an objective set of circumstances, independent of and external to a person" (p, 633). Nelson emphasized that performance can only be understood in terms of the occupational form. Moreover, occupations are characterized as occurring at different levels.

Christiansen (1991) discussed the effect that general systems theory has had on organizing the complex concepts involved in occupational therapy. General systems theory has allowed these complexities to be understood while avoiding reductionistic views that oversimplify phenomena.

General systems theory is congruous with the EHP. However, the conceptualization of the EHP is distinguished by a nonlinear, dynamic perspective. Dynamic principles describe systems as multiply determined, complex, and self-organizing (Thelen, 1992). They eschew schemas and static programs and emphasize variability. Persons may tend toward certain modes, behaviors, or patterns; however, small changes in the person or context alter these tendencies. Persons self-organize by adapting to these changes. When persons are unable to successfully self-organize, the occupational therapist provides interventions that encompass the complex relationship of the person and his or her context. In dynamic systems, hierarchies can exist to suggest patterns but are not requisite parts of the system.

The EHP provides a framework for examining situations that occupational therapists encounter every day. For example, the framework illustrates why some people in the intermediate stages of Alzheimer's disease may be able to live in a home environment, whereas others may be more comfortable in a nursing facility (i.e., the supports available to enable the person to function safely at home may be available to the first person, but not to the second one). The framework also illustrates why not all persons require prevocational training before they can work competitively (i.e., the contextual supports and cues available in the actual work environment may enable the person to perform the work task more consistently than in simulated task performance, which does not contain these supports). The EHP deciphers the variance in disruption of daily life that persons experience with disability, illness, or stress from a contextual perspective.

Recently, context's significance has received more attention in the occupational therapy literature. Mosey (1992) included context as one of three categories in occupational therapy's domain of concern. She classified age and environment as the components of context that "provide the perspective from which performance components and occupational areas are viewed relative to the individual" (1992, p. 260). Schkade and Schultz (1992) described occupational adaptation as a frame of reference that gives equal importance to the environment and the person. Occupational adaptation is organized by a holistic, nonhierarchical approach; however, the linear perspective of occupational adaptation distinguishes it from the nonlinear view of the EHP framework.

Several authors have strongly advocated the inclusion of context in occupational therapy assessment. Dunn (1993) recommended using a contextual approach to assessment so that the assessment is relevant to the person and addresses the person's wants and needs. Kiernat (1990) stated that environment is a factor in disability and must be considered when assessing function. Fisher (1992) advocated for the recognition of occupational therapy's unique perspective of function in the assessment process. She emphasized the importance of considering the meaningfulness of the measure and placing the assessment within context. Ethnographic methods have been proposed as a means of including context in occupational therapy assessment (Spencer, Krefting, & Mattingly, 1993). Proponents of ethnography have suggested that these methods can present a more realistic analysis of the person relative to the expectations within a setting.

The current literature has also discussed the application of contextual elements. Spencer (1991a) studied the relationship of social and cultural factors to independent living alternatives. Barney (1991) identified culture as a basic contextual determinant when providing services to older adults in need of assisted living.

In summary, although the occupational therapy literature has consistently included environment as a salient feature of performance, no author has proposed a framework for systematic consideration of environment–context. It is imperative that occupational therapy begin to directly address the features of context; this knowledge will broaden perspectives on successful intervention possibilities.

The EHP Framework

The EHP was developed to provide a framework for investigating the relationship between important constructs in the practice of occupational therapy: person, context (temporal, physical, social, and cultural [American Occupational Therapy Association, 1995) (see Appendix), tasks, performance, and therapeutic intervention, to better understand the domain of human performance. The primary theoretical postulate fundamental to the EHP framework is that ecology, or the interaction between person and the environment, affects human behavior and performance, and that performance cannot be understood outside of context.

The person in this framework includes one's experiences and sensorimotor, cognitive, and psychosocial skills and abilities. The person is represented by a simple stick figure in the circle (see Figure 1). The circle surrounding the person represents the person's context (physical, temporal, social, and cultural features); the only way to see the person is to look through the context. In Figure 1, a wedge has been cut out of the context to make the person easier to view. The ellipse in the diagram is the cut edge, enabling the reader to see the person. In this model, it is impossible to see the person without first seeing the context.

The circles with the Ts inside represent the tasks that are available to persons. *Tasks* are defined as objective sets of behaviors necessary to accomplish a goal. Everyone has the opportunity or the possibility of performing myriad tasks. Persons use their skills and abilities to focus attention on specific tasks from these possibilities.

When persons use their skills and abilities to perform tasks, they use environmental cues and features to support performance. Figure 2 illustrates a typical person embedded in a context supporting regular behavior, who has a particular focus on a particular area of performance. For example, a person may notice that the red light is on at the street corner, indicating the need to stop. A person's

contexts are continuously shifting; as contexts shift, the behaviors necessary to accomplish a goal also change.

When persons use their context to support performance, it is like using the lens within the eye to get a perspective on the world. As Figure 2 indicates, the contextual lens interacts with persons' skills and abilities to enable persons to perform certain tasks. The resulting scope of action is called the performance range (see Appendix). Persons view different potential tasks through their contextual filter, the accumulation of their experiences, and their perceptions about the physical, social, and cultural features of their current performance setting. One person might look toward being a downhill skier and another might look toward being a writer or a cook, but everyone looks through a context to derive meaning about needs or desires.

Occupational therapy also considers a person's life roles. Figure 3 illustrates how roles may be characterized in this model: it displays three roles (cook, mother, and wife) as a constellation of tasks; some of these roles overlap. Each person who has the roles of wife, cook, and mother includes a unique configuration of tasks in each role as a consequence of her skills and experiences and the demands of her context. For example, if one person is a gourmet cook, she might have more tasks in the cook configuration than another person who uses a microwave oven to prepare meals or goes to restaurants.

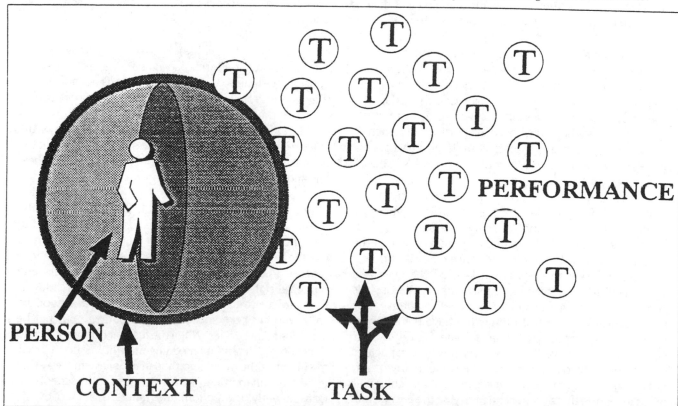

Figure 1. Schemata for the Ecology of Human Performance framework. Persons are embedded in their contexts. An infinite variety of tasks exists around every person. Performance results when the person interacts with context to engage in tasks.

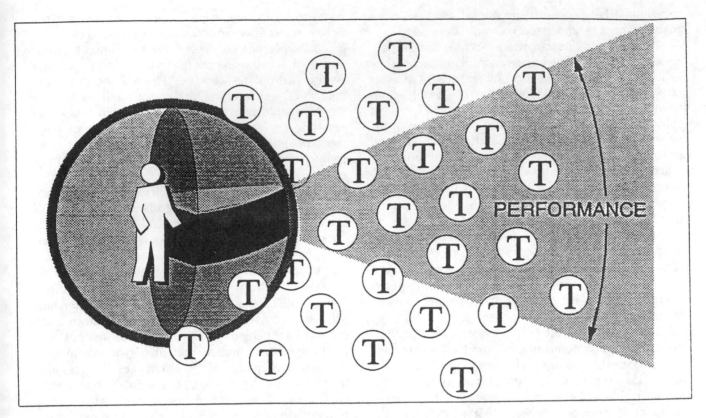

Figure 2. Schemata of a typical person within the Ecology of Human Performance framework. Persons use their skills and abilities to look through the context at the tasks they need or want to do. They derive meaning from this process. Performance range is the configuration of tasks that the persons execute.

The temporal context is also relevant to role characterization. For example, a child's role as cook might involve simpler recipes than an adult's. A person who has sustained an acute injury, such as a broken leg, may adapt the role of cook until it is possible to go out to restaurants again, whereas a person with a chronic disability, such as a head injury, may need to learn completely new cooking strategies. A person's configuration of the roles is based on the person's skills, abilities, context, and desires.

A person may have more limited skills and abilities but be embedded in a regular context that typically supports performance. This person may have the same possible cues and supports available in the context as that of the person in Figure 2, but the performance range is narrower because this person does not notice all the cues and supports. When a person has a more limited set of skills and abilities, then the person may either derive less meaning from the context or may not have the personal resources to support performance (see Figure 4). This person may not have the necessary physical capacities (e.g., a person who is blind may not be able to drive), may not pick up the cues the context provides (e.g., a child may fail to recognize that another child is trying the engage him or her in play), or may not know how to take advantage of contextual features (e.g., a person may stand in a full-service lane at the grocery store with only four items when

an express lane is available). Each condition may result in a more limited performance range. The tasks that are possible are limited because the person is not able to use the resources that might be available to support performance in the context.

For example, if a person is learning to ski, all of the contextual features are available to support skiing but the person initially lacks the skills to perform the skiing behaviors and so has a more limited performance range. An adult with developmental disabilities may need transportation to work. The bus system is available in the context; all the features are there to allow persons to use the bus to get to work, but the person may not have the skills necessary to use those features to an advantage, so the performance range is limited. A child may have attentional deficits and limited social skills. Although the context for this child has the same cues that it has for every other child at school, the child who has poor social skill development may not be sensitive to these cues. When the teacher frowns, this child may not understand its meaning, may not notice, or may misinterpret the frown and thus may behave in a way that is viewed as inappropriate for the context of the school day. Consequently, the performance range is limited by the inability to take advantage of the cues or by the irrelevance of the cues to the person. When a person has limited skills and abilities, these limitations can be compounded by

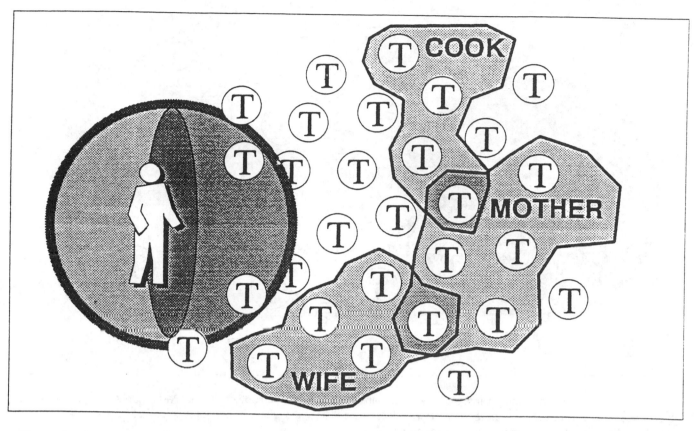

Figure 3. Illustration of roles in the Ecology of Human Performance framework. Life roles are a constellation of tasks. Persons have many roles; some tasks fall into more than one role. These role configurations are unique for each person.

inability to use contextual features to an advantage in support of performance.

Sometimes, there is a more limited contextual environment available to the person, but the person possesses typical skills and abilities (see Figure 5). For example, a gourmet cook may have extensive cooking skills, but in a kitchen with only a toaster oven, that cook has limited ability to demonstrate those skills and abilities. A skillful downhill skier has a difficult time demonstrating those skills in the tropics; the person must travel to a more contextually relevant location.

Persons with disabilities sometimes have limited skills and abilities and are also in an impoverished context (e.g., a person with severe mental illness who is also homeless). They do not have a context that provides them with the salient cues and the objects or events that are relevant to them to support performance. Performance of daily life tasks, work, or leisure activities in this situation becomes even more complex.

Therapeutic Intervention Within the EHP

Occupational therapy is most effective when it is imbedded in real life. If occupational therapists evaluate

individual performance without considering the context of the performance, there is a great risk of interpreting the behavior inappropriately. Misinterpretation can lead to inappropriate choices about therapeutic intervention. For example, consider an occupational therapist working with a young woman and her daughter, who was physically ready to feed herself. The woman resisted the occupational therapist's repeated suggestions to use more independent eating strategies. Upon completing a home visit, the occupational therapist discovered that the mother only knew how to interact with her daughter during mealtime. At other times, the child sat on the floor with toys, but with no direction or interaction. The home visit made it clear to the occupational therapist that the mother was reluctant to give up her only time of interaction with her daughter. This new insight helped the occupational therapist redirect therapeutic efforts so that the mother and child could play together in a manner that was satisfying to both. By not considering context, this occupational therapist would have put this mother in the difficult situation of having to compromise her relationship with her daughter by following the therapist's suggestions. Additionally, by not considering context, the therapist would have taken the risk that

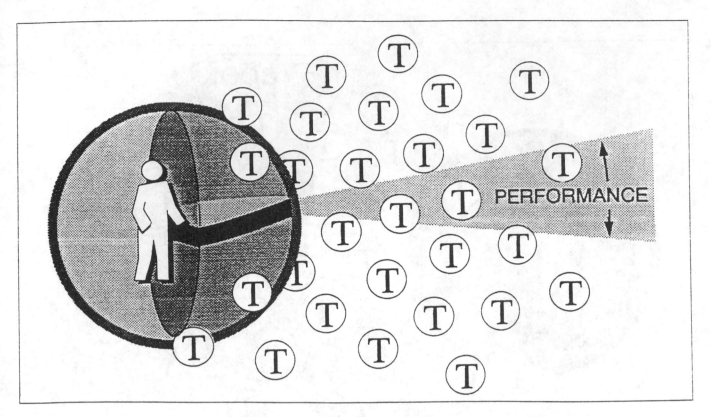

Figure 4. Schemata of a person with limited skills and abilities within the Ecology of Human Performance framework. Although context is still useful, the person has fewer skills and abilities with which to look through context and derive meaning. This lack limits the person's performance range.

the child would not make progress because the mother might not have followed her suggestions.

A naturalistic study by deVries & Delespaul (1989) examined context and the experiences of persons with schizophrenia. They concluded that knowledge of context provided a new clinical tool. In one example, a man with schizophrenia was having severe problems with hypertensive illness. Clinical investigation to determine the cause of his high blood pressure was puzzling. An analysis of this man's context revealed that he worked as a dishwasher and became extremely anxious when he had to sort silverware during the lunch rush. The clinician was able to use this contextual information to convince the employer to change the employee's work tasks. Consequently, the man's blood pressure decreased to near normal.

Relationships among the EHP framework and the variety of interventions available to the occupational therapist are shown in Figure 6. Within this framework, therapeutic intervention is a collaboration among the person, the family, and the occupational therapist directed at meeting performance needs. Figure 6 displays five alternatives for therapeutic intervention; the Appendix contains definitions of each therapeutic intervention.

Establish or Restore

The first therapeutic intervention alternative is to establish or restore (remediate) the person's skills and abilities. In this category, the occupational therapist identifies the person's skills and the barriers to performance and designs interventions that improve the person's skills and abilities. The occupational therapist, person, and family might be concerned with reestablishing the person's role in the family, and so might work on coping skills or physical endurance to enable the person to perform tasks related to the family role. Restorative approaches are common options chosen by therapists, particularly within the medical model, which considers what is wrong with the person and sets a plan to correct the problem. This approach is adapted, especially with young children, to include establishing needed skills for function. For example, a therapist might work on the muscle tone of a child with Down syndrome so that the child can move about to play with friends. Adults use these approaches within their own lives when they learn a new skill or when they work to restore a lost function (e.g., increasing range of motion in a joint after removing a cast).

Even when the focus of intervention is on skill development, context is still important. For example, Abreu and Hinojosa (1992) suggested that predictable environments provide the feedback necessary to correct motor behaviors. Toglia (1992) explained that an understanding of the interactions of person, task, and environment is essential to effective cognitive rehabilitation strategies.

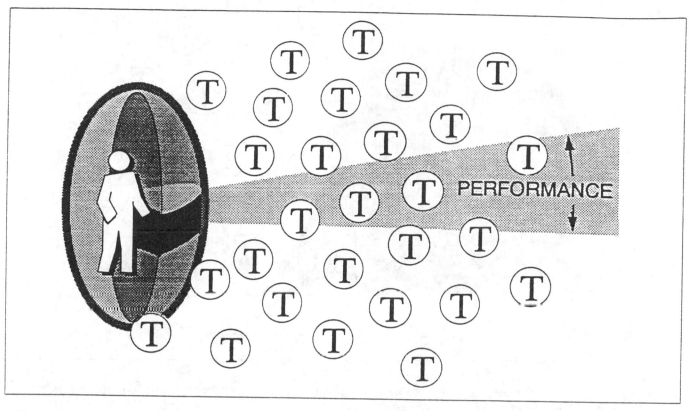

Figure 5. Schemata of a limited context within the Ecology of Human Performance framework. The person has adequate skills and abilities, but the context does not provide resources needed to perform. In this situation, performance range is limited.

Alter

The second therapeutic intervention alternative is to alter the actual context in which persons perform. This intervention emphasizes selecting a context that enables the person to perform with current skills and abilities. The person can be placed in a different setting that more closely matches his or her current skills and abilities, rather than changing the present setting to accommodate the person's needs. The occupational therapist would consider the person's skills, abilities, and difficulties and find a context that was compatible with this performance profile. The important feature of the alter intervention is that the therapist does not set out to correct the person or the environment; instead, the therapist is looking for the best match between the person and current contextual features available. Allen (1992) acknowledged the lack of direction for occupational therapists working with persons beyond the acute phase of illness who must live with functional limitations. Her frame of reference provides guidelines for making the best fit for persons with cognitive disabilities and available contexts.

Fairweather (1980) used the alter strategy in his Lodge Society, a community program for persons with severe mental illness. He was concerned that persons who were able to succeed in jobs at the hospital were unsuccessful at work in the community because of the intolerance for behavior that was viewed as deviant. One strategy was to create janitorial crews that worked at times and in settings where their contact with others was limited.

Another example involves a person who has low assertiveness ability and needs to buy a car. Although the therapist could work on assertiveness skill development or visit the car dealer to offer some adaptations to the process to facilitate the person's purchase, an alternative that uses the alter intervention option would be for the therapist to suggest that the person buy a car at a dealership that employs the no-haggling approach. Some manufacturers market their sales strategy as one that minimizes the need for assertiveness because there is one price for their cars and no negotiating is necessary. The therapist does not have to change the context and the person can succeed with current skills to purchase the car.

Adapt

The occupational therapist can also adapt the contextual features and task demands to support performance in context. When therapists adapt, they design a more supportive context for the person's performance.

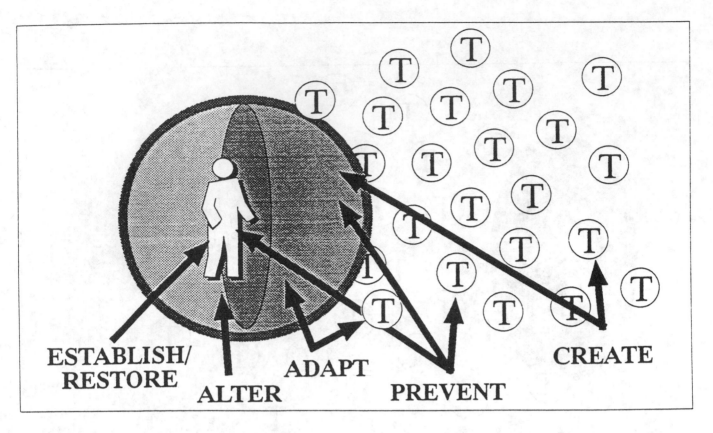

Figure 6. Illustration of therapeutic interventions within the Ecology of Human Performance framework. The arrows indicate the variables that are affected by each intervention.

Therapists might enhance some contextual features to provide cues and reduce other features to minimize distractibility and make the task more possible for the person. When children are distractible, therapists suggest shorter assignments for their seat work in class. When an adult with severe disabilities needs to manage the home environment, the therapist might select an environmental control unit. Therapists adjust desk and table configurations to meet individual needs. They might change a desk's height to match the person's postural support needs or might find a lower table in the dining area for someone whose ethnic background suggests preference for a lower eating surface. Many persons use stick-on notes to help them remember things they need to do. Persons whose vision is failing may purchase hard-cover novels because they have huger print than paperbacks. Buning and Hanzlik (1993) reported a single-subject study in which the person's context was considered in technological adaptations. In this case, computer technologies were used so that a doctoral student with severe visual impairments could complete her dissertation.

Prevent

The fourth therapeutic intervention option is to prevent the occurrence or evolution of maladaptive perfor-

mance in context. Sometimes, therapists can predict that certain negative outcomes are likely unless intervention is provided. Therapists can create interventions to change the course of events by addressing person, context, and task variables to enable functional performance to emerge. This view is supported by Coulter (1992) who proposed that prevention efforts in mental retardation must take an ecological approach that focuses on the interaction between persons and their environment. Department managers employ a prevention approach when they provide an orientation for newly hired employees; managers do not wait until the employee faces a problem to instruct them in proper procedures. Runners who stretch before running are employing a prevention approach. Occupational therapists teach persons with spinal cord injuries how to adjust their position frequently to prevent contractures and decubitus ulcers. Therapists also provide lifting classes in industrial settings to prevent work injuries. Therapists can construct a map of community services for a person with severe mental illness who is moving to a new apartment area to prevent him or her from feeling socially isolated. Prevention approaches anticipate possible and likely problems and change the course of activities to increase positive outcomes. Prevention approaches are good options for persons with long-term conditions that lead to secondary problems; the temporal context is relevant to these person's outcomes.

Create

The fifth therapeutic intervention option is creating circumstances that promote more adaptable or complex performance in context. This therapeutic intervention does not assume that a disability is present or that a disability has the potential to interfere with performance. The person or family seeking assistance may see the problem from a functional performance standpoint, not from a disability standpoint. The therapist participates by providing expertise to enrich contextual and task experiences that will enhance performance. Circumstances that do not presume disability are constructed; this is what distinguishes the create intervention from the prevent intervention, which addresses precluding the occurrence of a problem that is likely to arise. Early intervention programs are common examples of community-based programs that have an enriching philosophy; therapists use their expertise to plan age-appropriate tasks that embellish the young children's development. Therapists might also participate in the development of living communities for elders that provide varied and stimulating activities. These community settings do not presume their consumers have disabilities. They are designed to make the best possible use of environment to enhance living and development. For example, a large building complex may have many signs to lead visitors and workers to correct locations efficiently, not because there are presumed disabilities, but because signs make the environment easier for everyone. When adults play an icebreaker game at the beginning of a party they are creating an enriched environment for socialization.

Occupational therapists have many therapeutic choices with each person they serve, and at each point along the therapeutic relationship. Therapists often employ several intervention approaches either simultaneously or across time. Table 1 shows two examples of how an occupational therapist might deal with a person and family who need occupational therapy services from all of these approaches. When occupational therapists include context in the total perspective, it creates possibilities; when persons are viewed out of context, viable options are lost.

Directions for Future Work

The EHP proposes the relationships among the key variables of person, context, tasks, and performance. Within the domain of concern of occupational therapy, context is only relevant as it relates to human performance.

Mosey (1981) indicated that a frame of reference must describe postulates that allow application to prac-

Table 1
Case Examples Applying the Ecology of Human Performance Framework

Area Addressed	Strategy Employed/Information
	CASE 1
Background	M is 15 months old; he has two older siblings and both of his parents living in his home. He has very low muscle tone and a developmental delay and his family wants him to play and socialize.
Establish/Restore	The therapist decides to work on M's eye contact and vocalizing as ways for the family to know that M is paying attention to them.
Alter	The therapist suggests that the family enroll M in a part-time day care program so he can have the stimulation of the other children playing as a way to learn play skills.
Adapt	The therapist talks to the family about moving the toys closer, having the siblings move closer when they play with M. The therapist works with the siblings to help them learn how to change their voice tone so that M can pay attention easier.
Prevent	The therapist decides to work on functional communication strategies to prevent M's frustration at socializing. The therapist works with the family to pick some simple gestures and sounds that everyone recognizes as communication signals from M, so he can get some basic needs met.
Create	The therapist and parents discuss the usefulness of getting together with other families from the church that have similar aged children for a family gathering. This will be a positive socialization experience for all members, and involve M in a typical socialization opportunity.
	CASE 2
Background	Ms. T is a 75-year-old who has had a right hemisphere stroke. She lives with her son and daughter-in-law and two grandchildren.
Establish/Restore	The therapist decides to work on functional range of motion for reaching and stepping.
Alter	The therapist and Ms. T discuss her need to socialize and Ms. T expresses concern over her usual socializing in the quilting club, which expects a certain level of performance. The therapist suggests Sunday school as a place to socialize that doesn't require the fine motor control.
Adapt	The therapist brings clamps to help her with her stitching so that she could still do some stitching. The therapist brings her a stocking darner and velcro to attach to key items in the bathroom when she expressed desire to dress and complete personal hygiene.
Prevent	The therapist helps Ms. T to establish a daily routine to prevent joint, muscle, and skin breakdowns.
Create	The therapist helps her plan regular times to play with her grandchildren as part of the family routine.

lice and offer specific guidance for intervention. Scholars will therefore need to refine these constructs by assessing their adequacy and answering practice-oriented questions. Several lines of study provide important initial information that will refine current frames of reference that affect occupational therapy, develop new frames of reference, and create new assessment and intervention strategies.

Several questions emerge as fundamental to the investigation of basic relationships proposed in this framework. A primary question is: How do we capture contextual features objectively, and how do we then decide which features are salient for particular performance situations? We must also determine how a contextual feature becomes relevant for a particular person. There are many more contextual features available to persons in a particular context than are noticed or used by a person for successful performance. In particular performance situations, we need to determine which contextual features support or create barriers to performance. Are there particular contextual features that contribute to a person's resilience?

Occupational therapy assessment strategies also need to consider context. It will be important to determine whether standardized functional assessments are valid for capturing what is actually known about the person's performance in the natural context. For example, does the dressing item on a standardized test rate the person the same way that a therapist would rate the person if watching the person's morning dressing routine? This information will enable occupational therapists to construct initial data about persons so that planning can be individualized and relevant to their needs. It will also be important to create new, contextually relevant assessments in the future.

There are also questions that need to be answered about the proposed therapeutic interventions. For example, which interventions are the best choices for which performance problems? What is the effect of the proposed therapeutic interventions on performance outcomes? What is the difference in functional outcomes when therapeutic interventions occur in natural and contrived contexts? It is not likely that all the intervention options described here will be equally useful for all performance problems. Therefore, it will be important to test the relationships among particular performance problems and various intervention options.

The tendency to take ideas created through professional dialogue in the literature and regard them as certainty is tempting; in fact, in dialogue this is easy to do. Ideas must be tested, and it seems only fitting that ideas proposed about context be evaluated in that setting. As knowledge and understanding grow about the role of context in human performance, these initial proposals will need adaptation, a suitable outcome for a set of ideas about ecological relationships.

Appendix

Ecology of Human Performance: Definitions

Person: An individual with a unique configuration of abilities, experiences, and sensorimotor, cognitive, and psychosocial skills.

A. Persons are unique and complex and therefore precise predictability about their performance is impossible.

B. The meaning a person attaches to task and contextual variables strongly influences performance.

Task: An objective set of behaviors necessary to accomplish a goal.

A. An infinite variety of tasks exists around every person.

B. Constellations of tasks form a person's roles.

Performance: Both the process and the result of the person interacting with context to engage in tasks.

A. The performance range is determined by the interaction between the person and the context.

B. Performance in natural contexts is different from performance in contrived contexts (ecological validity, Bronfenbrenner, 1979).

Context: (adapted from Uniform Terminology for Occupational Therapy, 3rd edition):

Temporal Aspects (note: although temporal aspects are determined by the person, they become contextual due to the social and cultural meaning attached to the temporal features)

1. Chronological: person's age
2. Developmental: stage or phase of maturation.
3. Life cycle: place in important life phases, such as career cycle, parenting cycle, educational process.
4. Health status: place in continuum of disability, such as acuteness of injury, chronicity of disability, or terminal nature of illness.
5. Period: the measurable span of time during which a task exists or continues.

Environment

1. Physical: nonhuman aspects of context (includes the natural terrain, buildings, furniture, objects, tools, and devices).
2. Social: availability and expectations of important persons, such as spouses, friends and caregivers (also includes larger social groups that are influential in establishing norms, role expectations, and social routines).
3. Cultural: customs, beliefs, activity patterns, behavior standards, and expectations accepted by the society of which the person is a member

(includes political aspects such as laws that shape access to resources and affirm personal rights; also includes opportunities for education, employment, and economic support).

Therapeutic intervention: A collaboration between the person/family and the occupational therapist directed at meeting performance needs.

Therapeutic interventions in occupational therapy are multifaceted and can be designed to accomplish any or all of the following.

Establish/restore a person's abilities to perform in context. Therapeutic intervention can establish or restore person's abilities to perform in context. This emphasis is on identifying a person's skills and barriers to performance, and designing interventions that improve the person's skills and experiences.

Alter actual context in which people perform. Therapeutic interventions can alter the context within which the person performs. This intervention emphasizes selecting a context that enables the person to perform with current skills and abilities. This can include placing the person in a different setting that more closely matches current skills and abilities, rather than changing the present setting to accommodate needs.

Adapt contextual features and task demands so they support performance in context. Therapeutic interventions can adapt contextual features and task demands so they are more supportive to the person's performance. In this intervention, the therapist changes aspects of context and/or tasks so performance is more possible. This can include enhancing some features to provide cues, or reducing other features to reduce distractibility.

Prevent the occurrence or evolution of malpractice performance in context. Therapeutic interventions can prevent the occurrence or evolution of barriers to performance in context. Sometimes, therapists can predict that certain negative outcomes are likely without intervention to change the course of events. Therapists can create intervention to change the course of events. Therapists can create interventions that address person, context, and task variables to change the course, thus enabling functional performance to emerge.

Create circumstances that promote more adaptable/complex performance in context. Therapeutic interventions can create circumstances which promote more adaptable performance in context. This therapeutic intervention does not assume a disability is present or has the potential to interfere with performance. This therapeutic choice focuses on providing enriched contextual and task experiences that will enhance performance.

References

Abreu, B.C., & Hinojosa, J. (1992). The process approach for cognitive—perceptual and postural control dysfunction for adults with brain injuries. In N. Katz (Ed.), *Cognitive rehabilitation: Models for intervention in occupational therapy* (pp. 167–194). Stoneham, MA: Andover Medical.

Allen, D. K. (1992). *Occupational therapy treatment goals for the physically and cognitively disabled.* Rockville, MD: American Occupational Therapy Association.

American Occupational Therapy Association. (1995). Uniform terminology for occupational therapy—third edition. *American Journal of Occupational Therapy.* (Reprinted as Appendix I).

Auerswald, E. H. (1971). Families, change, and the ecological perspective. *Family Process, 10,* 263–280.

Barney, K. F. (1991). From Ellis island to assisted living: Meeting the needs of older adults from diverse cultures. *American Journal of Occupational Therapy, 45,* 486–593.

Barris, R. (1982). Environmental interactions: An extension of the model of occupation. *American Journal of Occupational Therapy, 36,* 637–644.

Bronfenbrenner, U. (1979). *The ecology of human development.* Cambridge, MA: Harvard University Press.

Bruner J. (1989). *Acts of meaning.* Cambridge, MA: Harvard University Press.

Buning, M. E., & Hanzlik, J. R. (1993). Adaptive computer use for a person with visual impairment. *American Journal of Occupational Therapy, 47,* 998–1007.

Christiansen, C. (1991). Occupational therapy: Intervention for life performance. In C. Christiansen & C. Baum (Eds.), *Occupational therapy: Overcoming human performance deficits* (pp. 3–44). New York: McGraw-Hill.

Clark, F. A., Parham, D., Carlson, M. E., Frank, G., Jackson, J., Pierce, D., Wolfe, R. J., & Zemke, R. (1991). Occupational science: Academic innovation in the service of occupational therapy's future. *American Journal of Occupational Therapy, 45,* 300–310.

Coulter, D. L. (1992). An ecology of prevention for the future. *Mental Retardation, 30,* 363–369.

Csikszentmihalyi, M. (1990). *Flow: The psychology of optimal experience.* New York: Harper Perennial.

deVries, M. W., & Delespaul, P. A. E. G. (1989). Time, context, and subjective experiences in schizophrenia. *Schizophrenia Bulletin, 15,* 233–244.

Dunn, W. (1993). The Issue Is—Measurement of function: Actions for the future. *American Journal of Occupational Therapy, 47,* 357–359.

Fairweather, G. W., (1980). The prototype lodge society: Instituting group process principles. *New Directions for Mental Health Services, 7,* 13–32.

Fidler, G. S., & Fidler, F. W. (1978). Doing and becoming: Purposeful action and self actualization. *American Journal of Occupational Therapy, 32,* 305–310. (Reprinted as Chapter 7.)

Fisher, A. (1992). Functional measure, Part 1: What is function, what should we measure, and how should we measure it? *American Journal of Occupational Therapy, 46,* 183–185.

Gibson, J. J. (1986). *An ecological approach to visual perception,* Hilldale, NJ: Erlbaum.

Hall, E. T. (1983). *The dance of life.* New York: Doubleday.

Hart, R. (1979). *Children's experience of place.* New York: Irvington.

Holahan, C. J. (1986). Environmental psychology. *Annual Review of Psychology, 37,* 381–407.

Howe, M. C., & Briggs, A. K. (1982). Ecological systems model for occupational therapy. *American Journal of Occupational Therapy, 36,* 322–327.

Kielhofner, G., & Burke, J. P. (1980). A model of human occupation, Part 1. Conceptual framework and content. *American Journal of Occupational Therapy, 34,* 572–581.

Kiernat, J. M. (1990). Considering the environment. In C. B. Royeen (Ed.), *AOTA Self Study Series: Assessing function (Lesson 6).* Rockville, MD: American Occupational Therapy Association.

Kiernat, J. M. (1992). Environment: The hidden modality. *Journal of Physical and Occupational Therapy in Geriatrics, 21,* 3–12.

King, L. J. (1978). Toward a science of adaptive responses. *American Journal of Occupational Therapy, 32,* 429–437. (Reprinted as Chapter 8.)

Lawton, M. P. (1982). Competence, environmental press, and the adaptation of older people. In M. P. Lawton, P. G. Windley, & T. O. Byerts (Eds.), *Aging and the environment* (pp 33–59). New York: Springer.

Llorens, L. A. (1970). Facilitating growth and development: The promise of occupational therapy. *American Journal of Occupational Therapy, 24,* 93–101.

Mosey, A. C. (1981). *Occupational therapy: Configuration of a profession.* New York: Raven.

Mosey, A. C. (1992). *Applied scientific inquiry in the health professions: An epistemological orientation.* Rockville: American Occupational Therapy Association.

Murray, H. A. (1938). *Explorations in personality.* New York: Oxford.

Nelson, D. L. (1988). Occupation: Form and performance. *American Journal of Occupational Therapy, 42,* 633–641. (Reprinted as Chapter 41.)

Reilly, M. (1962). Occupational therapy can be one of the great ideas of 20th century medicine. *American Journal of Occupational Therapy, 16,* 1–9. (Reprinted as Chapter 6.)

Schkade, J. K., & Schultz, S. (1992). Occupational adaptation: Toward a holistic approach for contemporary practice, Part 1. *American Journal of Occupational Therapy, 46,* 829–837.

Spencer, J. C. (1991a). An ethnographic study of independent living alternatives. *American Journal of Occupational Therapy, 45,* 243–251.

Spencer, J. C. (1991b). The physical environment and performance. In C. Christiansen & C. Baum (Eds.), *Occupational therapy: Overcoming human performance deficits* (pp. 125–140). New York: Slack.

Spencer, J., Krefting, L., & Mattingly, C. (1993). Incorporation of ethnographic methods in occupational therapy assessment. *American Journal of Occupational Therapy, 47,* 303–309.

Thelen, E. (1992). Development as a dynamic system. *Current Directions in Psychological Science, 1,* 189–193.

Toglia, J. P. (1992). A dynamical approach to cognitive rehabilitation. In N. Katz (Ed), *Cognitive rehabilitation: Models for intervention in occupational therapy* (pp. 104–143). Stoneham, MA: Andover Medical.

Wicker, A. W. (1979). *An introduction to ecological psychology.* Cambridge, MA: Cambridge University Press.

Wertsch, J. V. (1985). *Vygotsky and the social formation of mind.* Cambridge, MA: Harvard University Press.

Vygotsky, L. S. (1978). *Mind in society: The development of higher psychological processes.* Cambridge, MA: Harvard University Press.

Zerubavel, E. (1981). *Hidden rhythms: Schedules and calendars in social life.* Berkeley: University of California Press.

Chapter 14

Safety for Older Adults: The Role of Technology and the Home Environment

James R. Watzke, PhD

Bryan Kemp, PhD

Although an accident-free life style by no means guarantees the older adult a healthier life, there can be no disputing that accidents do seriously threaten quality of life for those older adults who experience them. The accomplishment of safety is a complicated enterprise. Most investigators would agree that the majority of accidents for older adults are a result of some combination of age-related changes, pathologic states, and environmental hazards. To complicate matters further, other host factors, such as psychologic states, may also contribute to the accident event. Also, any adequate study of accidents must include the activity in which the person is engaged, that is, the analysis must be dynamic.

Sattin et al. provide an excellent summary of this point: ". . . the most frequent fall [accident] in the elderly is a consequence of persons with diminished capacity attempting to meet the intrinsic and external demands of mobility [or any task] within specific environments."[1(p3)] Years ago, Lawton and Nahemow[2] put forth the personal competence–environmental press model of adaptation and aging, which proposed a similar view of behavior for older persons (ie, as a person–environment transaction). Another way of stating this is that older persons who do not adjust their activities and environmental demands to meet their particular level of capacities (whether they are declining or not) are at increased risk for falls or other accidents. Indeed, the health care professional's challenge is to help his or her client accomplish such a person–activity– environment congruence. Before turning to the role that technology and the built environment might play in this challenge, a brief review of some of the existing information justifying the fundamental concern with senior safety is indicated.

Human factors professionals have shown the most interest in accidents and aging as a general research topic; even so, there is a sparsity of literature in the area.[3,4] By and large, the work to date has used traditional human factors approaches (eg, age-related speed of response and visual acuity) and/or public epidemiologic databases (eg, the National Safety Council[5] and the Consumer Product Safety Commission[6,7]) to study older persons and occupational accidents,[8,9] automobile accidents,[10,11] and, most recently, home accidents with consumer products (S.J. Czaja, C.G. Drury, K. Hammond, M. Brill, V. Lotti, unpublished manuscript, 1987).

The literature generally agrees that in the United States, accidents are the fifth leading cause of death for persons older than 65 years of age; also, at least 800,000 seniors per year can be expected to receive disabling injuries from accidents.[5] Another piece of evidence of relatively higher accident rates for older adults is the fact that in a given year persons older than 65 years accounted for 43% of all documented home accidents.[3] There is also evidence that the consequences of accidents are more serious for seniors (eg, as measured by their disproportionally higher use of hospitals because of accidental injuries).[5,12]

No discussion of accidents and the older adult is complete without mention of the topic of falls. Indeed, falls deserve their status as the most studied accident in the older population. Falls, as a clinical and research topic, have found the most support in the medical community, and there is no shortage of publications in this area (for more comprehensive treatments see Sattin et al,[1] Rubenstein et al,[13] Tideiksaar,[14] and Woollacott[15]). The most common incidence statistic for falling in the elderly is about one-third; that is, for community-based persons over the age of 65 years, about one of every three can be expected to experience a fall each year.[16] Falls are estimated to account for two thirds of all fatal accidents to seniors;[13] this is around 9,500 deaths each year.[17] The vast majority of elderly falls do not result in severe injury. Only about 5% of falls result in serious injury; 1% to 2% are estimated to result in hip fractures.[1,18] For those approximately 200,000 elderly individuals who do receive fall fractures, however, the prognosis is quite bleak and comes at a cost of billions of medical dollars each year.[1,18,19]

Although, as mentioned earlier, the causes of most falls are believed to be multifactorial, it is of particular relevance to note here that many investigators have reported sizeable percentages (17% to 50%) of in-home falls as being attributable to environmental factors or hazards.[20,21] In other words, can the design and condition of one's environment as well as the products and equipment that one uses in that environment affect one's risk of falling? Inconsistent methodology in fall studies, especially in the assessment of environmental hazards, prevents a clear answer to this question. There is evidence, however, that environmental features that interfere with activities of daily living (eg, poor lighting, low seating, obstacles in walking paths, and stairs) contribute to many falls in older adults.[20–22] Concerning falls and accidents in general, the Consumer Product Safety Commission's National Electronic Injury Surveillance System data have shown that a disproportionate percentage of older adults

report accidents to hospital emergency departments involving the following products: stairs and steps, floors and floor coverings, beds, bathtubs and showers, and step stools.[4] Even though there are few hard data implicating environmental features in home accidents, manifest sense and clinical observation indicate that improved environmental safety and technology designed to increase senior safety should be important. Furthermore, such an axiom fits well with many of the underlying principles of the field of geriatric rehabilitation.[23]

In the remaining sections, a selection of environmental features, technologies, and equipment with the potential to enhance safety is highlighted. The focus is on both existing and developing technologies as well as on products that vary along the low- to high-technology continuum. The primary emphasis is in-home safety, especially safe mobility and environmental control. Because of space limitations some important safety areas are not emphasized here, namely burns, medication intake errors, driving hazards, and occupational safety hazards. For treatments of these topics, see Linn,[24] Ray and Griffin,[25] Williams and Carsten,[11] and Dillingham.[9]

Safe Mobility

Currently, most antifall interventions are not high technology. This may attest to the above mentioned complexity of the fall event. Therefore, most recommendations for safe mobility involve common sense and principles of good environmental design. For detailed treatises on this topic, see Koncelik,[26,27] Raschko,[28] Calkins,[29] and Christenson.[30]

Proper Lighting

Many older adults experience some loss in vision. One important compensation for decreased vision is the use of effective lighting. The authors' experience is that many older adults are not cognizant of effective task-lighting fit (ie, arranging lighting that is appropriate for each task performed in their daily lives). The most common lighting deficiencies found in seniors' homes are poor control of daylight (glare), too weak ambient lighting, lack of direct lighting for close-up tasks, and ineffective placement of light switches. Even a simple night light placed en route from the bedroom to the bathroom can prevent a trip or fall.

Several technologic developments have occurred in lighting in the last decade (eg, halogen bulbs and full-spectrum fluorescent bulbs), but from the perspective of safety the most crucial developments have been in the area of automatic and remote control of lighting. The safety goal here should be to light walking paths before the user even begins to walk in a given space. As a result of mass advertising a fair number of seniors seem to be aware of such products (eg, photosensitive night lights, lamps that come on by touching their base or by making a loud hand clap, or automatic lamp timers). More technologies that allow remote control of many appliances, including lamps, are discussed below.

Object-free Walking Paths

As mentioned earlier, tripping over an object is one of the major environmental reasons that older adults fall. Although common sense says to keep things out of the way of any walking path, it is quite common for a home to become cluttered. There is a set of such common objects that appears on many home safety checklists: unsecured electrical cords, throw rugs, toys, pet dishes, spilled liquids, and shoes. Less publicized but potentially hazardous are objects such as bedspreads that hang over to the floor, assistive devices, garbage (empty bottles, boxes, or cans), pets themselves, and legs and edges of furniture. The manifest solution to these hazards is organization, and there are several types of low-technology products (eg, accessible shelving and cupboard systems and hooks) that can increase safety and at the same time make the most of limited storage space in the home.

Appropriate Flooring

Inappropriate floor materials may be the most hazardous object in seniors' homes.[4] This make sense if one considers how much time is spent walking indoors. Some older adults are at particular risk because of gait and/or balance problems. Many professionals recommend the elimination of all throw rugs, even though many seniors may be attached to them. If rugs remain, they should contrast with the surrounding floor and have nonskid backing. Noncarpeted floors should have skid-proof texture; today many slate and linoleum manufacturers feature such textured tiles. Also, from a safety perspective, low pile carpets are preferred to plush, highly padded ones. Finally, appropriate door thresholds, if feasible, should be flat or cambered. Thresholds are a good example of a hazard created by a transition point. The obvious remedy is to eliminate the change in plane altogether or, by use of color, contrast, and lighting, to make the threshold as visible as possible.

Transfers

There are a variety of health-related reasons why an older adult might have difficulty transferring (eg, orthostatic hypotension or general weakness). All furniture is potentially used for support at one time or another. Thus, the furniture must be stable and of the proper height.[26,27,30] For this problem, leg extensions for chairs, tables, and beds are available in most medical supply catalogs. For egression from chairs there are several portable inflatable cushions as well as electric lounge chairs that can help lift a person to a standing position. However, there are no studies that evaluate the effectiveness or safety of such products. A fair number of older adults have fall accidents related to the bed.[4] In addition to being the wrong height for short-statured persons, traditional beds usually do not provide anything to grab onto if a person needs assistance getting up. A properly placed grab bar could provide the needed support.

Stairs and Steps

It is not surprising that older persons seem to hold stairs in special esteem from the perspective of safety.[31] One of the surest ways to reduce injury from stairs is to reduce one's use of them. Many older adults do just this by moving to a ground-floor apartment or changing their bedroom to the ground floor of their home.

Once again, attention to possible visual impairments in the older adult is a key to improving stair safety. Light switches should be located at the top and bottom of all stairwells. Stair treads should be skid-proof (with textured paint or adhesive strips), and, because most stair accidents occur at the first and last steps, increasing the visibility of those steps is recommended. If stairs are carpeted, it is imperative that the carpet fit snugly to the stair and not be worn and slippery. Even the best carpeting reduces the tread depth, however, which in many cases may already be too short.

Another crucial factor for stair safety is the functional handrail.[32] According to Pauls,[32] stairwells ideally should have handrails on both sides, and those handrails should be at the correct height (36 to 39 inches), graspable (the best handrail is round or oval, has a diameter between 1.25 and 1.75 inches, and is graspable from the side or below so that it can be grabbed in the course of a fall), and within reach (most adults can effectively grab a handrail that is around 24 inches from the center of their body). There is at least one handrail manufacturer that offers an extendable rail, one that can be left in a traditional position near the wall or pulled down and locked into a position that may allow a user to gain support from both arms while using stairs.[30]

Another reachability issue is whether or not the handrail extends far enough at the top and bottom of the stairs to provide proper support for safe landings. For a detailed discussion of effective stair design, see Pauls,[33] Archea et al,[34] and Templer et al.[35]

There are other more expensive technologies to help disabled persons conquer stairs: Elevators, chair lifts, and mini-stair climbing vehicles are all manufactured for use in residential environments. Such devices are still relatively rare, however, and there are no studies looking at safety issues surrounding these products.

Although separate sections discussing the kitchen and bathroom are not presented here, many of the same safe mobility issues discussed above also apply to these areas of the home. Both bathrooms and kitchens are particularly unforgiving environments because of the many hard materials (porcelain, plastics, and metals) required to make the products used in those environments durable (eg, toilets, bathtubs, stoves, and countertops). There are individual products such as automatic shut-off timers for stoves or antiscald devices for shower spigots that certainly increase safety, but the even greater need is to design these environments so that they are multiple-task sensitive, for example by placing sinks, toilets, and bathtubs in a configuration that facilitates safer transfers from and among all three products. Kitchen tasks, as well demonstrated in Faletti's work,[36] are even more complex. For instance, persons retrieve ingredients and utensils from many levels of cabinets, operate what is often a poorly designed stove, and then must transfer hot food or utensils from the stove to counters and/or tables, which may be at an unsuitable height. One could argue that this lack of holistic ergonomic design diminishes the functional potential of many older disabled persons, even if their environment contains one or two well-designed products or features.

Aside from products or environmental features that attempt to prevent the fall itself, a series of technologic devices has been developed aimed at preventing or reducing injury once an older person does fall. Under the direction of David Colvin, Triangle Research and Development Corporation in Raleigh, North Carolina has developed a number of such devices under the trademark of Fall-safe.[37] The most technical of these fall-intervention systems features a braking device connected to an overhead trolley. A tether runs between the ceiling tracking and a special vestlike garment worn by the person. In the fall event, the system catches and lowers the person to the floor, spreading the stress impact over the whole torso. This particular device is reported to absorb 98% of the energy from a fall.[37,38]

In addition to the tethered system, which has limited application for community dwelling older adults, Colvin's group has been working on other untethered devices whose goal is also to reduce injury from falls themselves. These devices include both active and passive air bags that are inserted into garments worn by the older person, the intention being to protect hips, knees, and other vulnerable impact points. The active air bags use carbon dioxide cartridges that eject gas into the bag when sensors detect the onset of a fall.[39] It is encouraging to note that some of these injury-prevention devices are being tested for psychosocial responses (eg, stigma effects), not just engineering and biomechanical performance.[40] These products are not yet commercially available.

Environmental Control

There is an established body of literature exploring the importance of sense of control for older adults (see, for example, Rodin and Langer[41] and Schultz[42]). Although empiric investigations of the effects of environmental control on well-being or functional status are lacking, Lawton[43] observed what he termed the *control center* in the home environments of disabled elderly. This indicates a person's attempt to center as many daily living features within a limited portion of their environment; an example is a living room area that has the favorite chair located with an outside view, chairside tables, television, hot plate, telephone, reading lamp, and hobby basket all within a small space. Such a control center is an understandable response to limited mobility. Today, thanks to electronic technology, in principle almost any movable feature and/or appliance in the home can be automated. Home automation has important implications for the independence, safety, and energy use of many disabled persons. The ability to turn lights on remotely before entering a dark hallway, to have an electric stove shut off automatically after 30 minutes, or to alert local police silently that an unwanted intruder is in the house are only a few of the safety applications of this technology. Even more attractive is the potential to integrate the control of several home appliances or features (this is known as intelligent distributed control in the electronics industry).

According to Birch,[44] home automation will eventually achieve mass consumer acceptance at least to the degree of personal computers. The market will fall into two categories. The first is retail-distributed products, such as the X-10 and other do-it-yourself products that automate assorted functions in the home (eg, security, lighting, and temperature). Rehabilitation professionals know these products as environmental control units, and their sophistication varies considerably from simple push-button to voice-recognition control. The second category is automation systems for the whole house. Right now, both categories of products are somewhat difficult to install for the average homeowner. From the engineering and marketing perspectives, the major obstacle to wider acceptance of home automation is lack of a standard communication protocol. Currently in North America there are two such competing standards: Consumer Electronic Bus and Smarthouse. Until there is one industry standard, manufacturers are reluctant to develop home automation products.[44] From the perspective of the older and/or disabled consumer, the critical issues, as with many new technologies, are affordability and user-friendly interface.

Two other expanding safety and technology areas are personal emergency response systems (PERS) and so-called antiwandering devices. The invention of PERS is credited to Andrew Dibner and resulted in Lifeline Systems, Inc, Watertown, Mass.[45] Although there are several manufacturers of PERS today,[46] the basic elements of many of the systems include portable help buttons (to be pushed by the subscriber in an emergency event, such as a fall), a help console that is integrated with the telephone, and some kind of response center (either locally or nationally based). There are more than 250,000 PERS subscribers in the United States and Canada,[47] and there is reason to believe that this market will grow.

Several reports assess the utility of PERS; for reviews see Watzke[48] and Dibner.[49] Most of these studies have looked at psychopersonal effects and/or cost–benefit/service utilization effects of PERS usage. Self-reports have shown high subscriber satisfaction with the technology as well as reduced anxiety about medical vulnerabilities. Nevertheless, PERS usage has not been shown significantly to affect other psychopersonal variables such as general anxiety, sleep, happiness, psychologic distress, or sense of mastery.[48,50,51] Effects on families have revealed no significant changes in sense of burden, although in one study the average number of visits to subscribers by family members declined during PERS usage.[51]

PERS studies of hospital, nursing home, and home care aide use have reported mixed outcomes. Some investigations have showed favorable effects for PERS users (eg, longer stays in the community and fewer days in nursing homes and/or hospitals).[48] As well, PERS acquisition has resulted in significant decreases in number of hours used for homemaking services.[52–54] Such reductions in services (formal and informal) have resulted in attractive cost–benefit ratios and reported dollar savings for some agencies; for example, $808,000 in savings was reported for only 34 home care aide clients during a 2-year demonstration project.[53]

The potential substitution of a technology (PERS) for human contact (home care aide) is a classic example of the kind of ethical–economic dilemma health care providers are now facing. Furthermore, in the interest of presenting PERS technology as comprehensively as possible, in a review of the literature Watzke[48] noted weaknesses in some study designs (eg, lack of matched control groups, small sample numbers, etc). It was also concluded that PERS acquisition is a selective phenomenon and that it often correlates with an older adult having had particularly bad previous months (or years) of health. This, together with the fact that PERS subscribers on the average do not continue using the system for more than 1 to 3 years because of failing health, makes it difficult to rule out Hawthorne-like effects and/or problems of regression toward the mean (eg, in hospital usage curves).[48]

A final technology to be discussed concerns safety and the cognitively impaired older adult. A host of antiwandering, antifall, and resident tracking devices is now on the market. These electronic systems vary in their sophistication but may contain any of the following components: electronic door locks and/or open door sensors, frequency transmitters (alert tags) that clip on the resident's clothing, video camera surveillance, pressure-sensitive strips placed on the resident's mattress or chair or under exit door mats, position change alarms that fasten to the resident's body, remote call/ alert receivers worn by staff, and a staff call/alert panel located at the nursing station. To date, these devices are primarily being marketed to health care facilities, but it is quite

likely that versions of these products will soon be adapted for home use by caregivers (and not only to those taking care of Alzheimer's patients).

Interestingly, compliance with Omnibus Budget Reconciliation Act (OBRA) regulations has become a major sales incentive for these devices, especially as an alternative to physical restraints. Although there is only one research center doing empiric studies of such devices,[55] there is a growing clinical awareness of them.[56–58] In addition to investigating whether such technologies in fact do what they are purported to do (eg, reduce falls and/or unwanted exiting from facilities), there is a need to study more qualitative issues surrounding these devices, especially with respect to care staff in facilities that use such devices. How often do care staff interact with or respond to such devices? Do nurses feel that such devices make their jobs easier? Have they been adequately trained to use such devices? Do they feel that these devices are an effective alternative to physical restraints? Do they think that such devices increase the confusion and/or agitation in some of their patients? These and other issues are currently being investigated in a Canadian study by Watzke and Wister.[59]

Future Needs

The fields of gerontology, human factors, environmental psychology, architecture, interior design, and geriatric rehabilitation are constantly noting the lack of rigorous data on how frail elders and disabled persons respond to and safely negotiate the demands of everyday tasks and products in the home environment (see, for example, Smith,[60] Czaja,[61] and Vanderheiden[62]). For example, there is little scientific information about how these groups do household cleaning, retrieve an object from a high shelf, perform such self-care activities as bathing and toileting, and regulate the lighting in their environment. Environments and products that are created without such information often do not suit users' needs and necessitate their reliance on others.

Positive efforts to begin filling these knowledge gaps are emerging. For example, human factors studies by Park[63] and Al-Awar Smither[64] and their colleagues looked at seniors and their use of over-the-counter medication organizers and automated banking teller machines, respectively. There have also been recent attempts to develop self-report scales to measure psychologic factors of older adults' safety behaviors (eg, the Falls Efficacy Scale,[65] the Safety Awareness Scale for the Elderly,[66] and the Home Hazard Ranking Survey[67]). It is also encouraging to find major research funding agencies in the United States, such as the National Institute on Disability Rehabilitation Research and the National Institute on Aging, calling for research proposals that specifically address problems of human factors, rehabilitation, and technology for older adults. The last few years have also seen the creation of two new journals particularly suited for these topics: the *Journal of Assistive Technology* and *Technology and Disability*.

In addition to the need for more empiric research, there continue to be formidable gaps in the product development, application, and marketing process (see, for example, Batavia and Hammer[68] and Koncelik[69]). According to La Buda,[70] evidence of the importance of this problem is the number of manufacturers of geriatrics products that go out of business annually, from the large-scale seniors housing developer to the manufacturer of a single jar lid opener. According to Koncelik, "Marketing professionals must take a pro-active as opposed to a reactive approach to developing information about aging. In relation to product development, marketing should precede product development—not the typical reliance on the experience of designers."[69(p7)] Further evidence of the recognition of such problems is seen in the development of several centers in both the United States and Canada that focus on issues of technology transfer (see the Box). Although such government-funded centers are a step in the right direction, it may be necessary for governments to play an even more direct role if the goal is to get the kinds of technologies discussed here into the homes and hands of senior users (eg, through broader health care equipment reimbursement policies).

A final need area concerns interventions, training, and information dissemination about safety and technology for older adults. In some ways the most progress has been made in this area. There are a variety of home safety checklists, safety videotapes, and environmental assessment protocols available.[71–73] Databases and clearinghouses also exist, such as ABLEDATA, the Adaptive Device Locator System, and the American Association of Homes for the Aging's newly funded National Clearinghouse on Aging and Environmental Design Codes (see the Box). Training and education programs are increasing, for example, in the form of a national survey and video training program by Somerville et al[74] on the assistive technology training needs of occupational therapists and the first international conference on technology and aging, which was held in The Netherlands in August 1991. Also worth noting are the *Product Reports* published by the American Association of Retired Persons on topics such as hearing aids, wheelchairs, and personal emergency response systems (see the Appendix). Those reports are one attempt to reach a large non–healthcare professional audience. Finally, on a local level, it is encouraging to see a multitude of falls prevention and home safety and security programs being offered by both private and public agencies of all sorts. Nevertheless, the role that technology might play in facilitating safe, independent living for older adults needs to be elevated in any such intervention program.

References

1. Sattin RW, Nevitt MC, Waller PF, Seiden RH. *Health Promotion and Aging "Injury Prevention."* Presented at Surgeon General's Workshop; March 1988; Washington. DC.

2. Lawton MP, Nahemow L. Ecology and the aging process. In: Eisdorfer C, Lawton MP, eds. *Psychology of Adult Development and Aging.* Washington, DC: American Psychological Association; 1973.

3. Sterns HL, Barrett GV, Alexander RA. Accidents and the aging individual. In: Birren JE, Schaie KW, eds. *Handbook of the Psychology of Aging.* 2nd ed. New York, NY: Van Nostrand Reinhold; 1985.

4. Smith DBD. *Safety and security: Human factors issues for older people.* Paper prepared for the National Research Panel on Human Factors for an Aged Population; 1987; Washington, DC.

5. National Safety Council. *Accident Facts.* Chicago, Ill: National Safety Council; 1981.

6. Consumer Product Safety Commission. *Hazard Identification and Analysis: Product Summary Report.* Washington, DC: National Information Clearing House; 1979.

7. Consumer Products Safety Commission. *National Electronic Injury Surveillance System (NEISS)—Product Summary Report.* Washington, DC: Government Printing Office; 1985.

8. Sparrow PR, Davies DR. Effects of age, tenure, training and job complexity on technical performance. *Psychol Aging.* 1988; 3:307–314.

9. Dillingham AE. Age and workplace injuries. *Aging Work.* 1981; 4:1–10.

10. Yanik AJ. *Vehicle Design Considerations for Older Drivers* (SAE 885090). Warrendale, Pa: Society of Automotive Engineers; 1988.

11. Williams AF, Carsten O. Driver age and crash involvement. *Am J Public Health.* 1989;79:326–327.

12. Hague CC. Injury in later life: Epidemiology. *J Am Geriatr Soc.* 1982; 30:183–190.

13. Rubenstein LZ, Robbins AS, Schulman BL, et al. Falls and instability in the elderly. *J Am Geriatr Soc.* 1988;36: 266–278.

14. Tideiksaar R. *Falling in Old Age: Its Prevention and Treatment.* New York, NY: Springer-Verlag; 1989.

15. Woollacott MH. Balance and falls. *Top Geriatr Rehabil.* 1990; 5:1–84.

16. Sorock G. Falls among the elderly: Epidemiology and prevention. *Am J Prev Med.* 1988;4:282–288.

17. Tinetti ME, Speechley M. Prevention of falls among the elderly. *N Engl J Med.* 1989;320:1055–1059.

18. Brummel-Smith K. Falls in the aged. *Primary Care*. 1989; 16:377–393.

19. Barclay A. Falls in the elderly. *Postgrad Med*. 1988; 83:241–248.

20. Tinetti ME, Speechley M, Ginter SF. Risk factors for falls among elderly persons living in the community. *N Engl J Med*. 1988;319:1701–1707.

21. Nevitt MC, Cummings SR, Kidd S, Black D. Risk factors for recurrent nonsyncopal falls: A prospective study. *JAMA*. 1989;261:2663–2668.

22. Archea JC. Environmental factors associated with stair accidents by the elderly. *Clin Geriatr Med*. 1989;261:555–569.

23. Kemp B, Brummel-Smith K, Ramsdell JW, eds. *Geriatric Rehabilitation*. Boston, Mass: College-Hill; 1990.

24. Linn BS. Outcome of burns. *J Am Geriatr Soc*. 1980;27:118–123.

25. Ray WA, Griffin MR. Prescribed medications and the risk of falling. *Top Geriatr Rehabil*. 1990;5:12–20.

26. Koncelik JA. *Designing the Open Nursing Home*. Stoudsburg, Pa: Dowden, Hutchinson & Ross; 1976.

27. Koncelik JA. *Aging and the Product Environment*. New York, NY: Van Nostrand Reinhold; 1982.

28. Raschko BB. *Housing Interiors for the Disabled and Elderly*. New York, NY: Van Nostrand Reinhold; 1982.

29. Calkins MP, *Design for Dementia*. Owings Mills, Md: National Health Publishing; 1988.

30. Christenson MA. *Aging in the Designed Environment*. New York, NY: Haworth; 1990.

31. Watzke JR, Smith DBD, Somerville NJ, Verran A. *The study of home safety problems for older disabled persons: A multidimensional approach*. Presented at the Human Factors Society's annual meeting; October 1989; Denver, Colo.

32. Pauls JL. Are functional handrails within our reach and our grasp? *South Build*. 1989:52:20–30.

33. Pauls JL. Review of stair-safety research with an emphasis on Canadian studies. *Ergonomics*. 1984;28:999–1010.

34. Archea J, Collins BL, Stahl FI. *Guidelines for Stair Safety*. (NBS building science series 120, National Bureau of Standards, Center for Building Technology). Washington, DC: National Engineering Laboratory, 1979.

35. Templer J, Mullet G, Archea J. *An Analysis of the Behavior of Stair Users*. Washington, DC: National Bureau of Standards; 1978. National Bureau of Standards publication NBSIR.78-1554.

36. Faletti MV. Human factors research and functional environments for the aged. In: Altman I, Wohwill JE, Lawton MP, eds. *Elderly People and the Environment*. New York: Plenum Press: 1984;7:191–237.

37. Colvin DP. *Fall-safe: A falls intervention and mobility aid system for elderly and handicapped rehabilitation populations*. Presented at the conference, Exploration: Technological Innovations for an Aging Population; January 1989; Lake Buena Vista, Fla.

38. Zylke JW. Medical news and perspectives. *JAMA*. 1990:263:2021–2023.

39. Rothman SA. Minimizing fall injuries to older patients. *Contemp Senior Health*. 1990;263:2021–2023.

40. Myers A. *Perception and acceptability of protective garments among high risk hip fracture patients*. Presented at the annual meeting of the Gerontological Society of America; November 1990; Boston. Mass.

41. Rodin J, Langer EJ. Long term effects of a control-relevant intervention with the institutionalized aged. *J Pers Soc Psychol*. 1977;35:897–902.

42. Schultz R. Effects of control and predictability on the physical and psychological well-being of the institutionalized aged. *J Pers Soc Psychol*. 1976;33:563–573.

43. Lawton MP. Residential environment and self-directedness among older people. *Am Psychol*. 1990; 45:638–640.

44. Birch G. Home automation: The potential for persons with severe mobility restrictions to achieve significant levels of independence. In: Watzke JR (ed), *Seniors Housing Update*. Vancouver, British Columbia: Gerontology Research Centre, Simon Fraser University; 1991;2.

45. Dibner AS, Lowy L, Morris J. Usage and acceptance of an emergency alarm system by the frail elderly. *Gerontologist*. 1982;22:538–539.

46. American Association of Retired Persons. *Meeting the Need for Security and Independence with Personal Emergency Response Systems*. Washington, DC: American Association of Retired Persons, Consumer Affairs Program, Department; 1987.

47. Stafford JL, Dibner AS. *Lifeline Programs in 1984: Stability and Growth*. Watertown, Mass: Lifeline Systems; 1984.

48. Watzke JR. *Personal response systems (PRS): A review of the research*. Presented at the annual meeting of the American Society on Aging; March 1991; New Orleans, La.

49. Dibner AS. Personal emergency response systems: Communication technology aids for elderly and their families. *J Appl Gerontol*. 1990;9:504–510.

50. Sherwood S, Morris JN. *A Study of the Effects of an Emergency Alert and Response System for the Aged: A Final Report*. Boston, Mass: Hebrew Rehabilitation Center for the Aged; 1981.

51. Gatz M, Pearson C. *Evaluation of an Emergency Alert Response System from the Point of View of Subscribers and Family Members*. Los Angeles, Calif: University of Southern California; 1988.

52. Ruchlin HS, Morris JN. Cost-benefit analysis of an emergency alarm and response system: A case study of a long-term care program. *Health Serv Res.* 1981;16:65–80.

53. Coordinated Care Management Corporation. *Emergency Response System Demonstration Project: Final Report.* Buffalo, NY: Coordinated Care Management Corp; 1989.

54. Dixon L. *Evaluation of the Electronic Call Device Pilot Project.* New York, NY: City of New York Human Resources Administration Medical Assistance Program; 1987.

55. Martino-Saltzman D, Blasch B, Morris R, McNeal LW. Travel behavior of nursing home residents perceived as wanderers and non-wanderers. *Gerontologist.* 1991:31:666–672.

56. Brower HT. The alternatives to restraints. *Gerontol Nurs.* 1991;17:18–22.

57. Rader J. Modifying the environment to decrease use of restraints. *Gerontol Nurs.* 1991;17:9–13.

58. Watzke JR. *Reduction of physical restraints: The role of the environment and technology.* Presented at the annual meeting of the American Society on Aging: March 1991; New Orleans, La.

59. Watzke JR, Wister AW. *Attitudes of nursing staff from different cultures toward use of higher technology in long term care facilities.* Presented at the annual meeting of the Canadian Association on Gerontology; October 1991; Toronto, Ontario.

60. Smith DBD. Human factors and aging: An overview of research needs and application opportunities. *Hum Factors.* 1990;32:509–526.

61. Czaja SJ, ed. *Human Factors Research Needs for an Aging Population.* Washington, DC: National Academy Press; 1990.

62. Vanderheiden GC. Thirty something million: Should they be exceptions? *Hum Factors.* 1990;32:383–396.

63. Park DC, Morrell RW, Frieske D, Blackburn AB, Birchmore D. Cognitive factors and the use of over-the-counter medication organizers by arthritis patients. *Hum Factors.* 1991;33:57–67.

64. Al-Awar Smither J, Smither RD, Braun CC. *Resistance by the elderly to technology: The case of the automatic teller machine.* Presented at the annual meeting of the American Society on Aging; March 1991; New Orleans, La.

65. Tinetti ME, Richman D, Powell L. Falls efficacy as a measure of fear of falling. *J Gerontol.* 1990;45:239–243.

66. Smith DBD, Watzke JR. Perception of safety hazards across the adult life-span. In: *Proceedings of the Human Factors Society Meeting.* Santa Monica, Calif: Human Factors Society, 1990.

67. Watzke JR, Smith DBD. *Perception and knowledge of safety hazards among seniors.* Presented at the annual meeting of the Gerontological Society of America; November 1990, Boston, Mass.

68. Batavia AI, Hammer GS. Toward the development of consumer-based criteria for the evaluation of assistive devices. *J Rehab Res Dev.* 1990;24:425–436.

69. Koncelik JA. *Appliance and furnishings design.* Presented at the Canadian Aging and Rehabilitation Product Development Corporation's workshop; May 1991; Winnipeg, Manitoba.

70. La Buda DR. *High technology and its benefits for an aging population.* Presented at a hearing of the Select Committee on Aging, House of Representatives; May 1984; Washington, DC.

71. Pynoos J, Cohen E, Lucas C. Environmental coping strategies for Alzheimer's caregivers. *Am J Alzheimers Care Relat Disord Res.* 1989,4:2–8.

72. Geriatric Environments for Living and Learning. *The "Safe Home."* Chicago, Ill: Geriatric Environments for Living and Learning; 1990.

73. Consumer Products Safety Commission. *Safety for Older Consumers, Home Safety Checklist.* Washington, DC: Consumer Product Safety Commission; 1986.

74. Somerville NJ, Wilson DJ, Shanfield KL, Mack W. A survey of the assistive technology training needs of occupational therapists. *Assistive Technol.* 1990;2:41–49.

Resources for Technology in Geriatrics

AARP Fulfillment
601 E Street, NW
Washington, DC 20049

ABLEDATA Assistive Technology Information Service
(Owned by National Institute on Disability and Reha-
  bilitation Research, Washington, DC)
Macro International
8455 Colesville Road, Suite 935
Silver Spring, Maryland, 20910-3319

Adaptive Device Locator System
Academic Software, Inc
331 W Second St at Broadway
Lexington, KY 40507

Center for Assistive Technology
State University of New York at Buffalo
515 Kimball Tower
Buffalo, NY 14214

Center for Therapeutic Applications of Technology
State University of New York at Buffalo
515 Kimball Tower
Buffalo, NY 14214

Center for Universal Design
School of Design
North Carolina State University
Box 8613
Raleigh, NC 27695-8613

Centre for Studies in Aging
Sunnybrook Health Science Centre
2075 Bayview Avenue
Toronto, Ontario, Canada M4N 3M5

Electronic Industries Foundation
Rehabilitation Engineering Center on
  Technology Transfer
1901 Pennsylvania Ave, NW, Suite 700
Washington, DC 20006

Gerontology Research Centre
Simon Fraser University
515 West Hastings Street
Vancouver, British Columbia, Canada V6B 5K3

Institute for Technology Development
Advanced Living Systems Division
428 N Lamar Blvd
Oxford, MI 38655

Kinsmen Rehabilitation Foundation of
  British Columbia
999 West Broadway, Suite 360
Vancouver, British Columbia, V5Z 4R1, Canada

Ontario Rehabilitation Technology Consortium
  (ORTC)
The Hugh ManMillan Rehabilitation Centre
350 Rumsey Road
Toronto, Ontario, Canada M4G 1R8

productABILITY
1010 Sinclair Street
Winnipeg, Manitoba, Canada R2V 3H7

ProNatura Group
Institute for Technology Development
428 North Lamar
Oxford, MS 38655

Rehabilitation Research & Training Center on Aging
Rancho Los Amigos Medical Center
7600 Consuelo Street
Downey, CA 90242

(Editor's note: This information has been updated because some resources that appeared in the original are no longer available. Some resources have been added that have come available since original publication.)

Chapter 15

Culture: A Factor Influencing the Outcomes of Occupational Therapy

Ruth Levine Schemm, EdD, OTR/L, FAOTA

Overview

People can accomplish seemingly impossible goals if invested in the outcome; on the other hand, few people are interested in activities that have no personal meaning. This paper will explore one of the factors that can make therapy more meaningful to our patients. The concept is a complex pattern of living which is called culture. As therapists, we search for activities that will stimulate and interest our patients as well as promote functional abilities. This is no easy task because few of our patients come from the same culture group that we do. This paper will define culture, review the importance of culture in occupational therapy practice, and describe how cultural beliefs and values affect assessment and treatment in occupational therapy.

Let us begin with a treatment vignette that offers an introduction to the concept of culture.

Case Study. Mrs. W., a 57 year old, attractive, upper-middle class, urban housewife, suffered from Guillian-Barre syndrome, was hospitalized and transferred to a rehabilitation center and then to home care. Mrs. W. occupied a first-floor bedroom suite in the newly purchased home of one of her daughters. The family reasoned that Mrs. W. could interact with family members, walk short distances and join the family for meals. The physical therapist felt that Mrs. W. was almost ready to return to her own home if it were adapted to accommodate Mrs. W.'s needs. Mrs. W. lived in a newly constructed three story townhouse in center city. Although the OTR felt that referral to occupational therapy was perhaps too late for best results, she decided to visit the patient anyway.

On the day of the scheduled evaluation visit, the OTR was admitted into the gracious house by the maid because the daughter was conferring with an interior decorator. The OTR was led to the first floor bedroom where Mrs. W. was propped up in bed while a full time attendant fussed over her sheets and cleared her breakfast dishes. Mrs. W. ignored the therapist and continued her conversation with the attendant. After a few minutes, Mrs. W. briefly acknowledged the OTR and spent the next fifteen minutes describing her symptoms as if the OTR was an unwanted, inexperienced newcomer. Mrs. W. praised "her" physical therapist and attributed her progress to his guidance and skill. The occupational therapist tried to guide their conversation toward the patient's previous interests and activities and her present views on self-care and independence, but Mrs. W. switched the conversation back to the physical therapist.

The OTR decided to define her role and the type of equipment that might improve Mrs. W.'s functional abilities. This seemed to make Mrs. W. act more defensively. The OTR tried to ameliorate her discomfort by pointing out useful safety rails and tub seats in an equipment catalog. Mrs. W. grew even more negative and told the OTR that she did not need adaptive equipment. The OTR soon realized that something was wrong with the interview but could not fathom why it was going so poorly. Mrs. W. became more upset as the therapist tried to win her approval by switching the topic to the other services offered by an occupational therapist including work simplification and analysis of architectural barriers. Unfortunately, this topic also proved difficult and Mrs. W. interrupted the OTR and told her that the physical therapist said that she was making excellent progress. The OTR tried to explain that she was impressed with Mrs. W.'s efforts but this praise did not impress Mrs. W.

The OTR decided there was nothing else to do so she concluded the evaluation by telling Mrs. W. that she would close the case since Mrs. W. had no interest in adaptive equipment. Mrs. W. said she hoped that she would never see the occupational therapist again and told the OTR that she planned to report her to the physical therapist.

Later, the physical therapist called the OTR to find out what had gone wrong with the evaluation. He reported that Mrs. W. was angry and upset and claimed that the OTR insisted that she would need "handicapped" equipment for the rest of her life. The OTR was both hurt and confused and wondered what she had done to infuriate Mrs. W. After all, she was doing exactly what she had been taught in her training for home health care.

The negative outcome of this evaluation visit affected all of the team members—patient, caretakers, physical therapist, nurse and the occupational therapist. Each person was interpreting events from their own perspective. The meaning of the communication was, in part, determined by the person's values, interests, goals, roles and habits. Each person's culture became a filter or screen that either passed information through or blocked it. The vignette demonstrates that even though the therapist's professional manner was similar to that prescribed during her professional training, the patient interpreted the visit as an attempt to jinx her hard won progress. In retrospect, the OTR may have realized that two different opinions about the value of adaptive equipment started the tangled communication. Within a short time, the OTR could not extricate herself from the negative meaning that "handicapped" things had for Mrs. W. The therapist moved her treatment agenda too quickly without hearing what the patient was really saying. Mrs. W. was frightened by her diagnosis and did not want to see, touch, own, or talk about anything that implied that she might not regain her independence. In Mrs. W.'s culture outward appearances were of vital importance, people who used adaptive equipment were handicapped and the thought that other people might regard her as disabled was more stressful than being dependent on an attendant.

Historical Overview

Occupational therapy founders first considered culture as an important aspect of treatment planning because of their belief in the interrelationship between mind and body. If an activity generated a patient's interests it could also promote functional independence. In the first occupations training course, Tracy identified activities that matched the patient's lifestyle[1] and Dunton agreed and emphasized the need to stimulate the patient's interests by prescribing activities based on personal and cultural values.[2] Hall and Buck claimed that "brain workers should be given work that was largely physical and those who worked with their hands, must have simpler, more primitive tasks."[3] Although the consideration of culture was not fully developed, the Founders searched for different ways to elicit a patient's interest through the use of novel experiences. In 1925 a committee of the American Occupational Therapy Association defined occupational therapy and formulated fifteen principles of which one-third emphasized the importance of considering the patient's interests and needs.[4] Thus, the early literature of the profession is filled with examples of attempts to consider the patient's culture during treatment.

As medical care became more scientific in the 1930's and 1940's, therapists began to concentrate more on the patient's pathology than on residual strengths; thus, decreasing their initial commitment to linking the patient's goals, interests and values, habits and roles with the activity process. At the same time, many therapists were arts-and-crafts teachers who were committed to a philosophy that tended to encourage patients to refine their craft skills and produce an attractive end-product. It was believed that the quality product would enhance self-confidence. Other therapists concentrated on the benefits that occurred during the *doing* part of the activity process. Thus, ideological differences grew between the therapists and the diversionists.[5] Another factor that compromised initial consideration of culture during the Depression years was the scarcity of funds. Therapists had to treat large numbers of patients and market and sell patient projects in order to replenish department supply budgets. The patients' interests were subordinated to the department needs since some projects were more cost efficient than others.

The emphasis on arts-and-crafts with little concentration on the therapeutic use of activities may have prompted Eleanor Clarke Slagle to tell the 1930 graduating class at Sheppard and Enoch Pratt Hospital that "handicrafts are not enough" because " . . . the patient is being more and more considered in relation to his domestic and community life."[6]

Culture was as important in early practice as it must be today, because occupational therapy deals with goal-directed activities which are part and parcel of everyday life. Recently, modern therapists are rediscovering the importance of early beliefs that emphasized the interaction of mind and body during treatment. Theorists Mosey,[7] Fidler and Fidler (see Chapter 7),[8] Llorens,[9] Reilly,[10] Keilhofner and Burke,[11,12] Barris,[13] Nuse-Clark,[14] and Yerxa,[15] all address the influence of culture in treatment. Using basic concepts from our past, present-day theorists still emphasize the importance of the patient's motivation, interests, goals, interests, values, habits, time-orientation, roles, caretaker network and use of the non-human environment. All of these concepts are part of a person's culture.

Defining Culture

Culture has been described as a "blueprint" for human behavior, influencing individual thoughts, actions and collectively influencing a particular society.[16] Culture can be viewed as a multifaceted influence which is learned by direct and indirect daily experiences based on what people do (cultural behavior), say (speech messages), make and use (cultural artifacts). In short, a child learns a life pattern of beliefs and values which shape the way that he or she believes, thinks, perceives, feels and behaves.[17] Culture is a way of life which encompasses kinetic or overt behavior, psychological expressions and the material products of labor or industry. The major cultural transmission agents are behavioral and material elements simply because psychological states are not transferable.[18]

Kinetic or overt behaviors, the first elements of culture, are evident in actions performed by an individual and include: body motions, speech patterns, distance selected during communication with others and use of products and tools. People use their bodies in unique ways to indicate agreement, acceptance, rejection, discomfort and other reactions.

Speech patterns are also culturally determined; rate of speech, expression and emphasis, pronunciation, and choice of words are part of a person's culture. Even the distance preferred between people during different activities is also culturally determined.[19] Tool use, as part of one's behavior, is another factor indigenous to one's culture: some people use handtools exclusively, others rely on sophisticated gadgets and technology, some others prefer to use only their hands in doing tasks. In examining culture one must also consider how people employ objects and other artifacts. For example, consider a patient who uses the same hammer over and over and seems to derive pleasure from completing a task by using this object which almost seems like a non-human friend. In contrast, another patient may be careless with tools and abuse them without giving it a second thought. Still another patient may regard the use of tools with disdain since handmade objects can be purchased and "time is money."

Psychological aspects, the second elements of one's culture, include knowledge, attitudes and values that are shared by members of a given cultural group. These factors cannot be readily observed since they take place in a person's mind. Psychological factors are therefore more difficult for an observer to assess and observe. Although these factors are subjective they still deserve some of our attention since people exhibit different reactions to events in their daily lives. On the other hand, measurement of psychological factors is not precise and individual reactions may be inconsistent and variable even under the same circumstances. For example, if you introduce yourself to a patient using your first name only some people may feel right at home, welcome your informality and respond with warmth and humor. On the other hand, another person may find it annoying but tolerable and respond stiffly to requests for additional information. We can speculate that the first patient equates the informality with a type of relationship where the therapist and he are equal partners. The second patient may feel that she has just met the therapist and the use of first names indicates a forced familiarity that makes the patient feel guarded. Thus we see that the same event can take on different meaning for each participant depending on one's cultural background.

The last element associated with culture, the "material products of labor or industry," are the objects and artifacts that comprise *the non-human environment*. This category includes signs, symbols, objects, tasks, roles and social organizations used to create products in the environment. Consider the work produced by a given group of people, the way that ideas are transformed into reality and the type of organization that is needed to produce the goods and services. Members of a group teach their children how to participate in their culture through a complex system of rewards and punishments which are conveyed through thoughts, actions, social beliefs, attitudes, communication patterns, perceptions, time orientation and ways of handling animals, plants and objects. In effect, a child is exposed to a pattern of beliefs, attitudes, perceptions, meanings and emotions based on personal experiences in a particular setting.[20]

Culture imposes a conditioning variable that is internalized in the human psyche and not easily forgotten.[21] Values, interests, goals, habits, roles, time orientation, communication patterns, the ways in which one uses symbols and artifacts, selects non-human objects—all are well ingrained as one grows, making change difficult. In fact, Likroeber compared culture to the great coral reefs built by polyps. The polyps die but their secretions leave a permanent record of their former life.[22] Thus, culture establishes a filter through which individuals interpret daily events. At the same time, one's group establishes patterns that become "commonly defined meanings and sanctioned behaviors favored by the group."[23] Individuals are never free of the group influence—sometimes subtle and sometimes more specialized—to meet individual physical and psychological needs.[24]

The Relevance of Culture in Occupational Therapy

Culture is a central component of occupational therapy because people judge the quality of their therapy through a filter which is comprised, in part, of past learning and emotions and which is based on three levels of beliefs: (1) the patient's perception of illness and health, (2) the patient's perception of therapy, and (3) the patient's belief in the meaning of his own life and activities. These factors overlap and are not discrete.

Illness is not the same to all individuals. Sociologists have long identified significant differences in the ways that members of specific cultures decide to: seek health care, care for themselves, use family caretaker networks, take medication and follow prescribed remedies, participate in a healthful daily regime, assist other ill family members and endure pain and suffering.[25,26,27,28,29,30] Occupational therapists can not assume that people all react to the stress of illness, traumatic events or other life disruptions in the same way. "Illness behavior" refers to the ways in which symptoms may be differently perceived, evaluated and acted (or not acted) upon by different kinds of persons.[31] The behavior varies with a person's socioeconomic class, education level, community cohesiveness and ethnic origin. The higher the social status of a population, the better educated and informed they will be about signs and symptoms of illness.[32]

Being "ill" certainly is not the same to everyone. Some people are not ill until they are incapable of performing daily roles, others are ill as soon as they note a slight change in their body, still others are ill only if the illness is labeled by the medical establishment and therefore given "official" sanction. Therapists must consider the issue of illness behavior in rehabilitation because of diverse reactions such as a patient who does not want to participate in therapy because he is "ill" and therefore is not *capable* of participation. This type of behavior was described in a case study depicting the progress of an elderly Italian–American, with a left hemiparesis, who maintained that he could not dress or toilet himself until his arm "got well." This response is logical if you understand the culture of the first-generation, Southern Italian.[33,34]

Another question to consider is how well patients understand their treatment programs. Occupational therapy can only be perceived as meaningful, and deserving of the patient's interest and cooperation if it is relevant to patients and their caretakers. Treatment is valued only if patients believe that they have been helped by it. If not, services are judged as irrelevant and inconsequential. Chances are that therapists who are capable of attending

to the patient's cultural values by selecting relevant treatment activities are also able to convince the patient that therapy is important. Yet, it is difficult to tap into the interests of patients who have experienced a traumatic illness, accident or event which has drained their energies and made adaptation seem overwhelming and taxing. Sharrott maintained that occupational therapists "play a profound role in creation, affirmation and experience of meaning" since therapy provides opportunities for patients to redefine their previous experiences in light of their present abilities and needs.[35] Effective therapy alters the patient's perception of meaningful existence by offering concrete feedback on daily performance in activities that are important in a patient's life roles. Unlike other treatment, occupational therapy mirrors the painful limitations wrought by traumatic incident, aging, development or deprivation. But therapy sessions can alter the patient's perception of life by providing immediate evidence on what the patient CAN do rather than what is lost.[36]

Another factor, frequently overlooked when designing therapy programs is the patient's beliefs and values regarding the nonhuman environment. Barris discussed the importance of the treatment environment because it should provide "adequate but not overbearing stimulation."[37] Patients will express culturally determined values about their environment and these ideas should be respected. For example, some patients prefer to do their therapy activities alone and refuse to participate in a group project whereas other patients like to be involved in the social interactions that evolve during work on a collective project. Relevance or the link between therapy and the patient's reality, should become part of initial treatment planning because the therapist is responsible for developing a strong link between the patient's interests and the goals of the occupational therapy program. This is not to say that it is easy to develop therapy that is compatible with the patient's goals, values and interests. These three factors: the patient's perception of illness and health, the patient's perception of therapy and the patient's belief in the meaning of life and activities are all considered in a successful therapy program.

Factors to Consider During Evaluation and Treatment

This section will use information presented in the earlier case study to demonstrate how the OTR could have improved her assessment if cultural factors had been considered during the evaluation visit.

Conceptual Framework. One way to systematically include culture in one's daily treatment is to select a conceptual framework or model that includes culture. Although many occupational therapy theories and models mention culture, the Model of Human Occupation[38,39] includes a conceptual structure that integrates data about the patient's values, goals, interests, personal causation, habits and roles into occupational therapy.

Background. The next step is to observe and investigate the lifestyle of cultural group members. Consider the largest number of ethnic group members in your patient load and find out where group members live. Try to do a small-scale, informal ethnographic study by exploring a local store, restaurant, recreational center or religious sanctuary.[40] During your visit use your clinical skills to observe the human and non-human environment and the way that group members interact. Consider the values that are conveyed through all of these cues.

For instance, if the OTR had visited Mrs. W.'s neighborhood, she would have found a row of exclusive townhouses in a village within center city. The colonial-style, three-story, brick houses have narrow stairways and small rooms—in no way a barrier-free environment. Each house faced an attractive courtyard with a few trees and benches in the center. Garages were hidden underground and could only be accessed by an enclosed walkway. The houses were situated near a cluster of exclusive stores where one could buy things like gourmet take-out food, imported wine, custom made tiles, designer clothing or hand-made lampshades.

This uppermiddle-class neighborhood conveyed an air of cosmopolitan homogeneity. Although the OTR could not assume that Mrs. W. shared all of her neighbors' values, she could still learn something about her patient's lifestyle. It is not realistic to visit every patient's neighborhood; nonetheless, one can choose the largest group among one's patients and gather some background information about them. This data is as important as looking up medication side-effects and unfamiliar medical diagnoses.

Reading offers another source of information. Research on particular cultural groups appears in sociological, anthropological and historical journals. Books also depict life in a particular culture. For instance, Chute's novel about the pain, humiliation and rage of a poverty-stricken New England family[41] offers insight into rural deprivation. Factual accounts are also useful, such as the story told by Wideman, a Black-American Rhodes scholar and English professor, who searches for an answer to why his brother who was raised by the same parents in the same environment as the author is presently serving a life sentence for murder.[42] Television and film documentaries that portray family and community life are helpful in understanding different lifestyles. In short, the OTR should gather as much information as possible about a patient's cultural group before the evaluation visit.

Using the case-study as an example, the OTR did not adequately prepare for the evaluation visit. The nurse and the physical therapist could have been used as informants so the OTR could be introduced to the patient's lifestyle. The OTR tried to control the interview by taking charge and asking questions. Mrs. W. valued competition and outward appearances; moreover, it was important for her to act like the family matriarch. Thus, the OTR became a rival. During the first fifteen minutes of the interview, the OTR could have satisfied Mrs. W.'s need for attention by listening to her description of her progress and offering support for her efforts. At the same time, the OTR could have thoroughly observed the environment.

Evaluation. The initial evaluation is a crucial time to establish trust and gather cues from the human and the non-human environment. There are a number of evaluation tools that can be used to direct these observations. Use a guide to begin your search for an effective instrument. The Kielhofner text *The Model of Human Occupation*[43] includes an overview of assessment tools or Asher's *Annotated Index of Occupational Therapy Evaluation Tools*[44] which includes profiles on 87 occupational therapy instruments, as well as information on where to find the tool.

Since no instrument is perfect, consider elements of the patient's lifestyle by observing values concerning life, death, health, productivity, work, family relations, human nature, time, meaningful activities and religion. Be alert to ethnic myths and taboos which will impede care if misunderstood by the therapist. Use data gathered from the evaluation tools you use to refine your ideas about treatment. For example, Mrs. W. may have responded better if the OTR had explored one of her interests and then used the activity to observe Mrs. W.'s functional abilities.

Specific tools which could have been used in conjunction with other ADL, cognitive, perceptual or motor evaluations are the Occupational Role History,[45,46] a semi-structured interview on occupational choice, work experience and leisure satisfaction, or The Occupational Questionnaire[47] which collects data on the patient's use of time in daily activities and how that relates to the patient's values, interests and personal causation. Two other useful tools are The Role Checklist which assesses productive adult life-roles by indicating the individual's perceptions of past, present, and future roles[48] and the Time Battery for gathering qualitative and quantitative data on temporal adaptation and use of time.[49] The OTR should have selected a tool which seemed to provide appropriate ideas for treatment planning.

Even if the OTR had used better interviewing skills, completed an ADL Evaluation and administered an instrument such as the Occupational Questionnaire, she would still need to compare this data with cues from the environment. Thus, the OTR's observation skills are fundamental to evaluation and treatment planning because patients may not always mean what they say. Examine the "extent to which the patient's beliefs, values, and customs are congruent with a trifold set of standards: from the patient's culture or ethnic group, from the therapist's own culture, and from the setting in which the treatment takes place.[50] Consider the extent that the patient is "like all other humans, like some other humans, and like no other humans."[51] Take time to identify and label similarities and differences between the patient's culture and the therapist's. This will help to separate personal bias and needs from those of the patient. For example, not all patients want to be independent in self-care. Some want to direct their energies toward other activities and view assistance as a trade-off. This was certainly true for Mrs. W.

A final consideration is the setting in which treatment takes place. Is the therapist a guest in the patient's home or is the patient a visitor in the hospital? The answer to those questions will determine roles and relationships. Treatment must be appropriate for the setting. For example, the institution is not always the best place to teach cooking and toileting skills since the information must be retaught once the patient returns home. On the other hand, the home setting is not suitable for constructing complex equipment and hand splints.

Summary

This paper has explored the importance of culture in occupational therapy. Occupational therapy founders emphasized the need to consider the patient's interests in treatment. Today, we again realize that treatment must be meaningful to patients. Thus, cultural factors must be considered in evaluation and treatment. This is no easy task since we are all entrenched in our own value systems. However, although there are many differences among cultural groups there are also many similarities. Occupations can serve as a "common light among cultures."[52]

N.B. Throughout this paper the author has used the term "patient" to refer to the recipient of treatment. The term client was eschewed because it did not reflect people who were receiving medical services.

References

1. Tracy, SE: *Studies in invalid occupations.* Boston: Whitcomb and Barrows. 1912.

2. Dunton, WR: *Occupational Therapy: A manual for nurses.* Philadelphia: WB Saunders Co. 1918.

3. Hall, H and Buck, MMC: *Handicrafts for the Handicapped.* New York: Moffatt, Yard and Company. 1916, p. xii.

4. American Occupational Therapy Association Committee. An outline of lectures in Occupational Therapy to medical students and physicians. *Occupational Therapy and Rehabilitation. 5,* 1925, p. 278.

5. Doane, JC: Presidential address delivered at AOTA annual meeting. Toronto, Canada, September 28–30, 1931. Reprinted in *Occupational Therapy and Rehabilitation, 10* 1931, p. 365.

6. Slagle, EC: Address to Graduates, Sheppard and Enoch Pratt Hospital, Towson, Maryland, June 28, 1930. *Occupational Therapy and Rehabilitation, 9* 1930, p. 275.

7. Mosey, AC: *Occupational Therapy: Configuration of a Profession.* New York: Raven Press. 1981, p. 78.

8. Fidler, GS and Fidler, JW: Doing and becoming: the Occupational Therapy experience. In Kielhofner, G, *Health through occupation.* Philadelphia: FA Davis Company. 1983, p. 267–280. (Reprinted as Chapter 7).

9. Llorens, LA: *Application of a developmental theory for health and rehabilitation.* American Occupational Therapy Association. 1976.

10. Reilly, M: The modernization of Occupational Therapy. *Amer J Occup Ther 25,* 1971, p. 243–246.

11. Keilhofner, G and Burke, JP: Components and determinants of human occupation. In Kielhofner, G (Editor): *A model of human occupation: theory and application.* Baltimore, Maryland: Williams and Wilkins. 1985, p. 12–36.

12. Kielhofner, G and Burke, JP: A model of human occupation, Part I. Conceptual Framework and content. *Amer J Occup Ther 34,* 1980, pp. 572–581.

13. Barris, R: Environmental interactions: an extension of the model of occupation. *Amer J Occup Ther 36,* 1982, pp 637–644.

14. Nuse-Clark, P: Human development through occupation: A philosophy and conceptual model for practice, part 2. *Amer J Occup Ther 33,* 1979, pp. 577–585.

15. Yerxa, E: Audicious values: the energy source for occupational therapy practice. In Kielhofner, G. (Editor) *Health through occupation.* Philadelphia: FA Davis. 1983, pp. 149–162.

16. Leininger, M: *Transcultural nursing: concepts, theories and practices.* New York: John Wiley and Sons. 1978, p. 80.

17. Spradley, JP, McDurdy, DW (Editors): *Conformity and conflict.* Boston: Little, Brown. 1980, p. 2.

18. Linton, R. *The cultural background of personality.* New York: Appleton-Century-Crofts, Inc. 1945, p. 38.

19. Hall, ET: *The hidden dimension.* Garden City, New York: Anchor Books. 1969.

20. Laudin, H: *Victims of culture.* Columbus, Ohio: Charles E. Merrill Pub. Co. 1973.

21. Opler, M: *Culture and social psychiatry.* New York: Atherton Press. 1967, p. 14.

22. Likroeber, Al: quoted in Laudin, op. cit. p. 4.

23. Ibid. p. 184.

24. Ibid. p. 189.

25. Mechanic, D: Response factors in illness: the study of illness behavior. In Jaco, EG. (Editor): *Patients, physicians and illness.* New York: The Free Press. 1972, pp. 128–141.

26. Leininger, op. cit.

27. Saunders, L: *Cultural difference and medical care.* New York: Russell Sage Foundation. 1954.

28. Scott, CS: Health and healing practices among five ethnic groups in Miami, Florida. *Public Health Reports. 89* 1974, pp. 524–32.

29. Suchman, EA: Social patterns of illness and medical care. *Journal of health and human behavior. 6,* 1965, pp. 2–16.

30. Wolff, BB and Langley, S: Cultural factors and the response to pain. A review, In Weisenberg, M (Editor): *Pain: clinical and experimental perspectives.* Saint Louis: The CV Mosby Co. 1975, pp. 141–143.

31. Mechanic, D. Religion, religiosity, and illness behavior. *Human organization. 22,* 1963, p. 202.

32. Suchman, EA: Sociomedical variations among ethic groups. *American Journal of Sociology. 70* 1964–5, pp. 319–331.

33. Lopreato, J: *Italian Americans.* New York: Random House, 1970.

34. Levine, RE: The cultural aspects of home care delivery. *Amer J Occup Ther 38,* 1984, pp. 736–737.

35. Sharrott, G: Occupational therapy's role in the client's creation and affirmation of meaning. In Kielhofner, G: *Health through occupation.* Philadelphia: FA Davis. 1983, p. 215.

36. Rogers, JC: The spirit of independence: the evolution of a philosophy. *Amer J Occup Ther 36,* 1982 pp. 709–715.

37. Barris, op. cit.

38. Kielhofner and Burke, op. cit.

39. Kielhofner, G. op. cit.

40. Merrill, SC: Qualitative methods in occupational therapy research: an application. *The occupational therapy journal of research. 5* 1985, pp. 209–222.

41. Chute, C: *The Beans of Egypt, Maine.* New York: Ticknor & Fields, 1985.

42. Wideman, JE: *Brothers and keepers.* New York: Penguin Books. 1984.

43. Kielhofner, op. cit.

44. Asher, IE: *Annotated index of Occupational Therapy evaluation tools.* Thomas Jefferson University, Department of Occupational Therapy, 1985.

45. Moorehead, L: The occupational history. *Amer J Occup Ther 23,* 1969, pp. 329–334.

46. Florey, LL & Michelman, SM: Occupational role history: a screening tool for psychiatric occupational therapy. *Amer J Occup Ther 36,* 1982 pp. 301–308.

47. Riopel, N & Kielhofner, G: *Occupational questionnaire.* In Asher, op. cit. p. 57.

48. Oakley, F: *The role checklist.* In Asher. op. cit. p. 58.

49. Larrington, G: *Time Battery.* In Asher. op. cit. p. 59.

50. Tripp-Reimer, T., Brink, PJ, Saunders, JM: Cultural assessment: content and process. *Nursing Outlook. 32,* p. 81.

51. Kluckholn, C: quoted in Brill, NI: *Working with people: the helping process.* Philadelphia: JB Lippincott, 1976, p. 19.

52. Malinowski, B: *Argonauts of the western pacific.* New York: EP Dutton and Co., Inc., 1961. p. 25.

Chapter 16

The Culture Concept in the Everyday Practice of Occupational and Physical Therapy

Laura Krefting, PhD

Although the concept of culture is a central tenet in the social sciences, it is only recently that its relevance to the provision of health care has been widely acknowledged. The purpose of this article is to present a concept of culture that has application in everyday practice, to describe the hazards of avoiding culturally sensitive practice, and to present some ways to facilitate the use of the culture concept in clinical practice.

The Culture Concept

In anthropology, where culture is a central theoretical concept, entire books have been devoted to its definition, suggesting the richness and complexity of the concept (see for a discussion Geertz, 1973;[1] Keesing, 1981;[2] Kroeber & Kluckholn, 1963[3]). In fact, after decades of debate anthropologists have not agreed on a single definition. There are, however, certain commonalities among the definitions which provide a basis for understanding the concept. Most agree that it is a system of learned patterns of behavior.[4] The idea that culture is learned rather than inherited biologically is important. Learning occurs through the socialization process—it is transmitted to the young of the group by other group members. Another commonality in definitions of culture is that it is shared by other members of a group rather than being the property of an individual. Finally, in many definitions, culture includes the concept of providing the individual and the group with effective mechanisms for interacting both with others and with the surrounding environment. In this way culture can be seen as adaptive. A shorter capsular definition of culture refers to culture as a blueprint or organizing framework to guide daily behavior.

An important aspect of culture is that the influence of culture on behavior is not always conscious. Hall calls it the silent language and describes cultural traditions and convention as largely subconscious.[5] He argues that most people do not recognize the effect of culture on themselves, yet behavior is rigidly influenced by it. For example, some cultural groups have a less rigid definition of "appointment time" than do most Western-trained therapists. The client that arrives four hours late, in the company of a friend who has brought his two children along for an assessment as well, can present problems to the therapist.

Those who use culture in practical ways, as advocate, often adopt a multi-dimensional definition of culture. Figure 1 depicts the different dimensions of culture as concentric circles. In the preceding definitions, culture refers to common patterns held by larger groups, e.g., states or nations. This outer regional circle is the one most often seen in cross-cultural studies. It focuses on visible, commonly held patterns; an example would be a comparison of mental health patterns in Ireland and the United States. I chose that particular cross-cultural example from the book *Saints, Scholars and Schizophrenics* by Scheper-Hughes.[6] In this study she describes the dynamics behind the mental health patterns in Ireland and associates them with land tenure and customs related to family role. She focuses in particular on the custom of the youngest son staying on the small farm with aging parents while siblings emigrate to North America. The study illustrates that the life of these youngest "caretaker sons" is one that is conducive to the development of schizophrenia. In this example, types of industry, natural resources, and geographic diversity within the culture are pertinent factors. It is at this level that comparisons of health service delivery models are often made, e.g., comparing the more nationalized systems of Britain and Canada to that of the American health care system. The regional level also includes the popular definition of groups, such as the Navaho or Inuit culture. Within these cultures, however, there is also variation.

In considering culture at a *community* level, smaller and more refined commonalities between people are noted. For example, there might be similarity in type of housing, ethnicity, and economic background among Caucasian middle class suburbanites, particularly if compared to individuals in an inner city core. Similarities in health care practices might be seen at the community level in how frequently and for what reasons community members see family physicians.

Even within these communities, cultures differ as can be seen by comparing two neighboring families in the same community. Factors that might differ at the family level of culture include family power structure, style and frequency of worship, and ways that stress are demonstrated. Potential differences are apparent when comparing the family reaction to the birth of a neonate with severe physical disability in a family which has lived in the area for 10 years and has experience with the health care services to reactions in a family which has recently emigrated from a Latin American country and for whom the knowledge of appropriate services and how to access them is a major difficulty.

Finally, culture can be defined in terms of the individual, i.e., each person can be considered to have an *individual* culture. Although culture is a shared phenomenon, sharing is seen in the context of transmission and socialization. Moreover, individuals learn culture from a number of different people and places so that, in fact, each person's contact with and interpretation of the culture is unique. For instance, siblings brought up in the same home culture might differ in terms of food preference, coping style, and degree of interaction with peer group.

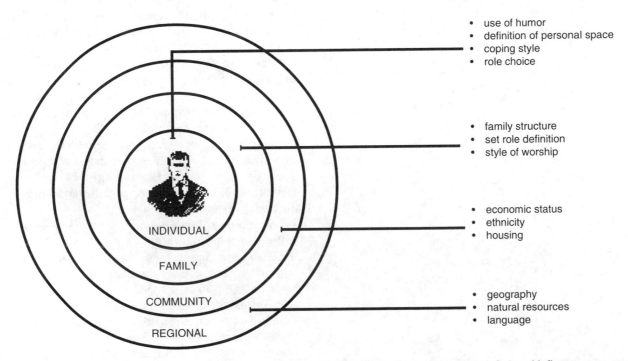

- use of humor
- definition of personal space
- coping style
- role choice

- family structure
- set role definition
- style of worship

- economic status
- ethnicity
- housing

- geography
- natural resources
- language

INDIVIDUAL

FAMILY

COMMUNITY

REGIONAL

Figure 1. Cultural Influence at Different Levels. (From Krefting, L. H. and Krefting, D. V. (1991) Cultural influences on performance. In Christiansen, C. and Baum, C. (Eds), *Occupational Therapy: Overcoming Human Performance Deficits*. Thorofare, NJ: Slack Incorporated, p. 103).

In looking at the different definitions of culture and the heterogeneity of cultural groups, it is important to consider the assimilation of cultures. Assimilation refers to the process whereby people of one culture lose their culturally unique characteristics and become more like those of the dominant culture.[7] Assimilation is the term often used in describing how well immigrants adapted to their new country. The degree of assimilation depends on such factors as length of residence in new country or region, residential area, language spoken at home and fluency in the new language or dialect, and amount of contact with country of origin. Variety amongst groups, even of recent immigrants, can be noted. Differing characteristics include whether they belong to official cultural organizations (such as the Korean Students' Sports Club or a children's language training group), their clothing style, food preference, and involvement with others of the same cultural group. This dilution of stronger cultural characteristics prevents therapists from making broad generalizations about how members of certain groups will behave.

Further complicating the issue of cultural identity is the fact that some individuals are bicultural. These are individuals who may adapt to the dominant culture in one role in life, e.g., at work, yet retain their own cultural values and customs at home.[8] This can also be seen at the family level in which one family member, usually the wife or grandmother who stays at home with young children, retains more of the original cultural characteristics than the primary wage earner, who has more contact with the new cultural group through work. Intergenerational comparisons also illustrate the process of assimilation. For example, in some groups elders are the authority because they are the repositories of knowledge (where knowledge was passed orally). This changes when they emigrate to a new country or region with a different culture. In this new setting the young may become powerful because they more quickly learn the knowledge that helps them adapt to the new culture through attending school or work and through peer contact.

To summarize, the concept of culture can be understood on multiple levels. Each individual is a product of the integration of multiple levels of culture and can be seen to have a unique cultural identity. It is at this level that the definition of culture is of most use to physical and occupational therapists.

What Culture Is Not

One way to help clarify the complex definition of culture is to describe what it is not. A common misinterpretation of culture is that it is the same as ethnicity. Ethnicity is that part of one's identify derived from membership, usually through birth, in a racial, religious, national or linguistic group or subgroup.[9] Ethnicity is an important component of culture but the terms are not synonymous. For example, two patients may come from the same neighborhood and share a strong Hispanic-American background but can differ in other cultural factors such as religion, family structure, ways of expressing pain or discomfort, and experience with the medical system. The broader concept of culture can be noted when considering the best approach to the families of two disabled children of Pakistani background: one a family of seven on social assistance whose members have had minimal contact with the formal medical system and another family of three in which one parent works in a hospital and the other is involved in community politics.

Unfortunately, the most common way that culture has been addressed in the occupational and physical therapy literature is to equate it with ethnicity or race. In this approach writers attempt to provide background information on certain "cultural groups." For example, McCormack discussed characteristic health beliefs and practices of Hispanics, Indo-Chinese and African-Americans,[10] and Blakeney[8] used Appalachian peoples as a case example of the importance of addressing the values of a subculture.

As Litterst observes, such a narrow definition of culture neglects potential variation within groups.[11] Such articles imply a homogeneity among group members and can, if not carefully written, perpetuate stereotypes. Such anecdotal information provides a sort of practical definition of ethnic groups; without a cultural assessment at the individual level, therapists can easily develop preconceived ideas about how groups of people will manage their illness or disability.

Nor is culture synonymous with a geographic region. Culture can be misrepresented in this way in articles such as "Rehabilitation in India" or "Lower Limb Prosthetics in Irian Jaya." This geographic definition often describes a small slice of the disability experience (children with upper limb amputations) or of professional services (mental health occupational therapy) in a particular country while making the assumption that these experiences or services are homogeneous throughout a country. Such cultural analyses (I use that term loosely) often result from what is known as "windscreen" medical anthropology in which only brief contact has been made with a small segment of the health care system.

A third way that the culture concept has been misrepresented is in limiting its relevance only to immigrant health. Clearly, immigrant health highlights the importance of cultural diversity. Changing immigration laws and refugee policies, as well as increased mobility within regions of North America, have created a situation in which it is quite feasible for a therapist to work with people from nearly every cultural group in the world.[12,13] The area of immigrant health also reveals new types of illnesses or disabilities or ones that are no longer common in North America, e.g., post-typhoid paralysis, polio, and nutritional-related disabilities such as blindness due to vitamin A deficiency. New arrivals to a culture are also at risk for stress-related disorders or complications because they often suffer social, economic, and cultural dislocation.[14] These factors result in an increased visibility of immigrants in the rehabilitation system.

Although I have emphasized the importance of immigrant health issues, I must stress that culture in health care is much more than that. The idea of culturally sensitive treatment should not come to mind only when a therapist hears an unfamiliar accent or sees a note on the patient history indicating that the person in the treatment room is a recent immigrant. It should come to mind *every time* the therapist enters that treatment room.

In relation to what culture is not, it is important to realize that no specific rules exist for working with members of any particular cultural group. Thus you will not find the definitive article on working with the first generation Ethiopian patient. As Baptiste notes, a shopping list of cultural traits is not the answer for developing culturally sensitive practice.[15] In fact, this is a challenge for clinical social scientists who are called in to consult about patients whose cultural background is different from that of the majority of the rehabilitation team. An example from my personal experience is a patient from Asia whose mother had moved into the hospital room, was sleeping on rugs by her daughter's bed and, in following her religious traditions, was ensuring that her daughter was awake for all five calls to prayer. Because there are no set rules that help you interpret particular cultures, it is critical to understand the basic components of culture and then assess the cultural identity of each patient.

Cultural Pespectives in Therapy

Culture is often considered from the perspective of the patient/client and the family members. In any therapeutic relationship, however, the culture of both the patient and the therapist must be considered. Not only do the cultural factors influencing the patient's behavior need to be identified but their interaction with the cultural background of the therapist is important.[16]

It is not surprising that therapists who are typically from white middle-class backgrounds and possess the inherent values, mores, and expectations of those experiences[17] can be in conflict with patients. A potential dilemma might arise in the case of the therapist brought up as a rugged individualist who is fiercely independent in interaction with a parent who never leaves the disabled child's side, helping him or her with every activity. This sort of cultural blindness is a good example of ethnocentricity, in which unfamiliar cultures are judged or defined in terms of the health professional's own, with the sense that the professional's culture is superior.

Therapists, then, must try to understand the background of the patient and to identify how their personal values and biases may interfere with assessment and treatment. At the same time therapists must recognize the nature of their own background and how it influences the therapeutic situation. In this way, both partners in the therapeutic relationship can arrive at a common understanding of the problem areas, their priority in treatment, and means of intervention.

The Cost of Culturally Insensitive Therapy

What is the cost of dismissing cultural factors in everyday practice of providing health care? First, rapport will be difficult to establish thereby decreasing the patient's trust in the therapist. Poor rapport can develop into major communication problems. The situation in which different perspectives regarding the preferred outcome of treatment exist but are not communicated is an illustration. Such a situation might be one in which a child is determined to attend a regular school, one parent supports special education, and the other a non-traditional Montessori type of education, and the therapist prefers an educational program in a school–hospital setting. Such communication problems can result in non-compliance and patient dissatisfaction with treatment.

One of the keys to cultural sensitivity is understanding that culture affects illness behavior. Illness behaviors are the ways in which people respond to bodily indication and conditions that they come to view as abnormal.[18] It is the way in which people monitor their health, define and interpret symptoms, take remedial action, and use sources of available help. One of the major factors in illness behavior, is whether patients and families adhere to various treatment regimes. Understanding the patient's culture helps the professional to influence health behavior in positive ways—whether that means following a schedule of home exercises or wearing a protective helmet.

Moreover, by ignoring cultural factors, the behavior of therapists can be affected. They can be left with feelings of helplessness, frustration and anger because of differences in perception with patients and/or families. Most therapists have probably experienced the frustration of either trying to dissuade parents from "doing for" their child with a disability or, on the other hand, to persuade parents to carry out home therapy programs.

In addition to the frustrations experienced by therapists and patients, family members can also be affected by cultural problems, becoming antagonists rather than facilitators in the treatment process. In the field of pediatrics, in which parents are key members of the rehabilitation team, their satisfaction with the therapeutic relationship is critical.

To summarize, recognizing the role of culture in assessment and treatment can improve rapport and communication and increase compliance, and perceived satisfaction with treatment, thereby creating treatment that is effective, efficient, and economical.

Culturally Sensitive Practice

The health care professions have responded to the issue of providing service in a multi-cultural society in a number of ways.[19] One approach focuses on language barriers and involves recruitment of translators for key linguistic groups. This approach is superficial because it reduces the culture concept to the issue of language differences. A second approach is to provide limited awareness training for staff members. This might include bringing in a speaker on multi-cultural communication or having a staff member of a different cultural background discuss cultural barriers s/he has encountered in the medical system. A third approach is to recruit bicultural health care professionals or at least ones with a different ethnic background. (I call this the "United Nations in one rehabilitation department" strategy.) Again, this reduces culture to ethnic background or skin color and does not really address cultural diversity.

The fourth approach is to develop culturally sensitive assessment and intervention strategies that can be used by any therapist person with any patient or family member regardless of the individual cultural background. The remainder of the paper will address a number of strategies that can be used to develop cultural sensitivity in occupational and physical therapy programs. An approach that is particularly useful in introducing cultural sensitivity is to involve a medical anthropologist or sociologist on a consultation basis, for example in weekly rounds in which cultural issues are discussed. This brings immediate relevance to the issues of multiculturalism and daily practice. Cultural sensitivity can also be encouraged by modifying the physical features of an occupational or physical therapy department. Multicultural prompts in orientation boards that include a number of religious and ethnic festivals (for example, the Duvali—the Indian Festival of Lights) might be used. Morse's article describing a non-traditional community program based in the Jewish cultural context illustrates the ways that cultural beliefs can be incorporated into a life skill program for those with developmental delay.[16] Examples of activities integrating principles of the Jewish faith included preparation of Bar and Bat Mizvahs, holiday cooking classes, and joining with other Jewish cultural groups.

A critical step in providing culturally sensitive service is to assess the cultural validity of standardized assessment instruments. The composition of the sample used to establish norms is one aspect to be evaluated. A perusal of most rehabilitation test norms will show that they are based on urban middle- and upper-middle-class subjects. Another factor in cultural validity is the relevance of the evaluation tools and tasks to children of different cultural background. The following situation illustrates how research efforts were frustrated because of poor cultural validity of an instrument. A team of experienced researchers was conducting a study of developmental delay in a northern Canadian community. Although the particular test had excellent psychometric properties, the common tasks children were expected to do were impossible to do in a harsh northern climate where, for example, riding tricycles on the pavement was impossible both because of the lack of pavement and of money to purchase tricycles.

Cultural relevance of diagnostic tests are particularly important when scores are used to determine whether a child is "normal" or in some way delayed and requires special services. A remarkable article by Edgerton describes how an individual labelled as "brain damaged" as a child spent his youth receiving special services for persons with developmental delay.[20] When retested at the age of 17 years, he was found to be of normal intelligence.

One of the ways of approaching the cultural validity of assessments is to compare the test scores of children of different cultural backgrounds. An example of this approach is a recent Master's thesis studying the Miller Assessment for Pre-schoolers (MAP). Hohl noted that Mexican American children in Texas scored significantly lower on the verbal index of the MAP when compared to normative data, emphasizing the potential for cultural differences between groups.[21]

An initial evaluation can be modified in several ways to ensure that culturally relevant data are gathered. The degree to which therapists, children and their families agree that a disability exists is one area to assess. The identification of a specific physical or mental impairment as "illness" or "disability" varies from one culture to another as well as among social classes or ethnic groups within a single culture. For example, variation in the definition of disability by social class is seen in the middle-class American view of asthma, stuttering, and learning disabilities as handicaps requiring treatment; other cultural groups view them as personal characteristics not directly related to health at all.[22] The labelling of these conditions as "disabilities" by the therapist, when the patient and/or family do not believe there is a problem, can lead to non-adherence to treatment as well as frustration of all concerned.

A second question to include in a culturally sensitive intake evaluation is "what caused the illness?" This relates not to pathophysiology but to social or supernatural causes of an illness or disability. The influence of beliefs about "why *my* child" or "why now" are clearly illustrated in the disability detection program with which I am associated in Indonesia. Figure 2 illustrates the kinds of beliefs that are attributed to the birth of an infant with cleft palate—all of the causes are related to behavior of the parents. Knowledge of such information would clearly help a therapist to understand parents who were reluctant to bring a child to a screening clinic or for treatment.

A third type of question to include in an initial evaluation is related to patterns of help-seeking. Patterns of help-seeking are the culturally distinct ways in which people go about finding help at particular times in their illness. Help-seeking refers both to the range of alternatives open to an individual and how and why choices are made between various alternatives.[23] Therapists usually think of help-seeking in terms of the professional health care network such as physicians, sports medicine clinicians, and rehabilitation counsellors. However, people seek help from a variety of nonmedical sources such as family and friends, naturopaths, faith healers, and acupuncturists.[24] Clinicians should not assume that health care professionals are the only alternative used by the patient.

Three studies illustrate the concept of help-seeking by describing different approaches to family caregiving for children with chronic illness. Anderson reports on caregiving patterns for chronically ill children in a Chinese-Canadian context.[25] She notes that immigrant families are often not able to integrate the ideological structures behind the Western health care system and that this may be reflected in non-adherence. A lack of understanding about "normalization" by immigrant families was evident in a tendency to discontinue the exercise program or medication at the least bit of discomfort shown by the children. The family members' goal was the "happiness and contentment" of children rather than normalization procedures advocated in Western medicine.

An article by Oremland describes an ethnographic approach to studying work dynamics in family care of hemophilic children.[26] The division of labor surrounding family caregiving is clearly sensitive to cultural variation; in this study the central role that siblings play in caregiving is described. A third study describes "parental entrepreneur-

ship"—activism among parents of children with a disability to promote better systems of professional caregiving.[27]

The concept of help-seeking has a number of practical implications for assessment and intervention. First, the history of help-seeking (including the perceived importance and success of each alternative) should be a part of any comprehensive assessment. Eliciting the child's and family's feelings about the use of informal sectors is often difficult because they may be reluctant to disclose "unmedical" or unsophisticated sources of help despite the fact that they have used them. One of the ways to facilitate communication is to convey an accepting attitude about the range of alternatives, perhaps by introducing the topic with a comment about the number of people you see in therapy who use non-medical options.

It is important to consider therapeutic networks in which two or more options from different sectors are used simultaneously because occupational and physical therapy assessment and intervention might conflict with other alternatives. An example is the situation in which an herbalist is advocating fasting and meditation for a chronic respiratory condition and the therapist is encouraging moderate exercise and postural drainage. Such a situation may create tension or anxiety for the child and family and may cause them to disregard the therapist's treatment choice. One approach is for therapists to try to incorporate non-traditional sources of help in his or her therapeutic program, for instance in preceding the therapy treatment sessions with relaxation or creative visualization.

The suggestions mentioned represent only a small number of examples of how therapists can begin to

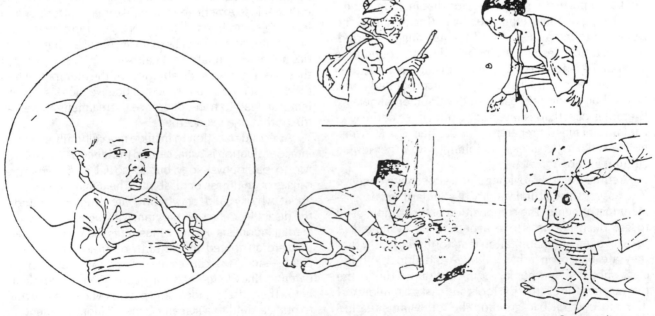

Figure 2. Cultural Understanding of the Cause of Cleft Palate. (Used with permission of Dr. Soeharso, Community Based Rehabilitation Centre, Surakarta, Indonesia).

develop more culturally sensitive treatment approaches. They are meant to illustrate how the rather vague culture concept can be incorporated into daily practice.

Conclusions

Culture is a complex concept that is of central importance to the provision of effective services for infants and children who are disabled and to their families. I have argued that therapists must consider the cultural identity of the individual and avoid cultural "rule books" that assume all people of a particular ethnic or racial background are similar in health beliefs and practices. It is also important for therapists to evaluate their own cultural values and beliefs and to be aware of how these influence practice. A reconceptualization of all aspects of assessment and treatment is needed if the multicultural nature of today's society is to be acknowledged in the rehabilitation field. This article presents some ways to begin this process.

References

1. Geertz, C. (1973). *The interpretation of cultures.* New York: Basic Books.

2. Keesing, R. (1981). Theories of cultures. In R Casson (ed): *Language, Culture and Cognition.* New York: MacMillan.

3. Kroeber, A. L. & Kluckholn, C. (1963). *Culture: a Critical Review.* New York: Vintage Books.

4. Low, S. M. (1984). The cultural basis of health, illness and disease. *Social Work in Health Care, 9,* 13–23.

5. Hall, E. (1959). *The Silent Language.* New York: Doubleday.

6. Scheper-Hughes, N. (1979). *Saints, Scholars, and Schizophrenics.* Berkeley: University of California Press.

7 Shawski, K. A. (1987). Ethnic/racial considerations in occupational therapy. *Occupational Therapy in Health Care, 4,* 37–49.

8. Blakeney A. B. (1987). Appalachian values: Implications for occupational therapists. *Occupational Therapy in Health Care, 4,* 57–72.

9. Hartog, J. & Hartog, E. E. (1983). Cultural aspects of health and illness behaviours in hospitals. *Western Journal of Medicine, 139,* 910–916.

10. McCormack, G.L. (1987). Culture and communication in the treatment planning for occupational therapy with minority patients. *Occupational Therapy in Health Care, 4,* 17–36.

11. Litterst, T. A. E. (1985). A reappraisal of anthropological fieldwork methods and concept of culture in occupational therapy research. *American Journal of Occupational Therapy, 39,* 602–604.

12. Dyck, I. (1989). The immigrant client: Issues in developing culturally sensitive practice. *Canadian Journal of Occupational Therapy, 56,* 248–255.

13. Health and Welfare Canada (1986). *Review of the Literature on Migrant Mental Health.* Ottawa: Department of National Health and Welfare.

14. Clarke, M. M. (1983). Cultural context of medical practice. *Western Journal of Medicine. 139,* 806–810.

15. Baptiste, S. (1988). Chronic pain, activity, and culture. *Canadian Journal of Occupational Therapy, 55,* 179–184.

16. Morse, A. (1987). A cultural intervention model for developmentally delayed adults: An expanded role for occupational therapy. *Occupational Therapy in Health Care, 4,* 103–113.

17. Robinson, L. (1987). Patient compliance in occupational therapy home health programs: Sociocultural considerations. *Occupational Therapy in Health Care, 4,* 127–137.

18. Mechanic, D. (1986). The concept of illness behaviour: Culture, situation, and personal predisposition. *Psychological Medicine, 16,* 1–7.

19. Cuellar, I., & Arnold, B. R. (1988). Cultural considerations and rehabilitation of disabled Mexican Americans. *Journal of Rehabilitation,* 35–41.

20. Edgerton, R. B. (1986). A case of delabeling: Some practical and theoretical implications. In L. Langness & H. Levine (Eds). *Culture and Retardation* pp 101–126. Norwell, MA: Kluwer Academic Press.

21. Hohl, M. R. (1990). *The Performance of Mexican–American Children in Texas on the Miller Assessment for Pre-schoolers.* Unpublished master's thesis. Chapel Hill, NC, University of North Carolina at Chapel Hill.

22. Gliedman, J. & Roth, W. (1980). *The Unexpected Minority: Handicapped Children in America.* New York: Harcourt Brace Jovanovich.

23. Helman, C. (1984). *Culture, Health and Illness.* Bristol: John Wright and Sons.

24. Kleinman, A. (1980). *Patients and Healers in the Context of Culture.* Berkeley: University of California Press, pp 104–118.

25. Anderson, J. (1986). Ethnicity and illness experience: Ideological structures and the health care delivery system. *Social Science and Medicine, 22,* 1277–1283.

26. Oremland, E. K. (1988). Work dynamics in family care of hemophiliac children. *Social Science and Medicine, 26,* 467–475.

27. Darling, R. (1988). Parental entrepreneurship: A consumerist response to professional dominance. *Journal of Social Issues, 44,* 141–158.

Chapter 17

Temporal Adaptation: A Conceptual Framework for Occupational Therapy

Gary Kielhofner, DrPH,OTR, FAOTA

In 1922, Adolf Meyer proposed a philosophy of practice for the newly formed profession of occupational therapy (see Chapter 2.) He maintained that the key to successful application of occupational therapy would lie in an awakening to:

> ... a full meaning of time as the biggest wonder and asset of our lives and the valuation of opportunity and performance as the greatest measure of time .... (1)

Eleanor Clarke Slagle pioneered the application of Meyer's proposal that occupational therapy should view patients within the context of time through the unfolding of their daily lives. She implemented a program of "habit training" based on the principle that the normal use of time in a purposeful daily routine would exert an organizing force on even the most regressed, unmedicated mentally ill patients (2). Slagle intuitively recognized habit as a critical regulator of man's use of time and consequently as a significant component of his adaptation.

From Meyer and Slagle the profession received the proposition that in the richness of man's daily routines and his purposeful use of time, there was both health-maintaining and health-regenerating potential. Further, the way in which disabled individuals used and organized their time in daily life was revealed as a measure of their adaptiveness. Health was revealed in how patients functioned on a day-by-day, hour-by-hour basis. The temporal dimension in human adaptation was installed as a legitimate concern for occupational therapists. This temporal perspective gave to occupational therapy a special caretaker position for patients' activities of daily living.

However, occupational therapy practice has subsequently evolved away from a concern for patients' temporal functioning (3). The full appreciation of the meaning of time, which Meyer so strongly advocated, never came to pass in occupational therapy. Consequently, the broad humanistic theme of activities of daily living suffered a substantial loss of content. Presently, the concept of activities of daily living conveys little more than a checklist for self-care (4).

At a time when occupational therapy must face the reality of its "derailment," as Shannon suggests in his paper, it is imperative that the profession scrutinize its underpinnings and carefully examine its philosophy and practice for critical concepts that have been lost. The task that lies before the profession is to reclaim and revitalize those elements which made occupational therapy such a viable and energizing idea for the founders and early leaders of the profession.

The theme of temporal adaptation is a valuable scheme for practice and should be reintroduced to occupational therapy. Therefore, this paper first provides support for temporal functioning as a useful conceptual base from which human adaptation and dysfunction of the disabled can be better understood. Second, it proposes a temporal conceptual framework that serves as a background from which to generate evaluations and interventions.

The Temporal Dimension in Adaptation

The elderly person whose abundant leisure has become painful monotony, the physically disabled person whose self-care has been expanded into a long and tedious procedure, the psychiatric patient whose personal helplessness makes the future an unwelcome burden, and the mentally subnormal person for whom the string of events in time seems a jumble ... each represent a special difficulty in temporal adaptation. Although occupational therapists are thoroughly acquainted with such temporal problems, the systematic application of clinical intervention aimed at temporal dysfunction is not formally or consistently part of the clinician's treatment. In order to reintroduce temporal adaptation to clinical practice, this section provides a general, theoretical overview. *Temporal adaptation* serves in this paper as a descriptive term for integration of an entire spectrum of activities, the organization of which supports health on an ongoing daily life basis. *Temporal dysfunction* will refer to problems that arise in this daily life organization. Temporal adaptation and dysfunction represent descriptive terms for talking about complex daily activity from the specific but universal dimension of time.

Time. Time is the inescapable boundary for human existence and activity. Hall describes it as the "unconscious determinant or frame upon which everything else is built," (5) and Henry states that for man time is a universal dimension, guiding and structuring his experience and his activity (6). Human adaptation is inextricably bound up in the conscious experience of time. Man's conscious placement in time is a function of the capacity to symbolize internally that which is perceived externally (7). Each man bears a complex symbolic model or image of himself located in time (8). His initial awareness of time results from the experience of change in the self and the environment (9). The model or image of external temporal reality is generated and continuously reorganized through the accumulated experience of changing events.

Armed with temporal consciousness, man is a supreme actor in time. Not only is he aware of changing events, but he is likewise conscious of the fact that he can have some effect on that course of events. The percep-

tion of the self as a cause comes from experiencing the results of one's own actions in time (10). Man's awareness of time, the awareness of his causative ability, and its potential for consequences are interrelated phenomena. The human condition is transformed by the awareness of the individual that he or she has acted, is acting, and will continue to act. Man's awareness of time makes possible this continuity of experience that transforms the nature of his adaptation. In John Dewey's words:

> Man differs from the lower animals because he preserves his past experiences .... With the animals, an experience perishes as it happens and each new doing or suffering stands alone. But man lives in a world where each occurrence is charged with echoes and reminiscences of what has gone before, where each event is a reminder of other things. Hence he lives not, like the beasts of the field, in a world of merely physical things, but in a world of signs and symbols. (11)

Although overt experiences occur as disconnected and episodic events, the inner symbolic experience is an uninterrupted flow in which past and future are orienting reference points for human adaptation. Man draws upon his past experiences as an information source for future action. He projects himself into the future, planning events, and setting goals that may not be realized for days, months, or even years. Through imagination, he can test alternative courses of action and contemplate their consequences (7). Once placed consciously in time, the human organism adapts through purposeful action. Man adapts through awareness of his own agenthood and placement in time that makes possible the conscious planning of action. Action and time are concomitant components of the human experience linked to purpose through hindsight and foresight.

The Conceptual Framework

The concepts of temporal adaptation can be put into operation through a conceptual framework designed to generate strategies of evaluation and treatment in occupational therapy. A preliminary framework was constructed as a series of propositions about temporal adaptation. The first four concern external factors and learning that influence temporal experience and activity. Propositions five and six concern the internal organization of temporal behavior. The seventh proposition concerns pathologies or dysfunctions of time.

Proposition 1: Each person bears a temporal frame of reference that is culturally constituted. Individuals carry an image of their placement in time that is a unique product of their culture (12). Their temporal frame of reference is maintained and transmitted within the culture in the form of norms and values and contains the basic notion and valuation of time (13).

In American society the notion of time is that of a straight line or path extending into the future. Time is experienced as a "supersensible medium or container, as a stream of infinitely extended warp upon which the woof of human happenings is woven ...." (14) It is sectioned off and takes on the nature of enclosed or finite space, the segments of which are to be filled with activity (12, 13). This notion of time is exhibited in the American habit of scheduling events. Random behavior that lacks a pattern of organization is not functional in the mainstream of American society (6). The American culture values time as a commodity; it can be bought, sold, saved, or wasted (13). This sense of time is captured in the phrase *time is money* and, understandably, wasting time has a strong negative connotation in the culture.

Although the orderly, punctual life of Americans is not an innate feature of human existence, it is largely considered a fact of nature. This notion and valuation of time is the framework of the culture that sets boundaries for competent action in daily life. In order to adapt to the society the individual must to some degree internalize and order behavior according to the culture's temporal frame of reference.

Proposition 2: A unique temporal frame of reference is accumulated through learning and socializing experiences that begin in childhood. Although the basic ability to perceive time is a cognitive developmental phenomenon, the particular culture frame of reference is a product of socialization (6). The transmission of the temporal frame of reference has been classified by Hall into three levels of socialization or learning: technical, informal, and formal (13).

The technical learning of time occurs in a didactic framework, as when a child is taught to tell time and to comprehend the division of seconds, minutes, and hours. Informal time is learned through imitation of role models and the learning comprises activities and mannerisms that are so much a part of daily life that they are performed almost unconsciously. An example of informal time is knowing that being 5 minutes late for an appointment is acceptable, whereas 20 minutes is not. Formal learning is taught by precept and admonition, and concerns traditions and values transmitted through the expectations and prohibitions of each culture. As an example, the prohibition of wasting time is passed on in American culture as an important value.

From this teaching, modeling, precept, and admonition, children's socialization is accomplished through the internalization of a complex temporal frame of reference. It is within the family that children first learn to organize time under this framework toward fulfillment of a social role. The role of children or siblings within the family bears with it a whole set of activities ordered in time. Learning to be on time for meals, to do chores when assigned, to habitually care for themselves, and to periodically clean their rooms are all part of the complex schema children must incorporate. Learning temporal organization, which occurs within the family, generalizes to other roles children must take

on later. Children not only know a particular set of behaviors ordered in time, but more importantly, also learn to organize activity in time.

In addition to learning how and when to behave, children learn a complex set of temporal expectations; Toffler gives the following poignant description.

From infancy on the child learns, for example, that when Daddy

> ... *leaves for work in the morning, it means that he will not return for many hours.... The child soon learns that "mealtime" is neither a one-minute nor a five-hour affair, but that it ordinarily lasts from fifteen minutes to an hour. He learns that going to a movie lasts two to four hours, but that a visit with the pediatrician seldom lasts more than one. He learns that the school day ordinarily lasts six hours. He learns that a relationship with a teacher ordinarily extends over a school year, but that his relationship with his grandparents is supposed to be of much longer duration. Indeed some relationships are supposed to last a lifetime. (15)*

Where the household temporal patterns are chaotic, children's learning of the temporal frame of reference may be maladaptive (6). Consequently, competent participation in the culture may be hindered as they falter in organizing tune to respond to other successive social institutions, such as school and the job setting.

Proposition 3: There is a natural temporal order to daily living organized around the life–space activities of self-maintenance, work, and play. Adolph Meyer pointed out that there is a natural rhythm in the organization of daily life around life spaces (1) (see Chapter 2). These life spaces are assigned to activities that represent a social order, determining appropriate times for role behavior. Reilly conceptualized daily living as divided into life spaces of existence, subsistence, and discretionary time (16). Existence is that time spent for eating, sleeping, personal hygiene, and other aspects of self-maintenance; subsistence is the life space devoted to working for an income; and discretionary time is that life space reserved for recreation and leisure. Recreation and leisure comprise dual aspects of play in adult life. Recreation is the period of time when man is made ready for the next cycle of work through relaxation. Leisure is earned time made possible by the satisfying performance of work.

Health consists of the proper balance of the life spaces that is both satisfying to individuals and appropriate for their roles within society. Balance refers to more than just so much work, play, and rest. Rather, balance recognizes an interdependence of these life spaces and their relationship to both internal values, interests, and goals, and external demands of the environment. It is the interrelated balance of self-maintenance, work, and play that comprises health.

While homeostasis is used to describe the biological health of the organism, a broader concept of balance in daily life describes the conditions for psychosocial health of the human organism. Occupational therapists are in a position to make critical statements about the health of their patients from both interrelated dimensions of homeostasis and balance. Far from being limited to the idea of self-care, activities of daily living refer to man's total state of health, which depends on both biological and psychosocial factors.

Proposition 4: Society requires its members to organize their use of time according to ascribed social roles. While cultural norms and values provide a contextual framework for man's use of time, his individual daily pattern must be organized around his occupational roles (17). Heard expands on this theme of role behavior in her paper. The sum total of man's activity within his life spaces has been referred to as occupational behavior (18). Life spaces are filled according to the occupational roles to which they are assigned. Within the daily routine, an individual's life spaces may be divided between several occupational roles such as the father, worker, and community volunteer. Adaptation requires individuals to use their time in a manner that supports their roles. The student must organize time for attendance at classes and homework, the worker for the job schedule, and the retiree for effective and satisfying use of leisure time.

The organization of time around one's roles is not a static skill. Occupational roles change and overlap; each individual passes through a succession of roles in a lifetime (19). Taking on a new role requires a new strategy for organizing one's time. When role change is abruptly forced upon an individual through an incurred disability, developing new temporal skills is a critical factor in adapting to the disability.

Proposition 5: An individual's use of time is a function of internalized values, interests, and goals. Values are commitments to action that organize an individual's use of time by establishing an internal order of what comes first and how much time will be allotted to various activities (20). An individual's values set priorities of actions, and their consequences create a personal valence that is ultimately translated into a life style. Values serve an important function in the choice an individual makes to take on various roles. Although values reflect more serious commitments, interests also guide the commitment process. They are states of readiness for choices and action (21). Interests sustain action and serve thereby to maintain commitments over time. Like values, interests prioritize activities and lend organization to temporal behavior.

Goals represent strategies toward the fulfillment of values and interests. Values and interests yield automatic goal-setting and consequent adjustment and organization of daily patterns of time use. This process occurs at various levels of awareness and is necessary for ordering daily life. The individual who has no goals or has difficulty setting goals cannot organize daily life to use existing skills effectively and will, consequently, feel frustrated or helpless (22, 23). Further, an individual must be able to identify and execute appropriate actions for goal-attainment. Problems arise when an individual cannot identify and carry out in proper sequence those activities that lead to successful goal achievement (23, 24). Robinson expands this notion, sequencing action in time, in her paper on rules.

Proposition 6: Habits are the basic structures by which daily behavior is ordered in time and psychosocial health is maintained. While habits are traditionally thought of in terms of vices and virtues, they extend a more subtle and profound influence on daily temporal functioning. All that is familiar, routine, and predictable in daily life bears a relationship to habit. Without habit structure, an individual's daily life would be a chaotic series of disjointed events.

Habits are instantaneous, automatic choices of action made throughout the day (3). Although organized into unconscious routines, they are the products of once conscious choices made until they become automatic (3). Habits reflect actions related to values and interests cemented over time in daily patterns. Further, habits provide a crucial service to adaptation by organizing temporal behavior to meet societal requirements for competence. Consequently, habits perform an important role in assuring that skills are used in an adaptive manner. Skills must not only be present, but also organized into a daily routine.

Proposition 7: Temporal dysfunction may exist in relationship to categories of pathology. Temporal dysfunction may occur as an integral part of some mental illness or as a consequence of imposed physical disability.

When viewing individuals from the perspective of temporal adaptation, it becomes obvious that strategies for intervention cannot begin and end with the physical, mental, or emotional pathology. Each may be integrally related to a broader and often more difficult set of problems in the person's temporal adaptation.

Persons who are so disoriented in time that they cannot give the day, month, or year are readily suspected of being afflicted with dementia, senility, or some psychotic disorder (12). Actual distortions of the perception of time have been shown to occur in some cases of mental illness (9). Further, when individuals cannot organize their time toward fulfillment of their social roles, they may become candidates for psychiatric care (24). Disorganization of time is associated with the subjective sense of helplessness and incompetence seen in mental illness.

Disorganization of temporal adaptation may also be identified in the reaction of an individual to residual physical disabilities. Maintaining a pace of life comparable to individuals without disability may be impossible for some persons whose motor performance is dysfunctional. The impact of sudden disability often imposes tremendous distortions of daily life spaces by increasing the amount of time required for routine activities. Further, where one or more roles change or end as a result of acquired physical disability, the individual may be unable to find new meaningful activities and roles to fill the life–spaces formerly occupied by old ones.

Implementation

Propositions were formulated as a guiding framework for incorporating temporal adaptation into clinical evaluation and treatment. The clinician may use the framework for integrating clinical data with points raised in the propositions. The framework gives the clinician another dimension for viewing patient problems and for generating and interpreting data. It thereby serves as a basis for developing new treatment strategies. Three principles should be adhered to in applying the conceptual framework to evaluation. First, data should be collected on several variables contained in the propositions. Relevant data include the patient's values, interests, goals, balance of play and work, habit structure, and temporal frame of reference. Second, the evaluation should take into consideration internal constraints on time as revealed in the nature of the patient's physical, mental, or emotional disability. Third, the evaluation should also consider the external factors influencing time use: the patient's roles, family expectations, cultural background, and the demands of time and physical space that affect the patient's daily living.

Treatment intervention will be based on the particular pattern of temporal dysfunction revealed by the evaluation. As data is interrelated and considered in light of the conceptual framework, dysfunctional patterns should become evident. For example, one patient's chaotic day may be a reflection of a lack of ability to prioritize interests and to set goals. Without the ability to set priorities and goals, the patient cannot generate habits for a normal, satisfactory daily routine. By using the conceptual framework of temporal adaptation, the clinician should be able to formulate a more comprehensive treatment plan.

Case Examples

Two case histories, together with examples of clinical interventions that follow the principles above, are presented to serve as examples of how the temporal adaptation framework can be applied. Treatments described speak only to the temporal framework and assume the inclusion of other traditional occupational therapy interventions.

Case H. B. H. B. is a 24-year-old, single male psychiatric patient. When admitted to the hospital, his presenting problems included depression and chronic repeated failures in work settings. H.B. graduated from college with a degree in music with plans to reenter college for graduate study in musicology. He not only has definite skills as a musician but has also demonstrated a strong commitment by voluntarily organizing a teenage choir in a local church.

However, H.B. has not managed during the last three years to hold down a steady job and save enough money to re-enter college. His recent occupational history includes such jobs as working in an electrical shop repairing fans, driving a school bus, and doing maintenance work in apartment complexes. H.B. was fired from each of these jobs because of his inability to concentrate on the work. He found the jobs uninteresting and had difficulty applying himself. He attempted to save money toward college, but used up his savings during periods of unemployment between jobs.

H.B. describes his daily life as highly variable and without routine. He has been unable to maintain any schedule and often finds himself late for work and appointments. Further, social activities have taken up a large part of his schedule so that he is negligent in doing many basic self-maintenance tasks. His housekeeping recently became so disorganized that he was evicted from his apartment. H.B. perceives his daily life as chaotic and complains that "there is so little time with so much to do, that I often get stuck on things and never get around to what I set out to do." He feels helpless and depressed since he is not close to his goal of reentering college and does not feel he is progressing toward it. At this point his response to this subjective state is to become inactive. He is without a job and recently does not even pursue his interests in music on a leisure basis.

When considered in light of the conceptual framework, H.B.'s temporal dysfunction can be outlined as follows. H.B. has internalized values and goals. He considers further education important and realistically has chosen an area of study within his capacities. His temporal dysfunction lies in the areas of: (a) identifying and pursuing reasonable short-term objectives that will bring him closer to his overall goal; (b) maintaining a satisfying daily schedule that would balance activities of work, play, and self-maintenance; and (c) organizing his time around present necessary role of being a worker. The temporal dysfunction that has eroded his competence in several areas augments his feelings of depression and helplessness.

Recommendations for treatment should include: 1. assisting H.B. in identifying how his present worker role will lead to the eventual goal of re–entering college and developing a strategy that balances his interest in music with the necessity of working on a daily basis; 2. practice in formulating a basic, balanced daily routine and adhering to it consistently; and 3. making beginning steps toward his overall goal, by gathering information on graduate programs in music, their requirements, and possible scholarships. By subdividing each of these goals into subroutines such as finding a new job or ways of pursuing his interest in music on a leisure basis, he may be able to overcome the vicious cycle of daily life incompetence, helplessness, and depression. Treatment would occur in graded steps toward the eventual reconstruction of daily living skills.

Case T.J.

T.J. is a 17-year-old male who sustained a spinal cord injury in an automobile accident. Five months after the injury, T.J., a paraplegic, remains depressed and withdrawn. When approached about his depressed state, T.J. responds that his life-plans have been destroyed. Prior to his injury he was an excellent athlete with a promise of an athletic scholarship to a university.

Beyond his college training, T.J. had hoped to become a high school coach. Further, T.J. points out that he is now forced to spend days in bed or a wheelchair, whereas formerly he was active in a variety of intramural and varsity sports. He describes the present as boring and sees little prospect for change in the future. Also, data from his family points out that T.J.'s former positive self-image revolved around his physical appearance and athletic prowess; he now views himself as an invalid.

In T.J.'s case it should be noted that: (a) his former values and interests focused on activities he can no longer engage in or he must learn to participate in with some modifications; (b) his self-image and prospects for the future revolved around skills and capacities no longer intact; (c) his former daily routine revolved around his athletic role. In summary, those values and habits that formerly maintained a satisfying daily routine and those skills and goals which made the future desirable are no longer intact.

T.J.'s treatment under the framework of temporal adaptation would focus on the following sequence of treatment strategies: 1. reconstruction of the self-image through successful experiences in areas related to his past interests; 2. exploration of new activities to develop interests (in the clinic and his own community); 3. reconstruction of his daily routine, which will have to accommodate different life spaces—such as the expanded space necessary for self-care and personal hygiene; and 4. refocusing on his career goals so that a viable and acceptable objective could at least be tentatively pursued.

Conclusion

Temporal adaptation was identified as an early theme in occupational therapy that has been dropped out of clinical practice. The concept of temporal adaptation was reintroduced and formulated in a preliminary framework for clinical intervention. Temporal adaptation serves as a conceptual schema to broaden the clinician's current perspective and repertoire of skills and, as such, does not replace traditional therapeutic efforts but expands them into a more comprehensive framework. Temporal adaptation is a rich conceptual schema for occupational therapy because it speaks to a class of dysfunction found in the entire range of patients seen by occupational therapists.

Acknowledgment

This article is based in part upon material submitted in partial fulfillment of the requirements for the Master of Arts Degree, University of Southern California, Los Angeles. Partial financial support for this study was provided by the Division of Allied Health Manpower, Department of Health, Education and Welfare.

References

1. Meyer A: The philosophy of occupational therapy. *Arch Occup Ther 1:*1–10, 1922, p 9 (Reprinted as Chapter 2).

2. Slagle EC: Training aides for mental patients. *Arch Occup Ther 1:*11–16, 1922.

3. Kielhofner GW: The evolution of knowledge in occupational therapy — understanding adaptation of the chronically disabled. Master's Thesis. Department of Occupational Therapy, University of Southern California, Los Angeles, 1973.

4. Reilly M: The modernization of occupational therapy. *Am J Occup Ther 25:*243–247, 1971.

5. Hall ET: The paradox of culture. In *In the Name of Life,* Bernard Landis and Edward S. Tauber, Editors, New York: Holt, Rinehart, and Winston, 1971, p 226.

6. Henry J: *Pathways to Madness,* New York: Vintage Books, Random House, 1971.

7. White R: Strategies of adaptation: an attempt at systematic description. In *Coping and Adaptation,* George Coelho, David Hamburg, and John E. Adams, Editors. New York: Basic Books, 1974.

8. Boulding K: *The Image,* Ann Arbor: University of Michigan Press, 1961.

9. Larrington G: An exploratory study of the temporal aspects of adaptive functioning. Master's Thesis. Department of Occupational Therapy, University of Southern California, Los Angeles, California, 1970.

10. DeCharms R.: *Personal Causation,* New York: Academic Press, 1968.

11. Dewey J: *Reconstruction in Philosophy,* New York: H. Holt and Company, 1920, p 36.

12. Hallowell I: *Culture and Experience,* New York: Schocken Books, 1955, p 217.

13. Hall ET: *The Silent Language,* Greenwich: Fawcett Publications, Inc., 1959.

14. Parkhurst HH: The cult of chronology. In *Essays in Honor of John Dewey,* New York: H. Holt and Company, 1929, p 23.

15. Toffler A: *Future Shock,* New York: Random House, 1970, p 360.

16. Reilly M: A psychiatric occupational therapy program as a teaching model. *Am J Occup Ther, 20:* 2–10, 1966.

17. Newcomb T: *Social Psychology,* New York: Henry Holt and Company, 1959.

18. Matsutsuyu J: Occupational behavior a perspective on work and play. *Am J Occup Ther 25:* 291–293, 1971.

19. Arensenian J: Life cycle factors in mental illness. *Ment Hyg 52:* 19–30, 1968.

20. Kluckhohn C: Values and value orientations in the theory of action: an exploration in definition and classification: In *Toward a General Theory of Action,* T. Parsons and E. Shils, Editors. Cambridge: Harvard University Press, 1951.

21. Matsutsuyu J: The interest checklist. *Am J Occup Ther 23:* 323–326, 1969.

22. Lakein A: *How to Get Control of Your Time and Your Life,* New York: The Signet, The New American Library, Inc., 1974.

23. Kiev A: *A Strategy of Daily Living,* New York: The Free Press, 1973.

24. Black MM: The evolution of social roles—a perspective on fantasy. Master's Thesis. Department of Occupational Therapy, University of Southern California, Los Angeles, 1973.

Chapter 18

Comparison of Temporal Patterns and Meaningfulness of the Daily Activities of Schizophrenic and Normal Adults

Timothy C. Weeder, MHS, OTR/L

Occupational therapists are just beginning to explore the useful framework of temporal adaptation for a more holistic examination of human health and illness. The proposition that an individual's use of time in productive and playful endeavors could be studied for evaluation and treatment purposes is one of the earliest concepts introduced into occupational therapy philosophy (Meyer, 1922) (see Chapter 2). It was thought that a balance among one's daily activities was crucial to sustaining good mental health. Although this theme is one of the profession's oldest, it has not commanded significant attention until recently (Kielhofner, 1977 [see Chapter 17], 1979, 1980; Neville, 1980; Rosenthal and Howe, 1984; Neville, Kreisberg, and Kielhofner, 1985).

Clinical interviews reveal that a frequent complaint of psychiatric patients with temporal dysfunction is a lack of meaningfulness in their daily activities. Unless individuals find meaning in their daily activities, it is doubtful that engagement in those behaviors will continue, resulting in an imbalance in their daily activities, hence temporal dysfunction. Since practitioners are responsible for assisting dysfunctional patients in reorganizing their use of time in a more adaptive manner, there is a vital need to better understand how time and meaning can influence state of health.

The disorder of schizophrenia was chosen for study since it is one of the most debilitating psychiatric disorders in the United States (President's Commission on Mental Health, 1978). The illness is marked by deterioration in the ability to function in work, social relations, and self-care activities. Additionally, disturbances in volition or the ability to initiate and carry out goal-directed action is quite characteristic of this population (American Psychiatric Association, 1980; Neville et al., 1985). The nature of the disorder would appear to make individuals with schizophrenia especially susceptible to dysfunction in use of time. In order to gain a perspective on what constitutes healthy use of time and meaningfulness of daily activities, a comparison to normal adults was made.

The objective of this study was threefold. The first objective was to determine whether or not the amount of time spent in daily activities is different for a sample of schizophrenic adults than it is for a sample of normal adults. The second objective was to determine whether or not the meaningfulness of those daily activities is different for a sample of schizophrenic adults than they are for a sample of normal adults. The final objective was to determine the relationship between the amount of time and meaningfulness of each activity for each of the two groups.

Literature Review

The conceptual frameworks of time and action are inseparable in early occupational therapy philosophy. These concepts were first introduced into the profession by Dr. Adolf Meyer (1922) (see Chapter 2). Since that time, significant variables have been identified in occupational therapy literature which serve to shape an individual's use of time. The internalized images of time which are shaped by the culture and personal experiences, give the individual certain inner definitions of time, values concerning time, and perspectives about the "proper" organization of time (Barris, Kielhofner, and Watts, 1983). Personal causation has been linked to how an individual uses time (Kielhofner and Burke, 1980; Neville et al., 1985). Two facets of personal causation, sense of autonomy and perceived competence, are believed to yield a self-image regarding efficacy. A negative self-image regarding efficacy may then preclude engagement in certain human activities. Level of interest has also been identified as a factor which helps to shape a person's configuration of time by increasing or decreasing participation in certain activities (Kielhofner, 1977 [see Chapter 17]; Kielhofner and Burke, 1980). Interest is in part determined by the enjoyability associated with a particular object or event. These factors, values, personal causation, and interests serve to guide how a person will actually perform in the temporal-action dimension. The themes of time and action are unquestionably interrelated, and they provide the profession with a unique foundation for understanding human's occupational nature.

It has been proposed by many (Meyer, 1922 [see Chapter 2]; Nystrom 1974; Kielhofner, 1977 [see Chapter 17], 1979, 1980; Cynkin, 1979; Neville, 1980; Reed and Sanderson, 1980; Mosey, 1981; Barris et al., 1983; Neville et al., 1985) that one's use of time is reflective of one's state of health. According to these authors, work and leisure time play important roles in developing and maintaining a healthy personality. They suggest that a balance of daily activities is necessary for good mental health. However, very little research has been conducted to verify this generally-held assumption. The idea that an individual's engagement in activities in an adaptive manner can be health promoting and regenerating, continues to be the essence of occupational therapy theory and practice. The need for further validation of this theory is clear.

Kielhofner defined temporal adaptation as "A descriptive term for the integration of an entire spectrum of activities, the organization of which supports health on an ongoing daily life basis" (Kielhofner, 1977, p. 236) (see Chapter 17). The term temporal adaptation, however, implies a healthy state of being; a state that is adaptive for the individual. Temporal patterns refer to the configuration of time spent in various human activities. It is important to note that no assignment of value is given concerning adaptation or maladaptation. For research purposes, this is obviously very important.

In occupational therapy, the literature that exists on temporal patterns is focused on dysfunctional patients and their maladaptive use of time. Most of the literature is in the form of theoretical statements or hypothetical case studies, with limited scientific backing. According to the literature, temporal disorganization is a typical problem for many people with psychosocial dysfunction. Neville (1980) reported temporal dysfunction in many of her patients. They may demonstrate chaotic patterns of time use, be unable to manage their time, or demonstrate imbalances in their life spaces (Barris et al., 1983). Temporal dysfunction and schizophrenia has been studied by Neville, et al. (1985). Simply stated, temporal dysfunction refers to "problems that arise in the daily life organization" (Kielhofner, 1977, p. 238) (see Chapter 17).

In addition to problems in the daily organization of activity, persons whose temporal practices do not provide meaning should be recognized as being in a state of temporal dysfunction (Barris et al., 1983). Nystrom (1974) in her study of the elderly and their activity patterns, asserted that no study of activity is sufficient unless the meaning associated with it is explored. Reilly (1960) further points out the importance of meaning in occupational therapy, "For us, in occupational therapy, the most fundamental area of research is, and probably always will be, the nature and meaning of activity" (Reilly, 1960, p. 208).

The relationship of meaningfulness and use of time, however, has been inadequately explored. The model of human occupation holds that personal causation, interests, and values are important organizers of occupational behavior, or how we use time, and that meaningfulness is a dimension of values (Barris et al., 1983). It is asserted that successful adaptation to the environment is dependent upon engagement in activities and relationships that have personal meaning and satisfy societal needs. While occupational therapy has always espoused the therapeutic value of meaningful activity, it is this investigator's contention that an indepth understanding of meaningfulness is often lacking. Sharott summed up the profession's relationship to meaning best:

Occupational therapists are not strangers to the notion of meaningful activity. Despite universal recognition of meaning, it remains an elusive concept. In the years since the founders of occupational therapy postulated the health giving effects of meaningful participation in occupations, little has been done to extend the field's appreciation of meaning as a feature of human existence or to augment understanding of how meaning is created and transmitted in human action and interaction. (Sharott, 1983, p. 213)

As mentioned above, a major problem encountered in studying meaningfulness, is how to make it more objective and concrete, and how to measure it reliably. Gregory (1983) operationalized meaningfulness of activity as: (1) enjoyability—how much one enjoys what he or she does, (2) autonomy—whether or not one chooses to do it, and (3) competency—how competent one feels in doing it. The scales were determined to have good reliability. Validity has not been determined. The Meaningfulness of Activity scales are similar to those developed by Watanabe (1968). Her inventory, the Activity Configuration, was developed for use with psychiatric patients. It consists of a daily time schedule and scales to measure autonomy and adequacy. It is her inventory of daily time use that was adapted and used in this researcher's study.

The null hypotheses of this study were as follows:
1. There is no significant difference in the temporal patterns of daily activities of schizophrenic and normal adults.
2. There is no significant difference in the meaningfulness of daily activities of schizophrenic and normal adults.
3. There is no significant relationship between the amount of time spent in each daily activity and the meaningfulness of that activity for schizophrenic adults.
4. There is no significant relationship between the amount of time spent in each daily activity and the meaningfulness of that activity for normal adults.

Methods

Sampling Procedures

The sample of schizophrenic adults who participated in the study were outpatients receiving day treatment at New Horizons Day Treatment Program in Gainesville, Florida. This program provides vocational, recreational, social, and self-maintenance services for the chronically mentally ill five days a week. Of the possible participants in the study, only twenty subjects met the requirements of age, voluntary consent, schizophrenic diagnosis, and sufficient reality orientation to complete a questionnaire. Persons with all types of schizophrenic disorders were admitted to the study. The sample contained the following types: nine undifferentiated types, nine paranoid types, one disorganized type, and one catatonic type. No residual types were represented.

The sample of normal adults was also volunteer sampled. These twenty subjects were required to meet the criteria of age, voluntary consent, no previous psychiatric history, and current employment status or student status. The group of normal subjects was also a convenience sample, solicited at Shands Teaching Hospital, University of Florida. They represented a wide variety of occupations such as blue collar, white collar, and student.

Data-Gathering Instruments

The data collection technique used in this study was a questionnaire adapted from two existing occupational therapy evaluation tools: Watanabe's Activity Configuration and Gregory's Meaningfulness of Activity Scale. Adaptations were necessary to quantify the temporal data and to study only the six daily activities of interest. The first part of the questionnaire addressed the background or demographic information needed to describe the two groups more accurately. The second part of the questionnaire was constructed by this investigator to measure the temporal patterns of the two groups (see Appendix 1).

To determine how much time is spent in an activity, the questionnaire has one-hour units representing a total of 24 hours. Next to each period of time are the six major activity categories of sleep, chores, work, active leisure, passive leisure, and socialization. The following definitions were provided each subject as follows; *Sleep* includes naps and nocturnal sleep. *Chores* include household tasks, shopping, meal preparation, eating, laundry, dressing, bathing, other personal hygiene, transportation, or yard maintenance. *Work* means salaried or volunteer work, education, childcare, or care of family member(s). *Active leisure* is defined as recreation, sports, hobbies, card playing, taking walks, dancing, reading, etc. *Passive Leisure* is watching television, listening to the radio or music, or just relaxing. *Socialization* are those activities done with other people, such as parties, get-togethers, church, or other groups, or family gatherings. The total amount of time spent in each activity is computed to yield time usage for a typical weekday, Saturday, and Sunday. To yield the total time spent in various activities for a five-day week, the totals from the typical weekday data were multiplied by five. To yield the time use for a weekend, the data from the Saturday and Sunday periods were added together. By adding the weekdays and weekend data, estimates of time use over a total seven-day period were arrived at for analysis. Reliability and validity for this scale were not determined, but face validity appears good.

The method utilized for measuring the meaningfulness of daily activities listed above was to use a questionnaire which measured self-reported enjoyability, autonomy, and competency. The scales are ordinal, providing a ranking of possible responses for each dimension (see Appendix 2). Reliability and validity for this population were not determined.

Procedure

To administer the questionnaire the subjects were asked to complete it as carefully and honestly as possible. The schizophrenic subjects were administered the questionnaire in either a small group of two to five persons, or on an individual basis. The difference in administration procedures was due to the fact that some persons had inadequate reading skills, required interpretation of the directions, or needed psychological support. The remaining subjects did not require direct assistance. The questionnaire was checked for completeness and accuracy before the subjects were dismissed. Completion time was approximately 30 minutes. The instructions were written and orally presented for each section of the questionnaire.

The normal sample was given the questionnaire to complete on their own time. No assistance was given or requested by this group. If any inaccuracies were discovered the subject was asked to correct his or her mistakes.

Statistical Treatment

To analyze the temporal pattern data, two-sample "t" tests were performed for each activity variable. Analysis of the time spent in daily activities was performed for the weekday, weekend, and the total week.

To analyze the meaningfulness data, Fisher's Exact test using a 2 x 2 contingency table was performed. Ideally, a Mann-Whitney U test would have been performed if so many ties in the rank data had not been present, making the use of this statistical procedure unreliable. The next best choice would have been a Chi Square test, but because of the small sample size, not all categories contained at least five responses, a requirement of this procedure. The Fisher's Exact test which requires use of a 2 x 2 contingency design was the next best option. However, in order to utilize this procedure the ordinal responses for enjoyability and competency had to be collapsed to form two groups of possible responses for each. The researcher chose to separate the strongest positive response from the weaker ones. Thus, the ability to discriminate subtle differences between the groups was reduced.

Finally, Pearson Product-Moment Correlations were performed to determine the relationship between the amount of time spent in the six activities and the meaningfulness (enjoyability, autonomy, and competency) of the activity, for each group.

Results

Table 1 represents the demographic characteristics of the schizophrenic and normal adults making up the

Table 1
Demographic Characteristics of the
Schizophrenic and Normal Groups

Extraneous Variable	Schizophrenics	Normals
Number of subjects	N=20	N=20
Mean Age and Range	36.75 23 to 59	26.30 21 to 38
Sex	Male=14 Female=6	Male=13 Female=7
Race	White=15 Black=5	White=17 Black=3
Marital Status	Single=19 Married=1	Single=13 Married=7
Living Alone	Yes=4 No=16	Yes=3 No=17
Educational Level	11th Grade or less=7 12th Grade=12 College=1	11th Grade or less=0 12th Grade=4 College=16

two samples in this study. Excepting higher mean age and lower educational level of the schizophrenic sample all other demographic variables were comparable.

Temporal Patterns

Table 2 indicates the means, standard deviations, and test statistics when comparing the amount of time spent in daily activities for *weekdays* of the schizophrenic and normal adults.

Significant differences were found concerning sleep, work, and socialization. Schizophrenics as a group spent statistically significantly more time in sleep activities (p < .05) and socialization (p < .01). Normals spent more time in work activities (p < .01) during the week than did schizophrenics.

Table 3 represents the statistical analysis results comparing the amount of time spent in daily activities for *weekends* of the two groups.

Significant differences were found concerning the amount of time spent in work, active leisure, and passive leisure for the typical weekend. Normals spent more time in work-related activities (p < .05) and active leisure activities (p < .01) than the schizophrenics. Schizophrenic adults spent more time in passive leisure activities (p < .01) than did the normal adults.

Table 4 depicts the results of statistical analysis comparing time usage for the *entire week* for the two groups.

Significant differences were found concerning the amount of time spent in sleep, work, passive leisure, and socialization for a total week. The schizophrenic group spent significantly more hours in sleep (p < .05), passive

leisure (p < .05), and socialization activities (p < .01) than did the normal group. Normals spent significantly more time in work-related activities (p < .01) than did the schizophrenics.

Meaningfulness of Daily Activities

Analysis of the meaningfulness of activity responses yielded no significant differences between the proportion of responses for the enjoyability scale, autonomy scale, and the competency scale between the two groups for any of the daily activities. Table 5 depicts the proportion of responses by group and by activity.

Although no significant differences were found, several trends emerged. The schizophrenic sample saw themselves as less autonomous in active leisure (p > .05) and socialization (p > .05) than did the normal sample. In the area of social competency, the schizophrenic sample reported less competency (p > .05). Concerning chore activities, the schizophrenic adults expressed greater enjoyability (p > .05) than did the normal adults.

Correlates of Temporal Patterns and Meaningfulness

Correlation procedures were used to study the relationship between the amount of time spent in each of the six daily activities and measures of meaningfulness for the schizophrenic and normal group. Table 6 and Table 7 depict the results of the analysis for each group.

The results depicted in Table 6 indicate that there was a significant moderate, negative correlation be-

Table 2
Comparison of Schizophrenic and Normal Groups in Terms of Average Number of Hours Spent in Daily Activities for Weekdays Assessed by Means of "t" Tests

Activity Variable	Schizophrenics		Normals		t
	H	SD	H	SD	
Sleep	43.50	9.74	38.50	4.89	2.05*
Chores	21.50	8.59	18.25	6.93	1.31
Work	16.50	6.50	39.25	9.49	8.83**
Active Leisure	4.25	6.93	4.50	5.10	0.12
Passive Leisure	24.00	13.53	17.50	11.52	1.63
Socialization	10.25	10.06	1.50	3.66	3.65**

*p < .05.
**p < .01.

Table 3
Comparison of Schizophrenic and Normal Groups in Terms of Average Number of Hours Spent in Daily Activities for Weekend Assessed by Means of "t" Tests

Activity Variable	Schizophrenics		Normals		
	H	SD	H	SD	t
Sleep	19.65	5.07	17.65	2.66	1.56
Chores	8.55	4.47	9.00	4.16	0.32
Work	.50	2.23	2.70	3.90	2.18*
Active Leisure	2.60	3.01	5.45	3.70	2.66**
Passive Leisure	13.20	7.12	8.60	4.15	2.49**
Socialization	3.50	3.26	5.10	4.24	1.33

*p < .05.
**p < .01.

tween the amount of time spent in active leisure and the perceived autonomy (p < .05) for the schizophrenic group and a moderate, positive correlation for sleep and competency of that activity (p > .05) for the schizophrenic group. No other significant correlations were found.

Table 7 revealed only one moderate, positive correlation between sleep and perceived competency (p > .05) of that activity for the normal group. No other significant or nearly significant correlations were found.

Table 4
Comparison of Schizophrenic and Normal Groups in Terms of Average Number of Hours Spent in Daily Activities for Total Week Assessed by Means of "t" Tests

Activity Variable	Schizophrenics		Normals		
	H	SD	H	SD	t
Sleep	63.15	13.71	56.15	6.60	2.05*
Chores	30.05	11.61	27.25	9.77	0.82
Work	17.00	7.14	41.95	11.27	8.35**
Active Leisure	6.85	8.22	9.95	7.05	1.27
Passive Leisure	37.20	17.49	26.10	14.80	2.16*
Socialization	13.75	10.76	6.60	6.76	2.51**

*p < .05.
**p < .01.

Table 5
2 x 2 Contingency Tables for Proportion of Meaningfulness
Responses by Groups Using Fisher's Exact Tests

	Enjoyability		Autonomy		Competency	
	Very Much	Somewhat/ Little/ Not At All	Want To	Have To	Very Well	Well Enough/ Do Not Do Well
	Sleep		**Sleep**		**Sleep**	
N	12	8	10	10	11	9
S	13	7	8	12	10	10
	p=1.0000		p=.7512		p=1.000	
	Chores		**Chores**		**Chores**	
N	1	19	7	13	9	11
S	6	14	7	13	9	11
	p=.0915		p=1.0000		p=1.0000	
	Work		**Work**		**Work**	
N	6	14	10	10	14	6
S	9	11	7	13	10	10
	p=.5154		p=.5231		p=.3332	
	Active Leisure		**Active Leisure**		**Active Leisure**	
N	14	6	20	0	11	9
S	13	7	16	4	9	11
	p=1.0000		p=.1060		p=.7524	
	Passive Leisure		**Passive Leisure**		**Passive Leisure**	
N	15	5	19	1	14	6
S	16	4	17	3	10	10
	P=1.0000		p=.6050		p=.3332	
	Socialization		**Socialization**		**Socialization**	
N	13	7	18	2	13	7
S	15	5	12	8	8	12
	p=.7311		p=.0648		p=.2049	

Note. N = Normal group; S = Schizophrenic group. Numbers represent number of responses for each category.

Discussion

Major Findings

The results indicate that the temporal patterns of schizophrenic adults were different concerning four aspects: the amount of time spent in the activities of sleep, work, passive leisure, and socialization, for the total week. The greater amount spent by the schizo- phrenic group in sleep and passive leisure activities suggests that inactivity may be characteristic of this group as was suspected. The greater occurrence of socialization time for the schizophrenic group during the weekdays possibly reflects participation in planned social opportunities which are available at the day treatment center on a routine basis, particularly since on the weekends they spent fewer hours in social activities than the normal group. Had no program been

Table 6
Pearson Product-Moment Correlations Between Measures of Amount of Time Spent in Each Activity and Measures of Meaningfulness for the Schizophrenic Group

Activity Variable	Enjoyability	Autonomy	Competency
Sleep	.08	-.04	.43
Chores	.21	.37	.10
Work	.18	-.13	-.15
Active Leisure	-.17	-.49*	-.07
Passive Leisure	.23	-.04	-.25
Socialization	.05	.24	-.05

*p < .05.

available, one could hypothesize that the schizophrenic persons, on the average, would have spent considerably less time. Not surprisingly, the normal sample spent more than two times the amount of time pursuing work related tasks than did the schizophrenic sample. This may be attributable, in part, to the fact that the schizophrenics participate in a part-time vocational training program, which limits their productive opportunities. Nonetheless, they did spend considerably less time in work activities than their counterparts. Although not statistically significant, time use regarding chores and active leisure indicates the schizophrenic sample, on the average, spent more time on chores, and the normal sample, on the average, spent more time engaging in active leisure. Several possibilities exist to explain these results. Self-maintenance routines may provide greater structure in terms of familiar-

Table 7
Pearson Product-Moment Correlations Between Measures of Amount of Time Spent in Each Activity and Measures of Meaningfulness for the Normal Group

Activity Variable	Enjoyability	Autonomy	Competency
Sleep	.27	.03	.44
Chores	.18	.31	.00
Work	.23	.21	.25
Active Leisure	.29	.00	.31
Passive Leisure	.25	-.01	-.07
Socialization	.14	.23	.08

Note. No significant correlations were found.

ity of habits than other forms of occupation, offer more direct cause and effect, provide greater satisfaction, or simply require greater length of time to perform.

The null hypothesis that meaningfulness of daily activities will not differ significantly for the two groups was accepted. Disappointingly, no significant differences between the proportion of responses on the enjoyability, autonomy, and competency scales between the two groups for any of the daily activities emerged. Several noteworthy trends, however, were observed. The schizophrenic sample viewed themselves as more externally controlled regarding active leisure and socialization pursuits than did the normal sample. This may be due largely to the structure of the day treatment program which strongly encourages participation in these two areas. Engaging in occupations one perceives as having little control over, theoretically would have some negative effect on the quality of mental health. In the area of social competency, the schizophrenic sample reported less belief in skill than did their counterparts, which may reflect actual skill deficiency of which they are cognizant. Concerning chore activities, the schizophrenic sample expressed greater enjoyability than did the normal sample, possibly reflecting greater pleasure derived from more productive forms of occupation.

Turning to the relationship between the amount of time spent in each daily activity and the meaningfulness of that activity, only two clear relationships were apparent for either group. Based on the results, there was a statistically significant discrepancy between sense of control and participation in active leisure for the schizophrenic group. The findings suggest that despite the nearly seven hours performing leisure of an active nature, they felt externally controlled in determining whether or not to participate. This situation presents a serious problem in which sense of autonomy and engagement in an activity are diametrically opposed. Concerning the normal group, the results indicated a nearly significant positive correlation between sleep and perceived competency of that activity. This suggests that the greater amount of time participating in sleep activities is congruent with greater perceived competence of that activity, which appears to be a highly desirable situation.

Conclusions

Based on the results of this study, the generally-held belief that persons who exhibit psychosocial dysfunction may demonstrate abnormal temporal patterns appears to have some validity. The schizophrenic disordered sample in this research study demonstrated significant differences when compared to a normal sample. The inactive states of sleep and passive leisure, in which the schizophrenics spent more time, indicates that there is an interaction between schizophrenia and inactivity. Whether the inactivity is a causal factor of the mental illness, or whether the mental illness caused the inactivity is unclear and beyond the scope of this research study. The fact that the schizophrenic sample spent great amounts of time in social activities, but viewed themselves as less competent and less autonomous indicates a problematic concern. A day treatment program which provides little opportunity for its patients to obtain a sense of control, obtain planned social skills, and promotes excessive socialization time would appear to be countertherapeutic. Less autonomy in active leisure, expressed by the schizophrenic sample, further suggests the importance of patient involvement in determining the kinds of active leisure and frequency of involvement. Not surprisingly, the normal sample spent more time engaging in work-related and active leisure activities than did the schizophrenic sample. This pattern further suggests a relationship between productive and active playful pursuits and good mental health.

Finally, the relationship between the amount of time spent in each daily activity and the meaningfulness of that activity was studied resulting in disappointing findings. Occupational therapists would expect to find strong, positive correlations between these two measures. The only significant correlation which emerged was between external locus of control and active leisure, suggesting the schizophrenics were experiencing a serious lack of control considering the amount of time spent in that activity. Caution should be exercised in generalizing from these findings. The limitations inherent in a cross-sectional design and non-random subject selection should be considered when examining the results.

Implications for treatment include:
1. Help patients to achieve a greater sense of autonomy in all areas of daily living when possible, particularly social and active leisure pursuits.
2. Increase efforts to improve interpersonal skills, recognizing that participation in socialization opportunities does not necessarily imply improved skill level.
3. Continue to assist patients in developing more healthy patterns of time use through the use of time management approaches and experiential opportunities to establish better habits.

Recommendations

As noted in the review of the literature, there have been a limited number of studies performed by occupational therapists in the area of temporal patterns and its relationship to meaningfulness of activity. It appears to this investigator that this area is one which needs more extensive study to determine the validity of some of the profession's most basic tenets concerning mental health.

This study needs to be replicated with a larger sample of schizophrenic and normal adults so that the loss of valuable ranking information on the meaningfulness of activity scale would not occur, thus permitting more fine discrimination. Reliability and validity of the tool need to be established.

Further study as to the relationship between other psychiatric diagnoses and use of time and meaningfulness of activity is also indicated. Longitudinal studies on normals and the mentally ill may yield informative data on how use of time changes over age and over the course of the psychosocial disorder.

High priority should be placed on study of temporal patterns and meaningfulness of activity by the national association. It behooves occupational therapists to substantiate their most basic claims of uniqueness.

References

American Psychiatric Association. (1980). *Diagnostic and statistical manual of mental disorders* (3rd ed.) Washington, DC: Author.

Barris, R., Kielhofner, G., & Watts, J.H. (1983). *Psychosocial occupational therapy: Practice in a pluralistic arena.* Laurel, Maryland: Ramsco.

Cynkin, S. (1979). *Occupational therapy: Toward health through activities* (pp. 24–29). Boston: Little, Brown and Company.

Gregory M. (1983). Occupational behavior and life satisfaction among retirees. *American Journal of Occupational Therapy, 37,* 548–553.

Kielhofner, G. (1977). Temporal adaptation: A conceptual framework for occupational therapy. *American Journal of Occupational Therapy, 31,* 235–242. (Reprinted as Chapter 17.)

Kielhofner, G. (1979). The temporal dimension in the lives of retarded adults: A problem of interaction and intervention. *American Journal of Occupational Therapy, 33,* 161–168.

Kielhofner, G. (1980). A model of human occupation, part 2: Ontogenesis from the perspective of temporal adaptation. *American Journal of Occupational Therapy, 34,* 657–663.

Kielhofner, G., & Burke, J.P. (1980). A model of human occupation, part 1: Conceptual framework and content. *American Journal of Occupational Therapy, 34,* 572–581.

Meyer, A. (1922). The philosophy of occupation therapy. *Archives of Occupational Therapy, 1,* 1–10. (Reprinted as Chapter 2.)

Mosey, A.C. (1981). *Occupational therapy: Configuration of a profession* (pp. 77–78). New York: Raven Press.

Neville, A. (1980). Temporal adaptation: Application with short-term psychiatric patients. *American Journal of Occupational Therapy, 34,* 328–331.

Neville, A., Kreisberg, A., & Kielhofner, G. (1985). Temporal dysfunction in schizophrenia. *Occupational Therapy in Mental Health, 5* (1), 1–19.

Nystrom, E.P. (1974). Activity patterns and leisure concepts among the elderly. *American Journal of Occupational Therapy, 28,* 337–345.

President's Commission on Mental Health. (1978). *Report to the President.* Washington, DC: U.S. Government Printing Office.

Reed, K.L. (1984). *Models of practice in occupational therapy* (pp. 163–177). Baltimore: Williams and Wilkins.

Reed, K. & Sanderson, S.R. (1980). *Concepts of occupational therapy* (pp. 99–103). Baltimore: Williams and Wilkins.

Reilly, M. (1960). Research potentiality of occupational therapy. *American Journal of Occupational Therapy, 14,* 202–209.

Rosenthall, L.A. & Howe, M.C. (1984). Activity patterns and leisure concepts: A comparison of temporal adaptation among day versus night shift workers. *Occupational Therapy in Mental Health, 4* (2), 59–79.

Schwartzberg, S.L. (1982). Motivation for activities of daily living: A study of selected psychiatric patient's self-reports. *Occupational Therapy in Mental Health, 2* (3), 1–26.

Sharrott, G.W. (1983). Occupational therapy's role in the client's creation and affirmation of meaning. In G. Kielhofner (Ed.), *Health through occupation: Theory and practice in occupational therapy* (pp. 213–235). Philadelphia: F.A. Davis.

Watanabe, S. (1968). *Final Report RSA-123-T-68.* A paper presented at the American Occupational Therapy Association sponsored Regional Institute on the Evaluation Process, (pp. 46–47). New York.

Appendix 1
Temporal Pattern Questionnaire

Please circle which activity you typically engage for each one-hour of the day. Remember to refer to the definitions as often as you need. Answer this part as if it were a typical or usual weekday.

Morning

6-7 am	Sleep	Chores	Work	Active Leisure	Passive Leisure	Socialization
7-8 am	Sleep	Chores	Work	Active Leisure	Passive Leisure	Socialization
8-9 am	Sleep	Chores	Work	Active Leisure	Passive Leisure	Socialization
9-10 am	Sleep	Chores	Work	Active Leisure	Passive Leisure	Socialization
10-11 am	Sleep	Chores	Work	Active Leisure	Passive Leisure	Socialization
11-12 am	Sleep	Chores	Work	Active Leisure	Passive Leisure	Socialization

Afternoon

12-1 pm	Sleep	Chores	Work	Active Leisure	Passive Leisure	Socialization
1-2 pm	Sleep	Chores	Work	Active Leisure	Passive Leisure	Socialization
2-3 pm	Sleep	Chores	Work	Active Leisure	Passive Leisure	Socialization
3-4 pm	Sleep	Chores	Work	Active Leisure	Passive Leisure	Socialization
4-5 pm	Sleep	Chores	Work	Active Leisure	Passive Leisure	Socialization
5-6 pm	Sleep	Chores	Work	Active Leisure	Passive Leisure	Socialization

Night

6-7 pm	Sleep	Chores	Work	Active Leisure	Passive Leisure	Socialization
7-8 pm	Sleep	Chores	Work	Active Leisure	Passive Leisure	Socialization
8-9 pm	Sleep	Chores	Work	Active Leisure	Passive Leisure	Socialization
9-10 pm	Sleep	Chores	Work	Active Leisure	Passive Leisure	Socialization
10-11 pm	Sleep	Chores	Work	Active Leisure	Passive Leisure	Socialization
11-12 pm	Sleep	Chores	Work	Active Leisure	Passive Leisure	Socialization
12-1 am	Sleep	Chores	Work	Active Leisure	Passive Leisure	Socialization
1-2 am	Sleep	Chores	Work	Active Leisure	Passive Leisure	Socialization
2-3 am	Sleep	Chores	Work	Active Leisure	Passive Leisure	Socialization
3-4 am	Sleep	Chores	Work	Active Leisure	Passive Leisure	Socialization
4-5 am	Sleep	Chores	Work	Active Leisure	Passive Leisure	Socialization
5-6 am	Sleep	Chores	Work	Active Leisure	Passive Leisure	Socialization

Appendix 2
Meaningfulness of Activity Scale

For each activity below, place a mark (x) in each of the three columns that best describes it.

Activity	How Much You Enjoy It				Why You Do It		How Well You Do It		
	Very Much	Somewhat	Very Little	Not At All	Want To	Have To	Very Well	Well Enough	Do Not Do Well
Sleep									
Chores									
Work									
Active Leisure									
Passive Leisure									
Social									

Chapter 19

Quality of Time Use by Adults with Spinal Cord Injuries

Elizabeth J. Yerxa, EdD, OTR, FAOTA
Susan Baum Locker, MS

This chapter was previously published in the *American Journal of Occupational Therapy, 44*, 318–326. Copyright © 1990, American Occupational Therapy Association.

Occupational therapy has a 70-year tradition of interest in how patients organize and use their time (Meyer, 1922) (see Chapter 2). Scientists today are increasingly recognizing the importance of the study of time, for example, as *chronobiology* (Campbell, 1986), the exploration of the biological rhythms of humans, or as *chronosociology* (Young, 1988), the study of the rhythms and habits of society. Occupational science, which supports the practice of occupational therapy, is concerned with understanding the patterns of occupation that humans use to meet environmental challenges and demonstrate efficacy. *Occupation*, as defined by the occupational therapy department at the University of Southern California, refers to the chunks of activity within the ongoing stream of behavior that are named in the lexicon of the culture and that are self-initiated, goal directed, organized, composed of adaptive skills, and personally satisfying. A person chooses what he or she will do daily and organizes personal and environmental resources to accomplish these goals.

Little is known about what people do with their time and, especially, how they feel about their daily occupations. Even less of this information is known concerning persons with disabilities who are living in the community. Occupational therapists strongly emphasize independence in daily living as a treatment goal for patients undergoing rehabilitation (Trombly, 1983). But what happens to those patients when they leave occupational therapy and return to the community? How do their daily lives compare to those of persons who are not disabled?

This paper reports a study of the self-perceived quality of time use of 15 community-based adults with spinal cord injuries compared with that of 12 age- and sex-matched nondisabled adults. The purposes of the study were to determine (a) how the subjects classified their daily occupations, (b) how they felt while engaged in these occupations, and (c) the quality of their future orientation. We previously reported the quantitative results from the first phase of the study (Yerxa & Baum, 1986).

Research Questions

We analyzed the data that we had gathered in our previous study (Yerxa & Baum, 1986) through a content analysis (Fox, 1969) to answer the following research questions:

1. How did the disabled and nondisabled subjects classify their occupations into categories of Work, Rest, Sleep, Play, Self-Maintenance, or Other, based on the Activity Configuration Log?
2. How did their categorization compare with that of a group of experienced occupational therapists using the raw data from the disabled subjects? (This was done to assess the degree to which occupational therapists' classifications agreed with those of subjects with spinal cord injuries. Occupational therapists often analyze activity patterns in treatment and draw conclusions about their significance to patients, which may or may not be valid.)
3. What occupations (e.g., watching TV, reading) were most often rated as *very good*, *good*, *fair*, or *poor* in quality?
4. In which occupations did the disabled and nondisabled subjects spend the greatest amount of time?
5. Concerning future orientation, what were the content and number of goals as well as the wishes and hopes and fears and worries for both groups?
6. How did the quality ratings of occupations relate to the overall daily quality ratings for each group?

Method

Subjects. One hundred and fifty-two persons with spinal cord injuries who were living in the greater Los Angeles area in noninstitutional settings were invited to participate. Fifty-eight who agreed to participate were sent a packet of instruments and a consent form. Each of these participants was asked to contact a nondisabled friend of the same age and sex to serve as a comparison subject. Fifteen subjects with spinal cord injuries and 15 matched adults completed all of the instruments. Three participants from the nondisabled group were eliminated because they, too, had chronic disabilities. The final sample, therefore, comprised 15 subjects with spinal cord injuries and 12 nondisabled subjects. Each subject received $10 for participating.

Instrument. Three instruments were used in this aspect of the study. The Activity Configuration Log (mod-

ified from an unpublished clinical assessment developed by Claudia Allen) required that subjects record all of their occupations for 8 days and 8 nights, beginning on a Monday and ending on a Monday (see Figure 1). The subjects entered each activity that they actually did. Then they classified that activity into one of six categories: Self-Maintenance, Work, Rest, Sleep, Play or Other. The subjects also answered two questions modified from the Cantril Ladder (Cantril, 1965), following these instructions: "Here is a picture of a ladder. At the top, write in your wishes and hopes for the future. At the bottom, write in your fears and worries about the future." Other data from the ladder reflecting degree of life satisfaction were reported in a previous study and showed no significant differences between the disabled and nondisabled subjects (Yerxa & Baum, 1986). A single item from the General Questionnaire (Yerxa & Baum, 1986) incorporated the following question based on a study by Kemp and Vash (1971): "What are your goals for the future? List as many as you wish."

Results

Subjects' Characteristics

The disabled and nondisabled subjects were similar demographically. The mean age for the disabled group was 38.1 years; for the nondisabled group, 38.4 years. Ten men and 5 women constituted the disabled group; 8 men and 4 women, the nondisabled group. Ethnic characteristics (most subjects were Caucasian) and geographic location of the groups were almost identical. The majority of subjects in both groups were educated beyond the high school level. A major difference, however, was found in employment and income. Only 5 subjects (33%) in the disabled group were employed, whereas all but 1 (a retiree) of the nondisabled subjects were employed. Sixty percent (9) of the disabled group had annual incomes below $10,000, whereas only 17% (2) of the nondisabled group had annual incomes below that level. The 5 disabled subjects who were employed held the following positions: nurse-coordinator, executive secretary, community liaison (for spinal cord-injured patients), computer operator, and teacher for a disabled students' service.

Eleven of the spinal cord-injured subjects had quadriplegia. The mean time since injury, was 15.64 years (range = 6 to 31 years). Fourteen of the 15 spinal cord-injured subjects had previously received occupational therapy, but only as inpatients. None lived alone, and the majority lived with a family member or spouse. Thirteen of the 15 disabled subjects received help in their daily activities. The mean amount of help provided per day was 5.67 hr (range 0 to 24 hr). Fourteen were mobile in both the home and community. Eight considered themselves to be independent through the use of a manual wheelchair, 5 were independent through the use

ACTIVITY CONFIGURATION LOG

Last 4 digits Soc. Sec. No. / __ __ __ __   Two sheets per 24 hours

DATE   DAY OF THE WEEK   (Start on Monday please)

Activity Characteristics

(Write in for each activity)   (Check column)

PRIMARY _DAY_ ACTIVITIES	1. Sleep 2. Self-main. 3. Work 4. Rest 5. Play 6. Other	(Write in each activity) V Good Good Fair Poor	Useful	Not useful	For now	For the future	Alone	With others	For $	Not for $
What I Did										
6–7 A.M.										
7–8 A.M.										
8–9 A.M.										
9–10 A.M.										
10–11 A.M.										
11–12 A.M.										
12 noon– 1P.M.										
1–2 P.M.										
2–3 P.M.										
3–4 P.M.										
4–5 P.M.										
5–6 P.M.										

Overall rating of the day (Circle one):   V Good   Fair

Good   Poor

ACTIVITY CONFIGURATION LOG

Last 4 digits Soc. Sec. No. / __ __ __ __   Two sheets per 24 hours

DATE   DAY OF THE WEEK

Activity Characteristics

(Write in for each activity)   (Check column)

PRIMARY _NIGHT_ ACTIVITIES	1. Sleep 2. Self-main. 3. Work 4. Rest 5. Play 6. Other	(Write in each activity) V Good Good Fair Poor	Useful	Not useful	For now	For the future	Alone	With others	For $	Not for $
What I Did										
6–7 P.M.										
7–8 P.M.										
8–9 P.M.										
9–10 P.M.										
10–11 P.M.										
11–12 P.M.										
12 midnight– 1A.M.										
1–2 A.M.										
2–3 A.M.										
3–4 A.M.										
4–5 A.M.										
5–6 A.M.										

Overall rating of the night (Circle one):   V Good   Fair

Good   Poor

Instructions to Subjects

We want to find out what you do with your time and how you feel about what you do. Please start filling out your _Activity Configuration Log_ next Monday morning starting with 6:00 A.M. It should be filled out each day until the following Tuesday morning, ending at 5:00 A.M. (8 24-hour logs total).

Two sheets are needed for each 24-hour period, one day sheet and one night sheet. During the day, at the end of each 4-hour period, please fill in the primary activity or activities you have done for each hour of that 4 hours. For example, "went shopping," "write a letter," "took a nap," "ate dinner." Then write whether you felt the main purpose of each activity was for sleep, self-maintenance (taking care of your self), work (as you define work), rest, play/leisure (for fun) or for some other purpose. Next, write in how you felt about what you did. Did you feel very good, good, fair, or poor as you were doing it? Next check whether it was useful or not useful; check whether you did it for now or primarily for the future; check whether you did it alone or with others. Finally, check whether it was for pay or not for pay. Around 6:00 P.M. circle the overall rating you gave the day. In other words, how did you feel about how you spent the entire day?

During the evening do the same thing until you go to bed. Record the amount of time you spent in sleep the next morning and give an overall rating for the 12 hours spent during the evening and nighttime hours. Be sure that you fill in the last four digits of your social security number and the date and day of the week on _every sheet_.

Figure 1. Activity Configuration Log (24 hr). Modified from an unpublished clinical assessment developed by Claudia Allen.

of an electric wheelchair, and 4 needed assistance in wheelchair activities (some subjects used both manual and electric wheelchairs). Nine were _pretty satisfied_ with their ability, to function in the community, 3 were _completely satisfied_, and 2 were _not very satisfied_. One subject did not answer. Obstacles to community functioning that were identified by 11 of the spinal cord-injured subjects were architectural barriers (5); lack of social resources, that is, lack of friends or social activities (3); lack of accessible transportation (2); lack of physical ability (2); and lack of financial resources (1) (subjects could identify more than one obstacle).

Previous Findings

Significant differences between subjects in the disabled and nondisabled groups were previously reported for the amount of time used for Work and for Other (i.e., activities other than sleep, rest, self-maintenance, and play) (Yerxa & Baum, 1986). The subjects with spinal cord injuries spent less time in work and more in other activities. The subjects with spinal cord injuries also had lower levels of satisfaction with their performance of home management and their community problem-solving skills. A significant relationship between satisfaction with performance in these two areas and overall life satisfaction was found for the total sample (N = 27). No significant differences were found in overall life satisfaction or locus of control (Yerxa & Baum, 1986), as measured by the I-E Scale (Rotter, 1966).

Answers to Research Questions

How did the disabled and nondisabled subjects categorize their daily activities as Work, Rest, Sleep, Play, Self-Maintenance, or Other based on the Activity Configuration Log? We performed a content analysis by listing all of the occupations (discrete activities) that the subjects had placed into each of the six categories. Then the number of subjects classifying the same activity into the same category was tallied for both groups. The rank order of subjects classifying activities into each of the six categories was then compared between the disabled and nondisabled groups. For example, for Self-Maintenance, each occupation categorized as self-maintenance was listed first. Then the number of subjects who classified the same occupation as self-maintenance was tallied for both groups of subjects (see Table 1). The results showed that Rest, Sleep, and Play had more similarities in classification of occupations between the groups, whereas Work, Self-Maintenance, and Other showed greater differences. Occupations in which fewer than 3 subjects used the same category were not included. The spinal cord-injured subjects were more detailed in their descriptions of occupations categorized as self-maintenance. Employment-related work was the occupation most often classified as work by the nondisabled subjects, whereas making phone calls was rated highest by the disabled subjects. The Other category was of particular interest, because the first phase of this study (Yerxa & Baum, 1986) showed that the amount of time that would have been spent on work was shifted to this category by the unemployed disabled subjects (*n* = 10). The disabled

subjects categorized 14 activities as Other, 12 of which were not included in Other by the nondisabled subjects.

The same occupation was often classified into several different categories. In our analysis, occupations were rank ordered again, this time according to the categories into which each had been placed. Eating was categorized as Self-Maintenance (11 subjects), Rest (9 subjects), Other (8 subjects), and Play (2 subjects) by the disabled subjects and as Self-Maintenance (11 Subjects), Rest (6 subjects), and Play (4 subjects) by the nondisabled subjects. Watching TV was categorized as Rest (10 subjects), Other (7 subjects), Play (5 subjects), and Self-Maintenance (4 subjects) by the disabled subjects and as Rest (6 subjects) and Play (3 subjects) by the nondisabled subjects. Visiting friends or family was categorized as Play (6 subjects), Other (4 subjects), and Self-maintenance (3 subjects) by the disabled subjects and as Play (6 subjects) and Other (5 subjects) by the nondisabled subjects. Reading was categorized as Rest (8 subjects), Other (6 subjects), Work (3 subjects), and Play (2 subjects) by the disabled subjects and as Rest (3 subjects) by the nondisabled subjects. The categorization of an occupation seemed to vary according to its context or purpose. The disabled subjects used a greater number of categories for eating, watching TV, visiting friends or family, and reading than did the nondisabled subjects.

How did the disabled subjects' classification of occupations compare with that of a group of occupational therapists? To see how similarly the two groups perceived the occupations, a random selection of one 24-hour Activity Configuration Log from each of the disabled subjects was presented to 10 experienced occupational therapists from a large rehabilitation center. The subjects' daily occupations were listed in their own words, but their categorizations of these activities (e.g., Work, Rest, Sleep) were removed. The occupational therapists were asked to categorize all of the occupations listed, following the instructions on the log. The generalized weighted kappa was used to compare the categories used by the disabled subjects with those of the occupational therapists, based on the same raw data (Thomas, Spitzer, & MacFarlane, 1981). A statistically significant but minimal amount of agreement of categorization was found between the occupational therapists and the disabled subjects (*k* = .37, *p* < .0001). A second analysis assessed the agreement of the categorizations used by the 10 occupational therapists among themselves (*k* = .58, *p* < .0001). The occupational therapists agreed more strongly with each other than they did with the disabled subjects in classifying the subjects' daily occupations. This shows that occupational therapists may have different perspectives on patients' occupations than do the patients themselves.

What occupations were most often rated by the 15 disabled and 12 nondisabled subjects as very good, good, fair, or poor? These were tallied from the Activity Configuration Log. The top

Table 1
Rank Order of Subjects' Categorization of Occupations

Category	Disabled Group (*n* = 15)		Nondisabled Group (*n* = 12)	
	Occupation	Total No. of Subjects Using Category	Occupation	Total No. of Subjects Using Category
Work	Phone calls (5)[a] Read (3)[a] Write letters (3)[a] Clean house (3)[a] Work (employment) (3)	10	Work (employment)(10) Clean house (4) Yard work (4)[a] Drive to work (3)[a] Clean up (3)[a]	10
Rest	Watch TV (10) Eat (9) Rest, take it easy (8) Read (8) Go to bed (5)[a] Take nap (4)[a] Eat out (3)[a] Listen to music (3)[a] Read paper (3)[a]	14	Eat (6) Watch TV (6) Relax at home (4) Read (3)	11
Sleep	Sleep (14)	14	Sleep (11)	11
Play	Visit friends (6) Watch TV (5) Play games (4)[a] Eat out (4)[a] Listen to stereo (3)[a]	14	Eat (4)[a] Prepare meal (3)[a] Watch TV(3) Visit friends (3) Visit family (3)[a]	10
Self-Maintenance	Eat (11) Get up/get out of bed (7) Dress (7)[a] Wash face and teeth (6)[a] Get ready for bed/go to bed (6)[a] Wash hair (5)[a] Bathe (4)[a] Bowel program (4)[a] Driving (task-oriented) (4) Watch TV (documentary) (4)[a] Visit friends (3)[a] Exercise, range of motion (3)[a] Medical activities (3)[a]	13	Eat (11) Prepare for work (8)[a] Shower (6)[a] Meal preparation (4)[a] Shopping (4)[a] Driving (task-oriented) (4) Eat out (3)[a] Get up (3)	11
Other	Eat (8)[a] Watch TV (7)[a] Read (6)[a] Driving (task-oriented) (6)[a] Grocery shopping (4) Had visitors (4) Go to church (4) Auto/van maintenance (4)[a] Read paper (3)[a] Drive home (3)[a] Get gas (3)[a] Eat out (3)[a] Phone calls (3)[a] Bible study (3)[a]	14	Visit friends/family (5) Work in yard (4)[a] Go to church (3)	10

Note. Parentheses indicate number of subjects who listed this activity.
[a]Activity listed in category by that group only.

five occupations were then ranked according to the number of subjects who rated them in each of the four quality categories (see Table 2). The rankings between the groups appeared similar except that no nondisabled subject rated watching TV as *very good*, whereas 5 disabled subjects rated watching TV as *very good*. Sex was mentioned and rated only by the disabled subjects. Ten of the disabled subjects rated at least one occupation as *poor*, compared with only 2 of the nondisabled subjects.

In which occupations did both groups spend the greatest amounts of time? To examine this question, we first categorized the occupations by content. Then, we computed time spent in each occupation by mean hours per day per subject, based on the 7-day time log (Monday through Sunday). These data were then rank ordered.

Both the nondisabled and disabled groups spent the greatest amount of time per day sleeping (7.49 and 7.12 hr, respectively). The rankings differed after that, however. The disabled subjects spent much more time watching TV (2.91 hr), relaxing (2.17 hr), talking (1.10 hr), and partying (1.00 hr)—all leisure activities. The nondisabled subjects spent more time in paid employment (5.07 hr), in self-maintenance (2.83 hr), in community organizations (1.39 hr), and in traveling to work (1.11 hr).

The data from the sample for this study were then compared which data gathered by Robinson (1977), a social psychologist, who studied the time use of a national sample of more than 2,000 nondisabled persons. This was done to determine the comparability of the time use by our subjects with a large sample from a wider geographic area. Robinson's (1977) data were generated from one 24-hr log. Occupations were classified by researchers, not by subjects. The occupations from this sample were recategorized according to Robinson's classification and put into rank order according to mean minutes per day (see Table 3.). Using these new categories, we found that both groups in the present study spent the greatest amount of time in the category of personal needs (693 min per day for the disabled group; 635 min per day for the nondisabled group). Robinson defined personal needs as personal care, eating, and sleeping.

The disabled group spent only 109 min per day in work, whereas the nondisabled group averaged 350 min per day in work, leaving less time for leisure (175 min per day) and mass media activities (e.g., watching TV, listening to the radio or to records) (96 min per day). In comparison, the disabled group spent the second and third highest amounts of time in leisure and mass media activities. Robinson's (1977) sample of 508 employed men spent much less time in leisure and mass media activities and much more time in work activities than did the disabled group in our study. The amount of time Robinson's subjects spent in work, housework, and personal needs activities was comparable to that found for the present study's nondisabled group. Robinson's sub-

jects spent more time than each of our groups in non-work-related travel and child care activities. When the bottom four categories of non-work-related travel, study and community participation, mass media, and leisure

Table 2
Rank Order of Subjects' Ratings of Specific Occupations

Disabled Group	n	Nondisabled Group	n
POOR			
Watch TV (4)[a]	10	Work (1)[a]	2
Sleep (4)		Sleep (1)	
Tried to sleep (2)[a]			
Library (2)[a]			
Get up (2)[a]			
Eat (2)[a]			
FAIR			
Watch TV (12)	13	Drive to work (3)[a]	8
Up/out of bed (6)[a]		Study (3)[a]	
Eat (5)		Work (3)	
Sleep (5)[a]		Eat (3)	
Go to bed (5)[a]		Watch TV (2)	
Start work (5)		Drive home (2)[a]	
Shop (5)		Ready for work (2)[a]	
		Clean house (2)[a]	
		Shop (2)	
GOOD			
Eat (14)	14	Eat (11)	11
Watch TV (14)		Work (employment)(11)	
Go to bed (11)		Sleep (9)	
Sleep (10)		Watch TV (8)	
Get up (8)[a]		Drive home (7)	
Read (8)		Ready for work (7)[a]	
Visit friends (8)			
Talk with friends/family (8)[a]			
VERY GOOD			
Sleep (8)	13	Eat (7)	11
Eat out (6)		Sleep (6)	
Eat (6)		Visit friends (5)	
Watch TV (5)[a]		Go to church (4)[a]	
Friends visit (5)		Relax at home (3)	
		Prepare for work (3)[a]	
		Eat out (3)	

Note. Parentheses indicate number of subjects who listed this activity.
[a] Classified as such by this group only.

Table 3
Comparison of Minutes per Day Spent in Occupations

| Occupation | Minutes (M) | | |
	Robinson's Group[a] (N = 508)	Disabled Group (n = 14)	Nondisabled Group (n = 11)
Work	436	109	350
Housework	30	20	32
Household obligations	36	52	53
Child care	12	3	0
Personal needs[b]	611	693	635
Free time			
Non-work-related travel	44	26	24
Study and community participation	20	70	75
Mass media activities	148	238	96
Leisure	100	227	175
Total free time	312	561	370

Note.   Mass media activities refer to watching TV or listening to the radio or to records.
[a]From Robinson's (1977) study, which, for this comparison, looked at 508 employed, nondisabled men nationwide.
[b]Personal care, eating, and sleeping, as defined by Robinson (1977).

were combined into free time (nonobligatory activities), the disabled group had much more free time (561 min per day) than either of the nondisabled groups (i.e., Robinson's (1977) and our groups).

What were the content and number of goals as well as wishes and hopes and fears and worries of both groups? These were determined with a content analysis of the goals question from the General Questionnaire and the two future-oriented questions from the Cantril Ladder (Cantril, 1965). The mean number of goals was 3.13 for the disabled group and 3.17 for the nondisabled group (see Table 4). The content of the goals was similar except that slightly more of the disabled group had goals in the vocational area (e.g., earning a living, new job), and more of the nondisabled subjects wanted to travel. In analyzing the content of the goals according to Kemp and Vash's (1971) theory of which types of goals are more related to subject productivity, we found that the goals related to higher productivity (vocational, materialistic, and familial) were about equal to those related to lower productivity (avocational, materialistic, and physical) in both groups. Wishes and dreams for the future were similar except that 7 of the disabled subjects wished for independence in new areas (e.g., driving, better access to home, becoming more active) and 3 for recovery of physical function. Both groups ranked highly in the wish for an improved vocational outlook.

The most frequently named category of fears for the nondisabled group was none (5). The most frequently named category for the disabled group was ill health. Other fears that were health or disability related were

ending up in a nursing home, needing surgery, losing independence, losing a needed family member, and dying without dignity.

What relationship, if any, appeared between the affective quality of individual occupations within 12 hr and the overall quality ratings for the entire 12-hr period? We answered this question by using an analysis of variance of repeated measures on the mode of the ratings of each occupation within each 12-hr log and the overall rating of that entire 12-hr period (*poor, fair, good,* and *very good*). The results showed that there was no significant difference in these sets of ratings ($F = .57, p = .4592$). Thus, the affective quality of each 12-hr period seemed to be related to the qualitative ratings of the specific occupations constituting it.

Discussion

The classifications of occupations into categories of Work, Rest, Sleep, Play, Self-Maintenance, and Other differed within and between groups. The disabled and nondisabled subjects included different occupations in all categories except Sleep. The divergence in occupations categorized as Work, Self-Maintenance, and Other might stem from the fact that 10 of the 15 disabled subjects were unemployed. Work and Other consisted of occupations that substituted for employment among disabled subjects. The shift of time from Work to Other, rather than to Play, Sleep, Rest, or Self-Maintenance, seems to support the inherent human drive for competence and efficacy, which is expressed in adults by work and other productive occupations (Reilly, 1962) (see Chapter 6).

The fact that the same occupation was classified into four different categories supports the need for a phe-

Table 4
Rank Order for Subjects' Reporting of Goals for the Future

Disabled Group (n = 15)		Nondisabled Group (n = 12)	
Earn living/new job	(6)	Travel	(4)
Better family relations	(5)	Better family relations	(3)
Avocational	(4)	New job	(3)
Camper/car to drive	(3)[a]	Exercise/health	(3)
Financial independence	(3)	Avocational	(3)
Good health	(3)	Vocational advancement	(2)[a]
Travel	(2)	Live Christian life	(2)[a]
New home	(2)[a]	Financial independence	(2)
Find girlfriend/ boyfriend	(2)[a]	None	(1)
Live independently	(2)[a]	Miscellaneous/ unclassified	(15)
None	(2)		
Miscellaneous/ unclassified	(13)		
Total	47		38

Note. Parentheses indicate number of subjects who listed this goal.
[a] Named by this group only.

nomenological perspective on the meaning or purpose attributed to activities. It refutes analysis of activities according to their inherent qualities and suggests instead that the occupational therapist needs to understand the patient's goals for engagement in occupations. It also raises a question about whether occupation can be understood from a behavioristic approach, that is, by only observing what people do. This study emphasizes the significance of the subject's experience as important information in all activity analysis.

The data from the present study were supported by Robinson's (1977) data. The similarity in the amounts of time spent in a variety of categories between our nondisabled sample and Robinson's sample of 508 urban American employed men validates the findings of this study and lends support to the nondisabled subsample, though small, as a reasonable comparison group.

Occupational therapists agreed more with each other than they did with persons with disabilities regarding how occupations are categorized. This suggests that the individual patient may be the most valid source of information regarding the classification of activities and interpretation of their meaning.

The category of Work has particular significance for occupational therapists. Although the instructions on the

Activity Configuration Log asked subjects to classify activities such as work as they defined them, 5 of the disabled subjects did not classify any occupation as work. Work seemed to be perceived primarily as paid employment (Anderson, 1961). If a person in the prime of life who is disabled and living in the community is unemployed, can any other occupation fulfill the role of paid employment in organizing the daily round of occupations or of creating a balance among work, rest, sleep, and play in daily life (Meyer, 1922) (see Chapter 2)? Occupational therapists seeking to enable patients to achieve such a balance will first have to determine how the patient views these categories. The Activity Configuration Log may help the therapist discover the patient's view.

In classifying specific occupations affectively, more subjects with disabilities experienced at least one activity as *poor*, thus implying that the Activity Configuration Log might be a useful clinical tool to help pinpoint occupations that are low in satisfaction. According to Robinson (1977), asking people to report how they feel while they are performing an activity may be a more valid measure of their affective response than asking them how they feel in general about the activity. Thus, the Activity Configuration Log might serve as a useful adjunct to other more general assessments such as the Interest Check List (Matsutsuyu, 1969).

The fact that 5 subjects with disabilities rated watching TV as *very good* whereas 4 rated it as *poor* and 12 as *fair* supports Robinson's (1977) finding that the same activity may be classified as both enjoyable and not enjoyable. In this case, the number of disabled subjects who rated watching TV as *poor* and *fair* is important to compare with the large amount of time spent watching TV in the disabled group.

In the present study, an important question remains: Was the amount of time spent watching TV related to the degree of satisfaction derived from it or because it was available and required little effort? Robinson (1977) observed that television is likely to be used when people have excessive time on their hands. Although seldom listed as "least satisfying," it is often below average in satisfaction when compared with other free time activities.

Occupational therapists could explore whether alternatives to television might be more satisfying and goal-related for community-based subjects with spinal cord injuries. Such alternatives might include the use of computers, VCRs, and electronic classrooms without walls, all of which could be related to the high incidence of vocational goals in this sample.

This study demonstrated that the affective quality of particular occupations seemed to be related to the affective quality of an entire day, thus supporting the relationship between satisfaction with occupations and a more general satisfaction with use of time, a primary premise of occupational therapy (Kielhofner, 1977) (see Chapter 17).

The group with spinal cord injuries spent significantly less time on self-maintenance than did the nondisabled group, probably because helpers provided assistance in these areas. The assumption that disabled persons will automatically spend more time in self-care and less in other pursuits (Kielhofner, 1977) (see Chapter 17) is questionable. Perhaps we should prepare people with severe and chronic disabilities to be effective managers of their time and environmental resources rather than expect them to spend time on their own self-maintenance activities, especially when that time and energy could be used for more rewarding pursuits.

The disabled group had a higher number of goals in the vocational area than did the nondisabled group, reflecting the high unemployment rate in the disabled group. After their inpatient rehabilitation, the disabled subjects received no occupational therapy as outpatients. They wanted to join the work force but appeared to be lost in the community. To be without an occupational role is to be without a major social role in this culture (Parker, Brown, Child, & Smith, 1977). Occupational therapists must ensure that their services are provided in the community, where people with disabilities encounter barriers to adaptation, including a lack of skills and social constraints on paid employment.

Lack of employment also means more free time, a commodity that Robinson and Shaver (1973) and Nystrom (1974) showed was related to lower, not higher, life satisfaction. In fact, the disabled subjects spent 3 to 4 more hours per day in free time activities than either of the nondisabled comparison groups. Occupational therapists in the community need to explore ways in which such patients might organize and use their time in more satisfying occupations.

Finally, the disabled subjects' fears for the future contrasted strongly with those of the nondisabled group. Fears of ill health, surgery, ending up in a nursing home, or dying without dignity may be realistic when one has a spinal cord injury and lives in the community.

Conclusion

Due to this study's small sample size and limited geographic area, one should exercise caution in generalizing its results. The similarity of time use by the nondisabled group and Robinson's (1977) national sample, however, lends credibility to these results.

Additional research is needed to assess to what extent physical disability is a major factor influencing the quality of time use. Robinson's (1977) studies on Americans' use of time need to be replicated to include samples of persons who have disabilities. Studies are needed that look at subjects' assessments and categorizations of time use rather than researchers' classifications. Additional studies are needed with other samples in other geographic locations, to replicate the results of this study. Occupational therapists must explore the extent to which the context (Bateson, 1979) of occupations influences their categorization. The present study suggests that the study of occupations must consider the meaning that these occupations hold for individuals.

A final challenge for occupational therapists is to discover alternative satisfying uses of time to replace the excessive free time experienced by disabled persons who live in the community.

Acknowledgments

We appreciate the contributions of the 27 subjects, of Wendy Mack, PhD, OTR, of our biometry consultant, and of the American Occupational Therapy Foundation, which supported this research.

References

Anderson, N. (1961). *Work and leisure*. New York: Free Press of Glencoe.

Bateson, G. (1979). *Mind and nature: A necessary unity*. New York: Bantam.

Campbell, J. (1986). *Winston Churchill's afternoon nap*. New York: Simon & Schuster.

Cantril, H. (1965). *The pattern of human concern*. New Brunswick, NJ: Rutgers University Press.

Fox, D.J. (1969). *The research process in education*. New York: Holt, Rinehart & Winston.

Kemp, B.J., & Vash, C.L. (1971). Productivity after injury in a sample of spinal cord injured persons: A pilot study. *Journal of Chronic Disability, 24*, 259–275.

Kielhofner, G. (1977). Temporal adaptation: A conceptual framework for occupational therapy. *American Journal of Occupational Therapy, 31*, 235–242. (Reprinted as Chapter 17.)

Matsutsuyu, J.S. (1969). The Interest Check List. *American Journal of Occupational Therapy, 23*, 323–328.

Meyer, A. (1922). The philosophy of occupational therapy. *Archives of Occupational Therapy, 1*, 1–10. (Reprinted as Chapter 2.)

Nystrom, E.P. (1974). Activity patterns and leisure concepts among the elderly. *American Journal of Occupational Therapy, 28*, 337–345.

Parker, S.R., Brown, R.K., Child, J., & Smith, M.A. (1977). *The sociology of industry*. London: George Allen & Unwin.

Reilly, M. (1962). The Eleanor Clarke Slagle Lecture—Occupational therapy can be one or the great ideas of 20th century medicine. *American Journal of Occupational Therapy, 16*, 1–9. (Reprinted as Chapter 6.)

Robinson, J.P. (1977). *How Americans use their time*. New York: Praeger.

Robinson, J.P., & Shaver, P.R. (1973). *Measures of social psychological attitudes.* Ann Arbor, MI: University of Michigan, Survey Research Center, Institute of Social Research.

Rotter, S.B. (1966). Generalized expectancies for internal versus external control of reinforcement. *Psychological Monographs, 80,* 609.

Thomas, D.C., Spitzer, W.O., & MacFarlane, J.K. (1981). Interobserver error among surgeons and nurses in pre-symptomatic detection of breast disease. *Journal of Chronic Disease, 34,* 616–626.

Trombly, C. (1983). Activities of daily living. In C. Trombly (Ed.), *Occupational therapy for physical dysfunction* (pp 458–479). Baltimore: Williams & Wilkins.

Yerxa, E.J., & Baum, S. (1986). Engagement in daily occupations and life satisfaction among people with spinal cord injuries. *Occupational Therapy Journal of Research, 6,* 271–283.

Young, M. (1988). *The metronomic society.* Cambridge, MA: Harvard University Press.

Chapter 20

Beyond Performance: Being in Place as a Component of Occupational Therapy

Graham D. Rowles, PhD

This chapter was previously published in the *American Journal of Occupational Therapy, 45,* 265–271. Copyright © 1991, American Occupational Therapy Association.

The essence of becoming and remaining human is a combination of *knowing, doing,* and *being* (Knos, 1977). An accumulation of information results in our knowing everything from how to brush our teeth through how to prepare a salad to more complex tasks such as servicing an automobile. Knowing also involves expertise acquired through practice, as we apply learned skills in activities of self-care, work, and play. We learn and achieve a sense of accomplishment by doing (Fidler & Fidler, 1978) (see Chapter 7) Finally, to live as a fully self-actualizing person involves the process of being, of simply experiencing life and the environment around us, frequently in an accepting, noninstrumental way. Being, in this sense, involves the realms of meaning, value, and intentionality that imbue our lives with a richness and diversity that transcends what we know and what we do (Maslow, 1966). Appreciation of the beauty and fragrance of a rose, the meaning of a home as distinguished from the house where one resides, the warmth of a lifelong relationship with a friend, one's sense of self, and one's perspective on the meaning of existence all fall within this rubric.

In recent decades, occupational therapy has tended to emphasize knowing and doing as focal concerns. The purpose of this article is to suggest that occupational therapists may significantly enhance their contribution to improving the quality of life by more explicitly incorporating within everyday practice and research an increased concern with understanding *being in place,* which is one important aspect of their clients' being. Such a reorientation may be especially useful in working with and understanding elderly people and other less mobile populations for whom the environment may have come to assume particular significance.

An expanded, more experientially grounded focus would seem to be timely in view of several trends in occupational therapy. These trends include (a) a growing concern with differentiating occupational therapy from a purely medical model (Kielhofner & Burke, 1977; Mosey, 1974, 1980; Reilly, 1969; Rogers, 1982); (b) increased interest in promulgating basic research; (c) the quest for a dominant research paradigm and for theory, a science of human occupation (Christiansen, 1981; Kielhofner & Nicol, 1989; Llorens, 1984); and (d) a rediscovered concern with the evolution of a holistic perspective on human occupation that places emphasis on the role of the environment as an influence on capacity for functional independence (Barris, 1986; Kiernat, 1982, 1987).

In developing this perspective, I focus on three themes: the need for increased emphasis on the nature of being in place; some methodological implications of adopting such an expanded philosophy in terms of the need for naturalistic and qualitative research; and illustrations, drawn from my own research as a social geographer and gerontologist, of the kind of basic insights that can emerge from such a perspective.

Adding Being to Knowing and Doing

Emphasis in occupational therapy on knowing and doing as cornerstones of practice and research is the outcome of a philosophy premised on maximizing individual competence and autonomy in activities of daily living. Such a perspective involves a number of limiting assumptions about individual needs and the nature of well-being that are deeply embedded in western industrial and postindustrial culture. First, this perspective places an emphasis on performance and productivity as life goals (for a notable exception, see Reilly, 1974). Often this translates into a therapeutic focus on instrumental relationships and activities rather than on interpersonal and socioemotional aspects of identity—the belief that people's sense of worth and fulfillment arises from what they do or how they perform rather than from who they are and who they have been. A second implicit assumption is an underestimation of persons' ability to respond creatively to incapacity and to compensate without occupational therapy intervention for particular dysfunctions through life-style adjustments, psychological accommodation, or enhancement of other domains of their lives. Third is a pervasive assumption that an orientation toward knowing and doing is invariant over the life span—in short, that there are no developmental changes in the degree to which people are or wish to be passive and contemplative rather than active and productive. For example, children at play characteristically spend lots of time "hanging around" with their peers. They engage in seemingly nonproductive activities that generate the familiar response of "Nothing!" to the "What are you doing?" of an inquisitive adult. At the other end of the life cycle, people who are growing older may have an increasing propensity for reminiscence, life review, and more reflective modes of being in the world (Butler, 1963; Coleman, 1986).

Finally, there is an underestimation of the role of a person's environment as a source of identity and well-being. In this article, environment is viewed as far more than the physical or social setting. Environment is the *lifeworld*—the culturally defined spatiotemporal setting or horizon of everyday life (Buttimer, 1976). This phenomenological perspective embraces physical, social, cultural, and historical dimensions of an environment of lived experience. Thus, the lifeworld not only includes the person's current setting but also has a space–time depth that is uniquely experienced within the framework of personal history. Being in place expresses immersion within such a lifeworld.

Increased understanding of clients' being in place can be achieved by exploration of the meanings, values, and intentionalities that underlie their experience of particular environments. Through this process, it will be possible to develop insights that both contribute to theory and enhance practice. Such an endeavor has significant epistemological implications.

Implications for Epistemology

There is a need for basic research on normative populations that explores the nature of being in place. How do healthy people experience their lives in different environmental contexts? Clearly, in an increasingly multidisciplinary world, much can be learned from insights developed in other disciplines. Such borrowing needs to be complemented by original research with an explicitly occupational therapy focus that probes the underlying meanings, values, and intentionalities associated with adaptations healthy people normally make in the way they use their homes and conduct activities of self-care, work, and play as they pass through various phases of their lives (King, 1978) (see Chapter 8). Basic research is also necessary on the way in which people cope experientially with illness and reduced competence in different environments, both with and without occupational therapy intervention.

To develop such insight, it is important to nurture growing acceptance within occupational therapy of the value of qualitative research (Kielhofner, 1982a, 1982b; Merrill, 1985; Philips & Pierson, 1982; Schmid, 1981). A major feature of such research is an imperative to study people's experience in naturalistic context outside the laboratory. As Barris, Kielhofner, Levine, and Neville (1985) noted,

Because persons both shape and are shaped by their environments, occupational function and dysfunction reflect the individual's history of environmental interactions.

As a result, no attempt to understand a person's behavior will ever be complete without some understanding (or assessment) of the environments from which the person came and the behavior patterns that were encouraged by these environments. (p. 60)

Implicit within this observation is an acknowledgment that each person's response to a situation is uniquely conditioned by personal history and temporal context. A person's handling of recovery from a stroke may be as dependent on previous patterns of response to personal crises or the prevalent values of his or her age cohort as upon physical and occupational therapy regimens (Kaufman, 1988). Finally, qualitative research focuses on the phenomenological world of the individual to reveal experience as he or she actually understands it rather than as externally interpreted. Such research delves into the experiential meaning of having a stroke and the way this meaning impinges on the path to recovery and the effectiveness of interventions.

What does this mean in practical terms? There are now many sources of information on both philosophies and methodologies of qualitative research (Bogdan & Taylor, 1975; Kielhofner, 1982a, 1982b. Lofland & Lofland, 1984; Miles & Huberman, 1984; Reinharz & Rowles, 1988; Spradley, 1979; Van Maanan, 1983–1989). Although this information will not be reviewed in detail, several underlying themes are worth highlighting.

The quest for depth of insight frequently necessitates the use of limited numbers of subjects selected through purposive or theoretical sampling procedures (Glaser & Strauss, 1967). Emphasis is placed on the establishment of strong interpersonal relationships with these subjects. In developing such relationships, the researcher endeavors to be open to the sociocultural and environmental context and to develop a sense of empathy and mutual trust that will enable the subject to reveal dimensions of experience that might otherwise remain taken for granted and unexpressed (Von Eckartsberg, 1971). This process often entails a lengthy investment of time by the research participants (researcher and subject) in developing a shared language. By developing such a lexicon, the researcher is able to assume the role of translator of the subject's experience.

Significant contamination of the research situation can result from such intimate and potentially intense involvement by the researcher. In qualitative research, however, this is not a problem, because the focus of inquiry is descriptive and oriented toward the development of hypotheses and the generation of original insight. Such insight arises through inductive generalization from case studies. In contrast with traditional experimental and survey research, the criteria for verification are intuitive: They rely on the degree to which the researcher can authentically convey the essence of the research experience, rather than on measures of statistical significance. The presentation of qualitative findings becomes a crucial determinant of their usefulness. Presentation is characteristically detailed and descriptive. It relies on the researcher's ability to write, not only in a way that evokes the nuances of the research situation, but also in a manner that effectively conveys the environmental context and the process involved in arriving at conclusions—the natural history of the project.

Having provided the outlines of a methodology for exploring people's being in place, a study of elderly people living in a rural Appalachian environment will be used to illustrate the value of such an approach in occupational therapy.

The Colton Study

In the spring of 1978, I began a 3-year ethnographic study of 15 elderly residents of Colton,[1] a community of approximately 400 people (Rowles, 1980, 1981, 1983a, 1983b, 1983c). The subjects, 11 women and 4 men, ranged in age from 62 to 91 years at the outset of the study. Most were lifelong residents of Colton or its vicinity.

Close interpersonal relationships were developed with each participant to explore their involvement with the places of their lives. Particular emphasis was placed on attempting to reveal their relationship with the Colton environment. This involved learning about their daily activity patterns, identifying social networks, assessing perceptions of local space, and trying to reveal the phenomenological meaning of the setting that had been their home for so many years. In addition to observation and both unstructured and semistructured tape-recorded interviews, data gathering included time–space activity diaries, mental mapping procedures, aerial photography of the space around each participant's residence, social network measures, and a variety of morale and life-satisfaction scales. The overall objective was to develop a comprehensive understanding of each participant's lifeworld and the role of being in place in conditioning their experience of growing old.

Analysis involved both ongoing interpretation during interactions with the participants and inductive sorting of material following the fieldwork. Descriptive case studies were developed on each person. In addition, the dossiers compiled on each of the participants were carefully reviewed in a search for common themes. A clear image of what it is like to live and grow old in Colton gradually emerged through this process. Three themes in particular carry implications for occupational therapy.

The Rhythm and Routine of Taken-for-Granted Behavior

Each participant inhabited a highly individualistic lifeworld characterized by distinctive patterns of daily activity, a unique set of social relationships, and a highly

[1]Pseudonyms are employed for all persons and locations referred to in this account.

personalized emotional affinity with the Colton environment. Early in the research, it became apparent that there were a number of shared underlying motifs that characterized elderly Colton residents' being in place. One of these was the way daily behavior had become highly routinized and taken for granted. There are two aspects of this phenomenon.

First is the concept of body awareness, an implicit sensitivity to the physical context that allows the person to effectively negotiate space on a preconscious level. This phenomenon, originally identified by French phenomenologists and elaborated by Seamon (1979), involves the way the repetition of actions within a familiar environment may allow a person to transcend sensory capabilities. For example, typing proficiency developed by practice enables us to produce a memorandum on our personal computers without having to identify each letter; our fingers seem to know where to place themselves. We climb the stairs many times in our residences without being conscious of the number of steps involved. When driving on the freeway, we may suddenly become aware that we have traveled 20 miles while daydreaming and yet have not driven off the pavement. In each case the body's "automatic pilot," or learned awareness of the context, has guided our actions. This phenomenon is clearly manifested in the lives of the Colton elderly. Walter, 82 years of age when my research began, had lived with his 81-year-old wife, Beatrice, in the same house for more than 57 years. He did not have to think about the location of the throw rugs or about the camber on the porch steps that made them particularly treacherous following a rainstorm. Intimate familiarity with the layout of his home had served him well as he had grown increasingly constrained by failing vision. Beatrice's use of this environment was also facilitated by her body awareness of the placement of furniture. The configuration of furniture had gradually evolved over the years in a manner that provided places for her to hold on should she experience one of the dizzy spells to which she had become prone. Body awareness may become particularly adaptive in old age. It may compensate for sensory decrements and allow elderly people to continue functioning effectively in residences that might otherwise preclude independent living. Such familiarity may be a factor in the strong attachment to home and reluctance to leave displayed by many elderly people (O'Bryant, 1983).

Body awareness of the larger environment beyond the residence may contribute to the rhythm and routine that characterizes elderly Colton residents' everyday use of space within the community. Every morning, shortly before 10:00 a.m., Walter takes a leisurely 400-yd stroll down the hill from his house to the trailer that serves as the post office to "pick up the mail." He traces exactly the same path each day. Several male age peers from different locations within Colton embark on the same trip at about the same time. Of course, there is often no mail to be collected, but that is not the point. Rather, picking up the mail provides a rationale for an informal gathering of the elderly men of the community at the bench outside the Colton Store, which is located adjacent to the post office. The men generally linger throughout the morning. They watch the passing traffic, converse with patrons of the store, and discuss events of the day. Then, around lunchtime, the group disperses and Walter wends his way home again. There is also a spatiotemporal rhythm to the way in which the elderly women of Colton use community space. Their activity patterns tend to be focused on the Senior Center during the noontime hour when lunch is served. Indeed, most elderly Colton residents exhibit highly regular and routinized activity patterns focused on a limited number of behavior settings (Barker, 1968; Barker & Barker, 1961). Considered together, this regular interaction of diverse activity patterns reveals an ongoing "place ballet" (Seamon & Nordin, 1981). The spatiotemporal consistency of this place ballet may be highly adaptive. It provides a sense of security, because deviation from the regular pattern (e.g., the failure of Walter to appear at the bench outside the Colton Store) is characteristically noted and investigated.

Recognition of taken-for-granted and routinized behavior as a component of normative adaptation is not new (King, 1978; Meyer, 1922) (see Chapters 8 and 2, respectively), but it is a theme that merits reemphasis in occupational therapy. To what extent is it possible to enrich practice through exploring interventions that build on these aspects of being in place? Recognizing the importance of taken-for-granted behavior also suggests that individual functioning—the freedom and confidence to participate in the environment beyond the home—may be closely related to the sociocultural ambience (accepted rules and norms of behavior) of the community environment. It becomes important to study not only actual behavior but also the underlying premises that condition such behavior—premises that include community expectations with respect to the assumption of mutual responsibility for the welfare of the vulnerable.

The Surveillance Zone

A second theme concerns the importance of certain zones of space as components of many elderly people's being in place. There is now a large and growing literature on the meaning and significance of home (Altman & Werner, 1985; Rybczynski, 1987). Most occupational therapists are at least implicitly aware of the significance of this space to many of their clients. Only a few, I suspect, are equally cognizant of the significance of space immediately beyond the threshold. In Colton, the surveillance zone (space within the visual field of home) assumed increasing importance in many elderly persons' lives as they grew older (Rowles, 1981). For some, particularly the homebound, this space became the arena of their lives—space that could be viewed from the window or from the porch. Several of the study participants spent many hours each day watching events as they transpired on the street below. In some cases this involved the development of unspoken relationships with those who passed by. In turn, this was the zone of space in which they were watched by concerned neighbors. Some of the participants had developed a system of signals whereby they would open their shades or switch on the porch light at prearranged times each day. They gained a sense of security from the knowledge that they would be checked on should they fail to follow this procedure.

The surveillance zone often becomes the focus of both practical and social support relationships between neighbors. Some of the participants engaged in a process of setting up for surveillance. They would position a favorite chair by the window and place their telephone, television remote control, sewing, lunch tray, and other needed items within arm's reach. The significance of the surveillance zone is illustrated by 68-year-old Peggy, who perceived herself as virtually housebound. Following the death of her husband, she had the window by which she spent much of her time replaced with a larger picture window affording a better view.

The surveillance zone view from the window may have therapeutic value not only for elderly people but also for those who are sick (Ulrich, 1984). Occupational therapists may significantly enrich their clients' lives by showing increased sensitivity to the potential of this space. This might be accomplished by facilitating the process of setting up for surveillance, recommending the removal, where feasible, of obstacles to vision (e.g., trees or high sills), and engaging in efforts to enhance communication with neighbors within the visual field.

Environment as a Component of Self

One of the most important findings from the research was that for many of Colton's older residents, particularly persons 75 years of age and older, the environment had become almost literally a part of the self (Rowles, 1983c). Over many decades of residence, the environment had developed a time-depth as it accumulated layer upon layer of meaning. Participants in the study had known the setting in a variety of different contexts. They had known it in childhood as a bustling and vibrant railroad and coal town of more than 800 residents. They could visualize the excitement of the annual Oyster Day when one of the local businessmen would arrange for oysters to be brought in from Baltimore and the whole community would celebrate an unofficial holiday. They could recall the first kiss of adolescence, stolen by the pond in Raccoon Hollow, a favorite teenage haunt. They had also known this place during the hard times of the Great Depres-

sion. They remembered the day in 1931 when the bank closed its doors; they remembered the stores that had gone out of business, the abandonment of homes, and the departure of the young in search of employment in cities beyond Appalachia. Indeed, over the years, they had accumulated memories of incidents and events within a series of different Coltons that had evolved during their lifetimes.

For each person the reservoir of memories was unique. It represented a collage of incident places, that is, locations where particular events transpired, that are grounded in personal history and suffused with emotional significance. Each participant was able to vicariously immerse himself or herself within the places of the past and in so doing was able to transcend the bounds of both physical competence and the contemporary environment. Acknowledging this ability enables us to understand how the environment, particularly for those who have lived in the same setting for many years, may become a repository of meaning, a part of the self that is inextricably linked to self-identity.

Such fusion with the environment is well illustrated by the way many older people, and young ones too, manipulate their physical setting in a way that transforms it into an expression of who they are and have been. For example, Walter had assembled a working set of railroad lights and signals in his front yard. The trains no longer stopped in Colton, but these memorabilia served not only to remind him of the focus of his working life as a railroader but also presented a statement of his enduring identity to all who passed by.

Similar insight can be gleaned from the environment that Dan, a burly 86-year-old former coal miner, had created for himself. Dan shared a home with one of his daughters and her husband; it was located on a hillside overlooking the center of Colton. During our early meetings, I met with Dan in his bedroom or in the living room of the house. His sparsely decorated room contained many of the artifacts one might expect to find in the home of a rugged person who had enjoyed hunting. There was a gun rack on the wall and photographs recording successful fishing exploits. During our initial conversations, Dan would sometimes refer to his "rooms." I assumed that he was referring to his bedroom. One day, after I had come to know him a little better, he decided to show me the rooms. There were two of them, interconnected and located on the second floor of the house. As we entered, I was surprised to be confronted with a blaze of color. The walls were covered with decorated china plates and the tables, cabinets, and shelves were crammed with neatly arranged vases, china dolls, and ceramic and glass ornaments. When Dan was in his early 30s his wife had died, leaving him alone to raise five children. He had been obliged to adopt a more conventionally feminine role. In the process, he had begun to accumulate the artifacts, and gradually his interest had evolved to the point where he would search out such items at yard sales and local fairs. His rooms both reflected and symbolized an important aspect of an unusual life experience that had become a part of his identity and a source of feelings of accomplishment in his old age.

By attempting to reveal and become sensitive to the spatiotemporal meaning and significance of the environment to their clients, occupational therapists may be able to identify intervention strategies more attuned to the experiential worlds of those they seek to serve. Such sensitivity may be especially important in dealing with people who have resided for many years in the same setting or who recently relocated from such a familiar environment. From a pragmatic perspective, developing deeper understanding of being in place will necessitate research. In-depth qualitative studies may be valuable in developing a clearer understanding of why some people respond positively to specific occupational therapy interventions and conscientiously follow recommendations but others seem resistant to efforts to assist them (Merrill, 1985). Such research may suggest ways in which environmental manipulation may be used to substitute or compensate for losses and to foster a continued sense of self-identity. This may be an important complement to more traditional skill- and competence-building interventions. Finally, research into the existential meaning of environment to clients may contribute significantly to the development of more sophisticated theory in occupational therapy.

Conclusion

In developing my thesis, I am not suggesting that knowing, doing, and being are discrete and mutually exclusive components of human occupation. They are intimately interrelated. Indeed, implicit within the illustrations from Colton are elements of knowing and doing. Physical routines of moving around within the environment, the process of scanning the surveillance zone, and accumulating artifacts to reinforce a sense of identity are all active components of occupying place. They undergird the person's experience of being in place and are prerequisite to it.

My argument is that widely accepted and internalized tenets of contemporary occupational therapy philosophy may be compromising and limiting the potential of the field. Emphasis on performance, as manifested by knowing and doing, has tended to relegate the notion of being (as a component of well-being and a fulfilling life) to an ancillary role. One outcome of this has been inadequate consideration, at least until recently, of the role of the person's experienced spatiotemporal environment in conditioning his or her response to dysfunctions and to the intervention strategies designed to remedy them.

More explicit incorporation of concern for understanding the person's being in place will enrich occupational therapy research and practice in several domains.

First, it becomes possible by employing naturalistic and qualitative methodologies to more directly incorporate within emergent theory, consideration of the influence of the environmental context as a component of the meanings, values, and intentionalities with which clients imbue their occupation (be it self-care, work, or play).

Revelation of the nature of being in place in all of its space–time complexity in both normative and therapeutic situations facilitates discovery of ways in which compensatory strengths may be manifest in both the person and his or her environmental context (Rogers, 1982). Such strengths may emanate from dimensions of human experience that are neither productivity nor performance driven. They may arise through the identity-reinforcing potential of reminiscence, through vicarious immersion in spatially or temporally displaced environments, or through other noninstrumental aspects of being in place that are part of the context in which occupational therapy is practiced.

Finally, concern with an exploration of the nature of being in place offers the potential for improved understanding of the way in which many people function as their own occupational therapists or as therapists for their peers. They may accomplish this by developing an invariant daily routine in their use of the environment, by increasing the size of a picture window, or by surrounding themselves with artifacts and memorabilia that provide a constant reminder of their enduring identity—who they are and who they have been. Such simple and frequently taken-for-granted facets of being in place may assume great importance in persons' striving for continuing independence and autonomy as they accommodate to changing abilities and personal circumstances.

In making these observations, I am not suggesting that occupational therapy should turn away from other aspects of its mission—for example, from concern for increasing a person's range of motion, or for enhancing a person's ability to cope with or overcome physical or sensory losses. Rather, I am reinforcing recent arguments for a return to the more holistic perspective that characterized the origins of occupational therapy in the early part of this century as the field evolved out of a Moral Treatment tradition (Kielhofner & Nicol, 1989). I am advocating that efforts to enhance performance be framed within the broader context of increased sensitivity to and concern for clients' being in place. It is these sometimes subtle components of a person's lifeworld that may continue to sustain him or her as a fully self-actualizing human being in spite of the circumstances that have necessitated occupational therapy intervention.

Acknowledgment

I thank Gary Kielhofner, DrPH, OTR, of the University of Illinois at Chicago for his helpful comments on an earlier version of this article.

References

Altman, I., & Werner, C. M. (Eds.). (1985). *Home environments.* New York: Plenum.

Barker, R. G. (1968). *Ecological psychology.* Stanford: Stanford University Press.

Barker, R. G., & Barker, L. S. (1961). The psychological ecology of old people in Midwest, Kansas and Yoredale, Yorkshire. *Journal of Gerontology, 61,* 231–239.

Barris, R. (1986). Activity: The interface between person and environment. *Physical and Occupational Therapy in Geriatrics, 5,* 39–49.

Barris, R., Kielhofner, G., Levine, R. E., & Neville, A. M. (1985). Occupation as interaction with the environment. In G. Kielhofner (Ed.), *A Model of Human Occupation: Theory and application* (pp. 42–62). Baltimore: Williams & Wilkins.

Bogdan, R., & Taylor, S. J. (1975). *Introduction to qualitative research methods.* New York: Wiley Interscience.

Butler, R. N. (1963). The life review: An interpretation of reminiscence in the aged. *Psychiatry, 26,* 65–76.

Buttimer, A. (1976). Grasping the dynamism of lifeworld. *Annals of the Association of American Geographers, 66,* 277–292.

Christiansen, C. H. (1981). Editorial: Toward resolution of crisis: Research requisites in occupational therapy. *Occupational Therapy Journal of Research, 1,* 115–124.

Coleman, P. G. (1986). *Aging and reminiscence processes: Social and clinical implications.* New York: Wiley.

Fidler, G. S., & Fidler, J. W. (1978). Doing and becoming: Purposeful action and self-actualization. *American Journal of Occupational Therapy, 32,* 305–310. (Reprinted as Chapter 7.)

Glaser, B. G., & Strauss, A. (1967). *The discovery of grounded theory: Strategies for qualitative research.* New York: Aldine.

Kaufman, S. R. (1988). Stroke rehabilitation and the negotiation of identity. In S. Reinharz & G. D. Rowles (Eds.), *Qualitative gerontology.* New York: Springer.

Kielhofner, G. (1982a). Qualitative research: Part One—Paradigmatic grounds and issues of reliability and validity. *Occupational Therapy Journal of Research, 2,* 67–79.

Kielhofner, G. (1982b). Qualitative research: Part Two—Methodological approaches and relevance to occupational therapy. *Occupational Therapy Journal of Research, 2,* 150–164.

Kielhofner, G., & Burke, J. P. (1977). Occupational therapy after 60 years: An account of changing identity and knowledge. *American Journal of Occupational Therapy, 31,* 675–689.

Kielhofner, G., & Nicol, M. (1989). The model of human occupation: A developing conceptual tool for clinicians. *British Journal of Occupational Therapy, 52,* 210–214.

Kiernat, J. M. (1982). Environment: The hidden modality. *Physical and Occupational Therapy in Geriatrics, 2,* 3–12.

Kiernat, J. M. (1987). Promoting independence and autonomy through environmental approaches. *Topics in Geriatric Rehabilitation, 3,* 1–6.

King, L. J. (1978). 1978 Eleanor Clarke Slagle Lecture: Toward a science of adaptive responses. *American Journal of Occupational Therapy, 32,* 429–437. (Reprinted as Chapter 8.)

Knos, D. S. (1977). On learning. In M. Sarris (Ed.), *New perspectives on geographic education: Putting theory into practice.* (pp. 1–11). Dubuque, IA: Kendall/Hunt.

Llorens, L. A. (1984). Theoretical conceptualizations of occupational therapy: 1960–1982. *Occupational Therapy in Mental Health, 4* (2), 1–14.

Lofland, J., & Lofland, L. (1984). *Analyzing social settings. A guide to qualitative observation and analysis.* Belmont, CA: Wadsworth.

Maslow, A. (1966). *The psychology of science; A reconnaissance.* Chicago: Henry Regnery.

Merrill, S. C. (1985). Qualitative methods in occupational therapy research: An application. *Occupational Therapy Journal of Research, 5,* 209–222,

Meyer, A. (1922). The philosophy of occupation therapy. *Archives of Occupational Therapy, 1,* 1–10. (Reprinted as Chapter 2.)

Miles, M. B., & Huberman, A. M. (1984). *Qualitative data analysis.* Beverly Hills, CA: Sage.

Mosey, A. C. (1974). An alternative: The biopsychosocial model. *American Journal of Occupational Therapy, 28,* 137–140.

Mosey, A. C. (1980). A model for occupational therapy. *Occupational Therapy in Mental Health, 1* (1), 11–31.

O'Bryant, S. L. (1983). The subjective value of "home" to older homeowners. *Journal of Housing for the Elderly, 1,* 29–43.

Philips, B. U., & Pierson, W. P. (1982). Commentary: Qualitative research in occupational therapy. *Occupational Therapy Journal of Research, 2,* 165–170.

Reilly, M. (1969). The educational process. *American Journal of Occupational Therapy, 23,* 299–307.

Reilly, M. (Ed.). (1974). *Play as exploratory learning.* Beverly Hills, CA: Sage.

Reinharz, S., & Rowles, G. D. (Eds.). (1988). *Qualitative gerontology.* New York: Springer.

Rogers, J. C. (1982). Order and disorder in medicine and occupational therapy. *American Journal of Occupational Therapy, 36,* 29–35.

Rowles, G. D. (1980). Growing old "inside": Aging and attachment to place in an Appalachian community. In N. Datan & N. Lohmann

(Eds.), *Transitions of aging* (pp. 153–170). New York: Academic Press.

Rowles, G. D. (1981). The surveillance zone as meaningful space for the aged. *Gerontologist, 23,* 304–311.

Rowles, G. D. (1983a). Between worlds: A relocation dilemma for the Appalachian elderly. *International Journal of Aging and Human Development, 17,* 301–314.

Rowles, G. D. (1983b). Geographical dimensions of social support in rural Appalachia. In G. D. Rowles & R. J. Ohta (Eds.), *Aging and milieu: Environmental perspectives on growing old* (pp. 111–130). New York: Academic Press.

Rowles, G. D. (1983c). Place and personal identity in old age: Observations from Appalachia. *Journal of Environmental Psychology, 3,* 299–313.

Rybczynski, W. (1987). *Home: A short history of an idea.* London: Penguin.

Schmid, H. (1981). Qualitative research and occupational therapy. *American Journal of Occupational Therapy, 35,* 105–106.

Seamon, D. (1979). *A geography of the lifeworld: Movement, rest and encounter.* New York: St. Martin's.

Seamon, D., & Nordin, C. (1981). Marketplace as place ballet: A Swedish example, *Landscape 24,* 35–41.

Spradley, J. (1979). *The ethnographic interview.* New York: Holt, Rinehart & Winston.

Ulrich, R. (1984). View through a window may influence recovery from surgery. *Science, 224,* 420–421.

Van Maanan, J (Ed.). (1983–1989). *Qualitative methodology.* Beverly Hills, CA: Sage.

Von Eckartsberg, R. (1971). On experiential methodology. In A. Georgi, W. F. Fischer, & R. Von Eckartsberg (Eds.), *Duquesne studies in phenomenological psychology.* (Vol.1, pp. 66–79). Pittsburgh, PA: Duquesne University Press/Humanities Press.

Chapter 21

The Lazarus Project: The Politics of Empowerment

Nancy Kari, MPH

Peg Michels

This chapter was previously published in the *American Journal of Occupational Therapy, 45,* 719–725. Copyright © 1991, American Occupational Therapy Association.

Our vision for long-term care describes a possibility for reshaping institutional aging in this society. The creation of an empowering environment requires the involvement of diverse groups: institutionalized elderly who receive human services, their families, the staff who work in nursing homes, and staff in administrative and policy-making positions. The vision is one of fundamental change that requires both a political process and a conceptual framework, or road map (see this chapter's Appendix).

This paper discusses current nursing home models of governance and the conceptual development of an alternative model for institutional long-term care. The community model is interdisciplinary in nature and was influenced by a group of people from a broad range of disciplines and practices, such as sociology, psychology, theology, political theory, public policy, economics, nursing, education, and occupational therapy. This model is being implemented in a pilot study called the Lazarus Project. The conceptual development of the community model comes from the Lazarus Project.

The Lazarus Project

The Lazarus Project is a 3-year pilot project that is co-directed by an occupational therapist and a political educator (i.e., the first and second authors, respectively). It is being done in collaboration with the Augustana Home of Minneapolis, a nursing home that employs an administrator, an assistant administrator, 12 managers, and 400 staff members for its 360 residents. The facility is part of a larger campus of 700 apartments in four adjoining high-rise building. The apartments and nursing home share a variety of services, including a grocery store, post office, bank, beauty shop, and health clinic.

The intent of the Lazarus Project is to develop and evaluate the feasibility of an alternative model for the existing hierarchical models of governance that organize service provision and institutional living for elderly persons. In hierarchical models, power and authority are held by those at the top of the organization. Decisions are made by the administrator and managers for the good of the organization. Limited opportunity exists for nonmanagerial staff, residents, and families to access information or to influence important decisions affecting them. We believe that hierarchical models of governance are not sufficient to deal with the difficult issues facing institutional long-term care, such as meeting physical needs without diminishing the autonomy of the frail elderly; recruiting and sustaining a competent, well-trained work force; or providing quality care in the face of diminishing economic resources.

The community model proposed by the Lazarus Project is based on democratic principles. *Democratic governance* means that all members of the community have a voice in shaping the environment in which they live or work, thereby creating a broader, more flexible base for problem solving. The community model should not be confused with a resident enrichment program, which provides more choices or services for people. What democratic governance does mean is that the residents and staff can choose among options that they have helped create rather than from among options offered by others in authority. Our assumption that residents wish to participate in shaping their lives was verified through public discussions held in the nursing home. In these discussions, the residents indicated that they would like opportunities to create meaningful rituals for death and loss. They suggested possible solutions for maintaining privacy. They stated that they wanted to help create ways in which they could assume meaningful roles in their daily lives.

Effects of Institutionalization on Elderly Residents

The problems associated with institutional care of elderly people are documented (Cohen, 1989; Rosenfelt, 1965; Vladeck, 1980). Many persons experience nursing home placement in terms of loss, that is, loss of individuality and privacy, loss of connectedness to earlier lives, loss of meaningful roles, and loss of control over the living environment. Resulting behaviors may include hostility, withdrawal, depression, passivity, and incapacitation. In addition, the frail elderly have physical deficits related to chronic health conditions. In health care institutions these problems are framed and treated from a medical perspective, thus emphasizing disease and functional loss. Ultimately, the elderly person internalizes the identity of dysfunction (Kalish, 1979). Incapacity and powerlessness become self-fulfilling prophecies when institutionalized persons acquiesce and accommodate to the limited roles of patient and recipient of services rather than the fuller role of community resident. Caregivers who believe that disabled elderly persons are victims and are unable to change their situation assume paternalistic attitudes, thus reinforcing powerlessness. Decision-making structures that distribute power unequally so that professionals and staff in authority have most of the power help maintain residents in a powerless situation.

Powerlessness of Staff in Nursing Homes

Nursing home staff members, including health professionals and nurse's aides, can also experience disempowerment. Williams (1988) described a powerlessness that many staff feel in their inability to bring about change in the long-term-care system. Several problems related to nursing home staff were identified by Tellis-Nayak and Tellis-Nayak (1989) and Vladeck (1980), including low morale, a low-level commitment to the organization, and a high rate of turnover. Aides in nursing homes are often associated in the media with an apparent lack of care for residents. The media, however, often ignore the morass of mixed expectations that the elderly, families, and society, place on long-term-care staff. Complex nursing home regulations reflect this ambiguity. Is it the nursing home staff's responsibility to make decisions on behalf of residents, or should the staff members respect the residents' autonomy? If an injury occurs, the legal system makes it clear that the staff is responsible. Negotiating this ambiguity falls most heavily on nurse's aides, who constitute about 70% of the personnel within nursing homes. These workers earn low wages and often do not have adequate training (Tellis-Nayak & Tellis-Nayak, 1989). Like the residents, aides are at the low end of the organization's hierarchical structure and, therefore, have little access to policy-making or decision making, yet they have essential knowledge of residents' lives. Their lack of influence affects the institution's ability to provide quality care. Furthermore, their low position in the hierarchy encourages turnover, which is costly. Society ultimately pays this addition to the price of nursing home care.

Nursing home aides and residents are not alone in perceiving themselves as unable to influence forces shaping their work and their daily lives. For example, many occupational therapists in long-term care are unable to develop a practice that reflects the broad, holistic philosophy of the profession, primarily because their practice has been narrowly redefined by parties outside the field, such as third-party reimbursers and state and federal regulators. Additionally, they see themselves as unable to make change within the existing organizational structure. But influencing changes within systems is a political process that requires one to learn how to analyze and affect power relationships and decision making within an organization. Political skills are usually not part of the preparation for work in long-term care. Most students are taught the necessary professional skills to practice their work within the existing governing structures of long-term care institutions.

Traditional Models of Governance in Long-Term Care

Models of governance have great influence in shaping the mission, procedures, and interactions within an organization. The model of governance is embedded within the institution's philosophy and decision-making processes. Models carry with them a powerful language that is used to frame problems, define solutions, and guide what can be imagined as appropriate possibilities.

Most nursing homes embody the medical or therapeutic model (see Table 1). The medical model emphasizes the isolation and treatment of residents' problems related to disease and dysfunction, and medical personnel have the greatest authority. The roles of other staff members, residents, and family members carry less authority and are ancillary to medical roles. Although we acknowledge that the medical model is essential in acute care settings, we question its adequacy as a governing structure that organizes the whole of daily life of the institutionalized elderly. If as a democratic society we believe that each person is capable of creating a common good and exercising decision making to that end, then a hierarchical model that highly values decisions made by experts does not allow residents to create a meaningful life for themselves.

The therapeutic model is a derivative or a modification of the medical model. It is used by rehabilitative and therapeutic personnel to identify needs and provide appropriate health services. In this model, health (sometimes referred to as *wellness*) can be viewed more holistically, with consideration given to the person's emotional and spiritual dimensions. Although rehabilitative approaches are generally problem oriented (i.e., focusing on skill deficits), they also consider individual strengths and capacity for adaptation. The therapeutic model is effective when the person needs an enhanced environment or a specific program to facilitate individual change. We question, however, whether this model promotes the skills needed to create and maintain an empowering environment. If residents and other staff are to have an active voice in shaping their environment, the skills that allow people to make public contributions are required (e.g., agenda setting, decision making, role negotiation, management of conflict arising from diverse interests).

When a living environment is organized according to either of these two models, a hierarchy of relationships is created. The staff are the experts who have the knowledge and techniques to identify the needs, name the problems, and provide the solutions. Those served become the recipients. Although skilled clinicians collaborate in goal setting and provide choices for their patients, the institution's organizational structure still defines the parameters and expectations for role behaviors of both the service providers and the residents. These two traditional governing models exclude the concept of reciprocity. Daily life for those living within the institution can become compartmentalized and focused on receiving services to alleviate dysfunction or participating in activities that primarily fill time.

Table 1
Models of Organizational Governance

Medical Model	Therapeutic Model	Community Model
Focuses on acute care, disease, and disability.	Focuses on the provision of a variety of services.	Focuses on capacities and the ability to contribute.
Facilitates dependency on staff.	Facilitates dependency on staff.	Encourages interdependency among all members.
Information and knowledge are seen as technical expertise.	Information and knowledge are compartmentalized and perceived as servicing the client.	Information and knowledge are perceived as wisdom gained from experience.
Uses specialized language, which creates dependency.	Uses specialized language, which creates dependency.	Uses a common language accessible to all.
Focuses on patients' rights.	Focuses on clients' consumer needs.	Focuses on contribution and reciprocity among staff and resident members.
Uses a reductionistic, scientific approach.	Uses a programmatic approach that tends to fragment spiritual, physical, and social well-being.	Uses a holistic approach that addresses physical, social, and spiritual well-being.
Creates a social structure based on a hierarchy.	Creates a social structure based on a hierarchy.	Creates a democratic, egalitarian social structure.
Is staff intensive.	Is staff intensive.	Includes nonprofessional and mutual caregiving.
Activities geared toward improved physical functioning	Activities geared toward personal development and contentment.	Opportunities for public decision making and contribution.
Holds staff responsible.	Holds staff responsible.	Holds all accountable.
Empowers staff.	Empowers staff.	Encourages relational empowerment.

Note. Copyright 1989 by the Lazarus Project. Reprinted by permission.

A model of democratic governance was introduced in the Lazarus Project. In this model, residents, staff, and families learn to collaborate in creating their institutional community. This project proposes fundamental changes in the institution's philosophy, from providing an enriching environment and quality services for residents to empowering residents and staff members to create an environment reflective of their interests. For this to be accomplished, decision-making structures must shift from hierarchical to collaborative processes.

Theory Base of the Lazarus Project

The conceptual framework of the Lazarus Project is based on social support theory (Gottlieb, 1985; Minkler, 1981, 1984; Minkler, Frantz, & Wechsler, 1982; Pilisuk & Minkler, 1980, 1985), which is used by human service disciplines to understand the role of the community in promoting health, and on a political theory called *citizen politics*, developed from the work of Project Public Life, a national initiative to engage citizens in governance of their communities. Project Public Life is based at the Humphrey Institute of Public Affairs at the University of Minnesota, Minneapolis.

Social Support Theory

Social support theory describes relationships between social support and a person's sense of control and health status. A social support network was defined by Minkler (1981) as the network of people through which a person's social identity is maintained. This network is also a resource base that provides emotional support, material and information resources, services, and new social contacts. Social support theory has three primary hypotheses (Minkler et al., 1982):

1. Support networks positively influence a person's health behaviors.
2. Social support increases one's ability to cope with problems of living and, in this way, may influence resistance to disease.
3. The person's experience of support from others leads to a generalized sense of perceived control over his or her environment.

Social support theory identifies key ways in which a person maintains health within a social environment. The Lazarus Project uses these insights from social support theory to explain the need for a strong community within a health care institution.

Citizen Politics

Politics is the process by which a person becomes critically aware of power and control in relationships and social structures and then uses that knowledge to work collectively for change (Brookfield, 1988). Citizen politics, defined as the work of the citizen, assumes that citizens are at the center of decision making and problem solving. The core concepts that define citizen politics are self-interest (i.e., the person's direct concerns), public (i.e., the problem-solving arena in which people debate, render collective judgment, and learn to shape their environment), power (i.e., a dynamic relationship rather than a one-way force), and diversity, (i.e., the variety of people, interests, cultures, and ideas found in public life that are needed to define and solve public problems) (Boyte & Lappe, 1990).

Citizen politics differs from partisan politics in that the former views community members as active participants in public decision making rather than as spectators who leave problem solving to such experts as lobbyists, politicians, or special-interest groups. Citizen politics has a deep respect for persons' capacities to determine their own destinies. These capacities are rooted in their histories, cultures, and understandings of their experiences. This knowledge is as necessary as professional expertise in solving the problems of a specific community.

It is important that we distinguish citizen politics of the Lazarus Project from the residents' rights movement. The residents' rights movement, which began in the late 1960s, offers impressive examples of the kinds of public involvement and influence that institutionalized elderly people can undertake (Holder & Frank, 1984; Kautzer, 1983). The establishment of resident councils, the legislation of a residents' bill of rights, and the creation of various citizen advocacy organizations are results of this movement. We believe that resident councils do not generate a form of politics that can create and maintain community by ensuring that diverse interests work together in naming and solving common problems; resident councils work within the established hierarchy to address grievances or advocate for particular resident issues. They focus on policy change but not on governance and therefore do not systematically alter power relationships.

Citizen politics defines a public arena, in which diverse self-interests are required to address the complexity of issues affecting society. It is within this arena that the public good is defined and used to guide the process of empowerment (Boyte & Lappe, 1990). The word *power* means "to be able." Empowerment, therefore, is not something one does to or for another person, but rather, is the ability to act collectively to solve problems and influence important issues. Empowerment occurs when parties influence each other. Citizen politics and social support theory form the framework for the community model used in the Lazarus Project.

The Community Model

The community model builds a collaborative rather than a hierarchical relationship and employs democratic governance in an institution's structures (e.g., decision-making processes and procedures for policy development). In this model, professionals have technical information required for problem solving, but all members of the community have part of the knowledge that contributes to the understanding and solving of problems. The concept of *community* refers to an interdependent, diverse group of persons who have a common purpose. Each member of the community has a role recognized by others. All members have the opportunity to participate in decision making, and all are accountable to the community. A community can influence a larger public world through the practice of public politics.

Distinctions exist between this concept of community and a *therapeutic* community. Although the Lazarus Project community recognizes the legitimate need for therapeutic and medical interventions, its primary function is not to accomplish individual therapeutic goals within a group setting. The Lazarus Project community is not designed or controlled by service providers, and members of this community are not categorized as patients, residents, health professionals, or staff members, but as citizens who govern.

The definition of *community* used in the Lazarus Project was influenced by the writings of Tuan (1986), Boyte (1984, 1989), Boyte and Lappe (1990), and Evans and Boyte (1986). Tuan, a geographer, described community as embodying an agreed-on "good life" (Tuan, 1986, p.9). This good life has three dimensions: a physical dimension based on the sensory experiences of sight, sound, smell, taste, and touch; a meaningful social connection; and an ethical purpose, or a power greater than oneself.

In a complex, diverse world, the creation of the good life is highly dependent on a conscious knowledge of the function of public values. Communities, whether they occur within institutions or neighborhoods, are composed of persons who have both public and private dimensions to their lives and who have the capacity to create a mutually agreed-on good life. The concepts of public and private are linked, yet distinct. This integration allows one to imagine politics capable of creating a meaningful community of institutionalized citizens. Residents would have clearly defined private lives and spaces as well as public arenas in which they could assume leadership in shaping their immediate environment and, ultimately, the broader public. Private lives generally center on friends and family—people with similar views and values. Private relationships are based on loyalty and tend to be spontaneous and less reserved. The outcome of a healthy private life is unconditional love. The public aspect of life differs, although private values often initiate one's movement toward a public arena. Diverse relationships are established for the purpose of task accomplishment and problem solving. A public relationship assumes accountability rather than loyalty. The result of a well-crafted public life is empowerment (Boyte, 1989).

The Lazarus Project community model is broadly inclusive. Its membership includes residents, family members, volunteers, and those who work within the institution (i.e., professional service providers, housekeepers and other staff, managers, and nurse's aides). To function effectively, each of these groups must have access to information and the ability to influence decision making. Members learn and use public skills, such as negotiation, collaborative decision making, and evaluation. The anticipated outcomes are many: New friendships and peer relationships are established; meaningful rituals are created and celebrated; and persons expand and strengthen their ability to act on their values, shape the ethical purpose of their community, and influence the public world.

Implementation of the Lazarus Project

The Lazarus Project, consisting of three phases, is expected to last 3 years. At the time of this writing, only Phase 1, that is, the first year, had been completed.

Phase 1: Concept Development and Training of the Management Team

Planning began in 1989. A national group of interdisciplinary advisors was assembled and a 3-day retreat held in June 1989. The purpose of this meeting was to critique and deepen the interdisciplinary conceptual base and review strategies for implementation. A second advisory meeting was held 6 months later to critique the overall research design for the project. The project uses an action–research model, which applies the knowledge gained through practice and reflection on the concepts of citizen politics to shape subsequent strategies. Descriptive data are collected from journals, interviews, interactions occurring in training workshops, and conversations recorded from public forums to track learning of the concepts and events that trigger change.

Our focus in Phase 1 was to train the nursing home's administrators and management team how to incorporate the concepts of the community model. The training began with the creation of a common mission statement, which was used to guide strategies for implementation of the community model. The initial statement read, "The purpose of Augustana is to create and sustain a wholistic [sic] community which supports and promotes the opportunity for growth and ownership through contribution, for the enhancement of residents." The word *enhancement* was later replaced with *empowerment*.

During this first year, the management team at the Augustana Home worked together to establish a collaborative, public environment for problem solving. Their training was presented within the context of issues affecting daily work, and strategies were generated to address tasks such as budgeting, fund-raising, planning and conducting more effective meetings, and negotiating roles for new positions. They learned the concepts of citizen politics (i.e., self-interest, public, diversity, and power), and they practiced such skills as collaborative decision making, conflict negotiation, public debate, role clarification and negotiation, and work evaluation. Because they were able to begin creating a public, open process using a public language, the Augustana management team made some changes in its practice of decision making within the institution. When problems were raised, members of the management team requested information so that the problem could be collectively defined, and they worked together to generate strategies for solutions. Management meetings went beyond information exchanges to later include debates and discussions. Most important, some of the managers began to integrate a deeper understanding of power relationships. Their own experience of working to create a public decision-making environment in which they were expected to influence and practice power allowed them to consider what role they would play as residents experienced empowerment. These changes have helped establish the environment for the next phase.

Key to Phase 1 was the development of a strong relationship with an on-site staff person who could develop the role of internal organizer. This person plays an important role in integrating the community model by adapting training workshops to fit the unique culture of the nursing home. The person selected was the director of the therapeutic activities program.

Conclusions from the first year of the project concerning the person filling the internal organizer role were that this organizer have the following characteristics: (a) experience managing educational programs, (b) intellectual curiosity about the Lazarus concepts and the ability to think conceptually, (c) openness to change, (d) a high level of commitment to the mission of the Lazarus Project, (e) respect for everyone involved (i.e., residents, administration, managers, and all staff members), and (f) access to authority.

The decision to begin the project by training the Augustana management team was a strategic one given the reality of power relationships in a hierarchical structure. Without involvement and modeling from the nursing home managers and administrator, it would be difficult to access information to influence decision making from lower positions within the hierarchy. Although Phase 1 of the project focused on the training of managers, these managers will not unilaterally determine the process for implementing the community model.

The first year of the project provided important insights: (a) The project could not occur without administrative support and the willingness of people with authority to look critically at decision-making processes, (b) fundamental change from a hierarchical to a community model cannot be imposed or rushed—It requires time, (c) institutional change involves both personal struggle and conflict over professional turf, and (d) new knowledge and an agreed-on mission statement are motivators for change.

Phase 2: Building the Community Model

The goal of Phase 2 of the Lazarus Project is to build the community model. Implementation of this phase is in progress. The questions that guide this phase are (a) Can the staff imagine new roles? (b) What capacities do residents have to contribute to governance? and (c) Can the residents' family members create important roles for themselves in the governance of the institution? The

answers to these questions will continue to shape the understanding of the community model.

Phase 2 of implementation begins with the selection of a steering committee composed of an equal number of staff and nonstaff members. This group will represent all subgroups associated with the nursing home community. The selection process will occur through a series of public forums and interviews designed to identify important issues, potential leadership, and existing support networks among residents. The purpose of the steering committee will be to establish a democratic governing body within the institution. An important function of the steering committee will be to teach the conceptual knowledge of the Lazarus Project, so that members can provide leadership in extending the model throughout the nursing home community.

Phase 3: Influencing the Broader Public

Phase 3 of implementation will address the capacity of the Lazarus Project community to influence the broader public (i.e., media, legislators, regulatory agencies, professional organizations, and educational institutions) on issues of aging. Effective public leadership must first be developed within the community before members can be successful with powerfully organized groups outside their community. This does not, however, preclude smaller scale public strategies implemented during Phase 2 that allow members to practice influencing the broader public.

Occupational Therapy and the Community Model

Why should occupational therapy challenge the constraints of the medical and therapeutic models in long-term-care institutions? How can occupational therapists assume leadership in the broader long-term-care system?

Adaptation; mastery of one's environment; fulfillment of meaningful roles; and engagement in purposeful, goal-directed actions have always been the focus of occupational therapy. Empowerment is the ultimate goal. Occupational therapists have strongly argued that the therapeutic relationship must involve *doing with*, not *doing for* or *doing to*, the patient. Yet most occupational therapy practice in nursing homes is directed by the medical and therapeutic models. Thus, the primary role of occupational therapy is the provision of treatment to improve or compensate for dysfunction. The broader goal of the creation of an empowering environment in which persons can assume control over their lives and establish meaningful roles cannot be easily achieved. Traditional health models define limited expectations and roles for residents. They also limit the possibility for occupational therapists to act on their commitment to the improvement of the quality of life in nursing homes. The community model recognizes the need for medical intervention and therapeutic programming in nursing homes, but the provision of health care services is not its primary focus. Occupational therapy personnel can use the community model to reconceptualize and expand their roles within long-term-care institutions.

Challenging institutional governance is an interdisciplinary task and cannot be accomplished by occupational therapists alone. Occupational therapy does not currently have a theoretical framework that can bring about change in the governing structures of nursing homes. Health care professions generally do not explicitly address issues of power and governance. The Lazarus Project defines a political process for change that results in empowerment.

Occupational therapy personnel who gain political knowledge and skills can collectively extend their leadership to the broader health care environment. Such leadership can give the profession a stronger voice in shaping the decisions that affect health care for the elderly and even in changing the way in which society views aging.

Appendix: The Lazarus Project's Vision for Long-Term Care

The Lazarus Project believes that the frail elderly can be contributing members to society. It is through contribution that persons exercise power and are able to live a life of meaning and dignity. Empowerment happens when communities are created—communities that govern themselves by drawing on the diverse strengths of their members to address common problems.

The Lazarus Project believes this kind of community can be created in nursing home environments. This requires a broad, holistic understanding of health that goes beyond physical and emotional health. It must include the ability to have authority in one's life, to shape one's environment and to extend influence within a broader public world.

Aging is a public issue; it is not simply an individual experience. When people become older and more frail, their ability to be contributing members in society changes. In a society that measures worth in terms of contributions and influence, the loss of physical and cognitive capacity quickly defines the frail elderly as "a problem." One of the ways the public has chosen to address this "problem" is to separate itself from chronically ill and disabled elderly persons by institutionalizing aging.

The authors of the Lazarus Project believe that the focus on the medical and service missions of long-term-care institutions views residents as incapacitated rather than as productive contributors. When this assumption becomes embedded in the institution's governing system, it can lead to a loss of influence and power for all involved—the residents, staff, administrators, and families. This loss of influence constrains an institution's ability to effectively respond to the "problems of aging" in a creative way.

Ultimately, the public is separated from the insights that come from the struggles in growing old. The lack of wisdom in public policies on aging reflects the loss of those insights.

Acknowledgments

We thank Pam Hayle, Lazarus Project liaison and organizer, for her insights and commitment to the project; Harry Boyte, director of Project Public Life; and Louise Fawcett, Jean Kalscheur, and Sharon Stoffel for editorial assistance. We are also grateful for the encouragement and financial support from the American Occupational Therapy Foundation.

References

Boyte, H. (1984). *Community is possible: Repairing America's roots.* New York: Harper & Row.

Boyte, H. (1989). *The commonwealth: A return to citizen politics.* New York: Free Press.

Boyte, H., & Lappe, F. (1990). The language of citizen democracy. *National Civic Review, 79,* 417–425.

Brookfield, S. (1988). *Developing critical thinkers: Challenging adults to explore alternative ways of thinking and acting.* San Francisco: Jossey-Bass.

Cohen, E. (1989). The elderly mystique: Constraints on the autonomy of the elderly with disabilities. *Gerontologist, 28* (Suppl.), 24–31.

Evans, S., & Boyte, H. (1986). *Free spaces.* New York: Harper & Row.

Gottlieb, B. (1985). Social networks and social support: An overview of research, practice, and policy implications. *Health Education Quarterly, 12,* 15–22.

Holder, E., & Frank, B. (1984). *Resident participation in nursing homes: A key to the improvement of life in nursing homes and improvement in the nursing home regulatory system.* Paper prepared for the Institute of Medicine Committee on Nursing Home Regulation and presented at a workshop entitled "Consumer Role in Quality Assurance in Nursing Homes," Fredericksburg, VA.

Kalish, R. (1979). The new ageism and the failure models: A polemic. *Gerontologist, 19,* 398–402.

Kautzer, K. (1983). Empowering nursing home residents: A case study of "Living is for the Elderly," an activist nursing home organization. In S.R. Reinharz & G.D. Rowles (Eds.), *Qualitative gerontology* (pp. 163–183). New York: Springer.

Minkler, M. (1981). Applications of social support theory to health education: Implications for work with the elderly. *Health Education Quarterly, 8,* 147–165.

Minkler, M. (1984). Health promotion in long-term care: A contradiction in terms? *Health Education Quarterly, 11,* 77–89.

Minkler, M., Frantz, S., & Wechsler, R. (1982). Social support theory and social action organizing in a "grey ghetto": The tenderloin experience. *International Quarterly of Community Health Education, 3,* 3–15.

Pilisuk, M., & Minkler, M. (1980). Supportive networks: Life ties for the elderly. *Journal of Social Issues, 36,* 95–115.

Pilisuk, M., & Minkler, M. (1985). Supportive ties: A political economy perspective. *Health Education Quarterly, 12,* 93–106.

Rosenfelt, R. (1965). The elderly mystique. *Journal of Social Issues, 21,* 37–42.

Tellis-Nayak, V., & Tellis-Nayak, M. (1989). Quality of care and the burden of two coutures: When the world of the nurse's aide enters the world of the nursing home. *Gerontologist, 29,* 307–313.

Tuan, Y.F. (1986). *The good life.* Madison, WI: University of Wisconsin Press.

Vladeck, B. (1980). *Unloving care.* New York: Basic.

Williams, C. (1988). *Power, politics, and advocacy: Issues that influence the care of older people.* Keynote address presented at the Second Annual Student Day, Community College of Philadelphia.

Chapter 22

The Americans With Disabilities Act of 1990 and Employees with Mental Impairments: Personal Efficacy and the Environment

Patricia A. H. Crist, PhD, FAOTA
Virginia C. Stoffel

Paid employment carries both practical and symbolic significance, because work results in compensation for basic needs, provides resources for community participation and giving, and is a symbol of full citizenship (Mancuso, 1990; Rhodes, Ramsing, & Bellamy, 1988). Productive work is highly valued in our society and is often the focal point around which self-care, leisure, and rest pursuits are selected and planned; it is one of the two determinants of our socioeconomic status. Unfortunately, many qualified Americans who have a mental disability may have been denied employment because of their mental health problems. Fortunately, we now have Title I of the Americans With Disabilities Act of 1990 (ADA) (Public Law 101-336), which mandates that qualified persons with physical or mental impairments not be excluded from employment and work activities because of disability.

When President Bush signed the ADA on July 26, 1990, he referred to the law as the new "Declaration of Independence" for 43 million Americans with disabilities (Staff, 1990). Occupational therapy philosophy, values, and rehabilitation goals are supported by the ADA, and our professionals can serve a central role in the implementation of this legislation. Recently, Townsend (1991) discussed a vision for the profession's future:

> I do not believe that it is enough to treat our patients in the confines of our hospitals and clinics without regard to factors outside that realm that influence their right to life and happiness.... As we look beyond our clinics out into the larger world and make our presence felt in a broad and meaningful way, we become instruments of change for our patients and the greater society. Occupational therapy is grounded in the respect for, search for, and achievement of maximum human potential for all of those we serve. (p. 873)

The ADA provides a mechanism for occupational therapists to be the "instruments of change" in helping persons with mental health impairments realize their potential as employees and productive citizens. Because the environment influences job performance and personal competence (Christiansen, 1991), occupational therapists can adapt individual job skills or the work site or both.

The purpose of this paper is to describe the role of occupational therapy in implementing the ADA to enhance the employment of persons with mental health problems. To achieve this goal, aspects of the ADA necessitating special attention for psychosocial disabilities are reviewed, and the influence of personal competence (self-efficacy) and the environment on performance are discussed. For the purposes of this paper, the job environment consists of four environmental components:

1. Employer and co-worker attitudes toward persons with mental health impairments.
2. Definition of essential job functions related to mental health.
3. Reasonable accommodations for employment skills associated with dysfunctional employee behavior resulting from mental impairments.
4. Access to employee functions.

Each of these components is necessary to fully comply with the ADA for employment processes (Lotito & Pimental, 1990).

The ADA and Mental Health

Under the ADA, mental or psychological disorders include mental retardation, organic brain syndrome, emotional or mental illness, and specific learning disabilities (National Mental Health Association, 1990). Excluded conditions include current illegal use of alcohol or drugs, homosexuality and bisexuality, sexual behavior disorders not resulting from physical impairments, compulsive gambling, kleptomania, and pyromania. Human immunodeficiency virus, AIDS, and other communicable diseases are protected under the ADA.

Persons disabled by drug addiction or alcoholism are covered under the law as long as the person is not currently abusing drugs or alcohol. Persons entitled to protection in the workplace are those who are (a) former users who have successfully completed a supervised rehabilitation program and no longer use illegal substances, (b) participants in a supervised drug rehabilitation program who no longer use illegal substances, and (c) persons using alcohol or drugs who are erroneously regarded as engaging in illegal drug use (i.e., using a drug that is illegal unless prescribed by a physician) (ADA, Title 1, § 104).

Legal drug use is that which occurs under the care of a licensed health care professional. A person who is currently abusing drugs is protected against discrimination under the ADA only if the present disability is not related to the illegal drug use. Protection is only for the defined disability and is not concurrent with drug- or alcohol-related disability problems. Employers may require a drug-free workplace and hold illegal drug users and alcoholics to the same performance standards as other employees, as established pursuant to the Drug-Free Workplace Act of 1988 (National Mental Health Association, 1990; Watson, 1990). Drug testing to identify illegal drugs during preemployment screenings is permitted, as are employment decisions made solely on drug test results. Termination and disciplinary actions can be taken, and no reasonable accommodations are required under the ADA for active drug and alcohol users.

Employers are not required to offer mental health coverage as part of their insurance benefits. An employer could not use the ADA to justify not employing a qualified applicant because the employer's current insurance plan does not cover the person's disability or because the cost of insurance benefits to the employer may increase. This is true for both health and liability insurance. Reasonable accommodation does not require that the employer provide alcohol or drug rehabilitation. A person with a drug addiction cannot be denied health and rehabilitation services if he or she was otherwise entitled to such coverage under the employer's medical plan.

The ADA protects persons with mental impairments from discrimination and supports inclusion in employment (Title 1) as well as access to public accommodations and services (Title III) that enhance employability and employee's rights. For successful engagement in productive work roles, a person with mental health problems must experience personal competence or self-efficacy in performing employment-related tasks.

Personal Self-Efficacy and Employment Readiness

To be successfully employed, one must view oneself as employable. Employability is a match between work-related skill, one's judgments regarding work abilities, and the job itself. According to the ADA, skills required to perform a job are delineated in the job description and referred to as *essential job functions*. Work skill is the ability to do work tasks. However, one's judgment regarding one's ability to work may be an even more important contributor to employability than work skills themselves.

Bandura (1977) described this judgment about one's skills or competence as *self-efficacy*. Efficacy allows a person to competently engage with the environment using multiple subskills and to execute courses of action required to deal with situations. Bandura stated that perceived self-efficacy influences a person's choice of activities and environmental settings, the effort expended, and persistence. Through research, he demonstrated that perceived self-efficacy is a better predictor of subsequent behavior than are performance skills (Bandura, 1982). Success as an employee is the result of perceived self-efficacy. Because persons with mental impairments often have low self-esteem, Bandura's theory can be used to develop strategies for persons with mental health problems to acquire self-efficacy. The self-efficacy will then allow them to perform the essential functions of a job, with or without accommodation, as addressed in the ADA.

Bandura's (1977) theory is based on the assumption that psychological procedures create and strengthen expectations of personal efficacy. In this model, two personal efficacy expectations are differentiated—efficacy expectations and outcome expectations:

> An efficacy expectation is the conviction that one can successfully execute the behavior required to produce the outcomes. An outcome expectation is defined as the person's estimate that a given behavior will lead to certain outcomes. Individuals can believe that a particular course of action will produce certain outcomes, but if they entertain serious doubts about whether they can perform the necessary activities, such information does not influence their behavior. Expectations of personal mastery affect both initiation and persistence of coping behavior. (Bandura, 1977, p. 193)

For persons with mental impairments to successfully engage in employment, both components of self-efficacy need to be developed, reinforced, and maintained to achieve the desired outcome, which is appropriate work behaviors. Persons with mental impairments are unlikely to report self-efficacy beliefs. Despite possessing the skills to perform the essential functions of a job, a person will not succeed if he or she has poor self-efficacy beliefs. Thus, development of positive work-related self-efficacy judgments is critical for employability. Occupational therapists can assist with the development of positive self-efficacy beliefs. Employability of persons with mental health problems can be enhanced through an understanding of the criteria used to judge employability. Therapists can then implement activities that enhance the employee's self-efficacy.

Bandura (1977, 1986) identified four sources of judgements about one's self-efficacy and, ultimately, the ability to perform: (a) emotional arousal, (b) verbal or social persuasion, (c) vicarious experience, and (d) performance accomplishments. These are hierarchically ordered from least influential to most influential in the development and maintenance of competency behavior.

As stated by Bandura (1977), *emotional arousal* is a source of physiological information used to judge anxiety and vulnerability to stress. Experience with stressful situations enables the development of coping skills and competency to deal effectively with fearful situations. *Verbal persuasion* involves leading people to believe that they can cope successfully with what has overwhelmed them in the past. Verbal persuasion can contribute to the successes achieved through performance, because peo-

ple can be socially persuaded that they possess the capabilities to master difficult situations. *Social persuasion*, without arrangements for conditions to facilitate effective performance, will most likely lead to failures that discredit the persuaders and further undermine self-efficacy. *Vicarious experience* involves seeing others perform difficult activities without adverse consequences. This experience can generate expectations of the observers that they too will improve if they persist in their efforts. Vicarious experience relies on inferences from social comparison used to model another person's behavior. Modeled behavior with clear outcomes conveys efficacy information. Observing another's performance, which results in repeated successes with evident consequences, enhances the observer's efficacy expectations. *Performance accomplishments*, the most influential and enduring sense of personal efficacy, involve personal mastery experiences. Successes raise mastery expectations; failures lower them. Mishaps that occur early in the course of events erode self-efficacy beliefs more than later failures during the development of self-efficacy. Repeated success lessens the negative effect of occasional failures, which in themselves can reinforce self-efficacy if failures are overcome. Performance exposure with a model present conveys powerful efficacy information, because verbal persuasion, vicarious experiences, and performance accomplishments are available to develop self-efficacy judgments. Opportunities to translate personal behavioral conceptions into appropriate successful actions and to make corrective refinements toward the perfection of skills are essential to the development of self-efficacy.

Psychological self-efficacy is probably acquired through more than one type of efficacy experience. Efficacy results from capability, which is the result of cognitive, social, and behavioral skill organization; but capability is only as good as its execution (Bandura, 1982). Once established, enhanced self-efficacy will generalize to other performance.

Bandura's (1977, 1982) self-efficacy model and occupational therapy are mutually supportive. Occupational therapists value all four types of efficacy experiences, and Bandura's emphasis on the importance of performance accomplishments is consistent with our focus on the doing process in treatment using purposeful activity. The importance of selected functional activities is to provide actual performance experience, the preferred facilitator for self-efficacy beliefs. Simulation, modeling, observation, and repeated movement exercises are only preliminary or underpinning experiences to the development of self-efficacy through actual performance. In occupational therapy, the value of actually performing the functional activity combined with using the three other forms of efficacy experiences is underscored.

Occupational therapists in mental health are aware of the importance of the emerging trend called *supported and transitional employment* in providing work-related efficacy expectations in their clients. Supported and transitional employment approaches assume that all people can do meaningful, productive work in competitive employment settings, if it is what people choose to do and if they are given necessary supports or accommodation appropriate for the setting (Anthony & Blanch, 1987). ADA outcomes will include the increased use of supported or transitional employment and opportunities to engage in regular work roles with reasonable accommodations. An example follows:

A 51-year-old woman with mental retardation who had never gone to school or worked lived at home with her 92-year-old mother until her mother's increasing age required both of them to move to a nursing home together. The head nurse at the nursing home requested that this woman engage in more productive work than that offered by the activity specialist. Both the client and her mother did not believe that she was employable.

Initial observation by the occupational therapist during a 3-hr trial in the workshop revealed that the client was able to do the essential job functions for several tasks in the sheltered workshop with minimal support from a female staff member. However, when a male supervisor or male co-worker addressed her or stood nearby, she became angry, hostile, and unable to keep working. The issue of tolerance for the opposite sex was considered to be a marginal job function.

The treatment plan, which was also a reasonable accommodation for a marginal job function, was simply to place the client in a work room with other women only. As expected, her work skills developed. Modeling by peers and the therapist, verbal persuasion by the therapist and others, and practice facilitated the development of her self-efficacy as a worker.

The outcome of the treatment plan was to have this client successfully employed in nearby industry. The treatment program incorporated the behavioral approach of desensitization, so that she would be able to work alongside men and talk with them without it disrupting her work. This would be less isolating for the client in the workplace. A second alternative, if not successful, was to seek reasonable accommodation in the workplace.

A person's perceived self-efficacy influences choice and structures needs for specific types of support and transition. Frequently, persons with mental health problems are not able to accurately report their job abilities. However, coupling one of the self-efficacy approaches with a person's job expectations may reveal the person's true abilities and decrease the influence of negative or limiting perceived expectations. The following case exemplifies the importance of self-efficacy experiences:

In the television show "L.A. Law," the character named Benny has developmental disabilities and started working at the law firm by helping with mail delivery, performing relatively simple filing, and making deliveries. His view of his own skills was narrow, based on living in a loving home environment with his mother, who provided for all of Benny's's needs but not for the development of work attitudes or behaviors. The work environment was new to him. As Benny's strengths were reinforced by performance experiences and accommodation, he got clear, strong, powerful feedback from his supervisors and other personnel as to the importance of the service he provided. His confidence in his skills increased to the point where when accused of losing a file, he would respond with "No, I know exactly where that file is" and would produce it. He demonstrated mastery and accompanying self-efficacy and participated in employee activities and work-related social events.

Important aspects of the work environments described in the above examples were the employers' positive attitude regarding each person's employability, accurate definitions of essential job functions, appropriate accommodations for both marginal and essential job functions, and full access to employee privileges. Each of these aspects is described below.

Attitudes Toward Mental Impairment

The ADA does not require a person to disclose a disability. Information regarding an identified disability must remain confidential, except in employment situations where supervisors and managers need to be informed regarding restrictions or accommodations. The greatest challenge for persons with mental impairments may be the decision to disclose a mental health impairment to a potential employer. On the one hand, disclosure can provide protection under the law; on the other hand, many psychosocial disabilities are invisible or just considered eccentric behaviors, making disclosure of mental impairment a matter of individual choice. The decision to report a mental impairment can be difficult because of the stigma associated with mental health problems:

The stigma associated with mental illness often results in attitudinal barriers that hinder a person's ability to work or enjoy life. Concerns by employers regarding productivity, safety, insurance, ability, attendance, and acceptance by co-workers and customers have been identified as common barriers that frequently result in the exclusion of persons who have sought mental health care from the work force. (National Mental Health Association, 1990, p. 7)

A person cannot be rejected from a job because of stereotypes, stigma, myths, or fear associated with mental illness. Stigma and stereotypic expectations regarding the ability of persons with mental impairments to be suitable employees are often founded in bias and a lack of knowledge by both the public and employers (Combs & Omvig, 1986; Howard, 1975). Just as with attitudes about race, culture, and sex, assumptions and attitudes toward any minority group not only define our perceptions, but also direct our actions toward the group (Lotito & Pimental, 1990). Hartlage and Roland (1971) reported that employers viewed persons with mental health problems as less desirable employees and as having behavioral problems that lead to poor work abilities. Such negative attitudes are a serious impediment to the successful employment of many persons with psychiatric disabilities. These persons are being deprived of the opportunity to restore their mental health through engagement in productive work roles (Howard, 1975). These attitudes and perceptions are counterproductive to the intent of the ADA and are cause for action.

Persons with psychosocial disabilities can be educated to become self-advocates. Ultimately, the decision to disclose information about one's mental impairment is the employee's. Advocacy training may allow the person to disclose this information in order to assist with beneficial accommodations instead of continuing negative patterns of behavior, which might limit or prevent full participation in work roles. Personal advocacy training should begin before the need for job accommodation arises. Self-advocates are able to share concerns regarding their mental impairments with employers and suggest beneficial accommodations.

The reduction of stigma associated with mental illness will also require the education of people in the workplace and the community regarding appropriate attitudes and behaviors toward persons with mental impairments. Common strategies to use in assisting with attitude change include personnel training for managers and supervisors, advocacy training for staff and persons with mental health problems, visibility of successful employees with mental health impairments, employee counseling and consultation, and modeling of normal interactions between co-workers. Occupational therapists can provide information, encouragement, counseling, and suggestions to employers and co-workers regarding employment of persons with mental health problems. Training sessions that focus on capabilities, understanding, and acceptance of the employee with a mental impairment can help create a work environment where reasonable accommodation is understood and the employee is able to work more effectively.

Occupational therapists might use the following format for employer and co-worker training. This information could be included for self-advocacy training also.

1. Self-assessment of common myths and expectations regarding mental impairments.
2. Group discussion of self-assessment and information to dispel myths.
3. Information regarding mental impairments.
4. Discussion of the ADA regarding employment.

5. Presentation of successful employees with mental impairments either through personal testimony or audiovisual resources.
6. Identification of workers' behaviors and related reasonable accommodations needed by persons with mental impairments.
7. Protection of confidential information and civil rights during preemployment interviewing and employment.

When this general foundation is in place in co-workers, employment practices can be reviewed and accommodations designed to meet the specific individualized needs of the employee with mental impairments.

The individual qualified for a job is not required to prove that the employer's concerns regarding the influence of mental impairment on job performance are invalid. Under the ADA, a person's employability is established through assessment of his or her fitness for duty using the essential functions of a job.

Essential Job Functions

Every job in society, regardless of skill level and perceived efficacy, can be described in great detail (Lotito & Pimental, 1990). The ADA stipulates that job functions can be divided into two categories: essential and marginal. These two categories become the basis for the job description, preemployment screening, medical examination, and employment processes. The focus during these activities is on the person's abilities, not the disability. Job descriptions guide the other processes, because they provide a clear explanation of each job, its performance expectations, and its relation to other jobs.

The employer determines what needs to be done, what each job will look like, how jobs interrelate, and the employee qualifications needed in each job. The ADA mandates that hiring and employment policies not discriminate against qualified employees on the basis of their disability. These job descriptions must differentiate between essential and marginal performance requirements.

Essential job functions are work tasks that are critical, fundamental, indispensable, required, and necessary. A person who, through reasonable accommodation, can demonstrate the ability to perform essential job functions is considered to be qualified for the job. *Marginal job functions* are work tasks that are nonessential, peripheral, extra, or incidental; they cannot be used to disqualify an otherwise qualified person with mental health impairment. All marginal job functions require reasonable accommodation. The following is an example of mental impairment that requires accommodation of marginal, not essential, job functions:

A worker with a history of depression is employed as a cashier in a fast-food restaurant. Essential job functions include taking accurate orders, handling money, and providing change to customers with accuracy and in a timely manner. Marginal functions included smiling at each customer and making positive, energetic statements to customers when greeting them. The worker found that after 2 hr at the counter, he was unable to maintain accuracy and speed in the essential job functions as well as fulfill the marginal job functions. The worker's self-esteem was affected, and he consulted with an occupational therapist. The therapist recognized this situation as contributing to low self-efficacy and discussed with the worker how to adapt the situation. Following a supervisory session between the worker and supervisor, reasonable accommodations were made by scheduling the worker for $1/2$ hr at the counter followed by 45 min of cleanup duties, a break, and then a repeat of that schedule. The worker was coached by the therapist to alert the supervisor to fatigue and to an increase in his negative thoughts that might precede a potential negative interaction with a customer. The supervisor also provided the worker with verbal praise at $1/2$-hr intervals throughout the work shift.

The accommodations in the case above qualify as reasonable accommodations under the ADA.

Occupational therapists are familiar with job analysis in work settings that have physical, emotional, cognitive, or social requirements. A job analysis is unique to each work environment and job description. Occupational therapists can use their skills in job analysis to assist employers with defining job descriptions and potential reasonable accommodations. An important task will be defining essential job functions related to emotional and psychosocial performance and differentiating the essential ones from the marginal. in the process of developing job descriptions, therapists can identify attitudes needing to be changed.

In the following situation, Bowman (1991) demonstrated that mental or emotional health can be identified as an essential job function.

> An occupational therapy position is available in a psychiatric treatment program that is behaviorally oriented. The therapist working in the program is expected to model appropriate social behavior. A new therapist is hired who has an emotional problem resulting in her exhibiting irrational, inappropriate social behavior when she is in stressful situations. The occupational therapist is terminated and files suit against the manager and facility for discrimination. The evidence used to determine if the [therapist] has been discriminated against is the job description. If the job description did not include "modeling appropriate social behavior" as an essential job function, the manager could not claim it was essential. Unwritten assumptions about what a job requires no longer apply. The performance skills required must be outlined in the job description, which must be shown to the applicant. (p. 2)

In this situation, two critical parts were present that are necessary under the ADA. First, the modeling of appropriate social behavior was defined as an essential function in the job description for this position, and, second, there was no suitable, reasonable accommodation that could substitute for this essential job requirement.

Reasonable Accommodation

There is pressing need for widespread education regarding reasonable accommodations within the mental health field (Mancuso, 1990). Reasonable accommodations reduce the gap between a worker's capabilities and job demands. In planning for employment, one must examine both elements. Occupational therapists can assist both the employee and employer with this planning, as demonstrated below:

> A computer programmer with a mental disability and related problems with fatigue was seen by an occupational therapist during outpatient sessions. Assessment revealed that the fatigue increased in relation to the amount of stress associated with programming responsibilities and with the client's sleeping patterns. Recently, she had been working overtime for 2 weeks to solve problems in a new inventory system. She reported that the increased hours disrupted her normal sleep cycle and that previously discussed adaptations were not helping. An adaptation was planned to prevent this fatigue.
>
> She requested from her supervisor 3 days of sick leave to work with her physician and to get the necessary rest to get back into a normal awake-sleep cycle. She informed the supervisor of the employer's policy for employees to use paid sick time to see their physician. The supervisor agreed to her sick leave. The supervisor will use two other programmers to solve any computer problems that occur during the client's 3-day absence. Upon her return, both parties agreed to discuss other job accommodations to prevent this level of fatigue from occurring in the future.

A person is qualified for accommodation whether the disability is a condition that exists prior to employment or develops during employment, as indicated in the following example:

> An employee recovering from alcohol dependence (i.e., he has not had a drink for $1^1/2$ months) has been a sales and delivery person for 3 years with a company that sells and distributes snack products. Of the 100 customers in the employee's sales territory, 7 are liquor stores or taverns that the employee used to frequent. He reported to his occupational therapist how stressful it was to continue to serve these accounts.
>
> The employee was a participant in an employer-sponsored alcohol rehabilitation program. The employer wanted the employee to return to work as soon as possible and asked for a planning meeting. The occupational therapist from the rehabilitation program was asked to assist in the

decision-making process, and the problems with the assigned territory were discussed. A reasonable accommodation involved transferring these accounts to another salesperson in a nearby territory. In exchange, this employee would service appropriate accounts from the nearby territory. Thus, the employee was able to return to work sooner than expected, and the employer was able to continue business.

Accommodation must also reflect limitations that are static or changing. For example, job accommodation for people with personality disorder behaviors may need to be implemented only once and are predictable, whereas for people with bipolar disorders, accommodation may need to vary depending on the current behavior pattern.

Reasonable accommodation may include (a) making existing employment facilities accessible to and usable by persons with disabilities; (b) job restructuring; (c) part-time or modified work schedules; (d) reassignment to a vacant position; (e) acquisition or modification of equipment or devices; (f) appropriate adjustment or modification of examinations, training materials, or policies; and (g) provision of qualified readers or interpreters and other similar accommodations for persons with disabilities [ADA, Title I, § 101.9.(A)]. Reasonable accommodation for persons with mental disabilities might include the following:

- Part-time or flexible work schedules to allow for medical appointments.
- Provision of unpaid leave days.
- Re-delegating assignments.
- Exchanging assignments with another employee.
- Reassignment to a vacant position if this would prevent the employee from being unemployed or the employer from losing a valuable employee. (National Mental Health Association, 1990, p. 13)

Under the ADA, reasonable accommodation is expected of the employer; it is usual or typical and not an exception, as seen in the following situation.

A job is open for a purchasing clerk in a large, open work space that has 16 purchasing clerks. A person with an anxiety disorder is able to meet all the essential job functions for the clerk position except that she has difficulty concentrating on multiple tasks. The occupational therapist reviewed the situation and made suggestions.

Reasonable accommodations included placing the employee's desk within a three-sided portable wall system to decrease general office distractions and developing an in-out work basket system outside this immediate work area to decrease interruptions. Follow-up by the occupational therapist indicated that these accommodations supported satisfactory work behaviors.

These two accommodations are not exceptional because they are also appropriate for a nondisabled employee with poor concentration on the job (e.g., the office socializer). Implied is the fact that persons with disabilities cannot be disqualified because of their inability to perform nonessential, or marginal, functions of the job and that reasonable accommodation be made to help such persons meet legitimate criteria (National Mental Health Association, 1990). As of July 1, 1992, employers will have to defend discrimination charges related to their standards, selection criteria, tests, and refusal to accommodate in employment-related decisions (ADA, Title I, § 107).

According to the ADA, employers who interview a potential employee or consider an employee's continued employment are not allowed to focus on what a person cannot do or on the diagnosis itself. They must focus instead on essential job functions and the capability of the person in question to perform the job tasks. An occupational therapist could assist the employer in making plans to address potential problems, such as in the following scenario:

A certified public accountant for a medium-sized business, whose condition is diagnosed as bipolar affective disorder, appears agitated at tax time and highly sensitive to the supervisor's questions about the time line for submitting tax documents. Instead of confronting the worker and requesting immediate documentation, the employer along with the occupational therapist could plan a reasonable accommodation that would entail asking the worker to meet the supervisor the next day with a time line and to be prepared to identify the need for additional help or personnel. Additionally, at the meeting, the supervisor could offer the employee support for his diligent efforts. The supervisor could also encourage the employee to take time to see a physician to make sure his medications are conducive to his work responsibilities. These actions demonstrate positive regard for the employee's work and facilitate the employee's performance and self-efficacy beliefs.

Occupational therapists can help the employer and employee identify desired work behaviors and plan reasonable accommodations to facilitate essential work behaviors. Psychiatric disabilities present functional limitations that recur and require adaptation during employment. Mancuso (1990) identified these limitations as (a) duration of concentration, (b) screening out environmental stimuli, (c) maintaining stamina throughout the workday, (d) managing time pressures and deadlines, (e) initiating interpersonal contact, (f) focusing on multiple tasks simultaneously, (g) responding to negative feedback, and (h) physical and emotional side effects of psychotropic medications. (See the Appendix of this chapter for an expanded list and reasonable accommodations for work-related behaviors associated with mental impairment.) This list may be useful for employers who, in good faith, want to employ persons with mental impairments, for occupational therapists who will oversee the work site, and for persons with mental health problems to identify potentially beneficial accommodations that allow them to successfully engage in work.) The selection of accommodation must reflect the person's functional abilities, his or her self-efficacy, and the work environment. For example, if a person cannot do word processing for more than 90 min, then the accommodation may be to require a 10-min break every 90 min, and the software package itself could notify the employee when it is time for a break.

Not providing reasonable accommodations to a qualified person with a disability is prohibited discrimination, unless the change would be unreasonably burdensome. The legal term for this employer burden is *undue hardship*. Undue hardship is an action requiring significant difficulty or expense when considered in light of the nature and cost of the accommodation needed and the overall operational, financial, and personnel resources of the facility. Accommodation is required unless it creates a significant difficulty or expense. Employers must provide evidence to support their undue hardship decisions when denying employment to a qualified individual with a mental impairment. If there is more than one way for an employer to provide accommodation, he or she may choose the easiest one to implement or the least expensive. The following example describes a potential undue hardship.

An aging day-care worker has shown signs of cognitive deterioration, forgetfulness, and shortened concentration. The day-care center meets the strict state-mandated standards for number of personnel assigned to care for the various age groups. The employee continues to be a warm, gentle person who wants to maintain her full-time job and denies any cognitive problems. Because she has developed such a good, long-standing relationship with the children and their parents, the supervisor consulted with an occupational therapist and decided to add part-time workers to assist the day-care worker in her assigned room.

The agency suffered a significant financial loss due to the increased personnel costs of providing for the safety of the children and the worker. During the consultation, the supervisor said that this increased financial outlay could not be continued. The worker was aware of the change in her abilities and agreed to resign her position. Knowing that the worker enjoys children the therapist helped her find a church-based nursery to volunteer her services.

In this case, the employer could claim undue hardship as long as access to adequate financial resources to cover the financial loss were not available. For example, a small, privately owned day-care center could claim undue hardship, whereas a facility owned by a large corporate entity would need to prove undue hardship based on total corporate assets.

Two related important factors influence decisions regarding reasonable accommodation for persons with mental impairment under this law—direct threat and fitness for duty. If direct threat or fitness for duty are used in employment decisions, either must be shown to be job related and consistent with business necessity. Mental illness is hard to define, and the stability of an emotionally disturbed person is difficult to assess and predict (Strasser, 1991). Strasser said that not only should a person be able to perform a job, but the person should perform it safely and, in doing so, not endanger himself or herself, his or her co-workers, or society.

Essential job functions regarding safety should be included in the job description, and occupational therapists, physicians, and job interviewers should be instructed to assess for this ability. According to Section 103 of Title 1, employers may write and screen for job qualifications that exclude persons with mental health conditions from consideration if they pose a significant safety risk for other employees (Verville, 1990). A person with a history of aggressive, violent behavior in the work environment, for example, could be excluded from jobs where the behavior could create an unsafe working environment. The following example reviews such an instance:

A slaughterer from a local meat-packing company was hospitalized because he had been swinging meat cleavers at fellow workers, saying he was going to kill them. Clearly, this behavior is life threatening. The employer with a carefully constructed job description could justify excluding this person from this job and show that the company was not violating the employee's civil rights by not providing reasonable accommodation. The occupational therapist could inform the worker and employer of their rights and return-to-work expectations.

Direct threat is defined in the law as a significant risk to health or safety of others that cannot be eliminated by reasonable accommodation. Direct threat can be used as a qualification standard when screening a person for a specific job. Regarding mental illness, this section of the law ensures that decisions pertaining to a person's qualifications for a job are based on current, objective evaluation rather than on misconceptions and stereotypes (National Mental Health Association, 1990). To disqualify a person for a job, an employer must obtain objective evidence that an applicant or employee has recently made threats that threatened injury or has committed overt, threatening, or harmful acts. The specific risk and behavior posed by the disability must be identified. The perceived threat of harmful actions in the future is not a factor. The following case exemplifies the direct-threat issue.

In the process of interviewing a person for hire as a bank clerk, the manager discovered that the applicant had been treated for cocaine addiction 2 years earlier. The applicant openly talked about his recovery and his current involvement in support groups. The manager's previous experience with cocaine addicts was negative and assumed that this employee could not be trusted with cash, would try to steal money for cocaine, or might have cocaine-addicted friends who would use the applicant to rob the bank in the future. The employer is considering not hiring him to work at the bank.

In the above example, the employer would be in conflict with the ADA, because these conclusions had no objective basis or no current behavioral indicators related to this employee's ability to perform the essential job functions; they were based on misconceptions or stereotypes. An occupational therapist who offered seminars for employers regarding cocaine addiction and rehabilitation could increase this employer's understanding and maybe his acceptance of addiction.

A second qualification standard related to direct threat is fitness for duty, which also requires individualized, objective assessment. In the ADA, *fitness for duty* is defined as the degree of risk justifying disqualification that demonstrates reasonable probability of serious or substantial harm. The likelihood, seriousness, and imminence of injury are factors that one would consider in determining the legality of exclusion. The recurrence of a clinical condition could be used to estimate this standard for each person in a specific job. Both individual factors and job-related factors should be considered (Maffeo, 1990). Additionally, established scientific bases for determining risk may contribute to fitness-for-duty decisions. For example, Maffeo (1990) stated that an employer who is concerned about an applicant who has threatened suicide in the past must assess (a) both the applicant and the requirements of the job, with attention to the applicant's current and past mental health problems; (b) the published data on suicide risk, general nature, and specific hazards in the target job; and (c) adequacy of the applicant's performance at previous jobs. The final decision must be based on information from objective data about known risk factors and possible accommodations to permit essential and marginal job functions.

Employers are reminded that concerns regarding direct threat and fitness for duty cannot circumvent the prohibition against preemployment inquiries into a person's disability (ADA, 1990). This includes generalized requests or inquiries related to medical records, mental health history, or mental disability under the guise of wanting to ascertain the possibility of direct threat posed by the applicant. Instead, employers must focus on the ability of the applicant or employee to perform the essential functions of a job with or without reasonable accommodation.

Access to Employee Functions

Employees with mental health disabilities are entitled to attend any function provided to any other employee. Any public accommodation or service provided to other employees must be accessible to them as well. Employees cannot be excluded from annual office re-

treats, use of the corporate condominium, or business trips, as shown in the example below:

> The company holiday party for employees and their families has been announced and the personnel department is taking reservations. An employee who has a 14-year-old daughter with mental disabilities made her reservation. Personnel is aware that this daughter has been known to be loud and distracting in her speech, and they are concerned about her behavior being disruptive and inappropriate in the restaurant's elegant setting. The company is considering asking this employee not to bring her daughter.

Under ADA protection, the company cannot make such a request. The employee's right to equal access for her family to join in the employer's holiday party is protected by Title III.

Employers must ensure that employees have access to employment-related activities that may occur off the job site. For example, a business with a total staff of 75 employees offers supported employment for 12 mentally retarded persons. A bowling league is being set up for interested employees, and 7 of the supported employees wish to join the bowling league. Under the ADA, it is discriminatory not to offer the persons with mental disabilities access to the integrated bowling league.

Clearly, Titles I and III work in concert with each other when addressing access to employment-related activities, whether these activities are at the work site or are related to employer-sponsored activities.

Implications for Occupational Therapy

The focus on employment and reasonable accommodations for clients with mental disabilities focuses more on abstract psychosocial components of employment, including interpersonal behaviors and personal beliefs, and less on assistive technology. Occupational therapists can help persons with mental disabilities become a part of the work force by doing the following:

- Providing attitude and advocacy training for persons with disabilities as well as for employers and co-workers.
- Preparing persons with mental impairments to be successful employees through training programs to promote self-efficacy as a worker.
- Collaborating with employers who want to employ persons with mental impairments by helping them to identify the essential functions of jobs and determine reasonable accommodations for persons with mental disabilities.

If employment is a goal of any mental health rehabilitation program, then occupational therapists should plan meaningful treatment activities that simulate work and provide opportunity to acquire self-efficacy as a worker. Bandura's (1977, 1982) model, which is consistent with occupational therapy philosophy, provides a mechanism for returning clients to work roles. This model also has implications for keeping persons with mental impairments on the job. Thus, the self-efficacy model provides a mechanism to ensure successful employability within the guidelines of the ADA.

Occupational therapists in mental health will see numerous related roles emerge as the ADA is implemented, including those of advocate, educator, designer, provider of reasonable accommodations, and, perhaps, liaison between employers and employees with disabilities. We hope that implementing the suggestions made in this paper will direct ADA-related decisions about those with mental disabilities toward access and participation in life roles, especially the most meaningful role—that of worker—for persons with mental impairments (Gonzalez & Gordon, 1990). Occupational therapists can facilitate the process of integrating Americans with mental disabilities into the mainstream of life and be instrumental in providing leadership to assist in the full implementation of this new civil rights legislation. As agents of both personal and environmental change, we as occupational therapists can demonstrate application of our knowledge in a timely way to help persons with mental disabilities attain their employment rights and support this declaration of independence.

References

Americans With Disabilities Act of 1990 (Public Law 101–336), 42 U.S.C. § 12101.

Anthony W. A., & Blanch, A. (1987). Supported employment for persons who are psychiatrically disabled: An historical and conceptual perspective. *Psychosocial Rehabilitation, 11* (2), 5-23.

Bandura, A. (1977). Self-efficacy: Toward a unifying theory of behavioral change. *Psychological Review, 84,* 191-215.

Bandura, A. (1982). Self-efficacy mechanism in human agency. *American Psychologist, 37,* 122-147.

Bandura, A. (1986). Fearful expectations and avoidance actions as coeffects of perceived self-efficacy. *American Psychologist, 41,* 1389-1391.

Bowman, O. J. (1991, September). Managers to play an important role in implementing the Americans With Disabilities Act. *Administration and Management Special Interest Section Newsletter,* pp. 1-2.

Christiansen, C. (1991). Occupational therapy: Intervention for life performance. In C. Christiansen & C. Baum (Eds.), *Occupational therapy: Overcoming human performance deficits* (pp. 2-43). Thorofare, NJ: Slack.

Combs, I. H., & Omvig, C. P. (1986). Accommodation of disabled people into employment: Perceptions of employers. *Journal of Rehabilitation, 52,* 42-45.

Gonzalez, E. G., & Gordon, D. M. (1990). Americans With Disabilities Act: The crumbling of another wall. *Archives of Physical Medicine and Rehabilitation, 71,* 951.

Hartlage, L., & Roland, P. (1971). Attitudes of employers toward different types of handicapped workers. *Journal of Applied Rehabilitation Counseling, 2,* 115-120.

Howard, G. (1975). The ex-mental patient as an employee: An on-the-job evaluation. *American Journal of Orthopsychiatry, 45,* 479-483.

Lotito, M. J., & Pimental, R. (1990). *The American With Disabilities Act: Making the ADA work for you.* Northridge, CA: Milt Wright.

Maffeo, P. A. (1990). Making non-discriminatory fitness-for-duty decisions about persons with disabilities under the Rehabilitation Act and the Americans With Disabilities Act. *American Journal of Law and Medicine, 14,* 279-326.

Mancuso, L. L. (1990). Reasonable accommodation for workers with psychiatric disabilities. *Psychosocial Rehabilitation Journal, 14,* 3-19.

National Mental Health Association. (1990). *ADA. Americans With Disabilities Act of 1990 (Public Law 101-336): Legislative summary series.* Alexandria, VA: Author.

Rhodes, L. E., Ramsing, K. D., & Bellamy, G. T. (1988). Business participation in supported employment. In G. T. Bellamy, L. E. Rhodes, D. M. Mank, & J. M. Albin (Eds.), *Supported employment: A community implementation guide* (pp. 247-261). Baltimore: Brookes.

Staff. (1990, July-August). Americans With Disabilities Act signing: "Declaration of Independence" for 43 million. *Quality of Care,* pp. 8-9.

Strasser, A.L. (1991). Americans With Disabilities Act raises ethical considerations for physicians. *Occupational Health and Safety, 60* (2), 26.

Townsend, B. (1991). Nationally Speaking—Beyond our clinics: A vision for the future. *American Journal of Occupational Therapy, 45,* 871-873.

Verville, R. E. (1990). The Americans With Disabilities Act: An analysis. *Archives of Physical Medicine and Rehabilitation, 71,* 1010-1013.

Watson, P. G. (1990). The Americans With Disabilities Act: More rights for people with disabilities. *Rehabilitation Nursing, 15,* 325-328.

[a] These headings are adopted from Mancuso (1990).

Appendix
Reasonable Accommodations for Recurrent Functional Problems Among Persons With Psychiatric Disorders

Personal self-efficacy

Reinforce or coach appropriate behaviors.
Test for job skills on the job and avoid self-report of abilities.
Place in job where there is a model to follow or imitate.
Teach self-advocacy skills.
Provide successful job experiences. Use positive feedback.
Begin with close supervision and then cut back slowly as skills are maintained.
Maintain similarity or consistency in work tasks.
Encourage positive self-talk and eliminate negative self-talk.

Duration of concentration [a]

Put each work request in writing and leave in "to do" box to avoid interruptions.
Provide ongoing consultation, mediation, problem solving and conflict resolution.
Provide good working conditions, such as adequate light, smoke-free environment, and reduced noise.
Provide directive commands on a regular basis.

Screening out environmental stimuli [a]

Place in a separate office.
Provide opaque room dividers between workstations.
Allow person to work after hours or when others are not around.
Ensure that workstation facilitates work production and organization.

Maintaining stamina throughout the workday [a]

Provide additional breaks or shortened workday.
Allow an extended day to allow for breaks or rest periods.
Avoid work during lunch, such as answering the phone; buy an answering machine instead.
Distribute tasks throughout the day according to energy level.
Job share with another employee.
Develop work simplification techniques, such as collect all copying to be done at one time or use a wheeled cart to move supplies.
Have a liberal leave policy for health problems, flexible hours, and back-up coverage.
Individualize work agreements.
Verify employees' efficacy regarding their ability to sustain effort or persist with a task.
Teach on-the-job relaxation and stress reduction techniques.

Managing time pressure and deadlines [a]

Maintain structure through a daily time and task schedule using hourly goals.
Provide positive reinforcement when tasks are completed within the expected time lines.
Arrange a separate work area to reduce noise and interruptions.
Screen out unnecessary business.

Initiating interpersonal contact [a]

Purposely plan orientation to meet and work alongside co-workers.
Allow sufficient time to make good, unhurried contacts.
Make contacts during work, break, and even lunch times, adjusting the conversation to the situation.
When standing, instead of facing each other, try standing at a 90° angle to each other.
Allow the person to work at home.
Have an advocate to advise and support the person.

Communicate honestly.
Plan supervision times and maintain them.
Develop tolerance for and helpful responses to unusual behaviors.
Provide awareness and advocacy training for all workers.

Focusing on multiple tasks simultaneously [a]

Eliminate the number of simultaneous tasks.
Redistribute tasks among employees with the same responsibilities, so each can do more of one type of job task than a lot of different tasks.
Establish priorities for task completion.
Arrange for all work tasks to be put in writing with due dates or times.

Responding to negative feedback [a]

Have employee prepare own work appraisal to compare with supervisor's.
Work together to establish methods employee can use to change negative behavior.
Provide positive reinforcement for observed behavioral change.
Provide on-site crisis intervention and counseling services to develop self-esteem, provide emotional support, and promote comfort with accommodations.
Establish guidelines for feedback.

Symptoms secondary to prescribed psychotropic medications [a]

Provide release time to see psychiatrist or primary physician.
Encourage employee to work with physician to establish a time schedule to take medications that are conducive to work responsibilities.
Provide release time or changes in job tasks that match condition.

[a] From: Mancuso (1990)

Chapter 23

Building Inclusive Community: A Challenge for Occupational Therapy

1994 Eleanor Clarke Slagle Lecture

Ann P. Grady, MA, OTR, FAOTA

This chapter was previously published in the *American Journal of Occupational Therapy, 49*, 300–310. Copyright © 1995, American Occupational Therapy Association.

Preparation of the Eleanor Clarke Slagle Lecture promotes reflection on the values and philosophy of occupational therapy. I chose the topic *Building Inclusive Community: A Challenge for Occupational Therapy* because it provided me with an opportunity to explore my own values and the values of the profession regarding inclusion of all persons into the community they choose and into the world community at large. The topic particularly led me to review my own work in adaptation theory developed with Elnora Gilfoyle (Gilfoyle, Grady, & Moore, 1990) In light of changes occurring or being promoted in society regarding opportunities for inclusion of all persons in all aspects of living.

Ideas about inclusion; the meaning of community; the relationship between environment and community; the interaction between a person's past experience, present situation, and future hopes and dreams and its effect on the relationship that develops between an occupational therapist and a person seeking therapy services all became focal points for exploring our role in building inclusive community. The result has been some expansion of our understanding of the environment category of the spatiotemporal adaptation theory and exploration of the relationship between environment and community. In addition, exploring the concepts of the theory led to consideration of its relevance for enhancing our ability to plan with consumers of service who are creating or returning to their own community. Focal points for exploring the challenges related to building inclusive community, include

- An understanding of the meaning of community building within a person's own environment and according to his or her choices.
- A review of current ideas about the nature of disability in relation to both philosophy and mandates for inclusion.
- An expansion of ideas about the role of environment in a person's adaptation to community living.
- A consideration of strategies for promoting choice and inclusion.

For as far back in time as we know, human beings have gathered together to share—in daily living and use some form of symbols as means for communicating with each other, hence the building of community (Dance & Larson, 1972). To this day, we share meaning in our communities through symbols composed of pictures, words spoken in our own culturally determined language, and gestures or nonverbal expressions of our thoughts or feelings. Native Americans in the southwestern regions of our country choose to tell the stories of their community living and beliefs through petroglyphs, or rock art (Patterson–Rudolph, 1993). One expert in petroglyphs compared attempts at identifying subject matter and its significance to cloud watching in that no two people will interpret what they see in the same way. Petroglyphs were apparently not intended to represent words of a language as we know it, but instead were meant to convey more general concepts or global ideas about the society, such as ideas about religion, medicine, governance, art, war, and peace. An artist's rendition of petroglyphs titled "Circle of Friends" (see Figure 1) is chosen to represent ideas about community and inclusion that are central to the themes of this article. In rock art, spirals, concentric circles, and other geometric shapes are interpreted to be universal symbols used to convey conceptual ideas (Patterson, 1992). There are dozens of possible interpretations connected to each figure in the circle because rock art is interpreted not only according to the individual symbols present, but also by the figures that are combined in a panel, just like words in spoken language. For me, the Circle of Friends represents the encompassing nature of a community whether it is the community that each of us constructs for ourselves or the

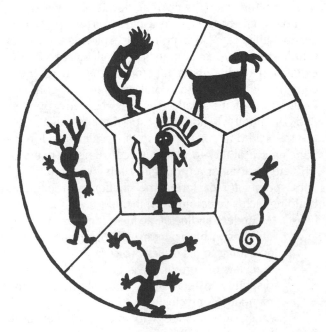

Figure 1. Circle of Friends petroglyph. Original metal sculpute by Kevin Smith, Golden, Colorado. Appears with permission of Kevin Smith.

larger environment in which we discover ourselves. The circle represents the wholeness of a community, and the figures relate to diversity that can exist within the community. Just as the circle is considered a symbol of inclusion and wholeness, the extension of the circle as a spiral is well known as a symbol of growth and continuity. Spirals frequently appear as symbols of continuity in Native American culture (Patterson, 1992). The spiral reflects evolution and renewal with growth emanating from continuous learning and new challenges. The spiral and its embedded circles will be used in this article to represent change and continuity.

Why is the idea of building inclusive community important to us as people and as occupational therapists? The idea is both profound and simple. Simply, we believe that people belong together regardless of real or perceived differences. All persons have the right to choose where they wish to live, work, learn, and play and with whom they wish to spend time. On a deeper level, we believe that people belong together *because* of differences. There is a richness that characterizes a community constructed with appreciation for both differences and similarities among its members. The idea is not new, but as Winston Churchill said, "Men [and women] stumble over the truth from time to time, but most pick themselves up and hurry off as if nothing had happened" (McWilliams, 1994, p. 413).

The Nature of Community and Choice

Community provides a context for actualizing individual potential and experiencing oneness with others (McLaughlin & Davidson, 1985). The human condition yearns for a greater sense of connectedness, expressed as a need to reach out, deeply touch others, and throw off the pain and loneliness of separation. The term *community* encompasses *communication* and *unity*. Yankelovitch said that the community evokes in the individual the feeling that "here is where I belong—these are my people, I care for them, they care for me, I am part of them, I know what they expect from me and I from them, they share my concerns. I know this place, I am on familiar ground, I am at home" (1981, p. 224).

There are established communities such as towns, neighborhoods, schools, and workplaces, and there are personal communities we create for ourselves, which include family, friends, acquaintances, how and where we spend our time formally or informally, and the relationships we build over time. Our personal communities do not necessarily depend on specific location or specific time, although they are often embedded in established communities. Building inclusive community refers to both the larger, more formal community context and the smaller, informal community that a person identifies as a personal community. Ideas about diversity and inclusion in community in this article apply to all people, but we as occupational therapists have particular concerns for assuring choice in community living for persons with disabilities and chronic health problems, as well as persons for whom disability and health issues can be prevented.

Personal community building begins at the center of the circle, where the person is embedded in family and close relationships (see Figure 2). Networks of informal support develop in the center of a personal community. Relationships grow because persons choose to be connected. The unique culture of personal community is created from family experience. Values are established; heritage, myths, and traditions are communicated. The foundation for building personal community is established within the family.

> We all come from families. Families are big, small, extended, nuclear, multigenerational, with one parent. two parents, and grandparents. We live under one roof or many. A family can be as temporary as a few weeks, as permanent as forever. We become part of a family by birth, adoption, marriage, or from a desire for mutual support. Families are dynamic and are cultures unto themselves, with different values and unique ways of realizing dreams. Our families create neighborhoods, communities, states, and nations. (Shelton & Stepanek 1994, p. 6)

For both children and adults, family provides a personal culture of embeddedness. Each person creates a community of family culture in the broadest sense of the concept of community. Like all cultures, each culture we create within our community is based on our values and may differ substantially from another's uniquely consummated community. However the family is constituted, whether we judge it adequate or not according to our value system, a person is embedded in his or her family and that is our starting place for inclusion. A *challenge for occupational therapy practitioners is understanding each person's unique community, including its culture and the context in which it was formed.*

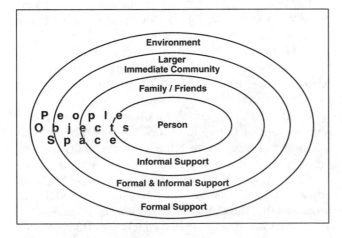

Figure 2. Personal community building.

The concept of community is broadened to include relations with acquaintances, coworkers, and schoolmates as well as locations like neighborhoods, workplace, and town. The community circle includes both formal and informal sources of support. The environment provides the context in which communities are formed. It is composed of persons, objects, and space—all of which can be combined for personal or formal community building. The environment generally provides formal support to persons in community. Community is not a static structure in the environment, but an ongoing process of interaction among persons, objects, and space. Community provides familiarity with daily interactions that reduces the uncertainty experienced in new and challenging situations and creates a sense of belonging.

A sense of belonging in a community provides the comfort and security needed to explore and use one's gifts. According to Maslow's hierarchy, belonging is an important component in the development of self-esteem. Building blocks to self-esteem include a sense of safety in one's immediate community, a sense of self-acceptance, identity, affiliation with others and a sense of competence and mission. In some instances, we seem to expect children and adults with disabilities to demonstrate a sense of self-esteem before they can be included in a typical classroom or work or living environment. forgetting that belonging to a typical community is the means by which a person develops a sense of self (Kunc, 1994). *One of the challenges we often face is resolution of the conflict we have over the need for persons with disabilities to prove themselves capable before they are included in typical communities of their choice rather than creating opportunities for them to develop their capacities in their community with appropriate supports.*

Choice is a valued dimension of our community life. Choice means having alternatives from which to make a selection. As occupational therapists, we recognize the importance of choice in every person's pursuit of self-actualization, particularly as he or she fulfills occupational roles of daily living, work, school, and play and leisure. Choice in occupational therapy has traditionally meant that the person seeking services takes an active part in planning and carrying out a therapy program. Yerxa (1966) maintained that one of the most important roles an occupational therapist plays is providing choice in selection of therapeutic activities, interaction with the activities and, most important, establishment of objectives for a therapy program. Exercising choice in a therapeutic environment provides opportunities to explore capabilities and options for life outside the therapy setting. Making choices is another way of exploring personal values about daily living, relationships, roles, and the physical, psychological, social, and spiritual communities in which living needs to occur to pursue self-actualization. Making choices in therapy is only a prelude to the choices people need to make regarding their life in the community. How will I make a living?

Where will I live? Where will my child go to school? What supports will I need to live fully in the community of my choice? A *challenge for occupational therapy, practitioners is fostering choice that reflects their consumer's priorities for living and accomplishing occupational tasks, even if there are differences between them regarding values or perceptions of expertise.* Schön (1983) wrote that the interactive practitioner realizes that he or she is not the only one in the situation to have relevant and important knowledge. The consumer interacts by joining with a service provider to make sense of the situation and, by doing so, gains a sense of increased involvement and action—or choice.

Being part of a community provides opportunities for lifelong development. Persons with disabilities and their family members have a right to pursue and participate in all levels of their community, whether it is one they have known well or one they wish to build to accommodate new circumstances and fulfill new or old dreams. Each person creates a community of his or her own culture in the broadest sense of the concept. Like all cultures, each culture we create within our community is based in our values and may differ substantially from another's uniquely consummated community. Creating community opens doors to new cultural vistas with opportunities to cooperate with each other and participate in community activities. Inclusion in an community also means an end to loneliness and helplessness and the beginning of empowerment to fulfill dreams (McLaughlin & Davidson, 1985). Building inclusive communities with all persons provides opportunities for members of the community to experience different relationships. Each of us has the capacity for creating inclusive community through our work with individuals as well as our ability to influence society and its established institutions.

The Nature of Disability and Inclusion

A new sociopolitical environment is developing in which persons with disabilities are taking or creating social and political actions on their own behalf. Changing perceptions of disability and the histories of the civil rights movement in the 1960s and the women's rights movement in the 1970s resulted in substantial legislative action for disability rights. In his book *No Pity,* Shapiro (1993) chronicled the course of the disability rights movement in the United States. Shapiro stated that persons with disabilities insist simply on common respect and the opportunity to build bonds to their community as fully accepted participants in everyday life. In the past, disability was usually viewed as a medical problem with the expectation that, to be accepted, persons with disabilities needed to be as much like persons without disabilities as possible without regard for their own uniqueness. Now, persons with disabilities are thinking differently about themselves. Many no longer think of their physical or mental differences as a

source of shame or something to overcome in order to be like others or inspire others. In *Flying Without Wings,* Beisser, who contracted polio as an adult, said "When I stopped struggling, working to change, and found means of accepting what I had already become, I discovered that changed me. Rather than feeling disabled and inadequate, I felt whole again" (1989, p. 169). Beisser views disability as a difference among people. Considering disability as a difference is in itself neutral and changes the way persons with disabilities view themselves and are viewed by others. For example, in the village of Chilmark on Martha's Vineyard Island in Massachusetts, more than half the residents in the 1800s were genetically deaf (Groce, 1985). All the people in the village were fluent in sign language. It has been reported that spoken and sign language were used simultaneously or, if a person who was deaf joined a speaking group, group members immediately started to use sign as well as speech. Deafness was not a disability in Chilmark. Disability is a dimension of diversity not unlike ethnic background, color, religious, or gender differences (Shapiro, 1993). Differences do not necessarily equal limitations, but rather create opportunities for meaningful interaction (J. Snow, personal communication, 1994) as long as people are living together naturally.

Just as perceptions of disability are changing, so are the reasons that disability was so often seen as a limitation. The difference within the person is no longer viewed as the main problem; instead, the environment that cannot accommodate the person is considered responsible for society's failure to include persons with disabilities in the mainstream. Social considerations have led to a shift from the traditional medical view of disability to an interactional model that accounts for the relationship between person and environment. Gill (1987) summarized this shift in perspective as follows:

According to the medical view, disability is considered a deficit or abnormality. In an interactional model, disability is a difference.

In the medical view, being disabled is perceived as negative. In an interactional model, being disabled is in itself neutral.

Medicine views disability as residing in the individual. In an interactional model, disability is derived from problems encountered during interaction between the individual and their environment.

In medicine, the remedy for disability-related problems is cure or normalization of the individual. In an interactional model, the remedy for disability-related problems is a change in the environmental interaction.

Finally, the medical view identifies the agent of remedy as the professional. An interactional model has proposed that the agent of remedy may be the individual, an advocate, or anyone who affects the arrangements between the individual and society.

The last interactional category in Gill's summary can have a significant effect on the roles for occupational therapists. The shift from a medical perspective to an environmental framework is not difficult for us to understand. Occupational therapists have always recognized that disability was not an illness that could be cured by medicine. *The challenge for us is to promote the interactive model for practice regardless of the venue of our practice. A concurrent challenge is to increase support for more practice venues in the community were engagement in real occupation takes place.*

Change in perception of disability has fostered the disability rights movement and legislative action. The disability rights movement has focused on the rights of persons with disabilities to be included in society according to the choices they make for themselves and their families. The rights movement could also be called an *inclusion* movement. Inclusion in community means that all persons regardless of differences participate in natural environments for living, learning, playing, working, resting, and recreating. For persons with disabilities, participation may be with specific support from others or with adaptations to the environment. According to Gill (1987), inclusion means removal of barriers to power, which results in a greater number of alternatives or choices.

Shapiro (1993) identified the 1960s as the beginning of the disability independent living movement started by Ed Roberts and other students at the University of California–Berkeley. The movement spread to include action in Washington, DC, that initiated funding for independent living. Groups of parents of children with disabilities began to form around the country at about the same time, primarily to provide support to other parents in the same situations. The groups were often connected to existing organizations like United Cerebral Palsy or the Easter Seal Society. Later, parent organizations would emerge as independent, social change groups.

The 1970s saw adoption of Section 504 of the Rehabilitation Act (Public Law 93–112) prohibiting discrimination on the basis of disability. But Section 504 was not implemented for nearly 5 years after its adoption and was implemented only after a group led by Roberts and others staged a sit-in at Department of Health, Education and Welfare office in San Francisco. Besides succeeding in obtaining regulations for Section 504, the event in San Francisco created an awareness that linked groups of adults around the country in a civil rights movement. Also in the 1970s, Public Law 94–142 was adopted as the Education for All Handicapped Children Act (1975), mandating public education in the least restrictive environment for children with disabilities who were 5 years of age and older.

In the 1980s, support was provided for that act through the establishment of statewide parent information and advocacy centers in every state. The legislation was expanded to include infants and toddlers with passage of the Education of the Handicapped Act Amendments of 1986 (Public Law 99–457). With this expanded legislation for education came the components of family-centered care, or respect for a family's central role as decision maker for a child, or support for an adult, which is now considered best practice across the life span. Public Law 94–142 and Public Law 99–457 were combined and expanded in reauthorization as the Individuals With Disabilities Education Act of 1990 (IDEA) (Public Law 101–476). Meanwhile, the Technology-Related Assistance for Individuals With Disabilities Act (Public Law 100–407) (1988) began the process of changing policy and availability of assistive technology for persons with disabilities in all states. The legislative decade of the 1980s culminated with the Americans With Disabilities Act of 1990 (ADA) (Public Law 101–336). ADA encompasses ideology from all previous legislation by ensuring that the barriers to inclusion be eliminated for persons with disabilities. Although far-reaching disability rights legislation was officially adopted in the 1980s, we are still struggling with implementation of all the laws in the 1990s.

The disability rights movement and legislation has focused primarily on removing physical and legal barriers to inclusion. Legislative mandates serve the purpose of forcing inclusion. The spirit of inclusion only comes with attitude change supported by community preparation and relationship building. In a midwestern city, 9-year-old Amy, who has cerebral palsy, visited Santa Claus last year and had only one wish for Christmas-just one day in school when the kids did not tease her about her cerebral palsy. Clearly, Amy was present in school with her typical peers, and being there is a start. But she is not truly included since a community that accepts her for who she is has not been created. She needed a school community that gave her a sense of familiarity, caring, and belonging. She needed relationships that she could depend upon for support ("Disabled Girl Asks Santa," 1993). In another city, 14-year-old Kevin, who has Down's syndrome, has been with typical peers from the beginning of his school career. His inclusion has focused on preparation and relationship building that included Kevin along with the teachers and children in the building. When asked what it would be like if he was not included in typical school, he replied that he'd feel sad. "I like to be in school with my friends—I learn from them and they learn from me" (Kevin, personal communication, February 1993).

Inclusion is about relationships. Judith Snow, a consumer advocate in Canada, has said that the only real disability, is having no relationships (personal communication. January 1994). Inclusion means participation. Inclusion in school is only the prelude to inclusion in life. Participation may require support not only in the traditional sense of personal assistance and adaptations, but also in terms of preparing the persons in the community to welcome differences into their community and help develop natural support systems. A *challenge for occupation-*

al therapy is development of programs that prepare persons and their families for life in the community while working to prepare the community and persons in it to welcome the gifts of diversity. If we espouse the interactive model of disability, we can affect the arrangements between the individual and society and make unique contributions to the interactive model of change. We can assist with remediation of the person's physical or psychological problem to the extent that the manifestations of the problem can be changed. We can participate in modification of the person's environment so that it can accommodate the needs. We can assist with building community with the person or family in order to create a place for belonging that includes both the formal and informal sources of support. We can continue to promote inclusion as a value through our sociopolitical systems.

Building inclusive community sometimes requires change in value-based practices. The spiral (see Figure 3) serves as a model to illustrate that when we recognize differences in values, we may experience conflicts within ourselves or with others. If we cannot move beyond the downward spiral between values and differences, we will not be able to move beyond conflict. But if we move upward to change our perspective to one of appreciating differences, we can make a commitment to using differences in ways that productively build community. The spiral begins with a small, defined center focusing on personal values about differences. These values were established with past experience. As the spiral moves upward and widens, new experiences are included. The person uses past experience to respond to new situations. The response may be use of past behavior or of a new behavior that will modify old behaviors. For example, Bobbie wants to live alone in an apartment, but he cannot tie his shoes, button his shirt, prepare meals very well, or use the telephone to summon help. If your values about independence mean a person can only choose between doing everything alone or living in a segregated community, then Bobbie's proposal is different, causes conflict,

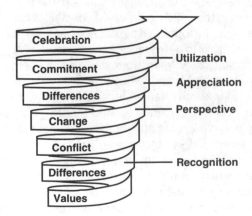

Figure 3.   Celebrating diversity: Individual and Society.

and probably elicits a negative response. If you stay in a downward spiral of conflict between values and differences, you will continue to respond negatively to full inclusion for persons who cannot perform all tasks independently. But if you take an interactive view of disability, your perspective changes. You appreciate that Bobbie's disability resides in the community that cannot accommodate his differences. A change in perspective leads to modification of old behavior by new responses. A commitment to using rather than rejecting differences creates new possibilities for removing the barriers to inclusion. *The challenge for individual occupational therapists and the profession is making a commitment to inclusion in community for all persons with disabilities and chronic health problems.* The following values are proposed for occupational therapy:

- Every person has a right to be an integrated member of a community of choice.
- Every person has a right to active participation in decision making for self and family
- Every person has a right to information and options as part of decision making.
- Every person has a right to choice of services delivered in natural environments in order to maximize success in occupational roles.

The Nature of Adaptation and Environment

To explore means for occupational therapists to meet the challenges of building inclusive community, I would like to turn to the spatiotemporal adaptation theory developed with my colleague Elnora Gilfoyle. The theory was developed when we were both involved in pediatric practice and education. During those years, pediatric occupational therapy and other disciplines focused knowledge development and research on typical child development as a means for designing programs for children who were not developing typically. Although the spatiotemporal adaptation theory articulated the importance of interaction between the child and the environment, it emphasized ways in which therapists could influence the child's development rather than ways in which the environment could be prepared to accommodate the child's function. In light of the shift from medical to interactive approach to disability, it seems appropriate to reexamine the categories of the theory, especially the environmental category of the model. The original categories in the theory included *movement, environment, adaptation, and spiraling continuum of development* (Gilfoyle et al., 1990).

In the theory, both development in children and ongoing functioning of adults is seen as a transactional process between a person and the environment; for example, movement provides a means for action and the environment presents a reason to act. The person influences and is influenced by the environment through a process of adaptation. According to Kegan, "adaptation is not just a process of coping or adjusting to events (of the environment) as they are, but an active process of increasingly organizing the relationship of self to the environment"(1982, p.113). The relationship is transactional because persons organize themselves around events of the environment while simultaneously organizing environmental events to meet their needs (Yerxa, 1992). Adaptation as a category of the theory is viewed as an ongoing process of change in behavior. The spiral again provides the model for the adaptation process (see Figure 4). Throughout the life span, a person uses past experience, including values established in early life, to adapt to current situations and prepare for future adaptations. Through adaptation, more complex behaviors evolve to respond to more extensive demands from the environment. If the demands of the current or future situations exceed the ability to adapt, the person may recall past behavior to respond until environmental events can be reorganized to elicit a higher level response. With adaptation as a process for organizing one's self and environment, interaction between person and environment sets up a system of relationships.

Environment as a category in the adaptation theory is all-inclusive. Environment represents the complete setting or surrounding in which a person lives, including self, other persons, objects, space, and relationships between all components in the environment (see Figure 2). According to Winnicott, a "good enough" (1965, p. 67) environment meets and challenges a person's need to grow and develop by adapting to stimulation from continually changing situations. Yerxa (1994) (see Chapter 68) noted that persons need just the right challenge to make an adaptive response. Daloz said that

> how readily we grow—indeed whether we grow at all—has a great deal to do with the nature of the world in which we transact our lives' business. To understand human development, we must understand the environment's part, how it confirms us, contradicts us and provides continuity (1986, p. 68).

Environment–person relationships (see Figure 5) are conceptualized on a spiraling continuum from a *holding environment*, which promotes inclusion, to a *facilitating environment*, which promotes independence, to a *challenging environment*, which increases independence, to an *interactive environment*, which fosters interdependence. The holding environment begins in infancy and provides support through physical and psychological holding. Winnicott maintained that the holding environment is the context in which early development takes place. The infant experience can influence a lifetime. Kegan referred to holding as the "culture of embeddedness" (1982, p. 115), which means an environment that is for growth as well as for accumulating history and mythology. In the holding environment, the infant begins to acquire a culture based on values and traditions communicated during this phase. According to Kegan, there is no single holding environment in early life, but a succession of holding environments, a life history of embeddedness. Holding environments are psychosocial environments that hold us and let go of us. If the infant's experience is satisfactory, it becomes a reference point whenever holding or support is needed later in life. The holding environment promotes a sense of inclusion or belonging, which usually precedes movement away from sources of support and is vital for all persons' development of independence.

The facilitating environment motivates a person to move beyond a familiar setting and on to new challenges and independence. It provides just enough support for moving, literally or figuratively, into new situations.

The challenging environment focuses on separating the person from embeddedness in order to develop and test potential. Just the right amount of challenge is needed if the person is to make an adaptive response to the situation. Increased independence evolves from successful adaptation to challenges.

Finally, the interactive environment promotes interplay between person and environment by combining a sense of self with an appreciation for relationships with

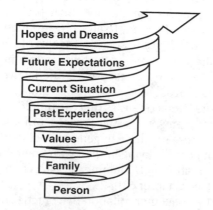

Figure 4. The person in life span.

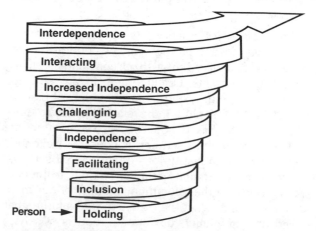

Figure 5. Environment–person relationships.

others. Interactive environment supports interdependence. Winnicott stated that independence is never absolute. The healthy person does not become isolated, but relates to the environment in such a way that person and environment can be considered interdependent. The different functions of environment and the spiraling sequence of relating to environment can be useful for helping persons identity, the environment they need to seek or create for their own health and well-being.

The role of the therapist is construction of Winnicott's "good enough" environment, depending on the person's adaptation needs (Letts et al., 1994). A new parent of a child with significant health problems may need a supportive holding environment to learn the special care that will be given at home. A teenager with a spinal cord injury may seek a facilitating environment when he decides to go to college. He may begin assembling the sources for assistance and adaptations he will need to live independently as well as the advocacy skills he will need to act on his own behalf. A woman recovering from a head injury may have regained considerable function in a rehabilitation setting, but may be fearful of being back in her community. She will need challenge to regain her independence but with enough support and facilitation to ensure progressively successful adaptation. She may want to reconstruct the life she led before the accident, or she may construct a new community and need resources for her new life. An infant may literally require a supportive environment to learn sensorimotor skills or speech or to focus on learning through play. For all of us, gaining and maintaining a balanced interaction between self and environment is a work in progress. We often need to challenge ourselves if we wish to move ahead. Or we seek facilitation for new situations, or support in difficult times. A challenge for occupational therapy practitioners is development of skill in analyzing environments and helping consumers to identify the type of environmental milieu that will facilitate their adaptation process.

Interactive Strategies for Choice and Inclusion

The promise of occupational therapy lies in our ability to continuously combine the mandates put forth in the early tenets of our discipline with our constantly changing practice environments. Occupational therapy emerged from both community, and medical models of practice although our philosophy is more related to what we know, as the community-based model because occupations are practiced in community settings. For decades we tended to practice more in institutions or specialized settings, usually trying to simulate real-life settings to prepare persons to live in their community. Some of our more visionary colleagues set the course toward a future that focused on community consultation models of service delivery. The founders and leaders in our profession have fostered the importance of providing services in a person's own setting and according to the person's own choices and priorities for gaining or regaining specific skills for living. Our philosophy from the beginning of our profession has included the value of choice, relevance, and active participation through engagement in meaningful occupations. Occupation provides a context for organizing one's self and one's environment, thus promoting the transactional process of adaptation within a community setting (Engelhardt, 1977; Gilfoyle et al., 1990; Grady, 1992; Meyer, 1922 [see Chapter 2]; Schwartz, 1992; Yerxa, 1966). Therapy programs are designed to prevent or remediate the effects of disability, or health issues and promote independent living in the community through occupations such as self-care and daily care of others, ability to play independently or with other children, ability to learn as a child and engage in lifelong learning as an adult, ability to be engaged in meaningful work to make a living or for one's own satisfaction or both, ability to balance work and recreation, and ability to blend all occupational activity with rest. Although models for community service delivery have been promoted from within the profession, external mandates for change have also influenced expansion of our practice environments. The voices heard from our consumers, our colleagues, legislation at state and national levels, and rapidly changing payment systems direct us toward service delivery that focuses on consumers' priorities for goals and naturally occurring venues for activities. The new directions in practice allow us to combine our past experience and founders' mandates with the current realities of practice in ways that lead us to realize the future hopes and dreams of our consumers, ourselves as individuals, and the profession as a whole.

To build collaborative models of consumer-driven, community-based practice, we need to focus on a communication process that helps us understand other persons' unique culture and priorities for life occupations as well as meaning associated with past experiences, current situations, and hopes for the future. Recent developments in the field support a focus on communication that enhances a shift from medically focused to interactive models of practice in which the therapist serves as an agent of remedy to affect the arrangements between the individual and society. The use of narrative for storytelling has increased our understanding of a person's past and present experience. Reflective practice and clinical reasoning support our ability to gain insight into the interactive roles that can unfold between a therapist and a person seeking services. Ethnographic approaches to research have in general heightened our knowledge of persons living in their own environments (Clark, 1993; Mattingly & Fleming, 1994; Schön, 1983; Yerxa, 1994 [see Chapter 68]).

Therapist—consumer collaborative practice models mean that communication among the therapist, the person seeking services, the family members, and the close community members is critical. From the beginning, it is the relationships we build that are critical to our ability to collaborate effectively. Listening, talking, reflecting, informing, and demonstrating are all part of the ways we establish relationships. Human beings are uniquely constituted for giving and receiving information, making and sharing meaning. We have the capacity to use intrapersonal communication skills to explore the meaning of our own values and experiences, and interpersonal communication skills to link with another person's values and experiences. *Intrapersonal communication* refers to the creating, functioning, and evaluating of symbolic processes that operate within us. Such activities as thinking, reflecting, solving some problems, and talking with oneself are part of our unique intrapersonal communication system (Dance & Larson, 1972). Intrapersonal communication is active within us whenever meaning is attached to an internally or externally generated source of stimulation. Meaning associated with past events and current situations is deeply embedded in the intrapersonal system of both the persons seeking services and the service provider. Interpersonal communication serves to link us through verbal and nonverbal expression so that we can more explicitly share information and meaning. Through interpersonal communication, we can tell our stories; explore the meaning of relationships, events, and circumstances; reflect on similarities, differences, strengths, and challenges; and develop plans for working together toward future goals. Kegan said, "If you want to understand another person in some fundamental way, you must know where the person is in his or her evolution. You need to understand his or her underlying structure for making meaning" (1982, p. 113). The context in which we as therapists seek and receive the information shared by persons seeking services can enhance our communication and collaborative planning. A communication model of collaboration can be illustrated by the spiraling model of person in life span (see Figure 4). If we place spirals side by side and let one spiral represent the consultant therapist and the other represent a person seeking services, we can visualize the communication sequences that occur. Communication moves from intrapersonal reflection to interpersonal linking through listening and speaking (see Figure 6). A closer look at the circle representing past experience provides details that can be shared about the meaning embedded in values and culture of childhood, family, and personal community (see Figure 7). We can discuss past experiences in terms of activities and relationships with family and close friends, with personal community, and with the larger environment. Exploring the past provides insight into the values that have directed past choices and the types of environments that the person has experienced. Discussing the current situation (see Figures 8 and 9) in the same context allows the therapist to understand the extent and meaning of

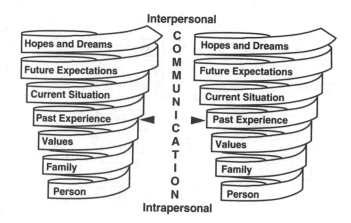

Figure 6. Linking past experiences.

the change that has occurred in the person's life as well as the priorities and types of environments that need to be foremost in planning together. The persons can glean considerable information about the therapist's perspective on the current situation on the basis of past experience. The interpersonal linking increases understanding and promotes collaborative goal setting between person and therapist. As much as we have moved toward collaboration in family-centered and person-centered planning, we are still sometimes heard to say that we are having difficulty with a person receiving services accepting the goals we have set for their therapy. Interactive strategies mean that persons receiving services set the goals and therapists collaborate to design programs with them that will help address the goals. Information shared and the meaning it holds for both consumer and therapist provide the basis for collaboratively planning the future (see Figures 10 and 11). According to Schön (1983), there is gratification and anxiety for the reflective, interactive practitioner in becoming an active participant in a process of shared inquiry. For a therapist or consumer who wishes to move from traditional to reflective communication, there is the task of reshaping expectations for the relationship. But if we are to be agents of remedy in the arrangements between a person and the

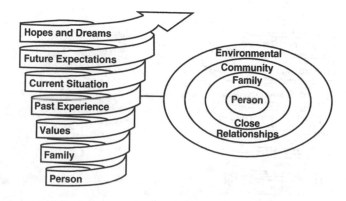

Figure 7. The link of past experience with personal community.

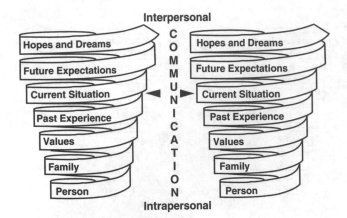

Figure 8. Linking current information.

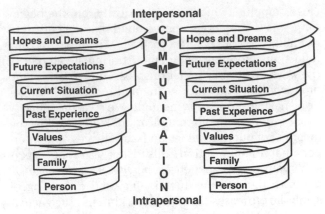

Figure 10. Exploring future possibilities.

environment, we need to be able to share with and receive comprehensive information from the persons who are seeking choices for inclusion in their community.

Summary

We have had an opportunity to focus on the challenges and opportunities for building inclusive community with the persons with whom we work in occupational therapy. We have gained understanding about the meaning of community and choice, reviewed current ideas about the nature of disability and mandates for inclusion, expanded ideas about environment and adaptation, considered strategies for promoting choice and inclusion, and related these concepts to the philosophy of occupational therapy. I had the extraordinary opportunity to explore my own values, past experience, current situation, and hopes for the future and I am forever changed by the experience. As Emily Brontë reflected, "I've dreamt in my life—dreams that have stayed with me ever after, and changed my ideas: they've gone through and through me, like wine through water, and altered the color of my mind." (cited in *The Quotable Woman*, 1991, p. 185) Leading the development of inclusive community is right for occupational therapy and we all have it in us to do it. The challenges before us are as follows:

1. Understanding each person's unique community, including its culture and the context in which it was formed.
2. Resolving the conflict we have over the need for persons with disabilities to prove themselves capable before being included in typical communities of choice rather than creating opportunities for developing capabilities in the community with appropriate supports.
3. Fostering choice that reflects a person's priorities for living and accomplishing occupational tasks, even when there are differences regarding values or perceptions of expertise.
4. Promoting the interactive model for practice, regardless of the venue of practice.
5. Increasing support for more practice venues in the community where engagement in real occupation takes place.
6. Developing programs that prepare people and their families for life in the community while working to prepare the community to welcome the gifts of diversity.
7. Making a commitment to inclusion in community for all persons.

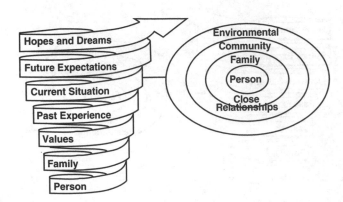

Figure 9. The link of current situation with personal community.

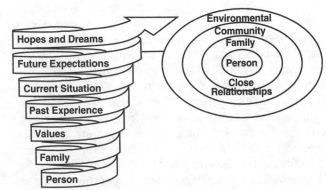

Figure 11. The link of hopes, dreams, and future expectations with personal community.

8. Developing skill in analyzing environments and helping people identify the type of environmental milieu that will facilitate their adaptation process.

Acknowledgments

I thank Ellie Gilfoyle for leading the Eleanor Clarke Slagle nomination process and for a lifetime of creative collaboration; my colleagues who supported the nomination and by doing so offered focus for the topic; Lou Shannon for ongoing support and inspiration; my colleagues at The Children's Hospital for their support; Anita Wagner, Jackie Brand, and all the other parents who enlightened me with their perspectives and changed the course of my professional life; Betty Yerxa, whose philosophy and writings have influenced my thinking for many years; and my family, who are in the center of my personal community. I also thank Carol Wassell from Instructional Services at Colorado State University for creating beautiful slides for the presentation and graphics for this article and Diane Brians for drawing the Circle of Friends.

This lectureship is dedicated to my parents, the late Marion and James Grady, with deep love and appreciation for the strong focus on family and community that they lived and instilled in their children.

References

Americans With Disabilities Act of 1990 (Public Law 101–336)42 U.S.C. § 12101.

Beisser, A. (1989). *Flying without wings.* New York:Doubleday

Brontë, E. (1991). Cited in *The quotable woman.* Philadelphia: Running Press.

Clark, F. (1993). Occupation embedded in a real life: Interweaving occupational science and occupational therapy. 1993 Eleanor Clarke Slagle Lecture. *American Journal of Occupational Therapy, 47,* 1067–1078.

Daloz, L. (1986). *Effective mentoring and teaching.* San Francisco: Jossey–Bass.

Dance, F., & Larson, C. (1972). *Speech communication: Concepts and behavior.* New York: Holt, Rhinehart, & Winston.

Disabled girl asks Santa to end teasing. (1993, December 14). *The Denver Post,* p. 1,

Education for All Handicapped Children Act of 1975 (Public Law 94–142).

Education of the Handicapped Act Amendments of 1986 (Public Law 99–457).

Engelhardt, H. (1977). Defining occupational therapy: The meaning of therapy and the virtues of occupation. *American Journal of Occupational Therapy, 31,* 666–672.

Gilfoyle, E., Grady A., & Moore, J. (1990). *Children adapt* (2nd ed.). Thorofare, NJ: Slack.

Gill, C. (19877). A new social perspective on disability and its implication for rehabilitation. *Occupational Therapy in Health Care, 7,* 1.

Grady A. (1992). Nationally Speaking—Occupation as vision. *American Journal of Occupational Therapy, 46,* 1062–1065.

Groce, N. *(1985). Everyone here spoke sign language: Hereditary deafness on Martha's Vineyard.* Cambridge. MA: Harvard University Press.

Individuals With Disabilities Education Act of 1990. (Public Law 101–476).

Kegan, R. (1982). *The evolving self.* Cambridge, MA: Harvard University Press.

Kunc, N. (1994). *The other side of therapy.* Port Alberni, BC: Axis Consultation and Training.

Letts, L., Law, M., Rigby, P., Cooper, B., Stewart, D., & Strong, S. (1994). Person-environment assessments in occupational therapy. *American Journal of Occupational Therapy, 48,* 608–618.

Mattingly, C., & Fleming, M. (1994). *Clinical reasoning: Forms of inquiry in a therapeutic practice.* Philadelphia: F. A. Davis.

Meyer, A. (1922). The philosophy of occupation therapy. *Archives of Occupational Therapy, 1,* 1. (Reprinted as Chapter 2).

McLaughlin, C., & Davidson, G. (1985). *Builders of the dawn.* Summertown, TN: Book Publishing.

McWilliams, P. (1994). *Do it again!* Los Angeles. Prelude.

Patterson, A. (1992). *Rock art symbols of the greater Southwest.* Boulder, CO: Johnson.

Patterson–Rudolph, C. (1993). *Petroglyphs and Pueblo myths of the Rio Grande* (2nd ed.). Albuquerque, NM: Avanyu.

Rehabilitation Act of 1973 (Public Law 93–112), 29 U.S.C. § 794.

Schön, D. (1983). *The reflective practitioner.* New York: Basic.

Schwartz, K. (1992). Occupational therapy and education: A shared vision. *American Journal of Occupational Therapy, 46,* 12–18.

Shapiro, J. (1993). *No pity.* New York: Times.

Shelton, T., & Stepanek, J. *(1994). Family-centered care for children needing specialized health and developmental services.* Bethesda, MD: Association for the Care of Children's Health.

Technology-Related Assistance for individuals With Disabilities Act (Public Law 100–407) (1988).

Winnicott, D. (1965). *The maturational processes and the facilitating environment.* New York: International Universities Press.

Yankelovitch, D. (1981). *New rules.* New York: Random House.

Yerxa, E. (1966). Eleanor Clarke Slagle lecture—Authentic occupational therapy. *American Journal of Occupational Therapy, 21,* 1–9.

Yerxa, E. (1992). Some implications of occupational therapy's history for its epistemology, values, and relation to medicine. *American Journal of Occupational Therapy, 46,* 79–83.

Yerxa, E. (1994). Dreams, dilemmas, and decisions for occupational therapy practice in a new millennium: An American perspective. *American Journal of Occupational Therapy, 48,* 586–589. (Reprinted as Chapter 68).

Section III

The Developmental Continuum: Purposeful Activities across the Lifespan

Introduction

Developmental theories have strongly influenced occupational therapy (OT) models of practice and frames of reference with most, if not all, integrating concepts and principles of human development (Coster, 1995; Kramer and Hinojosa, 1993; Trombly, 1995). However, identifying and analyzing developmental milestones in the performance components does not result in a complete understanding of a person's overall pattern of activity performance or level of adaptation (Coster, 1995). One must also consider the environmental contexts of development and the personal meaning of activity performance to obtain a true picture of the individual throughout his or her life span. Many OT theorists and scholars have considered these holistic aspects of development as evident in Sections I and II of this text; however, further study and research on the contextual aspects and personal meaning of developmental activities is needed (Coster, 1995); the importance of purposeful activity across the life span cannot be underestimated (Gregory, 1983).

The chapters in this section were selected for their holistic view of the role of purposeful activity during the different stages of human development and their clinical applicability to OT practice. They do not attempt to provide a presentation of developmental theory; rather, they aim to give a broad overview of developmental concepts and principles as applied to purposeful activity across the life span from the perspective of OT. In Chapter 24, Breines begins this section with an analysis of the human need to contribute to one's own well-being and the well-being of others through meaningful activity. She explores the developmental continuum of activity performance and discusses how the developmental sequence is repeated throughout life as one develops new skills or relearns skills that had been restricted or lost. To enhance skill level, OT intervention across the

developmental continuum must include the patient's view of meaningfulness to maximize his or her engagement in purposeful activity. Breines emphasizes that the need to influence the world and make a difference for oneself and others continues as one ages and is a prime motivator for the attainment and maintenance of health.

To assist children in attaining and maintaining health, self-initiated, free play experiences must be readily available for play as the principal purposeful activity that contributes to a child's normal growth and development. Chapter 25 by Missiuna and Pollock explores the nature, purpose, and benefits of play, emphasizing the need for occupational therapists to help children with disabilities develop free play skills. They postulate that children with disabilities who are deprived of normal play opportunities develop secondary social, emotional, and psychological disabilities. These secondary disabilities hinder development and may limit potential for independence and adaptive functioning throughout the life span. Missiuna and Pollock explore barriers to free play for children with disabilities including restrictions set by caregivers; the physical, sensory, and personal limitations of the child and physical and social environmental barriers. They advocate that occupational therapists assume an active role in developing and maintaining free play for the child with disabilities in many settings. Guidelines for comprehensively assessing developmental play levels, principles for collaborating with parents, teachers and caregivers, and recommendations for a multitude of interventions are provided. The authors emphasize the need for occupational therapists to consider the child's developmental abilities, familial and peer relationships, adaptations of play materials, and environmental modifications. They conclude that the promotion and provision of active, self-initiated play in the home, school, and community will provide children with disabilities the developmental experiences needed to become productive members of society.

The theme of prevention of disability in children is continued in Chapter 26 by Olsen, Heaney, and Soppas-Hoffman. They describe the role of OT in preventing the development of psychiatric disorders in preschool children attending a community day care center and considered psychologically at risk. A review of the literature of the inherent value of play to a child's development and a comprehensive analysis of the characteristics of the mother–child relationship that influence the child's development of coping skills is provided. Based on attachment and play theory, they designed a parent–child activity group that used play as a therapeutic tool. They emphasize that play is an integral part of parent–child interaction and it can provide opportunities for immediate feedback, the practice of new behaviors, and the integration of adaptive skills. This prevention program is clearly described, with straightforward information on staffing, participants, reimbursement, group structure, therapeutic interventions, and methods for monitoring change provided. A case study supports the value of this OT intervention, documenting the child's increased adaptive functioning and the improved relationship between parent and child resulting from engagement in mutually satisfying and pleasurable play activities. This unique collaboration between a hospital-based treatment team and a community day care provider is an excellent example of the benefits of OT community outreach, and it clearly substantiates the role of OT in preventing psychosocial dysfunction.

Chapter 27, by Gorski and Miyake, describes another unique community-based prevention program in which OT made a significant contribution by providing preventive services to a well population. This outpatient life/work planning group at a community health care agency was designed to assist adolescents without disabilities in making effective transitions to adult roles. Gorski and Miyake review issues relevant to adolescence and the adolescent passage to adulthood, recognizing that this period is often confusing and difficult for the teenager (and for caring parents and teachers) in today's turbulent society. They focus on the particularly complex problems of occupational choice, career planning, and employment preparation, given the viewpoint that decisions made during adolescence can effect future life satisfaction. Components for a successful transition to employment and positive adolescent development are reviewed. Characteristics of adolescents at risk who are considered appropriate for this prevention program are identified along with group leader characteristics and program structure. Their program plan organizes group activities into five stages. They clearly describe each stage and its goal; providing the reader with realistic format guidelines and relevant activity suggestions to facilitate goal attainment. Their focus on real-life pur-

poseful activities and functional community living skills, rather than an emphasis on performance components and simulated tasks, is a welcome one and critical for the adolescent developing an identity as a productive contributing member of society.

As clearly described by Gorski and Miyake, the transitional phase of adolescence is often difficult, requiring a great deal of decision making and a large amount of personal growth. This normal transition can be further complicated when the adolescent is not completely well but has a limiting disability. Therefore, there is a critical need to develop interventions for adolescents with disabilities designed to facilitate healthy transitions from adolescence to adulthood. Chapter 28 by Broiller, Shephard, and Markley addresses this vital need by discussing the use of Individualized Transition Plans (ITP) for students with disabilities to enable them to successfully move from a school setting into employment and community living. They describe the assessment and intervention process, focusing on functional activities within the home, school, community, recreational, and vocational environments. Standards for realistic, relevant goal setting, intervention principles, and service characteristics are provided. A strong emphasis is placed on developing those skills needed for safe, healthy productive living and in fostering community integration and adult activities. Their presentation is supported by a review of OT and special education literature on occupational performance, functional activities, and transitional planning. Federal initiatives and legislative mandates concerning vocational transition for youths with disabilities are also reviewed. The role of the ITP team in collaborating with the student and parent to develop and implement a comprehensive transition plan is discussed. Potential barriers to collaborative planning are explored, with suggestions to reduce these barriers and increase parental and student participation provided. The role of the occupational therapist in adapting activities, modifying the environment, and providing technological aids to implement ITPs and develop adolescents' social, self-care, home management, work, school, and leisure skills to live and work within the community is clearly discussed.

This role of OT, collaborating with persons with disabilities to develop the skills needed to live, work, and play within communities, is an invaluable one. However, the need for play and meaningful leisure is often neglected once a person with disabilities reaches adulthood. Chapter 29 by Kielhofner and Miyake addresses this vital need by describing a pilot study that used games to increase the play skills of adults with mental retardation. A literature review of the theoretical principles and empirical research supporting the inherent value of play in the development of self-identity and adaptive behavior and in the acquisition of social roles is presented. The impact of mental retardation, environmental deprivation, and lack of opportunities on the play behavior of adults is also explored. The program of games used in this study and the dual role of the occupational therapist as service provider and participant–observer is described. Strategies and procedures, including grading complexity, leveling relationships, coaching and modeling, and keeping up the game's continuity, are explained in an understandable manner. The effectiveness of these interventions in maximizing clients' game behavior and improving play skills is well documented and substantiated with numerous case examples. The resulting improvements in motor, cognitive, psychological, and social skills and the enhanced quality of life for the program's participants is clearly evident, validating the inherent worth of play. The finding that normal play and games can increase functional skills, improve quality of life, and help develop positive, personal adult identities is relevant to male and female populations with, or without, mental retardation.

The relationship among purposeful activity, adult self-identity, and quality of life is evident in Kielhofner's and Miyake's portrayal of adult men with mental retardation. The use of purposeful activity to develop a positive personal identity and to increase social skills in the adult is further explored in Chapter 30 by Donohue, who focuses her study on adult women with psychiatric illnesses. Donohue presents a theoretical model for an identification group based on concepts from sociological theories of groups. The benefits of shaping the members of an identification group by fostering a sense of kinship and "we-ness" are explored. Suggestions for developing and maintaining this kinship through group structure and process are provided. OT principles used to develop social skills within the environment are also reviewed. Donohue discusses the effective use of purposeful activities, life simulation tasks, topical discussions, and aerobic exercises in developing an affirmative female identification and adult social role. The historical and cultural nature of adult women from a given era is discussed with implications for group goals and process identified. Concrete information on the group's referral process, membership, session structure, purpose, activity ideas, discussion topics, and leadership style is provided. Suggestions for developing and structuring a men's reference group are also briefly reviewed. Donohue's discussion clearly highlights the personal relevance of meaningful, satisfying growth-producing activity.

Chapter 31 by Smith, Kielhofner, and Watts continues to examine the relationships between developmental stages and life satisfaction. They present a study of 60 elderly individuals that sought to determine whether the interests, values, personal causation, and activity pattern of an elderly person's daily occupation correlated with his or her life satisfaction. A review of the Model of Human Occupation is provided, because this served as a framework for the study. A comprehensive analysis of

the impact of aging on a person is presented with an emphasis on the volition subsystem components of interest, values, and personal causation. Smith, Kielhofner, and Watts describe the three research instruments used to measure study's variables and the research procedures employed to gather and analyze data. They present and discuss the results of the study. Most noteworthy was the finding of a significant relationship between the volitional characteristics of interests, values, personal causation, and life satisfaction. Time spent in work and leisure correlated more highly with life satisfaction than time spent in rest and daily living tasks. These findings have relevant implications for occupational therapists, because they suggest that OT interventions should emphasize interests, values, personal causation, work, and leisure rather than self-care tasks. The authors postulate that purposeful activities related to recreation and work may contribute to enhanced life satisfaction, whereas a focus on rest and daily living tasks may diminish life satisfaction. Although this is only one study, with no causal relationship established, the clear correlations between daily activities and life satisfaction warrant careful consideration and further study.

The meaning of purposeful activity in one's daily life is analyzed from the perspective of family caregivers of elderly individuals in this section's final chapter. To understand the significance of activity in caregiving, she conducted 60 ethnographic interviews with 15 family caregivers for frail elderly people living in the community. From this comprehensive research three goals of caregiving activity were derived: (1) getting things done, (2) achieving a sense of health and well-being for the care-receiver, and (3) achieving a sense of health and well-being for caregiver. Hasselkus conceptualizes the family caregiver as a lay practitioner who is faced with clinical reasoning and ethical dilemmas regarding the provision of care for a family member on a day-to-day basis. Caregivers' judgments regarding the prioritization of goals determines the form of caregiver activity. Implications for OT practice and the relationship between the family caregiver and professional are discussed with focus placed on the therapeutic relationship. The need for a reflective contract between the OT and the caregiver to ensure the contexts and meaning of activities are considered, and the need to validate the caregiver's need for balance and variety in daily activities is emphasized. This knowledge will enable occupational therapists to assist caregivers in a manner meaningful to and supportive of the family as a caring unit.

Although patterns of purposeful activity in daily life obviously change as one ages and develops new life roles, the inherent value of purposeful activity throughout all stages of development is clearly illustrated by each chapter in this section. Occupational therapists are challenged to consider the personal meaning and relevance of purposeful activity to its environmental contexts across the life span, in all areas of OT practice. This section provides an introduction to the development aspects of purposeful activity. The reader is referred to Appendix M for a listing of publications and articles that further explore theories, concepts, and principles of purposeful activity, human development, and OT practice.

Questions to Consider

1. Construct an activities history for yourself from early childhood to the present. Identify the purposeful activities that were meaningful to you in each stage of your life. Ask family members for their recollection of your daily activity patterns and your favorite activities from your early childhood. Reflect on your later childhood, adolescence, early adulthood, and present activities. How did your activity pattern change as you developed new life roles (e.g., student, club member, worker)? What changes occurred in the tasks associated with these roles as you aged? Which activities remained meaningful to you as you developed? Which activities lost their meaning for you? Why? How did play influence the development and maintenance of your skills, self-identity, and social roles? What other purposeful activities were most important to your development?

2. Visit a playground that has diversity of children reflective of a variety of age groups playing. Observe and document the children's free play. How does the play of the younger children differ from the older children? What are the developmental reasons for these differences? How would the acquisition of a disability affect this self-initiated free play? What would be the affect of this change in free play on development? How could this play environment be modified to meet the free play developmental needs of children with disabilities?

3. Interview two retirees, one who had expected and preplanned his or her retirement and one who did not expect to retire at this stage of life and who had no time for planning (i.e., a forced retirement because of company downsizing). How has each person's daily activity pattern changed as a result of his or her retirement? Is the person satisfied or dissatisfied with this change? What are factors influencing this level of satisfaction with daily activities? What purposeful activities provide meaning in his or her retirement? Are there meaningful purposeful activities that are no longer pursued in retirement? What factors influence the pursuit of purposeful activities? Did preplanning or the lack of it influence adaptation to retirement? Explain the nature of this influence.

References

Coster, W. (1995). Developmental aspects of occupation. In C. B. Royeen (Ed.), *The Practice of the Future: Putting Occupation Back Into Therapy* (Lesson 10). Bethesda, MD: American Occupational Therapy Association.

Gregory, M. D. (1983). Occupational behavior and life satisfaction among retirees. *American Journal of Occupational Therapy, 37,* 548–553.

Kramer, P., & Hinojosa, J. (1993). *Frames of Reference for Pediatric Occupational Therapy.* Baltimore, MD: Williams & Wilkins.

Miller, R. J., & Walker, K. F. (1993). *Perspectives on Theory for the Practice of Occupational Therapy.* Gaithersburg, MD: Aspen Publishers.

Mosey, A. (1986). *Psychosocial Components of Occupational Therapy.* New York, NY: Raven Press.

Trombly, C. A. (Ed). (1995). *Occupational Therapy for Physical Dysfunction.* Baltimore, MD: Williams & Wilkins.

Chapter 24

Making a Difference: A Premise of Occupation and Health

Estelle B. Breines, PhD, OTR, FAOTA

uman beings engage in many activities during their lives, but their engagement depends on a variety of conditions. One condition is that the activity must be meaningful in some way. When people attempt to interact with or influence their surroundings, whether for themselves or for others, they need to see results that allow them to perceive themselves as effective. Causal intent is a direct precipitant of action; purpose, action, and occupation are inextricable. The will to "make a difference" pervades human beings. People feel that they must influence their world. This compelling feature of human behavior permeates human occupation. Making a difference is a way of describing the influence a person has on the concrete and social worlds. This influence can be described in terms of development or evolution (Darwin, 1914; Dewey, 1916).

Human development and occupation replicate their ancestral origins in their sequence of growth and acquisition. Development and occupation are innately and acquisitionally dedicated to the survival of the individual and the species (Freud, 1918/1946). People are motivated by their inherent nature and the demands of their world to act on their own behalf and on behalf of their kin or society. The need to make a difference remains as evolution and development proceed; only the level of involvement alters. The continuation of the evolutional and developmental genetic process depends on the feedback received. Whether feedback is described in terms of proprioception (Trombly, 1982a, 1982b), feelings of efficacy (Fidler, 1981; Fidler & Fidler, 1978 [see Chapter 7]; White, 1963), or group dynamics, people act on the assumption that the action they take will make a difference for themselves or others. An environmental response is sought and must be perceived, for without response, there is no connection between the person and the world. Making a difference refers to a person's involvement, response, and occupation in the sense of occupying or taking one's place in the world (Breines, 1986; Mead, 1932). In other words, human performance is restricted and enhanced by the forces and influences of the person's surroundings; therefore, human action can be understood only in terms of the relationships it generates with the world. Whether the action is devoted to solving problems of the self or problems of society, it is directed at making things happen. The simple expectation that action results in reaction is the factor that steams the engine of performance. Without such an expectation, a person's motivation to act disappears, leaving individual or societal needs unmet.

I believe this is the principle upon which occupational therapy is built, the foundational concept for our profession's principles of occupation. Human beings need to be active and, by that action, to contribute to their own well-being and the well-being of others. When a person is unable to act, it is the therapist's role to facilitate performance, enabling that person to function without intervention, and by functioning, to make a contribution to the world. People must make a difference for themselves or others in order to function and continue to grow. This is the rationale for our philosophy, our science, our art, and our practice.

The synthesis of automatic performance with purpose leads to active occupation, which is directed at creating change and altering experience throughout life. By virtue of both nature and nurture, our evolution, our development, and our history provide a foundation of automatic performance phenomena. These automatic elements of performance enable deliberate, purposeful activity to meet human needs. Active occupation is possible because of the synchrony of its automatic and deliberate elements.

This interaction of automation and intention occurs throughout life at many levels of performance; the actions themselves span a developmental continuum. Initial action is primarily egocentric; subsequent action is influenced by the environment of space and objects; and mature action is influenced by the social environment (achieved through consensus with other people) while retaining aspects of all that has gone before (Breines, 1986). This sequence is repeated every time a new skill is acquired. The person interacts with the environment, ultimately using newly acquired skills to meet society's needs. This sequence is pertinent to (a) the development of humankind, (b) individual lifelong development, and (c) the development of contributory skills within each phase of life. It is also pertinent to the redevelopment of skills. For example, the infant, with its instinctive rooting reflex, searches and suckles; the child, unbound by primitive reflexes, runs and climbs and plays. All of these activities prepare children for the adult roles of hunter/gatherer, farmer, industrialist, computer technologist, or parent, as history and environment require. When

these skills are restricted by circumstance, they must be relearned. In essence, the themes of evolution and development are repeated throughout life, as observed in the actions people make not only on their own behalf, but also on behalf of society.

Viewing the developmental and relational aspects of active occupation, one can begin to ascertain the significance of these concepts in terms of health. A person who perceives or comprehends his or her own actions in relation to the environment remains engaged with that environment, which results in further involvement. Were one's action or one's ability to perceive the relationship between actions to be impaired, function and development would be diminished or even cease. Occupational therapy addresses the implications of this phenomenon. One must demonstrate skill on preliminary levels of performance to be able to act purposefully upon one's surroundings, that is, one must walk before one can hunt. Furthermore, this interaction between the self and the environment occurs at all levels of body action, self-care, skill building, social interaction, work, and leisure. When learning the skills of life, human beings must anticipate reactions, gain control, and achieve rewards in the form of success, or they will not continue to strive. It is this condition of continued striving to make a contribution, to make a difference, that occupational therapists help patients to achieve. This, in fact, is a measure of health, for the person and for society. I believe it is also the principle for which occupational therapy stands.

This treatment philosophy has many implications. If the purpose of one's engagement in active occupation is to be healthful, then the activity must be perceived as contributory. The arguments about the usefulness of crafts, exercise, or biofeedback (Breines, 1984 [see Chapter 12]; Fidler, 1981; Huss, 1981; and Trombly, 1982a) are secondary to the patient's view of the meaningfulness of the involvement. If patients view their activities as contributory to themselves, their families, or society, they will continue their involvement. If they perceive tasks as meaningless, they are apt to disengage and can be expected to decline in function. Therefore, competent therapists will identify tasks and occupations that patients view as meaningful, using creative adaptation to further enhance skill levels. If patients do not view their actions as making a difference, the goal of health through active occupation (Addams, 1910; Addams, 1935; Cohen, 1983; Meyer, 1922 [see Chapter 2]), upon which occupational therapy is built, will not be met.

Active occupation as a tool for health has a broad evolutional and developmental perspective. To engage in activities at any level of development, humans need to see their actions as meaningful. Therapists should keep this principle in mind when guiding patients in the selection of tasks that will contribute to their continued development and health.

References

Addams, J. (1910). *Twenty years at Hull House.* New York: Macmillan.

Addams, J. (1935). *My friend Julia Lathrop.* New York: Macmillan.

Breines, E. (1984). An attempt to define purposeful activity. *American Journal of Occupational Therapy, 38,* 543–544. (Reprinted as Chapter 12).

Breines, E. (1986). *Origins and adaptations: A philosophy of practice.* Lebanon, NJ: Geri-Rehab.

Cohen, S. (1983). The mental hygiene movement; the development of personality and the school: The medicalization of American education. *History of Education Quarterly, 23,* 123–149.

Darwin, C. R. (1914). *The origin of species by means of natural selection.* Philadelphia: R. West.

Dewey, J. (1916). *Democracy and education: An introduction to philosophy of education.* Toronto: Collier-Macmillan.

Fidler, G. S. (1981). From crafts to competence. *American Journal of Occupational Therapy, 35,* 567–573.

Fidler, G. S., & Fidler, J. W. (1978). Doing and becoming: Purposeful action and self-actualization. *American Journal of Occupational Therapy, 32,* 305–310. (Reprinted as Chapter 7).

Freud, S. (1946). *Totem and taboo* (A. A. Brill, Trans.). New York: Vintage Books. (Original work published 1918).

Huss, A. J. (1981). From kinesiology to adaptation. *American Journal of Occupational Therapy, 35,* 574–580.

Mead, G. H. (1932). *The philosophy of the present.* Chicago: Open Court.

Meyer, A. (1922). The philosophy of occupation therapy. *Archives of Occupational Therapy, 1,* 1–10. (Reprinted as Chapter 2).

Trombly, C. A. (1982a). Include exercise in 'purposeful activity' [letter to the editor]. *American Journal of Occupational Therapy, 36,* 467–468.

Trombly, C. A. (1982b). *Occupational therapy for physical dysfunction* (2nd ed.). Baltimore: Williams & Wilkins.

White, R. (1963). Ego and reality in psychoanalytic theory. *Psychological Issues, 3,* 3.

Chapter 25

Play Deprivation in Children with Physical Disabilities: The Role of the Occupational Therapist in Preventing Secondary Disability

Cheryl Missiuna

Nancy Pollock

Self-initiated free play experiences are vital for the normal growth and development of all children. In this chapter, children with physical disabilities who are deprived of normal play opportunities are viewed as having a second disability that hinders their potential for independent behavior and performance. Physical, social, personal, and environmental barriers that may limit the play experiences of children with physical disabilities are delineated. Studies of the interactions of these children during play are discussed, and a case is made for the promotion of active, free play in the home, the school, and the community. As facilitators of this process, occupational therapists must consider a variety of factors, including the unique capabilities of the child, the influence of parent-child and peer relationships, the role of other caregiving adults, the adaptation of toys and materials, and the impact of the environment and setting.

Occupational therapists are unique in their emphasis on productive activity. A primary productive activity for young children is play (Bundy, 1989). In therapy, we frequently use play activities to achieve treatment objectives such as fine motor skill development, postural control, and concept development. This widely accepted use of toys and playful activity can be contrasted with another less evident function of play: the value of free play for its own sake. Rast (1986) noted, "Play and therapy almost appear to be mutually exclusive. A child's play is an intrinsically motivating activity done voluntarily and for its own sake; therapy proceeds according to the therapist's plan to achieve definite treatment objectives" (p. 30). If we consider play to be the primary productive activity for children, then the development of play skills becomes, in itself, an important goal for therapeutic intervention. Play acts as an antecedent for work and adult recreation and also serves to develop competence. We need to concern ourselves with play skills and also with the child's playfulness and motivation to engage in play.

In this paper, literature is used to demonstrate the purpose and benefit of free play experiences and to outline some of the barriers to free play that may be encountered by children with physical disabilities. The role of occupational therapists working with parents in preventing play deprivation and secondary disability is explored.

What Is Play?

Play is a complex, multifaceted behavior that is relatively easy to observe and describe but difficult to define theoretically (Rubin, Fein, & Vandenberg, 1983). Two characteristics that would be considered by most to be essential to the construct of play are that it be intrinsically motivated and that it be pleasurable (Ellis, 1973; Lindquist, Mack, & Parham, 1982; Mack, Lindquist, & Parham, 1982). In an occupational behavior framework, play is considered to be the primary activity of the child, a prerequisite to competence in occupational roles later in life (Reilly, 1974). Play has an exploratory component that is engaged in for its own sake and a competency component that results from an inner drive to master the environment (Reilly, 1974). Work and play are viewed along a developmental continuum, with play continuing to serve an adaptive function in adulthood (Kielhofner & Barris, 1984; Matsutsuyu, 1971). Sheridan (1975) elaborated on this work-play distinction by defining play as "eager engagement in pleasurable, physical or mental effort to obtain emotional satisfaction" (p. 5). Work, in contrast, is defined as "voluntary engagement in disciplined physical or mental effort to obtain material benefit" (p. 5).

The benefits of play are well-established (Ayres, 1981; Ellis, 1973; Erikson, 1963; Garvey, 1977; Gralewicz, 1973; Kielhofner & Barris, 1984; McHale & Olley, 1982; Piaget, 1951, 1952; Reilly, 1974; Vandenberg & Kielhofner, 1982). During play, children have the opportunity to discover what effect they can have on objects and people in their environment and to develop and test social and occupational roles. As children move around and explore their world, they receive information through their senses, gain knowledge about the nature and properties of objects, and develop rules about their own location in time and space (Robinson, 1977). The skills that are developed during play permit children to interact with and respond to the demands of their environment (Anderson, Hinojosa, & Strauch, 1987) (see Chapter 46). This, in turn, leads to perceptual, conceptual, intellectual, and language development and, it has been argued, to the eventual integration of cognitive abilities (Levitt, 1975; Weininger, 1979, 1980, 1988; Weininger & Fitzgerald, 1988).

Occupational therapists working within sensory integrative, neurodevelopmental, occupational behavior, and developmental perspectives have recognized the sensorimotor, social, and constructive benefits of play and have justified its wide use in therapy as a treatment modality (Anderson et al., 1987) (see Chapter 46). It is important for us, as therapists, to examine whether or not the benefits that may be attributed to the playful use of activity can be equated to the definition of play as a pleasurable activity that is emotionally satisfying. The distinction between the two forms of play can be highlighted by referring to the latter form as free play. In contrast to planned therapy sessions that are designed to produce specific responses through play, free play is spontaneous, intrinsically motivated, and self-regulated and requires the expressive personal involvement of the child (Calder, 1980; Garvey, 1977; Gunn, 1975; Yawkey, Dank, & Glossenger, 1986).

Primary and Secondary Forms of Play Deprivation

The designation, children with physical disabilities, is used in this paper to refer to children with sensory impairments, multiple handicaps, or limitations in voluntary movement or mobility. The impact of any of these disabilities can range from mild to severe in the degree to which the disability interferes with the child's ability to function independently. A child with mild cerebral palsy may have poor hand function, limiting his or her ability to manipulate a toy as desired; a child with a more severe impairment may be unable even to communicate his or her interest in a toy. Regardless of the individual circumstances, Mogford (1977) has proposed that the ability of children with physical disabilities to "explore, interact with, and master their environment is impaired with a consequent distortion or deprivation of normal childhood experiences" (p. 171).

The deprivation described by Mogford can be considered from two perspectives. First, a physical disability often implies an absence of, or deficiency in, sensory and motor information being received by the child. A child will inevitably be deprived of the play experiences that cannot be made available to him or her due to the disabling condition. For example, a child with a visual impairment will not be able to experience directly the effect of play with lights or colors, nor will a child with a hearing impairment have the opportunity to play with voices and musical sounds. Alternative forms of play can be substituted, but this primary form of deprivation will remain unchanged.

Second, the occupational therapist is concerned with the secondary disabilities that may arise as an indirect result of play deprivation. Children with physical disabilities are often more dependent on their caregivers and other people than are nondisabled children (Rubin et al., 1983). Brown and Gordon (1987), in a study of the activity patterns of children with physical disabilities, found that disabled children spent more time in self-care and passive activities in their own homes than did nondisabled children. The child who is unable to experience normal childhood play because of a physical disability may encounter secondary social, emotional, and psychological disabilities. Examples of this form of play deprivation are children with visual impairments who are not permitted to climb monkey bars because they might fall, children with hearing impairments who are not allowed to play outside because they might not hear a car, and children in wheelchairs who are unable to cross the street to get to a park.

Free play provides a forum for children to explore their own capacities, to experiment with objects, to make decisions, to understand cause-and-effect relationships, to learn, to persist, and to understand consequences. This type of play also fosters creativity and allows a child to develop social skills when the play involves peers. Cotton (1984) suggested that, in addition to developing competence through play, the child also learns to cope with anxiety, frustration, and failure.

If children with physical disabilities are deprived of the opportunity to regularly engage in free play, it seems plausible that particular types of secondary disabilities are likely to result. Increased dependence on others, decreased motivation, lack of assertiveness, poorly developed social skills in unstructured situations, and lowered self-esteem are a few of the difficulties that may be experienced by children with disabilities (Clarke, Riach, & Cheyne, 1977/1982; Levitt & Cohen, 1977; Mogford, 1977; Philip & Duckworth, 1982). These secondary disabilities have an impact not only on the child's play and development, but also on later functioning in the school setting, the community, and the workplace. It is in the prevention of secondary disabilities that the role of the occupational therapist becomes important.

Barriers to Free Play

Play deprivation, primary and secondary, may occur as a result of many different forms of barriers. For children with physical disabilities, the areas that have been addressed most frequently in the literature are limitations imposed by caregivers, physical and personal limitations of the child, environmental barriers, and social barriers.

Limitations Imposed by Caregivers

Children need the freedom to initiate and engage actively in activities, the chance to make decisions and take risks, and the opportunity to master their physical selves or to accomplish a task they have chosen (Diamond, 1981). Well-meaning parents and teachers frequently overprotect children who have disabilities and may not permit their participation in normal activities (Calder, 1980; Hewett, Newson, & Newson, 1970; Philip & Duckworth, 1982; Williams & Matesi, 1988). Whether due to fear of injury, pity, compassion, or lack of knowledge about a child's abilities, adults may intervene too quickly and may unnecessarily limit the child's opportunity to play (Diamond, 1981; Levitt, 1975). In addition, concern for the child's physical development and progress may lead caregivers to fail to appreciate his or her need for play, with the result that free time may be used for therapy or for catching up on schoolwork (Calder, 1980; Mogford, 1977).

Physical and Personal Limitations of the Child

The natural exploration of the environment observed even in infancy in nondisabled children may not be possible for the child with a physical disability. Lack of mobility, limited communication, difficulty with reach and grasp, and impaired sensory responses may all interfere with the child's ability to play with toys or household objects. Children with physical disabilities may not be provided with chances to engage in nonstructured forms of play, such as launching an assault on the kitchen cupboards, bouncing on the bed, roughhousing, and participating actively in the neighborhood, at the park, and on the playground (Levitt, 1975; Russell, 1978). Csikszentmihalyi (1975) stressed the importance of matching a person's skills to the challenges of the environment. In the case of the child with a physical disability, environmental challenges often exceed the child's skills, leading to anxiety and frustration.

In addition to the apparent physical and sensory limitations, a number of authors have suggested that there may be factors within the child that limit participation in play. Limited intrinsic motivation (Levitt & Cohen, 1977; Mogford, 1977), lack of drive and decreased concentration (Salomon, 1983; Sheridan, 1975), and withdrawal due to lack of skill or frustration (Calder, 1980) have all been proposed as problems that maybe inherent in the disabled child. It is not possible to state with certainty whether these problems originate within the child or arise secondarily due to a lack of opportunity for participation in self-initiated play activities.

Environmental Barriers

Barriers imposed by the physical environment (e.g., steps, narrow doorways) may severely limit the disabled child's opportunities for free play. These barriers may be present in the home as well as in the community (e.g., schools, recreational facilities, and playgrounds). The physical structure of toys, materials, and equipment may limit children's ability to express themselves and to explore objects (Rubin et al., 1983). Changes within the child's home environment may have been made to suit the child's individual needs; however, in the authors' experience, these modifications are rarely extended to the broader community environment. For the most part, buildings and playgrounds have been constructed to meet the needs of the young person without physical disabilities. A safe environment that allows opportunity for freedom of movement and that is filled with familiar play materials is considered to be optimal for free play (Knox, 1989). How often is this type of environment available for the child with physical disabilities?

Social Barriers

Interaction with peers. Most normal free-play experiences center around interaction with peers. Parten (1932), in the now-familiar hierarchy of social interaction during play, described the increasingly complex stages of play ranging from parallel play to cooperation among players to achieve a common goal. Through these increasingly sophisticated interactions, the child learns societal norms and rules of behavior, is given the chance to experiment with different roles (e.g., leader, organizer), and models the social behaviors of other children. Children with physical disabilities are often limited in their interactions with other players due to both physical limitations and exclusion by their peer group. With decreased opportunities for interaction during the early years, the child with a disability may have a limited repertoire of social skills, which further increases his or her isolation. To illustrate this point, consider the presence of a child with physical disabilities in a mainstreamed kindergarten program. The child may not know how to initiate play with another child or how to join a group of children already playing at an activity center. It is no wonder that studies have repeatedly demonstrated that children with physical disabilities have poorly developed social skills (Clarke et al., 1977/1982; Philip & Duckworth, 1982).

Interaction with parents. The lack of playfulness present in many parental interactions is another potential area of social deprivation during play (Kogan, Tyler, & Turner, 1974; Oster, 1984). Therapists may ask parents to become the child's teacher-therapist in the home environment. Although consistency and carryover of treatment ideas and approaches are beneficial to achieve therapy objectives, the question of the cost to the parent-child relationship must be raised. The interaction of a parent functioning as a therapist can be very different from normal parent-child interaction, and professionals have recently begun to question the effect of this interaction on the social development of the child with a disability (Rogers, 1988). It has further been proposed that the role of home therapist may produce an emotional conflict for the nurturing, accepting parent (Foster, Berger, & McLean, 1981). If parents are asked to follow a regimen established by a therapist, then their unique role and interaction with the child may be diminished (Kaiser & Hayden, 1984).

A number of studies performed in recent years have addressed this issue through an examination of the play of mothers with children who have physical disabilities. In contrast to nondisabled children, results suggest that mothers of disabled children perceive play and teaching situations as similar (Oster, 1984); show more negative affect and perceive the play situation as unrewarding (Kogan, 1980; Kogan et al., 1974); and are more directive and controlling (Brooks-Gunn & Lewis, 1982a, 1982b; Crawley & Spiker, 1983; Cunningham & Barkley, 1979; Hanzlik, 1989; Hanzlik & Stevenson, 1986; Oster, 1984). Many parents have expressed concern about the "one good hour" that they may have with their child: Their desire to simply cuddle and play with the child is rapidly extinguished when they recall the necessity to perform a home program (Kaiser, 1982). Similarly, several adults with cerebral palsy reported to Kibele (1989) that therapy had a negative effect on their relationships with their mothers. The demands of home programs limited their leisure time and, in some cases, led to the impression that they were disappointing their parents, particularly when skill development did not improve. It is essential for a parent to have positive interactions with his or her child, yet it is also important for the child's development to be stimulated whenever possible. Free play, not disguised therapy, may achieve similar objectives with less stress on the family.

Overcoming Barriers to Play: The Role of the Occupational Therapist

Occupational therapists may be in an ideal position to develop and maximize the free play opportunities of the child with physical disabilities in many settings. As professionals who are concerned with the child's development in the areas of self-care, productivity, and leisure, occupational therapists have the opportunity to work with the child in the home, in a treatment facility, or in a wide variety of community settings. Awareness of the barriers that the child frequently encounters and an understanding of the child's capabilities may facilitate the consultative process.

Assessment

Naturalistic observation and appraisal of a child's developmental play level is as essential to an occupational therapy assessment as evaluation of other activities of daily living. The play history, the types of play engaged in (e.g., active, exploratory, imitative, constructive, dramatic), the stage of play (e.g., solitary, independent, parallel, associative), and the developmental progression of object play (e.g., functional, relational, symbolic, combinatory) may all receive consideration. (Good reviews of these areas can be found in Behnke & Fetkovich, 1984; Florey, 1981; Kielhofner & Barris, 1984; Sheridan, 1975; and Sparling, Walker, & Singdahlsen, 1984.) Other important parts of a complete assessment are the frequency of play times, the variety of toys available, the physical location, and the opportunities for social interaction with peers and caregivers during these times.

Intervention

Providing opportunities for free play. Children with physical disabilities often have much less time available for play than do their nondisabled peers, in part due to the time spent in therapeutic programs (Brown & Gordon, 1987). If play is believed to be an important component of the child's life, then time must be built in to allow for free play experiences in the classroom, the therapeutic setting, the home, and the community.

In any play situation, a child needs to have the opportunity to choose, to explore, to create, and to respond to change if the result is truly to be called free play, Consideration can be given to the play space, recognizing the child's need for both personal play space and free ranging space in contact with other people (Stout, 1988) 'Whenever possible, caregiving adults can be encouraged by the therapist to let the child explore and interact independently. Numerous studies have indicated that adults working with physically disabled children tend to intervene too quickly, with the result that the children become highly dependent on this intervention during play (Federlein, 1979; Field, 1980; Field, Roseman, de Stefano, & Koewler, 1982; Levitt, 1975).

Consultation with parents. The therapist's expectations of, and recommendations to, the parent in the home environment must be thoughtfully considered. Parental participation in a child's play is not only positive but may be essential for children with more severe impairments. Many parents view this play time, however, as a time to "learn to use materials and to learn to use them correctly" (Oster, 1984, p. 156). To maximize play opportunities, parents may first need to be convinced of the importance of free play to the total health and development of the child. Understanding the educational value of play as well as the sequence of development that occurs in play may help parents view play as more than a pastime. Henderson and Bryan (1984) have suggested that parents must believe that self-direction is important and must trust their child's ability to learn from his or her own play experiences. The parent-child relationship is reciprocal, and parental expectations and beliefs will have an impact on the quality of the play. In addition, some of the apparent benefits of play—increased motivation, improved self-concept, and more active participation—may be viewed negatively by parents. For example, children who were previously satisfied with the vicarious experiences provided by television may become more demanding in their desire to have an active play life. In these instances, increasing the involvement of siblings or peers at home or in a play setting may be beneficial.

Consultation with teachers and caregivers. When therapists talk to teachers or caregivers about play and make recommendations for toys and play activities, the specific barriers that may limit the child's play in that setting must be addressed. The limitations imposed by caregivers are usually grounded in a genuine concern for the safety and welfare of the child. It is important for the therapist to acknowledge these concerns and to discuss with caregivers or teachers the extent to which their fears are realistic. Suggestions can be provided regarding the child's optimal positions for play and the extent to which he or she may need assistance. The child's capabilities, not limitations, should be stressed for two reasons: First, a child can demonstrate unique abilities and be remarkably creative when motivated to move or perform an activity, and second, a child needs to be enjoyed as a child, not as a child with a disability. Free play periods may offer this opportunity.

Integrated preschool and school settings offer ideal opportunities for peer interactions. Both the therapist and the caregiver should maximize the child's opportunities to be involved with his or her peers, without interfering with the spontaneity of these situations. Children with physical disabilities may need assistance with mobility, positioning, and access to playthings and equipment in order to allow them to participate to their maximum potential; however, dependence on the presence of an adult should be discouraged. The child may need some instructions on how to enter a play group, but this skill can also be learned from peer models. The role of the adult is to structure the environment, both physically and socially, and then allow play to happen.

Recommendations about playthings. The toys and activities that are made available for the child will influence both the type and quality of play. Sensitivity must be shown to social, emotional, physical, and educational needs and also to the interests of the child. A toy that is suitable for one child may be extremely unsuitable for another because of differences in temperament, motivation, and previous life experiences. To maximize the play experience, careful consideration must be given to the child's current developmental level. Toys of intermediate novelty are usually optimal: A toy should have an element of familiarity to the child but be sufficiently novel to induce exploration. Gradual pacing of activities will encourage the child to experiment and take risks but will ensure that the resulting information can be integrated into knowledge acquired previously. For example, familiarity with pouring water from cups into the bathtub might lead to the introduction of a funnel, a sieve, or a can with holes punched in it. The same items carried to the sandbox will produce entirely new results for the child. As a guideline for the development of intrinsic motivation, Ellis (1973) proposed that activities should be paced to the next developmental level, possess sufficient complexity to require investigation, be manipulable and responsive, and pose questions to be pondered by the child.

Advances in technology and computer applications have opened up a new world of play for even the most severely disabled child. Langley (1990) provided a thorough review of many toys that are suitable for children with physical disabilities. More traditional toys and materials, however, may still require modification by the occupational therapist (Lemire, 1988). The size, shape, weight, and consistency of materials may need to be adapted to suit the individual child (Anderson et al, 1987). A toy library may be helpful, allowing parents to borrow the more expensive electronic toys or to test adapted toys on a trial basis. Equipment modifications (e.g., an adapted playground, foot straps and back rests for a tricycle) may also serve to make an out-of-bounds activity accessible to the child. The "toys" that normal children discover in cupboards, basements, and backyards (e.g., pots and pans, insects, cardboard boxes, sticks) must not be overlooked for the child with a disability. As Diamond (1981), a physically disabled adult, pointed out, spitting 3 ft away and playing in the mud are also accomplishments for the child.

Summary

Free play has been proposed in this paper as a vitalizing element in the development of the whole child. The experiences derived from childhood play include exploration, mastery, decision making, achievement, increased motivation, and competency—qualities that will, eventually help children to develop occupational roles and to become more productive members of society (Bundy, 1989). Children—already restricted by physical limitations who are not given adequate opportunities to engage in free play may be acquiring secondary disabilities, including diminished motivation, imagination, and creativity; poorly developed social skills; and increased dependence. The occupational therapist may be able to prevent some of these secondary problems by enhancing free play opportunities for the child who has a physical disability.

Acknowledgments

The development of this paper was supported in part by scholarships awarded to the first author by the Easter Seal Research Institute and the Social Sciences and Humanities Research Council of Canada.

References

Anderson, J., Hinojosa, J., & Strauch, C. (1987). Integrating play in neurodevelopmental treatment. *American Journal of Occupational Therapy, 41*, 421–426. (Reprinted as Chapter 46).

Ayres, A. J. (1981). *Sensory integration and the child.* Los Angeles: Western Psychological Services.

Behnke, C. J., & Fetkovich, M. M. (1984). Examining the reliability and validity of The Play History. *American Journal of Occupational Therapy, 38*, 94–100.

Brooks-Gunn, J., & Lewis, M. (1982a). Affective exchanges between normal and handicapped infants and their mothers. In T. Field & A. Fogel (Eds.), *Emotion and early interaction* (pp. 161–188). Hillsdale, NJ: Erlbaum.

Brooks-Gunn, J., & Lewis, M. (1982b). Development of play behavior in handicapped and normal infants. *Topics in Early Childhood Special Education, 2* (3), 14–27.

Brown, M., & Gordon, W. A. (1987). Impact of impairment on activity patterns of children. *Archives of Physical Medicine and Rehabilitation, 68*, 828–832.

Bundy, A. (1989, November). Play: The occupation of childhood. Workshop presented to the Occupational Therapy Play Research Group, Hamilton, Ontario.

Calder, J. E. (1980). Learn to play –Play to learn. In J. K. Atkinson (Ed.), *Too late at eight. Prevention and intervention, young children's learning difficulties* (pp. 163–188). Brisbane, Australia: Fred & Eleanor Schonell Educational Research Centre.

Clarke, M. M., Riach, J., & Cheyne, W. M. (1982). Handicapped children and pre-school education [Report to Warnock Committee on Special Education, University of Strathclyde]. Cited in M. Philip & D. Duckworth (Eds.), *Children with disabilities and their families*. Windsor, England: NFER-Nelson. (Original report published 1977).

Cotton, N. (1984). Childhood play as an analog to adult capacity to work. *Child Psychiatry and Human Development, 14*, 135–144.

Crawley, S. B., & Spiker, D. (1983). Mother-child interactions involving two-year-olds with Down syndrome: A look at individual differences. *Child Development, 54*, 1312–1323.

Csikszentmihalyi, M. (1975). Play and intrinsic rewards. *Humanistic Psychology, 15*, 41–63.

Cunningham, C. E., & Barkley, R. A. (1979). The interactions of normal and hyperactive children with their mothers in free play and structured tasks. *Child Development, 50*, 217–224.

Diamond, S. (1981). Growing up with parents of a handicapped child: A handicapped person's perspective. In J. L. Paul (Ed.), *Understanding and working with parents of children with special needs* (pp. 23–50). New York: Holt, Rinehart & Winston.

Ellis, M. J. (1973). *Why people play.* Englewood Cliffs, NJ: Prentice-Hall.

Erikson, E. (1963). *Childhood and society.* New York: Norton.

Federlein, A. C. (1979, April). *A study of play behavior and interactions of preschool handicapped children in mainstreamed and segregated settings*. Paper presented at the annual meeting of the Council for Exceptional Children, Dallas, TX.

Field, T. (1980). Self, teacher, toy, and peer-directed behaviors of handicapped preschool children. In T. Field, S. Goldberg, D. Stein, & A. Sostek (Eds.), *High-risk infants and children: Adult and peer interactions* (pp. 313–360). New York: Academic Press.

Field, T., Roseman, S., de Stefano, L. J., & Koewler, J. (1982). The play of handicapped preschool children with handicapped and nonhandicapped peers in integrated and nonintegrated settings. *Topics in Early Childhood Special Education, 2* (3), 28–38.

Florey, L. L. (1981). Studies of play: Implications for growth, development, and for clinical practice. *American Journal of Occupational Therapy, 35,* 519–524.

Foster, M., Berger, M., & McLean, M. (1981). Rethinking a good idea: A reassessment of parent involvement. *Topics in Early Childhood Special Education, 1* (3), 55–65.

Garvey, C. (1977). *Play.* Cambridge, MA: Harvard University Press.

Gralewicz, A. (1973). Play deprivation in multihandicapped children. *American Journal of Occupational Therapy, 27,* 7072.

Gunn, S. L. (1975). Play as occupation: Implications for the handicapped. *American Journal of Occupational Therapy, 29,* 222–225.

Hanzlik, J. (1989). The effect of intervention on the free play experience for mothers and their infants with developmental delay and cerebral palsy. *Physical and Occupational Therapy in Pediatrics, 2* (2), 33–51.

Hanzlik, J., & Stevenson, M. (1986). Mother-infant interaction in families with infants who are mentally retarded, mentally retarded with cerebral palsy or nonretarded. *American Journal of Mental Deficiency, 77,* 492–497.

Henderson, G., & Bryan, W. V. (1984). *Psychosocial aspects of disability.* Springfield, IL: Charles C Thomas.

Hewett, S., Newson, J., & Newson, E. (1970). *The family and the handicapped child.* Chicago: Aldine Publishing.

Kaiser, C. F. (1982). *Young and special.* Baltimore: University Park Press.

Kaiser, C. E., & Hayden, A. H. (1984). Clinical research and policy issues in parenting severely handicapped infants. In J. Blacher (Ed.), *Severely handicapped young children and their families* (pp. 275–317). Orlando: Academic Press.

Kibele, A. (1989). Occupational therapy's role in improving the quality of life for persons with cerebral palsy. *American Journal of Occupational Therapy, 43,* 371–377.

Kielhofner, G., & Barris, R. (1984). Collecting data on play: A critique of available methods. *Occupational Therapy Journal of Research, 4,* 150–180.

Knox, S. (1989, April). *The power of play as therapeutic media.* Paper presented at the 69th Annual Conference of the American Occupational Therapy Association, Baltimore, MD.

Kogan, K. L. (1980). Interaction systems between preschool handicapped or developmentally delayed children and their parents. In T. Field, S. Goldberg, D. Stein, & A. Sostek (Eds.), *High-risk infants and children: Adult and peer interactions* (pp. 227–247). New York: Academic Press.

Kogan, K. L., Tyler, N., & Turner, P. (1974). The process of interpersonal adaptation between mothers and their cerebral palsied children. *Developmental Medicine and Child Neurology, 16,* 518–527.

Langley, M. B. (1990). A developmental approach to the use of toys for facilitation of environmental control. *Physical and Occupational Therapy in Pediatrics, 10* (2), 69–91,

Lemire, E. (1988). Toy adaptations in pediatrics. *Occupational Therapy in Health Care, 5,* 87–93.

Levitt, E., & Cohen, S. (1977). Parents as teachers: A rationale for involving parents in the education of their young handicapped children. In L. G. Katz (Ed.), *Current topics in early childhood education* (Vol. 1, pp. 165–178). Norwood, NJ: Ablex.

Levitt, S. (1975). A study of the gross-motor skills of cerebral palsied children in an adventure playground for handicapped children. *Child: Care, Health and Development, 1,* 2943.

Lindquist, J. E., Mack, W., & Parham, L. D. (1982). A synthesis of occupational behavior and sensory integration concepts in theory and practice, part 2: Clinical applications. *American Journal of Occupational Therapy, 36,* 433–437.

Mack, W., Lindquist, J. E., & Parham, L. D. (1982). A synthesis of occupational behavior and sensory integration concepts in theory and practice, part 1. Theoretical foundations. *American Journal of Occupational Therapy, 36,* 365–374.

Matsutsuyu, J. (1971). Occupational behavior -A perspective on work and play. *American Journal of Occupational Therapy, 25,* 291–294.

McHale, S. M., & Olley, J. G. (1982). Using play to facilitate the social development of handicapped children. *Topics in Early Childhood Special Education, 2* (3), 76–86.

Mogford, K. (1977). The play of handicapped children. In B. Tizard & D. Harvey (Eds.), *Biology of play* (pp. 170–184). London: Spastics International.

Oster, K (1984). *Physical disabilities in children: An exploratory study in mother and child interactions.* Unpublished doctoral dissertation, University of Toronto.

Parten, M. B. (1932). Social participation among preschool children. *Journal of Abnormal Psychology, 27,* 243–269.

Philip, M., & Duckworth, D. (1982). *Children with disabilities and their families.* Windsor, England: NFER-Nelson.

Piaget, J. (1951). *Play, dreams and imitation in childhood.* New York: Norton.

Piaget, J. (1952). *The origins of intelligence in children.* New York: Norton.

Rast, M. (1986). Play and therapy, play or therapy.? In The American Occupational Therapy Association, Inc., *Play. A skill for life* [Monograph] (pp. 29–4 1). Rockville, MD: American Occupational Therapy Association.

Reilly, M. (1974). *Play as exploratory learning.* Beverly Hills, CA: Sage.

Robinson, A. L. (1977). Play: The arena for acquisition of rules for competent behavior. *American Journal of Occupational Therapy, 31,* 248–253.

Rogers, S. J. (1988). Characteristics of social interactions between mothers and their disabled infants: A review. *Child: Care, Health and Development, 14,* 301–317.

Rubin, K. H., Fein, G. G., & Vandenberg, B. (1983). Play. In P. H. Mussen & E. M. Hetherington (Eds.), *Handbook of child psychology* (Vol. 4, pp. 693–774). New York: Wiley.

Russell, P. (1978). *The wheelchair child.* London: Souvenir Press.

Salomon, M. K. (1983). Play therapy with the physically handicapped. In C. E. Schaeffer & K. J. O'Connor (Eds.), *Handbook of play therapy* (pp. 455–469). New York: Wiley.

Sheridan, M. D. (1975). The importance of spontaneous play in the fundamental learning of handicapped children. *Child: Care, Health and Development, 1,* 3–17.

Sparling, J. W., Walker, D. F., & Singdahlsen, J. (1984). Play techniques with neurologically impaired preschoolers. *American Journal of Occupational Therapy, 38,* 603–612.

Stout, J. (1988). Planning playgrounds for children with disabilities. *American Journal of Occupational Therapy, 42,* 653–657.

Vandenberg, B., & Kielhofner, G. (1982). Play in evolution, culture, and individual adaptation: Implications for therapy. *American Journal of Occupational Therapy, 36,* 20–28.

Weininger, 0. (1979). *Play and education: The basic tool for early childhood learning.* Springfield, IL: Charles C Thomas.

Weininger, 0. (1980). The learning potential of play. *Canadian Journal of Early Childhood Education, 1,* 21–28.

Weininger, 0. (1988). "What if" and "as if": Imagination and pretend play in early childhood. In K. Egan & D. Nadaner (Eds.), *Imagination and education* (pp. 141–149). New York: Teachers College Press.

Weininger, O., & Fitzgerald, D. (1988). Symbolic play and interhemispheric integration: Some thoughts on a neuropsychological model of play. *Journal of Research and Development in Education, 21* (4), 23–40.

Williams, S. E., & Matesi, D. V. (1988). Therapeutic intervention with an adapted toy. *American Journal of Occupational Therapy, 42,* 673–676.

Yawkey, T. D., Dank, H. L., & Glossenger, F. L. (1986). *Playing. Inside and out.* Lancaster, PA: Technomic Publishing.

Chapter 26

Parent-Child Activity Group Treatment in Preventive Psychiatry

Laurette Olson, MA, OTR
Colleen Heaney, MS
Bettye Soppas-Hoffman, MA, OTR

This chapter was previously published jointly in *Health Promotion and Preventive Programs: Models of Occupational Therapy Practice*, (Haworth Press, 1989) and *Occupational Therapy in Health Care*, 6 (1):29–43. Copyright © 1989, The Haworth Press, Inc.

The New York Hospital-Cornell Medical Center, Westchester Division, and a local day care center engaged in a contract to offer a comprehensive psychiatric treatment program for at-risk families. In addition to the mutual recognition of a need for psychiatric services, the hospital administration was eager to increase its profile in the community by engaging in outreach projects. Additionally, the day care administration was eager to participate in a program that would support parents while assisting the center in managing and maintaining children who were beginning to display behavioral problems.

This chapter will focus on the role that an occupational therapist and a counseling therapist had in proposing and co-leading a parent-child activity group. The rationale, goals, and methods were based on theories of attachment, play, and occupational therapy. The goals of this activity group were to shape the child's behavior so that his approach to his parent would most likely elicit positive attention and to shape the parent's response so that the child's needs were addressed effectively. The method included a mother's prediscussion group that focused on parent-child activity interactions at home and throughout the activity group. The leaders then facilitated play between the mothers and children. The activities were planned and structured to enhance the adaptive capacities of the families to interact in ways that promote growth and satisfaction.

As secondary prevention, this service was designed to inhibit dysfunction through the development of better coping skills within the parent and child relationship. Attachment theory emphasizes the importance of a secure and mutually pleasurable parent-child relationship in a child's development.

Environment and Systems Influenes

The primary author was invited to join a consultation and service planning group consisting of administrators from the day care center, and a psychiatrist and a nurse practitioner from the medical center. Occupational therapy services were recruited because occupational therapy was recognized as offering concrete and pragmatic services to improve parent-child interaction. The primary author had developed parent-child activity groups on the Child Inpatient Unit. Therapeutic Activities staff had continuously led the groups for three years with acknowledgment and support within the hospital system. The day care administrators were interested in contracting for this type of service, as it was easily understood by educators and more easily explained to parents than was psychotherapy.

The day care educational coordinator, with the help of her teachers, identified those children who were developing major behavior problems in day care and who had negative interaction patterns with their parents. She referred each parent and child to the hospital team after getting parental agreement to accept services.

Frame of Reference

Of great importance to a child's development is his ability to play. Reilly (1974) theorizes that play is the vehicle through which a child learns the rules of sensorimotor activities, then the rules of objects and people, and finally, the rules of thinking.

Cotton (1984) discusses the major strides of children in their problem-solving abilities through play. Play is also the medium through which specific activity skills, ego strength, and the capacity to cope with anxiety are developed. But, most importantly, play fosters the child's development of an investment in life. This is central for human adaptation and success in life roles (e.g., student, worker, parent).

As a child plays, he is learning what he can do. As he is challenged in play, he is at times overwhelmed and retreats. A parent who is "quietly available" to engage in the play is important (Mahler, 1975). Winnicott (1971) discusses the importance of a parent being available to "hold the situation." "Holding" play involves offering physical comfort, verbal assurance, encouragement, direction or engaging in the activity. The goal is to enable the child to maintain his play.

In a series of longitudinal studies, Murphy and Moriarty (1976) examined characteristics of the mother-child relationship which seemed to help or hinder the child's development of coping skills. They defined coping as the child's way of dealing with new and difficult situations resulting in competence or mastery. When a child can cope, he has a range of resources for gratification. He is invested in figuring out and interacting with his environment. He finds many types of experiences pleasurable and seeks stimulation rather than avoiding it. Murphy and Moriarty stressed that the quality of the mother's enjoyment of her child is the most critical variable. Her active support and encouragement and her accurate understanding of the child's unique way of coping are also important factors.

Attachment is an enduring, emotional, discriminating bond between a parent and child which develops through interaction. According to Bowlby (1969), attachment promotes a relationship which protects a child from danger. It also provides the opportunity to socialize him progressively for the biological advantage of the human group. Stroufe (1977) expanded this theory by emphasizing the role of attachment in supporting the child's exploration of the environment as flexibility and, problem solving are major advantages for human beings. He discusses attachment as the flexible organization of behavior in both parent and child that supports the child's development.

Ainsworth (1967) developed the concept of the parent as a secure base. Her classic studies examined the quality of the relationship between parent and child by examining the behavior of the child at reunion with his mother after a brief separation. Children were classified as securely or insecurely attached with sub-classifications in each category. A securely attached child seeks out the parent for comfort upon reunion but then can re-engage in a separate activity or continue to explore the environment.

The secure child develops a working model in which the parent is perceived as responsive and readily available. Secure attachment promotes the child's independence, facilitating rather than restricting separation and fostering exploratory and other adaptive responses even in unfamiliar settings. More recent investigations by Ainsworth et al., (1978) have also shown that aspects of maternal behavior, specifically the mother's responsiveness and expression of positive affect, differentiate the securely attached child from the insecurely attached. The insecurely attached child, in contrast, is less readily comforted, may avoid the parent at reunion or may display ambivalent behavior such as alternately moving toward or away from the parent.

Studies exploring the outcome of secure attachment in infancy have suggested a positive correlation with the child's later development of competence. In followup studies, Matas (1978) investigated the relationship between the quality of attachment in infancy and the problem-solving skills of two-year olds. His study demonstrated that toddlers who showed more secure attachment relationships as infants were more enthusiastic, persistent and cooperative during play involving tool use and problem solving. Toddlers who were more insecurely attached infants were more easily frustrated by challenges, could not use their parents as resources and demonstrated more resistant behaviors (e.g., hitting and kicking).

Arend (1979) examined the relationship between the quality of infant-mother attachment at eighteen months and measures of competence at five years. Children who had been more securely attached as infants scored higher on measures related to the child's resourcefulness, flexibility, and engagement during difficult, challenging tasks. Arend suggested that effective infant-mother attachment supports toddlers' early attempts at exploration and mastery which, in turn, support continued positive engagement and development of confidence.

Lieberman (1977) and Waters (1979) found correlations between secure attachment in infancy and competence and social comfort with peers. Children who had been classified as insecurely attached were, at three and a half years, more socially withdrawn and more hesitant to engage with peers than securely attached children.

In a 1983 study by Stroufe et al., preschool children who were classified as securely attached at twelve and eighteen months were found to be more competent in seeking instrumental assistance from their teachers when their own resources were insufficient. The authors interpreted this as skill in being effectively dependent. In contrast, children who were rated as insecurely attached were highly dependent on their teachers; they sought significantly more guidance and physical contact and were disciplined more frequently.

Bowlby (1969) posits a range of intensity of the attachment behaviors. The child uses low-intensity attachment behavior to gain parental attention for play and stimulation. The child smiles, talks, initiates playful interchanges in ways appropriate to his developmental age to seduce the parent or caretaker. Most often, the parent responds to the child's initiation, elaborates on the play, and communicates interest, pleasure and approval of the child at concrete and symbolic levels. Low-intensity attachment behavior comprises the highest proportion of behavior that a young child directs toward attachment figures over the course of a day. Such behaviors cement the reciprocal bond between the parent and child.

High-intensity attachment behavior is elicited in response to fearful events and situational or biological distress in the child. The child attracts the care giver, for example, by crying, clinging, or running to her to relieve the distress. The parent soothes the infant by rocking and feeding him, for example. The parental response is dependent upon the situation and the age of the child. The goal of both parent and child in these situations is to lessen the level of distress so that the child's internal emotional equilibrium is restored, and both parent and child can return to their separate activities.

Heard (1987) wrote that Winnicott's concept of parental "holding" (1971) is consistent with attachment theory. The behavior that a child displays to elicit parental "holding" of play fits on the continuum between high- and low-intensity attachment behavior. When a child becomes frustrated or overwhelmed by challenges faced in play, he withdraws from it. He attracts the parent by a change in affect and by seeking parental contact and instrumental assistance. Optimal parent-child interaction in this situation of moderate intensity enables the child to develop the most adaptive coping skills (Murphy and Moriarty, 1976).

Main, in a 1987 presentation for the National Center for Clinical Infant Programs, stated that the quality of an attachment relationship is dynamic and has the potential to change as the child develops. Changes in the stresses or coping skills of family members affect the security of the attachment.

The basic theoretical concepts of occupational therapy were fundamental to the inception of the program. The activity of play served as an integral part of the parent-child interaction and provided opportunity for immediate integration and practice of new behaviors. The parent and child were actively engaged in the learning process with the resultant opportunity to learn from the immediate reinforcement. The selection of activities for the group was based on task analysis of the cognitive, perceptual and interpersonal components relative to the developmental skills of the three- and four-year olds.

Program Description

Organization

The hospital team responsible for this project had a traditional medical model organization. The psychiatrist and the medical residents that he supervised were responsible for the overall coordination of the cases. The residents provided the initial assessments and individual play or psychotherapy as needed. Only those families receiving psychiatric services by a resident could be referred to the group. Reimbursement for outpatient services in this teaching hospital is based on resident involvement in each case.

The services offered by the occupational therapist and the counseling therapist who co-led the group were directly coordinated with the day care administrator for educational services. The occupational therapist met with the administrator to discuss outreach, the specific cases and the organization of the service.

Support

As the Therapeutic Activities supervisor for child and adolescent services at the hospital, the primary author was encouraged to increase the breadth of the services offered and to be responsive to the trends in community outreach. Since this was a newly developing project, the primary author led the group with a counseling therapist experienced in community outreach. Financial support was provided through Medicaid and private insurance.

Participants

The liaison between the hospital and the day care center was initiated by the Medical Director of the Child and Adolescent Division at the New York Hospital-Cornell Medical Center, Westchester Division in White Plains, New York and the administrator of the White Plains Day Care Center. A psychiatrist and nurse practitioner from the hospital and administrator, educational coordinator, psychologist and other day care staff met to develop the direction for the program. After initial meetings where priorities were established, the primary author joined these meetings to discuss a parent child activity group. She and the counseling therapist then met with the educational coordinator to plan specifically for the implementation of the group.

The group members included four single mothers in their twenties and their preschool children. Two mothers were divorced from reportedly abusive men; two had never married. Only one child consistently saw his father. One mother attended the group with two children; the others had one child each. The racial, ethnic and educational backgrounds of the members were varied. One parent worked sporadically at blue collar jobs, and one did not work. Two families received public assistance.

The children, two boys and three girls, ranged in age from two and one-half years to four and one-half years old at the start of the group.

Services Provided

The parent-child activity group was conceptualized with attachment and play theories as frames of reference. The group format was selected based upon Yalom's concepts of the curative factors in group treatment. Yalom (1970) suggests that groups provide opportunity for participants to imitate, observe, and integrate the adaptive behavior of others. Groups also provide a safe environment to examine negative behaviors since the participants share common concerns.

The use of activity is intrinsic to occupational therapy. Fidler and Fidler (1978) (see Chapter 7) discussed the value of "learning by doing." Feedback from meaningful activity allows a person to recognize his potential and limitations. With this information, he can master and/or adapt to life situations.

Play was the chosen activity since it is the primary mode of communication and learning for a child. Mutual play between parent and child is also proposed to cement the attachment bond (Bowlby 1969). The play within the group was divided into two distinct periods. During the first period, parents assisted their child in constructional play. During the second period, each parent–child dyad engaged in free play.

Constructional play is activity in which a child builds, contrives or elaborates on materials or objects from his own mental images or ideas for no purpose other than the pleasure derived from the activity. It is one of the most effective types of play to develop concentration, problem solving, and imagination in a child (Sylva 1984). The parent frequently was provided with opportunities to assist in the play activities. During constructional play, the parent was helped to guide her child's play through support, structure, guidance and modeling from the leaders and by observing other group members.

Guided play utilizes encouragement, demonstration, and assistance, not control. During constructional play, a child frequently seeks out praise and positive regard for his work; his excitement and pride are infectious. Following a child's success, parents expressed similar emotions over their success in helping their children create something that was appealing.

The subsequent free play period afforded each parent-child dyad an opportunity to practice negotiating the choice of a mutual play activity. The choices in the day care playroom were varied. Puzzles, building toys, games, dolls and other items for imaginary play were available. This phase permitted enhanced opportunities for the parent-child dyad to learn to attract, engage, and enjoy one another through play.

Through these play experiences, children learned that they could depend upon their parents to share interest and excitement, to consistently help and praise, and to engage in a reciprocal and satisfying relationship, at least within the group. The strength of the children's investment in this group was striking to all members of the team.

Consistent with Yalom's discussion of interpersonal learning (1970), these families were reexposed to a situation (mutual play) which they had not handled successfully in the past. In a benign and supportive environment, they learned that parent-child play was possible and could be mutually pleasurable, satisfying, and growth promoting for both parties. The acquisition of positive attachment and caretaking behaviors within the group, along with persistent vigilance in the application of that behavior, led to some transfer of the skill to the home environment.

Case Study

The following case example will describe a typical parent-child interaction and interventions of the group leaders.

Presenting Problems

Ms. Carlton,* a twenty-six-year-old, single, fully employed woman and her three and one-half-year-old daughter, Laura, attended the group. The day care educational coordinator, as well as Ms. Carlton, were concerned with Laura's obstreperous attention seeking behavior, poor interaction skills with other children, inability to respond to limit setting and impaired relationships with teachers and other authority figures. Ms. Carlton reluctantly agreed to the suggested services as she recognized that the problem was worsening.

Treatment

During the first several sessions, significant problems with attachment were evident. Ms. Carlton often was uninvolved, made minimal efforts to discipline, minimal

*All names of parents and children are fictitious.

or no efforts to assist her child with activity, and offered neither positive nor negative reinforcement. Laura, in an effort to get attention, consistently became disruptive.

In subsequent sessions, however, some change was noted. Both Ms. Carlton and Laura made efforts to engage with one another and with the group. Ms. Carlton, though, became quickly critical of Laura during interactions, permitting the child no opportunity for experimentation or independence. She demanded perfection in the activity project, anticipated that Laura would make a mess of things and exhibited no pleasure in the encounter or in the end product. When Laura was unable or unwilling to do the task absolutely in accordance with her mother's expectations, Ms. Carlton would simply exclude her and work on the project independently. On one occasion, she struck Laura for not following her activity directions .

During all of the sessions, leaders provided role modeling for Ms. Carlton. They disciplined Laura when indicated, praised her for positive behavior, and took over the interaction when Ms. Carlton was overwhelmed. Ms. Carlton was requested to observe the leader interventions and try to emulate them. The mother and child were constantly reminded of the group goals.

Over time, Laura engaged in the group more qualitatively. The turning point was evident in one session when Laura became very interested in a tee shirt painting project. She was enthusiastic about her mother's presence; she demonstrated interest in working on a task with her mother ; and she slowly began to respond to leader intervention. However, whenever power struggles evolved over the task, Laura would fulfill her mother's prophecy and resort to disruptive behavior that included temper tantrums, whining, wandering, refusal to interact and resistance to authority. Ms. Carlton would express her annoyance and appreared humiliated and resigned to what she felt was a willfully provacative child, determined to undermine her mother.

Subsequently, Laura was redirected to her mother during the group and Ms. Carlton increasingly was making efforts to follow the leaders' interaction style. Slowly, the mother and child interacted in a more positive manner, appeared to enjoy their time together, expressed pride in the projects and in one another, and began to do similar play activities at home. Ms. Carlton verbalized that she thought th egroup was helping because Laura was becoming more cooperative.

During one of the final sessions, Ms. Carlton stated that she had gained insight into how her negative, unnurturing, impatient behavior toward Laura triggered the child's disruptive behavior, leading to a vicious cycle. She recalled her earlier experiences inthe group and articulated changes in the interaction pattern. She also stated with pleasure and pride, "Laura is not a bad kid."

Outcome

The method of monitoring change within the parent-child activity group was through examining extensive weekly progress notes on each family. The leaders met immediately following the group session. Process notes provided a non-intrusive way of studying phenomena and generating hypotheses. Vasta (1979) in his book, *Studying Children: An Introduction to Research Methods* describes systematic descriptive observations as valid to the extent that what is observed is clearly identified and representative. Notes were organized around concerns related to the child attachment behaviors and the parents' reciprocal responses. Parents' reports of interactions at home were also noted. The written recordings were made over the entire period of treatment.

The educators provided feedback on a regular basis in formal and informal meetings related to the progress of these families in the day care center. Although feedback was very positive, the group was not evaluated in a formalized manner.

Positive changes were noted in the target population treated by the group. Day care staff reported that the children's behavior stabilized and was less problematic. More positive parent-child interchanges at the day care center were reported by the educational coordinator. For example, one mother who in the past generally ignored her daughter and was not observed offering the child praise, brought her parent-child project to the day care center a few days after a group meeting. Both parent and child sought the praise of the educational coordinator with enthusiasm and animation.

The parent participants also expressed more pleasure in their children. They discussed successful attempts to engage with their offspring in mutual activity at home. They also demonstrated more concern and interest in providing appropriate play materials and space for the children's solitary play at home.

Additional assessment measures would be of use in clearly establishing the efficacy of the parent child activity group. Videotaping these sessions and analyzing the tapes to examine the competency of the parent's caretaking skills and the child's coping skills would be attempted. Those behaviors most commonly cited in the literature as signifying competency would be rated. In this way, those behaviors most amenable to change by this treatment method would be identified. The Teaching Scale and the Home Observation for Measurement of the Home Environment of the Nursing Child Assessment (1978) would provide useful pre- and post-testing data, though it was designed to be used with mothers and their children who are under the age of three. Most of the items are still applicable throughout the preschool years, but some items should be added or adjusted to reflect the child's further development during the third, fourth, and fifth years and the parent's reciprocal changes in approach to the child.

Conclusion

The occupational therapist became a participant in the community outreach program because of an identified need. Once initiated, the parent-child activity group was embraced readily by the day care center. It was the least threatening and most easily understood service for parents. The viability of occupational therapy as a preventive service within a day care program was very clear. As reimbursement was tied to Resident training, services were limited by that training program.

References

1. Ainsworth, M. (1967), "Object relations, dependency and attachment: A theoretical review of the infant-mother relationship." *Child Development, 40,* 969–1025.

2. Ainsworth, M., Blehar, M., Waters, E., Wall, S. (1978), *Patterns of Attachment—A Psychological Study of the Strange Situation.* Hillsdale, NJ: Lawrence Erlbaum Associates, Publisher.

3. Arend, R., Gore, F.L., Stroufe, L.A. (1979), "Continuity of individual adaptation from infancy to kindergarten: A predictive study of ego resilience and curiosity in pre-schoolers." *Child Development, 50,* 950–957.

4. Barnard, Kathryn (1978), Nursing Child Assessment Satellite Training. University of Washington, School of Nursing.

5. Bowlby, John (1969), *Attachment and Loss* (Vol. 1). New York: Basic Books, Inc.

6. Cotton, Nancy (1984), "Childhood play as an analog to adult capacity to work." *Child Psychiatry and Human Development, 14* (31), 135–144.

7. Dowdney, L., Mrazek, D., Quinton, D., Rutter, M. (1984), "Observation of parent-child interaction with two to three year olds." *Journal of Child Psychology and Psychiatry.* July, 379–407.

8. Fidler, G.S. and Fidler, J.W., (1978), "Doing and becoming: Purposeful action and self actualization." *American Journal of Occupational Therapy, 32* (5), 305–310. (Reprinted as Chapter 7).

9. Fine, S. (1983), "Occupational therapy: The role of rehabilitation and purposeful activity in mental health practice." Statement of practice approved as a White Paper by the Executive Board of American Occupational Therapy Association.

10. Heard, D.H. (1978), "From object relations to attachment theory: A basis for family therapy." *British Journal of Medical Psychology, 51,* 67–76.

11. Heard, D.H. (1981), "The relevance of attachment theory to child psychiatric practice." *Journal of Child Psychology and Psychiatry, 22,* 89–96.

12. Kiser, L., Bates, J., et al. (1986), "Mother-infant play at six months as a predictor of attachment security at thirteen months." *Journal of the American Academy of Child Psychiatry.* January, 68–75.

13. Lieberman, A.F. (1977), "Pre-schoolers' competence with a peer: Influence of attachment and social experience." *Child Development, 48,* 1277–1287.

14. Lytton, H., (1980), *Attachment in Parent-Child Interaction,* New York: Plenum Press.

15. Mahler, M.S., Pine, F., Bergman, A. (1975), *The Psychological Birth of the Human Infant,* New York: Basic Books.

16. Main, M. (Dec. 1987), Presentation titled "Influencing and interrupting cycles of maladaptation—Insights from attachment and object relations theory and research" at the Fifth Biennial National Training Institute of the National Center for Clinical and Infant Programs, Washington, DC.

17. Matas, L., Arend, R., Stroufe, L.A. (1978), "Continuity of adaptation in the second year: The relationship of the quality of attachment and later competence." *Child Development, 49,* 547–556.

18. Murphy, L. (I 967), *The Widening World of Childhood.* New York: Basic Books, Inc.

19. Murphy, L., Moriarty, A. (1976), *Vulnerability, Coping and Growth from Infancy to Adolescence.* New Haven and London: Yale University Press.

20. Parker, G. (1983), "The mother-child tie: Its nature and factors influencing its evolution" in *Parental Overprotection, A Risk Factor in Psychosocial Development.* New York: Grune and Stratton, Inc.

21. Reilly, M. (1974), *Play as Exploratory Learning.* Beverly Hills: Sage Publications.

22. Siegel, I., Dreyer, A., McGillicuddy-Delisi, A. (1984), "Psychological perspectives of the family" in *The Family Review of Child Development Research #7.* Edited by Ross Parke, Chicago and London: The University of Chicago Press.

23. Smale, S. et al. (1980), "Evolving concepts of attachment" in *The Child in His Family,* edited by E. James Anthony and Colette Chiland, John Wiley and Sons, Inc.

24. Stroufe, L.A., Fox, N.E., Pancake, V.R. (1983), "Attachment and dependency in developmental perspective," *Child Development, 54,* 1615–1627.

25. Stroufe, L.A., Waters, E. (1977), "Attachment as an organizational construct," *Child Development, 48,* 1184–1199.

26. Stern, D. (1977), *The First Relationship—Infant and Mother.* Cambridge, MA: Harvard University Press.

27. Sylva, K. (1984), "A hard-headed look at the fruits of play," *Early Child Development and Care, 15,* 171–184.

28. Vasta, R. (1979), *Studying Children: An Introduction to Research Methods.* San Francisco: W. H. Freeman.

29. Waters, E., Wittman, J., Stroufe, L.A. (1979), "Attachment, positive affect and competence in the peer group: Two studies in construct validation." *Child Development, 50,* 821–829.

30. Winnicott, D.W. (1971), *Playing and Reality.* London: Tavistock Publications.

31. Yalom, I. (1974), *The Theory, and Practice of Group Psychotherapy.* New York: Basic Books, Inc.

Chapter 27

The Adolescent Life/Work Planning Group: A Prevention Model

Grace Gorski, OTR

Shawn Miyake, MA, OTR

This chapter was previously published jointly in *Occupational Therapy and Adolescents with Disability*, (Haworth Press, 1985) and *Occupational Therapy in Health Care, 2*, (3), 139-150 Copyright © 1985, The Haworth Press, Inc.

The adolescent passage has traditionally been viewed as a very turbulent period in the individual life span.[1,2,3] This view continues to be prevalent, especially today, as concerned parents and professionals watch young people struggle to find an adult role in an increasingly complex society. Various developmental tasks need to be accomplished and choices made that often critically influence future life satisfaction.[4,5] Now, more than ever adolescents are experiencing confusion and lack of direction for their lives; parents voice concern but feel helpless in offering guidance. Some suggest the schools have somehow been unsuccessful in providing the vital link between education and an effective transition into adult life.[2,3] This paper focuses on the adolescent passage, the issues relevant to the developmental period and offers suggestions for an outpatient life/work planning group designed to assist adolescents from the well population in making a more effective transition into adulthood. In implementing such a program occupational therapy has an opportunity to widen its service base by assuming a preventive role in health care.

The Adolescent Passage

Adolescence can be basically defined as a time when the dependence of childhood is left behind and the independence of adulthood is embraced.[4] Because this is a transitional phase of life, social expectations are often unclear as the adolescent strives to find his own societal niche. Adolescents wonder about who they are and where they are headed.[5] Recent magazine reports have pointed to the ever present need for adolescents to attach themselves to various movements for self-identity. The "punk" and "religious" movements are two such modern examples. This need by adolescents for discovering their identity and place in society is the same yesterday, today and will continue into tomorrow.

A recent television newscast[6] pointed out the lack of connectedness adolescents feel from their school experience and their upcoming adult life. Despite the fact the educational system is a supposed preparatory ground for successful adaptation to adult life, young people sometimes fail to grasp important connections. On this particular newscast an adolescent was heard to say, "mathematics, who needs to study mathematics, after all what job uses mathematics?" Educator Maurice Gibbons[7] emphasizes this apparent irrelevancy of education to later adult life in his pointed article based on a film called "Walkabout", a story of a primitive people's rite of passage into adulthood.

Today, adolescents are no longer steeped in the pretwentieth century work life where opportunities existed to learn about and practice various roles. For example, in the past a boy who wanted to learn about becoming a farmer like his father, merely worked alongside dad in a kind of apprenticeship position.

In contrast to the more practical opportunities of the past, today's youth are educated and then released into an adult working world to perform sometimes rather sophisticated roles.[3] Curiously enough, the educational process often occurs in isolation of the very context the adolescent is expected to progress into and perform within. The formal educational process, supposedly the vehicle by which opportunities for role selection and preparation are provided, is having trouble meeting the current challenge of teaching toward a broad spectrum of worker roles. To complicate the picture further these roles offer very vague if not altogether unclear pathways to their achievement. In the 1980's, the adolescent pursuing a possible career in nuclear engineering is not readily able to discern what interests, abilities and skills are necessary to perform such a job or how one's school experience necessarily ties in with that particular occupation. The job goal seems very distant. The trajectory to reach the goal is often not clear. Consequently, there is little understanding of how time spent in non-academic pursuits (e.g., leisure activities) relates to successful adult role performance.

Preparing for Employment

The central feature in the transition from adolescence to adulthood is preparation for employment.8 The major components of a successful transition are identified as: "education; opportunities to acquire a degree of personal autonomy; preparation for a social lifestyle, including personal and recreational pursuits; experiences to ac-

quire the skills for optimal independent living; and training and services to enhance the ability to earn one's own living. Maintaining employment and a satisfying adult lifestyle require more than just work content skills." [8,2]

In addition to the previous components, conclusions from a 1970 conference on delinquency prevention and controls outlined conditions necessary for positive youth development. They are as follows:

1. young people need to perceive that they have access to roles which give them a stake in the life of their community and they need opportunities to exercise these roles;
2. they need opportunities in communities whereby they can come to see themselves as competent and worthwhile;
3. they need real and perceived access to socially gratifying and desirable roles from which self-identity is developed.

It has been established that adolescents need to build skills in order to develop a stable foundation from which a satisfying and productive adult lifestyle can ensue. But equally important, adolescents need the perception that they have access to adult work roles.[1,3] From this perceived access, there derives a sense of identity and of meaning and value in society. Then adolescents feel that they have a place, a social niche to fit into which gives them hope for the future and expectations to work toward.

Prevention Programs

The components delineated above as necessary, for successful transition into adulthood can be the focus for a preventive program in occupational therapy in an outpatient setting. The following discussion describes a proposed life/work planning group targeted for adolescents from the well community. While most inpatient facilities offer remedial programs for a sick population, this kind of focus on the well adolescent can be considered preventive health care. The specific outpatient setting in consideration for this group serves outpatients with mental illness, but also people from its well community. Promoting itself as a 'wellness center', the institution is serving people with many special, health related needs with, for example, programs in assertiveness training and to stop smoking. As a part of a wellness concept the proposed adolescent group fits nicely. Funding now comes from private insurance for some of the wellness services; others are paid for out-of-pocket. With ever greater patient-paid shares of cost in health care, especially for additional services, wellness groups are increasingly well received by the community.

In addition, current statistics support the need for a group of this kind. It has been estimated that for every one percent rise in unemployment, an exponential increase occurs in mental hospital admissions, homicides, suicides and arrests. Clinical evidence exists that high school drop-out rates and youth unemployment are related closely to crimes of violence, vandalism, suicide, heavy drug abuse and delinquency.[1] While not all of these statistics can be linked to adolescents, youth are certainly well represented in them. This planned wellness group is designed to assist the adolescent in maximizing his potentials so that he views himself as a productive member of the community. The group may also be viewed as a welcome relief for parents at a loss for how best to help their child through these difficult years.

While it is not the purpose of this paper to present a complete picture in detail of what the adolescent group would be like, some basic guidelines and principles, and a possible format that others might use are suggested. The adolescent group as proposed would assist adolescents in making a smoother and more effective transition into an eventual occupational role and consequently prevent poor or very restricted decisions of occupational choice.

Characteristics of Persons Sought for the Group

The group would be composed of adolescents aged 14 to 20 years who are encountering one or several obstacles in making immediate and/or long range decisions concerning career choice. Problems may be reflective of basic lack of experience or information. Among those targeted for participation would be the adolescent who is confused and overwhelmed with the number of decisions he needs to make (e.g., how much education do I need? what skills must I have or acquire?), or the adolescent who is painfully aware of the expectation that he choose a possible career but who is struggling still with learning prerequisite skills (e.g., how to find a part-time job, or even how to fill out a job application and participate in a job interview).[1] Some adolescents, feeling immobilized, may overestimate their abilities such as by identifying a possible career which demands a higher level of intelligence than they possess. On the other hand, other adolescents may underestimate their potentials because they lack information about their personal assets or of the steps they must take to reach a certain goal. Others may prefer just not to think about career choice, hoping things will eventually fall into place.

Some adolescents may need additional support and guidance concerning their current interpersonal functioning with authority figures such as job supervisors or with peers. They may be able to find jobs but are not able to hold them due to run-ins with supervisors or trouble getting along with others on the job. Still others may be experiencing marginal academic success (poor grades) and may therefore view themselves as potential failures as workers. These are the types of concerns which would be addressed in an adolescent life/work planning group such as the one proposed.

Prerequisites for acceptance in the group would be evidence of adequate functioning in a high school setting or possession of a high school diploma, and a stable living situation such as with parents or some other caretaker. Since group members would be expected to engage in exploration and assignments outside of group sessions, it would also be necessary to have evidence of their ability to follow through and benefit from such routines. This could be determined through discussion with the adolescent himself and by collecting information from significant others, e.g., parents, teachers, community referral sources. Individuals motivated to engage in purposeful exploration rather than to depend on trial and error methods to make vocational decisions are the persons who would most benefit from this group.

Since leader(s) of the group would strive to provide general guidelines for all members as well as giving individualized support, the size of such a group should be small, perhaps 8 to 10 persons, male and female. Sessions, each lasting, an hour, would continue on a weekly basis for total of 10 to 12 weeks.

Characteristics of the Group Leader(s)

An occupational therapist, as a group leader for this kind of activity needs to be flexible and knowledgeable enough to function in several roles simultaneously during the course of the sessions. He will need to function as an information resource with extensive knowledge of jobs and of the community. He will also be a teacher of new skills. As a source of encouragement he will motivate individuals to grow. He will need to offer guidance and suggestions for specific courses of action based on individual, personal characteristics of participants as well as the realities of the work, school and community environments And finally, he will need to possess interpersonal sensitivity resulting from a broad knowledge of human behavior and adolescence in order to support and guide each participant according to their developmental needs.

Program Plan

It is proposed that the group activities be organized into five stages: (1) learning about oneself, (2) learning about the work world, (3) goal planning, (4) maximizing one's potentials and (5) closure. A description of each stage follows, including the primary goal for that stage along with examples of activities or exercises that could be used to move group members toward that goal. Flexibility in applying the proposed progression would be necessary to match the needs of participants. In addition, not all information and activities suggested are to be carried out in the 10- 12 week time frame, but are presented as a possible menu from which one could select options when organizing sessions.

Stage 1: Learning About Oneself (2 to 3 Sessions)

Goal: To have each participant explore his own individual characteristics, interests, values, special talents, hobbies, relationships and use of time ending in an assessment of both one's personal strengths and problem areas.

The opening session would focus on getting group leader(s) and group members to know each other. Also included would be descriptions of what the group is about, what subject areas are to be covered, an overview of the entire five stages as well as discussions among group members regarding their expectations from participating.

Group leader(s) will reflect with the group on the similarities and differences among group members and will encourage each participant to feel comfortable with growing at his own pace regardless of what others may be doing. Group members will also be encouraged to ask questions and to let their own needs and wants be known.

Possible Format: The activities in these early sessions will involve both paper and pencil exercises and group discussions.

Possible Exercises–Activities:
1. Getting-to-know-you exercise: every member talks for two minutes to a partner about himself, including such things as his name, school, what he likes to do, etc.[10]
2. Group members write one page about themselves including interests, goals in attending the classes, attitudes, abilities, limitations about career planning,[10] or Group leader(s) may pass out a sheet called 'personal self-evaluation' which contains structured questions to be answered concerning personal attributes, goals and such.
3. Given a list of personality characteristics, members will check those qualities they think they possess and will identify how they believe other people view them as individuals. They will also be asked to discriminate between personal characteristics they view as desirable and undesirable.
4. In a group discussion led by the leader(s) questions will be raised to get at content relevant to the goal which has not yet been revealed: are there strengths the members have not identified? things they would like to change? talents not mentioned? Leader(s) will assist each member in identifying his own personal characteristics.[10]

Overall the result should be that each group member ends up with a more realistic view of his assets and skills as well as of things he may wish to work on as he looks ahead to career and life roles.

Stage 2: Learning About the Realities of the Work World (As Many As 3-4 Sessions)

Goal. To increase knowledge concerning the world of work for the group members.

This stage emphasizes exploring the realities of the work world through having members bridge the gap between their stated interests and abilities and the actual requirements of various jobs.

Possible Format: There are many strategies one could use in achieving this goal. Certainly among them would be lectures, reading materials, role playing, films, guest speakers, out-of-class assignments.

Possible Exercises/Activities:
1. Providing, information on various categories of jobs (service, technical, etc.), labor market trends, educational or training requirements for specific jobs, implications for job selection of differences between one's interests and one's abilities, where to find occupational information, how to fill out job applications, how to prepare for and conduct job interviews.
2. Assignment of homework exercises, such as visiting one or two places of employment to talk with people in worker roles. Participants use a questionnaire to fill in as they interview workers, but in general obtain information such as how long the person has worked in the job, what educational background he has had to qualify for the job, what training he needed to get.
3. Another homework assignment: visit one community resource concerned with vocational information, such as a library or college/career center to obtain facts regarding one or more specific occupations.

In general participants would be helped by leader(s) to explore areas of work that might fit with their own stated interests or known skills and abilities so that each ends the stage with a clearer idea of the directions he wishes to move in.

Stage 3: Goal Planning (Approximately 2 Sessions)

Goal: To have each participant identify possible short and long term goals toward his occupational development.

This stage emphasizes establishing a more specific course of action by each group member. Based on the broader understandings of personal characteristics and of the work world, each member is helped in understanding how to set and implement career goals, to establish priorities for reaching them and to adapt to changes in plans that may occur.

Goals actually established may take various forms based on the needs of each individual. Examples of short term goals might range from increasing involvement in school social activities to increase the ability to get along cooperatively with others, to searching for and applying for a particular part-time job. If possible, these short term goals would facilitate the acquisition of skills necessary to accomplishing a long-term goal, such as working in a service oriented occupation. Group members will have an opportunity to try out new roles based on their goals and will be guided in making changes and further advancements as a result of their experiences.

Possible Format: These steps are necessarily individualized so that individual counseling should accompany group discussion.

Possible Exercises–Activities:

1. Group leader(s) may offer individual guidance and suggestions: for example, one member may state a tentative occupational choice of becoming a landscape gardener. A suggestion might be made that he get involved in activities/classes to obtain necessary skills such as in horticulture/agriculture classes, or woodworking or machine shop.

2. Or a group leader may suggest further exploration of a specific gardener-related job and use of community resources to gain more information about employment possibilities, such as the skills necessary for different levels of responsibility in gardening, or the pay scales for various kinds of gardening.

3. Or an individual might be ready to begin searching for or applying for a specific job. The leader may suggest part-time job possibilities which would enable the individual to obtain experience in his field of interest.

Stage 4. Maximizing One's Potentials (Up to Two Sessions)

Goal: To provide encouragement and support for group members as they plan and pursue specific courses of action. Continue to teach skills that address specific problems or concerns that arise at this stage.

In this stage, for example, the group leader(s) might plan a special session on how to improve communication skills, assertiveness skills or time management skills to emphasize their importance in job success. Focus for discussions would depend upon the group as well as individual needs, but special problems can lead to good session content, e.g., a member having interpersonal difficulties with a peer at a new job.

Possible Format: At this stage role playing of different work-related situations would be valuable along with lectures and discussions.

Possible Exercises–Activities:

1. The group leader might arrange a role play of a specific problem situation or a typical problem encountered on a job, such as what to do if you do not know how to do certain operations/ tasks of the job you are assigned. Group members having the opportunity to play the various roles in such a situation generate strategies to solve the problem.[9]

2. Pre-made videotapes of individuals dealing effectively and ineffectively in typical work situations involving relationships, job-related behaviors, etc., could be good vehicles for discussions. From them group members would identify effective/ ineffective approaches and discuss the different outcomes.

Stage 5: Closure (One Session)

Goal: To provide a review of strategies learned during the sessions as well as the information about how to locate and access additional resources in the community. This would focus on counselors or agencies/institutions that provide assistance in career planning, job training.

In the final session major points of the program will be reviewed and re-emphasized. Further, group members would be provided with lists of resources of helping agencies or bibliographies of materials available in local libraries that might be helpful for future planning. Strategies for locating and accessing helping agencies will also be provided. Arrangements for future feedback to leader(s) might be outlined so that some continued access to familiar help is assured.

Possible Format: This session will be largely lecture and discussion.

Possible Exercises–Activities:

1. Review principal steps in the process of career exploration for life/work planning which have been covered in previous sessions.

2. Go over resource lists of community agencies/ institutions to clarify the kinds of help available to group members.

3. Have group members verbally share all of the positive points they can list about participating in the group. In addition, they might list all the new things they have learned about themselves as a result of being in the group.

Summary

This paper has provided an overview of the adolescent passage and the current problems and needs of this age group. It has also described a proposed preventive occupational therapy outpatient program based in the community and designed to address problems of life/ work planning. The ideas offered in the paper are not new to occupational therapy, but rather are inherent to its philosophies. The plan, the setting and the population proposed are seen as a logical extension of occupational therapy, services into a potentially new market arena for health care.

The use of a community-based outpatient setting for offering a program for adolescents focused on occupational choice has its distinct advantages. All of the resources and experiences available in the community can be utilized in programming. Emphasizing experiential learning, the program strategies offer adolescents the chance to try out new ideas and roles within their communities while having a continuous, safe base of support in a peer group. Thus true growth and change can occur.

References

1. Levine, Saul V. The Psychological and Social Effects of Youth Unemployment. *Children Today.* Nov-Dec 1979. Pp 6-9.

2. A Nation of Runaway Kids. *Newsweek.* Oct 1982. New York.

3. Youth as a National Resource. *Children Today.* Nov-Dec 1979. Pp 2-5.

4. Black, Maureen. Adolescent Role Assessment. *AJOT.* Feb 1976, Vol. 30, #2. Pp 73-79.

5. Shannon, Phillip D. The Adolescent Experience. *AJOT* 1972, Vol. 26, #6. Pp 294-287.

6. ABC-TV. *World News Tonight.* November 1984.

7. Gibbons, Maurice. Walkabout: Searching for the Right Passage From Childhood and School. *Phi Delta Kappa.* May 1974. Pp 596-602.

8. Transition From School to Work: An International Perspective. *Rehab Briefs.* April 1984.

9. Cartledge, Gwendolyn. *Teaching Social Skills to Children.* Pergamon Press, N.Y. 1980.

10. *Personal Resources for Employment-Handbook.* Cassandra Sheard. Copyright 1981.

Chapter 28

Transition from School to Community Living

Chestina Brollier, PhD, OTR, FAOTA
Jayne Shepherd, MS, OTR
Kerri Flick Markley, MS, OTR

This chapter was previously published in the *American Journal of Occupational Therapy, 48*, 346–353. Copyright © 1994, American Occupational Therapy Association.

The education and services for children with disabilities have improved since the Education of All Handicapped Children Act of 1975 (Public Law 94–142) (U.S. Department of Education Office of Special Education and Rehabilitative Services, 1991). Yet between 50% and 75% of persons with disabilities remain unemployed (Harris, 1986; Hasazi, Gordon, & Roe, 1985; Wehman, 1992a). Nearly the same percentage of the 250,000 to 300,000 students with disabilities who have left the public schools each year had no jobs or independent living arrangements (Wehman, 1992a). These statistics suggest that transition planning for special education students deserves the attention of professionals such as school-based occupational therapists. *Transition planning* is the process by which a student is prepared to leave the school setting and enter into employment and community living (Wehman, 1992a). A literature search on this topic revealed little occupational therapy coverage.

Because the emphasis in transition programs is on functional daily life skills, occupational therapists' knowledge of activities of daily living, work, and leisure is applicable. The literature review, our clinical experiences, and research have led us to question whether some school system occupational therapists may be underemphasizing occupational performance areas while overemphasizing a developmental approach and sensorimotor occupational performance components (Barber, McInerney, & Struck, 1993; Spencer & Sample, 1993). This paper synthesizes some key issues for the transition process by reviewing occupational therapy and special education literature on functional activities and transition planning. The following key issues for the transition process are highlighted: federal initiatives, team efforts, parental involvement, assessment, goal setting, service characteristics, and roles for occupational therapy.

Federal Initiatives

The Office of Special Education and Rehabilitative Services (OSERS) has made vocational transition for students who have moderate to severe disabilities a national priority (Will, 1984). OSERS calls for the availability of services necessary for transition from school to work for all persons with disabilities and for a goal of sustained employment.

Additionally, the federal government has passed numerous laws concerning transition. The Education of the Handicapped Act Amendments of 1983 (Public Law 98–199) and 1986 (Public Law 99–457) mandated secondary education and transition services for youth with disabilities between the ages of 12 and 22 years and authorized funding for research on the transition process. The Carl D. Perkins Vocational Education Act of 1984 (Public Law 98–524) provided funding for vocational education and legislated that students and their parents be made aware of vocational opportunities in the school one year before services are provided, or by the time the student reaches the ninth grade. The 1986 amendments to this act (Public Law 99–506) funded supported employment services in all states (Wehman, Moon, Everson, Wood, & Barcus, 1988). The Carl D. Perkins Vocational and Applied Technology Education Act of 1990 (Public Law 101–392) guaranteed full vocational education for youth with disabilities (National Information Center for Children and Youth with Disabilities [NICHCY], 1991).

In 1990, Congress passed the Education of the Handicapped Act Amendments of 1990 (Public Law 101–476), called the Individuals with Disabilities Education Act (IDEA). This law includes transition services and assistive technology as new definitions of special education services that must be included in a student's individualized education program (IEP) (NICHCY, 1991).

The Individualized Transition Planning Team

An individualized transition planning (ITP) team is essential to establishing a comprehensive transition plan (Giangreco, 1992; Rainforth, York, & MacDonald, 1992). The team may include special educators, occupational therapists, physical therapists, speech and language pathologists, representatives from adult service agencies, a vocational rehabilitation counselor, parents, the student, and, often, an employer. With this many team members, collaboration between agencies is essential to avoid duplication of services (Wehman, 1992a).

IDEA requires formal transition planning as part of the IEP process for all 16-year old special education students (and those at a younger age, if considered appropriate) (Code of Federal Regulations, 1992). For many students with moderate to severe disabilities, transition planning and community living experiences are needed in the elementary and middle school years even if a formal ITP team has not been developed (Spencer & Sample, 1993).

Parental Involvement

A key issue in transition planning is active involvement by parents. First, they have the legal right to be involved in the education of their children. Second, they know their children better than anyone and are a significant source of information regarding skills needed by the student (Bates, Renzaglia, & Wehman, 1981; Wehman, 1992a). Third, after completing mandatory education, the former student and his or her family are responsible for carrying out the goals of an ITP. If they are not invested in these future plans, the targeted outcomes for transition may fail.

Studies on parental involvement in ITP development (Karge, Patton, & de la Garza, 1992) and IEP conferences (Vaughn, Bos, Harrell, & Lasky, 1988) found that parents took a passive role. Vacc and colleagues (1985) had similar results. They found that academic and social functioning were the most discussed IEP topics; topics receiving relatively little attention included planning for parental involvement, learning about student preferences and future environments, and integration of the student into real life settings. These confirmed those of Lynch and Stein's (1982) study, in which only 18% of 400 parents of students with disabilities reported participating in the development of the IEP. Additionally, Lynch and Stein found that parents of 13- to 14-year-old students participated significantly less in IEP meetings than parents of younger students. This study warrants current replication because transition planning for teenagers is legally required.

Parental input may be affected by several obstacles: logistical problems lack of transportation, lack of child care, and inconvenient times), communication problems (language barriers and misunderstanding of terminology), inferiority feelings, and uncertainty about their child's disability (Lynch & Stein, 1982; Turnbull & Turnbull, 1990). Parents may resist transition planning due to concerns about their child's safety or about the questionable potential for success. They may worry about the attitudes of others, the school district's commitment to this programming, and the quality of the program (Hanline & Halvorsen, 1989). Parents also may have difficulty accepting the change in therapy programming from remediating medical problems to developing life skills; they may have difficulty thinking about the future and seeing their children in more adult roles (Turnbull & Turnbull, 1990). Therefore, transition planning may be an emotional event for families that influences their level of participation in the ITP.

There are several ways to reduce the barriers to parental participation in ITP meetings. Parents can be given a choice about when and where to meet. They, along with their child, can help select the specific professionals to be involved in the ITP process (Turnbull & Turnbull, 1990). Depending on their wishes and abilities, they can be given a list of possible topics to prepare for discussion at the ITP meeting. A few sample topics are living arrangements, jobs, guardianship, social security benefits, sexuality, fitness, and medical access (Sample, Spencer, & Bean, 1990). Besides preparation time, parents can be given information on what services are currently available and about the need for changes in service provision. Respect for cultural preference and open communication can promote effective working relationships between all team members, including the parents.

Functional, Environmentally Referenced Assessments

Before the ITP meeting, each member of the team uses functional, environmentally referenced assessments to determine the student's current levels of functioning relative to the previous year's IEP goals (Spencer & Sample, 1993). Dividing duties, the team evaluates the student's performance at home, in school, in the community, during recreation, and during temporary job placements (Brown et al., 1991; Spencer, Murphy, Bean, & Schelly, 1991). Functional performance, environmental demands and expectations, performance gaps, and support or training needs are noted (Spencer & Sample, 1993). Parents, teachers, and other key people are also interviewed for their input.

To determine which activities to assess within various environments, team members ask, "If the student does not learn this activity, will someone else have to do it for him or her?" (Brown et al., 1986; LaVesser & Shealey, 1986). If the answer is yes, the activity is functional and should be evaluated. For example, the ability to use a toilet is a functional skill and may be evaluated in multiple environments (e.g., school, a restaurant, a work site, a movie theater). Additional activities considered for the evaluation are those the student and parents prefer, those that reflect his or her culture, and those that influence safety or health (Brown et al., 1991; NICHCY, 1990).

After completion of the functional, environmentally referenced assessments, a discrepancy analysis is performed. This analysis determines what part of a desired skill the student can perform, what specific aspect of a skill is difficult for the student and why, and whether assistive technology could help this student.

Compared to functional, environmentally referenced assessments, standardized developmental tests often used in school system occupational therapy practice may have several shortcomings in transition programming for students with severe disabilities. Many of these assessments test isolated skills that may not be used in a student's home, community, or work (Rainforth & York, 1987), and they do not provide clear information on the student's and parent's priorities. Furthermore, because students with severe disabilities do not necessarily develop skills in the "normal" sequence (Orelove & Sobsey, 1991), an emphasis on performance components may not be appropriate. Additionally, developmental tests often lack information about a student's learning style (Falvey, 1986; Lehr, 1989).

Goal Setting

After completing the evaluation, the ITP team discusses long-term transition goals. These focus on the student's desired life-style after the school years in terms of domestic or home life, ability to function out in the community, and leisure and vocational activities (Spencer & Sample, 1993). The student's current levels of functioning and needs influence the IEP goals. Each annual goal addresses some need related to a long-term goal.

There are six areas to examine when setting goals: (a) preference, (b) number of environments in which the skills are used, (c) number of occurrences, (d) social significance, (e) probability of skill acquisition, and (f) safety and health issues (Brown et al., 1986; Meyer, Peck, & Brown, 1991). Preference refers to the judgments of all team members, especially those of parents and students. Each person comes to the ITP meeting with opinions about what skills are most important.

Determining the number of environments in which a skill is to be used is important in prioritizing goals. For example, many special education students have been taught to sort cubes or cones by color, a prereadiness activity not usually required in many environments. In contrast, matching clothes by color is a skill used in dressing at home or in doing laundry at home or at a work placement (Brown et al., 1986; Wehman et al., 1988; Wehman, 1992a).

The more a skill is practiced throughout life, the more likely it is that the skill will be learned and used (Billingsley, 1986; Brown et al., 1986). For example, washing dishes or loading a dishwasher may only be used in a home or vocational setting, but they are skills used several times a day for years. Therefore, these skills often will be of high priority.

Social significance refers to how a skill affects the social acceptance of the student. According to Brown and associates (1986), failing to teach the student some skills may hinder peer acceptance. For example, although a student may be instructed in ordering food from a restaurant, if he or she acts out by yelling or throwing food, he or she is less likely to be accepted by peers. However, teaching a 16 year old how to operate an age-appropriate device, such as a switch to a radio rather than one connected to an infant's toy, may influence social acceptance by peers. Even the choice of equipment or assistive devices the student will need has social significance. For example, children and teens may reject a deltoid sling because of its appearance even though it can make eating easier.

Probability of skill acquisition is another area to be appraised when setting goals. Is the development of a skill worth the time and effort of instruction? (Brown et al., 1986; Wehman, 1992a). For example, independence in dressing may not be an appropriate goal for many students with severe physical disabilities.

When distinguishing which skills or activities are important for the student to acquire, the team must emphasize those that will assist the student in learning safety measures and that promote healthful living (Brown et al., 1986; Wehman et al., 1988; Wehman, 1992a). Because students with disabilities have typically been taught in sheltered environments, they may not have experience in dealing with environmental obstacles or potential dangers (e.g., stairs, toilets without railings, street crossing, cooking).

Service Characteristics

Each annual ITP goal is accompanied by a list that identifies who will be responsible for goal attainment, who will provide consultation, what adaptations or supports are needed by the student, when the goal is to be achieved, and what environments will be used for training (Spencer & Sample, 1993). Several team members may be responsible for different aspects of the same goal. The student's responsibilities are also delineated (Ward, 1992).

A number of authors (Brown et al., 1991; Chandler, 1992; Sailor et al., 1986; Wehman, 1992a) have successfully implemented a functional life skills curriculum. Such curricula use the classroom in a regular public school or an integrated private school; nonclassroom areas such as the cafeteria, library, hallways, and playground; community areas such as parks, restaurants, work environments, and residential settings; and other age-appropriate community environments or areas in which to teach life skills. These curricula require careful planning for the needs of each student and increased time for community-based instruction as the student gets older. Students from 12 to 16 years old may spend as much as 75% of their time out of school in community-centered instruction (Brown et al., 1991, Sailor et al., 1986). The work force for community training programs can be provided by occupational therapy personnel, teachers, teacher's aides, physical therapists, speech and language pathologists, and parents and volunteers (Giangreco, York, & Rainforth, 1989). One adult to three students is the recommended ratio for effective community training and integration (Hutchins & Talarico, 1985). Examples of functional assessment and intervention activities that may be used in a life–skills curriculum are shown in Table 1.

Intervention Principles

There are several key principles of intervention for effective transition services. These are
- Teach at natural times, using naturally occurring cues, reinforcers, and consequences
- Teach in natural environments
- Use real materials
- Teach all day and across environments to promote generalization
- Use partial participation (What part of a task can the student do?)
- Keep student data to determine effectiveness of intervention
- Integrate student with nondisabled peers
- Use functional activities

Intervention concentrates on specific skills that help to integrate the student into the community and ensures participation in adult activities (Bellamy & Wilcox, 1982; Brown et al., 1991: Spencer, 1989; Wehman, 1992b).

Roles for Occupational Therapy

IDEA mandates that transition services address work, education, independent living, and community participation. These domains are synonymous with the occupational performance areas delineated by the American Occupational Therapy Association's (AOTA) *Uniform Terminology* (AOTA, 1989) (see Appendix I for most recent edition of *Uniform Terminology*). Occupational therapists in transition programs can address these performance areas by providing direct or indirect therapy, consultation, and monitoring while offering services in school and community environments (Dunn, 1991; Giangreco, 1986; Giangrceco, Edelman, & Dennis, 1991; Niehues, Bundy, Mattingly, & Lawlor, 1991).

Occupational therapy transition services concentrate on functional life skills programming. In Table 2, functional activities are contrasted with less functional activity choices and simulations that may not be generalized to natural environments. Occupational therapists use the tasks of everyday living to help students develop the self-care, home management, work, school, and leisure skills necessary to live and work in their community.

Occupational therapists can structure the physical environment to facilitate the learning of functional life skills. This process may lead to task or environmental modifications and the use of technological assistive devices (TADs). The physical environment may be modified to promote accessibility, work simplification, appropriate positioning of the student, the effective level of sensory stimulation, or combinations of the above.

Environmental modification often involves the use of technological assistive devices. Speech pathologists and occupational therapists frequently are the primary ITP members with expertise in assistive technology (Spencer & Sample, 1993) and often recommend equipment

Table 1
Examples of functional assessment and intervention activities for life-skill programs.

Student	Domestic	Community	Leisure	Vocational
TB, 10 years old, autistic-like behaviors, considered to be at trainable mentally retarded level	Picking up toys, washing dishes, making beds, dressing, grooming, eating skills, toileting skills, sorting clothes, emptying trash (lives at home with parents)	Eating meals in a restaurant, using restroom in a local restaurant, putting trash into container, giving the clerk money for an item he wants to purchase, recognizing and reading pedestrian safety signs, participating in local scout troop, going to neighbor's house for lunch	Climbing on swing set, playing simple board games, playing tag with neighbors, tumbling activities, running, playing kickball, riding bicycles, playing with age-appropriate toys	Cleaning the room at the end of the day, working on a task for designated period (15–30 min), wiping table after meals, following 2- to 4-step oral instructions, taking messages to people
JS, 17 years old, post brain injury, right hemiplegia with behavioral problems. Ambulates with a walker	Sweeping and dusting at place of residence, cooking simple meals (bowl of cereal, sandwich), operating simple machines (microwave, TV, stereo, tape recorder), putting the groceries away, caring for personal hygiene, dressing independently Ready to leave parents and live within a group residence	Using bus system to get around community; getting in and out of community stores and restaurants; negotiating steps, curbs, and revolving doorways; simple comparative shopping; using community health facilities (physician, pharmacist); interacting courteously with public	Watching college basketball, playing card games, listening to and recording music, going to movies with friends, playing video games	Performing janitorial duties at local store, food stocking duties at grocery store, inventory and reshelving videos duties at video store, ticket-taking duties at local movie theater

Adapted with permission from Wehman, P., Moon, M. S., Everson, J. M., Wood, W., & Barcus, J. M. (1988). *Transition from school to work: New challenges for youth with severe disabilities.* Baltimore: Brookes.

for students to become more integrated within their environments (Bain, 1989). Besides assessing and recommending TADs, the therapist can be responsible for instructing the student, parent, or teacher in proper use and maintenance of the equipment (Trefler, 1987).

A variety of technological aids are available to assist students with severe disabilities, including augmentative communication devices, computers, telephones, power wheelchairs, environmental control units, and adaptive aids (Mann & Lane, 1991; Vanderheiden, 1987). The same criteria used for selecting transition goals (listed above) help in prioritizing which technological aids to use.

One technological aid frequently used is the computer. Computer games are used to help improve visual perceptual skills. However, these games may not be adequate for an older student who has severe disabilities because the skills may not transfer to doing schoolwork or a job placement even though they may provide appropriate recreation. For example, skills learned in using the Muppet Learning Keys[1] do not transfer easily to those needed for word processing skills because the letter configuration on the Muppet Learning Keys keyboard is not similar to other computer keyboards found in work and home environments. With team input, the occupational therapist can carefully select the hardware, software, and peripherals to increase the student's functional outcomes in multiple environments (e.g., postschool training, employment, and home management).

Table 2
Contrasting activity choices for students with severe disabilities.

Community Living Functional Activities	Less Functional Activities
Sorting silverware	Working with pegs and patterns
Setting table	Working with block designs
Clipping coupons	Cutting predrawn shapes
Dressing and undressing self for gym and outdoors	Using activities of daily living (ADL) button, lacing and zipper boards
Using money to purchase items in cafeteria, school store, fast-food restaurant, drugstore	Practicing simulated shopping with play money
Using real washer and dryer at home, laundromat, or in work setting	Using simulated washing machine
Applying telephone skills, making real business and social calls	Practicing telephone skills by talking to occupational therapist
Completing application for desired part-time job	Using simulated copies of job application
Finding a specific classified advertisement or telephone number	Using figure–ground worksheets (e.g., "circle all the Es")
Practicing specific social skills with peers without disabilities and non-staff adults	Practicing social skills training with a special needs group
Using computers to do school assignments, write letters, etc.	Playing computer games or using visual–perceptual training programs
Practicing wheelchair mobility in school, home, and community environments	Practicing wheelchair mobility only in school or classroom environment

Occupational therapists can also structure the temporal environment while teaching functional life skills. This allows students to work at peak performance times. Temporal cues may aid a student's performance. For example, watches or clocks with alarms can be placed in the environment to cue students to begin, change, or end tasks. Or students may be taught when to perform a job or a self-care task according to the time of day when it is needed.

Structuring the social environment can facilitate the development of interpersonal and social skills likely to prove beneficial across many domains of adult life (NICHCY, 1993). This social structuring may include positioning the student with peers or role models who support appropriate behaviors and assisting students in determining the appropriate time and place for socialization. Besides structuring the environment, knowledge of psychosocial performance components (AOTA, 1989) helps occupational therapists teach skills such as stress management, time management, and self-management techniques. For example, if a student is having difficulty behaving in socially appropriate ways, ITP objectives may include learning appropriate greetings; knowing differences between strangers, friends, and employers and how each should be treated; or developing conversational skills appropriate for job or social settings.

When modifying environments, task analysis and adaptation can be the basis for teaching functional skills. Task analysis identifies not only all the steps necessary for successful performance of a task, but also the intellectual,

[1]Manufactured by Sunburst Communications, 39 Washington Avenue, Pleasantville, NY 10570.

psychosocial, perceptual, and motor skills required. Information gained from the analysis of a task is placed into a step-by-step learning sequence. The transition team often relies on the occupational therapist to adapt the activity, or the learning sequence (Spencer & Sample, 1993). Physical and verbal cuing, cue cards, or photo reminders can be used to prompt the learning of complex tasks. For example, a teenage student with mental retardation who is unable to follow verbal three-step directions may be taught feminine hygiene skills through photo cue cards and an adaptive aid.

Roles for occupational therapy in transition programming are multifaceted. Occupational therapists not only teach functional daily living skills, but also help structure the physical, temporal, and social environments. Through task analysis and adaptation, therapists help modify the student's skills to meet environmental demands.

Conclusion

Transition programming for a student with moderate to severe disabilities involves an appropriate life-centered, functional school-based program, formalized plans involving the parents and the entire array of community agencies that are responsible for providing services, and multiple quality options for gainful employment or meaningful postschool training and appropriate community living arrangements. School-based occupational therapists have much to offer the transition process when they concentrate on real-life functional activities.

Acknowledgments

This paper is based in part on a faculty-designed research project conducted by the third author while a professional master's degree student in occupational therapy at Virginia Commonwealth University. Presentations on this topic have been given at the 1991 Great Southern Occupational Therapy Conference and the 72nd Annual Conference of the American Occupational Therapy Association Conference, Houston, Texas, March 1992.

We thank the following organizations for their participation in the ongoing transition project, of which this paper is a part: The Richmond Cerebral Palsy Center, The Chesterfield County Public Schools, and The Virginia Commonwealth University Rehabilitation Research and Training Center.

References

American Occupational Therapy Association. (1989). Uniform terminology, for occupational therapy—second edition. *American Journal of Occupational Therapy, 43*, 808–815. (Third edition reprinted as Appendix I.)

Bain, B. (1989). Assessment of clients for technological assistive devices. In *Technology review '89: Perspectives on occupational therapy practice* (pp. 55–59). Rockville, MD: American Occupational Therapy Association.

Barber, M., McInerney, C., & Struck, M. (1993, June). Training for independence: Transition from school to work. *Work Programs Special Interest Section Newsletter*, pp. 1–2.

Bates, P., Renzaglia, A., & Wehman, P. (1981, April). Characteristics of an appropriate education for the severely and profoundly handicapped. *Education and Training of the Mentally Retarded, 16*, 142–148.

Bellamy, G. T., & Wilcox, B. (1982). Secondary education for severely handicapped students: Guidelines for quality services. In K. P. Lynch, W. E. Kiernan, & J. A. Stark, *Prevocational and vocational education for special needs youth: A blueprint for the 1980's* (pp, 65–80). Baltimore: Brookes.

Billingsley, F. (1986). Where are the generalized outcomes? An examination of instructional objectives. In H. Powell (Ed.). *PILOT: Project for independent living in occupational therapy* (pp. 96–103). Rockville, MD: American Occupational Therapy Association.

Brown, L., Falvey, M., Vincent, L., Kaye, N., Johnson, F., Ferrara–Parrish, P., & Gruenewald, L. (1986). Strategies for generating comprehensive, longitudinal and chronological–age-appropriate individualized education programs for adolescent and young adult severely handicapped students. In H. Powell (Ed.). *PILOT: Project for independent living in occupational therapy* (pp. 104–115). Rockville, MD: American Occupational Therapy Association.

Brown, L., Schwarz, P., Udvari–Solner, A., Kampschroer, E., Johnson, F., Jorgensen, J., & Gruenewald, L. (1991). How much time should students with severe intellectual disabilities spend in regular education classrooms and elsewhere? *Journal of the Association for Persons with Severe Handicaps, 16*, 39–47.

Carl D. Perkins Vocational Education Act of 1984 (Public Law 98–524).

Carl D. Perkins Vocational Education Act Amendments. (Public Law 99–506), (1986).

Carl D. Perkins Vocational and Applied Technology Education Act of 1990 (Public Law 101–392).

Chandler, B. (1992). How to design and implement classroom programming. In C. Royeen (Ed.), American Occupational Therapy Association Self-Study Series, *Classroom applications for school-based practice*. Rockville, MD: AOTA.

Code of Federal Regulations 300–301 (1992, October). Final Regulations; Correction: Assistance to states for the education of children with disabilities program and preschool grants for children with disabilities. *Federal Register, 57* (208).

Education of All Handicapped Children Act (Public Law 94–142). (1975).

Education of the Handicapped Act Amendments of 1983 (Public Law 98–199).

Education of the Handicapped Act Amendments of 1986 (Public Law 99–457), 20 U.S.C., § 1400.

Dunn, W. (Ed.). (1991). *Pediatric occupational therapy: Facilitating effective service provision.* Thorofare, NJ.: Slack.

Falvey, M. (1986). *Community-based curriculum: Instructional strategies for students with severe handicaps.* Baltimore: Brookes.

Giangreco, M. F. (1986). Delivery of therapeutic services in special education programs for learners with severe handicaps. *Physical and Occupational Therapy in Pediatrics, 6* (2), 5–15.

Giangreco, M. F. (1992, February). *Integrating related services in the education of students with disabilities.* Symposium on using the transdisciplinary approach to related services in classrooms, Williamsburg, Virginia.

Giangreco, M., Edelman, S., & Dennis, R. (1991). Common professional practices that interfere with the integrated delivery of services. *Remedial and Special Education, 12* (2), 16–24.

Giangreco, M., York, R., & Rainforth, B. (1989). Providing related services to learners with severe handicaps in educational settings: Pursuing the least restrictive option. *Pediatric Physical Therapy, 1* (2), 55–63.

Hanline, M., & Halvorsen, A. (1989). Parent perceptions of the integration transition process: Overcoming artificial barriers. *Exceptional Children, 55,* 487–492.

Harris, L. (1986). *International center for the disabled survey of disabled Americans. Bringing disabled Americans into the mainstream: A nationwide survey of 1, 000 disabled people.* New York: International Center for the Disabled.

Hasazi, S., Gordon, L., & Roe, C. (1985). Factors associated with the employment status of handicapped youth exiting high school from 1973–1983. *Exceptional Children, 51,* 455–469.

Hutchins, M., & Talarico, D. (1985). Administrative considerations in providing community integrated training programs. In P. McCarthy, J. Everson, M. S. Moon, & M. Barcus (Eds.), *School-to-work transition for youth with severe disabilities.* Project Transition into Employment, Rehabilitation Research & Training Center, School of Education, Virginia Commonwealth University, Richmond, Virginia.

Individuals With Disabilities Education Act (Public Law 101–476). (1990).

Karge, B. D., Patton, P. L., & de la Garza, B. (1992). Transition services for youth with mild disabilities: Do they exist, are they needed? *Career Development for Exceptional Individuals, 15,* 47–68.

LaVesser, P., & Shealey, S. (1986). The occupational therapy process. In H. Powell (Ed.), *PILOT: Project for independent living in occupational therapy* (pp. 87–95). Rockville, MD: American Occupational Therapy Association.

Lehr, D. (1989). Educational programming for young children with the most severe disabilities. In F. Brown & D. Lehr (Eds.), *Persons with profound disabilities: Issues and practices* (pp. 213–237). Baltimore: Brookes.

Lynch, E. W., & Stein, R. (1982). Perspectives on parent participation in special education. *Exceptional Education Quarterly, 3* (2), 56–63.

Mann, W. C., & Lane, J. P. (1991). *Assistive technology for persons with disabilities: The role of occupational therapy.* Rockville, MD: American Occupational Therapy Association.

Meyer, L., Peck, C., & Brown, L. (1991). *Critical issues in the lives of people with severe disabilities.* Baltimore: Brookes.

National Information Center for Children and Youth with Disabilities. (1990, December). Transition summary. *NICHCY 6,* 1–13.

National Information Center for Children and Youth with Disabilities. (1991). The education of children and youth with special needs: What do the laws say? *NICHCY, 1* (1),1–11.

National Information Center for Children and Youth with Disabilities. (1993, March). Transition summary. *NICHCY, 3* (1), 1–20.

Niehues, A., Bundy, A., Mattingly, C., & Lawlor, M. (1991). Making a difference: Occupational therapy in the public schools. *Occupational Therapy Journal of Research, 11,* 195–211.

Orelove, F., & Sobsey, D. (1991). *Educating children with multiple disabilities: A transdisciplinary approach* (pp. 231–258). Baltimore: Brookes.

Rainforth, B., & York, J. (1987). Integrating related services in community instruction. *Journal of the Association for Persons with Severe Handicaps, 12,* 190–198.

Rainforth, B., York, J., & MacDonald, C. (1992). *Collaborative teams for students with severe disabilities: Integrating therapy and educational services.* Baltimore: Brookes.

Sailor, W., Halvorsen, A., Anderson, J., Goetz, L., Gee, K., Doering, K., & Hunt, P. (1986). Community intensive instruction. In R. Homer, L. Meyer, & B. Fredericks (Eds.), *Education of learners with severe handicaps* (pp. 251–288). Baltimore: Brookes.

Sample, P., Spencer, K., & Bean, G. (1990). *Transition planning: Creating a positive future for students with disabilities.* Fort Collins, CO: Office of Transition Services, Department of Occupational Therapy, Colorado State University.

Spencer, K. (1989). The transition from school to adult life. In S. Hertfelder, & C. Gwin (Eds.). *Work in progress: Occupational therapy in work programs* (pp. 157–179). Rockville, MD: American Occupational Therapy Association.

Spencer, K., Murphy, M., Bean, G., & Schelly, C. (1991). Vocational needs assessment: A functional, community referenced approach. In K. Spencer (Ed.)., *From school to adult life: The role of occupational therapy in the transition process* (pp. 185–213). Fort Collins, CO: Department of Occupational Therapy, Colorado State University.

Spencer, K., & Sample, P. (1993). Transition planning and services. In C. Royeen (Ed.), *Classroom applications for school based practice* (pp. 6–48). Rockville, MD: American Occupational Therapy Association.

Trefler, E. (1987). Technology applications. *American Journal of Occupational Therapy, 41,* 697–700.

Turnbull, A., & Turnbull, R. (1990). *Families, professionals, and exceptionality: A special partnership.* Columbus: Merrill.

U.S. Department of Education, Office of Special Education and Rehabilitative Services. (1991). *Thirteenth annual report to Congress on the implementation of the Education of the Handicapped Act.* Washington, DC: U.S. Government Printing Office.

Vacc, N. A., Vallecorsa, A. L., Parker, A., Bonner, S., Lester, C., Richardson, S., & Yates, C. (1985). Parents and educators' participation in IEP conferences. *Education and Treatment of Children, 8* (2), 153–162.

Vanderheiden, G. (1987). Service delivery mechanisms in rehabilitation technology. *American Journal of Occupational Therapy, 41,* 703–710.

Vaughn, S., Bos, C., Harrell, J., & Lasky, B. (1988). Parent participation in the initial placement/IEP conference ten years after mandated involvement. *Journal of Learning Disabilities, 21* (2), 82–89.

Ward, M. J. (1992). Introduction to secondary special education and transition issues. In F. R. Rusch, L. DeStefano, J. Chadsey-Rusch, L. A. Phelps, & E. Szymanshi (Eds.), *Transition from school to adult life: Models, linkages, and policy* (pp 387–389). Sycamore, IL: Sycamore.

Wehman, P. (1992a). *Life beyond the classroom: Transition strategies for young people with disabilities.* Baltimore: Brookes.

Wehman, P. (1992b, Summer). Transition from school to adulthood for young people with disabilities. *Rehabilitation Research and Training Center Newsletter,* p. 1.

Wehman, P., Moon, M. S., Everson, J. M., Wood, W., & Barcus, J. M. (1988). *Transition from school to work: New challenges for youth with severe disabilities.* Baltimore: Brookes.

Will, M. C. (1984). *OSERS programming for the transition of youth with disabilities: Bridges from school to working life.* Washington, DC: Office of Special Education and Rehabilitative Service, U.S. Department of Education.

Chapter 29

The Therapeutic Use of Games with Mentally Retarded Adults

Gary Kielhofner, DrPH, OTR, FAOTA
Shawn Miyake, MA, OTR

This chapter was previously published in the *American Journal of Occupational Therapy, 35,* 375–382. Copyright © 1981, American Occupational Therapy Association.

Games considered essential in early occupational therapy practice are not currently in widespread use. However, games are consistent with the "art and science" of occupational therapy (1) and should be included as legitimate media for practice. It has always been the central concept of occupational therapy that humans' use of themselves in everyday activities, in self-care, in work, and in play has the power to maintain, restore, and increase health. This art and science of the field suggests the use of multiple media as therapy, including games. A theoretical rationale for and findings from a study of the use of games as a form of occupational therapy for mentally retarded adults will be presented.

Theoretical and Empirical Support for Play as Survival Behavior

Play, a central human characteristic, is responsible for both individual learning and the very fabric of social and cultural life (2). Evidence suggests that play is a prerequisite to behavioral flexibility necessary for higher species to survive (3). Among living species, those who play most exhibit the greatest ability to adapt their behavior for survival in a wide variety of ecologies, rather than exhibiting specialized behaviors for narrow ecologies. Man is the best example of this relationship between play and flexibility for adaptation in multiple ecologies.

Experiments convincingly point to social play deprivation as the key feature of social isolation; the absence of play assures that the adult will be an inflexible and poor survivor (3). It is not only *what* one learns in play, but also *how* one learns *to* adapt behavior to emerging and changing circumstances that is important. The player, besides learning what is necessary to adapt in a particular circumstance—a game, for example—also learns how to adapt to external conditions. If such learning were to take place in a more serious arena where the consequences could threaten survival, it would be rather ineffectual and inefficient.

Play also allows the player to process latent learning by increasing the general stock of knowledge that the person can draw upon in later circumstances (4). For instance, studies show that children who play with objects have more information later about possible ways to use those objects and are more successful in solving problems involving the manipulation of such objects than their peers who had the same information demonstrated to them by an adult (5). Such research suggests that play is a form of learning by doing.

Play is a behavioral mechanism that processes learning of rules (6). Rules are symbols that inform the person about the world and how to act in that world. These rules or symbols inform the person of constraints on action (7). As such, rules tell the person what to do and how to do it. Thus, in play, the player generates his or her own rules for doing, which are in concordance with the constraints of the physical and social world. Without normal play, it is theorized that the organism is a poor learner and a poor doer, lacking information and competence for survival (6, 7).

The play and games of childhood and adolescence form a context in which an individual develops an operational concept of self within an organized social group (8). Prior to game behavior, children practice taking on social roles in dramatic play, symbolically becoming doctors, firemen, parents, and teachers. Within the game, the player takes on a role with organized consequences. In the game, the player exercises a group of responses and organizes them into a pattern of behavior.

The player is also able to perceive himself or herself performing under some acquired identity while playing a role (8). The player learns self-organization by enacting various characters or roles in the game. In this manner, the player begins the process of gathering a generalized notion on self-identity in relation to others, and the player learns how to enact role identities in a social context (9).

The organized game provides a special set of social conditions. The player who plays a game must take on the attitude of everyone who is involved in the game. For example, to behave as a pitcher in a game of baseball, a player must know the purpose, plan, and intentions of the batter, catcher, and the team. A player projects himself or herself into a social scene and becomes a member of a meaningful social context. He or she must understand how roles of various players (e.g., in a baseball or football game) have a definite interrelationship to each other. The player must know what everyone else in the game is going to do in order to play competently. The responses of others are organized so that the attitude and actions of one calls out the appropriate attitudes and actions in the others (8). Such organization is a manifestation of the rules of the game.

For competent behavior, the individual must take into account phases and aspects of a common social activity or set of social understandings about the process in which all are engaged. The organized functioning of any person requires incorporating both a general sense of social rules and the special meanings of any social event. The game is a critical step toward social competence since it allows the player to experience and participate in a complex phenomenon of organized social life. In the game one learns to *be* social and to *do* social behavior.

From this theoretical perspective, it was judged appropriate to use the game situation as a modality to help retarded adults adapt to the social life of the community. Besides being valued for all the above reasons, play can be valued for its own sake, as an essential component of human life, not just a means to an end. Any improvement in the context of play is a sufficient gain for quality of life.

Play and the Retarded Person

Mentally retarded children and adults may have delayed and suppressed patterns of play (10). Several etiological factors are implicated. The severity of retardation is correlated with a decreased response to stimuli that ordinarily arouses the person and evokes play (11). Retarded persons also may suffer from environmental deprivation, thus receiving insufficient stimuli to evoke playful responses (12). In addition, the lack of adults to encourage and participate in play, is implicated in the inability for normal play of institutionalized retarded persons. The lack of normal play among mentally retarded persons may well lead to further disability since it represents suppression or distortion of a crucial learning mechanism in an individual whose capacity to learn is already limited. Further, since play is part and parcel of human experience, its absence signals a lesser quality of life (6).

Theoretical and empirical literature support the concept that play is an environmental behavior. Conditions in the environment (especially human conditions) can greatly influence the amount, duration, and nature of play (13, 14). Ways a therapist defines the activity, role models the behavior and attitude of play, delineates times and places for play, and participates in the play itself are all important influences (14–16). In this study, we asked whether and how the occupational therapist can influence the play of clients who may demonstrate delayed, disturbed, or suppressed patterns of play.

The Study

This exploratory study examined both how therapists were able to implement a program of games and listed effects observed from such intervention (1). The study described here was part of a larger 3-year ethnographic study of retarded adults in the community supporting the development and evaluation of a program of relevant services.

Occupational therapists in the study assumed roles both as service providers and as observers who became immersed as participants in the games being studied and in the everyday lives of the subjects outside the therapeutic program. Participant observation is increasingly used and recognized as a legitimate research method (18–21). Methodologists argue that the researcher who is a practitioner intervening with the subjects cannot only maintain, but also can enhance the validity of findings (22). Intersubjectivity between the researcher and subjects through participation is a new but legitimate criterion for validity of social science research.

The study method also takes a different approach to the degrees of freedom problem in generalization of results so that case studies or studies of few subjects are generalizable. Campbell (23) points out that ethnographic studies in which multiple questions are asked must be conceptualized differently and must not be critiqued from specific perspectives that set parameters on other study methods. Thus small samples subjected to long-term multiple observations in several heuristic categories are often used.

The major form of data collection included taking field notes, supplemented by audiotape and videotape. The data included what was done while carrying out the program and the visible impact of the program on clients. The report describes findings using a program of games implemented with seven males (three Mexican-American and four Caucasian), in an activity center for developmentally disabled persons. The subjects, aged 21 to 50, had a mean age of 30. All had retardation from moderate to severe; three had Down's Syndrome. None of the men had major physical disabilities.

Findings

The findings focus on the strategies and procedures therapists had to employ to maintain the games effectively and on areas of improvement in the men's behavior.

Strategies for Maximizing Game Behavior

While engaging the retarded men in various games, therapists (participant observers) discovered that they were using "natural strategies" for maximizing game behavior. These strategies were initially unreflexive since the games proceeded as ongoing situated encounters rather than as preplanned episodes. By examining field notes and videotapes, the therapists discovered themselves engaging in instances of what were only later identified as categories of strategies. Eventually the therapists more consciously enacted these procedures. Still, the application of these strategies was always situated and could not totally be pre-planned.

The strategies are organized into categories here to enhance their utility in other clinical applications and in order to lead to more systematic delineation and testing in the future. Each discussion of a strategy includes a description of why the strategy was needed, why it worked, and what was involved in carrying it out.

Grading complexity Observations revealed early in the project that it was not possible to engage these men immediately into complex games. Rather, the complex-

ity of a game needed to be graded both over a series of sessions and within a single session. During the program, the progression was from simple games of catch, to keep away and tag, to more complex and organized games such as baseball, basketball, and football. Within a single session it was fruitful to begin with simple routines and then work toward more complex forms of interaction and play. The following field note describes a typical course of progress during a session:

> On the basketball court it was clear in the beginning that the men expected us to tell them exactly what to do. I suggested we pass the ball around just to get used to it and to limber up. Things went slowly at first with everyone obediently passing the ball as they understood my directive. Then I asked Dan to suggest how we might pass the ball around and he suggested that we toss it in a circle. Shawn modeled for the men how to do a fancy pass, whereupon I suggested that the men try their own variations of passing the ball. Following this we threw baskets. Things really got going. Michael could do a very unconventional but successful lay-up, while Ralph did mostly free-throws. Dan initially had difficulty tossing the ball toward the basket. He would lift it far over and behind his head and heave it toward the basket while looking down. I suggested that he reverse the process, throwing from his knees while looking up. Voila! Instant success; he made the basket on the first try and had good luck thereafter. Each of the men got increasingly involved and began to interact with each other. Further, they verbally exhorted each other and commented on the other's relative success at making shots. The activity seemed to be quite pleasurable for them. They were all visibly more alert, mobile, and verbal by the end of the hour.

Grading the sessions from simple to complex allowed the men to organize their behavior in a meaningful hierarchy. Each step or skill along the way could be integrated into a higher level of organization or new set of rules. Over time the men learned not only a sense of what rules were about, but had acquired facility in following and using rules. In this way they were able to engage in more and more complex games. In addition, grading the complexity was a means of maintaining arousal and interest. Often the men's attention wandered during repetitive exercises in other settings. By slowly allowing the game session to become increasingly complex, the men remained engaged and interested.

The principle of grading complexity also had two implications for the arrangements of groups and the entering of individuals into types of games. Because the men had heterogeneous abilities, there was a problem of keeping the game at an optimum level of complexity for everyone. If a man entered a game he did not understand, or if he were overwhelmed with the amount of excitement, he would not become playful or exhibit a sense of pleasure. Similarly, more competent persons were bored by engaging in sports and games clearly below their ability.

These problems could be overcome by having two different groups with games of different complexity and by carefully observing an individual's level of skills. For example:

Chuck had shown some indication last week that he was picking up the nature of the tag game so that he was allowed to join us this week. The tag game required that the individual understand that by being hit with a soft ball that he was "it." He had to realize that "being it" means he would be expected to chase another person and tag him with a ball by throwing it at the person. Also, the person had to have the physical skill to run and to throw the ball accurately while either running or standing still. Further, he had to use deceptive tactics in chasing someone, use evasive tactics in avoiding the person who was "it," and so forth.

When someone needed to learn skills before entering into a game, he would be worked with first in a very small group or on a one-to-one basis. As the note indicates, therapists had to pay careful attention to the requirements of the game in assessing and preparing a person for readiness to enter the game. If someone entered the game with too few or no prerequisite skills, he would have difficulty acquiring a total sense, or ultimate purpose, of the game. Further, he would not have fun and thus not be playing.

Leveling relationships   Whenever possible, therapists joined the men in the game. This allowed the men an opportunity to take charge and more importantly to experience a sense of personal status and worth as they became "equals" with therapists in an activity. This leveling occurred more readily within the context of sports since the men had difficulty performing many symbolic functions, but were more likely to excel in physical skill. For example:

In the past Charles was quite good at throwing the Frisbee. Larry surprised me with his abilities, but it was Michael who surprised both Shawn and myself. Michael ordinarily appears fragile and docile, often assuming postures that look like he is ducking from danger. However, he was truly excellent with the Frisbee, making long and unbelievably accurate tosses and nearly spectacular catches. Shawn and I were impressed with everyone's abilities and had a good time with the three men. They all, especially Michael, seemed to enjoy themselves. Shawn and I both complimented Michael on his prowess afterwards. Throughout the Frisbee game we were all "leveled or averaged." The ordinary differences that existed between us were erased. Shawn and I were no longer obviously superior to the rest. In fact, Michael emerged as the best Frisbee player.

This leveling phenomenon allowed the men to experience competence and excellence, which they rarely ex-

perienced elsewhere. They could also autonomously determine outcomes and processes. Gradually, within the games, the men demonstrated more confidence and independence in making choices and controlling events. Their patterns of looking to a teacher or therapist for direction or help started to be replaced with responsibility for their immediate affairs. This included simple behaviors such as crossing the street or keeping track of one's own jacket.

Coaching and modeling   Throughout the program it was critical to provide these men with information concerning the actions and strategies they could profitably employ in the games. When coaching, therapists verbalized and displayed feedback to the men concerning the results of their performance. This often meant demonstrating what the man was doing and what the effect was together with an explanation or demonstration of why it did not work or was not the best strategy.

Modeling appropriate behaviors was extremely beneficial. Therapists provided models of affect, attitude, and behavior that the men could originally imitate and later integrate into their own participation in the game. This required that the therapists remain genuinely involved in the games so that they were always available to the men as models of what was appropriate or effective within the context of the game.

Keeping the game context and continuity   There was always the need to keep the game going, particularly in the beginning of the program. Later, the men more and more shared in keeping up the pace, emotion and organization of the game. At first the therapists had to orchestrate the game through substantial effort in order to maintain it as the men learned to become a part of it. Otherwise, there would have been no game for the men to enter. The following field note describes this orchestration:

My work is twofold. First I must work to be a competent player in the game. I often get chased and must avoid bing hit and also play the role of being "it" when I am hit. In addition, I must "orchestrate" the game and constantly watch it for problems that threaten its ongoing organization. I also do a fair amount of work to keep the excitement and pace of the game going.

Part of the game or play context was the attitude of playfulness. When an atmosphere of playfulness or fun replaced a more serious mood, it elicited participation, thus resolving many of the motivation problems acknowledged by others who were working with these men. The following field note illustrates this process:

In the park an activity center aide wanted to get the men to exercise. The aide took Larry and Bart by the hand and dragged them with her as she ran. She was expending much effort to get the men to run and they both had solemn looks on their faces. They did not enjoy it. I thought about our tag game and how naturally these men ran and the expressions of intense involvement and excitement that were displayed on their faces. I decided to experiment by trying it the aide's way. I took Dan and said, "Let's run, Dan." He started to walk fast never breaking into a run and his face was completely blank. I said, "Come on, Dan, run." I urged him to no avail. He just looked at me and said, "I want to play with the sporting goods; they're fun." I felt sorry for making him run like I did, but this confirmed the value of the fun element. I looked over and spotted Charles; he saw me and gestured to me to chase him (as we did in tag). I did and he ran. His run was of a much different quality. He looked excited and put more power behind his steps. This was in stark contrast to Dan's forced run.

After a couple months, a playful mood emerged spontaneously, which was contagious and elicited others' participation. For example:

> All of a sudden Dan gets a smile on his face and grabs the ball and hits the volunteer. He in turn hits Larry. Larry starts to laugh and chases down the volunteer and hits him. I chase Dan who is running and laughing and smiling. I give up pursuit and hit Chuck. I notice Dan hiding behind the volunteer and laughing. Larry ran just about the whole time chasing and avoiding people. In such a short time we achieved a very normal-looking game of tag, with minimal effort. George even got into the game. When the ball came near him he would grab it, run two or three steps, and throw it at someone. Larry started to employ a strategy of acting like he was going to throw the ball at someone just to get them going.

When the game context (i.e., some rule-bound procedures and attitude of fun or playfulness) was not maintained, the men would engage in random and unrelated actions, rather than mutually interacting.

Effects of the Games on the Retarded Men

This section discusses changes in the retarded men during the course of the game program. Each section describes early findings on the men together with changes observed within the games.

Motor behavior   One of the most notable characteristics of these men was their limited motor behavior. Many were overweight, moved only with difficulty, and in an uncoordinated fashion. They walked remarkably slowly and often were fatigued during brief and relatively nontaxing physical exertion. Few were able to run. Most managed a fast walk but demonstrated stiffness and pain at such physical exertion. In the activity center, frustrated staff often resorted to manipulating the men physically through exercise routines.

While the men initially demonstrated the same limitations and inabilities in the sports or games, the allure soon conquered the men's reluctance to physical exertion and diverted the men's attention from minor aches and pains. For instance, one man, who reportedly was unable to run and demonstrated his inability in early sessions, eventually became so engrossed in a game that he spontaneously burst into a run. Several weeks later a participant observer notes:

> I noticed Dan was pursuing the ball carrier this time much longer and more vigorously. In fact, half way through the game he became so exhausted from running that he fell down on his elbows and knees gasping for air. Despite fatigue he got up and started running again. A few months ago, getting Dan to run was almost impossible, since a fast walk would tire him out.

Throughout the program all the men showed progress in their motor behavior, most notably, increased coordination and stamina.

Cognitive abilities   These retarded men demonstrated poor cognitive abilities for practical problem solving and for using appropriate strategies within social situations. Our observations suggested that many of their cognitive limitations were caused by a lack of experience in situations using learning, problem-solving, and strategy generating skills.

One remarkable change in the men was their increased ability to generate and effectively use strategies of interaction and to problem solve around a game. For example:

> When we got more into playing tag, I was struck with how some of the people were already demonstrating remarkably improved skills. Dan was much more alert, ran more (both to avoid and chase people), and was throwing the ball much more accurately. I also noticed him picking out targets excitedly, whereas before he just threw at whoever was around. Michael was the most strikingly different player. He was no longer standing on the fringes of the game field but entered in actively, daring persons to chase him. When he was "it," he often chased Shawn who is difficult to hit because he runs fast and dodges shots. Michael laughed and smiled as he ran after his target, and demonstrated amazing accuracy as he threw the ball.

As the men became familiar with the game, its rules, and purposes, they attempted more elaborate and strategic ways of playing. Games served as meaningful and safe contexts in which to try out new ways of acting. By the end of the study, men who could barely play the simplest games gained sufficient understanding of complex games such as basketball and softball to strategically play with rules and keep other players in mind. These cognitive skills were not demonstrated by the men at the beginning of the study.

The men also improved in their organization of space and time. Early observations revealed that they had no sense of boundaries in games or knowledge of the temporal sequence of events that made up games. They also confined any activity to a small space as if afraid to venture any distance when a ball accidentally rolled away. During the program, the men became increasingly comfortable with large spaces and became able to organize themselves in a space of a football field and a baseball diamond. The games afforded opportunities for them to gain concepts of temporal organization as they had to take turns. At the end of the project, most of the men demonstrated a greatly increased ability to follow the sequence of events in a game and to understand their own relationship in time.

Affect and attention In the beginning of the study, the men usually appeared bored, lethargic, and disinterested in immediate events. Many expressed fear of engaging in behaviors outside a familiar and safe routine. This fear included physical activities and sports, usually manifested as a concern about getting hurt. For example:

> Michael mentioned, very seriously, on the way to the park that we must be very careful and not hit his head. I remarked that we would not "bounce the ball off his head," but he did not find it funny as I intended. In fact, he began to tell me about a world full of dangers and evils in which almost everything was to be avoided.

In addition to this frequent fear of unknown activity, many of the men became easily angered. Mild teasing from a peer might escalate quickly into a fist fight. This consequence appeared linked to a lack of social skill in expressing and negotiating feelings and in recognizing the affect expressed in the reactions of others to one's actions.

Games provided a context for the men to observe, express, experience, and integrate emotions into the rules of the ongoing situation. They learned acceptable expressions of anger and how to identify when someone was upset or angry. Those who had been lethargic became excited and invested in the games. For example:

> The intensity with which Dan plays the game is evident in his facial expressions. His face appears to be more alive on the playing field and he physically demonstrates more life. He also appears more alert. This is in stark contrast to the somewhat tired and slow–moving Dan I know in the center.... Larry understands the game and when he is hit, his face lights up and wears an expression, and he immediately and excitedly breaks into a run. This is so uncharacteristic of him in the center where he just slouches around all day. He gets so much into the emotion of the game that he actually yelled out to another player.

That the men were attending to their environment and to the events around them was remarkable. This increased attention often carried over after the game ended:

Today, I was surprised to see Chuck more aware of our presence. He remembered the game and wanted to go again to the park. He was holding the football with the appearance of being ready to go. He seemed more alert (something Nancy noted as we came back from the park and later mentioned to me) and more aware of things around him. He was looking about more and appeared purposeful in his demeanor.

The fact that the men were more alert meant that they had acquired more information about surrounding events and were less prone to act incompetently, because they lacked such information.

Self-confidence Observations revealed that these men were often hesitant, not self-assured, and always looking to persons in charge for direction. Many appeared incapable of engaging in spontaneous behavior. They were passive and followed requests and orders without fail. Their mode of self-presentation indicated a lack of personal confidence. In settings such as the classroom or restaurants where they had to count or read, they became flustered and often performed below their abilities.

Because in the games the men experienced the leveling phenomenon described earlier and because they experienced success and personal competence, their confidence increased remarkably. The following note exemplifies this:

> The Frisbee activity was interesting for all of us because we had to spread ourselves over great distances and it included a lot of running. Michael's finesse with the Frisbee became apparent. I was impressed most of all by his command over the activity. Here he was a competent self-assured sportsman. This picture is very different from that in the center. It is my impression that he plays the constant role of "court jester" in the activity center, acting very foolish.

As self-confidence accrued, the men assumed more and more demanding roles in games, becoming team captains or quarterbacks. In these roles, they had to make consequential decisions. As confidence increased, the men spontaneously sought out opportunities for playing a variety of roles in the games, requesting to be the pitcher or the catcher. Previously, they stayed within familiar and comfortable roles.

Social interaction Earliest observations of these mentally retarded men revealed that they lacked skills of social interaction. Most were unable to notice and use social cues to guide their behavior. They seemed to have little or no sense of how others perceived and reacted to their own social behavior. Finally, they were unaware of many socially normative means of entering conversation, such as greeting and leave taking, accomplishing these social events in awkward and socially inappropriate ways. For instance, greetings often consisted of prolonged hugs instead of the conventional handshake. Further, these men routinely interacted with each other and with therapists in a teasing and aggressive fashion. The field note describes a typical series of interactions involving Bart, who was famous for his teasing and aggression:

> There were a number of interesting reactions to Bart's maneuvers. Michael became flustered. but wouldn't talk directly to Bart. He would say things about Bart with his head turned away such as, "Shouldn't do that" or, "have to be a good boy." Bart just responded by stuffing the glasses down Michael's shirt. Robert, in response to being called a "punk" by Bart and referred to by him as "nuts" threatened to slug Bart in the face....

During games, the men were faced with the consequences of their behavior for others and had to gauge and direct their own behavior according to the actions and attitudes of others. They eventually demonstrated increased ability to interact in ways that were more socially acceptable. For example, Bart, who formerly only got attention through teasing, learned to evoke normal social responses by playing the game competently. This was dramatically illustrated in a final baseball game when his teammates cheered as he hit a double.

Conclusions

This article reports findings from an exploratory study that examined the use of games as therapeutic media with mentally retarded adults. The rationale for the games was the potential game behavior could have as an important learning mechanism and the importance of normal play for quality of life. Occupational therapists collected data as participant observers during a year while they implemented a program of games with the men. The focus of data collection was on therapists' strategies to make effective use of the games and on changes in the subjects. Data, consisting of field notes and videotapes, were reported here under categories generated from analysis of the data.

The strategies employed by occupational therapists to enhance the game behavior of the men included grading complexity, leveling relationships, coaching and modeling, and keeping up the game context and continuity. Grading complexity helped assure that each person was optimally challenged in the game and was able to perform according to his abilities. Leveling relationships allowed the therapist to assume a parallel role with the retarded person when the latter showed the ability to act competently and autonomously. Remaining in the role of therapist or instructor was often counterproductive since it kept retarded persons in a reciprocal dependent role. Coaching and modeling provided information to the retarded person to formulate his own behavior. Coaching provided feedback and modeling provided instances of behavior and affect for imitation. Maintaining the game context and continuity was an extremely important strategy. Keeping up a rule ordered sequence of playful behavior was necessary to provide a game or playful context in which the men could effectively participate.

Change in the men included motor behavior, cognitive abilities, affect and attention, self-confidence, and social interaction. Improvement was observed in the areas of coordination and stamina. The men showed an increase in their cognitive ability to employ purposeful strategies of behavior and to understand and competently use time and space. Lethargic and disoriented demeanor was replaced with increased joy, excitement, investment, and attention. The game provided a context in which the men gained self-confidence through success in areas within which they could excel and in which they learned strategies of interaction with social others.

The findings from this exploratory study support the assertion that therapists can influence the game behavior (play) of retarded men. The strategies of therapists described in the findings should serve as suggestions for further refinement of techniques of using games as therapy. Further study using control groups and standardized measures of dependent variables would also be desirable. Also, the form of investigation used here is an appropriate research model for developing programs and achieving a preliminary assessment of how they can be made effective.

References

1. Wiemer R: Traditional and nontraditional practice areas. In *Occupational Therapy: 2001 A.D.* Rockville, MD: American Occupational Therapy Association, 1979.

2. Bruner J: Introduction. In *Play: Its Role in Development and Evolution*, J Bruner, A Jolly, K Sylva, Editors. New York: Basic Books, 1976.

3. Einon D: The purpose of play. In *Not Work Alone*, J. Cherfas, R Lewin, Editors. Beverly Hills: Sage Publications, 1980.

4. Reynolds P: Play language and human evolution. In *Play: Its Role in Development and Evolution*, J Bruner, A Jolly, K Sylva, Editors. New York: Basic Books, 1976.

5. Sylva K, Bruner JS, Genova P: The role of play in the problem-solving of children 3–5 years old. In *Play: Its Role in Development and Evolution*, J Bruner, A Jolly, K Sylva, Editors. New York: Basic Books, 1976.

6. Reilly M: *Play as Exploratory Learning*, Beverly Hills: Sage Publications, 1974.

7. Robinson A: Play as an arena for acquisition of rules for competent behavior. *Am J Occup Ther, 31:* 248–253,1977.

8. Mead GH: *Mind, Self, and Society,* Chicago: University of Chicago Press, 1934.

9. Sutton-Smith B: A syntax for play and games. In *Child's Play,* RE Herron, B Sutton-Smith, Editors. New York: John Wiley and Sons, 1971.

10. Horne B, Philleo C: A comparative study of the spontaneous play activities of normal and mentally defective children. In *Play: Its Role in Development and Evolution,* J Bruner, A Jolly, K Sylva, Editors. New York: Basic Books, 1976.

11. Morgan SB: Responsiveness to stimulus novelty and complexity in mild, moderate, and severe retardates, *Am J Ment Defic 74:* 32–38, 1969.

12. Collard R: Exploratory and play behaviors of infants reared in an institution and in lower- and middle-class homes. *Child Dev 42:* 1003–1015, 1971.

13. Berlyne D: Laughter, humor and play. In *The Handbook of Social Psychology, Vol III,* G Lindzer, SE Aronson, Editors. Reading, MA: Addison-Wesley Co., 1969.

14. Ellis MJ: *Why People Play,* Englewood Cliffs, NJ: Prentice-Hall, 1973.

15. Freyburg JT: Increasing the imaginative play of urban disadvantaged kindergarten children through systematic training. In *The Child's World of Make–believe,* G. Singer, Editor. New York: Academic Press, 1973.

16. Ellis, MJ, Scholtz GJL: *Activity and Play in Childhood,* Englewood Cliffs, NJ: Prentice-Hall, Inc., 1978.

17. Berlyne D: *Conflict, Arousal and Curiosity,* New York: McGraw-Hill, 1960.

18. Johnson J: *Doing Field Research,* New York: Free Press, 1975.

19. Lofland J: *Doing Social Life,* New York: John Wiley and Sons, 1976.

20. Denzin N: The logic of naturalistic inquiry. *Social Forces 50:* 166–182, 1971.

21. Patton MQ: *Qualitative Evaluation Methods,* Beverly Hills: Sage Publications, 1980.

22. Bodernan M: A problem of sociological praxis: The case for interventive observation in fieldwork. *Theory and Society 5:* 387–419, 1978.

23. Campbell D: "Degrees of freedom" and the case study. In *Qualitative and Quantitative Methods in Evaluation Research,* T Cook, C Reichardt, Editors. Beverly Hills: Sage Publications, 1979.

Chapter 30

Designing Activities to Develop a Women's Identification Group

Mary V. Donohue, PhD, OTR

Successful socialization or resocialization of the psychiatric patient is a difficult undertaking, regardless of diagnosis. Individual and group therapies are often geared toward change of obvious, glaring deficits and a variety of problem behaviors in each patient. Most activity groups aim themselves at instituting or restoring activities of daily living, communal planning or occupational skills in a heterosexual and age-blended environment.

By contrast, in an identification group, with specifically designated age and sex groupings, an opportunity is provided for socialization activities that generally occur in club-style reference groups, a particular type of gathering which people still develop and enjoy.

This paper presents a theory and suggested activities for a women's identification group that can provide an experience of camaraderie and familial belonging for selected patients.

Part 1: Theoretical Basis

Observing the clusters of psychiatric patients who drift together in a lounge or cafeteria provides an opportunity to appraise the natural social needs of individuals in a relatively self-selective situation. Such observation suggests that patients frequently display a tendency to spend their free time gathering together along homogeneous age and self-identification lines. Ample opportunity is provided in most psychiatric settings for heterogeneous work, social, and community decision-making style meeting. Yet spontaneous gravitations tend to indicate an on-going desire for some social experiences in the relaxed atmosphere of homogeneous groupings.

Purpose of Article

Why are homogeneous groupings so attractive, and what is their potential value for social growth in a psychiatric setting? Attempting to understand what goes on in a homogeneous group and exploring possible ways to take advantage of this natural phenomenon could enhance our therapeutic effectiveness in working with psychiatric patients. Since the writer has been working with an adult women's reference group, ages 28 and up, the applications discussed will be illustrations appropriate to that membership group.

This chapter was previously published in *Occupational Therapy in Mental Health*, 2, (1), 1–19. Copyright © 1982, The Haworth Press, Inc.

Theoretical Model of the Group

The theoretical model for an identification group is based on concepts of sociological theories of groups such as 1) a *natural group*, 2) a *membership group*, 3) a *reference group* and 4) a *primary group*. By type, age and sex homogeneous groups classified as identification groups include elements of these concepts.[1,2] A *natural group* is one to which an individual belongs innately, inescapably, such as by family, sex, nationality.[1,2] A *membership group* is one to which a person presently belongs.[1] One's *reference group* may or may not be a membership group: it is a group to which an individual "aspires to attain or maintain membership."[2] In scope, this definition has a dual aspect, applying either to an existing state or to a desired one, both events, actively relating to the group as a societal anchorage point. By type, an age-and-sex homogeneous group is both a natural and a membership group, but it is not necessarily a reference group, though it may become so by reason of selection. Since the terms "natural group" and "membership group" are too broad in their scope and may denote more than an age-and-sex homogeneous group, this latter group could be designated an *identification group*. Age and sex are both generally used by the communications media as the first two defining characteristics of an individual's identification. The term *identification group* can bear the meaning of a natural, social membership group composed of time-sequenced and gender-specific persons, thus avoiding violations against the elective aspect of the term *reference group*.

Theory of Identification Group Development

One therapeutic goal for selecting a group of psychiatric patients who are time-slotted in a given age range and gender-cast of the same mold is to choose candidates who can, by association, shape a membership group into a reference/identification group. Both theoretically and practically speaking, however, one cannot assume that this would occur since movement toward this group choice must develop on an individual basis, in individuals prepared to respond to the appealing aspects of the group.

Shaping the members of an identification group toward acceptance of the group as a reference group can be brought about by fostering the "we-ness" of age and sex that is inherent in the group at its outset. Emphasizing the common life experiences of individuals can promote sympathy and mutuality among members which may enhance development of relations of a primary nature. *Primary relations* are characterized as a response to the person as a total entity or as a response to a non-replaceable, non-transferable personality. Communications in primary relationships include sharing expressions of emotion, so as to acknowledge the person-as-individual. As Charles Cooley explained the term: "By primary groups I mean those characterized by intimate face-to-face association and cooperation ... they are fundamental in forming the social nature and ideals of the individual. The result of intimate association, the primary group, psychologically is a certain fusion of individualities in a common whole, so that one's very self, for many purposes at least is the common life and purpose of the group. Perhaps the simplest way of describing this wholeness is by saying that it is a "we"; it involves the sort of ... identification for which "we" is a natural expression."[3] The unity of the primary group lies in allegiance to basic standards and the sharing of common experiences, and is, therefore, able to support some degree of lack of harmony. The feelings of kinship in a primary group are based on the commonalities of human nature.

In the case of the identification group whose basis is age and sex, the common fund of experiences of passage through a specific set of decades, plus the kindred life-space of male or female within that defined era, constitute fertile fields for exploration of common time and life-style sets for group members. It is hoped that by focusing the identification group on representative experiences, while at the same time using the mode of communications styled "primary," that the membership group will, by election, become a reference group.

A primary mode of communication, as contrasted with a formal mode, can be introduced by imitation of the group leader who relates to the members of the identification group as unique persons, capable of emotion and deserving of adequate life-satisfaction. The leader should be a member of the age and sex group, and be able to communicate the attractiveness of "reference" to the group as a desirable entity. In this manner the central person with the reference group provides an infectious influence integrating members into a group.[4] In fact, serious hang-ups about age and sexual identity in the leader are contraindicated in this group. Some conflict in the attitudes of the central person can, through joint examination of the leader's ambivalence during the group, develop group emotions,[4] expand awareness, and stimulate expression of individual stances on controversial issues. Ideally, the central person should, in addition, be expansive enough in outlook to be empathetic toward the conflicts of group members who find themselves on the periphery of the group, allowing them to maintain their position, encouraging them to express and develop their unique relationship to the group.

Theory of Reference Group Process

The mode of the reference group process is supportive in nature, and tries to provide opportunity for the expression of a variety of opinions and emotions in a manner that maintains a tone of acceptance.[5] Encouraging the manifestation and release of tension, the asking for and giving of suggestions, opinion and orientation, should provide an experience of solidarity that can leave the group members with a feeling of relative comfort and security. Reviewing members' out-group and in-group stereotypes and discussing their degree of social distance in relating to people can promote an awareness of existing social positions and consciousness of the possibility of selecting one, or a number of these positions, as points of reference.

While having an awareness that members of the group may not have elected it as a reference group, the central person can rely quite heavily on a majority holding an initial, moderate allegiance to the group. People tend to accept groups which, in their judgement, hold opinions similar to their own, who look similar to themselves, and whose experience and abilities are near their own.[6] The attractiveness of the reference-identification group can allow for the lowering of inner restraints, thus providing a climate likely to foster the expression of individual experience. At the same time, the comfortable atmosphere, created by the feeling of group identity permits a temporary deindividuation[7] to occur whereby the person can become less self-conscious and less inhibited by strong feelings of responsibility for every utterance. One of the tasks of the group leader is to allow these non-defensive expressions of opinion and feeling to be made, acknowledge their validity as emotion, and promote group reaction in order to evaluate each position.

Humans possess a strong tendency to appraise their opinions and abilities by association with and in comparison with others. This process of examination of contrasts provides a range of comparability where the individual can feel at ease since the reference group milieu promotes an environment of social acceptance. "The very organization of the self-conscious community is dependent upon individuals" trying on "the attitude of other individuals." This taking the role of the other ... is of importance in the development of cooperative activity."[8] Trying on the position of others and giving comparative feedback allows for a timeout process, a delayed response, a halt in behavior while consideration of various options of response is going on. Persons involved in this process are exposed to a new repertoire of behaviors possible in situations under discussion in the group. Joining to this the element of evaluation of behaviors and attitudes helps the individual become socially self-critical, thus providing a base for the cooperative social learning interaction mentioned above.

In essence, a two-fold inter-locking process of group and individual interaction is underway in which the gregariousness of human nature brings individuals together to temporarily de-individuate them, opening them up to expressions of self, which are confirmed or modified, so that both group and individual entities are strengthened. What makes this possible is a group allowing a range of human behaviors promoting both commonality and individuality. Once the cooperative spirit is established, " . . . the presence of a co-working group is distinctly favorable to the speed of the process of free association"[9] by the individual. More ideas are produced in a group than by the sum total of the same people working alone, since the group stimulates expression of a more expansive type[9] thus enlarging the scope of behaviors possible both to the group and to the individual.

With the group generating ideas, opinions, comparisons and suggestions, and experiencing a common pool of vicarious situations through sharing, the individual begins to enjoy the rewards of camaraderie. At the same time, limits and sanctions will emerge to influence the member to conform to certain agreed upon norms. If the individual sufficiently enjoys the rewards of the group, its companionship and approval, he will wish to conform to the group norms to the degree necessary to remain a member. It is at this point that the first conscious decision to make this a reference group, or to reject it as a reference group, arises. This selection process is ongoing, never final. When used with discretion, the ability of a reference group to encourage a degree of social conformity can be a workable method of shaping social behaviors as well as of developing individual identity, for the individual comes to see that he is not identical to any other group member. But which social behaviors are to be promoted? Who should make that decision? Looking at the nature of the particular group can provide some of the answers.

Historical and Cultural Nature of Women's Group

A cohort of women twenty-eight and older has a common heritage dating at least from 1950. By comparison with a younger women's group, their cultural upbringing and time–space may have been more restrictive: their philosophy of life, their mores, and the roles they see open to them for the future tend to be more conservative."[10] Women of this era grew toward maturity, in most instances, modeling themselves on a traditionally female perception of vocational roles, a feminine mode of social relationships and a "female" cognitive style. Specifically, this meant a globalized self-concept as "female," rather than a particular person with individualized abilities and experience.[11,12] The female self-concept has frequently been lacking both in motivation toward achievement[13,14] and in the ability to make far-reaching decisions.[15] The integration of talent and capacities as potentially functional and productive may have been neglected. Growing up for females of this age range meant initiation into a mode of relating socially which was lacking in confident assertiveness, in appropriate competitiveness, and in respect for, and trust in, other women. Instead, women of these decades were given the expectation of learning receptivity, reactivity, general passivity, and complementarity toward men.[16,17]

Their education most often did not include emphasis on comprehension, mechanical aptitude, exploration in risk-taking, mathematical reasoning, analytic and problem solving ability. Rather, the learning style encouraged among women was more often rote memory, recitation, verbal fluency and field dependency.[18, 19]

Unfortunately for these women, it is the traditional male cognitive style that provides adequate preparation for scientific, technical, professional, and administrative competence.[20–24]

For many women of this age group, marriage carried with it a manner of relating to other women as wives of one's husband's male friends. This eliminated the possibility of selecting female friends as individuals, rather than as members of a coupled pair. The majority of today's women twenty-eight years and older have completed their child-bearing and toddler-rearing years. Their children are school age. Issues that are meaningful for them within a reference group include questions such as: what plans do they have to occupy their free time? Do they have the psycho-social and cognitive tools needed to define goals for themselves, and, if they so desire, to restructure their lives? A reference group cannot bear the responsibility of providing solutions, but it can make suggestions.

Relationships in an Adult Women's Group

The principles of the relationships for the group as expressed in theory are recommended for as close an application to the practical situation as is possible.

The purpose of what hopefully will evolve into an adult women's reference group is viewed as a step in the further socialization or re-socialization of the members. In the case of psychiatric patients, their recent life style may have been socially isolating or alienating. Moving from a marginal social position to a comfortable and secure manner of relating to others is a difficult task and requires the restoration of primary-style modes of relating. The key to initiating and reinstating these kinds of relationships is the leader's use of the self. From the outset, the leader should be a member, active in participating in the group's undertaking. Aside from employing suggestions made earlier in discussing the theory of relationships in primary groups, the central member should be a role model, making a natural but measured use of the self as a vehicle for generating interaction. As Cohan has expressed it in a monograph entitled "Reference Groups," "The leader should also serve as an attainable, approachable and appealing role model ..." so that, in fact, the patient should be able to feel that this group has the potential for becoming a peer group, in the true sense of the term.

Goals for the Adult Women's Group

Extracting the goals that surface from the needs of a psychiatric population, the general female age group, and

the given purpose of an identification group, the following objectives emerge as most basic: (1) increased comfort, satisfaction, and self-confidence in the essence of identification as woman, individually, and as a member of that half of the human race called female, (2) clarification of aspirations and capabilities of women in a structured, cognitive manner, (3) ability to select and develop appropriate primary relationships inside and outside the hospital experience, (4) development of what is called "socialization" in general parlance, but sociologically should be labeled sociability and social presence.

Social Activity Club Concept

In searching for the place in society where this type of identification/reference group occurs naturally, the investigation would lead to clubs where people relate to each other socially around an activity. Interestingly, upon further examination, it would be found that many such clubs tend to be single-sex groups, or to be sub-grouped sexually.

How can this type group be simulated in a rehabilitation activity program? The women's and men's identification groups should be designed to provide a selected social and leisure environment, employing purposeful activities in the goal directed use of a client's resources, time, energy, interest and attention, in the traditional occupational therapy mode described by Reilly and Llorens (see Chapter 6).[25–27]

Clark further points out specifically that: "Role performance, involves the use of selected purposeful activities, including the various skills, habits, tasks and relationships acquired through the acculturation of the individual."[28 (p. 579)] Social role development activities of casual conversation, topical-cognitive discussion, imaginative risk-taking simulations, role playing, as well as body-image exercises of movement and sports in single sex groups seem best suited to this task and thus have been selected after careful analysis of their ability to promote a social activity club environment.

During the group meetings the leader promotes the shaping of social growth in each individual, encouraging practice at the level appropriate to current abilities and giving specific feedback in situ. As Fidler has clearly indicated: "The nature of the occupational therapy setting, which effects active involvement in doing, provides a microcosm of life-work situations which can be seen and explored as they occur rather than in retrospect (see Chapter 7)."[29 (p. 45, 30)] There is much of the occupational therapy process in social activity groups that utilizes an on-site teaching–learning process. Mosey cites this latter process as a "legitimate tool of the occupational therapy model."[31]

Part II: Methodology

This second section will be devoted to the concrete application of the above theoretical principles, discussing referral procedures, membership criteria, and activity designs.

Referrals

Referrals to the Adult Women's group are made by activity therapists who feel that their clients need to work on further development of the goals mentioned in Part 1: (1) positive female identification, (2) recognition of women's capabilities, (3) appropriate selection of companions, and (4) sociability and social presence.

Contraindicated are (1) women who are near either end of the age range *and* who identify with a younger or older group, and (2) women who are too anxious to tolerate a heavily verbal group. The decision as to what is best for the individual should be made in collaboration with her.

Membership

The members of the specific group with whom the author has been working are women aged 28 to 50, of middle class background, with a psychiatrically-caused dysfunction, who have the shared experience of a hospitalization averaging two or three months in an in-patient hospital, day hospital, or after-care program. Some of the members of the group have experienced all three in sequence, some have been in the hospital a number of times, but all need guidance in integrating the results of that experience into the social aspects of their lives.

Most group members have been diagnosed within some category of schizophrenia. The majority are of middle and upper middle class socioeconomic status, living in an "outer city" environment. They tend to be high school graduates with some college exposure, who are relatively well-informed despite a history of psychosocial dysfunction.

All discussions on any topic inclusive of social interaction need to be open to incorporating issues that touch on the social consequences of mental illness. In some instances, this common experience provides the group with a built-in mutual bond; in other instances, depending on current membership, a group may still need guidance in relating to this shared life-situation.

Frequency of Meetings

The Adult Women's group is currently meeting three days per week to provide an opportunity for a variety of social learning experiences. Day One, a Formal/Cognitive Day, is devoted to specific topic-centered discussion of social issues for women; Day Two, an Experiential/Innovative Day, provides an opportunity for behavioral experimentation; and Day Three, Informal/Problem-Solving Day, consists of a rap session. The remainder of this article will develop the daily activities in detail. The range of these activities is designed to offer the women some scope in experiencing paired, sub-group and group interactions, of structured and informal types within

traditional, moderate and liberal perspectives to allow for change in life space, or for a conscious selection of present life-styles.

Style of Leadership

The leader relates as a group member, role model and moderator/guide. As a group member she manifests a lively interest in being with the group, in the personal lives of the individual members, and in the community activities within the therapeutic milieu.

As a role model, she listens intently, reacts to tension in the group, promotes tension release, indicates agreement, disagreement, opinion, suggestion, gives and asks for information, and fosters solidarity.[32] At times the role model uses illustrations from her own life experience, insofar as they are of assistance to the individual and the group, without burdening the group with significant problem-solving for herself. Selective use of role modeling provides an opportunity for imitative learning, stimulates discussion and makes the leader an example of one possible life-style as opposed to an unattainable leader-prototype.

As a moderator/guide, the leader encourages group planning, prepared, however, to present and promote alternatives should a member be unable to carry out responsibilities for group preparation of an activity. In this capacity the leader promotes member to member interaction within the group, avoiding constant comment which would set up a dyadic "leader–group" interaction rather than the desired cooperative peer interaction.[33] This aspect of her leadership can reinforce assets of members and encourage attempts at new undertakings by acknowledging a member's shaping of new behaviors.

Day One: Topic-Centered Discussion For the Formal / Cognitive Day

The topic-centered discussion meetings have focused on occupational therapy's traditional areas of concern: activities of daily living—roles, life-styles, relationships, health, sexuality, child-bearing and child rearing, birth control, exercise, dieting, venereal disease, leisure, money-making, grooming, self-defense, emotions, and women role models. These are structured cognitive discussions where, at times, the group members have raised the topics or brought in articles to discuss; for most topic-centered meetings, the leader or members can provide copies of short articles on the above topics. These are read briefly at the opening of the hour-long meeting, followed by a free-flowing discussion.

For many women, unaccustomed to female discussion of a somewhat structured nature, these topics have provided a first opportunity to experience women approaching each other in a manner indicating that they are knowledgeable—that they have information and experiences to share with each other. Through participating on content focused discussion, some women have expressed surprise that other women could be interesting, instructive, even intelligent! Often there are quiet participants, too, who are obviously listening, unable at the moment to join in, even upon invitation, but who are absorbing the life-happenings and opinions of others with apparent relish. On occasion, women with a sheltered background may manifest distress at hearing material that might be frightening to them. In these cases, the individual's occupational therapist and primary therapist have been alerted to reviewing these issues on a one-to-one basis.

A group that presents a cognitive-focused discussion provides schizophrenic patients with an occasion to practice concentration and sequential thought processes, since ample opportunity exists in most therapeutic centers for emotive-focused group therapy. Limit-setting interventions are employed to re-focus wayward contributions that stray from the focus of the topic in much the same way as in a well-ordered classroom discussion.

Generally, the women have been enthusiastic about this cognitive-oriented discussion hour. Several have reported to the leader that they were coming to like women for the first time, since they now saw them as capable of participating in meaningful, intelligent discussion.

Day Two: Growth Intervention Exercises for the Experiential / Innovative Day

While researching areas where women need growth-expanding experiences, the following issues emerged: identity, risk-taking, assertiveness, decision-making, fantasy, achievement motivation, resourcefulness, competition, trust-building, respect among women, sex-role stereotyping, and critical and cooperative listening.[17-21] It has been observed by many analysts of women's development that as girl-children, women generally have not had as many opportunities for involvement with or expression of some of these ego-maturing activities. In selecting developmental activities for a hospital-based population, it was kept in mind that many of group members might be limited in their desire or capacity to participate. All who are felt appropriate for referral to the group are encouraged, in a general manner, to participate or take a risk—however, without coercion, as in the style of a support group. Participation is acknowledged for whatever degree of involvement the individual is able to muster.

In introducing each *life-simulation activity*, a brief explanation of the reason why the activity is pertinent for women is presented. One or two goals of the exercise are concisely described so as to provide an objective to work toward, without revealing all that the women can discover experientially for themselves. This prelude, in addition, is meant to offset resistance from some members stemming from a discomfort with an exercise as "childish." Consistent with the utilization of purposeful activity in occupational therapy, an enthusiastic and rational

mode of presentation carries intentionality in a fairly light-hearted, playful vein. Individuals are encouraged to try on non-standard behaviors in an experimental fashion, and to immerse themselves in the activity, temporarily suspending their disinclinations, saving comments and observations for the discussion period at the end. In addition, the women are asked to make a mental note of inner reactions to the exercise as it is happening, so that they can share these experiences at the conclusion, if they so desire. It is also made clear that no one is obliged to share any part of themselves: that the focus of discussion will be in the process of the experience, so as to develop the cognitive and emotional skill of selective sharing based on considered judgements, an ability that naive schizophrenic patients often lose in the process of being "overtherapized" to the point of indiscriminate trustfulness.

The general aim of these initial remarks is to create a relaxed atmosphere where spontaneity of inner experience can be allowed with a minimum of stress on shared revelations, so as to create the milieu described above: a primary group developed by a process that is basically respectful of privacy and responding to shared contributions in a supportive manner.

There are many activity exercises that could be selected for specific use in highlighting the need for a particular outlook or skill to be added to the repertoire of behaviors and interpersonal interactions of adult women patients. A few sources are listed in the bibliography,[34-40] and will be described here to illustrate the particular goals outlined for consideration by adult women patients.

Activity-exercises used to explore and develop individual identity have included making *collage-brochures* representing the self in an "advertisement"; writing down the past, present and future *role-configuration of one's identity*, including social roles, work roles and activity roles; listing briefly *strengths and weaknesses of one's personality*, labelling them as traditionally male or female.

Well-known *decision-making exercises* used have consisted of listing "*Who Should Survive?*" an atomic attack and "*What to do*" on a trip when your car breaks down or your purse is stolen.

Exercises in *assertiveness* which were popular with this age group included role playing of *maintaining a mood* in the face of opposition, and taking the part of a real or imaginary "*role model*" whose traits are to be identified by one's exercise-partner.

Fantasy-exercises have been aimed at broadening risk-taking, and expanding the realm of the "possible." Some of the more appealing ones have been the *cosmic-visitors arrival fantasy*, played out in self-selected pairs; an *adventure-fantasy* on an imaginary raft-journey.

Achievement motivation activities have included written goals, listed numerically by priority and an orally-expressed "*Hopes Whip*," brainstorming about wishes and satisfactions hoped for and already fulfilled.

Combination *cooperative-competitive exercises* selected were: standing *two-handed hand-wrestling* aimed at pitting strength, and sizing-up coordination without throwing the partner off balance; and *building decorative "towers"* around contrived frames, vying for height, stability and attractiveness, in small groups versus other small groups. Discussions here centered around the balance between cooperation and competition, an unexplored area for many women.

Experiences of *ability to abstract* visually focused on exercises in *building models* of styrofoam and sticks, then drawing a diagram of someone else's model; and *giving instructions* to someone who is blindfolded to "steer" them around an "obstacle course" in the room. The well-known *blind walk* can still spark a discussion on trust and taking of responsibility for another.

The *"assets and abilities pot"* consists of members identifying the characteristics of others in the group from slips of paper drawn from a pile in the center of the floor or table. As each paper is drawn from the "pot" members try to identify other members to whom the personality traits might belong.

In general, the more threatening activity-exercises are done in pairs, with partners selected by group members rather than in a large group. The discussion of the experience has been carried on in the large group by those wishing to make a contribution. Discussion can be both structured by questions and spontaneous in following the lead of the group's needs and experiences. One or two activities zeroing in on particular attributes are *not* expected to totally change behaviors. However, they can and do remind the members of human attributes that they may have exercises premorbidly, or may be acquainting them with experiences opening up to them for the first time. Furthermore, they provide the group with a common ground of experience to live through at the moment, discuss, recall and repeat in situations outside the group, thus adding to the development of an identification group.

In effect, a time-honored principle of occupational therapy, the employment of graduated, shaping-behaviors to enable "learning by doing" is utilized.

Day Three: Rap Session for the Informal / Problem Solving Day

Since the primary group most often gathers around food, one day's meeting per week encourages members to bring coffee and whatever else is desired for a relaxed, freewheeling verbal exchange. The atmosphere here is a casual rap session with discussion touching on trivia, comparing notes, gossip and woman-talk. This environment allows for acceptance of the more traditional elements of women's gatherings, thus rounding out the opportunities to experience a range of weekly meetings: conservative, moderate and innovative in nature.

In carrying out the on-going re-assessment of patients' needs, a few months ago a re-arrangement of the plan for activities for these three days was implemented. This involved adding a dance-aerobics/flexibility exercise day weekly, and alternating the components of topic-centered discussion and growth intervention exercises every other week. With physical exercise currently in the spotlight of personal care objectives, the adult women patients have been pleased with this weekly combination of activities.

Men's Reference Group

Men's reference group activities have been planned along the same lines described above for women, looking at the needs *men* have to dynamically develop areas of their personalities which have been neglected or stifled due to cultural circumstances. The men's group has been successful in attracting its members with its social activity club environment, similar to that of the women's group.

Since psychiatric patients often have not experienced even the usual opportunities for male identification development, the addition of meetings devoted to sports in a gym or outdoors, and playing favorite records or tapes have proven to be popular quasi-social activities among the men, providing them with a more traditional starting place for interaction, comparable to the women's coffee klatch. From here the men can move on to their weekly rap session discussing current roles for men as they are lived out and experimented with in our society. The tone of the men's group has been low-keyed and relatively conservative by comparison with the women's group, accurately reflecting the general status of contemporary social roles within the larger community where women are presently more involved than men in social transformation.

Discharge Planning

After discharge from the hospital, patients have often expressed a feeling of loss of the women's group when they return for a visit. From time to time notes and letters addressed to the group have been received from former patients who look back to the group as a positive experience—one which they would like to continue. For this reason, presently members are given information on local women's groups before they leave the hospital. The woman's individual preferences are discussed with her around making a decision as to the tone and mode of group suited to her immediate needs so that suggestions include a variety of groups: for example, child-care exchange groups, church and synagogue auxiliaries, and near-by chapters of the National Organization of Women (NOW). In this way it is hoped that the group members will find an on-going identification group for themselves in the community. In addition, members are encouraged to meet together outside the group, to exchange phone numbers with women whose company they enjoy in order to develop their spontaneous relationships, possibly forming their own support group.

Summary

The Sociological Framework

The value of reference group affiliation for the individual lies in its contribution to formation of personal identity by comparison with the group, construction of norms for behavior, a sense of belonging, an exploration of the nature of one's social associations, as well as an opportunity to shift one's social outlook if one so desires.

The Occupational Therapy Method

The activities described above—this combination of planned experiences, structured discussions, and casual get-togethers—have been adequate vehicles for rudimentary exchanges of interpersonal interaction for beginners in peer communications, and have been more than sufficient stimulation for the resumption of complex relationships in more mature individuals. In fact, though an enjoyable group for most participants, it is the more socially developed women who express strong attachment to the group and its opportunity for companionship. The group provides an environment for rounding out and supplementing the patient's primary or individual therapeutic experiences. The primary therapist is most often in the position of providing a primary relationship with the patient. The women's group leader has the potential for becoming one of a number of secondary relationships. In an initially parental position, who can then lead the patient on to other secondary relationships with peers who discuss planfully how they may interact in still other secondary relationships.

This marriage of a sociological framework with occupational therapy principles and methods has been successful in evoking the revival of social skills and in building further on the pleasurable interaction elicited.

References

1. Siegel AE and Siegel S: Reference groups, membership groups and attitude change. *J Abnorm Psychol 55:* 360–364, 1957.

2. Sherif M and Sherif C: *Groups in Harmony and Tension,* New York. Harper and Brothers, 1953.

3. Cooley C: *Social Organization,* New York: Charles Scribner's Sons. 1937.

4. Redl F: Group emotion and leadership. *Psychiatry 5:* 573–596, 1942.

5. Bales RF: The equilibrium problem in small groups. Abridged from Parsons T, Bales RF, and Shils EA: *Working Papers in the Theory of Action.* Glencoe. IL: Free Press, 1953.

6. Festinger L: A theory of social comparison processes. *Hum Rel 7:* 117–140. 1954.

7. Festinger L. Pepitone A. and Newcomb TM: Some consequences of de-individuation in a group. *J Abnor Psychol 47:* 382–389, 1952.

8. Mead GH: *Mind, Self and Society from the Standpoint of a Social Behaviorist,* Chicago: University of Chicago. 1934.

9. Allport FH: The influence of the group upon association and thought. *J Exp Psychol (Gen) 3:* 159–182, 1920.

10. Mead M: *Male and Female,* New York: William Morrow and Company. 1949.

11. Mitchel J: *Psychoanalysis and Feminism: Freud, Reich, Laing and Women,* New York: Pantheon Books, 1974.

12. Blum HP, ed., *Journal of the American Psychoanalytic Association Supplement—Female Psychology, 24:* 5, New York: Universities Press. 1976.

13. Alper TG: Achievement motivation in college women. *Am Psychol 3:* 29. 194–203, 1974.

14. Hoffman LW: Early childhood experiences and women's achievement motives. *J Soc Issues 28:* 2. 129–155, 1972.

15. Chodrow N: Being and doing, a cross-cultural examination of socialization of males and females. In Gornick V and Moran BK: *Women in Sexist Society,* New York: New American Library, 1971.

16. Erikson E: *Identity, Youth and Crisis.* New York: WW Norton. 1968.

17. Rohrbaugh JB: Femininity on the line, *Psych Today 13:* 3. Aug. 79: 30–42.

18. Kohlberg L: A cognitive-developmental analysis of children's sex role concepts and attitudes. In *The Development of Sex Differences.* Edited by Maccoby E. Stanford, CA: Stanford University Press, 1966.

19. Mischel W: A social learning view of sex differences in behavior. In *The Development of Sex Differences.* Edited by Maccoby E. Stanford, CA: Stanford University Press, 1966.

20. Bardwick JM and Douvan E: Ambivalence: The socialization of women. In *Readings on the Psychology of Women.* Edited by Bardwick JM. New York: Harper and Row 1972.

21. Douvan E: Sex differences in adolescent character processes. In *Readings on the Psychology of Women.* Edited by Bardwick JM. New York: Harper and Row, 1972.

22. Rossi A: Barriers to the career choice of engineering, medicine or science among American women. In *Readings on the Psychology of Women.* Edited by Bardwick, JM, New York: Harper and Row, 1972.

23. Harragan BL: *Games Mother Never Taught You.* New York: Warner Books, 1977.

24. Collette C: Women and appropriate technology. *Sun Times,* September, 1980:3.

25. Reilly M: An explanation of play. In *Play as Exploratory Learning: Studies in Curiosity Behavior,* M Reilly, Editor. Los Angeles: Sage Publications, 1974, pp. 117–149.

26. Reilly M: 1961 Eleanor Clark Slagle Lecture: Occupational therapy can be one of the great ideas of 20th century medicine. *Am J Occup Ther 16:* 1–9. 1962 (Reprinted as Chapter 6).

27. Llorens LA: 1969 Eleanor Clark Slagle Lecture: Facilitating growth and development: the promise of occupational therapy. *Am J Occup Ther 24:* 1–9. 1970.

28. Clark, Pat Nuse. Human development through occupation: a philosophy and conceptual model for practice, part 2. *Am J Occup Ther 33:* 577–585, 1979.

29. Fidler GS: The task-oriented group as a context for treatment. *Am J Occup Ther 23:* 43–48, 1969.

30. Fidler GS, Fidler JW: Doing and becoming: purposeful action and self-actualization. *Am J Occup Ther 32:* 305–310, 1978 (Reprinted as Chapter 7).

31. Mosey, AC: A model for occupational therapy. *Occup Ther in Mental Health 1:* 11–31, 1980.

32. Bales RF. *Interaction Process Analysis. A Method for the Study of Small Groups,* New York: Holt, Rinehart and Winston, 1950.

33. Mosey, AC: *Three Frames of Reference for Mental Health.* Thorofare, New Jersey: Charles B. Slack, Inc., 1970.

34. Pfeiffer JW and Jones JE: *Handbook of Structured Experiences for Human Relations Training,* I, II, III, IV, Iowa City: University Associates Press, P.O. Box 615, Iowa, 52240, 1971.

35. Otto, HA: *Fantasy Encounter Games,* New York: Harper and Row, 1972.

36. Otto HA: *Group Methods to Actualize Human Potential, A Handbook,* Beverly Hills, CA: The Holistic Press, 1973.

37. Sax S and Hollander S: *Reality Games,* New York: Popular Library, 1972.

38. Lew HR and Streitfeld HS: *Growth Games,* New York: Bantam Books, 1972.

39. Hawley R and Hawley I: *Handbook of Personal Growth Activities for Classroom Use,* Box 767, Amherst, MA 01002, 1972.

40. Rider BB and Gramlin JT: An activities approach to occupational therapy in a short-term acute mental health unit. *Mental Health Specialty Section Newsletter, 3:*4, Rockville, MD. AOTA, 1980.

Chapter 31

The Relationships between Volition, Activity Pattern, and Life Satisfaction in the Elderly

Nancy Riopel Smith
Gary Kielhofner, DrPH, OTR, FAOTA
Janet Hawkins Watts

Many factors influence the life satisfaction of the elderly. Of particular concern to occupational therapists is occupation, defined as the life span manifestations of work, daily living tasks, and play (1). According to the Model of Human Occupation, which served as a framework for this study, performance, habituation, and volition interact and influence occupation (2–5). Increasing age often leads to declines in the habituation and performance subsystems, such as the loss of life roles or a decrease in physical abilities. Changes in volition may compensate for these declines because the volition subsystem influences decisions that an individual makes concerning engagement in occupations (2). If the volition subsystem can lead individuals to engage in new and more adaptive occupations as they age, volition may have a large influence on life satisfaction. For this reason, volition was chosen as the major occupational variable to be examined in this study. An additional variable, the activity pattern, defined as the relative amount of work, daily living tasks, recreation, and rest in which an individual typically engages, was also examined.

Review of Literature

The volition subsystem consists of an urge to explore and master the environment and is differentiated into components of interests, values, and personal causation (2). Its overall function is to guide occupational choices.

Little research has been done on the relationship between the volition subsystem and life satisfaction in the elderly. This review first examines those gerontologic studies that address a single component of the volition subsystem. Information about the components' relationship to life satisfaction is included. The final section examines the few studies that considered more than one of the volition subsystem components and the relationship of these components to life satisfaction.

Interests

Interests are personal dispositions to find pleasure in certain objects, events, or people that lead an individual to initiate or maintain involvement in various occupations (2, 6). The occupational therapy literature considers the elderly person's interests important for structuring newly acquired free time after retirement. For example, Wong (7) found that 80% of the elderly she sampled felt that "having a hobby, a vital interest and recreation were the secrets of the sense of fulfillment in retirement" (p. 54). Another study (8) identified interests as a dimension of adjustment, noting that the elderly must be interested in their daily occupations if they are to maintain a high level of life satisfaction.

In developing programs to meet the needs of the elderly, it is important to identify any unique characteristics or determinants of the interests of the elderly. One factor that may influence the interests of the elderly is their cultural background. For example, Guttmann (9), in studying leisure interests, found large differences between native and foreign-born elderly Jewish citizens in cultural background, interests, and activity preferences. Even though some variation in interests can be attributed to cultural factors, the interests of the elderly have evolved throughout their lives and are therefore unique for each individual (9). Although further research is needed to clarify these studies, it appears that to provide optimal programming for the elderly, occupational therapists must identify and address the interests of unique cultural groups and ultimately each individual within their client population (10,11).

Values

Values are concepts of what is good or right, which greatly influence an individual's perception and choice of occupation (2). Many factors influence values, such as cultural background, socioeconomic status, age, sex, occupational or educational group, family membership, and psychological state (12, 13). At times the values expressed by the elderly may also represent their perception of available opportunities rather than their deepest beliefs. For example, the elderly may say they do not value work because they believe it is not an option available to them (13). Since there is such a wide range of factors that influence the values of the elderly, values are likely to vary considerably among individuals, which makes it difficult to characterize the values of the group as a whole.

Studies investigating whether values change from adulthood to old age have yielded contradictory results (13–15). Studies based on cross-sectional data may reflect cohort differences, creating a false impression that values change with age (12, 16, 17). In a longitudinal study, Rokeach (18) found that values did not change appreciably during a 3-year period, supporting the argument that values in old age are stable and reflect continuity with adult values.

Personal Causation

Personal causation refers to an individual's self-image as an actor in the world (2). This image includes individuals' expectation of success, belief in their skills, belief in the efficacy of their skills, and locus of control (i.e., whether they feel in control or controlled by external forces) (19). This inner image is based on routine actions that over time can produce areas of special competence. On retirement elderly individuals lose access to their work as an area where they are able to demonstrate competence. This loss may be especially problematic for individuals who held high status vocations and for whom work was important to their feeling of efficacy or for individuals who held low status vocations and for whom retirement resulted in economic hardships and feelings of external control (20). In spite of such potential difficulties, retirement appears to have little direct effect on self-ratings of control or autonomy for the majority of the elderly (21).

Physical and social environments may also influence personal causation. Research has shown that the elderlys' ability to maintain a sense of competence and self-reliance partially depends on the opportunities, rewards, and punishments they encounter in their physical and social environment (22). For example, patronizing remarks have been found to encourage the elderly to become increasingly helpless and to hold a negative view of themselves (22). In addition, institutions such as nursing homes, which promote helplessness and dependency and lack opportunities for mastery, often result in the residents' adopting an external locus of control (23–26). Other studies (23, 27–29) concluded that with increased opportunities for self-control, elderly individuals reduce their negative self-concepts, feel more in control, and improve their functional independence.

Physical decline may also influence personal causation for elderly individuals who view their physical problems as inevitable consequences of the aging process (26). When physical deterioration accelerates during the last few months of life, this feeling of loss of control may be accentuated (30).

The literature reviewed so far deals with the volitional variables of interests, values, and personal causation on an individual basis. The literature suggests that these variables may or may not change with increasing age, that they are influenced by the environment, and that they vary considerably among individuals. There is some evidence that at least interests and personal causation may influence life satisfaction.

Two gerontologic studies consider more than one of the volitional variables. Maguire (31) found that an elderly person's "perceived adequacy of participation in valued activities" (a variable that includes a values component and a personal causation component) was a significant predictor of life satisfaction. Gregory (32) found that both interests and personal causation were significantly and positively correlated with life satisfaction. A limitation of the Gregory study was its general measure of occupation: Respondents were given a list of 23 activities which they ranked according to whether they were done three times a week, once a week, or not at all. Further research is needed to confirm these results, assess the three volitional variables simultaneously, and provide a more detailed assessment of the relationship between volition and an individual's occupations.

Method

This descriptive study sought to determine whether the degree of interest, value, and personal causation reflected in daily occupations would correlate with life satisfaction and whether the activity pattern would correlate with life satisfaction.

Subjects

Sixty subjects, 30 from a senior center and 30 from a nursing home, participated in the study. Their mean age was 78 years, with a range from 65 to 99 years of age.

Instruments and Procedure

All of the subjects completed three questionnaires. The Demographic Information Questionnaire was used to gather information on the subjects' characteristics. The Attitude Index, a subscale of the Attitude Inventory developed by Cavan and others (33), was used to measure life satisfaction. The Occupational Questionnaire (OQ), which was developed for this study (see Figure 1) is based on an activity configuration (34). The OQ was used to measure occupation. It focuses on the components of the volition subsystem that are reflected in everyday occupational activities and on the respondents's view of the type of occupation that each activity represents. To complete the OQ, respondents indicate their main activity during each waking half hour on a typical day; classify each activity as either *work*, *daily living task*, *recreation*, or *rest* (Question 1); and then rate from 1 to 5 the degree of personal causation (Question 2), value (Question 3), and interest (Question 4) for each activity. The results from the OQ can be summarized by percentages. For example, the results indicate the percentage of time that the subject classified as work each day or the percentage of time that the subject was extremely interested in any of his or her activities each day.

Pilot Test of the OQ

The reliability and validity of the OQ were explored in a pilot study before it was used in this study. To assess the questionnaire's test-retest reliability, the OQ was administered two times, 2 weeks apart, to a convenience sample of 20 elderly adults. For the entire sample, 68% of a typical day's activities reported during the first administration were again reported during the same time period of the second administration. There was also 87% agreement for type of activity (i.e., work vs. recreation), 77% for personal causation, 81 % for values, and 77% for interests. These results indicate that the OQ has an acceptable level of reliability.

To assess the questionnaire's validity, the OQ and the Household Work Study Diary (35), a record of a specific day's activities, were administered to 18 senior college students. If the day on which the students recorded the diary of activities turned out to be atypical, they

For the Half Hour Beginning at:	Typical Activities	Question 1 I consider this activity to be: 1-Work 2-Daily living task 3-Recreation 4-Rest	Question 2 I think that I do this: 1-Very well 2-Well 3-About average 4-Pooly 5-Very poorly	Question 3 For me this activity is: 1-Extremely important 2-Important 3-Take it or leave it 4-Rather not do it 5-Total waste of time	Question 4 How much do you enjoy this activity: 1-Like it very much 2-Like it 3-Neither like or dislike it 4-Dislike it 5-Strongly dislike it
5:00 A.M.		1 2 3 4	1 2 3 4 5	1 2 3 4 5	1 2 3 4 5
5:30		1 2 3 4	1 2 3 4 5	1 2 3 4 5	1 2 3 4 5
6:00		1 2 3 4	1 2 3 4 5	1 2 3 4 5	1 2 3 4 5
6:30		1 2 3 4	1 2 3 4 5	1 2 3 4 5	1 2 3 4 5

Figure 1. Sample worksheet of the Occupational Questionnaire. For a copy of the instructions and the complete worksheet, please write to Nancy Riopel Smith, Rt. 2, Box 27, Earlysville, VA 22936

completed the diary a second time. When results of the two tests were compared, it was found that 82% of the typical daily activities reported on the OQ were reported during the same time period on the diary.

When the activities reported during the same time periods on both forms were categorized, 97% of the activities classified as work on the questionnaire were so designated on the diary, and 90% of activities classified as leisure on the questionnaire were so designated on the diary. A comparison between those activities that persons rated as pleasant and satisfying on the diary and their equivalent rating of the same activities in terms of their values, interests, and feelings of personal causation yielded 86%, 84%, and 92% agreement, respectively. The degree of agreement between the OQ and the diary suggests that the OQ gives a valid estimate of the occupational activities an individual pursues on a given (typical) day and of how they are viewed by the respondent.

Data Analysis

Spearman correlations were used to assess the relationship between volitional characteristics and life satisfaction. The relationship between activity pattern and life satisfaction was examined with two different approaches. In the first approach the subjects were divided into high and low life satisfaction groups. Using chi-square tests, these groups were compared to identify similarities and differences in the activity pattern. The second approach involved computing Spearman correlations between subjects' life satisfaction scores and the percentage of time they spent in the different categories of activity (i.e., their activity pattern).

Results

Demographic information appears in Table 1. A significant relationship was identified between the volitional characteristics and life satisfaction. The Spearman correlations were .26 ($p = .04$) for interests, .40 ($p = .002$) for values, and .39 ($p = .002$) for personal causation.

The overall activity pattern for the 60 subjects was 6% work, 7% rest, 20% daily living tasks, 27% recreation and 40% sleep. Many were not sure how to classify periods of time when they were "waiting" or "just passing time till meals." They usually selected the categories *rest* or *daily living tasks* to describe these activities.

Aside from sleep, recreation occupied the largest percentage of the elderly subjects' time, and work occupied the smallest percentage. Since the subjects used their own subjective definitions to classify their activities, many may have underestimated the amount of time they spent working. For example, a middle-aged woman who described herself as a housewife would probably classify vacuuming as work. Since elderly individuals often subscribe to the cultural view of the elderly as retired and noncontributing members of society (13, 36), the same

Table 1
Demographic Characteristics of 60 Subjects

Characteristics	%
Male	18
Female	82
Health problems	55
Illness or death in family	45
Few friends	20
Housewife	20
Business	19
Clerical Work	18
Health and teaching	25
Other	18
Retired less than 10 years	36
Retired 11–20 years	25
Retired more than 20 years	38
Voluntary retirement	81
Income less than adequate	9
Income adequate	75
Income more than adequate	16

woman might classify vacuuming and other types of housework as daily living tasks once she entered old age.

Interesting differences in activity pattern became apparent when the high and low life satisfaction groups were compared. Table 2 shows that the high life satisfaction group spent more time in recreation and work, whereas the low satisfaction group spent more time in rest and daily living tasks. These relationships were supported by the Spearman correlations computed between activity pattern and life satisfaction. Table 3 shows that work and recreation were positively correlated with life satisfaction and that daily living tasks and rest were negatively correlated (although the correlation with daily living tasks was not at the $p < .05$ level of significance). These results suggest that recreation and work may contribute to increased life satisfaction in old age, whereas a concentration on rest and daily living tasks may contribute to decreased life satisfaction.

Discussion

The results of this study indicate that interests, values, personal causation, recreation, and work are positively correlated with life satisfaction. These correlations do not imply cause and effect, but if cause-and-effect relationships can be demonstrated in future studies,

Table 2
Comparison of Activity Pattern of Low and High Life Satisfaction Groups

| Daily Occupation | Mean Percent of Time Spent on Occupations | | Degrees of Freedom | t Values | Probability Level |
	Low Life Satisfaction*	High Life Satisfaction+			
Work	3	7	42.4	−1.87	0.07
Daily living tasks	23	19	15.8	1.06	0.07
Recreation	18	31	17.8	−2.73	0.01
Rest	12	5	13.5	2.05	0.06

Note. *n = 13; +n = 40.

this finding would substantiate occupational therapists' use of occupations for treatment with the elderly. It would also direct occupational therapists to focus their treatment programs on the areas of occupation that increase life satisfaction by (a) using activities that address the interests and values of their clients; (b) using activities that promote the personal causation of their clients; and (c) emphasizing work and recreation.

Other factors may account for the pattern of relationships found in these subjects. Time in work and recreation, and the degree of interest, value, and competence in daily occupations are likely to be associated with socioeconomic status, health, retirement experience, death of a spouse, previous occupation, sex and age. Since all of these factors have been associated with life satisfaction (37–40), they may have a more direct impact on life satisfaction than variables related to occupation. However, the interrelationships between these variables are complex and difficult to unravel. For example, the association between work and life satisfaction may be mediated by increased socioeconomic status of those who are able to be employed. The particiaption in leisure activities is also likely to depend on health status and on whether a spouse is living or not. In these cases, the lack of sufficient funds, poor health, and the loss of a partner may have not only a direct influence on life satisfaction but also an indirect one through changes in the activity pattern and constraints in volitional components.

This study supports previous findings (31–32) of a positive correlation between interests, values and personal causation, and life satisfaction. It extends past research in that it examines the three volitional variables simultaneously and includes activity pattern variables. The OQ developed for this study provides a more precise method of analyzing the relationship between volition and daily occupations and therefore enhances the accuracy of comparisons between these variables and life satisfaction. Future studies should attempt to control for factors such as age and socio-economic status when examining relationships between occupational variables and life satisfaction. Additional limitations of this study include its relatively small sample and the use of convenience sampling to select subjects.

Summary

This study provides further evidence of relationships between volition, activity pattern, and life satisfaction in elderly persons. It also introduces an instrument, the OQ, which facilitates the measurement of volition and activity pattern. Further research is needed to refine and empirically investigate the OQ and to further investigate the relationship between types of occupations and their volitional traits and life satisfaction. Knowledge about how occupation influences life satisfaction in the elderly is essential for the occupational therapist who must make choices of occupations to be provided for elderly clients in therapy.

Acknowledgments

The authors thank the staff and participants at the senior center and nursing home and Thomas W. Smith. This study was supported by a grant from the American Occupational Therapy Foundation and is based on a research project submitted in partial fulfillment of the requirements for a master's of science degree from the Department of Occupational Therapy, Virginia Commonwealth University, Richmond.

Table 3
Correlation of Life Satisfaction with Percent of Time Spent in Daily Occupations

Daily Occupation	Spearman Correlation	Probability Level
Work	0.27	0.007
Daily living tasks	−0.11	0.21
Recreation	0.18	0.05
Rest	−0.23	0.02

References

1. Rogers JC: The study of human occupation. In *Health through Occupation,* G Kielhofner, Editor. Philadelphia: Davis, 1983.

2. Kielhofner G, Burke JP: A model of human occupation, Part 1. Conceptual framework and content. *Am J Occup Ther 34(9):* 572–581, 1980.

3. Kielhofner G: A model of human occupation, Part 2. Ontogenesis from the perspective of temporal adaptation. *Am J Occup Ther 34(10):* 657–663, 1980.

4. Kielhofner G: A model of human occupation, Part 3. Benign and vicious cycles. *Am J Occup Ther 34(11):* 731–737, 1980.

5. Kielhofner G, Burke JP. Igi CH: A model of human occupation, Part 4. Assessment and intervention. *Am J Occup Ther 34(12):* 777–788, 1980.

6. Matsutsuyu JS: The interest check list. *Am J Occup Ther 23(4):* 323–328, 1969.

7. Wong PK: *Toward an Occupational Therapy Gerontology Theory,* master's thesis. University of Southern California, Los Angeles, 1969.

8. McKensie SC: *Aging and Old Age.* Glenview, IL: Scott, Foresman 1980.

9. Guttmann D: Leisure–time activity interests of Jewish aged. *Gerontol 13(2):* 2I9–223, 1973.

10. Gordon C, Gaitz CM, Scott J: Leisure and lives: Personal expressivity across the life span. In *Handbook of Aging and the Social Sciences,* RH Brinstock, E Shanas, Editors. New York: Van Nostrand Reinhold, 1976.

11. Kimmel DC: *Adulthood and Aging: An Interdisciplinary Developmental View.* New York: Wiley, 1980.

12. Bengston VL, Lovejoy MC: Values, personality, social structure, an interpersonal analysis. *American Behavioral Scientist 16(6):* 880–912, 1973.

13. Christenson JA: Generational value differences. *Gerontologist 17(4):* 367–374, 1977.

14. Gordon C, Gaitz CM, Scott J: Value priorities and leisure activities among middle aged and older anglos. *Diseases of the Nervous System 34(1):* 13–26, 1973.

15. Voydanoff PG: An analysis of sources of job satisfaction by age. In *Research on Mental Health of the Aging.* Rockville, MD: National Institutes of Health, 1977.

16. Dowd JJ: The problems of generations: A generational analysis. *Int J Aging Hum Dev 10(3):* 213–229, 1980.

17. Webber IL, Coombs DW, Hollingsworth JS: Variations in value orientations by age in a developing society. *J Gerontol 29(6):* 676–683, 1974.

18. Rokeach R: Change and stability in American value systems, 1968–1971. *Public Opinion Q 38:* 222–238, 1974.

19. Burke JP: A clinical perspective on motivation: Pawn versus origin. *Am J Occup Ther 31(4):* 254–258, 1977.

20. Simpson IH, Back KW, McKinney JC: Orientation toward work and retirement and self-evaluation in retirement. In *Social Aspects of Aging,* IH Simpson, JC McKinney, Editors. Durham, NC: Duke Univ Press, 1966.

21. Back KW, Guptill CS: Retirement and self-ratings. In *Social Aspects of Aging,* IH Simpson, JC McKinney, Editors. Durham, NC: Duke Univ Press, 1966.

22. Romaniuk M, Hoyer FW, Romaniuk JG: Helpless self-attitudes of the elderly: The effect of patronizing statements. Read before the annual meeting of the Gerontological Society, San Francisco, November 1977.

23. Harrison C: The institutionally-deprived elderly. *Nursing Clinics of North America 3(4):* 697–707, 1968.

24. Lester PB, Baltes MM: Functional interdependence of the social environment and the behavior of the institutionalized aged. *Journal of Gerontological Nursing 4(2):* 23–27, 1978.

25. Palmore E, Luikart C: Health and social factors related to life satisfaction. *J Health Soc Behav 13:* 68–80, 1972.

26. Simmons S, Given B: Nursing care of the terminal patients. *Omega 3(3):* 217–225, 1972.

27. Langer EJ, Rodin J: The effects of choice and enhanced personal responsibility for the aged: A field experiment in an institutional setting. *J Pers Soc Psychol 34:* 191–198, 1976.

28. Baltes MM, Zerbe MD: Independence training in nursing-home residents. *Gerontologist 16(5):* 428–432, 1976.

29. Rodin J, Langer E: Aging labels: The decline of control and the fall of self-esteem. *Journal of Social Issues 36(2):* 12–29, 1980.

30. Lieberman MA: Observations on death and dying. *Gerontologist 6(2):* 70–72, 125, 1966.

31. Maguire CH: An exploratory study of the relationship of valued activities to the life satisfaction of the elderly persons. *Occup Ther J Research 3:* 164–172, 1983.

32. Gregory MD: Occupational behavior and life satisfaction among retirees. *Am J Occup Ther 37(8):* 548–553. 1983.

33. Cavan RS, Burges EW, Havighurst RJ, Goldhamer H: *Personal Adjustment in Old Age.* Chicago: Science Research Associated, 1949.

34. Smith HD, Tiffany EG: Assessment and evaluation. In *Willard and Spackman's Occupational Therapy,* HL Hopkins, HD Smith, Editors. Philadelphia: Lippincott, 1978.

35. Berk RA, Berk SF: *Labor and Leisure at Home.* Beverly Hills, CA: Sage, 1979.

36. Strauss H, Aldrich BW, Lipman A: Retirement and perceived status loss: An inquiry into some objective and subjective problems produced by aging. In *Time, Roles, and Self in Old Age,* JF Gubrium, Editor. New York: Arno, 1979.

37. Edwards JN, Klemmack DL: Correlates of life satisfaction: A re-examination. *J Gerontol 28(4):* 497–502, 1973.

38. Walker JW, Kimmel DC, Price KF: Retirement style and retirement satisfaction: Retirees aren't all alike. *Int J Aging Hum Dev 12(4):* 267–281, 1980–1981.

39. Morgan LA: A re-examination of widowhood and morale. *J Gerontol 31(6):* 687–695, 1976.

40. Medley ML: Life satisfaction across four stages of adult life. *Int J Aging Hum Dev 11(I):* 25–33, 1980.

Chapter 32

The Meaning of Daily Activity in Family Caregiving for the Elderly

Betty Risteen Hasselkus,
PhD, OTR, FAOTA

Family caregivers are the primary source of support for long-term care for frail older people living in the community (Shanas, 1979). Research to understand the subjective experience of family caregiving has focused on such variables as a feeling of burden (Montgomery, Gonyea, & Hooyman, 1985; Zarit, Todd, & Zarit, 1986) and a sense of strain (Cantor, 1983; Robinson, 1983). Using a grounded theory approach to study the intergenerational caregiving experience, Bowers (1987) found that daily activities were organized by the invisible work of caregiving, such as anticipatory caregiving (making decisions on the basis of anticipated possibilities).

Recent research has focused on the relationship between informal family caregiving and formal caregiving systems (Clark & Rakowski, 1983; Litwak, 1985; Simmons, Ivry, & Seltzer, 1985). Bowers (1988) and Chenoweth and Spencer (1986) found that family members believed that health professionals do not have adequate backgrounds or training to provide quality care. The family members perceived a need to teach health care professionals how to care for their relatives (Bowers, 1988). Similarly, in my ethnographic study of the meaning of caregiving (Hasselkus, 1988), family members described the need to critique the professionals' caregiving and to teach the professionals how to provide care.

These findings suggest the need for further research on the meaning of family caregiving for the elderly and on the relationship between formal and informal caregiving systems. Eighty percent of all family caregivers for the elderly provide unpaid help 7 days a week: of these caregivers, only 10% use formal services for assistance (Stone, Cafferata, & Sangl, 1986). Hofer (1985) called for better integration of the formal and informal care systems and for increased recognition by professionals of the family's authority: "The existing family caretaking system, however unstructured and cumbersome, is the focal point for assistance to the older person and should be relied upon in tailoring services to fit the family situation" (p. 12).

Occupational therapists have begun to develop programs and special services to support family caregivers who are learning the tasks and responsibilities of the caregiving role (Gessert, 1987; Hasselkus & Brown, 1983). This paper provides the results of an ethnographic study on the meaning of family caregiving for the elderly. The purpose of this analysis was to achieve a better understanding of the meaning of daily activity to family caregivers for the elderly. This knowledge will assist occupational therapists in helping caregivers enhance their skills, thereby better supporting the family as a caring unit.

Previous empirical studies on the meaning of activity have operationalized meaning through the use of standardized measures of affective meaning (Kremer, Nelson, & Duncombe, 1984; Nelson, Thompson, & Moore, 1982; Rocker & Nelson, 1987 [see Chapter 56]); frequency and patterns of activity types (Broderick & Glazer, 1983; Johnson & Deitz, 1985; Nystrom, 1974; Thornton & Collins, 1986); and relationships of activity to other variables, such as life satisfaction and morale (Arnetz, 1985; Gregory, 1983; Maguire, 1983; Marino-Schorn, 1985–1986; Ray & Heppe, 1986; Smith, Kielhofner, & Watts, 1986 [see Chapter 31]). Fewer investigators have qualitatively explored the meaning of activity from the actor's perspective (Schwartzberg, 1982).

In this study of caregiving, 60 ethnographic interviews were carried out with 15 family caregivers in the community. Schön's (1983) framework of reflective practice was used to organize the data into units of analysis. An analysis of the ethnographic data revealed three broad activity goals: (a) getting things done, (b) achieving a sense of health and well-being for the care receiver, and (c) achieving a sense of health and well-being for the caregiver. The caregiver's judgments regarding goal prioritization and goal attainment determined the forms of activity undertaken. This paper will discuss implications for occupational therapy practice with family caregivers.

Method

A series of four 1-hour ethnographic interviews (Spradley, 1979) was conducted with each of 15 family caregivers in their homes. The caregivers' ages ranged from 54 to 82 years, and all were related by blood or marriage to their care receivers. The care receivers all required daily personal care, instrumental care, or both. All interviews were audiotaped and transcribed by the author. (For further information on the characteristics of caregivers and care receivers and the ethnographic interview process, see Hasselkus, 1988.)

On the basis of a sense of fit for the data, Schön's (1983) reflection-in-action framework was used to organize the data for analysis. Originally proposed as a model of practice for professionals, reflection in action emerged as an appropriate model of practice for lay caregivers as well. The transcribed data were coded into 25 problem situations (see Table 1). The Notebook II software database management program for text (Pro-Tem Software, 1985) was then used to organize the verbatim transcripts into the fields of Schön's model—

Naming (those things to which the caregivers attended), Framing (the context in which these things were attended to), Action, and Judgment (judgments about the consequences of the action). The data were then analyzed for themes of meaning and patterns of activity. (See Hasselkus, 1988, for a more detailed description of the methodology.)

Results

Goals of Activity

Three broad goals of caregiving activity were generated from the data: (a) achieving a sense of getting things done, (b) achieving a sense of health and well-being for the care receiver, and (c) achieving a sense of health and well-being for the caregiver.

Getting things done. The ability to get things done depended partly on the caregiver's carefully made decisions about the assumption of new tasks:

> He had always done all the upkeep and improvements on the house. So after he couldn't do it anymore, then I became the apprentice. He was a really good instructor and would tell me what to do. I got so I could wire, and we put in another toilet in the basement and I did some soldering. (Caregiver 14)

Female caregivers sometimes described discomfort with assuming tasks they perceived to be masculine:

> Now I do all the driving, which before I was glad that he could do. I mean, I thought, well, that's a man's job to drive. (Caregiver 5)

The decision to give up certain customary activities was also a part of getting things done. Often, these decisions revolved around the caregiver's perceived lack of time and energy:

> I try to go to mass in the mornings, but I've been so tired. By the time you're up and down three or four times in the night.... I don't go out to lunch, I don't go to plays. I used to go to travelogues... (Caregiver 11)

Caregiver 6 poignantly described her decision to quit her job:

> Before that I went to work a couple times a week and I enjoyed that and looked forward to that. When this came, I knew I could never go back again, I had to stay here. And I'll tell you, I had a heavy heart.

Some caregivers described their efforts to persist with valued activities, despite caregiving demands. Said Caregiver 7, "We got the elderly bus to pick us up and take us to the football game and meet us and bring us back home. It takes a bit of doing but we really enjoy that." Caregiver 8 expressed his concerns about being able to continue to work:

Table I
Problem Situations in Caregiving

Problem Situation	Code	Definition
Activity change	AC/CH	Giving up an activity; taking on an activity or responsibility
Cleaning	CLEAN	Keeping the environment clean (e.g., laundry, bed linens); getting rid of germs; preventing infection
Communication	COMM	Speaking unintelligibly; having difficulty hearing
Dressing	DRESS	Helping care receiver with dressing; helping with brace; lifting
Eating	EAT	Requiring special diets; liking and disliking certain foods; care receiver's appetite
Feelings	FEEL	Caregiver's worrying about own feelings (e.g., impatience, giving up)
Finances	FIN	Meeting health care costs and payments; paying bills, taxes; banking
Future	FUT	Asking such questions as, What if caregiver gets sick or dies? What if care receiver gets worse?
Going out	GO	Getting around in the community with care receiver; finding transportation; receiving help from others
Getting ready	GR	Getting care receiver ready to go out; getting care receiver ready before someone comes in
Getting things done	GTD	Feeling that caregiving takes so much time; having no time to get things done
Health care	HC	Dealing with emergencies; working with professionals; perceptions about care receiver's illness; making decisions; medication; hospitalizations
Hygiene	HYG	Bathing, cleaning care receiver; caring for skin; preventing infection
Living situation	LIV	Needing a change (nursing home?); consequences of a change
Moving around	MA	Lifting; transferring; helping with exercises, walking; using equipment (e.g., walker, cane); falling
Mental state	MENT	Forgetfulness; anger; unpredictability; overly emotional; physical threat; bad thoughts; demanding
Relationships	NET	Receiving support or nonsupport of family, friends; changing roles; disagreeing with family about caregiving
Night problems	NOC	Suffering from broken sleep; care receiver wandering, falling out of bed; keeping the bed dry; going out at night
Daily activity	OCCUP	Thinking of things for care receiver to do; persuading and enabling care receiver to do things; caregiver's finding own time to do things
Own going in	OGI	Spending time with care receiver (when living apart); spending time with care receiver when in hospital
Own going out	OGO	Getting out of the house; getting away; getting time out; making arrangements if caregiver needs surgery, respite
Own health care	OHC	Needing relief; needing medical care for self; needing assistance
Personality change	PERS	Observing that care receiver used to be so talkative, outgoing; is like a different person; used to be mean
Risk	RISK	Falling; leaving cigarettes to burn; not leaving care receiver alone, not being far from doctor
Toileting	TOIL	Controlling bowels and bladder; getting to the toilet; bowel regularity

I'm trying to hang in there until I'm 65. I'll have to stop work if I can't get things done. If I did retire, jobs that I try to get done in the evening or on the weekend I could get done during the week if I wasn't working.

Leaving the care receiver alone briefly (often while the care receiver was in bed) was viewed by some caregivers as acceptable management in order to get things done. "I will go to the store or bank while she's in bed. My neighbor has a key to the house, so if I wouldn't get home, she could get in" (Caregiver 11). Caregiver 13 remarked, "I've learned to go to the grocery store on the fly." Arrangements for the care receiver to spend time at a community adult day center also provided the caregiver with time to get things done.

Health and well–being for the care receiver. Many of the activities aimed at health and well-being for the care receiver consisted of daily routines of caregiving:

I keep track of the blood sugar and the weight. I weigh him every week. I do the blood test every morning. I usually look at his feet every morning and cream them, and I soak his feet every so often and then take care of his toenails. I'm somewhat methodical; I want to be sure things are right. (Caregiver 14)

Extensive measures designed by the caregivers to prevent any worsening of the care receiver's condition were often incorporated into these daily routines. The caregivers were particularly concerned with preventing falls. "When he gets up, I get up. I'm behind him or beside him all the time 'cause I don't want him to fall" (Caregiver 13). Other routines were aimed at the prevention of infection, constipation, and skin breakdown. The diligence with which such precautions were maintained affirmed the caregiver's sense of providing excellent care and coincidentally, reinforced the caregiver's decision against nursing home placement:

> The nurses are all so surprised when they come that her bottom's as clean as it is. I use an antiseptic cream on her all the time after I wash her. So far, she doesn't have any bedsores, which she probably would have if she was in a nursing home. (Caregiver 11)

Monitoring for health changes was another component of health and well-being for the care receiver. Monitoring involved deciding whether a change had occurred and whether to call the doctor.

> This week, he complained some about his stomach, so I don't know what's developing now. I'll have to find out, if this continues. (Caregiver 14)

Besides attending to health care tasks, the caregivers felt responsible for helping the care receivers to experience a variety and balance of activities in their daily lives:

> All he does is just sit. He doesn't want to do anything. The occupational therapist, now she comes, but he'll say, "I can't do it." Last Christmas we got him making cookies. I said to the neighbor, "I have to keep him busy." (Caregiver 5)

> He doesn't get as much exercise as he should. The therapy after we got home was wonderful for him—That gave him something to look forward to, and that's probably what he's missing now. I try to have magazines and books around, but this is where I fall down—thinking of things for him to do. (Caregiver 7)

Caregiver 9 placed a high priority on increasing her mother's social activity:

> My mother is not a social person. She doesn't participate in a whole lot of activities unless I call her or something. Now I've asked the apartment office to send me a calendar of events and I call her to remind her, and I circle them on the calendar in her apartment.

Health and well-being for the caregiver. The caregivers' sense of responsibility for their own health care and their perceived need to have a balance and variety of activity in their own daily lives contributed to a sense of health and well-being for the caregiver. The caregivers' health concerns were both ongoing ("When she rests, I rest") and temporary ("I think I have to go in for a little surgery, and to make all those arrangements [for the care of the care receiver] is really something").

Caregiver 6, who had a heart condition, described the need to persuade her care receiver to hire someone to shovel snow from the driveway: "He didn't care about me hiring anybody, and I said, 'Dad, it's going to be cheaper for us to pay to have the drives cleared out than for me to have a heart attack or a stroke.'" Other caregivers felt the need to keep their concerns to themselves. Said one caregiver, "I pray every night that the Lord will let me take care of her."

The caregivers expressed almost apologetically their need to plan variety and change in their own lives. "This makes it kind of hard to do things that you normally used to do—It gets kind of boring. I always hated to be in the house. . . . Sometimes I just put on my hat and coat and go for a walk" (Caregiver 8). Caregiver 5 stated softly, "It just seems like it's the same, day after day—You're here all the time." Caregiver 12 remarked, "I know how to escape sometimes, but I try not to escape too often because it concerns me if [I'm away] too long."

Because of the cost of paying someone to stay with the care receiver, even for a few hours, many caregivers felt uncomfortable about going out, except on rare occasions. "How can you go any place and enjoy yourself when you know it's going to cost $40?" (Caregiver 5). For others, the cost was emotional: "If I go out and I'm gone too long, when I come back he's so angry it just spoils my day. So I've been trying to stay home so he doesn't get so angry" (Caregiver 13).

A sense of escape was sometimes achieved by the caregiver's simply retreating to another part of the house. Dining out often provided caregivers with social contact and a sense of relaxation. Attendance at a local stroke club provided a change of routine for Caregiver 13: "The stroke club met every Wednesday, and that was nice, and I think that gave me a lot of support. That was my outing."

Some caregivers, however, expressed the need for a more dramatic change. "Right now I'm in need of a vacation—I need a break from all of this. I'm just tired and I need to get away" (Caregiver 4).

Dilemmas of Caregiving

In every problem situation of caregiving, the caregiver was confronted with the need to make a judgment about the consequences of an action on his or her own well-being, on the well-being of the care receiver, and on getting things done. Dilemmas arose when actions were perceived to serve one goal but not another (e.g., "The therapist said to put sandbags on [his leg] every hour, but I wondered how I was ever going to get my work done" [Caregiver 1]) or when the caregiver's view of how to achieve a goal differed from another person's view (e.g., "The doctor said to give her Mellaril, but I don't believe in too much of that" [Caregiver 11]). Such dilemmas required the caregiver to judge which goal should take priority, whose view should prevail, or whether an action based on a compromise of views or goals would be satisfactory.

The activity of caregiving was driven by this tension between goals and between conflicting views regarding how to reach the goals. The least stressful situations seemed to be those in which the caregiver perceived the views of others (e.g., care receiver, professional, family) to be compatible with his or her own. Compromised activities often resulted from the caregiver's trying to achieve compatibility between goals or views. For example, instead of the hourly sandbags, Caregiver 1 substituted having the care receiver perform "exercises in bed in the morning so I'd know he could get [the leg] straightened out, and it seemed to work pretty well." In many instances, the caregiver's view clearly prevailed: "They told me to let him do some of that [washing up] himself, but it takes him so long—He'd be forever at it and he'd never get his breakfast. So I do it and I do a better job, use soap and that" (Caregiver 1).

In setting priorities between conflicting goals, the caregivers often subordinated their own needs for the health and well-being of their care receivers: "When he first came home, I decided it was the best thing for him to have me stay here. I felt that was one of my duties" (Caregiver 5). Caregiver 2 stated, "I don't have time to take care of myself. It's always him first and me second."

Discussion

In this study, the family caregiver was conceptualized as a practitioner, and Schön's (1983) model of reflection in action was used to organize and interpret the practice of the caregivers. Reflection in action provided a framework for analysis in which activity and context were not separated. The three primary goals of activity in caregiving—getting things done, health and well-being for the care receiver, and health and well-being for the caregiver—were derived from the meaning and context of the situation, that is, from the values, standards, and cultural beliefs represented in the Naming and Framing fields of the problem situations. How these goals were reached and prioritized differed among the caregivers, but the activity of caregiving was directed broadly toward the achievement of these overarching objectives.

The Therapeutic Relationship

The conceptualization of the family caregiver as a practitioner provides insight into the process of family caregiving and into the relationship between the professional and the caregiver. The therapist who wanted the patient to do the washing up by himself had not taken the time to learn the caregiver's standards for getting things done ("He'd be forever at it and he'd never get his breakfast"). Another caregiver modified the prescribed hourly use of sandbags to better fit the goals of getting things done and achieving a sense of health and well-being for the care receiver. Differences between the caregiver's and the professional's views of reaching caregiving goals sometimes led caregivers to drastic action:

> The occupational therapist wanted to come early and watch me, what I did and everything. When they come early like that it makes me so nervous. I'd get real irritated, so I asked the occupational therapist not to come anymore. (Caregiver 1)

Schön (1983) suggested the need for a reflective contract between the professional and the layperson. In a reflective contract, the client and the practitioner examine the problem situation together. Each person recognizes that his or her expertise is embedded in a context of meanings, and each person makes those meanings accessible to the other. Any action taken is the result of this reflective conversation.

Data from the present study suggest that, too often, reflective conversation never takes place. Meanings are not exchanged between the professional and the family caregiver, and the professional's initial advice is soon modified or simply ignored, unless it fits the caregiver's meaning.

Ethical Dilemmas

In the clinical reasoning of health care practice today, "there is not one right answer but, rather, multiple options, all of which may be resolutions or compromises and not solutions that are correct for all time" (Neuhaus, 1988, p. 289). Kyler-Hutchison (1988), in her paper on ethical reasoning in health care, concurred: "Actions and judgments are the final result of applying a certain code of ethics to a given situation" (p. 283).

Caregiving dilemmas are ethical, derived from conflicts in values and goals. Repeatedly, the family caregiver faces the three generic questions of clinical judgment (Pellegrino, 1979): What is wrong? What can be done? and What should be done? For example, Caregiver 14 said, "This week he's complained some about his stomach, so I don't know what's developing now. I'll have to find out if this continues." The ethical decision making mandated by the question, What should be done? encompasses utilitarian and moral foundations. The caregiver is constantly making judgements about the value of the consequences of all actions ("that seemed to work pretty well") and the fulfillment of the sense of obligation ("I felt that was one of my duties"). For the family caregiv-

---

er, then, as well as for the professional, there is seldom one right answer, and reasoning is adjusted as new information and experience are accumulated. Actions and judgments result from the caregiver's applying his or her own code of ethics to caregiving practices.

Therapists who work with family caregivers need to recognize the ethical decision making that pervades the caregiving role. To paraphrase Rogers (1983) (see Chapter 37), the goal of the clinical encounter must be to devise a therapeutic plan that preserves the caregiver's values and represents a mutual understanding between the therapist and the caregiver. Services must be tailored to fit the family caretaking system, "however unstructured and cumbersome" (Hofer, 1985, p. 12). Both the therapist and the family caregiver (a) bring knowledge and experience to the situation (What is wrong?); (b) produce clinical data to identify options appropriate to the care receiver's needs (What can be done?); and (c) bring their own codes of ethics to the selection of a course of action (What should be done?). If the therapist and the caregiver can collaborate on this clinical reasoning process, then tension can be minimized and a sense of shared responsibility and shared ethical decision making can result.

Balance of Activity

The pervasive cultural beliefs regarding the need for variety and balance in daily activity affirm a basic tenet of occupational therapy theory and practice (Clark, 1979; Kielhofner, 1980). Apparently, it is unnecessary for the therapist to persuade people that they need a balance of daily activities. However, it is necessary for the therapist to take the time to determine each caregiver's understanding of the meanings of *balance* and *variety*. Statements made by caregivers such as "I always hated to be in the house" and "It just seems like it's the same, day after day" reveal a sense of imbalance in daily activity.

The occupational therapist's validation of the caregiver's needs for balance and variety in daily activity might dispel some of the caregiver's guilt associated with escaping or with spending money to hire someone for respite care. "This is where I fall down—thinking of things for him to do" clearly communicated a caregiver's burden from her sense of responsibility for her care receiver's daily activities. An occupational therapist can play a major role in assisting that caregiver to be more comfortable and more effective with this responsibility.

Relationship to Other Research

These ethnographic data on family caregiving for the elderly provide a rich context for the study of meaning in daily activity. Commonalities between these findings and those of other research studies suggest a beginning typology of consistent themes of meaning in activity. For example, Johnson and Deitz (1985) described the spatial patterning of activities. The thick descriptive data in the present study, however, provides a spatial concept that surpasses the physical location of an activity. The caregivers went in and out of the caregiving, and the sense of being in, going out, getting away, or escaping from the caregiving reflected both psychological and physical spatial meanings of caregiving, as illustrated by such quotes as "Right now I'm in need of a vacation . . . I'm just tired and I need to get away" (Caregiver 4).

Kielhofner (1977) (see Chapter 19) described temporal adaptation as the integration of an entire spectrum of activities, the organization of which supports health on a daily basis. The caregiving day was organized around the goal of getting things done, a culturally constituted temporal framework derived from the caregiver's values and goals and from the perceived need to assume roles and tasks prescribed by society. The careful balancing of the tasks to be accomplished, discarded, or modified to get things done was the crux of the caregiver's day, week, month, and year. "I still plan to take her to the day care sometimes if I retire, because there's times I still want to get something done" (Caregiver 8).

The goals of health and well-being in caregiving are similar to research findings that have demonstrated positive relationships between participation in valued activities and such variables as morale (Marino–Schorn, 1985–1986), life satisfaction (Gregory, 1983; Maguire, 1983; Ray & Heppe, 1986; Smith et al., 1986; Thornton & Collins, 1986), positive body image (Donohue, 1982) (see Chapter 30), and perceived health and well-being (Maguire, 1983; Thornton & Collins, 1986). Thornton and Collins concluded from their study on activity among older adults, "There is no doubt that older adults pursue activity with purpose; 'being active' and 'promoting one's well-being' are essential reasons for both leisure and physical activity" (p. 23).

Schwartzberg (1982) found that gratification from activities was related to such themes as social integration and a sense of participation in valued activities. From this finding, one can extrapolate that, to the extent that the caregivers perceived these variables to be present in their situations (e.g., social integration), the caregiving activity would be gratifying and thus contribute to a sense of well-being. Note the stress that occurred when such a variable was not present, as with Caregiver 6, who finally "laid down the law" by telling her husband, "I have to see other people."

Several studies (Adelstein & Nelson, 1985; Froehlich & Nelson, 1986; Kremer et al., 1984; Nelson et al., 1982; Rocker & Nelson, 1987 [see Chapter 56]) have relied heavily on the use of a standardized measure of affective meaning (Osgood, 1952) to study the meaning of activity. Of Osgood's three factors of affective meaning—power, evaluation, and action—evaluation, seems closest to the themes of meaning in the present study. The ethical dilemmas of caregiving seem to stem from the caregiver's continual weighing of the positive and negative consequences of an action. Data from this study suggest that new understandings of the meaning of daily activity might be best gained from naturalistic research carried out within the natural context of the activity.

To understand the meaning of activity and to promote health through that meaning is the essence of occupational therapy. "For us, in occupational therapy, the most fundamental area for research is, and probably always will be, the nature and meaning of activity" (Reilly, 1960, p. 208). Findings from the present study have yielded new insights into the meaning of activity in family caregiving for the elderly. Recognition of the family caregiver as a lay practitioner engaged in clinical reasoning and the resolution of ethical dilemmas suggest a need to reconceptualize the professional-caregiver relationship. This relationship can be viewed as a partnership involving the exchange of expertise, values, and interests. Sensitivity to the spatial, temporal, and evaluative components of meaning in caregiving will enable professionals to work more comfortably with family caregivers and thereby be more supportive of the family unit's role as a health provider for frail elderly people in the community.

Acknowledgments

I express my appreciation to Stephanie Stetson, Project Assistant, for her valuable and diligent help with the library research and for her organization and analysis of the data in this study.

This research was supported by funds from the Graduate School, University of Wisconsin–Madison.

References

Adelstein, L. A., & Nelson, D. L. (1985). Effects of sharing versus non-sharing on affective meaning in collage activities. *Occupational Therapy in Mental Health, 5(2)*, 29–45.

Arnetz, B. B. (1985). Gerontic occupational therapy— Psychological and social predictors of participation and therapeutic benefits. *American Journal of Occupational Therapy, 39*, 460–465.

Bowers, B. J. (1987). Intergenerational caregiving: Adult caregivers and their aging parents. *Advanced Nursing Science, 9*, 20–31.

Bowers, B. J. (1988). Family perceptions of nursing home care: A grounded theory study of family work in a nursing home. *Gerontologist, 28*, 361–368.

Broderick, T., & Glazer, B. (1983). Leisure participation and the retirement process. *American Journal of Occupational Therapy, 37*, 15–22.

Cantor, M. (1983). Strain among caregivers: A study of experience in the United States. *Gerontologist, 23*, 597–603.

Chenoweth, B., & Spencer, B. (1986). Dementia: The experience of family caregivers. *Gerontologist, 26*, 267–272.

Clark, N. M., & Rakowski, W. (1983). Family caregivers of older adults: Improving helping skills. *Gerontologist, 23*, 637–642.

Clark, P. N. (1979). Human development through occupation: A philosophy and conceptual model for practice, part 2. *American Journal of Occupational Therapy, 33*, 577–585.

Donohue, M. V. (1982). Designing activities to develop a women's identification group. *Occupational Therapy in Mental Health, 2(1)*, 1–19. (Reprinted as Chapter 30).

Froehlich, J., & Nelson, D. L. (1986). Affective meanings of life review through activities and discussion. *American Journal of Occupational Therapy, 40*, 27–33.

Gessert, V. G. (1987, December). Living room: A support group for families with aging relatives. *Gerontology Special Interest Section Newsletter*, pp. 1, 3.

Gregory, M. D. (1983). Occupational behavior and life satisfaction among retirees. *American Journal of Occupational Therapy, 37*, 548–553.

Hasselkus, B. R. (1988). Meaning in family caregiving: Perspectives on caregiver/professional relationships. *Gerontologist. 28*, 686–691.

Hasselkus, B. R., & Brown, M. (1983). Respite care for community elderly. *American Journal of Occupational Therapy, 37*, 83–88.

Hofer, A. (1985). *The caretaker family as the integrating agent.* (Available from A. Hofer, Consultant, Aging Programs, 1141 Loxford Terrace, Silver Spring, MD 20901).

Johnson, C. B., & Deitz, J. C. (1985). Activity patterns of mothers of handicapped and non-handicapped children. *Physical and Occupational Therapy in Pediatrics, 5(1)*, 17–25.

Kielhofner, G. (1977). Temporal adaptation: A conceptual framework for occupational therapy. *American Journal of Occupational Therapy, 31*, 235–242. (Reprinted as Chapter 17).

Kielhofner, G. (1980). Model of Human Occupation, part 3. Benign and vicious cycles. *American Journal of Occupational Therapy, 34*, 731–737.

Kremer, E. R. H., Nelson, D. L., & Duncombe, L. W. (1984). Effects of selected activities on affective meaning in psychiatric patients. *American Journal of Occupational Therapy, 38*, 522–528.

Kyler-Hutchison, P. (1988). Ethical reasoning and informed consent in occupational therapy. *American Journal of Occupational Therapy, 42*, 283–287.

Litwak, E. (1985). *Helping the elderly. The complementary roles of informal networks and formal systems.* New York: Guilford Press.

Maguire, G. H. (1983). An exploratory study of the relationship of valued activities to the life satisfaction of elderly persons. *Occupational Therapy Journal of Research, 3*, 164–172.

Marino-Schorn, J. A. (1985–1986). Morale, work and leisure in retirement. *Physical and Occupational Therapy in Geriatrics, 4(2)*, 49–59.

Montgomery, R. J. V., Gonyea, J. G., & Hooyman, N. R. (1985). Caregiving and the experience of subjective and objective burden. *Family Relations, 34,* 19–26.

Nelson, D. L., Thompson, G., & Moore, J. A. (1982). Identification of factors of affective meaning in four selected activities. *American Journal of Occupational Therapy, 36,* 381–387.

Neuhaus, B. E. (1988). Ethical considerations in clinical reasoning: The impact of technology and cost containment. *American Journal of Occupational Therapy, 42,* 288–294.

Nystrom, E. P. (1974). Activity patterns and leisure concepts among the elderly. *American Journal of Occupational Therapy, 28,* 337–345.

Osgood, C. E. (1952). The nature and measurement of meaning. *Psychological Bulletin, 49,* 197–237.

Pellegrino, E. D. (1979). The anatomy of clinical judgment. In H. T. Engelhardt, S. F. Spicker, & B. Towers (Eds.), *Clinical judgment: A critical appraisal* (pp. 169–194). Dordrecht, Holland: D. Reidel Publishing.

ProTem Software. (1985). *Notebook II* [Computer program]. (Available from Protem Software Inc., 2363 Boulevard Circle, Walnut Creek, CA 94595).

Ray, R. O., & Heppe, G. (1986). Older adult happiness: The contributions of activity breadth and intensity. *Physical and Occupational Therapy in Geriatrics, 4(4),* 31–43.

Reilly, M. (1960). Research potentiality of occupational therapy. *American Journal of Occupational Therapy, 14,* 206–209.

Robinson, B. (1983). Validation of a caregiver strain index. *Journal of Gerontology, 38,* 344–348.

Rocker, J. D., & Nelson, D. L. (1987). Affective responses to keeping and not keeping an activity product. *American Journal of Occupational Therapy, 41,*152–157. (Reprinted as Chapter 56.)

Rogers, J. C. (1983). Eleanor Clarke Slagle Lectureship—1983; Clinical reasoning: The ethics, science, and art. *American Journal of Occupational Therapy, 37,*601–616. (Reprinted as Chapter 34).

Schön, D. A. (1983). *The reflective practitioner.* New York: Basic Books.

Schwartzberg, S. L. (1982). Motivation for activities of daily living: A study of selected psychiatric patients' self-reports. *Occupational Therapy in Mental Health, 2(3),* 1–26.

Shanas, E. (1979). The family as a social support system in old age. *Gerontologist, 19,* 169–174.

Simmons, K. H., Ivry, J., & Seltzer, M. M. (1985). Agency–family collaboration. *Gerontologist, 25,* 343–346.

Smith, N. R., Kielhofner, G., & Watts, J. H. (1986). The relationships between volition, activity pattern, and life satisfaction in the elderly. *American Journal of Occupational Therapy, 40,* 278–283. (Reprinted as Chapter 31).

Spradley, J. P. (1979). *The ethnographic interview.* Chicago: Holt, Rinehart & Winston.

Stone, R., Cafferata, G. L., & Sangl, J. (1986). *Caregivers of the frail elderly. A national profile.* Rockville, MD: National Center for Health Services Research.

Thornton, J. E., & Collins, J. B. (1986). Patterns of leisure and physical activities among older adults. *Activities, Adaptation & Aging, 8(2),* 5–27.

Zarit, S. H., Todd, P. A., & Zarit, J. M. (1986). Subjective burden of husbands and wives as caregivers: A longitudinal study. *Gerontologist, 26,* 260–266.

Section IV

The Therapeutic Relationship:Facilitating Engagement in Purposeful Activity

Introduction

As Hasselkus clearly emphasized in Chapter 32, the interrelationships between the therapist, the consumer, and purposeful activity cannot be ignored. One cannot adequately understand the personal meaning of daily activity if one has not developed a positive therapeutic relationship. The therapist may consider an activity to be therapeutic and purposeful, yet the client may not be motivated to participate in the selected activity (Arnsten, 1990). As therapists, we do not apply activity or "do" an activity "on" or "to" a person; rather, we do activity with a person, thereby facilitating a therapeutic relationship (Gilfoyle, 1980). A partnership and a mutual cooperation develops (Yerxa, 1980) enabling the therapist to use him- or herself therapeutically (Sachs and Labovitz, 1994). This partnership is the art of occupational therapy (OT) practice (Gilfoyle, 1980; Mosey, 1986).

However, there are many forces that challenge our ability to practice this art. Shorter lengths of stay, reimbursement-driven practice, demands for productivity, and staff shortages are several of the trends that place pressure on occupational therapists to use mechanistic and technological techniques, rather than humanistic and holistic approaches (Peloquin, 1994; Yerxa, 1980). It is hoped that the chapters in this section will provide a solid foundation for the recognition of the vital importance of forming therapeutic relationships, along with the necessary skills and tools for implementing this philosophy into practice. This appreciation and skill development is essential to keeping the art of practice in OT.

In Chapter 33 Devereux begins this section with a thoughtful analysis of the caring relationship, which she presents as the basis for our profession's philosophy and practice. She emphasizes that the development of a caring relationship between the client and the therapist reinforces the holistic approach of occupational thera-

pists and enables them to make a unique societal contribution by being a caring profession. Devereux explores the therapeutic relationship and discusses how to develop a caring relationship with clients to assist them in reconnecting to activities that are meaningful. Equally important is her analysis of how the therapist can care for himself or herself to be able to enter into and maintain caring therapeutic relationships. She concludes with an exploration of how OT can maintain its caring focus in a complex and challenging health care system. The benefits of forming therapeutic relationships are strongly identified, and efforts made to deal with health care system constraints are clearly worthwhile and an inherent part of the art of practice.

The health care system challenges identified by Devereux as beginning in the 1980s have mushroomed in the 1990s, and the next millennium will likely bring increased complexities. Therefore, occupational therapists must develop knowledge, skills, and attitudes for effectively dealing with these challenges and for managing these complexities. The next three chapters in this section explore the clinical reasoning process that is essential to the development of the critical thinking skills that will enable occupational therapists to organize their assessments and prioritize their treatment while maintaining a caring, holistic approach with each client in a health care system loaded with constraints.

Rogers begins Chapter 34 with a discussion on the ethics, science, and art of clinical reasoning along with a strong call for the individuation of the treatment process. She poses a series of three fundamental questions, which each therapist should ask to ensure that interventions are congruent with the patient's needs, values, goals, and lifestyle. Each question is explored in terms of the knowledge needed to answer it and the processes used to obtain this essential knowledge; providing the reader with clear guidelines and concrete suggestions for improving clinical reasoning skills. Rogers acknowledges that there is no cookbook of clinical solutions and proposes the use of general systems theory as a framework for integrating data relevant to the uniqueness of each patient and pertinent to the complexities of clinical problems. She comprehensively explores the scientific, ethical, and artistic dimensions of clinical reasoning, substantiating these issues with a number of clinical examples that highlight benefits of becoming an "inquisitive practitioner."

Fleming and Mattingly in Chapters 35 and 36, respectively, expand on Rogers' exploration of the clinical reasoning process by reporting results of the American Occupational Therapy Association's and American Occupational Therapy Foundation's Clinical Reasoning study. This landmark research project analyzed the reasoning processes used by therapists in solving problems in their day-to-day practice. After extensive study, four types of reasoning—procedural, interactive, conditional, and narrative—were identified. The first three are discussed extensively in Fleming's chapter, with the last being explored in depth in the chapter by Mattingly. Each type of reasoning is defined with its major characteristics, purposes, methods, values, and benefits discussed. Case examples substantiate the implementation of these principles into clinical practice and add a humanness to the discussions. These chapters support the notion that therapists can "walk and chew gum" at the same time and that we can work with a person holistically using a "multi-track" mind. This ability to use a diversity of perspectives in a health care system that devalues holism and only values concrete reductionist procedures is a critical skill for occupational therapists to develop. Experienced occupational thereapists in this study appeared to move smoothly and sometimes rapidly between the different types of reasoning or simultaneously used multiple types of reasoning as they analyzed, interpreted, and resolved different types of clinical problems and selected meaningful, relevant, purposeful activities for OT interventions. The employment of these four different types of clinical reasoning also provides the occupational therapist with the knowledge, skills, and attitudes needed to form positive therapeutic relationships with clients.

One of the main purposes of establishing a therapeutic relationship with a client is to facilitate the client's active engagement in purposeful activity during OT intervention. However, the ability to enter into a relationship focused on "doing" can be influenced by one's judgment of his or her capabilities. A person is less likely to engage in an activity that is viewed as beyond his or her capability. Therefore, therapists must consider the client's perceived self-efficacy when selecting activities and planning OT intervention. Gage and Polatajko ex-plore the construct of perceived self-efficacy in Chapter 37, which considers the effects of perceived self-efficacy on activity selection, engagement, and performance. Perceived self-efficacy's origin, history, definition, parameters, and relationship to self-esteem, behavior, treatment outcome, and psychological well-being are discussed in a comprehensive manner. A literature review highlights relevant research and clinical examples support the impact of perceived self-efficacy on performance. Gage and Polatajko postulate that assessing and monitoring perceived self-efficacy and using activities that closely approximate community and similar real-life activities will result in better treatment outcomes and enhanced occupational performance. The benefits of considering perceived self-efficacy in OT assessment, treatment, planning, and intervention are clear. The authors challenge occupational therapists to identify and incorporate this construct into daily clinical practice. We can structure task experiences to be successful and provide a therapeutic relationship supportive of clients having a "real" voice about their treatment, thereby strengthening clients' perceived self-efficacy.

Perceived self-efficacy is one of the personal beliefs that shape the therapeutic relationship; there are many others. The therapeutic relationship is influenced by countless interpersonal, professional, societal, and cultural beliefs. In closing this section, Peloquin in Chapter 38 explores societal beliefs that shape the patient–therapist relationship and our ability to provide care. While Gage's and Polatajko's chapter emphasized the need for clients to have a "real" voice in the therapeutic process, Peloquin explores many of these voices through the presentation of a number of stories that reflect caring practice and, unfortunately, numerous stories that reflect depersonalized practice. In her presentation of these stories she examines three societal constructs that devalue caring and the formation of a therapeutic relationship. These constructs—an emphasis on the rationale fixing of the health care problem, overreliance on methods and protocols, and a health care system driven by business, efficacy, and profit—are carefully analyzed by Peloquin and strongly substantiated by comprehensive narrative data. Her thoughtful and sensitive analysis of these societal constructs is invaluable to the therapist struggling to maintain a level of caring in the current health care system that is largely unsupportive of therapeutic caring.

The impact of sociopolitical forces on the art of OT practice cannot be discounted. In 1980, Baum and Yerxa asserted that occupational therapists must exert their control and influence in shaping the health care system so that it remains humanistic. As Yerxa (1980) so eloquently stated, "The challenge of the future will be to preserve and enhance a climate of caring for our patients in the face of a society increasingly dominated by technique and objectivism, a culture of narcissism that depersonalizes work and trivializes play, in which medical science views Man as an object and the disabled as forever chronically ill, in which disabled persons while increasing in number might be provided with less of society's resources, and in which individuals are alienated and without social conscience because they have lost hope in creating change" (p. 532). Sixteen years later it is sad to note that although several important inroads have been made to improve the quality of life for persons with disabilities (e.g., passage of the ADA) the major challenges identified by Yerxa remain. Her call for the creation of a climate of caring needs to become a battle cry for occupational therapists, because we are in an era of health care "reform" that is largely dominated by cost-containment concerns and profit margins. As a caring profession, OT has an ethical responsibility to be concerned with the quality of life of those with whom we work and to advocate for sociopolitical change that will support the formation of therapeutic relationships, which are so critical to the provision of quality care.

Questions to Consider

1. What are your personal values regarding caring? How does your culture view caring? How do these values influence your ability to formulate caring therapeutic relationships with others?
2. What are societal views of caring? What is the market value of caring? Does the fact that OT is a predominately female profession influence the profession's view of caring and society's view of the profession?
3. Given current health care system trends, how can an occupational therapist maintain a focus on caring? How can an occupational therapist create a humanizing environment in an often dehumanizing, medical model health care system? How can you care for yourself in this demanding and evolving time in health care?

References

Arnsten, S. M. (1990). Intrinsic motivation. *American Journal of Occupational Therapy, 44,* 462–463.

Baum, C. M. (1980). Occupational therapists put care in the health care system. *American Journal of Occupational Therapy, 34,* 505–516.

Gilfoyle, E. M. (1980). Caring: A philosophy of practice. *American Journal of Occupational Therapy, 34,* 517–521.

Mosey, A. C. (1986). *Psychosocial Components of Occupational Therapy.* New York, NY: Raven Press.

Peloquin, S. M. (1994). Occupational therapy as art and science: Should the older definition be reclaimed? *American Journal of Occupational Therapy, 48,* 1093–1096.

Sachs, D., & Labovitz, D. R. (1994). The caring occupational therapist: Scope of professional roles and boundaries. *American Journal of Occupational Therapy, 48,* 997–1005.

Yerxa, E. J. (1980). Occupational therapy's role in creating a future climate of caring. *American Journal of Occupational Therapy, 34,* 529–534.

Chapter 33

Occupational Therapy's Challenge: The Caring Relationship

Elizabeth B. Devereaux,
MSW, ACSW/L, OTR/L, FAOTA

Caring exists only in relation to something; caring simply does not exist alone or in a vacuum. Before caring can exist or be relevant, it must be in relation to a living organism, a thing, or a thought. The relationship object may be tangible or intangible, the person may be self or other, and the living organism may be animal or human.

Occupational therapists are concerned about caring. We talk about this concern and act on it. In this paper my initial focus is on developing a caring relationship with the patient; this is followed by a discussion of the need to care for self as an integral part of developing any caring relationship with another and of the elements of therapeutic relationships. Finally, our functioning as caring professionals within the context and constraints of today's health care environment is explored.

Relationship with the Patient

We are all attracted to a health care profession because we are caring people. We value caring relationships, and the health care arena provides the structure within which our natural feelings and skills can find expression. Of even greater importance is the fact that we chose occupational therapy as the profession within the total health care field. Occupational therapy does not do to, or for, the patient, but it instead does with. Through our treatment, we facilitate the patient's doing for him- or herself. When we treat a patient, it is with the awareness of the person, first, and the person who may have problems, second (1, p 787). All health care practitioners recognize the pathology when they look at a patient; however, occupational therapists not only see the pathology and deal with it as a part of the treatment process, but we also recognize and focus on what is healthy about the individual. What is there to build on? What do we have to work with that can help this person learn, or relearn, the skills necessary to perform life tasks? We deal with the whole person, described by West (2) as "the mind-body-environment interrelationships activated through occupation." (p 22) The concept of wholism is expressed eloquently in the report of the *Project to Identify the Philosophy of Occupational Therapy* (3).

...Embodiment or wholism is that perspective where mind and body are perceived as inextricably connected, integrated as one entity, in contrast to the dualistic perspective where mind and body are perceived as separate and hierarchically related entities (one entity superior to the other).... (p 21)

To discuss a patient as "the kidney in room 319" or "the hand in the second treatment room" represents, to me, the height of dualism. Where and who are the people to whom these anatomic parts are vital? What right does anyone have to depersonalize them so? Ciardi (4) says, "If you don't really care, any reason is good enough." (p 158) Menninger (5) and Thomas (6) advised that physicians and health care providers should periodically become patients to experience, or reexperience, the patient role, to enhance sensitivity to what it's like to be a patient, and to see the effect of various provider behaviors on the patient's illness. Thomas said the following.

> One of the hard things to teach, is what it feels like lo be a patient ... (p 22) being a patient is hard work ... (p 223) The nearest thing to a personal education in illness is the grippe. It is almost all we have left in the way of on-the-job training.... (p 221)

There is, of course, an emotional, or psychological, component to every physical illness. During the stress of illness, a person reverts to a dependent role, to the wish—the need—to be taken care of. The awareness of this wish sets up an inner struggle, a push–pull relationship, an ambivalence between dependence and independence. Not only do we want to be cared for, we also want to remain in control of (as much as possible) our lives and our relationships.

Patients sometimes resent both the need to be cared for and the people who fill the need. As caring professionals, it is our responsibility to know and understand the emotions of illness, to be sensitive to the many variations of these emotional manifestations in patient behavior, and to acknowledge this in empathic, yet therapeutic, responses as an integral part of our treatment. This is the essence of the holistic approach to treatment. Although we may know the complete history of the patient (e.g., employment, family, economic, interests, developmental, medical), if we do not in some way communicate to the patient our *understanding* of what his or her illness means to his or her life, our treatment reflects the dualistic mind–body dichotomy; thus, we are treating only "the kidney in room 319" or "the hand in the second treatment room." When patients know that we care enough to understand them as people, then we are contributing to their drive toward action (7), toward the reawakening, of their drive for mastery of their environment. We then have helped patients to accept whatever level of dependency must be there for however long, and we have helped them reach for independence. This is an integral part of Reilly's (7) "nurturing of the spirit of man for action." (See Chapter 6.)

Several years ago a colleague and I were asked to consult with an occupational therapist working in a renal dialysis unit. This was the therapist's first job, and little about the role of occupational therapy treatment with renal dialysis patients had been published at that time. This pioneering therapist was questioning why she was there, her effectiveness, and whether she was actually "doing occupational therapy." She was particularly distressed about one patient, Charlotte (fictitious name), because Charlotte had been generally angry, hostile, and uncooperative, and was resistant to involvement in the discussion groups and other activities the therapist initiated. However, the therapist persisted in her attempts to engage Charlotte, and eventually Charlotte's behavior changed a great deal; Charlotte was involved and pleasant, and she even seemed to enjoy the activities and talked with the therapist and the other patients. The therapist was pleased but puzzled with this change in Charlotte's behavior. My colleague and I talked with the therapist about issues such as when is help helpful, patient resistance, and the concept of each patient having his or her own timing. We then went to talk with Charlotte. Charlotte told us about her husband at home who was even more seriously ill than she. She was concerned that her dialysis treatment three days each week took her away from caring for him. She told us about their two sons: one who had died from the same type of kidney disease Charlotte had and the other who was recently diagnosed as having this same disease. Charlotte talked of her anger, her despair, her feeling of hopelessness and helplessness, her inability even to drive a car, and her dependency on others for the trips to the dialysis unit. Charlotte said that each time she came for treatment, it reinforced the losses in her life caused by the illness. [Let me point out two important points here: (a) that being compliant by coming to treatment can have a negative and a positive component for the patient, that this action (of coming for treatment) prevents the denial of the illness, and (b) that the use of occupation during the treatment period helps the patient avoid getting caught in the emotional flooding of feeling the losses resulting from the illness and then connecting them to all the losses in his or her life.] She said that everything was out of control in her life but that she kept coming to dialysis because she could not function without it. She said the therapist accepted her in spite of her anger; one day, Charlotte reluctantly started working on a needlepoint project offered to her by the therapist, and an amazing thing happened. Charlotte said, "As I got involved, suddenly, I realized that this little piece of needlepoint was the only place I had any control in my life, but that I did have control here! Then I started looking around to see what other little things I could control. I knew I could not control my illness or that of my son or husband, and I couldn't drive, but I could control my behavior and I could become a more pleasant person and I could try to get and give more pleasure out of my time here. And that's what occupational therapy has meant to me so far, and I'm still looking for other places for me to control."

The story of Charlotte introduces another situation: some patients are simply not very lovable. We therapists dread the next treatment session of these patients, and we feel guilty that we do not like them. These patients are often noncompliant with treatment but are constantly demanding, and we frequently feel the impulse to grab them by both shoulders and say, "Hold still while I help you!" The therapist's anger and resentment may result in his or her becoming noncompliant also, if he or she becomes noncaring. As contradictory as it may seem, some manipulative patients learn to be powerful within the context of the dependent patient role; they have few behaviors that permit dependence and cooperation, while maintaining a sense of independence and coping within the patient role. As in Charlotte's case, a patient's resistance is often stirred by the mixture of emotions surrounding the disruptions in his or her life caused by the illness, the feelings of fear, anger, powerlessness, and the despair of having no hope for the future. In this type of situation, it is generally possible for the therapist to get under or around the resistance by empathetically understanding and acknowledging what the patient is experiencing.

Patients have their own timing for change, and we can facilitate this change, not by pushing, but by being supportive while they become sensitive to and in touch with that timing. We need to acknowledge that we cannot care for every patient. We need to accept that we cannot turn our caring feelings on and off at will. It is sometimes possible to refer a patient that we dislike to another therapist who can feel more positively for the patient, but at times this possibility is not an option. Whatever the situation, our responsibility is to deliver the best professional care. This ". . . in itself, is a kind of caring." (8, p 235)

The same colleague who participated in the renal dialysis consultation (B. Bennett) recently commented (in a discussion, March 1984) that she wondered if the importance of what we do lies in our awareness. In her view, occupational therapy allows for and promotes "connectedness." Our patients are human beings who have had some aspect of human functioning taken away from them. They have been deprived of the mechanisms for connectedness in some part of their relationships. Occupational therapy may invent connectedness where perhaps none existed or create opportunities for reconnecting the patient to other human beings and the environment. We reawaken the patient's capacity to care. Often the patients are unattached to people and institutions. Daily life activities are often the connectors between people; that is, the mechanisms of caring. Occupational therapists care by helping people disengage from despair and dysfunction and by helping them look forward, to see their loss as being able to be ameliorated through adaptation and occupation.

Occupational therapists are specialists in making caring happen. We know how to enrich all the transactions in the relationship with the patient. These become caring gestures. We augment the power of individuals to achieve their own objectives. In the same discussion mentioned earlier, Bennett continued that part of caring is knowing when to stop caring, to stop what she calls "emotional hemorrhaging"; walking the fine line between the two frequently becomes a balancing act. Finally, she added, when the structure of the treatment plan has been followed without the "spirit" of the plan, caring has been abandoned. (9) Caring implies quality of care and for us quality of life.

Occupational therapy is not the only caring profession. It demonstrates caring differently. To illustrate, a surgeon excised a malignant sarcoma from the hip joint of a middle-aged man and also removed about half the muscle tissue forming the buttocks on that side; the psychotherapist used family therapy to help the patient and his family deal with their fears of cancer, the changes in their lives, and the overwhelming feelings focused on his illness; the occupational therapist molded a special cushion allowing the patient to sit more comfortably while he drove a car and while he pursued his hobby of tinkering with cars. These "helpers" were all important to this patient, to his life and to his quality of life. The occupational therapist's intervention was different in that it helped the patient reconnect to those occupations meaningful to him.

What is the market value of caring and who pays for it? Fromm (9) said, "... human energy and skill are without exchange value if there is no demand for them under existing market conditions." (9, p 70-71) In discussing employment settings for occupational therapists, Jantzen (10) said, "Caring for others and other altruistic motives seem to me rarely sufficient to generate dollars for salaries." (p 72) The relationship between caring, *along with* the competence of the health care professional, and patient treatment compliance and its effect on malpractice litigation is well documented. Menninger (5) stated the following:

> ... more often than not, the breakdown has been in the "caring" aspect the physician–patient relationship—not in the quality of technical care and treatment provided ... Caring is an important aspect of health care quality. (p 837)

He further advocated including an assessment of caring within the professional standards review.

So far, caring has not been a part of the professional standards review. I do not believe that it ever will be, because the quality of caring is difficult to measure. However, every patient knows whether or not it is present. The ability of the health professional to develop a caring relationship with patients falls within the art rather, than the science of health care. I am convinced that a profession that consistently provides treatment giving patients a clear sense of having both their physical and psychological needs well tended and contributed to will not only survive, but will also experience an increase in the demand for their services. Occupational therapy is such a profession.

Relationships with Self

The emphasis so far has been on the patient and on the development of the caring relationship as an integral part of the treatment. The focus now shifts to another relationship: that which we have with ourselves. Is it a caring relationship?

If I am not for myself, who will be?
If I am for myself alone, what am I?
If not now, when? (11, p 237)

The meaning of these lines may be quite different for each person who hears them. Each individual's concept of self ". . . is composed of the thousands of perceptions varying in clarity, precision, and importance ..." gathered since birth (12). Our own perceptions screen every experience in our world and interpret that experience uniquely for each of us, thus constantly shaping our self-concept. "The most important single factor affecting behavior is the self-concept." (8, p 39) What we do at every moment in our lives is a product of how we see ourselves and the situations we are in. While situations may change, the beliefs, values, and purposes we have about ourselves are ever-present factors in determining our behavior. "Freud defined the ego (or the self) as that part of the mind which is aware of reality, stores up experiences (in the memory), avoids excessively strong stimuli (through flight), deals with moderate stimuli (through adaptation), and causes changes in the external world to its own advantage (through activity)." (12, p 86) The self is the star of every performance, the central figure in every act (8, p 39). Therefore, we who are engaged in a helping profession need the broadest possible understanding of the nature, origins, and functions of the self-concept, not only for our own benefit but for that of our patients (8, pp 6, 39).

The ability to develop caring relationships with others is in direct proportion to the ability to care for self. This caring for self is not an egocentric, narcissistic focus on self, but rather it is the sensitivity and knowledge of self that leads to personal growth. Just as Thomas (6) advocated a good case of the grippe to sensitize medical students to what it's like to be a patient (p 222), I recommend that we occupational therapists perform an Activity Configuration on ourselves to gain a more objective view of how we use ourselves. How many "shoulds" have we grown up with that are no longer valid in our lives? Once when I was agonizing over whether or not to attend a meeting that I felt I "should" but did not really want to, a friend offered the perspective that "the world is not minimized by your lack of participation in it."

The process of helping others helps one's self: it is satisfying, therapeutic, and curative. There is an exhilaration in helping others that "is the result of something deeper than the power involved or the satisfaction of professional pride and a job well done." It is "the curative power of being human." The response of patients to genuine caring is enormous. It mobilizes "assets and self-curative resources on the part of a person being helped which too often he cannot tap on his own." Helping others increases our own self-esteem as we become aware of the strength and resources being mobilized for this effort and the power they activate in relationships (13, pp 214-216).

Caring, for self and for others, ". . . orders other values around itself." (14, p 51) A life that is ordered through caring has some telling features. It acquires a special kind of certainty, not a stewing need to feel certain and to seek guarantees. It is restful, yet dynamic, as opposed to static, giving security that retains vulnerability (14). "Such inclusive ordering requires giving up certain things and activities, and may thus be said to include an element of submission. But this submission, like the voluntary submission of the craftsman to his discipline and the requirements of his materials is basically liberating and affirming." (14, p 53) Caring brings an order to our lives and relationships that frees our energy to be creative and productive, and provides parameters for our daily decisions. The energy thus freed, converted from negative to positive energy, has a direct effect on our productivity. Caring for self means choosing to attend to my needs first sometimes, not always second or third, because the less I give to me, the less I have to give to others.

We use relationships to define ourselves. As we look inward we see certain things about ourselves, but in the reflections from relationships we begin to see other facets of ourselves. Through relationships with our mothers, fathers, and others, we experience different levels of caring; our perceptions of that caring and how we use that information determine the kind of person we become. It is through this lifelong process that we learn to care for self and others. Our capacity to care and our ability to show we care are dependent on the kinds and quality of caring we receive. This is an ever-changing process for us, because once a word is spoken or an action has occurred, it becomes a part of our experience of the world. It is, in a psychic sense similar to the law of nature that for every action there is an equal and opposite reaction: we receive, we give; we give, we receive.

"One's actions are a part of one's existence" according to Pablo Casals (15). ". . . One feels it a duty to act, and whatever comes one does it—that's all—a very simple thing. I feel the capacity to care is the thing which gives life its deepest significance and meaning." (15, p 156)

If I am not for myself, who will be?

If I am for myself alone, what am I?

If not now, when? (11, p 237)

The Elements of Therapeutic Relationships

It is self-evident that caring alone is not enough to establish an effective therapeutic relationship. Caring is the base; its presence enriches all other aspects of the relationship. The following are additional elements essential to the development of such a relationship:

1. *Competence.* We may be the most caring therapists in existence, but without the knowledge, skill, and ability to provide the needed treatment, we may develop only minimally therapeutic relationships. We have the responsibility to develop an ongoing continuing education program for ourselves. This personalized program should include studying the research being reported and translating treatment efficacy into treatment effectiveness. It should include studying the literature of related fields and studying our own. Developing and maintaining competence is also a part of caring . . . for ourselves and for our patients.
2. *Belief in the dignity and worth of the individual.* This element is conveyed in mostly subtle ways. It involves believing in the integrity of the individual, including his or her need for mastery and control, which we must not violate, but preserve as important.
3. *Belief that each individual has the potential for change and growth.* The individual already has the capacity to adapt and grow. The occupational therapist provides a road map in a sense and facilitates th journey of adaptation through "occupation to improve health and performance." (16)
4. *Communication.* True communication involves listening, hearing the words and the feelings behind the words, making sensitive observations, and sending clear messages.
5. *Values.* Values are reflected in our beliefs. They are our standards for living, and provide stability and meaning in our lives and parameters for our behavior. Values are the foundations of our selectivity, for saying, "This is good, this I believe; that is not good, that is not the way I will go."
6. *Touch.* Rather than elaborating on the use of this powerful therapeutic element here, I urge you to read again Huss's 1976 Slagle Lecture (17, pp 11–18).
7. *Sense of humor.* A judicious use of humor can do much to bypass resistance or defuse a tense situation. It can introduce perspective for both patient and therapist. And it promotes health. In

the introduction to Cousins' book, Bernard Lown, Harvard professor of cardiology, quoted the famous 17th-century physician Thomas Sydenham: "The arrival of a good clown exercises more beneficial influence upon the health of a town than twenty asses laden with drugs." (18, p 24)

These are some of the elements necessary to therapeutic relationships. Individual therapists can expand this list by adding important elements from their experience. Taken individually, these elements are splinter skills; used collectively, they enable and enhance the use of self as a therapeutic tool. These elements become a part of us and a part of the treatment process; and, rather than requiring extra time to include, most often they save time, because we and our patients are in synchrony, and our actions and reactions are mutually supportive of our goals.

These same elements are eminently transferable to our relationships with coworkers, whether lateral, hierarchical, or interdisciplinary. Before staff members can relate to patients in a humanistic way, they have to be dealt with that way. How difficult it is for staff members to create a humanizing environment for patients within a setting where staff are being dealt with in a dehumanizing manner. I have observed that it is difficult to increase or even maintain productivity in situations like this.

Relationships within Today's Health Care Environment

No discussion of relationships in health care today is complete without some mention of how these relationships are affected by the complexity of the health care system. The push for productivity makes it necessary for us to cut costs of providing services and maintain larger caseloads. At the same time, we are being asked to increase documentation. All of these demands make it difficult for us to retain our motivation to develop relationships with our patients that go beyond a superficial level.

Additionally, we are experiencing the initial impact of the prospective payment system. Patients are leaving health facilities before their complete rehabilitation needs have been addressed. We are participating in a health care system that, for the first time, views our service as a cost as opposed to something directed toward supporting human function. Our educational programs face enrollment problems and decreased federal funding. These are definitely challenging times.

Along with the thrust for increased productivity and accountability in the health care arena, a new round of regulation has emerged. "Health care costs have been growing out of control and threaten to consume larger and larger shares of our national wealth. Even more perplexing is the fact that while we outspend other nations on health care we do not enjoy the best of health. We're clearly not getting our money's worth." (19, p 6)

Not only is the federal government sending the message to the health care system to do more, faster and better, with less, but also many states have enacted cost-containment legislation, and third party payers are strictly following their criteria for reimbursement in the effort to control their risks. Now patients—the health care consumers—are demanding more active participation in their own health care; that is, less dependence on and more accountability from their health care providers. One of the fastest growing consumer groups is the 35,000-member People's Medical Society, which has been in existence for just one year but adds 1,000 members each week. This past January, the organization asked all the physicians of West Palm Beach to sign a ten-point Code of Practice, which would include fees posting, complete and open discussion of proposed treatment, and the physician's particular competency to perform that treatment. Charles Inlander, the organization's executive director, said that the Code of Practice "simply affirms basic patient rights. We're only asking doctors the same questions they ask their Mercedes dealer's service department—up-front costs, prognosis, and 'You can't go ahead and do anything until I give you my full approval.' The only difference is we're not asking for the parts back." (20, p D-2)

The shifting relationships in today's health care environment are yet another phase of the action–reaction process that has its roots, at least in American medicine, in the beginning of this country. However, for our purposes, a few comments about the past decade will illustrate the pattern.

According to Starr (21), "Medicine, like many other American institutions, suffered a stunning loss of confidence in the 1970s!" (p 379) Until then, the federal government had supported the beliefs that more medical services were needed and decisions regarding the delivery of these services should be made by the private medical sector. As costs continued to rise, but with no proportionate improvement in health care, government regulations and constraints increased as never before. This reaction was more than an economic one, because it included concern about the rights of patients, about the effectiveness of medical treatment, and about the moral values of medicine. Women, in particular, began to assume more responsibility for their own health, thereby diminishing the power, influence, and control of the medical profession (21, pp 379, 380). It was no longer just a question of whether hospitalizations and surgery were necessary; rather, whether medical care made any difference in the health of the American people. "The nineteenth century doctrine of therapeutic nihilism—that existing drugs and therapies were useless—was revived in a new form. Now the net effectiveness of the medical system as a whole was [questioned]." (21, p 408)

Starr's (21) comments indicate that the pendulum does swing—action, reaction—and that the "doctrine of therapeutic nihilism" (p 408) appeared in both the nineteenth and twentieth centuries, although in a different form the second time around. That pendulum will certainly swing again. While Starr's book focuses on the medical profession, we, as associates of that profession, must closely evaluate our capacity to address the effectiveness of our services and maintain the relationships that give us a position within the system itself. The turbulence within the health care system today is but a reflection of the turbulence within society as it struggles to hold onto the old ways while also reaching to the new that are unknown. "One important characteristic to recognize is that if any one part of the system is changed, then all other parts within the system and any related system are changed as a result." (22, p 800) Thus, the restructuring of society, from the changing profile of the labor force to the graying of America, affects the health care system. Those of us who are in the health care arena are scrambling to find our new place, to restore balance and security to our environment. In this competitive environment, it is important to do what we do well and maintain the relationships that will support our patients' needs, along with our own.

The greater the use of technology, the greater the depersonalization of the individual. Caring is the counterbalance: the "high touch" human response to the introduction of "high tech." (23, p 39) From its beginning, occupational therapy treatment has been inextricably involved with high touch. We have helped our patients to do, participate, work, and enjoy, despite their dysfunction. Baum (24) has stated that, "As a profession, occupational therapy harnesses will and gives the individual control through activity. That is human, that is care." (p 515)

Summary

The constraints in today's health care environment make it extremely difficult to do the job we've been trained to do. With the possible exception of continuing competency, the elements of a therapeutic relationship described earlier do not increase the cost of health care, do not require additional time in the treatment process, and give the patient a clear sense of having both his or her physical and psychological needs well tended and contributed to. As occupational therapists, we have superb skills for developing and tending caring relationships. Let us continue to use them well.

Acknowledgments

The author thanks Carolyn Baum, MA, OTR, FAOTA, Binni Bennett, MSW, and Wanda Ellis-Webb for their invaluable support and assistance.

References

1. Devereaux E: Community home health care—in the rural setting. In *Willard and Spackman's Occupational Therapy,* 6th edition, Hopkins and H Smith, Editors. Philadelphia: Lippincott, 1983, p 787.

2. West W: A reaffirmed philosophy and practice of occupational therapy for the 1980s. *Am J Occup Ther 38:* 22, 1984.

3. *Project to Identify the Philosophy of Occupational Therapy.* Rockville, MD: AOTA, Jan 1983, p 21.

4. Ciardi J: In *Choose Life,* B Mandelbaum, Editor. New York: Random House, 1968, p 158.

5. Menninger W: "Caring" as part of health care quality. *JAMA 234:* 836–837, 1975.

6. Thomas L: *The Youngest Science: Notes of a Medicine-Watcher.* New York: Viking, 1983, pp 220–223.

7. Reilly M: Occupational therapy can be one of the great ideas of 20th century medicine. *Am J Occup Ther 16:* 1–9, 1962. (Reprinted as Chapter 6).

8. Combs A, Avila D, Purkey W: *Helping Relationships: Basic Concept for the Helping Professions.* Boston; Allyn & Bacon, 1971, pp 6, 39.

9. Fromm E: *The Art of Loving.* New York: Bantam Books, 1956, pp 70–71.

10. Jantzen A: The current profile of occupational therapy and the future professional or vocational? In *Occupational Therapy: 20001 AD.* Rockville, MD: AOTA, 1978, p 72.

11. Ethics of the fathers (chapt 1, verse 14). In *Choose Life,* B Mandelbaum, Editor. New York: Random House, 1968, p 237.

12. Appelton W: *Fathers and Daughters.* New York: Doubleday, 1981, p 86.

13. Rubin T: *Through My Own Eyes.* New York: Macmillan, 1982, pp 214–216.

14. Mayeroff M: *On Caring.* New York: Perennial Library, Harper & Row, 1971.

15. Casals P: In *Choose Life,* B Mandelbaum, Editor. New York: Random House, 1968, p 156.

16. Representative Assembly: Occupation as the common core of occupational therapy. In *Policies of the AOTA, Inc.* Rockville, MD: AOTA, 1979, #1.12.

17. Huss J: Touch with care or a caring touch? *Am J Occup Ther 31:* 11–18, 1977.

18. Cousin: Introduction. In *The Healing Heart, Antidotes to Panic and Helplessness.* New York: Norton, 1983, p 24.

19. Schneiderman L: The "Molting" of America's welfare system. In *NASW News.* Silver Spring, MD: National Association of Social Workers, Sept 1983, p 6.

20. Peirce N: Citizen's group going after more medical accountability. In *The Herald Dispatch.* Huntington, WV: Gannett Feb 19, 1984, p D-2.

21. Starr P: *The Social Transformation of American Medicine.* New York: Basic Books, 1982, pp 379–380, 408.

22. Baum C, Devereaux E: A systems perspective—Conceptualizing and implementing occupational therapy in a complex environment. In *Willard and Spackman's Occupational Therapy,* 6th edition, Hopkins and Smith, Editors. Philadelphia: Lippincott, 1983, p 800.

23. Naisbitt J: *Megatrends.* New York: Warner Books, 1982, p 39.

24. Baum C: Occupational therapists put care in the health system. *Am J Occup Ther 34:* 515, 1980.

Chapter 34

Clinical Reasoning: The Ethics, Science, and Art

Joan C. Rogers, PhD, OTR/L

A therapist, employed at a regional rehabilitation center, extracts cues from the records of acute hospitals, to judge the rehabilitation potential of patients referred for admission. Another therapist, working with persons with mental retardation, selects a treatment approach based on task analysis to teach self-care skills. A third therapist, serving on a geriatric assessment team, uses scores on a mental status examination and performance ratings in daily living activities to estimate patients' ability to continue living alone in their homes. A fourth therapist reviews patients' progress in manual dexterity to formulate a recommendation for or against hand surgery. These four therapists are using their clinical reasoning skills to collect and transform data about patients into decisions that have critical implications for the quality of life of their patients.

If we questioned the therapists about their decisions, each would probably comment on their potential fallibility. Some patients, denied occupational therapy because of a perceived lack of potential for rehabilitation, would make substantial gains in functional skills if intervention were initiated. Some patients with mental retardation will not benefit from the task breakdown approach to self-care training. Some geriatric patients admitted for institutional living could have been supported adequately in the community. Some patients undergoing hand surgery will lose functional abilities. The possibility of error in our clinical judgments and the potential ensuing negative consequences urge us to develop ways of improving our assessment and treatment decisions.

Despite the obvious importance of clinical judgment in the occupational therapy process, little attention has been given to explicating the thinking that guides practice. My research, albeit with a small number of occupational therapists, suggests that our cognitive processes are regarded as intuitive and ineffable. For example, when therapists were asked how they arrived at their treatment decisions, they commonly responded by saying, "I have never really thought about it." or "I don't know how I reached that conclusion. I just know." Cognitive activity constitutes the heart of the clinical enterprise. Our failure to study the process of knowing and understanding that underlies practice precludes an adequate description of clinical reasoning. This in turn prevents the development of a methodology for systematically improving it and for teaching it.

I intend to explore here the reasoning process through which we learn about patients so that we may help them through engagement in occupation. I will construct an intellectual device for viewing clinical reasoning from the perspective of the basic questions the therapist seeks to answer through clinical inquiry. The scientific, ethical, and artistic dimensions of clinical reasoning will be elucidated as these questions are explored. The device will be useful for directing and appraising our thoughts about treating patients and for developing a clinical science of occupational therapy. In developing my thoughts, I have relied on the basic scheme of clinical judgment presented by Pellegrino (1) for medicine and have adapted it to the occupational therapy process.

The Goal of Clinical Reasoning

The goal of the clinical reasoning process has an impact on each of the steps taken to achieve the goal. Hence, an appreciation of this goal provides insight on the whole process.

Patients come to occupational therapy when they, their physicians, family members, or caregivers perceive that they are not adequately performing their daily activities. Performance in self-care, work, and leisure occupations has been compromised because of the consequences of disease, trauma, abnormal development, age-related changes, or environmental restrictions. The disruptions in occupational functions are characteristically severe and enduring as opposed to transitory. To regain a former level of performance, maintain the current level, or achieve a more optimal one, the patient enlists the aid of the therapist. The therapist's task, therefore, is to select a right therapeutic action for the patient (1). In other words, the goal of clinical reasoning is a treatment recommendation issued in the interests of a particular patient. Decision making is highly individualized.

The occupational therapy treatment plan details what a particular patient should do to enhance occupational role performance. The therapeutic action must be the right action for this individual. This implies that it must be as congruent as possible with the patient's concept of the "good life." Treatment should be in concert with the patient's needs, goals, life style, and personal and cultural values. A therapeutic program that is right for one patient is not necessarily right for another. The ultimate question we, as clinicians, are challenged to answer is: What, among the many things that could be done for this patient, ought to be done. This is an ethical question. It involves a judgment to which facts contribute but that must be decided by weighing values. A salient criterion of an ethical action is its agreement with the patient's valued goals. The clinical reasoning process terminates in an ethical decision, rather than in a scientific one, and the ethical nature of the goal of clinical reasoning projects itself over the entire sequence.

Ethical decisions regarding treatment are not made in isolation from scientific knowledge. The patient comes to the therapist for expert advice regarding adaptation to chronic dysfunction. The factual basis for decision making is provided by the therapist. When therapists set out to solve clinical problems, they are confronted with an unknown—the patient. Scientific methodologies are used to learn about the patient. Once the patient's condition is adequately understood, scientific and empirical knowledge is applied in the efforts to enhance occupational status. Although ethical considerations can override scientific ones, they do not displace the need to secure a scientific opinion.

Clinical Questions

To ascertain the right action for each patient, clinical inquiry focuses on three questions: What is the patient's current status in occupational role performance? What could be done to enhance the patient's performance? And what ought to be done to enhance occupational competence? These are the fundamental questions that I previously alluded to as guiding the clinical process. Each question will be considered first in terms of the knowledge needed to answer it, and, subsequently, in terms of the cognitive processes used to obtain the knowledge.

What Is the Patient's Status?

Assessment. The first question to be considered is the assessment question: What is the patient's occupational status? The occupational therapy assessment is a concise and accurate summary of a patient's occupational role performance that arises from an investigation of the patient. The occupational therapy assessment tells us what we need to know about the patient to plan a sound intervention or prevention program. To serve this function, the assessment includes several features: it indicates what is wrong with the patient, it indicates the patient's strengths, and it indicates the patient's motivation for occupation.

The word *assessment* is preferable to the terms *diagnosis* or *problem definition* for the evaluation of occupational status because it has a much broader meaning. Diagnosis and problem definition connote the identification of pathological, abnormal, dysfunctional, or problematic processes or states. To assess means to rate the value of property for the purpose of taxation. The word *assessment*, then, with its emphasis on the evaluation of the worth of something, is an appropriate term to apply to the process of collecting information to resolve clinical problems and to the statement that summarizes the results of that process. Occupational therapy is concerned with helping disabled persons to adapt to chronic disability more effectively. This may be accomplished by enhancing abilities as well as by remediating or reducing dysfunction. The occupational therapy assessment serves as the end point of evaluation and the starting point for treatment planning. To serve this pivotal function, the assessment must specify both assets and liabilities. Thus, diagnosis, or the determination of what is wrong with the patient, is only a part of the assessment.

Knowledge. The assessment process usually begins with diagnosis, since knowledge of dysfunction tells us what is wrong and requires correction or amelioration. The therapist seeks to ascertain the specific problems the patient is having in performing self-care, work, and leisure occupations. Disruptions in occupational role are commonly of two major types: an inability to perform socially defined age-appropriate tasks and an inability to coordinate these tasks effectively in daily life. To the extent that a person has disruptions in occupational role, or impairments that we can predict will result in such disruptions, that person is an appropriate candidate for occupational therapy. The occupational therapy diagnosis clearly articulates the disruption in occupational role that is of concern for treatment. For example, we might state that Tom Smith is totally dependent in hygiene and dressing and requires physical assistance with feeding. This diagnosis indicates that these are the major problems at this time.

The occupational therapy diagnosis has a temporal quality. Participation in daily living tasks may change over the course of an illness or other disorder. For example, as Tom Smith gains competence in self-care, the diagnosis may switch to dysfunctions in home management. Similarly, as an individual matures and needs and interests change, the occupational therapy diagnosis changes, and intervention is refocused. Thus, the range of problems that comprise the occupational therapy diagnosis is broad and variable, and the diagnosis may change over time.

Often, the occupational therapy diagnosis indicates not only the disruption in occupational role, but also the suspected cause or causes for this disruption. This is the etiological component of the diagnostic statement and it offers an explanation of why the individual behaves or fails to behave in some way.

The most prevalent perspective for defining the etiology of occupational role dysfunctions is based on the biopsychosocial model. This enables us to pinpoint the causes of performance dysfunctions in terms of biological, psychological, and social variables. For example, we might state that Ida Cox cannot dress herself because she has contractures in her upper extremities, thus attributing the cause to a biological variable. Or, we might suggest that she cannot dress herself because of a memory problem, thus attributing the cause to a psychological variable. Or, we might conclude that the reason she is unable to dress herself is because she cannot reach her clothes from a wheelchair. In this case, the dressing dysfunction is attributed to the interaction of a biological variable, motor impairment, and a social variable, the man-made environment. Such attributions allow us to plan appropriate treatment. We can plan to remediate the contracture or memory deficit or to circumvent their effects on performance. We can remove the architectural barriers.

An occupational therapy diagnosis stemming from the biopsychosocial model is so specific that it is applicable to only one patient. For instance, an occupational therapy diagnosis might state: Homemaking disability secondary to a lack of endurance for shopping to procure groceries, and postural instability in negotiating the stairs to the laundry facilities in the basement; ability is complicated by blurred vision in both eyes as a consequence of cataracts. Such a diagnosis is unlikely to be appropriate for more than one patient. Although the diagnostic statement is highly descriptive, it is also highly prescriptive. For example, the above diagnosis suggests such interventions as: employing homemaker services, scheduling and performing activities in such a way as to control fatigue, using good light with no glare, and using mobility aids or environmental supports.

In addition to a description of what the patient cannot do and why, the occupational therapy assessment includes a description of what the patient can do and how well it can be done. Although the problem is diagnosed, it is the person who is assessed. The need to acknowledge positive factors was well expressed by the little boy who reacted to the scolding he received about his report card by saying, "Daddy, I think your eyes need fixing. You only saw the D and not the four As." Knowing a person's problems or deficits tells us little about his or her strengths. The image of the patient drawn from problem behaviors is distorted. It needs to be supplemented with snapshots of the patient's occupational competencies and strengths to enable the therapist to construct a fair and valid impression of the patient.

The assessment of occupational competence requires a wide-angled lens. Occupational performance emerges from a complex network of transactions between the internal characteristics of the individual and the external properties of the surrounding environment. Just as features of a particular situation may account for a limitation of ability, so they may also allow the expression of ability. The qualities of the environment are important enablers of human performance. You cannot swim without water or play tennis without a partner. Both the physical and the social environments influence the patient's ability to occupy time productively. To assess occupational competence, the therapist evaluates the people, places, and objects associated with the patient's occupational endeavors to determine the extent to which they support occupation.

The final requirement of the occupational therapy assessment is to summarize the patient's motivation to engage in occupation. Who among us has never pondered over the patients with excellent potential who fail to achieve and those with intractable conditions who surpass all expectations. We cannot understand the patient without an appreciation of the way in which the urge toward competence has been habitually satisfied. The ontogenetic aspects of occupation have critical implications for recovery and growth. The patient's history of occupation informs us whether the present dysfunction is extenuated by a pattern of adaptive behavior or augmented by a career of maladaptive behavior. The patient's mastery of the environment is documented in occupational achievement, while exploration of the environment is recorded in the use of time. Since time is occupied by doing things of value, the patient's use of time provides insight into the varieties of occupations that are meaningful to him or her. The patient's past is reviewed to shed light on how occupational behavior is organized and to lend perspective to activities that are important and incidental to the life plan.

Historical assessment is directed toward a deeper understanding of the patient's occupational nature. The normative sequence of occupational endeavors begins in childhood play and self-care. Participation in arts and crafts, games, academics, chores, and part-time work are added to the repertoire through young adulthood. Productive occupation in the form of employment predominates in adulthood. This often changes to leisure pursuits during later maturity. The therapist thus captures the development and balance of self-care, work, and leisure occupations in studying the sequence of preschool, school age, worker, and retiree roles.

The yield of the occupational therapy assessment is a model of the patient that describes and explains his or her unique functioning in occupation. The model superimposes current functional abilities on disabilities, and relates these to environmental demands and to past performance. It is from this comprehensive model of the patient that future capacity is predicted and treatment goals are recommended.

Process. Having described the requirements of the occupational therapy assessment. I will now turn to the cognitive processes used to formulate it. What is involved in clinical inquiry? How do we go about the task of constructing a model of the patient? The approach used here for looking at the cognitive processes that undergird practice reflects an information-processing view of cognition. The human mind is thus conceptualized as a computer that has certain information processing capabilities. It can do some things better than others and uses certain labor-saving strategies to overcome its limitations. A primary limitation of the human mind is its small capacity for short-term or working memory. Because of this limitation, data must be selected judiciously, processed serially, and managed through simplifying strategies (2). In assessment, the clinician has as intake to the information-processing system cues gathered from the patient or about the patient. The output is the conclusions summarized in the occupational therapy assessment. The conversion of intake data to output conclusions is a critical feature of clinical reasoning.

The therapist begins the assessment by choosing a plan for studying the patient. We say to ourselves, "Of all things that I could consider about this patient, what am I going to think about?" We typically respond to this question by constructing an image of the patient from the pre-assessment data and use this image to direct our plan. Our pre-assessment image tells us what to include and what to exclude as we observe the patient. Thus, the first labor-saving device the therapist uses is to limit the parameters within which the patient will be studied.

The pre-assessment image of the patient is derived from the conceptual frame of reference or postulate system of the therapist. A conceptual frame of reference represents a therapist's unique view of occupational therapy. It consists of facts derived from research studies, empirical generalizations drawn from experience, theories and models accepted by the therapist, and principles of practice obtained from instructors and colleagues. My frame of reference represents what I believe about occupational therapy practice. A frame of reference operates largely as a nonconscious ideology in forming the pre-assessment image. The therapist links his or her frame of reference with the pre-assessment data to construct an image of the patient that furnishes the outline for the clinical investigation.

Two salient pre-assessment factors are the medical diagnosis and age. By knowing even these elementary facts. we can predict certain things about a patient. For example, if we know that a patient's dominant arm has been amputated, we can anticipate problems in manual dexterity and bilateral coordination. If, in addition, we know that the patient is 6 years of age, rather than 76, we can expect to direct treatment toward habilitation of hand skills as opposed to rehabilitation.

The pre-assessment image of the patient is used to generate a series of testable working hypotheses. The therapist reasons that, if a particular hypothesis is valid, then it should follow that such and such will be found in further study of the case. For example, a therapist learns from the occupational therapy referral that the patient is a 40-year-old woman with depression. The therapist reasons that, if this patient is depressed, she is likely to be disheveled, to have a low level of involvement in activities, and to concentrate on events associated with negative affect. In other words, by knowing that the patient is depressed, the therapist is able to view the patient as a representative of the class of depressed patients, and, thus, hypothesizes that she will exhibit characteristics of depression. The therapist then sets out to perform the procedures needed to substantiate the hypothesis.

Up to this point, the reasoning process is essentially deductive in nature. The therapist recalls some general postulates from memory and applies them to a specific patient. The open-ended question of what is wrong with the patient has now been refined to a set of better-defined problems for exploration and resolution.

The working hypotheses provide a plan for acquiring cues from the patient to test the hypotheses. A cue is any bit of information that guides or directs the assessment (3). Cues arise from the observational process that employs three general types of data-gathering methodologies: testing or measurement; questioning, including history taking and interviewing; and observation. Accurate clinical decisions are dependent on the collection of good cues. Two tests of the goodness of cues are reliability and validity.

Cues can be used to test the working hypotheses developed from deductive reasoning. By comparing each cue to the working hypotheses, sense may be made of the data. The therapist reasons, "This is what I expect to find, now what do I find?" A cue may be interpreted as confirming a hypothesis, disconfirming a hypothesis, or noncontributary to a hypothesis. Thus, as information is collected about the patient, the therapist decides repeatedly whether or not a finding is related to the patient's problems. Confidence in each hypothesis increases or decreases, based on the interpretation of additional data. Extensive case data are reduced by eliminating, or holding in reserve, data that do not appear significant. Hypothesis testing is thus another of the mind's strategies for simplifying data management. Hypotheses direct the collection of data and determine how they are organized and filed in memory. This organization prevents the mind from becoming overloaded with irrelevant facts and assists the therapist in retrieving information from memory.

Cues may also be combined to formulate new hypotheses. As cues are collected to test the validity of the deduced hypotheses, some cues may not fit well. Some of the performance problems we had expected to find will not be found, and others that we had not anticipated will become manifest. Our thinking begins to move from the classical, textbook picture of the disorder, to the disorder as it is uniquely manifested in this patient. The reasoning process now becomes inductive, with problem definition induced from empirical study of the patient, rather than deduced from the therapist's frame of reference. Additional cues may then be collected to test the inductively derived hypotheses. Clinical reasoning proceeds by developing hypotheses that pull together several inferences into a broader pattern or model of the patient.

After gleaning a clear perception of the patient's problems, the therapist then begins to search for cues indicative of the health of the patient as avidly as the search was conducted to identify dysfunction. Inductive reasoning and hypothesis testing are the basic processes through which the clinician assesses the patient's competencies, motivation for occupational achievement, and the environments in which the patient operates or will operate. These kinds of data are highly personal and hence are less likely to be deduced from knowledge of disease or disorder.

Data collection cannot continue indefinitely, and at some point the therapist decides that adequate information has been collected. How much data constitutes adequate data is dependent on the ethical consequences of an error in judgment (2,4). A recommendation to institutionalize a patient because he or she is unable to look after his or her self-care needs would require more evidence than that required for the prescription of a rocker knife. Regardless of how many data are collected, however, the data base remains incomplete. The data base represents only a sampling of the patient's behavior. The therapist's task is to use this incomplete information to make a judicious decision. Decision making takes place under conditions of uncertainty.

Throughout the process of data collection, the therapist's pre-assessment image of the patient has been revised and elaborated, based on the accumulated cues. Once cue collection is stopped and no new information is being generated, hypothesis testing also ceases. The clinical reasoning of the therapist now resembles the dialectical process in which the therapist argues or defends the interpretation of the data in much the same way as a lawyer pleads a case in court. Does the patient have a dressing problem that is of concern? Is the cause of the patient's performance difficulties visual–perceptual problems? Is the mental status of the patient adequate for self-care? The evidence supporting or opposing each alternative is weighed with the objective of rendering one explanation more cogent than another. Inferences that are compatible are retained and others are rejected or modified as contradictions appear. Through the dialectical process the model of the individual patient is polished and repolished. In this way, the therapist arrives at a cohesive conception of the patient, and, having grasped the whole, re-interprets the parts in the light of this understanding. Once a holistic picture of the patient has been devised, the function of the assessment moves from model building to decision making.

What Are the Available Options?

The second of the three general questions guiding clinical inquiry is the therapeutic question: What can be done for this patient? Having proposed a model of the patient's occupational status, we then begin to explore the actions that could be taken to enhance occupational role performance. The intent is to generate a list of the treatment options available for the problems and assets presented by this patient. For example, suppose a patient's problems in self-care were attributed to hemiplegia subsequent to a cerebral vascular accident. To treat this problem, we might consider a neurological approach aimed at regaining controlled action in the involved arm, or a rehabilitative approach aimed at training the uninvolved arm to perform skilled activities, or a combination of these approaches. The aim, at this stage of clinical reasoning, is to foster an awareness of the range and kind of treatment possibilities. In effect, the therapist uses the model of the patient to construct a theory of practice for the patient.

Knowledge. The therapist's consideration of what could be done includes a review of the relative effectiveness of each treatment approach. If a particular treatment option is initiated, what results can be expected, and how long will it take to achieve them? Any hazards associated with the various treatments, or with no treatment, are evaluated in the light of the potential benefits.

Decision making concerning the appropriate action can approach certitude if the deleterious effects of a disorder without treatment are known, and if there is substantial evidence of how these effects can be altered by a particular treatment. We know, for instance, that if joints are not moved, contractures develop and the joints become immobile. Thus, movement becomes the scientifically acceptable treatment for preventing contractures.

For most occupational therapy approaches or procedures, however, the scientific evidence is not definitive. Rarely are the outcomes of research so specific that they allow us to know with 100 percent accuracy what will happen. Scientific findings generally emerge as probabilities rather than as certainties. They may, for example, tell us that 95 percent of the patients with right hemiplegia receiving self-care training will become independent in self-care. But when we apply this finding to Edith Jones, we do so with the recognition that her chances of becoming independent remain 50–50. The response of a patient to treatment cannot be predicted with certitude. Scientific knowledge can improve our chances of making accurate technical decisions but it cannot assure this. When the scientific evidence is inconclusive, the therapist has considerable leeway in devising treatment recommendations.

In the absence of scientific knowledge about the effectiveness of treatment options, clinicians rely on knowledge gleaned from their own clinical experience or from the experiences of others. Knowledge derived from practice rather than research indicates what works but may not indicate what works best.

Process. To draw up a list of the patient's treatment options, the therapist searches memory for relevant scientific and practice knowledge. Clinical experiences are stored and classified in memory and retrieved as needed for application to new patients. Each time a therapist treats a patient, a clinical experiment is performed in which the objective is to replicate a successful outcome of a past experiment (5). As a first step in reproducing the experiment, the therapist mentally reviews previous patients whose occupational status resembled the patient at hand. Although no two patients are exactly alike, the therapist assembles a subgroup of patients who are most similar to the patient under study (6). Treatment is selected for the new patient by analyzing and comparing the therapeutic actions and outcomes of the patients in the reference group. If there is a high degree of similarity between the patient being treated and previous patients, the therapist will select a treatment that is highly replicative. If the similarity is low, or if previous treatment was not very effective, the therapist will propose a treatment that is more inventive.

The cognitive process involved in the selection of treatment is again that of dialectical reasoning. The therapist argues one treatment option against another without recourse to new clinical data. The process of enumerating the patient's treatment alternatives relies heavily on the content of long-term memory. The more clinical experience therapists have, the more empirical data are available to guide decision making. It is impossible for therapists to consider a treatment with which they have no familiarity. Similarly, clinicians cannot debate the scientific merits of one procedure over another, unless the procedure has been scientifically investigated and the research has been assimilated.

What Ought to Be Done?

The third and final question to be considered is the ethical question: What ought to be done to enhance occupational competence? Simply because a goal appears technically feasible for the patient does not mean that it should be set as a goal. And, simply because a treatment approach can be initiated does not imply that it should be instituted. We must avoid confusing action that can be taken with action that ought to be taken. From an ethical standpoint, decisive action must take the patient's valued goals into account. It must conform to the patient's definition of health, accomplishment, and the "good life."

Knowledge. Ethical principles arise from reflection on the nature of humanity and human dignity. Respect for individuals requires that each individual be regarded as autonomous. Each individual has a definite pattern and characteristic style for mastering the environment in the pursuit of occupational competence. The life plan is guided by personal and cultural values. Values give meaning and direction to one's life by inciting future goals and sustaining involvement in activity.

The concept of respect for the individual implies that the occupational therapy treatment plan should not interfere with the patient's intentions for recovery. To develop an appropriate plan, the patient's values are distilled from the thematic continuity of the assessment of occupational status and taken into account in the review of technically feasible treatment options. When there is a range of possibilities for treatment goals and substantial lack of certitude concerning the technical merits of treatment alternatives, the therapist has considerable latitude in shaping recommendations. Expert advice is based more on opinion than fact. Ethical decision making requires the therapist to search for an understanding of the patient's life rather than to make an evaluation of it. This understanding facilitates the selection of options to be discussed with the patient.

The goal of the clinical encounter is to devise a therapeutic plan that preserves the patient's values and represents a mutual understanding between the therapist and patient. Occupational therapy involves habit training and often requires major restructuring of the way in which personal values are to be satisfied. If habits are to be developed, patients must choose the objects and processes that they want to master in occupational therapy. Worthwhile achievement is the end product of personally deliberated decision making. Occupational achievement begins with the choice to develop one's capabilities. It is the patient who restores, maintains, and enhances occupational performance. The patient, not the therapist, is the agent of change. The patient's active participation is required not only in determining and prioritizing the goals of treatment, but also in deciding on the methods to be used to achieve the goals. As a result of assuming personal responsibility for treatment decisions, the patient emerges from the assessment with an increased sense of self-determination and control, and a sense of commitment to accomplishing planned goals. In the capacity of expert advisor, the therapist guides patients through the decision-making process, and helps them fuse the intellectual and emotional aspects of decision making into choices that are right for them.

It cannot be assumed that the goals selected by a patient for himself or herself will match those the therapist would select. Each may have a different view of the "good life." Because most persons with quadriplegia secondary to a spinal cord lesion at the level of the 6th and 7th cervical vertebrae can relearn dressing skills, the therapist may reason that Tim Robbins should work toward this goal. However, Tim may conclude that he would prefer to spend his limited energy relearning how to manage his home computer.

When the therapist and patient have different goals, the potential for conflict is high, and the resolution of conflict can easily be tipped in favor of the therapist's view. Two factors contribute significantly, to the therapist holding the balance of power (1). First, the therapist has the knowledge and skills to alleviate the problems facing the patient. The patient is thus dependent on the therapist for help. Second, the patient's position of dependency is compounded by the patient's vulnerability. As a result of disease or other disorders, patients sustain insults to functions regarded as integral to human life and living. The very fact that they need help may diminish their sense of autonomy. Adaptive functioning in basic life tasks, such as eating and dressing, may be impeded. Patients may even be unable to express their own values or make rational choices. Such impairments place a patient's moral agency at risk, and often make it easy to take advantage of the patient's right to control his or her life.

Process. The methods used to answer ethical questions differ from those used in science. While scientific questions are answered by accumulating data and testing hypotheses, ethical questions are resolved by coming to grips with values and making value judgments (7). To empower the patient to act as his or her own moral agent, the therapist provides the patient with the knowledge needed to participate effectively in decision making. The patient's choice must not only be autonomous, it must also be informed. Patients are not adequately informed to make choices, unless they can anticipate the results of their choices. The ethical and scientific dimensions of clinical reasoning are closely intermingled. The therapist presents the possible options for treatment, projects the outcomes of each option, explains how the outcomes are achieved, and outlines a time sequence for goal attainment. Together the therapist and patient consider each recommendation and evaluate the consequences of each alternative in terms of the patient's occupational potential and goals. If necessary, the therapist tempers unrealistic expectations, corrects inaccurate information, and points out any inconsistencies in rationalization. In effect, the therapist assists the patient in imagining what might occur, if treatment is to be undertaken or rejected. The strength of arguments for one action over another is assessed by dialectic. Greater weight is assigned a position according to the importance it holds for the patient. The selection of treatment becomes more difficult as the merits of one action over other actions become more ambiguous, The therapist makes known his or her preferences for the patient's treatment as well as the rationale for this decision. The patient ends the deliberation by making a choice.

Once the patient has determined the course of action, the therapist supports or confirms the decision. The therapist captures the persuasive elements of the dialectical argument, and uses them to instill in the patient a belief that treatment X is the best course of action and should be undertaken. At the same time, the therapist strives to bolster the patient's belief that he or she can carry out the treatment and achieve the goals. The reasoning process ends, therefore, in persuasive rhetoric, which we call "motivating the patient." In situations where therapists judge that they cannot lend support to the patient's choice, responsibility for providing occupational therapy services is terminated.

The therapist is privileged to help the patient select from the available opportunities those that are to be brought to fruition. As the patient executes and fulfills his or her choice, the therapist learns about the healing power of occupation. Occupational choice rekindles the will to live, and mobilizes the mind to discipline the body, in enacting the creative processes associated with reversing disability. The subtle wisdom of participation in self-initiated and self-directed occupation becomes apparent as confidence is rebuilt and hope is restored. Choices are not confined to the outset of treatment. Assessment and planning are on-going processes and there are repeated occasions to consider if treatment should be continued, terminated, modified, or supplemented.

This discussion of the ethical dimension of clinical reasoning has been based on three cogent assumptions: 1. that patients can serve as their own moral agents; 2. that the patient's choice is the ultimate one; and 3. that the therapist acts independently. None of these conditions may be met in a particular situation, which introduces further complications into the already complex process of ethical decision making. Surrogates may substitute for patients in the planning process because patients are too young, too impaired mentally, or too emotionally disturbed to participate in decision making. The rights of family members and the values and resources of society may limit the choices patients can make. The conjoint decision of therapist and patient may be modified or set aside by the health care team. These are vital issues that cannot be avoided in clinical decisions.

In summary, the data collected in clinical inquiry play three roles in clinical reasoning. First, clinical data are used to describe the patient's occupational status. This description includes an indication of the patient's adaptive skills, performance dysfunctions and their presumed causes, and competency motivation. Second, clinical data are used to conjure up a group of patients who have an occupational status and history comparable to the patient under consideration. These patients serve as a reference group for the identification of treatment options and prediction of treatment outcomes. Third, clinical data are used to identify therapeutic options appropriate to the specific needs of the patient, and to recommend a course of action consistent with the patient's values. As the clinical reasoning process moves from an assessment of occupational status, to a review of treatment options, to a selection of the right action, the scientific mode of reasoning gives way to nonscientific intellectual processes. Choosing a course of action involves many value considerations. The closer we come to making a clinical judgment, the less use is made of facts and hypothesis testing, and the more reliance is placed on the dialectical process, opinion, and persuasion.

Perfecting Clinical Inquiry

Now that what is involved in clinical study has been considered, it seem appropriate to ponder how our habits of inquiry can be improved. My suggestions are intended to be directional rather than comprehensive.

Model of the Patient. The therapist's understanding of the patient is highly dependent on the development of a model of the patient. It is pertinent to point out that studies conducted with counseling professionals have consistently supported the value of inductive theory building for practice, as opposed to the application of deductive theory. McArthur (8), for example, found that psychologists who applied existing theories in a doctrinary fashion turned out to be the poorest appraisers of personality. The critical element in devising a model of the patient is meticulous attention to the cues obtained from the patient. The ability to use assessment-related data to develop hypotheses is a vital professional skill.

Although hypotheses have adaptive value for organizing and managing data, they represent strong conceptual biases. In collecting and interpreting data, we have a tendency to overlook evidence that does not support our hypotheses. This is accompanied by an inclination to overemphasize positive evidence. In other words, we are psychologically prone to affirm our ideas and, feel less compelled to refute them (4, 9). Agnew and Pyke (10) drew a salient comparison between the blindness imposed by hypotheses and that generated by love. They commented: "The rejection of a theory once accepted is like the rejection of a girlfriend or boyfriend once loved—it takes more than a bit of negative evidence. In fact, the rest of the community can shake their collective heads in amazement at your blindness, your utter failure to recognize the glaring array of differences between your picture of the girl or boy, and the data." (p 128) The rigid application of a conceptual bias emerged as a major concern in my study of occupational therapists' thinking (11). The medical diagnosis was used to formulate the pre-assessment image of the patient and that image remained stable, even in the face of cues portending a revision.

Once cognizant of the pitfalls involved in hypothesis use, the therapist can initiate steps to avoid them. Obtaining a second opinion through consultation is one method commonly used to check the validity of one's interpretation. Consultants should perform their own assessments without reference to the patient's data base. Objectivity will be destroyed if consultants read reports or participate in discussions about the patient before conducting their own evaluations. The consultant's final opinion, however, should be based on the total available data (5).

A fixed data collection schedule is another mechanism used to prevent premature closure of hypothesis generation. The Occupational Therapy Uniform Evaluation Checklist (12) is an example of a fixed data collection schedule. It specifies the boundaries of occupational therapy practice and lists the variables to be reviewed for assessment. The Checklist forces the therapist to examine occupational performance from a panoramic view rather than microscopically. In so doing, it fosters the search for information that might suggest hypotheses the therapist might not otherwise have entertained. Adherence to a fixed routine assures the therapist that observations will be conducted that afford a fair and adequate opportunity to disprove as well as to confirm favorite hypotheses (13).

Research on the assessment process suggests that practitioners' "favorite" hypotheses concentrate on the dysfunctional aspects of patient performance (14, 15). We seem to be more interested in exploring why Alice Thompson falls so often than in ascertaining why she maintains her balance for so long. This preoccupation with problematic behaviors probably stems from the fact that they are the reason for the patient's referral to occupational therapy and constitute the focus of interventive efforts. Our first response to the question concerning the patient's occupational status is that it is dysfunctional. Our image of the patient changes as we collect additional cues and make adjustments in the initial picture. However, once our thoughts are anchored in dysfunction, it becomes difficult to switch our focus and too few modifications may be made in the image (16). Wright and Fletcher (14) point out that the perception of strengths and weaknesses as a unit, that is, as belonging to one person, requires the therapist to integrate two dissimilar qualities and that such synthesis is difficult. The same rationale may also be used to explain why practitioners are prone to see more pathology in their patients than the patients themselves perceive. Patients live with disability and adapt to it. Professionals regard disability as something to be eliminated. From this vantage point it is hard for professionals to see how disability can have any positive implications. Unfortunately, an emphasis on negative perceptions results in a skewed image of the patient. Dysfunctions are overestimated and abilities are under-estimated (14).

Research also indicates that practitioners are more likely to hypothesize that a patient's problems are caused by factors within the patient as opposed to factors in the patient's physical and social milieu (14, 15). For instance, we are more apt to attribute a patient's distress to an inability to deal with authority figures than to an unreasonable supervisor. One reason for this tendency is that we generally have a clearer picture of patients than we do of the situations in which they live, work, and play. We generally see patients in health care settings and rarely sample their behaviors in natural settings. Thus, the patient's environment has a quality of vagueness about it compared to the patient, who appears more real. Another explanation for our neglect of the environment is that it is often impossible or very difficult to change the environment. Even if the patient's supervisor is irrational, the patient still has to learn to manage the situation or to find another job. Nevertheless, it should be recognized that our "clinic-bound" view of the patient may lead us to ignore or underestimate impediments to occupational performance residing in the environment. Furthermore, since patients often attribute their difficulties to situations rather than to themselves, there is a potential conflict between the therapist's and patient's perceptions of causation. The validity of the patient's causal attribution should not be dismissed lightly by the therapist because patients are attuned to situational exigencies by their struggle for occupational competence.

Recognizing the distortion that may occur because of the exploration of hypotheses oriented toward dysfunction rather than function, and emphasis on the person as opposed to the environment, the therapist can take steps to countermand these biases. The data collection schedule can be arranged to include both assets and liabilities for every aspect of occupational performance evaluated. Since a patient's self-perceptions of competence are as important for participation in activity as is competence itself, the checklist should also highlight the patient's subjective impressions of occupational status. The schedule can also be extended to include the physical and social environments. These additions will serve to remind us of the significance of these variables for occupation and to foster the habit of routinely evaluating them.

Integration of Data. The challenge presented to the mind by the occupational therapy assessment is intensified by the need to integrate the wide variety of information gathered about the patient. Although we may isolate aspects of human functioning for the purposes of data management, humans function as unities or wholes. Competence requires the individual to function as an integrated organism, with the physical, mental, emotional, and social dimensions of occupational behavior interacting with the surrounding human and nonhuman environment. The selection of treatment proceeds from a holistic conception of the patient. If the therapist is to manage the array of complex clinical data required to understand occupational behavior, a simplifying strategy is needed to ward off chaos in the information processing capabilities of the human mind. Clinical judgments are not made on the basis of one or two test scores. And, although the statistical integration of clinical data may be possible in some situations, it is impractical in most. We need a labor-saving device to assist the mind in integrating data. General systems theory provides such assistance.

According to the systems metaphor, data are framed in terms of relationships between systems and systems

---

are ordered hierarchically based on increasing levels of complexity. In the assessment of a patient with a traumatic spinal cord injury, for example, we would look at the effects of disorder on other biological systems, such as the musculoskeletal and integumentary. At the same time, the rules of systems hierarchy would direct our attention to factors in the psychological system, such as competency motivation, which will strongly influence the recovery of the biological system as well as the social re-integration of the patient. Although the assessment checklist is useful for reminding us of the spectrum of occupational performance, general systems theory provides rules for organizing the list so that the assessment data can be meaningfully related and stored in memory.

Occupational Therapy Assessment. Once an occupational therapy assessment has been made, viable therapeutic approaches are selected. The selection of treatment rests on a comparison between the patient under consideration and similar patients previously treated. Thus, the effective application of treatment requires that patients be accurately identified and grouped together according to characteristics that are salient for occupation. If the results of a clinical experiment are to be replicated, we must begin with a patient who closely resembles those used in the original experiment.

At the present time, occupational therapy has no meaningful way of systematically describing occupational role performance and of differentiating homogeneous subgroups based on occupational characteristics. The medical diagnosis is inadequate for delineating the diverse levels of occupational performance that occur in patients with the same diagnosis. It also lacks utility for identifying the similar levels of occupational performance that occur in patients with different medical diagnoses. Occupational therapy lacks a standardized way of classifying the functional disabilities that result from disease and other disorders. In the absence of an agreed upon system for thinking about, remembering, and expressing our clinical observations, each therapist develops his or her own idiosyncratic system for describing occupational performance. To the extent that these informal descriptions facilitate a comparison of patients, based on salient occupational characteristics, the inferences resulting from the comparison will be valid. However, until a systematic scheme for describing and organizing clinical data is developed, we will not be able to communicate meaningfully with each other, either in informal exchanges in the clinic, or in more scientific dialogue in our journals.

Selection of Treatment. We have seen that a treatment recommendation is largely based on the therapist's recall of similar cases. Some memories are more easily recalled than others (6). We are more likely to think of patients treated recently than those treated in the past. It is easier to remember patients who are seen frequently than those

treated less often. Exceptional cases, either of success or failure, make strong impressions. Inferences gleaned from patients who happen to come to mind are likely to be less accurate than those derived from systematic analysis. Although we can all recount our brilliant successes, how many of us know what our batting average is? How good are we as judges of occupational potential? By keeping a score of the accuracy of our clinical predictions, our judgmental abilities can be improved. Checking our initial predictions against discharge data is something that can be readily incorporated into the clinic routine. Did the patient accomplish what I predicted he or she would? If not, why not? Since the ultimate test of treatment is what happens after discharge, mechanisms should also be sought for testing the accuracy of our discharge predictions with follow-up data.

A common error made by therapists in arriving at a clinical judgment is to assume that the patient is like oneself (17). This assumption enables us to know the patient through ourselves. In using the self as a referent, one rationalizes, "I will treat the patient as I would wish to be treated if I were in this situation." This kind of reasoning risks denying the validity of the patient's values. The therapist ascribes meaning to the patient's situation according to his or her own criteria. The patient is presented with a decision, rather than a list of options, and the choice of occupation is denied. Respect for the individual implies giving the patient the same opportunity to express and achieve what the patient sees as worthwhile as one would desire for oneself. We must be sensitive to the human spirit and curb the offering of pseudo choices of activity that have little meaning for the patient.

Instrumentation. The validity of clinical reasoning is grounded in the collection of good cues. This is a critical point to consider as we concentrate our energies on developing assessment instruments for practice. The nature of the phenomena we are interested in evaluating dictates the appropriate kind of instrumentation. As clinicians, our primary interest lies in evaluating performance in self-care, work, and leisure occupations. Our concern is with the ability to do and that doing is observable. You do not need to infer that I can dress from my grip strength, or mental acuity. You can observe my ability. Performance is not an abstract construct as is intelligence, anxiety, or sensory integration. We can see performance. Furthermore, we know that performance in occupation depends on the environment or situation as much as it does on the patient. Recognizing the interplay between the patient and the environment leaves us with two fundamental ways of evaluating occupational performance. First, we can go into the environments where our patients live, work, play, and observe their performance. Second, we can simulate the occupational environments of our patients by providing test stimuli, such as beds, chairs, games, arts and crafts, and work and collect a series of behavior samples in our clinics. In this case, the validity of our evaluation depends on how well we approximate the places where function is to occur.

There is inherently little uniformity in the occupational environments of our patients and, if we try to establish that uniformity, we will obscure the validity of our evaluation. The strength of occupational therapy assessment lies not in placing patients in contrived and standardized situations and recording their responses, but rather, in observing them in real life settings and evaluating their adaptive competence. Thus, development of occupational therapy instrumentation depends on a conceptualization of the task environment, since this constitutes the test stimulus that evokes behavior. Our description of occupational behavior will be incomplete until we can mesh it with a description of the task environment.

The Art

Our exploration of the intellectual technology of clinical reasoning has focused on the scientific and ethical aspects. We have not considered the art except by implication and innuendo. In the peroration, I return to the therapist who says, "I don't know how I know, I just know that I know." While the scientific dimension of clinical reasoning is directed toward specifying the correct treatment from a technical standpoint, and the ethical dimension is geared toward selecting the treatment that meets the patient's criteria of right occupational role performance, the artistic dimension pursues excellence in achieving a right action—and it does this in the face of individuality, indeterminacy, and complexity (6). Artistry involves the orchestration of broad strategies for grappling effectively with the uncertainties inherent in clinical practice.

Skill in Thinking. Artistry is knowing as it is revealed in our actions (6). It is exhibited in knowing what to do and how to do it, rather than in knowing about something. In the early stages of acquiring a skill, such as dressing or piano playing, our actions are slow and clumsy. We have to think a lot about what we are doing and we make a lot of errors. But as skill develops, our actions become smooth, flexible, and spontaneous, and our thinking becomes automatic. We get a feel for the skill and that feeling allows us to repeat our performance. You know how to touch the piano keys to play a Mozart piano concerto, and your artistry is apparent in your music. If you were to describe your "knowing how to" play the piano, you would find this difficult, if not impossible, just as someone else would find it difficult to acquire the skill of piano playing by following your instructions.

Clinical reasoning may be viewed as a skill akin to piano playing. The skill consists of reducing the ambiguities inherent in clinical practice to manageable risks, and by so doing, enabling the formulation of prudent

decisions (6). In each clinical transaction, the therapist is challenged to apply the theories and techniques of occupational therapy to a particular patient. Our textbooks inform us of the implications of blindness, hemiplegia, and age-related changes, but the hiatus between theory and practice becomes readily apparent when 90-year-old John Green, accompanied by his loving wife and devoted daughter, stands before us with hemiplegia, blindness, and the beginning signs of brain failure. Who among us has not experienced the gap between what we learned in school and what we need to know in the clinic.

Clinical problems are not neat. They are messy and complex. Everything that could be known about the patient is not known and much of the data collected are flawed and imperfect. Clinical problems deal with the uniqueness of patients rather than with their similarities. And, as Gordon Allport (18) reminds us, uniqueness is not equivalent to the sum of the ways in which a person deviates from the hypothetical average human. Unlike the simple cause and effect problems associated with basic science, clinical problems involve a complex interplay of multiple variables, the effects of which are largely unpredictable. The outcomes of occupational therapy treatment cannot be guaranteed. Clinical problems change as patient's progress and regress and as the occupational opportunities provided by the environment fluctuate.

No one can provide "cookbook" recipes for dealing with situations in which uniqueness, uncertainty, complexity, and instability are the chief characteristics. There are no formulas or algorithms that tell us how to use the interneuronal processes associated with perception, memory, reasoning, and argument. In the clinical situation, the therapist is under pressure to act and to act now. One cannot interrupt an assessment to go to the library and read up on a critical point. In handling the uncertainties contained in clinical practice, therapists rely on their accumulated experience, conceptual and judgmental heuristics, intuition, and insight to "apply their knowledge" and make clinical judgments. In spite of defective data and incomplete information, artistic inquiry enables the therapist to make prudent decisions and to know why a treatment will work for a particular patient.

The artistry of clinical reasoning is exhibited in the craftsmanship with which the therapist executes the series of steps that culminates in a clinical decision. It is expressed in the interpersonal skills through which the therapist invites involvement in decision making, builds trust, explains treatment alternatives, and offers encouragement. Artistry manifests itself in the adeptness with which the therapist gathers cues: by selecting questions, probing for information not volunteered, clarifying discrepancies, administering tests, and observing performance. The degree of perfection with which the data to be processed are obtained influences the reliability and validity of the data, and hence sets limits on the quality of the final judgment. The art extends to grouping cues effectively, recognizing patterns, and depositing in memory organized reference images. The knowing derived from perceptual acuity, such as that needed to discern spasticity and achievement motivation, is also contained in the art of clinical reasoning. Linking the model of the patient with the appropriate memory structures to build a theory of practice for the patient requires considerable acumen. Artistic insight reaches its peak in combining evidence and opinion to support arguments convincingly, thus bringing closure to the decision-making process. Although each of these processes is difficult to master in and of itself, getting them coordinated and "on line" so that one can think "on one's feet" is an even vaster task.

Experts and Novices. The automation of clinical reasoning is not merely a matter of thinking faster. Experts think differently from novices. Because of the limited capacity of short-term memory, the human mind can only consider five to nine units of information at a time (16). This is why we find it difficult to remember telephone numbers. If I asked you to remember 9 1 9 9 6 6 2 4 5 1, chances are you would have forgotten the number long before you arrived at a telephone to dial it. However, if you knew that the area code for Chapel Hill is 919, and that all university numbers begin with the prefix 966, it is likely that you would have remembered the number 919-966-2451 correctly. Memory is aided by organizing and chunking information into larger units. By chunking telephone digits into familiar patterns, the number of units to be remembered is reduced and falls within the capacity of working memory.

Evidence is accumulating that expert and novice problem solvers differ in their use of problem-solving strategies, such as chunking (19). The expert sees and stores cues in patterns and configurations, whereas the novice records individual cues. Experts chunk data into larger information units than novices do. The expert creates memory structures by classifying data according to how they are to be applied in practice. The novice's memory structures, on the other hand, arise from features more peripheral to functional usage. The novice relies on conceptual principles to get things out of memory. The expert retrieves knowledge on the basis of situational cues as well as on conceptual stimuli. As the reasoning process unfolds, experts monitor their own thinking and understanding, which enables them to curtail errors and omissions. The ability to think faster is thus a result of thinking more efficiently, more functionally, and more critically.

Simply because our knowledge is in our action does not mean that we cannot think about it. When skill breaks down, and we strike a discordant note, drop a stitch, or fall off a bicycle, we step back, slow down our pace, and reflect on our actions. In clinical reasoning, skill breakdown occurs when clinical data are incongruous with our expectations and experience. Artistic inquiry is spurred by perplexity. As long as we are assessing patients whom we perceive as highly similar to those we have treated in the past, the clinical encounter presents no challenges, our intuitive understanding of the situation remains tacit. However, when we are no longer able to see things as we previously saw them, or do things as we previously did them, our curiosity is engaged, our anxiety is aroused, and we become inquisitive practitioners.

Expert clinicians are those who are competent in action and, simultaneously, reflect on this action to learn from it (6). They create opportunities for introspection by critically examining their reasoning to disclose bias and inconsistency. Artistic inquiry is also initiated through reframing, that is, by looking at the clinical situation from a new perspective. For example, a therapist might reason, "What would happen if this patient with low back pain were treated by diverting attention from back pain to pleasurable activity, instead of with exercises to improve body mechanics."

As thinking becomes less automatic and more conscious, through self-criticism and reframing, it also becomes more accessible to explanation. Although our explanations and descriptions of clinical reasoning may never be complete, they can become progressively more adequate through reflection, and the artistic dimension can be better understood. The conversion of our practice into theory revolves around a cycle of concrete experience, reflective thinking, conceptual integration, and active experimentation.

In conclusion, the clinician functions as a scientist, ethicist and artist. The scientific, ethical, and artistic dimensions of clinical reasoning are inextricably intertwined, and each strand is needed to strengthen the line of thought leading to understanding. Without science, clinical inquiry is not systematic; without ethics, it is not responsible; without art, it is not convincing. The intentions and potentials of chronically disabled patients are difficult to discern, but a therapist of understanding will elicit them, and use them to help patients discover health within themselves.

Acknowledgments

Sincere appreciation is expressed to the following individuals for their critical review of the ideas presented in this paper: Anne Blakeney, David Hollingsworth, Teena Snow, and Joyce Sparling.

References

1. Pellegrino ED, Thomasma DC: *A Philosophical Basis of Medical Practice*, New York: Oxford University Press, 1981.

2. Scriven M: Clinical judgment. In *Clinical Judgment: A Critical Appraisal*, HT Engelhardt, SF Spicker, B Towers, Editors. Dordrecht, Holland: D. Reidel Publishing Co., 1979, pp 3–16.

3. Cutler P: *Problem Solving in Clinical Medicine: From Data to Diagnosis,* New York: Basic Books, Inc., 1979.

4. Sober E: The art of science of clinical judgment: An informational approach. In *Clinical Judgment: A Critical Appraisal,* HT Engelhardt, SF Spicker, B Towers, Editors. Dordrecht, Holland: D. Reidel Publishing Co., 1979, pp 29–44.

5. Feinstein AR: Scientific methodology in clinical medicine, III. The evaluation of therapeutic response. *Am Intern Med 61:* 944–966, 1964.

6. Schön DA: *The Reflective Practitioner: How Professionals Think in Action,* New York: Basic Books, Inc., 1983.

7. Brody H: *Ethical Decisions in Medicine,* Boston: Little, Brown, and Co., 1981.

8. McArthur C: Analyzing the clinical process. *J Counseling Psychol 1:* 203–208, 1954.

9. Koester GA: A study of diagnostic reasoning. *Educ Psychol Measurement 14:* 473–486, 1954.

10. Agnew NM, Pyke SW: *The Science Game,* Englewood Cliffs, NJ: Prentice Hall, 1969.

11. Rogers JC, Masagatani G: Clinical reasoning of occupational therapists during the initial assessment of physically disabled patients. *Occup Ther Res 2:* 195–219,1982.

12. Shriver D, Mitcham M, Schwartzberg S, Ranucci M: Uniform occupational therapy evaluation checklist. In *Reference Manual of the Official Documents of The American Occupational Therapy Association,* 1983.

13. Elstein AS, Shulman LS, Sprafka SA: *Problem Solving: An Analysis of Clinical Reasoning,* Cambridge, MA: Harvard University Press, 1978.

14. Wright BA, Fletcher BL: Uncovering hidden resources; A challenge in assessment. *Prof Psychol 13:* 229–235, 1982.

15. Bateson CD, O'Quin K, Pych V: An attribution theory analysis of trained helpers' inferences about clients' needs. In *Basic Processes in Helping Relationships,* TA Wills, Editor. New York: Academic Press, 1982, pp 59–80.

16. Matlin M: *Cognition,* New York: Holt, Rinehart and Winston, 1983.

17. Sarbin TR, Taft R, Bailey DE: *Clinical Inference and Cognitive Theory,* New York: Holt, Rinehart and Winston, 1960.

18. Allport GW: *Pattern and Growth in Personality,* New York: Holt, Rinehart, and Winston, 1961.

19. Feltovich PJ: Expertise: reorganizing and refining knowledge for use. *Professional Education Researcher Notes,* December 1982/January 1983, pp 5–9.

Chapter 35

The Therapist with the Three-Track Mind

Maureen Hayes Fleming,
EdD, OTR, FAOTA

This chapter was previously published in the *American Journal of Occupational Therapy, 45*, 1007–1014 Copyright © 1991, American Occupational Therapy Association.

The primary purpose of the American Occupational Therapy Association/American Occupational Therapy Foundation Clinical Reasoning Study was to identify the reasoning strategy that occupational therapists used to guide their practice. The designers of this study assumed that there was one reasoning style that is typical of clinical reasoning in occupational therapy. They decided that ethnography was the research method (Gillette & Mattingly, 1987) most likely to enable them to identify this typical or best reasoning style. However, as investigators, Mattingly and I soon realized that the occupational therapists in the study employed a variety of reasoning strategies.

During the early stages of the research project, when we were still searching for a single reasoning style, the apparent use of several forms of reasoning led us to believe that the therapists' thinking was inconsistent or scattered. Further analysis of the videotapes of treatment sessions, interviews, and group discussions with the therapist-subjects gave us deeper insight into their reasoning processes. They employed different modes of thinking for different purposes or in response to particular features of the clinical problem. The occupational therapists in the study seemed to use at least four different types of reasoning: narrative reasoning (Mattingly, 1989, 1991), procedural reasoning, interactive reasoning, and conditional reasoning (Fleming, 1989). These last three types of reasoning are discussed in the present chapter.

Another insight was that each type of reasoning seemed to be employed to address different aspects of the whole problem. Eventually, we realized that the therapist–subjects attended to the patient at three levels: (a) the physical ailment, (b) the patient as a person, and (c) the person as a social being in the context of family, environment, and culture. We then saw that each type of reasoning was employed to address a particular level of concern. The procedural reasoning strategy was used when the therapist thought about the person's physical ailments and what procedures were appropriate to alleviate them. Interactive reasoning was used to help the therapist interact with and understand the person better. Conditional reasoning, a complex form of social reasoning, was used to help the patient in the difficult process of reconstructing a life now permanently changed by injury or disease.

These three reasoning strategies appeared to be distinctly different, yet the therapist–subjects seemed to shift rapidly from one form of reasoning to another. They changed reasoning styles as their attention was drawn from the original concern to treat the physical ailment to other features of the problem, such as the particular person's response to the present activity. Using procedural reasoning, the therapist–subjects readily moved back to the physical problem that they had been pursuing earlier. They analyzed different aspects of the problem simultaneously. They used different thinking styles without losing track of some aspects of the problem while they temporarily shifted attention to another feature of the problem. We began to think about these styles of reasoning as different operations that interacted with each other in the therapist's mind. We referred to these operations as different *tracks* for guiding thinking. Thus, we developed the notion of the occupational therapist as a therapist with a three-track mind. The track analogy helped us envision how a therapist thought about the multiple and diverse issues that pertained to the patient's problems and the therapist's ability to influence them.

Procedural Reasoning

The therapist–subjects used what we called *procedural reasoning* when they were thinking about the disease or disability and deciding on which treatment activities (procedures) they might employ to remediate the person's functional performance problems. In this mode, the therapists' dual search was for problem definition and treatment selection. In situations where problem identification and treatment selection were seen as the central task, the therapists' thinking strategies demonstrated many parallels to the patterns identified by other researchers interested in problem solving in general and clinical problem solving in particular (Coughlin & Patel, 1987; Elstein, Shulman, & Sprafka, 1978; Newell & Simon, 1972; Rogers & Masagatani, 1982). The problem-solving sequence of diagnosis, prognosis, and prescription, which is typical of physicians' reasoning, was commonly used. However, the words the therapists used to describe this sequence were *problem identification, goal setting*, and *treatment planning*.

Experienced therapists in the study used forms of reasoning similar to the problem-solving strategies identified by many investigators who study physicians. For example, therapists used all three problem-solving methods described by Newell and Simon (1972)—recognition, generation and testing, and heuristic search. They also displayed characteristics identified by Elstein et al.

(1978), such as cue identification, hypothesis generation, cue interpretation, and hypothesis evaluation. They interpreted patterns of cues, much like the ones that Coughlin and Patel (1987) identified among physicians and medical students. The structural features of the hypotheses generated by the therapists were similar to those of medical students in a study by Allal (as cited by Elstein et al., 1978), that is, hierarchical organization, competing formulations, multiple subspaces, and functional relationships.

One characteristic of reasoning common to all of the physicians and medical students in the studies by Elstein et al. (1978) was generation and evaluation of competing hypotheses. Physicians always looked for more than one potential cause of the problem presented. They devoted a considerable portion of their reasoning efforts to seeking additional cues and rearranging hypotheses in their minds in order to either support or negate more than one possible cause of the presenting ailment. Competing hypothesis generation was also a strategy commonly used by the occupational therapists. The experienced therapists in this study typically generated two to four possible hypotheses regarding the cause and nature of aspects of the person's problem. They generated several hypotheses about potential treatment activities as well. However, there was a tendency among the newer therapists to seek the right answer rather than to generate hypotheses about possibilities. When they generated hypotheses, they tended to consider only one or two of them.

Elstein et al. (1978) noticed a phenomenon that they referred to as *early hypothesis generation*, which they interpreted as being an attempt on the part of the physician to define, or mentally enter, the appropriate problem space, as theorized by Newell and Simon (1972). Newell and Simon hypothesized that abstract thinkers categorized problems or phenomena in different spaces or areas of the possible source of the problem or avenue of inquiry. A similar notion was advanced by Feinstein (1973), who suggested that physicians' thinking would be improved if they systematically searched for sources of the problem using a reverse hierarchical method. Using this method, physicians would think of what area of the body was involved, then what system, then what organ, then what process, until the problem space was sufficiently defined and specific problems could be identified. Experienced therapists seemed to quickly identify and search within the appropriate problem spaces. Novice therapists had more difficulty with this task.

It makes sense that occupational therapists who work in a medical center, as did the subjects in the Clinical Reasoning Study, and for whom part of their education contained long hours of medical lectures, would use a thinking style similar to that used in medical decision making. That therapists frequently used these logical reasoning styles was expected. However, it was surprising that therapists often did not use these styles. This phenomenon led us to search for other modes of thought that the therapist–subjects might be using.

In discussions with the therapists, a few persistent themes emerged. At first, these themes did not seem to be explicitly linked to clinical reasoning. Some seemed to be distractions from discussing reasoning. Later, we found that these seeming distractions were important to the therapists' thinking about clinical problems. Our misunderstanding of these possible distractions was a result of our initial failure to recognize that therapists viewed clinical problems from more than one perspective. After examining these perspectives, we achieved a greater understanding of how therapists think in general and how they think differently about different aspects of the patient's situation.

We were able to identify these perspectives by analyzing several of the persistent themes that flowed through the therapists' conversations. One such theme was that the therapist–subjects often questioned what aspects of the person and the disability were appropriate for them to treat. In one group discussion, we were analyzing a videotape in which a therapist was attempting to encourage an outpatient to solve a problem. The personal care attendants he hired all quit after only a few weeks of working with him. The therapist was unable to convince the patient that this was a problem. He engaged in a wide range of what therapists referred to as avoidance tactics. Clearly the therapist and the patient had differing points of view on this issue. As the problem was discussed, many therapists in the group interpreted it as a value conflict between the patient and the therapist. There were at least two value conflicts here. One was that the therapist thought it was unsafe for the patient to live alone without someone to assist him in accessing the bed, the tub, the toilet, or his wheelchair. The patient had fallen many times while attempting these moves by himself, and his solution was to call the fire department in his small town and have someone come to his house and pick him up. The patient viewed this as a simple solution, whereas the therapist viewed it as poor judgment and irresponsibility. Another conflict was that the therapist believed that the patient should keep himself and his home cleaner. The patient did not agree with this. The group of therapists focused on whether the therapist should have pursued the discussion. The concern was whether or not the therapist, who specialized in treating physical disabilities, should have been discussing personal issues with the patient. Some group members believed that discussions of personal issues were under the aegis of psychiatric therapists only. A therapist who worked in a psychiatric setting then said that in her hospital, occupational therapists were not supposed to discuss personal issues; only psychiatrists were to discuss personal issues. In her setting, therapists could only discuss observable behaviors and relate them back to possible implications for such

concerns as how one behaves at work. The discussion became more intense regarding the role of the different types of occupational therapists and what they could and could not do or discuss with their patients. It was clear that the group members had different opinions regarding the appropriate depth and range of their interaction with patients. This difference was not divided along specialty lines. One therapist said, "Well, I work in physical disabilities and I talk about all sorts of things with my patients." Others confirmed her position. The therapists were not in agreement regarding their role in discussing the more personal issues and what they considered to be intimate or embarrassing aspects of the person's thoughts, feelings, bodily functions, or history. Some believed that therapists should treat the whole person. However, others believed that their role was to treat only the physical aspects of the person's disability or functional limitation. Still other therapists were undecided about their stance on these issues.

A related issue came up weeks later in a discussion group with experienced therapists. Their concern was to identify exactly what constitutes treatment. They wanted to define which of the therapist's actions were part of the therapeutic process and which were not. These therapists were generally comfortable with the notion of treating the whole patient, but they were not sure whether their conversations with patients were part of the treatment. Because the therapists in this particular hospital tended to see patients on a fairly long-term basis, they knew the patients as individuals quite well. There seemed to be confusion regarding whether the therapist's understanding of the individual person and his or her concerns was part of therapy or simply an artifact of the therapist's personality. Some therapists felt strongly that the relationship with the patient was an essential element of the therapy. Others saw it as an adjunct to therapy. Still others saw it as not a part of therapy. Some believed that personal discussions were inappropriate.

It seemed that these two related issues of what aspects of the person an occupational therapist treats and what actions of the occupational therapist constitute the therapeutic process were sources of conflict for the therapists. There were two types of conflict. The opinion held by some therapists that occupational therapists should treat the whole person conflicted with the opinion that therapists should treat only the physical problems. Another conflict was that some therapists were uncertain about which of these two points of view or perspectives was the right one. This conflict seemed to be created, at least in part, by a perceived conflict between the medical model perspective and the humanistic perspective.

Therapists who had strong beliefs that their relationship with patients was an effective part of therapy thought that those beliefs were in conflict with the perspective of the medical setting. Issues such as what constitutes therapy, the role of the therapist, turf boundaries, and the necessity for scientific evidence as a validation of practice all served to deny or devalue the importance of therapists' concerns for the patient as a person. This feeling was so pervasive that some therapists had difficulty appreciating the depth and complexity of their practice. They seemed confused and wondered whether they should accept their own interpretations of their practice or the interpretations of individuals and groups around them. The discussions were full of comments like the following:

Well, I know I was supposed to be teaching the lady bathing techniques. After all, that's my job—that's what I get paid for. But she really wanted to talk to me about her grandchild. So I did and she felt better and we understood each other better. Besides, what was I going to say? "Don't talk to me while you take a bath"? She has been much better at learning the bathing since that session, by the way. Of course, I put on the chart, "bathing training," but I sort of felt guilty even though I know I did the right thing. I know I wasn't wasting time chatting, but it could have looked that way.

The therapists believed that the physicians, administrators, and especially the insurance companies did not value their interactions with patients. They further believed that these various authorities would criticize them for interacting with patients and taking time away from what the authorities considered the real treatment. It soon became clear that those therapists who valued their relationship with the patient persisted in interacting with them as people regardless of the requirements of the hospital and reimbursement agencies. Therapists talked to, listened to, understood, and were respected by their patients. Therapists and patients valued these interactions. Most therapists valued interacting with patients but did not report talking with patients.

This process of conducting essentially two types of practice, one focused on the procedural treatment of the person's physical body and the other focused on the phenomenological person as an individual, is discussed by Mattingly (1991). The point here is that while two practices were conducted, only one was reported—the procedural practice. The interactive practice, which was the unreported practice, we called the underground practice. Later, we saw that although often underground, this sort of practice was important both to patients and therapists. It also had a logic or reasoning strategy of its own and a particular ways of guiding therapists' thoughts and actions. We called this *interactive reasoning*.

Interactive Reasoning

Interactive reasoning took place during face-to-face encounters between the therapist and the patient. It was the form of reasoning that therapists employed when they wanted to understand the patient as an individual. There were many reasons why a therapist might want to

know the person better. The therapist might want to know how the person felt about the treatment at the moment or what the patient was like as a person, either out of sheer interest or in order to more finely tailor the treatment to his or her specific needs or preferences. Further, the therapist might be interested in this patient in order to better understand the experience of the disability from the person's own point of view. This is what Kleinman (1980) called the *illness perspective*, as contrasted with *the disease perspective*. The therapists wanted to know what the illness experience was like for a person. They wanted to understand the patients from their own point of view. Interactive reasoning occurred when therapists took the phenomenological perspective (Kestenbaum, 1982), although the therapists did not typically use that term to explain a shift to the humanistic point of view.

Several people have been interested in the clinical reasoning study and have analyzed various videotapes made during the data-gathering stage. Some have examined different aspects of interactive reasoning. The depth of these analyses is impressive, as is the complexity of the interactive reasoning strategies discovered. A compilation of those analyses shows us that therapists appeared to employ interactive reasoning for at least eight reasons or purposes, as follows:

1. To engage the person in the treatment session (Mattingly, 1989, identified six such strategies).
2. To know the person as a person (Cohn, 1989).
3. To understand a disability from the patient's point of view (Mattingly, 1989).
4. To finely match the treatment goals and strategies to this patient with this disability and this experience. Therapists call this process *individualizing treatment* (Fleming, 1989).
5. To communicate a sense of acceptance, trust, or hope to the patient (Langthaler, 1990).
6. To use humor to relieve tension (Siegler, 1087).
7. To construct a shared language of actions and meanings (Crepeau, 1991).
8. To determine if the treatment session is going well (Fleming, 1990).

It seems that although the therapists did not initially recognize interaction and interactive reasoning as central to their practice, they used it at least as an adjunct to practice on many occasions for various reasons. Perhaps particular interactive strategies were used for particular therapeutic reasons. Some of the reasoning styles or strategies identified and the hypothesized reasons for their use are similar to new concepts about reasoning that have been proposed by various psychologists and philosophers. Gardner (1985), for example, proposed that there are many useful ways to think and that hypothetical deductive reasoning is not necessarily the only, or even the best, way to think. Many forms of reasoning have been suggested by investigators who study how persons think about themselves and their experience within the cultural context (Berger & Luckman, 1967; Bruner, 1986, 1990). Many are concerned with how such elusive processes as values, norms (Perry, 1979), and symbolic meanings (Koestler, 1948) are used to guide, gauge, frame, and formulate thought and action (Bernstein, 1971; Dreyfus & Dreyfus, 1986; Geertz, 1983; Schön, 1983). Others examine properties of problems and relate them to particular problem-solving strategies. Some propose that features of the problem will influence individuals and, in effect, direct them to select a particular problem-solving method. Such features may include salient characteristics of a task or problem (Hammond, 1988), the context (Greeno, 1989), individual interests and talents (Gardner, 1985), or experience (Dewey, 1915).

The notion that characteristics of the presumed problem will prompt a particular thinking process seemed to be borne out in our observations of the therapists in the clinical reasoning study. The therapists shifted from one form of thinking to another. They often noted subtle cues and responded to them rapidly, then returned to another task and thinking mode without "skipping a beat," as one observer commented.

If such numerous reasoning strategies exist, and if the therapists had different purposes in mind for using interaction as a therapeutic medium, then it also seems likely that the purpose of the interaction would prompt the use of a particular reasoning strategy. For example, in trying to understand the person as a person, therapists' reasoning resembled what Belenky, Clinchy, Goldberger, and Tarule (1986) described as connected knowing, which they linked to empathy. In trying to understand the disability from the patient's point of view, therapists used a phenomenological approach similar to that advocated by Paget (1988). Therapists' interactions with patients created an understanding of the person as an individual within a culturally constructed point of view, or what Schutz (1975) called a reciprocity of motives.

When individualizing treatment, therapists appeared to be functioning intuitively rather than analytically. Hammond (1988) proposed, however, that intuitive reasoning is as effective and complex as analytical reasoning. Intuitive reasoning is employed in response to problems that are not well defined. Tasks in which there are many cues from several sources and that require perceptual rather than instrumental measurement, Hammond argued, induce the person to use intuitive methods of problem solving. He further asserted that in these situations, analytical reasoning would be less effective than intuitive reasoning.

The interactive reasoning strategies that Mattingly (1989) identified indicate that therapists use several ways to engage the patient in treatment. To be effective, some of these strategies require complex interpretations of subtle interactive cues. The 23 interactive strategies that one therapist used in treatment, which were identified by Langthaler (1990), seem to suggest that the therapist was partially influenced by psychoanalytic theorists such as Rogers (1961) and occupational therapy theorists such as Fidler and Fidler (1963) and Mosey (1970). This finding is not surprising, because occupational therapy students are required to read the works of these theorists. The complexity, subtlety, and facility with which some therapists used numerous interaction forms, however, suggest processes far more complex than could be accounted for by professional education alone.

We also had a strong sense that the therapists' reasoning about and interaction with patients was directly related to their values. Their sense of the importance of patients as individuals leads one to draw parallels to beliefs about ethical and moral decision making, such as those expressed by Gilligan (1982), Kegan (1982), and Perry (1979). The task of monitoring the patient's feelings about the treatment and yet managing that treatment, which is often difficult and sometimes painful or distasteful, seems to require a considerable amount of what Gardner (1985) referred to as *interpersonal intelligence*. Gardner postulated two kinds of interpersonal intelligence: "The capacity to access one's own feeling life" and the "ability to notice and make distinctions among other individuals in particular among their moods, temperaments, motivations and intentions" (p. 239). Interactive reasoning requires active judgment (Buchler, 1955) on several levels simultaneously. This requires that the therapist analyze cues from the patient, transmit his or her interpretation of the patient, and interpret the patient's interpretations of the therapist's interpretations quickly and accurately. This reciprocal process is one that Erikson (1968) considered essential to identity formation and future social interaction capabilities. Possibly, the therapist's ability to interact successfully and therapeutically is strongly linked to his or her personal and professional identify. Gardner hypothesized that interpersonal intelligence is based on a well-developed sense of self. Certainly it is linked to professional self-confidence. Novice therapists reported that in their first year of practice they did not have the confidence, nor did they believe they had the right, to interact with patients as individuals. They reported that they "stuck to the procedural" until they were confident in their use of those skills. We observed therapists even in the second year of practice going back and forth between the procedural and interactive modes of treating their patients. In the experienced senior therapists, procedural and interactive forms seemed to flow together, each enhancing the other.

We therefore found that interaction, which at first seemed like a distraction from treatment or, at best, an adjunct to it, was a necessary and legitimate form of therapy. Interactive reasoning was used effectively by most therapists to guide this aspect of their treatment. It appears that procedural reasoning guides treatment and interactive reasoning guides therapy. Although interactive reasoning is far less easy to map than procedural reasoning, we will continue to make observations and develop theory in this area.

Conditional Reasoning

The concept of conditional reasoning is perhaps the most elusive notion in our proposed theory of a three-track mind. Yet we are firmly, if intuitively, convinced that there is a third form of reasoning that many therapists used. This reasoning style moves beyond specific concerns about the person and the physical problems placed on them to broader social and temporal contexts. The term *conditional* was used in three different ways. First, the therapist thought about the whole condition, which involved the person, the illness, the meanings the illness had for the person, the family, and the social and physical contexts in which the person lived. Second, the therapist needed to imagine how the condition could change. The imagined new state was a conditional (i.e., temporary) state that might or might not be achieved. Third, the success or failure of treatment was contingent on the patient's participation. The patient must participate not only in the therapeutic activities themselves, but also in the construction of the image of the possible outcome, that is, the revised condition.

Conditional reasoning seems to be a multidimensional process involving complicated, but not strictly logical, forms of thinking. In using conditional reasoning, the therapist appears to reflect on the success or failure of the clinical encounter from both the procedural and interactive standpoints and attempts to integrate the two. Thinking then moves beyond those immediate concerns to a deeper level of interpretation of the whole problem. The therapist interprets the meaning of therapy in the context of a possible future for the person. The therapist imagines what that future would be like. This imagined future is a guide to bringing about a revised condition through therapy. This thinking process is essentially imagination tempered by clinical experience and expertise.

The therapists tried to imagine what the person was like before the injury. Similarly, they tried to estimate or imagine what the possibilities were for the person's future life. By imagining, therapists mentally placed the person in contexts of current, past, and future social worlds. The therapists used imagination in order to best match the treatment selections to the specific interests, capacities, and goals of the person. Thus, the therapists were able to make their current treatment relevant to the individual patient. The present treatment, therefore, was not simply a link to future performance, but also, was imagined within the context of a life in process.

Perhaps this form of reasoning is best described by example. Cathy, a pediatric therapist, was the most articulate about using this form of reasoning. Cathy usually treated very young children who lived in the community and had come to an outpatient early intervention program. The child's mother or guardian was usually present, and Cathy invariably included the mother in the session. The mother might be enlisted to hold the baby in an advantageous position or to help sustain the child's interest. Cathy would often talk to the mother while simultaneously working with the child. She often asked questions like, "Does he do this at home?" "Does he usually cry in this sort of situation?" "What does he like to do?" "Does he usually have difficulty calming himself down?" These were not diagnostic history-taking questions in the medical procedural sense. Cathy said she asked these questions to construct an image of what the child was really like on a day-to-day basis. She told us that she used this image to structure her treatment and imagine possible goals for the child. As she said,

> I see this little child and his movement patterns and his difficulties, and then I imagine what he will be like in 2 years and then when he is 5 (years old) and maybe going to school. I think of what I can do to help him develop the skills that he will need to function in school and in the community and what he will be like and how his family will be with him.

Here Cathy describes a process of imagining and integrating images of the past, present, and future for this child given the variables of the child himself, his developmental delays and disabilities, his family situation, the social and educational opportunities available to him, what he might be able to do in the future, and how she might enable that future condition to come about.

Clearly, it takes professional experience to be able to project the possible developmental pattern and potential rate of success in attaining a future developmental level. It also requires a mind that is imaginative, curious, and interested in future possibilities. Conditional reasoning involves a way of thinking that may include a systems perspective and that extends to the future (Mattingly, 1989), yet it moves beyond this perspective to an analysis of present interactions (Kielhofner, 1978; Mattingly, 1989), so that one can envision how these interactions might help create a better life for the child.

Having constructed these images, which changed slightly over time and throughout the course of treatment, the therapists used images as a way of interpreting the importance of the patient's treatment. Therapists would mentally compare the patient's abilities today and the relative success of today's treatment session against images of what the person was like before. They also compared where the patient was today to where they wanted the patient to be in the future. Each therapist would envision the patient today and estimate how close that was to where he or she thought the patient should be at this point in the course of treatment. They would mentally check to see how far the patient had come toward attaining the future the therapist had in mind. The evaluation of today's treatment was made in the context of past and future possibilities. Therefore, the particular state of things today would serve as a mental mile marker for indicating progress toward a distant, and perhaps only dimly perceived, future.

One reason that we called this conditional reasoning was because a change in the present condition was conditional on the therapist's and the patient's participation in effective therapy. This condition was dependent not only on the therapist's ability to engage the patient in treatment in the sense discussed in the interactive section, but also on building a shared image of the person's future self. This image building was often accomplished through stories or narrative, as described by Mattingly (1991). However, in many aspects of therapeutic interaction, the images that the therapists helped to build were often based in action. Pediatric therapists often included the mother in creating a mental image of the child in the future. This image was projected into the distant future, such as when a therapist wondered what an infant she was treating would be like in school several years later. Therapists projected images into the near future as well. They also used images as a way of extending therapy into the home setting. Cathy said to the child's mother, "Would he do this at home? Could he just sit quietly and look at something and have this nice position? Could the kids maybe hold him like I am doing while they watch TV?" Here she created a visual image, based on action in the present, of the child in a near-future situation. This was done not only to enhance the therapy, but also to build an image of the child as a participant in the family, rather than just as a disabled baby.

One technique for conveying these images that therapists often used was to tell patients that they were getting better and to produce evidence of this by saying such things as, "Remember when you could not do this? Now you can." Sometimes the therapists would also use this technique for themselves. Therapists commented that when they were discouraged with a patient's progress, they found it helpful to remind themselves of how far the patient had come. This technique helped both the patient and the therapist focus on the importance of their joint participation in this enterprise of treatment. It helped them through difficult, frustrating, and boring times and allowed them to place the moment in a more positive, though abstract and distant, context. Most importantly, it seemed to remind them that the condition was changing. Such changes were often quantitative, such as increased range of motion, and would be noted in the person's chart. But qualitative changes and their meanings were equally important to therapists and

patients. Although these changes were not reported in the patient's chart, they did indicate progress toward that shared future image that the therapist and patient jointly constructed and worked toward. Meaningful progress was best measured through the therapist's and patient's collective memory. Therapists were not simply saying, "This is progress. Remember how bad things were before?" Instead, they were saying, "If you have come this far, maybe we will get to where you imagined you would be, even though you are discouraged today."

Putting It All Together: Treating the Whole Person

The therapists in the Clinical Reasoning Study often used two phrases to describe their treatment—*putting it all together* and *treating the whole person*. Treating the whole person did not mean that the therapists were in charge of the patient's whole medical and psychological treatment. In fact, in the traditional medical sense of the word *treatment*, occupational therapists are peripheral to the patient's treatment. The phrase was intended to convey the belief that therapists concern themselves with the patient as a person, that is, as an individual with many facets, interests, and concerns. By saying that they treat the whole person, therapists mean that they treat the person as a whole, not as the sum of ill and healthy parts.

The phrase *putting it all together* seemed to mean that although the therapists often had to think only about the disability or only of the individual patient at a given moment, they were concerned that they eventually thought and did something about the patient as a whole person, that is, person, illness, and condition. Although they used several types of reasoning and addressed several different types of concerns, therapists always wanted their reasoning to track back to making a better life for the patient as a person. Their ultimate goal was to use as many strategies as necessary to improve the individual functional performance of the person. Because functional performance requires intentionality, physical action, and social meaning, it is not surprising that persons who concern themselves with enabling function would have to address problems of the person's sense of self and future, the physical body, and meanings and social and cultural contexts—contexts in which actions are taken and meanings are made. Because these areas of inquiry are typically guided by different types of thinking, it seems necessary that therapists become facile in thinking about different aspects of human beings using various styles of reasoning. Perhaps these multiple ways of thinking guide the therapists in accomplishing and evaluating the mysterious process of "putting it all together" for the person. This process, which enables the whole person to function as a new self in the future, seemed to be guided by a complex yet unidentified form of reasoning that was both directed and conditional.

Conclusion

The Clinical Reasoning Study showed that therapists use several different types of reasoning to solve problems and to design and conduct therapeutic processes. Further, the particular reasoning processes are selected to guide inquiry into different aspects of the person's problem or of the therapist's intervention. As part of this research process, we developed a theory about these reasoning processes and constructed concepts to which we added terminology in order to discuss these concepts among ourselves and with the therapists. Thus, we referred to the type of reasoning that was used to guide those aspects of practice that are concerned with the treatment of the patient's physical ailment as *procedural reasoning*. *Interactive reasoning*, we propose, is a type of reasoning that therapists used to guide their interactions with the person. *Conditional reasoning* is both an imaginative and an integrative form of reasoning that the more proficient therapists used to think about the patient and his or her future, given the constraints of the physical condition within the patient's personal and social context. The therapists who were part of this study confirmed our assumptions that they use different forms of reasoning for different parts of the problem and found these concepts and terms useful in understanding and explaining their reasoning and practice.

References

Belenky, M. F., Clinchy, B. M., Goldberger, N. R., & Tarule, J.M. (1986). *Women's ways of knowing.* New York: Basic.

Berger, P., & Luckman, T. (1967). *The social construction of reality.* Garden City, NJ: Anchor.

Bernstein, R. J. (1971). *Praxis and action.* Philadelphia: University of Pennsylvania Press.

Bruner, J. (1986). *Actual minds, possible worlds.* Cambridge, MA: Harvard University Press.

Bruner, J. (1990). *Acts of meaning.* Cambridge, MA: Harvard University Press.

Buchler, J. (1955). *Nature and judgement.* New York: Columbia University Press.

Cohn, E. S. (1989). Fieldwork education: Shaping a foundation for clinical reasoning. *American Journal of Occupational Therapy, 43,* 240–244.

Coughlin, L. D., & Patel, V. L. (1987). Processing of critical information by physicians and medical students. *Journal of Medical Education 62,* 818–828.

Creapeau, E. B. (1991). Achieving intersubjective understanding: Examples from an occupational therapy treatment session. *American Journal of Occupational Therapy, 45,* 1016–1025.

Dewey, J. (1915). The logic of judgements of practice. *Journal of Philosophy, 12,* 505.

Dreyfus, H. L., & Dreyfus, S. E. (1986). *Mind over machine.* New York: Macmillan.

Elstein, A., Shulman, L., & Sprafka, A. (1978). *Medical problem solving. An analysis of clinical reasoning.* Boston: Harvard University Press.

Erikson, E. H. (1968). *Identity, youth and crisis.* New York: Norton.

Feinstein, A. R. (1973). An analysis of diagnostic reasoning, Parts I &II. *Yale Journal of Biology and Medicine, 46,* 212–232, 264–283.

Fidler, G., & Fidler, J. (1963). *Occupational therapy: A communication process in psychiatry.* New York: Macmillan.

Fleming, M. H. (1989). The therapist with the three track mind. In *The AOTA Practice Symposium program guide* (pp. 70–75). Bethesda, MD: American Occupational Therapy Association.

Fleming, M. (Ed.). (1990). *Proceedings of the Clinical Reasoning Institute for occupational therapy educators.* Medford, MA: Tufts University.

Gardner, H. (1985). *Frames of mind: The theory of multiple intelligences.* New York: Basic.

Geertz, C. (1983). *Local knowledge: Further essays in interpretive anthropology.* New York: Basic.

Gillette, N. P., & Mattingly, C. (1987). The Foundation—Clinical reasoning in occupational therapy. *American Journal of Occupational Therapy, 41,* 399–400.

Gilligan, C. (1982). *In a different voice: Psychological theory and women's development.* Cambridge, MA: Harvard University Press.

Greeno, J. (1989). A perspective on thinking. *American Psychologist, 44,* 134–141.

Hammond, K. H. (1988). Judgment and decision making in dynamic tasks. *Information and Decision Technologies, 14,* 3–14.

Kegan, R. (1982). *The evolving self: Problems and process in human development.* Cambridge, MA: Harvard University Press.

Kestenbaum, V. (1982). *The humanity of the ill: Phenomenological perspectives.* Knoxville, TN: University of Tennessee Press.

Kielhofner, G. (1978). General systems theory: Implications for theory and action in occupational therapy. *American Journal of Occupational Therapy, 32,* 637–645.

Kleinman, A. (1980). *Patients and healers in the context of culture.* Los Angeles: University of California Press.

Koestler, A. (1948). *Insight and outlook: An inquiry into the common foundations of science, art and social ethics.* Lincoln, NE: University of Nebraska Press.

Langthaler, M. (1990). *The components of therapeutic relationship in occupational therapy.* Unpublished master's thesis. Tufts University, Medford, MA.

Mattingly, C. (1989), *Thinking with stories: Story and experience in a clinical practice.* Unpublished doctoral dissertation, Massachusetts Institute of Technology, Cambridge, MA.

Mattingly, C. (1991). What is clinical reasoning? *American Journal of Occupational Therapy 45,* 979–986.

Mosey, A. C. (1970). *Three frames of reference for mental health.* Thorofare, NJ: Slack.

Newell, A., & Simon, H. (1972). *Human problem solving.* Englewood Cliffs, NJ: Prentice Hall.

Paget, M. (1988). *The unity of mistakes.* Philadelphia: Temple University Press.

Perry, W. (1979). *Forms of intellectual and ethical development in the college years.* New York: Holt, Rinehart & Winston.

Rogers, C. (1961). *On becoming a person.* Boston: Houghton Mifflin.

Rogers, J. C., & Masagatani, G. (1982). Clinical reasoning of occupational therapists during the initial assessment of physically disabled patients. *Occupational Therapy Journal of Research, 2,* 195–219.

Schön, D. (1983). *The reflective practitioner: How professionals think in action.* New York: Basic.

Schutz, A. (1975). *On phenomenology and social relations.* Chicago: University of Chicago Press.

Siegler, C. C. (1987). *Functions of humor in occupational therapy.* Unpublished master's thesis, Tufts University, Medford, MA.

Chapter 36

The Narrative Nature of Clinical Reasoning

Cheryl Mattingly, PhD

Many professions identify good thinking with a process that resembles the scientific method—an application in practice of empirically tested abstract knowledge (theories) and generalizable factual knowledge. Here reasoning involves the recognition of particular instances of behavior in terms of general laws that regulate the relationship between the cause and a caused state of affairs (see Mattingly, 1991, for a related discussion of this point). There are many debates within the philosophy of science about whether this model of objective knowledge characterizes even the hard sciences, such as physics (Kuhn, 1962; Putnam, 1979; Rorty, 1979). Also debated is whether the scientific method provides an appropriate model with which to characterize professional reasoning (Dreyfus & Dreyfus, 1986; Schön, 1983, 1987). I enter these debates in arguing that a narrative model of reasoning, as opposed to scientific reasoning in the traditional sense, is fundamental to the thinking of occupational therapists.

Therapists think with stories in two distinct, but equally important, ways—through storytelling and story creation. *Storytelling* constitutes an extremely important and underrated mode of discourse in occupational therapy. Recently, there has been a surge of interest in the health professions in eliciting stories from patients (Coles, 1989; Kleinman, 1988). It became clear in the course of the American Occupational Therapy Association/American Occupational Therapy Foundation Clinical Reasoning Study that therapists not only listen to the stories that their patients tell them, but also tell stories about their patients. Furthermore, an important part of this storytelling involves the therapist's understanding of the patient's way of dealing with disability and with puzzling about how to approach a problematic patient. The creation of clinical stories in clinical time is the second way in which occupational therapists use narrative in their reasoning process. I call such creation *therapeutic emplotment*.

Narrative Reasoning and Storytelling: Making Sense of the Illness Experience

What does it mean to say that occupational therapists think about their patients through the telling of stories and that this constitutes a primary form of thinking in their therapeutic practice? Jerome Bruner (1986, 1990), a psychologist noted for his studies of cognitive development, argued that humans think in two fundamentally different ways. He labeled the first type of thinking *paradigmatic*, that is, thinking through propositional argument and the second, *narrative*, that is, thinking through storytelling. The difference between these two kinds of thinking involves how we make sense of and explain what we see. When we look at something and try to understand it through propositional argument, we are trying to take a particular and see it in general terms, as an instance of a general type. For example, when we see a patient with a set of symptoms, we may note that we are seeing a severe case of Parkinson disease. According to Bruner, in linking the particular symptoms to a general disease category, we are thinking propositionally.

Conversely, when we are thinking narratively, we are trying to understand the particular case. Specifically, we are trying to understand a particular person's experience. Narrative thinking is our primary way of making sense of human experience. We do this primarily through an investigation of human motives (Burke, 1945; Gardner, 1982). We think narratively when we want to explain not whether someone has Parkinson disease, but rather, why this patient's wife is so unwilling to have her husband be discharged home. The difference between these two modes of thinking in occupational therapy is illustrated by the way in which therapists use storytelling to talk about their cases over lunch or to present cases to colleagues in weekly departmental staff meetings.

At University Hospital in Boston, where the Clinical Reasoning Study took place, the therapists drew on two modes of talking to discuss patients. Case presentations consisted of two distinct parts: "chart talk" and storytelling. The first, chart talk, involved a familiar biomedical presentation. When speaking chart talk, therapists focused on the pathology in general. The items ordinarily addressed were (a) key symptoms; (b) major typical physical impairments and primary needs, especially activities of daily living needs; (c) assessment goals and other ways of rating a patient's extent of impairment; and (d) typical treatment modalities and strategies.

The second form of case presentation was through storytelling. Here the therapists shifted their focus from a discussion based on pathology to one based on the specific patients they had worked with and their experiences of disability. One example of such storytelling comes from a staff meeting in which an affiliating student was doing a presentation of a patient with Parkinson disease. After discussing Parkinson disease as a pathology, she turned to describe her problems with a specific patient with Parkinson disease whom she was treating and how his wife was responding to her husband's disability. As part of her description of treating the patient, she recounted her interchanges with his wife. Here is part of the student's story:

> He [the patient] said that something would have to be changed because his bedroom was downstairs in the basement. His wife wanted to keep him downstairs but finally agreed that he could have a bedroom in the living room. He progressed rapidly, and after a week and a half he was smiling, becoming more social. His wife told me, "He does nothing at home." I don't know if she could hear what we were telling her. We said, "He is not just sitting around. Many times he simply can't do anything because of the disease." When the wife heard that he would be on medication and that this would improve his functioning, she said to him, "Good. There's a lot of chores around the house you can do," I don't know how much she heard of what we were telling her.

This story triggered a storytelling exchange in which others around the table offered their own experiences in treating patients with Parkinson disease, emphasizing how the disease was experienced by the patient, the family, or themselves rather than its general medical features. Nearly all of the speakers told stories that elaborated themes raised by the initial story. What does this storytelling have to do with clinical reasoning? When the student told her story about the wife of the patient with Parkinson disease, she identified a critical problem for clinical reasoning: What is she supposed to do with the patient's wife? How should she best treat this patient, given his wife's feelings? How does the wife really feel? What are this wife's denial and anger about? Or is the wife displaying something that is being mistaken for denial or anger? These are all narrative questions whose answers require a kind of clinical reasoning that is fundamentally narrative in form. To return to Bruner's (1986, 1990) distinction, when we think in propositional arguments, we try to transcend particulars and strive for abstraction (i.e., for truths that transcend any particular historical situation). But narrative is rooted in the particular. Whereas propositional arguments are concerned with understanding phenomena in terms of general causes, narratives are concerned with the likely connections among particular events.

Bruner gave a simple example to illustrate the difference. The statement "if x, then y" belongs to propositional argument. An occupational therapist is relying on propositional reasoning when she says, "If you see these symptoms, then you probably have a case of Parkinson disease." Such if–then statements are aimed at providing an abstract description of a causal relationship that holds up generally or, ideally, universally across concrete individual cases.

This genre of descriptive and explanatory statements can be contrasted with a very different mode of explanation. Bruner (1986) gave the following illustration, borrowed from E. M. Forster (1927). The statement, "The king died, and then the queen died" (pp. 11–12) is a narrative statement that not only concerns the particular, that is, some specific king and queen, but also, suggests causes that lead one to wonder about intentions. Did the queen die of grief? Was the queen murdered? We investigate the meaning of a narrative statement by trying out different motivational possibilities; we search for what guided the action that the statement reports. And human action, unlike a pathological process, is motivated. Narratives make sense of reality by linking the outward world of actions and events to the inner world of human intention and motivation. To ask in a narrative sense why something happened is to ask what motivated the actors to do what they did. In the philosophy of history, this mode of narrative explanation has been called "explanation by reason" (Dray, 1971, 1980). In a story, a person's actions are accounted for— or explained—by their placement in some specific historical context that shows how and why they were begun, what other actions unfolded as a result, and how they evolved over time. So when we hear about a particular patient with Parkinson disease whose wife complains that he does not do enough housework and we want to explain what is going on, we start asking the narrative questions enumerated earlier.

In moving between chart talk and storytelling, therapists present the clinical problem in different ways. The shift in presentation from an abstract discussion of Parkinson disease to a story of a patient with Parkinson disease who has an uncooperative wife involves much more than a move from the general to the concrete or from the objective to the subjective.

In chart talk, the focus is on a disease. The disease is the main character. But in storytelling, it is the patient's situation or experience with the disease that is the central clinical problem. The therapist might ask, What is the best way to treat the patient with Parkinson disease who is going home to this particular wife? The severity and nature of the patient's dysfunctions are still important, but they are only one part of the picture that the therapist has to put together with the unique features of one patient's situation.

Therapists often speak of expert practice as involving the ability to "put it all together" for a particular patient. I suggest that what they mean by this involves a thinking that is essentially narrative. The therapist takes what he or she knows in general of a disease process, appropriate theoretical frames of reference, and relevant experience with similar patients and applies all of this generalized and abstract knowledge to a particular case, such as that of the patient whose wife thinks he should be able to do household chores and resists having his bed moved up to the first floor where he will have access to the bathroom.

Medical anthropologists have made an extremely useful distinction in looking at health care by separating disease from illness experience (Good, 1977; Good & Delvecchio-Good, 1980, 1985; Kleinman, 1988; Kleinman, Eisenberg, & Good, 1978). Although traditionally medicine has focused on the diagnosis and treatment of disease, anthropologists argue that much more attention needs to be given to treatment of the illness experience, which involves the way in which the disease affects the person's life. Physiologically, the same disease can result in a very different illness experience, depending on the patient's particular life history and life possibilities. The patient with Parkinson disease whose wife learns all she can about the disease and welcomes her husband home is likely to have quite a different illness experience than the patient whose wife wants to relegate him to the basement.

What anthropologists have argued to the medical community during the last decade or two, occupational therapists have known for a long time: To effectively treat persons with long-term disabilities, one must treat the whole patient, which involves looking beyond the disease to how that disease is experienced by that particular patient. Treatment of a patient's illness experience is integral to good occupational therapy and it is where the heart of clinical reasoning lies; it is also where the thorniest reasoning puzzles present themselves. Reasoning about how to treat the illness experience is often the most difficult thing to teach the affiliating student or new therapist. How does a supervisor help a novice therapist to examine what is going on with this patient's wife and what therapeutic approach would best help this patient make the transition back home to this wife? Notably, when one addresses the illness experience, as opposed to the disease alone, it is often hard to establish who has the disease. Although a disease obviously belongs to one person—the patient—the illness experience, especially in the case of serious life-changing illnesses, is likely to be shared by the whole family.

Puzzling over how to treat a patient with Parkinson disease, given how his wife is responding to the illness, involves narrative reasoning, because it involves consideration of the disease from the patient's and family's points of view. The therapist must try to imagine how it feels to the patient and to various family members to have this disease, how they are experiencing it, and how it enters and changes the life story of a patient and his or her family.

Narrative Reasoning and Story Making: Creating Clinical Stories

Therapists create as well as tell stories. The narrative nature of clinical reasoning manifests itself not only in the work therapists do to understand the effect of a disability in the life story of a particular patient, but also in the therapist's need to structure therapy in a narrative way, as an unfolding story. This is perhaps the most interesting and subtle use of narrative reasoning in occupational therapy practice. Therapy can be seen as a kind of short story within the patient's longer life story. The therapist enters and exits the patient's life, playing a part for only a short time. Often, this part occurs at a critical juncture in the patient's life, a turning point triggered by the onset or downturn of an illness. Sometimes it occurs at a critical juncture in an entire family's life, as is often true in pediatric therapy when a family is learning to adjust to a newborn with a disability or when a child with a disability begins school. If disability is considered in narrative terms as something that interrupts and irreversibly changes a person's life story, then work with a patient can be seen as one chapter in that life story.

Although this narrative language is not a familiar way for therapists to describe their own practice, it serves to highlight how intensely therapists want to make therapy itself an occasion for patients to remake life stories that can no longer continue as they once did when a disability was absent or less serious. The therapist enters the life story of a patient and has the task of negotiating with the patient what role therapy is going to play within the unfolding illness and rehabilitation story that the patient is living through. To be meaningful, occupational therapy must serve as a coherent short story within a larger narrative whole.

In each new clinical situation, then, the therapist must answer the question, What story am I in? To answer this question, the therapist must make some initial sense of the situation and then act on it. The process of treatment encourages, perhaps even compels, therapists to reason in a narrative mode. They must reason about how to guide their therapy with particular patients by imagining where the patient is now and where this patient might be at some future point after discharge. It is not enough for therapists to know how to do a set of tasks that have an abstract order based on a general or typical treatment plan; therapists must be able to picture a larger temporal whole, one that captures what they can see in a particular patient in the present and what

they can imagine seeing sometime in the future. This picturing process gives them a basis for organizing tasks.

In her study of clinical reasoning among nurses, Benner (1984) noticed this narrative mode of reasoning in her subjects, although she did not focus on its narrative nature per se. The need for a narrative framework was suggested by a nurse quoted in Benner's study who worked in an intensive care nursery. She described what she considered to be the most essential kind of thinking she wanted her newly graduated students to evince at the end of their 3-month affiliation with her:

> To my mind, moving the child from Point A to Point B is what nursing is all about. You have to perform tasks along the way to make that happen, but performing the task isn't nursing.... I wanted to see a light going on—that OK, here's this baby, this is where this baby is at, and here's where I want this baby to be in six weeks. What can I do today to make this baby go along the road to end up being better? It's that kind of thing that's just happening now. They're [the student nurses] just starting to see the whole thing as a picture and not as a list of tasks to do. (p. 28)

This example emphasizes both the imagistic character of what the clinician needs to know, in contrast with the knowledge of tasks, and the context-specific nature of those images. Therapists in the Clinical Reasoning Study spoke similarly about picturing the patient and especially about having future images of who the patient could be. They believed that what they often held most vividly in mind when treating patients was not plans or objectives, but rather, pictures of the potential patient, that is, the future patient. For example, one of the pediatric therapists said, "You know, when I treat that 18-month-old child, I see the child at 3, then I see the child at 6, learning to hold a pencil. I have all these pictures in my head." The therapists described their difficulty when the patients or their families held different images of the future and their dilemma about the extent to which they should give patients or families their therapeutically based pictures, which were often more pessimistic. The therapists were frequently in the difficult position of trying to give hope to a patient while also having to let the patient know of his or her dark prognosis. The patients and their families could be extremely depressed about conditions that were even worse than they had imagined. The therapists spoke of these images as necessary but dangerous: necessary because the therapist and patient needed some guiding pictures, but dangerous because these pictures could blind the therapist or patient to what was realistically possible.

The therapists in the Clinical Reasoning Study were, like Benner's (1984) nurses, also conscious of the need to create specific images appropriate to a particular patient. General treatment goals devised from general knowledge of functional deficits and developmental possibilities were insufficient guides to practice, in the therapists' view. Instead, they worked with much more concrete guides, images, and stories, which were the "wholes" that allowed them to selectively choose what aspects of their knowledge base were appropriate to the situation. These images were organized temporally and teleologically, thus giving the therapists a sense of an ending for which they could strive.

Although these images of the future were often not formulated in words, unless there was some need to explicitly communicate them, they were part of what I call a *prospective treatment story*. In this prospective story, the therapists envisioned a possible and desirable future for the patient and imagined how they might guide treatment to bring such a future about.

The treatment approaches and treatment paths that the therapists tried to follow were often guided by such stories. These stories, derived from particular experiences and stereotypical (collectivized) scenarios, were projected onto new clinical situations in order to help therapists make sense of what story they were in and where they might go with particular patients. The therapists then attempted to enact their projected stories in the new clinical situations, working improvisationally to narratively pull in and build on whatever happened in a clinical session so as to add to the story's plot line. The therapists saw a possible story, which they recognized as clinically meaningful, and they tried to make that story come true by taking the individual episodes of their clinical encounters and treating them as parts of a larger, narratively unfolding whole. Prospective treatment stories were based on what therapists observed and inferred about the patient's larger life history, which involved both the patient's past and future. The therapeutic stories that the therapists imagined took their power and plausibility as part of a larger historical context that included a past that began before therapy started and a future that would extend after therapy had ended.

Notably, the prospective story cannot be equated with treatment goals and plans, although these will be incorporated into the story. Therapists try to create significant therapeutic experiences and not simply reach a set of objectives in the most efficient way possible. They are concerned that the whole process of therapy unfold in such a way that patients will have powerful experiences of successfully met challenges; such challenges will motivate them to believe in therapy and work hard at it. In listening to therapy success stories, I found it rare for the success of therapy to have been measured by the reaching of the final goal. Rather, most of the therapists counted success as the generation of therapeutic experiences along the way, in which patients developed increasing confidence and commitment to take on challenges. The whole treatment story mattered.

Therapists in the Clinical Reasoning Study also worked to create significant experiences for their patients, ones worth telling stories about, because if therapy was to be effective, then the therapists had to find a way to make the therapeutic process matter to the patient. Each therapist faced the problem of constructing therapeutic activities that were meaningful enough to elicit the patient's active cooperation. The patients had to see something at stake in therapy. Otherwise, why should they bother to try? If the patient did not try, therapy did not work. This was partly because the therapists required the patients to do things in therapy that the patients did not necessarily feel ready to do or believe to be worth the effort. But more important, the patients had to become committed because they had to take up the therapeutic activities. Therapists were often with patients only a short time—just a few weeks or less. They might teach a few skills or improve the patient's strength a bit, but generally their effectiveness depended on the use of therapy as a catalyst to help patients begin to see how they might do for themselves even when the therapist was no longer present.

For example, a therapist is working with a spinal cord–injured patient, teaching him to move checkers pieces with a mouth stick. It is not enough for this patient to learn to move these checkers pieces for the therapy to be successful; he must also take up a point of view that comes with being committed to the tremendous concentration needed to perform this previously trivial task. He must absorb a vision about why he should work so hard at something that was once so easy. This is just as critical as the skills he acquires. The therapeutic time together itself must provide a kind of existential picture of how he might live his life in the future with his disability. Therapy will not ultimately work, not in any catalytic way that patients will take home when they leave the hospital, if they are not strongly committed to the process. Without experiencing treatment activities from a committed stance, they will not see any future in them. They will not see the point.

If the patient is to become committed to the therapeutic process, then both the patient and the therapist must share a view about why engaging in any particular set of treatment activities makes sense. Coming to share such a view requires that both the therapist and the patient see how these treatment activities are going to move the patient toward some future that he or she can care about. Such a view is not reducible to a general prognosis or even to a shared understanding of a treatment plan. The therapist and patient must come to share a story about the therapeutic process; they must come to see themselves as in the same story. This is a kind of future story, a story of what has not yet happened, or has only partly happened—an as yet unfinished story.

How is such a story constructed? Generally it is not constructed through any explicit storytelling, but rather, through the sharing of powerful therapeutic experiences that point to a prospective story—a path that therapy will take. Clinical reasoning requires that the therapist (a) see possibilities for creating important experiences in which the patient will be staked, (b) make moves to act on those possibilities, (c) respond to the moves the patient makes in return, and (d) build on the experience by showing the patient a future in which this therapeutic experience becomes one building block. In the language of narrative, the experience becomes one episode in a much longer story. The therapist tells the story not in words but in actions that create an experience the patient can care about.

I follow the work of the philosophers Ricoeur (1984) and White (1987) in describing this therapeutic work as "emplotment." The clinician's narrative task is to take the episodes of action within the clinical encounter and structure them into a coherent plot. A plot is what gives unity to an otherwise meaningless succession of events. Quite simply, "emplotment is the operation that draws a configuration out of a simple succession" (Ricoeur, 1984, p. 65). What we call a story is precisely this rendering and ordering of a succession of events (e.g., a series of treatment activities) into parts belonging to a larger narrative whole. When a therapeutic process has been successfully emplotted, it is driven and shaped by a sense of an ending (Kermode, 1966). To have a single story is to have made a whole out of a succession of actions. These actions then take their meaning by belonging and contributing to the story as a whole. A story, Ricoeur wrote, "must be more than just an enumeration of events in serial order: it must organize them into an intelligible whole, of a sort such that we can always ask what is the 'thought' of this story" (p. 65).

Narratives give meaningful structure to life through time. The told narrative builds, to borrow from Ricoeur's (1984) argument, on action understood as an as yet untold story. Or, in Ricoeur's provocative phrase, "action is in quest of narrative" (p. 74). Therapists are in a quest to transform their actions and the actions of their patients into as yet untold stories.

This can be translated into more familiar clinical language through a narrative reading of treatment goals. When an occupational therapist makes an assessment of the patient, the outcome is a set of treatment goals. Goals, according to Ricoeur (1984), are not predictions of what will happen; rather, they express the actor's intentions and preferences. These goals express a therapeutic commitment. They capture what the therapist intends to accomplish over the course of therapy. Treatment goals are an expression of what the therapist has committed himself or herself to care about with a particular patient.

As occupational therapists have argued (Rogers, 1983 [see Chapter 34]; Rogers & Kielhofner, 1985), a primary task of clinical reasoning is the individualization of treatment goals. Narratively, individualization involves the construction of a particular story of the treatment process rather than reliance on a generic line of action that strings together standard goals and activities.

Therapeutic Emplotment: A Case Example

A wonderful illustration of this process of narratively structured treatment is given by O'Reilly (1990), who, as part of the Clinical Reasoning Study, described her work with a head injury group. O'Reilly recounted a situation in which she was asked to take over a failing head injury group that was poorly attended. The first thing that bothered her was its name—the Upper Extremity Group. She described her first visit to the group, "I enter the large OT/PT treatment area where I see several residents scattered about at tables and exercise equipment.... At one table, a resident diligently puts small pegs into a pegboard.... What is most memorable is the silence. Except for the clang of the pulley weights, a dropped peg or the therapist's quiet voice, there is not a sound in this room" (p. 2).

O'Reilly noticed that several of the group members were not present, and when she went to inquire, they told her, "That [expletive deleted] group is a waste of time." She tried several strategies to entice members back, but nothing worked. She puzzled:

> I wonder, 'What's wrong with this group?' I make mental lists:
>
> 1. The name—I'll talk to the residents about that.
> 2. The activities—no meaning, no purpose, no life-related goals, no goals that belong to the patients.
> 3. No interaction among members with the therapist.
> 4. Nobody is having fun—the residents are bored and the therapist is bored (and boring?).
> 5. Is there any progress that the residents experience?
> 6. What are the reasons for attending or not attending? and There is no direction—no theme. (O'Reilly, 1990, p. 2)

Although O'Reilly did not use the language of story to describe the problems she noticed, this list could easily be restated in narrative terms. Her statement that the group has no direction and no theme could be recast to say that there is no plot to this group; there is no story for which the group members are a part. The group is not going anywhere, narratively speaking. Any particular group activity is not an episode in an unfolding story that members share. The activities of the group are focused on broken body parts, as the group name (Upper Extremity Group) implies. Although the exercises may help improve body functioning, they carry no intrinsic meaning to the group members, because group activities are in no sense a short story in the larger life story of the patients.

The therapist pondered what to do by beginning to think about individual group members. Her mode of puzzling represents a shift from a biomechanical framing of the members' disability to seeing their disability as having personal meaning in their lives. She described her reasoning in this way: "I think about the people. What do they want? What do they need? They are all so young; so far from home. They want to get out. They want to go home. HOME! They're all from New York. That's it! NEW YORK! I have a theme with which to begin" (O'Reilly, 1990, p. 2).

O'Reilly was reasoning in narrative terms. She was not telling a story, but she was beginning to envision a prospective story that all the group members could be a part of. She wrote:

> I have a theme with which to begin, but I don't know a thing about New York. The Program Director is from New York ... I dash to her office. "New York," I blurt. "The Upper Extremity Group, they're all from N.Y. Tell me something about N.Y., anything, everything". She lists: "Empire State Building, Statue of Liberty, Long Island Ferry, the subway." Laughingly, "You could have a New York Subway Group." I reply, "We could be *on the subway*. They can take me to New York. What does it look like—is there graffiti? We can do graffiti. I need a new room, away from the big treatment room. Can we use the small meeting room?" Program Director replies "yes" and adds that she has a map of the N.Y. subway and will bring it in. "I'll be the conductor ... I have a blue blazer." She says, "I think I have a funny little hat that will pass for a conductor's hat." We laugh through all the possibilities of this activity. This is going to be FUN! (O'Reilly, 1990, p. 3)

In deciding to create a therapy group around a New York theme, O'Reilly could not only locate therapy in the relevant past of these patients, but also locate it within the future that they desire. This study dealt with young people in a chronic long-term care facility in Massachusetts, one that residents rarely ever leave. These patients wanted to go home.

O'Reilly invented the ingenious idea of turning a therapy room into a New York subway station. She also devised a way of generating some interest in the group:

> I go straight to Mike's room and ask him to make sure everyone comes to group today. "I have a different type of activity planned, and I'd really like to talk to everyone so that we can make some plans together." Mike states that he hates the |expletive deleted| group. I tell him that I understand that and that perhaps he could gather everyone for me, and come for awhile. "Then, if you are really unhappy with the activity, you can leave." He agrees. I hand him a small bag containing poker chips and ask him to give one to each group member on the attached list and have them bring the chips to group. "Okay, but what the |expletive

deleted) are these for?" "It's a surprise. See you at 1:30." (O'Reilly, 1990, p. 3)

Notably, in announcing the group, she introduced a key narrative element critical to any dramatic story—the element of suspense. In any good story, the reader will want to know what will happen next. To prepare for the meeting of the group, the therapist lined three walls of the therapy room with white paper. She labeled spots with street names and subway stops and hung a subway map on the fourth wall.

Just as the group was scheduled to begin, O'Reilly stood outside the door in a subway conductor's uniform (trying not to feel too foolish in front of other surprised hospital colleagues) and waited for group members to arrive. She, herself, also felt unsure about what would happen:

> I put out materials, don my conductor's uniform and stand outside the door, on which a sign reads: NEW YORK THIS WAY. As I await the passengers, my stomach churns with anxiety and excitement, and I wonder where this subway ride will take us. (O'Reilly, 1990, p. 3)

She described the following scene:

> As the members arrive, escorted by Mike, I take their tokens, explaining that it's commuter fare for a ride on the New York Subway. Nancy grins, Eileen looks puzzled. Bobby shrugs. Mike says, with a great laugh, "You are crazy!" As these travelers enter the room, I hear snickers and queries like, "what the |expletive deleted| is she doing?" and comments like, "It's better than the other room." Then snickers, laughter, recognition. They go from stop to stop, reading, commenting, all smiling! |As they turn to her, she explains| "You folks are all from N.Y. Right? This is a N.Y. subway station. You've all ridden on the subway, right? M. tells me that there's graffiti, words and pictures on the walls, in the subway. We're going to do graffiti. You do remember graffiti, don't you?" "Yeah," laughs Mike, "but nothing I could write HERE!" With that, I close the door, and say, "You can draw or write anything you want in this room. The only rule is that you use the tools that I give you." These tools have been chosen with particular concern for the motor deficits of individual patients: "Large colored pencils and wrist weights for Mike who has a tremor, but brush and paint for Bobby who's working on gross motor skills, crayons for Nancy who needs to strengthen wrist and fingers, markers for Eileen who can't tolerate resistance." (O'Reilly, 1990, p. 4)

O'Reilly described the reaction of her "travelers" to this new activity:

> Eileen asks, "Where are we supposed to be?" "Anywhere you'd like to be, and when you finish working at one place, you can move to another. It's up to you." Nancy starts: "This is neat ... just like when I was a kid." We're off!

From this point on, drawing, writing, conversation and laughter, are continuous. So much activity fills this room that it is difficult to remember details. Words, pictures, memories and feelings cover the walls:

"This place sucks." "My ass is stuck in Mass." "Home sweet Home." And on and on.... I go from one participant to another, asking about their work or just watching. After 35 minutes, I ask the group to finish up their artwork so that we can talk a bit and plan for our next group session. Stickball wins unanimously. Since, I admit, I know nothing about stickball, I ask the group to write out rules and equipment we'll need and get it to me on Tuesday. They agree, and, in fact, begin to work immediately. As I leave to see my next client, I tell the group,"You guys can hang out here for awhile. Just be sure to take your words and pictures with you when you leave." Thinking ... clean up can wait. (O'Reilly, 1990. p. 4)

The end result of this therapeutic intervention was the beginning of the "New York Gang," as they came to call themselves. They met not only twice a week but also informally on the weekends, at which time they planned a series of events and activities. Their ventures included "making giant pretzels and cooking hot dogs to sell from a makeshift pushcart; taking a trip to a simulated Central Park; and filling a photo album with pictures of the group, home, drawings, postcards, and New York Times clippings" (O'Reilly, 1990, p. 4). The therapist had begun a story that spawned additional episodes. She set a therapeutic story in motion. The first group session that O'Reilly described in her case not only had a coherent plot, that is, a beginning, middle, and end (making graffiti), but also, because of her success, that session became just one episode in an unfolding therapeutic story in which patients became a cast of characters in the New York Gang. Even the name of the group came from the group members themselves. Specific biomechanical interventions were integrated in a meaningful way as activities that allowed group members to act their part in this drama, and the task of writing things on the wall allowed each person to express an individual voice as well.

When O'Reilly initially devised the idea of doing something with a New York theme, the prospective story that she had begun to envision (and that she had concretely begun when she fixed up a room and donned a conductor's uniform) was much more than a set of treatment goals. Specific goals were incorporated in the narrative plot that she started. The success of this therapeutic intervention was ensured when the patients themselves took the story up and began to create new episodes that the therapist could not have imagined.

Narratively speaking, the shift of names from the Upper Extremity Group to the New York Gang represents a shift from a series of interactions in which therapeutic time is treated as a mere succession of activities, that is, as a procedural movement not grounded in context or in a picture of the patient, to narrative shaping of the therapeutic interaction in which therapeutic time has been emplotted by the clinician's picture of how to create an important therapeutic experience for the patients. The therapeutic efficacy of this intervention is about much more than meeting specific treatment goals. It is about creating an experience that gives the participants a vision of themselves as actors in the world, that is, as more than just patients.

Conclusion

Narrative thinking is central in providing therapists with a way to consider disability in the phenomenological terms of injured lives. Narrative thinking especially guides therapists when they treat the phenomenological body; that is, when they are concerned with their patients' illness experience and how the disability is affecting their lives.

In this article, I examined two kinds of narrative thinking. One is narrative as a mode of talk that therapists rely on to consider certain kinds of clinical puzzles. Because narratives are predominantly about human actions, they provide a particular vantage point from which one can view the nature of clinical practice and pose clinical problems. The stories that the therapists told portrayed disability from an actor-centered point of view. They were personal, even individualistic, built on the structure of actors acting. Disability itself shifted from a physiological event to a personally meaningful one, that is, to an illness experience. General physiological conditions were shadowed as background context. What was brought to center stage were the ways that particular actors, with their own motivations and commitments, had done things for which they could be praised or blamed.

The second form of narrative thinking, which occurs in occupational therapy in a more subtle way, is story making, which involves the creation rather than the telling of stories. The telling of stories is always retrospective—a way of considering past events—whereas story making is largely prospective, playing out images that therapists have of what they would like to happen in therapy. Story making as therapeutic emplotment concerns the way in which therapists work to structure therapy narratively, thus creating dramatic therapeutic events that connect therapy to a patient's life. Often, the search for a meaningful therapeutic story appears to be triggered by resistance or alienation of the patient to the initial therapeutic activities offered, as in the case of the members of the Upper Extremity Group. Whatever the impetus, therapists try to create clinical experiences in which there is a significant occurrence or event for the patient in therapy, one in which the therapy itself is a meaningful short story in the larger life story of the patient.

References

Benner, P. (1984). *From novice to expert. Excellence and power in clinical nursing practice.* Reading, MA: Addison-Wesley.

Bruner, J. (1986). *Actual minds, possible worlds.* Cambridge, MA: Harvard University Press.

Bruner, J. (1990). *Acts of meaning.* Cambridge, MA: Harvard University Press.

Burke, K. (1945). *A grammar of motives.* Berkeley, CA: University of California.

Coles, R. (1989). *The call of stories.* Cambridge, MA: Harvard University Press.

Dray, H. (1971). On the nature and role of narrative in historiography. *History and Theory, 10,* 153–171.

Dray, W. (1980). *Perspectives on history.* London: Routledge & Keegan Paul.

Dreyfus, H., & Dreyfus, S. (1986). *Mind over machine: The power of human intuition and expertise in the era of the computer.* New York: Free Press.

Forster, E. M. (1927). *Aspects of the novel.* Harcourt Brace Jovanovich.

Gardner, H. (1982, March). The making of a storyteller. *Psychology Today,* pp. 49–63.

Good, B. (1977). The heart of what's the matter: The semantics of illness in Iran. *Culture, Medicine and Psychiatry, 1,* 25–28.

Good, B., & Delvecchio-Good, M.J. (1980). The meaning of symptoms: A cultural hermeneutic model for clinical practice. In I. Eisenberg and A. Kleinman (Eds.), *The relevance of social science for medicine* (pp. 165–196). Norwell, MA: D. Reidel.

Good, B., & Delvecchio-Good, M. J. (1985). *The cultural context of diagnosis and therapy.* Unpublished manuscript.

Kermode, F. (1966). *The sense of an ending: Studies in the theory of fiction.* London: Oxford University Press.

Kleinman, A. (1988). *The illness narratives. Suffering, healing and the human condition.* New York: Basic.

Kleinman, A., Eisenberg, L., & Good, B. (1978). Culture, illness and care: Clinical lessons from anthropologic and cross-cultural research. *Annals of Internal Medicine, 88,* 251–258.

Kuhn, T. (1962). *The structures of scientific revolutions.* Chicago: University of Chicago Press.

Mattingly, C. (1991). What is clinical reasoning? *American Journal of Occupational Therapy, 45,* 979–986.

O'Reilly, M. (1990). *The New York subway.* Unpublished data, Tufts University Clinical Reasoning Institute, Boston.

Putnam, H. (1979). *The meaning and the moral sciences.* Boston: Routledge & Keegan Paul.

Ricoeur, P. (1984). *Time and narrative* (Vol. 1). Chicago: University of Chicago Press.

Rogers, J. (1983). Clinical reasoning: The ethics, science and art. *American Journal of Occupational Therapy, 37,* 601–616. (Reprinted as Chapter 34).

Rogers J. C., & Kielhofner, G. (1985). Treatment planning. In G. Kielhofner (Ed.), *A model of human occupation* (pp. 136–155). Baltimore: Williams & Wilkins.

Rorty, R. (1979). *Philosophy and the mirror of nature.* Princeton, NJ: Princeton University Press.

Schön, D. (1983). *The reflective practitioner. How professionals think in action.* New York: Basic.

Schön, D. (1987). *Educating the reflective practitioner.* San Francisco: Jossey-Bass.

White, H. (1987). *The content of the form: Narrative discourse and historical representation.* Baltimore: Johns Hopkins University Press.

Chapter 37

Enhancing Occupational Performance through an Understanding of Perceived Self-Efficacy

Marie Gage
Helene Polatajko, PhD, OT(C)

Occupational therapists enable clients to develop occupational performance skills with the expectation that these skills will be used outside the treatment setting and that the use of these skills will enhance their clients' occupational competence and their ability to cope with the life stresses associated with their deficits. Therefore, it is important for occupational therapists to understand the role of any factor that influences their clients' occupational performance, or their resultant ability to cope with their deficit in the community. Perceived self-efficacy is one such factor.

It is postulated that perceived self-efficacy explains part of the variance between a person's skill and the quality of that person's actual performance outside the protected clinical environment (Bandura, 1977, 1986; Shaffer, 1978). Furthermore, according to the Appraisal Model of Coping, the concept of perceived self-efficacy is one of 12 factors that influence a person's manner of coping with stressful person–environment interactions, such as those encountered by people with occupational performance deficits (Gage, 1992). Perceived self-efficacy has been found to be a significant behavioral determinant of actual performance and to influence psychological well-being (Allen, Becker, & Swank, 1990; Bandura, 1977, 1986; Bandura & Adams, 1977; Bandura & Wood, 1989; Ewart et al., 1986; Seydel, Taal, & Wiegman, 1990; Shunk, 1982; Toshima, Kaplan, & Ries, 1990; Wang & Richarde, 1987; Wassem, 1992). The most effective means of enhancing perceived self-efficacy is deemed to be through performance-based procedures (Bandura, 1977): the procedures upon which occupational therapy practice is traditionally based.

This article explores the construct of perceived self-efficacy, including origin, definition, relationship to self-esteem, parameters, history, relationship to behavior, outcome expectancy, psychological well-being, and the means of enhancing a client's perceived self-efficacy. The purpose of our review is to help occupational therapists recognize the goodness of fit between perceived self-efficacy and occupational therapy practice and thereby to identify the potential benefits of incorporating the attributes of perceived self-efficacy into day-to-day clinical practice.

Perceived Self-Efficacy

Origins of Perceived Self-Efficacy

Perceived self-efficacy is a concept originally developed as part of Social Cognitive Theory. Social cognitive theorists view human functioning as the result of triadic reciprocality: "behavior, cognitive and other personal factors, and environmental events all act as interacting determinants of each other" (Bandura, 1986, p. 18). The relative influence of each of these three factors varies from situation to situation, from person to person, and from environment to environment. Within the framework of Social Cognitive Theory, people are attributed with six basic capacities.

1. Symbolizing capacity—the ability to use symbols to transform experiences into models that guide future actions, which in turn are guided by thoughts; thoughts are sometimes inaccurate due to misinterpretation of the incoming information.
2. Forethought capacity—the ability to anticipate the potential outcome of future actions, set goals, and develop action plans.
3. Vicarious capacity—the ability to learn through observation of others and thereby abbreviate the learning period; this ability is vital to survival.
4. Self-regulatory capacity—the ability to make choices based on personal beliefs, rather than on the expectations of the external environment. Internalized standards are used to guide behavioral choices.
5. Change capacity (Plasticity)—the ability to develop or change. The vast potential for human development is shaped by both direct and vicarious experiences into many forms, constrained only by biological limitations.
6. Self-reflective capacity—the ability to think about personal experiences and derive generic knowledge about oneself and the world in which one lives. One of the most powerful types of self-reflective thought is perceived self-efficacy (Bandura, 1986).

Each of these six capacities influences the degree of self-efficacy expressed for each task by any given person.

Definition of Perceived Self-Efficacy

The concept of perceived self-efficacy (or efficacy expectations) evolved primarily from the observation that traditional cognitive psychology models did not adequately explain the discrepancy between attained skills and the quality of performance output (Bandura, 1977). Traditional models attempted to explain the discrepancy between skills and performance as a function of the actors' expectation of outcomes or "action-outcome expectancy." Action-outcome expectancy theorists postulate that, given equivalent skills, performance differences are due to differences in the actor's belief that the response will lead to a desired goal. If this belief is strong, the actor will engage in the requisite behavior; if this belief is weak, the actor will not engage in the behavior even though he or she possesses the skill to do so.

Bandura (1977) suggested that a difference in outcome expectancy does not explain the total variance between skill and performance. He suggested that perceived self-efficacy is also a significant factor. Bandura (1986) defined perceived self-efficacy as

> people's judgments of their capabilities to organize and execute courses of action required to attain designated types of performances. It is concerned not with the skills one has but with the judgments of what one can do with whatever skills one possesses (p. 391).

Thus, Bandura (1977) asserted that one's belief in one's ability to use a specific skill partially explains why people of equivalent skill achieve at differing levels. This belief in one's ability to perform (i.e., perceived self-efficacy), develops as a result of the interaction of each of the six attributes of Social Cognitive Theory described earlier.

Relationship to Self-Esteem

Perceived self-efficacy should not be confused with the construct of self-esteem. *Self-esteem* is defined as "the dimension of self-concept that includes a negative and/or positive sense of self" (Daub, 1988, p. 57). Self-esteem is created by the person's analysis of his or her overall competency at factors that he or she considers to be socially relevant (Mayberry, 1990). Thus, a person may perceive himself or herself to be competent at many things but have low self-esteem due to a belief that these competencies are not socially relevant. Conversely, a person may express a low degree of perceived self-efficacy for one or more tasks yet have high self-esteem. Self-esteem and perceived self-efficacy should be highly correlated only when measuring perceived self-efficacy for a task that is highly socially relevant to the subject. A Nobel Prize winner may have high self-esteem in part due to the recognition of the value of his or her contribution to society. The same Nobel Prize winner may have low perceived self-efficacy for playing racquetball or gourmet cooking. However, his or her perceived self-efficacy for the activity that resulted in the Nobel Prize should be high and should correlate strongly with a measure of his or her self-esteem. Thus, perceived self-efficacy may contribute to a sense of self-esteem, but it is an independent construct.

Parameters of Self-Efficacy

Bandura (1977) identified three parameters of perceived self-efficacy: magnitude, strength, and generality. *Magnitude* refers to the relative level of difficulty of the task that is being rated. For example, Ewart and colleagues (1986) used different jogging distances to reflect differences in the magnitude of perceived self-efficacy for a group of subjects with postmyocardial infarction. Subjects who were completely confident that they could jog 1 mile were considered to have a greater magnitude of perceived self-efficacy than those who were completely confident that they could jog only a quarter of a mile and somewhat confident that they could jog 1 mile.

Strength of perceived self-efficacy refers to the degree to which people believe they can succeed at a given level of an activity; this degree can vary from total certainty to total uncertainty. The stronger the sense of efficacy, the more likely people are to persevere in the face of adversity and the less likely it is that failure will extinguish their efficacy expectations (Bandura, 1977).

Generality of perceived self-efficacy refers to the degree to which the person's perceived self-efficacy for one activity transfers to other similar or different activities. Successful performance of some tasks results in a strengthening of efficacy expectations for that task alone, whereas success at other tasks generalizes to tasks that are different from the original task (Bandura, 1977). Bandura does not identify the types of tasks that generalize or those that do not.

History of the Construct

Bandura postulated that, given the requisite skills and belief that the response will lead to a desired outcome, perceived self-efficacy would be an important determinant of successful performance. Bandura (1977; Bandura & Adams, 1977) tested the theory about perceived self-efficacy with an unspecified number of persons with snake phobias. Subjects were asked to state whether they were able to perform each of 18 tasks and to rate the strength of their expectations that they would succeed on a 100-point scale with 10-point intervals. The subjects were randomly assigned to one of three groups: vicarious experience, modeling (later called enactive experience), or no treatment. The subjects in the vicarious learning group observed an instructor handling snakes, while the enactive learning group first observed and then attempted the snake-handling techniques themselves. Of the subjects who achieved maximal performances during therapy (successfully achieved the snake-handling techniques), Bandura noted that not all expressed maximal efficacy expectations. Efficacy expectation and performance during the treatment sessions were examined as possible predictors of subsequent performance. Perceived self-efficacy was found to be the best predictor of subsequent performance. The higher the subjects' perceived self-efficacy at the completion of treatment, the better their performance when retested at a later date ($r = .75$, $p < .01$). This relationship existed regardless of whether the efficacy expectations were derived through vicarious or enactive experience. However, subjects who experienced enactive education produced higher, more generalized, and stronger efficacy expectations and increased performance attempts. Bandura (1977) stated that

> on the one hand, the mechanisms by which human behavior is acquired and regulated are increasingly formulated in terms of cognitive processes. On the other hand, it is the performance based procedures that are proving to be most powerful for effecting psychological changes. As a consequence, successful performance is replacing symbolically based experiences as the principal vehicle of change (p. 191).

Since his initial work, Bandura has examined the effect of perceived self-efficacy with a variety of subjects and found that perceived self-efficacy is a consistent predictor of performance (Bandura, 1982; Bandura, Cioffi, Taylor, & Brouillard, 1988; Bandura & Wood, 1989).

The construct of perceived self-efficacy has been applied in a variety of different clinical, educational, and organizational situations by many other authors. From January 1987 to December 1992, 933 articles referring to perceived self-efficacy have been printed in journals indexed by Psychlit alone. The following is a brief summary of the findings of a small sampling of these articles that were selected for their relevance to occupational therapy practice.

Clinical Examples

- Perceived self-efficacy for exercise was found to be correlated with an increase in exercise endurance in a sample of subjects ($n = 119$) with chronic obstructive lung disease (Toshima et al., 1990)
- Self-efficacy was found to explain 24% of the variance in adjustment to multiple sclerosis ($n = 62$) (Wassem, 1992)
- Self-efficacy for jogging proved superior to treadmill performance, depression, and type A personality in predicting adherence to exercise prescription in a sample ($n = 40$) of patients with coronary artery disease (Ewart et al., 1986)
- The results of a study of subjects ($n = 30$) diagnosed with arthritis indicated that a higher level of perceived self-efficacy for pain control after a cognitive behavioral education program was related to a lower level of perceived pain (O'Leary, Shoor, Lorig, & Holman, 1988)

Health Promotion Examples

- A scale, developed to measure perceived barriers to health-promotion activities, was found to be highly correlated (-.48) with perceived self-efficacy (Stuifbergen, Becker, & Sands, 1990)
- In a sample ($n = 600$) of subjects participating in the Stanford Heart Disease Prevention Program,

self-efficacy was found to be a better predictor of nutritional choices than demographic factors, social influences, and health knowledge (Slater, 1989). This study also found that cognitive control (the capacity to exercise control over one's own thinking and motivation) predicted the level of perceived self-efficacy

- Raising self-efficacy for health-promoting behaviors was found to be more effective than emphasizing the risk of not performing the health-promoting behavior in two separate studies (Seydel et al., 1990)

Education Examples

- Attributional feedback from the researcher (feedback about who was responsible for past successes), as opposed to feedback about future potential success or no feedback, was found to be related to faster mathematical skill development and higher perceived self-efficacy in a sample ($n = 40$) of children ranging in ages from 7 to 10 years (Shunk, 1982)
- Subjects who were successful using strategies taught in a "learning to learn" program led to enhanced perceived self-efficacy and generalized to other activities requiring similar learning skills for a group of 4th graders (Wang & Richarde, 1987)

Perceived Self-Efficacy as a Behavioral Determinant

A strong sense of perceived self-efficacy for an activity is crucial to successful performance because "it determines which activities people engage in, the amount of effort they expend before terminating the activity, and how long they will persevere in the face of adversity" (Bandura, 1981, p. 215). People are faced with frequent activity choices throughout their lives. The strength of their efficacy expectations for an activity affects whether they choose to engage in the activity or not. Strong efficacy expectations result in engagement in an activity; whereas weak efficacy expectations result in avoidance (Bandura, 1986). This process of activity selection has a profound effect on human development, in that activity choices enlarge or restrict one's opportunities to develop new skills, or to enhance existing ones (Bandura, 1986).

Errors in judgment regarding one's performance, whether too optimistic or too pessimistic, may result in significant consequences (Bandura, 1986). In activities with a small margin of error (e.g., driving a car), overly optimistic efficacy expectations may prove disastrous. However, in activities with a greater margin of error, activities that are unlikely to result in harm to oneself or others, appraisals of performance that exceed actual ability are quite functional (Bandura, 1989).

For example, when a patient is attempting to learn to maneuver a wheelchair, a high expectation that he or she is capable of learning to propel the chair will result in more frequent attempts and learning will advance more quickly. On the other hand, if the patient believes that he or she is unlikely to master propelling the wheelchair, he or she will avoid situations where this is a requirement and progress will be impeded. Bandura asserted (1989) that people must strive to exceed past performances, and that if efficacy expectations never exceeded past performance, the acquisition of new skills would not occur.

People with strong efficacy expectations will persevere in the face of adversity, due to a belief that they will ultimately succeed (Bandura, 1977). People with weaker efficacy expectations will quit when faced with obstacles, or refuse even to try. People who view themselves as efficacious are more likely to expect things to go right (Bandura, 1989). They approach difficult tasks as challenges to master rather than threats to avoid. People who experience success react by raising their personal goals and being more committed to the activity (Bandura & Wood, 1989). The stronger the sense of perceived self-efficacy, the higher the goals set and the stronger the commitment to attainment of the goals.

Although perceived self-efficacy is a crucial behavioral determinant, Bandura (1977) pointed out that perceived self-efficacy in the absence of skill, or a desire to perform, will not ensure successful performance. Attempts to enhance performance must be accompanied by an understanding of the influence of perceived self-efficacy on performance.

Outcome Expectations and Perceived Self-Efficacy

Perceived self-efficacy refers to a belief in one's ability to perform a certain task or behavior. It should not be confused with a belief that performance of a specified behavior will result in a specific outcome (Bandura, 1977). Rogers (1983) referred to a belief that performance of a specified behavior will result in a specified outcome as response efficacy. Both perceived self-efficacy and response efficacy affect whether or not the person will elect to perform a certain task; however, they are distinct behavioral determinants (Bandura, 1977). That is, one must believe both that a specific action will lead to a desired goal and that one is capable of performing the specific action, or one will not act.

Bandura (1986) argued that theories that emphasize outcome expectations are based on animal research where measurement of perceived self-efficacy was impossible. He stated that "convictions that outcomes are determined by one's own actions can be either demoralizing or heartening, depending on the level of self-judged efficacy" (Bandura, 1986, p. 413). Therefore an expectation that a certain behavior will result in a certain outcome is not sufficient to ensure successful performance unless one believes one has the skills to succeed at the required task.

Relationship to Psychological Well-Being

According to self-efficacy ideology, people can give up trying and become hopeless in two different ways: they may believe that their continued attempts will not bring positive results (response efficacy), or they may believe that they are unable to perform the tasks necessary to bring about the desired results (perceived self-efficacy) (Bandura, 1982). Different combinations of these two factors result in different self-assessments:

- If persons have a strong sense of perceived self-efficacy and a strong belief in the efficacy of the response, they will act in an assured manner and be dynamic.
- If persons have a strong sense of perceived self-efficacy but a weak sense of response efficacy, they will energize themselves to make changes in the system so that they can successfully attain their goal.
- If people have a weak sense of perceived self-efficacy and a weak sense of response efficacy, they will become resigned and apathetic.
- If people have a weak sense of perceived self-efficacy and a strong sense of response efficacy, they will become despondent and self-deprecating.

The relationship between perceived self-efficacy and psychological well-being was explored by Holahan, Holahan, and Belk (1984). Perceived self-efficacy was measured by asking a group of retired university faculty members how well they handled or could in the future handle each of the items on a list of daily hassles (self-efficacy / hassles scale) and a list of negative life events (self-efficacy / life events scale). The results indicated that higher levels of perceived self-efficacy were associated with lower levels of depression for both sexes. Additionally high levels of perceived self-efficacy were associated with lower levels of psychological distress for women and fewer psychosomatic complaints for men. Overall, the results indicate a significant association between perceived self-efficacy and psychological adjustment.

Perceived self-efficacy has also been shown to negatively correlate with depression. Davis-Berman (1990) administered the Physical Self-Efficacy Scale and the General Self-Efficacy Scale to a sample of 200 elderly residents of a retirement center. The Physical Self-Efficacy Scale consists of 22 items and includes questions about reflexes, muscle tone, and sports ability. The General Self-Efficacy Scale consists of two subscales, the General Scale and the Social Self-Efficacy Scale. The scale contains questions about one's general belief in one's ability to do things and one's ability to handle oneself in social situations. All three Self-Efficacy Scales were found to be inversely and significantly ($p > .01$) correlated to depression. (General Self-Efficacy $r = -.40$, Social Self-Efficacy $r = -.23$, and Physical Self-Efficacy $r = .50$.) That is, persons with lower self-efficacy scores were more likely to be depressed.

Influencing the Strength of Perceived Self-Efficacy

Perceived self-efficacy is influenced through an ongoing evaluation of success and failure with each task people participate in over the course of their lives (Bandura, 1986). Bandura (1982) stated that perceived self-efficacy develops through successful experiences that create high efficacy expectations and failure experiences that lower efficacy expectations. Thus, the development of perceived self-efficacy is a dynamic process.

Perceived self-efficacy is constantly affected by four sources of information: personal performance accomplishments, vicarious experience (watching others of similar skill perform a task), verbal persuasion, and the person's physiological state (Bandura, 1977).

Personal performance accomplishments. Personal performance accomplishments, also called *enactive experiences*, are the most influential source of information about one's perceived self-efficacy (Bandura, 1986). Success, as perceived by the person, enhances perceived self-efficacy and failure decreases it. Failure early in the development of a new skill is more likely to decrease perceived self-efficacy than failure after a firmly entrenched belief in the skill has been developed. When people believe they are efficacious, they attribute failure to the circumstances, poor effort on their part, or the use of poor strategies (Bandura, 1986).

Vicarious experience. A great deal of human learning begins with observing others perform tasks (Bandura, 1986). Vicarious learning is developed more readily when the observer considers the person being observed to have similar skills to himself or herself. Children watch and then imitate their parents. In this process of observing activities, some learning occurs before the person is required to attempt any of the requisite behaviors. For example, children observe their parents driving cars for years before they begin. They observe how the wheel is turned, how to start the car, what the highway signs mean, and so on. This learning decreases the number of new skills that must be learned when the children reach an appropriate age and actually begin to drive the car. They already understand the component skills and now need to learn to execute them independently (Bandura, 1986). Vicarious learning is not as powerful a source of information as enactive learning, but it is still very important.

Persuasion. Persuasion is a frequently used means of convincing someone that his or her self-assessment is incorrect. However, it is the weakest form of informa-

---

tion with respect to altering perceived self-efficacy (Bandura, 1986). Persuasion will be effective in altering beliefs only if the current belief is close to the belief that is being proposed. Subsequent performance quickly affirms or denies the new belief. Thus, accurate assessment of the other person's ability is required if persuasion is to succeed.

Physiological state. People read their level of somatic arousal as an indication of competency (Bandura, 1977). Thus, if your heart rate increases and you begin to sweat, you interpret these reactions as an indication that the activity you are approaching is in some way threatening. Strategies that decrease the level of arousal (relaxation techniques) have been found to enable people to feel more efficacious. This feeling of efficacy in turn leads to a willingness to attempt the behavior that had previously resulted in a state of physiological arousal, and to success experiences (Bandura, 1986).

Cognitive appraisal. Personal performance accomplishments, vicarious experience, persuasion, and physiological arousal are the types of experiences that affect perceived self-efficacy. However, the degree to which these experiences influence perceived self-efficacy is determined by the person's cognitive appraisal and integration of these experiences (Bandura, 1982; Gist & Mitchell, 1992).

Gist and Mitchell (1992) developed a model to explain the effect of these experiences on perceived self-efficacy. They suggested that the cognitive appraisal and integration process has three components. The first component is the analysis of the requirements of the task. The more complex the task and the less previous experience one has with a task, the harder it is to accurately assess one's perceived self-efficacy for the task. The second component is the analysis of the degree to which success or failure is attributed to oneself rather than others or to chance. If one believes that one is successful due to a skill one possesses, then perceived self-efficacy for the task will be heightened. However, if one believes that one was successful because of chance, the actions of others, or the environment, perceived self-efficacy will not be affected. The third component is the analysis of personal and situational resources and constraints that affect the task at hand. This appraisal process involves the assessment of personal factors such as skill, motivation, anxiety, and desire, as well as situational factors, such as distractions, support of influential others, and competing demands.

The three cognitive appraisal processes will result in the subjects' determination of the degree of perceived self-efficacy for a task, which in turn affects the person's willingness to participate or persevere with the task in the future, and hence will affect actual future performance.

Generalizability

The development of perceived self-efficacy is largely situation specific, with a tendency to generalize to similar activities (Ewart, Taylor, Reese, & DeBusk, 1983). Ewart and his colleagues studied the relationship between perceived self-efficacy and activity for a group of patients with postmyocardial infarction. These patients participated in treadmill testing and filled in a perceived self-efficacy questionnaire before the treadmill test, after the treadmill test, and after a counseling session that followed the treadmill test. The perceived self-efficacy questions covered walking, running, climbing stairs, engaging in sexual intercourse, lifting objects, and an overall estimate of ability to tolerate physical activity. Perceived self-efficacy ratings for the activities that used the same physical skills as the treadmill (walking, running, and climbing stairs) showed the greatest increase. With the addition of counseling (a form of verbal persuasion), the efficacy ratings for the other activities increased. Assistance with interpretation of the treadmill experience was necessary before generalization could occur.

Control

The degree of control the person perceives that he or she has alters the influence of success or failure on the development of perceived self-efficacy. Bandura and Wood (1989) studied the influence of perceived control on perceived self-efficacy in a simulated manufacturing environment. The degree of perceived control and the amount of success the subjects experienced were regulated through the design of the experiment. Subjects were randomly assigned to one of four groups. Each group received instructions designed to alter their perception of two constructs, personal control and performance expectations. The four groups were low perceived control with high performance expectations, low perceived control with low performance expectations, high perceived control with high performance expectations, and high perceived control with low performance expectations. The groups that were given high performance standards experienced less success than those with low performance standards. Subjects who viewed the organization as controllable, regardless of whether they were in the high or low performance expectations group, had higher mean self-efficacy scores than those who thought that they had little control over the organization ($p < .02$). Subjects in the high control, high performance standards group showed increases in perceived self-efficacy over three trials, whereas subjects in the high control, low success groups showed decreases in perceived self-efficacy ($p < .05$). Subjects who were led to believe that the organization was difficult to control demonstrated low self-efficacy regardless of whether they were in the high or low performance expectation group; that is, their perceived self-efficacy was low regardless of whether or not they were experiencing success.

Discussion of the Literature

Adolph Meyer, a major contributor to the philosophical basis of occupational therapy practice, recognized the value of the feelings of satisfaction and achievement associated with successful completion of a project (1922) (see Chapter 2). Thus, from the early days of occupational therapy practice, the value of successful experiences, that is, performance accomplishments, was recognized. Activity programs were structured to ensure success because success was believed to lead the patient to try another, more difficult task. Occupational therapists have often described this process as the enhancement of self-esteem (Christiansen, 1991; Meyer, 1922 [see Chapter 2]); yet the activities the occupational therapy client performs are not always socially relevant. Therefore, it is postulated that success with occupational therapy activities leads to an increase in perceived self-efficacy for these activities, which leads to a willingness to engage in and persist in future similar tasks. If the success experiences relate to socially relevant activities an elevation in self-esteem would also be predicted.

The occupational performance literature addresses the need to understand the effect of psychosocial factors on occupational performance (Christiansen, 1991; Pedretti & Pasquinelli-Estrada, 1985; Trombly, 1989). An underlying assumption appears to be that psychological factors affect only the acquisition of skill and that once the skill has been learned it will be used outside the protected clinical environment. However, just as Bandura (1977) noted that people do not always perform optimally even when they have the requisite skills, clinicians have stated that occupational therapy clients do not always perform at the level one might predict on the basis of clinical observation of skill (Gage, 1992).

The Model of Human Occupation, a model that guides occupational therapy practice, addresses the discrepancy between skill and performance through, among other things, a concept similar to perceived self-efficacy: personal causation (Oakley, Kielhofner, & Barris, 1985). *Personal causation* is defined as "the collective beliefs that an individual has efficacious skills, is personally in control, and will succeed in future endeavors" (Oakley et al., p. 148). This construct is equivalent to the construct of perceived self-efficacy.

When discussing the influence of inefficacy (a term that Kielhofner has used in the same view as perceived self-efficacy), Kielhofner stated that "occupational dysfunction is at the level of inefficacy when there is an interference with performing meaningful activity accompanied by dissatisfaction with performance" (1985, p. 69). He went on to state that "sources of inefficacy may be environmental constraints, disease processes, or imbalanced lifestyles" (p. 69).

The importance of the strength of the person's belief in his or her ability to perform the specific component parts of life roles is not articulated. One's perception of one's ability to perform is considered to be a major behavioral determinant (Allen et al., 1990; Bandura, 1977, 1986; Bandura & Adams, 1977; Bandura & Wood, 1989; Ewart et al., 1986; Seydel et al., 1990; Shunk, 1982; Toshima et al., 1990; Wang & Richarde, 1987; Wassem, 1992). Therefore, it is essential that the relationship of perceived self-efficacy to occupational performance be explored.

The terms *perceived self-efficacy* or *efficacy expectations* are beginning to appear in the occupational therapy literature. Crist and Stoffel (1992) (see Chapter 22), when discussing the Americans With Disabilities Act as it applies to persons with mental impairments, discussed the value of perceived self-efficacy with respect to successful employment of persons with mental disabilities. Christiansen (1991) acknowledged that the "single characteristic of the individual that has the greatest influence on performance is one's sense of competence" (p. 20), yet this concept is given only four paragraphs in the occupational therapy textbook written by Christiansen and Baum.

There is a growing recognition that clients' perceptions of performance (perceived self-efficacy) are important. In the March 1993 issue of the *American Journal of Occupational Therapy*, professional leaders discussed the needs of the profession with respect to assessment. Authors cited the need to measure client perception of performance (Law, 1993), the need to identify the psychological factors that contribute to performance deficits and strengths (Bonder, 1993), and the need to develop means of remediating these psychological factors once identified (Bonder, 1993). Trombly stated that the overall goal of occupational therapy is to "enable the client to gain a sense of efficacy" (1993, p. 254). The Canadian Occupational Performance Measure (Law et al., 1991) uses client perception of performance as one outcome variable. However, there is a need to incorporate this belief into occupational therapy practices.

The influence of perceived self-efficacy on the person's ability to cope with the effects of disability has also been articulated by Gage (1992). She was interested in determining why patients of equal physical impairment and rehabilitation potential do not progress at the same pace, and why, given similar goals, these patients attain different levels of independent function. After a review of the literature on coping, Gage formulated the Appraisal Model of Coping as a guide to assessment and intervention for occupational therapists. The Appraisal Model of Coping was based on the Cognitive Relational Theory of Coping and Emotion (Lazarus & Folkman, 1984) and Social Cognitive Theory (Bandura, 1977). *Coping* was defined by Lazarus and Folkman (1984) as the process through which people manage the demands and emotions generated by person–environment relationships.

The model presented by Gage identified 12 factors that influence the ability of persons to cope with their disability or any other life event that taxes personal resources. One of these 12 factors is perceived self-efficacy. In this model, perceived self-efficacy is considered by Gage to be particularly salient to the practice of occupational therapy because of its potential ability to explain the discrepancy between skill developed in therapy and occupational performance outside the protected clinical environment. However, the model is, as yet, conceptual and must be tested to determine the specific nature of the influence of perceived self-efficacy on coping with occupational performance deficits.

Enhancing Occupational Performance

A recognition that the client's level of perceived self-efficacy for a specific activity influences the likelihood of the client performing that activity outside the protected clinical environment has far-reaching implications for the practice of occupational therapy. This recognition brings with it an understanding that a client's ability to perform a specific skill in the clinical environment may not mean that the client will use the skill in his or her usual contextual environment. What good is treatment if it does not generalize to the use of the skill in the community?

Occupational therapists must learn how to evaluate their client's level of perceived self-efficacy and to develop techniques that not only improve clients' skills, but also enhance their self-efficacy for use of those skills in the community. As previously presented, empirical findings about the influence of perceived self-efficacy on clinical outcome are already available (Ewart et al., 1986; O'Leary et al., 1988; Toshima et al., 1990; Wassem, 1992). Although these studies do not specifically look at occupational performance activities or the influence of the occupational therapy process on perceived self-efficacy, they do provide information that is relevant to occupational therapy practice. Empirical studies have also investigated the relationship between perceived self-efficacy and the initiation or adherence to health-promoting behaviors (Seydel et al., 1990; Slater, 1989; Stuifbergen et al., 1990). The results of these studies are increasingly relevant to occupational therapists as more and more therapists become involved with primary and secondary prevention activities. In addition, the process of occupational therapy is often one of teaching new skills or teaching new ways to perform familiar activities. Thus, articles that present data about the relationship between perceived self-efficacy and learning are also relevant to occupational therapists (Shunk, 1982; Wang & Richarde, 1987).

It is important to remember that the articles cited in this paper are just a small sampling of the perceived self-efficacy literature available to occupational therapists. Occupational therapists working in various fields are encouraged to search the literature for articles that have valuable information about perceived self-efficacy within their area of practice. Occupational therapy research studies to add to this knowledge base are encouraged. There are many possible applications that arise from the attributes of perceived self-efficacy as presented in the section of this paper titled "History of the Construct." These themes can be categorized into three major categories: assessment, outcome, and therapeutic process.

Assessment and Outcome

Previous research has demonstrated a link between clinical outcomes and perceived self-efficacy (Allen et al., 1990; Bandura, 1977, 1986; Bandura &Adams, 1977; Bandura & Wood, 1989; Ewart et al., 1986; Seydel, Taal, & Wiegman, 1990; Shunk, 1982; Toshima et al., 1990; Wang & Richarde, 1987; Wassem, 1992). Thus, it is important to derive ways to measure perceived self-efficacy for occupational performance activities that will enable the exploration of its relationship to outcome. For example, perceived self-efficacy is thought to explain the variance between development of skill and performance of that skill in the community. It is, therefore, important to explore the influence of increases or decreases in perceived self-efficacy for occupational performance activities on treatment outcomes. The level of perceived self-efficacy that is required before a client will use the skill independently in the community must be determined. The belief that the development of a skill is not sufficient to ensure successful occupational performance in the absence of an adequate level of perceived self-efficacy leads to a need to monitor a client's perceived self-efficacy during the treatment process. The ability to demonstrate occupational competence in the clinical environment should no longer indicate successful treatment outcome. Therapists must find ways to determine whether their clients are using these skills in the community. Because perceived self-efficacy is believed to be a good predictor of future performance, therapists need to establish the level of perceived self-efficacy that is likely to result in use of the skill in the community. This level may then be useful in the determination of when to discharge from therapy. However, individual variation will always necessitate individual follow-up to ensure that a given client has been successful.

Therapeutic Process

The section of this paper titled "Influencing the Strength of Perceived Self-Efficacy" provides occupational therapists with specific strategies for increasing perceived self-efficacy in the clinical environment. For example, perceived self-efficacy is enhanced through personal performance accomplishments; that is, by actually doing the activity or very similar activities. In fact, it is suggested that perceived self-efficacy for an activity performed in the occupational therapy department will only generalize to very similar activities. Thus, occupational therapists must use realistic activities that simulate the contextual environment of the client. This will be easy for therapists working in the community who provide services in the client's home; it will be more difficult for therapists working in institutional environments. The relevance of reductionistic activities such as peg boards and puzzles must be questioned. How does the mastery of these component skills relate to changes in perceived self-efficacy and actual performance for personally important life activities?

The role of vicarious learning with respect to the development of occupational competence must also be explored. If, in fact, a great deal of human learning begins with observing others perform tasks, it would be important for clients to observe the successful performance attempts of their peers. Bandura (1977) suggested that vicarious experience is most powerful when the participants consider themselves to have similar skills. Thus, modeling by the therapist may be ineffective, and consumer self-help groups might be encouraged.

Gist and Mitchell (1992) suggest that self-efficacy beliefs are most accurate when clients are rating familiar activities because they understand the relationship between the skills required to perform the task and the skills they possess. For occupational therapy clients the knowledge of the skills they possess has often been affected by the onset of a disabling condition. Although the clients are aware of the skills required for occupational performance activities, they may believe that their disability has robbed them of these skills. Thus, the occupational therapist must provide them with a safe environment within which to experiment with their altered level of performance and to develop a new understanding of their efficacy.

Therapists often try to convince clients that they are able to go home and live independently, or return to work, only to be confronted with a barrage of reasons why the client is not yet ready. These patients are labeled as fearful or, worse yet, as malingerers. Perhaps it is simply their perceived self-efficacy for home management or work activities that has not yet reached the level necessary to engage in the activity independently. If one accepts that persuasion is the least influential method of raising efficacy expectations, then the therapist must devise new intervention techniques. The treatment plan must incorporate vicarious learning and relevant personal performance accomplishments if success is to occur. The use of such simulations as Easy Street,[1] a stay in an activities of daily living (ADL) apartment located in the protected

clinical environment, or a home visit with the therapist may be a better solution than attempts to persuade.

Perceived self-efficacy increases more when the client is in control. Thus, it is important for therapists to enable clients to articulate their needs and have a real voice in the therapeutic process. Tools such as the Canadian Occupational Performance Measure (Law et al., 1991) may create a feeling of control and enhance outcomes.

Summary

Perceived self-efficacy has great relevance to the practice of occupational therapy. It is consistent with the fundamental philosophical beliefs of the profession, may enhance and predict outcomes, and has a strong empirical basis that suggest specific changes to current occupational therapy treatment practice. Occupational therapists are challenged to develop, test, and publish these linkages.

Many of the attributes of perceived self-efficacy are relevant to occupational performance. By monitoring and working to enhance perceived self-efficacy, occupational therapists may be better able to explain the variance between development of skill and performance of that skill in the community, ensure successful occupational performance in the community, predict future performance, and enable occupational competence.

Acknowledgment

Funds for this study were obtained through a Health Services Research Grant awarded to the first author by Victoria Hospital, London, Ontario, Canada.

References

Allen, J. K., Becker, D. M., & Swank, R. T. (1990). Factors related to functional status after coronary artery bypass surgery. *Heart & Lung, 19,* 337–343.

Bandura, A. (1977). Toward a unifying theory of behavioral change. *Psychological Review, 84,* 101–215.

Bandura, A. (1981). Self-referent thought: A developmental analysis of self-efficacy. In J. H. Flavell & L. Ross (Eds.), *Social cognitive development: Frontiers and possible futures* (pp. 200–239). New York: Cambridge University Press.

Bandura, A. (1982). Self-efficacy mechanism in human agency. *American Psychologist, 37,* 122–147.

Bandura, A. (1986). *Social foundations of thought.* Englewood Cliffs, NJ: Prentice Hall.

Bandura, A. (1989). Regulation of cognitive processes through perceived self-efficacy. *Developmental Psychology, 25,* 729–735.

Bandura, A., & Adams, N. E. (1977). Analysis of self-efficacy theory of behavioral change. *Cognitive Therapy and Research, 1,* 287–310.

---

[1]Manufactured by Easy Street Environments, 6908 E. Thomas Road, Suite 201, Scottsdale, Arizona 85251.

Bandura, A., Cioffi, D., Taylor, C. B., & Brouillard (1988). Perceived self-efficacy in coping with cognitive stressors and opioid activation. *Journal of Personality and Social Psychology, 55,* 497–488.

Bandura, A., & Wood, R. (1989). Effect of perceived controllability and performance standards on self-regulation of complex decision making. *Journal of Personality and Social Psychology, 56,* 805–814.

Bonder, B. R. (1993). Issues in assessment of psychosocial components of function. *American Journal of Occupational Therapy, 47,* 211-216.

Christiansen, C. (1991). Occupational Therapy: Intervention for life performance. In C. Christiansen & C. Baum (Eds.), *Occupational therapy: Overcoming human performance deficits* (pp.3–43). Beckenham, Kent, England: Slack.

Crist, P. A. H., & Stoffel, V. C. (1992). The Americans With Disabilities Act of 1990 and employees with mental impairments: Personal efficacy and the environment. *American Journal of Occupational Therapy, 46,* 434–443. (Reprinted as Chapter 22).

Daub, M. (1988). Prenatal development through mid-adulthood. In H. L. Hopkins & H. D. Smith (Eds.), *Willard and Spackman's occupational therapy* (7th ed., pp. 50–75). Philadelphia: Lippincott.

Davis-Berman, J. (1990). Physical self-efficacy, perceived physical status, and depressive symptomatology in older adults. *Journal of Psychology, 124,* 207–215.

Ewart, C. K., Stewart, K. J., Gillilan, R. E., Kelemen, M. H., Valenti, S. A., Manley, J. D., & Kelemen, M. D. (1986). Usefulness of self-efficacy in predicting overexertion during programmed exercise in coronary artery disease. *American Journal of Cardiology, 57,* 557–561.

Ewart, C. K., Taylor, C. B., Reese, L. B., & DeBusk, R. F. (1983). Effects of early postmyocardial infarction exercise testing on self-perception and subsequent physical activity. *American Journal of Cardiology, 51,* 1076–1080.

Gage, M. (1992). The appraisal model of coping: An assessment and intervention model for occupational therapy. *American Journal of Occupational Therapy, 46,* 353–362.

Gist, M., & Mitchell, T. (1992). Self-efficacy: A theoretical analysis of its determinants and malleability. *Academy of Management Review, 17,* 183–211.

Holahan, C. K., Holahan, C. J., & Belk, S. S. (1984). Adjustment in aging: The roles of life stress, hassles, and self-efficacy. *Health Psychology, 3,* 315–328.

Kielhofner, G. (1985). Occupational function and dysfunction. In G. Kielhofner (Ed.), *A model of human occupation* (pp. 63–75). Baltimore: Williams & Wilkins.

Law, M. (1993). Evaluating activities of daily living: Directions for the future. *American Journal of Occupational Therapy, 47,* 233–237.

Law, M., Baptiste, S., Carswell-Opzoomer, A., McCall, M. A., Polatajko, H., & Pollock, N. (1991). *Canadian Occupational Performance Measure.* CAOT Publications ACE, Toronto, Canada.

Lazarus, R. S., & Folkman, S. (1984). *Stress appraisal and coping.* New York: Springer.

Mayberry, W. (1990). Self-esteem in children: Considerations for measurement and Intervention. *American Journal of Occupational Therapy, 44,* 729–734.

Meyer, A. (1922). The philosophy of occupation therapy. *American Journal of Occupational Therapy, 31,* 639–642. (Reprinted as Chapter 2.)

Oakley, F., Kielhofner, G., & Barris, R. (1985). An occupational therapy approach to assessing psychiatric patients' adaptive functioning. *American Journal of Occupational Therapy, 39,* 147–154.

O'Leary, A., Shoor, S., Lorig, K., & Holman, H. R. (1988). A cognitive-behavioral treatment for rheumatoid arthritis. *Health Psychology, 7,* 527–544.

Pedretti, L. W., & Pasquinelli-Estrada, S. (1985). Foundations for treatment of physical dysfunction. In L. Pedretti (Ed.), *Occupational therapy: Practice skills for physical dysfunction* (2nd ed., pp. 1–10). St. Louis: Mosby.

Rogers, R. W. (1983). Cognitive and physiological processes in fear appeals and attitude change: A revised theory of protection motivation. In J. T. Cacioppo, R. E. Petty, & D. Shapiro (Eds.), *Social psychophysiology* (pp. 153–176). New York: Guilford.

Seydel, E., Taal, E. & Wiegman, O. (1990). Risk-appraisal, outcome and self-efficacy expectancies: Cognitive factors in preventive behavior related to cancer. *Psychology and Health, 4,* 99–109.

Shaffer, H. (1978). Psychological rehabilitation, skills-building, and self-efficacy. *American Psychologist, 33,* 394–396.

Shunk, D. (1982). Effects of effort attributional feedback on children's perceived self-efficacy and achievement. *Journal of Educational Psychology, 74,* 548–556.

Slater, M. (1989). Social influences and cognitive control as predictors of self-efficacy and eating behavior. *Cognitive Therapy and Research, 13,* 231–245.

Stuifbergen, A., Becker, H., & Sands, D. (May 1990). Barriers to health promotion for individuals with disabilities. *Family and Community Health,* 11–22.

Toshima, M., Kaplan, R., & Ries, A. (1990). Experimental evaluation of rehabilitation in chronic obstructive pulmonary disease: Short-term effects on exercise endurance and health status. *Health Psychology, 9,* 237–252.

Trombly, C. A. (1989). *Occupational therapy for physical dysfunction* (3rd ed.) Baltimore: Williams & Wilkins.

Trombly, C. (1993). The Issue Is— Anticipating the future: Assessment of occupational function. *American Journal of Occupational Therapy, 47,* 253–257.

Wang, A., & Richarde, R. S. (1987). Development of memory monitoring and self-efficacy in children. *Psychological Reports, 60,* 647–658.

Wassem, R. (1992). Self-efficacy as a predictor of adjustment to multiple sclerosis. *Journal of Neuroscience Nursing, 24,* 224–229.

Chapter 38

The Patient-Therapist Relationship: Beliefs That Shape Care

Suzanne M. Peloquin, PhD, OTR

This chapter was previously published in the *American Journal of Occupational Therapy, 47,* 935–942. Copyright © 1993, American Occupational Therapy Association.

Occupational therapists can be with patients in many ways that reflect their various understandings of what it means to be competent and caring. Because the beliefs of a profession shape a therapist's sense of what it means to give care, the beliefs about competence and caring found in the occupational therapy tradition have warranted consideration (Peloquin, 1990). Three images of how occupational therapists act in practice dominate patients' stories: the images of technician, parent, and collaborator or friend. When therapists act as technicians or authoritarian parents, patients cast them negatively in stories that reflect their disappointment. When acting in either of these manners, therapists seem to value the competence articulated within the professional literature more than they value the caring aspects of *relationship* (Peloquin, 1990). Both of these enactments, however, reflect some understanding of what it means to care. The technical therapist, equating expertise with care, values the best method and the successful outcome. The parental therapist manipulates the decisions and methods that are in the patient's best interests and sees this action as caring. In each of these images of care, the therapist's competence dominates the encounter.

If choosing how to be among patients is a matter of some consideration, it follows that a number of societal beliefs and expectations also shape a therapist's choice. Those beliefs are the subject of this discussion. It seems apt for occupational therapists to consider the societal forces that surround practice. As Yerxa (1980) said, "Occupational therapy, which began in a climate of caring, has been influenced in its practice by social change" (p. 532). It is a growing truism that the current health care system is now perceived as "not oriented to the human being" (Baum, 1980, p. 514). What causes this disorientation to persons? King (1980) suggested that any sense of the meaning of caring is an intermingling of personal, professional, *and* societal beliefs. Any lack of caring that derives from a preferential valuation of competence must also reflect such an intermingling.

Nature and Scope of the Inquiry

This article constitutes part of a larger inquiry into the challenge of creating a climate of caring. Conducted between January 1990 and September 1991, the inquiry considered the following: (a) personal narratives that describe impersonal treatment; (b) the historical events and societal constructs that have shaped the patient–helper relationship; (c) empathy and the manner in which helpers learn to be empathic; (d) the nature, practice, and experience of art; and (f) the proposition that empathy might be cultivated through the use of art. Each step of the inquiry required an extensive literature review from which important themes emerged. These themes were then subjected to the reflection, analysis, and synthesis characteristic of studies in the medical humanities.

A number of phenomenological narratives about the impersonal treatment of patients served as subjects for an earlier discussion (Peloquin, 1993). That discussion produced a descriptive profile of those behaviors to which patients refer when they use the term *depersonalizing*. The central complaint found within those narratives was that when practitioners act impersonally their behaviors are discouraging. Patients say that helpers fail to see illness and disability as emotional events charged with personal meaning. They fail to attend to the experiences of patients; instead, they establish a distance that diminishes them. They withhold information, they use brusque manners, and they misuse their powers. They are insensitive, silent, and aloof. Patients conclude that their helpers may treat them, but they do not treat them well.

Alongside these descriptive narratives were a number not included in the discussion on depersonalization because they were more reflective than descriptive: (a) those written by patients who consider the beliefs that may cause their helpers to behave carelessly; (b) those written by caregivers who, after their own bout with illness and impersonal treatment, discuss societal expectations; and (c) those written by helpers who ponder the difficulties of caring. These reflections offer cues about the societal constructs that may have a hand in shaping care, and, as cues, they constitute assumptions that can direct further research.

This discussion does not address concerns in practice such as those that Bailey (1990) described as the "harmful variables" that cause therapists to leave the field (p. 23). Staff shortages, large caseloads, red tape, excessive paperwork, lack of job status, chronic conditions of the patient population, lack of respect for occupational therapy by other professionals, stress and overload, and the need to justify treatment also shape decisions about the manner in which helpers will choose to care. Many of these negative variables, although not the specific focus of this inquiry, can also be said to associate with the societal beliefs that are the subject of this discussion.

The Connections That Mean Care

A number of stories do portray helpers as caring persons who offer patients equal measures of competence and caring (Peloquin, 1989 [see Chapter 67]; Peloquin, 1990). These stories suggest that caring attitudes, gestures, and words give patients the courage to face illness and disability.

Pekkanen (1988) treated a 14-year-old boy whose electrical accident had warranted amputation of his legs; Pekkanen willed himself to feel the boy's injury from the inside out. He then understood:

> He was a tall, rangy black kid from the inner city and had been a very good junior high school basketball player. All he ever wanted to be was a basketball player, and I think that the young man took this news with more hurt, more disappointment, and more disbelief than any child I can remember. . . . I think it was one of the most crushing truths to come to a young man that I have ever seen. (p. 126)

A caring attitude can encourage patients. Lee (1987), a patient hospitalized with cancer, felt care in this small gesture:

> As I slept a nurse took the cloth wrapping off a sterile instrument. He smoothed out the material. He painted with a blue flow pen a moon face with wide eyes and an enormous crescent smile. He climbed over my bed. He climbed over my plants and hung this banner down from my window, using the extra-wide masking tape. It was the first thing I saw in the morning. (p. 111)

Patients also draw courage from caring words. Benziger (1969) remembered the encouragement that she took from this conversation with an occupational therapist:

> "You know, you go at your work too hard, too fast, too desperately—and too frenetically."
>
> "I guess I do, but that's the way I feel. Time stands still for me now, it is endless, and yet if I have something to do, I get the sense that there will not be time enough to finish it, or that someone will stop me."
>
> She said, "You are an intelligent person, and you will help yourself to get well quickly." "You know," I answered,

"you're the first person who has mentioned intelligence versus non-intelligence, instead of sanity. You make me feel like a human being." I was grateful. I should not forget her. (p.49)

The directness and the proffered confidence held in these words meant concern to Benziger; she would call this therapist *friend*.

Sarason's (1985) point of view is no doubt the most helpful. At the very least, he said, practitioners can *try*. Patients, he says, mostly ask helpers to try "in ways that say 'I am trying to understand because I want to be helpful.' It is those manifestations that are experienced as caring and compassionate, even though they may be more or less ineffective" (p. 188). And when "a patient, whether terminal or not, draws courage—courage to live or courage to die—from the man who stands at his bedside" (Hodgins, 1964, p. 843), surely they both feel the magic of care.

If practitioners can be both competent and caring among their patients, what societal beliefs cause them to act otherwise? Three constructs surface within the reflections of patients and practitioners as shaping forces that compromise caring expressions: (a) an emphasis on the rational fixing of problems; (b) an overreliance on methods and protocols; and (c) a health care provision system that is driven by business, efficiency, and profit.

The Emphasis on Rational Fixing

One societal belief that compromises caring actions is the emphasis on solving discrete health care problems in a logical and rational manner. When Hodgins wrote in 1964 after his stroke, he found a particular form of disregard at the heart of the problem. He described this picture of how the patient and the caregiver perceive illness:

> In stroke two basic sets of assumptions could govern treatment. One set proceeds from what the patient perceives or thinks he perceives; the other comes from what the doctor knows or thinks he knows. The two are very different sets of things. (p. 842)

Many health care narratives hold similar pictures, with helpers governing some aspects of care while neglecting others that their patients value. Sir Dominic Corrigan, a physician, argued as long as a century ago that the trouble with doctors is "not that they don't know enough, but that they don't see enough" (cited in Taylor, 1972, p. 6).

Van Eys (1988), also a physician, has regretted the hemisected worldview in which "diseases become problems, and patients become dissected into such problems" (p. 21). Patients resent this narrowness of focus because it feels uncaring. They complain that practitioners address their disease, the physiology and the mechanism of their bodies and dysfunctions, but not the experience of illness and unease, not its meaning, and surely not their feelings.

Disregard for parts of persons disturbs Murphy (1987), an anthropologist who wrote of his own disabling illness: "The full subjective states of the patient are of little concern in the medical model of disability, which holds that the problem arises wholly from some atomic or physiological disorder and is correctable by standard modes of therapy—drugs, surgery, radiation, or whatever" (p. 88). Sacks (1983), a neurologist who experienced impersonal care, considered this splitting insane:

> the madness of the last three centuries, the madness which so many of us—as individuals—go through, and by which all of us are tempted. It is the Newtonian-Lockean-Cartesian view—variously paraphrased in medicine, biology, politics, industry, etc.—which reduces men to machines, automata, puppets, dolls, blank tablets, formulae, ciphers, systems, and reflexes. (p. 205)

Sarton (1988) remembered in her journal that after a stroke she was made to feel like "so many pounds of meat, filled with potentially interesting mechanical parts and neurochemical combinations" (p. 106).

Leder (1984) argued while in medical school that a person is never so many pounds of meat, that the human body is "not a mere extrinsic machine but our living center" (p. 34). Paradoxically, however, it seems that the body, so prized in this narrow view of illness, matters little on a day-to-day basis. Most persons, said Leder, ignore the body until it malfunctions. Then when they are ill, they beg some practitioner to fix the complex mechanism that has disrupted the flow of their personal lives. And the picture of health care practice that one then sees is "an ironic fulfillment of Cartesian dualism—a mind (namely, that of the doctor) runs a passive and extrinsic body (that of the patient)" (p. 35). The image offered by Jourard (1964), a psychologist, illuminates this Orwellian disjunction:

> Each patient lies in his own cubicle, and there are attached to him all kinds of wires, connected to his brain, his muscles, his viscera. Every time these wires, which are actually electronic pick-ups, transmit signals to a computer indicating that the bladder is too full, a bowel stuffed, and patient hungry or in pain, before you could blink an eye, the computer sends signals to different kinds of apparatus which empty the bowel and bladder, fill the stomach, scratch the itch, massage the back and so on. We could even mount the bed on a slowly moving belt; the patient gets in at one end, and four or six days later his bed reaches the exit and the patient is healed—we hope. (p. 138)

If this reduction is a prevalent view, is it fair to expect practitioners to think divergently, to routinely see and treat a self embodied instead of a body? If the general population views the body as a mechanism controlled by higher functions, as something that one has instead of who one is, why the surprise that practitioners engage only their rational functions in practice? If imagining patient experiences, sensing patient needs, and expressing personal feelings seem actions incongruent with fixing, practitioners are quite reasonable in underusing these so-called lower functions. What is the problem, then, with treating bodies when they need fixing?

Most narratives answer that "when a patient appears as a physiological mechanism, the doctor may neglect personal communication in favor of the immediate scientific task at hand" (Leder, 1984, p. 36). The preference for fixing makes it easier for a helper to neglect feelings, easier to justify being silent, curt, or aloof. The resulting problem is impersonal care. Any caregiver can focus narrowly on fixing. Gebolys (1990) remembered this incident:

> A male therapist came in whistling and cheerfully setting up his equipment. He stuck the breathing tube into my mouth and told me to "breathe" which I did while he walked around the room admiring my flowers, gazing out the window and remarking at what a lovely day it was. (p. 13)

Mattingly (1991) (see Chapter 36) gave occupational therapists pause for reflection when she argued that "therapists can come to reduce their practice to a manipulation of the physical body, forgetting how much their interventions are directed to a person's life" (p. 986). Parham (1987) argued that there are such situations in occupational therapy when

> time, energy, and money are funneled into treating one small part of the total problem, a part that may be insignificant in comparison with complexities that are more difficult to understand but that have a profound impact on the life situation of the patient being served. (p. 556)

Schultz and Schkade (1992) shared a similar concern: "The current demand for therapists to base occupational therapy on acquisition of functional skills ... may actually limit the contribution of occupational therapy and may deny patients the opportunity to make vital changes in their occupational adaptation process" (p. 918). Certainly a patient's poem, "Some Other Day" (McClay, 1977), presents an occupational therapist bent on partial fixing:

> Preserve me from the occupational therapist, God
> She means well, but I'm too busy to make baskets ...
> "Please, open your eyes," the therapist says;
> You don't want to sleep the day away."
> She wants to know what I used to do,
> Knit? Crochet?
> Yes, I did those things, and cooked and cleaned, and raised
> five children and had things happen to me.
> Beautiful things, terrible things,
> I need to think about them, rearrange them on the shelves
> of my mind.
> The therapist is showing me glittery beads.
> She asks if I might like to make jewelry.
> She's a dear child and she means well,

> So I tell her I might.
> Some other day. (pp. 107–108)

The consequence of a strong commitment to rational fixing—of the disease, the body, or the dysfunction—is a disregard that feels careless. And although practitioners mean well, physician–educator Anthony Moore (1978) acknowledged the problem: "Professions tend to be right in what they affirm and wrong in what they ignore" (p. 3).

The Reliance on Method and Protocol

A second societal belief that compromises caring is an overreliance on the instruments of health care practice: the techniques, procedures, and modalities that solve the problem. When they are ill, patients seek concern in addition to solutions. They grieve that in health care practice they find something else. Hodgins (1964) regretted the find:

> For the physician, of course, it must have been wonderful, indeed, when true specifics began to arrive on the scene to supplant beef, iron, and wine or syrup of hypophosphates.... As so-called science more and more enters medicine, the heedless or routine physician will be accordingly tempted to withdraw his humanity and wait for specifics. (p. 843)

Hodgins considered the specifics needed for cure and the humanity needed for care different but inseparable aspects of care. Flagg (1923), a physician who practiced at the turn of the century, agreed; he regretted "the unwise employment of laboratory methods to the exclusion of personal attention" (p. 5).

When a drug or a procedure suffices, a practitioner may think less about the need to make meaningful connections with the patient. The problem becomes clear in Barbara Peabody's (1986) recollection of an incident that occurred during her son's hospitalization for acquired immunodeficiency syndrome (AIDS):

> Peter woke at two A.M., just as the intern was about to give him an injection in his left thigh.
> "What do you have there?" Peter asked.
> "What do you care?" the intern snapped back.
> "I care very much, and I hope that's not pentamidine."
> "What if it is?" the intern asked insolently.
> "Because if it is, I'm not supposed to get it anymore," Peter replied. "I think you better check my chart and you'll see that it was discontinued on Monday."
> "Oh, no, the orders are still on your chart."
> "I'm sure they're not," Peter insisted. "Go back and read them again, you'll see that I'm right."
> The intern left the room and never returned. (p. 51)

Reiser (1980) told the following story about helpers whose reliance on protocol precluded personal attention. A woman hospitalized with a diagnosis of acute granulocytic leukemia and severe anemia agreed to an aggressive course of chemotherapy that made her quite ill. She was discharged after remission, and when she was readmitted 4 months later she refused chemotherapy. The staff decided that if she continued to refuse this treatment, she would be discharged Against Medical Advice. She refused and was discharged. Reiser's perception was that she had "stepped out of the established 'system' and had to be punished for it" (p. 146).

Sacks (1983) rejected the argument that helpers must use only treatments or protocols. When facing surgery, he wondered,

> What sort of man would Swan be? I knew he was a good surgeon, but it was not the surgeon but the person that I would stand in relation to, or, rather, the man in whom, I hoped, the surgeon and the person would be wholly fused. (p. 92)

Cassell (1985), another physician, shared a similar belief: "Doctors who lack developed personal powers are inadequately trained.... Doctors are themselves instruments of patient care" (p. 1).

When they are effective, however, methods and protocols take the upper hand. Helpers side with what works, so that a challenge to the procedure also threatens them. Martha Lear (1980) remembered the upshot of such an identification when her husband Hal, a urologist, requested a milder painkiller: "The resident got angry. He said, 'There is a medication ordered for pain for you. If you want it, you can have it. If not, you'll get nothing.' And he walked out" (p. 41). But patients, wrote the physician Pellegrino (1979), do not want practitioners to fuse with their skills: "Physicians have a medical education, an M.D. degree, a set of skills, knowledge, prestige, titles. They possess many things by which they mistakenly identify themselves" (p. 228).

Helpers wrap themselves in their procedural authority, binding themselves so tightly in their concern for the right method, the latest technology, that it is no wonder that their actions then seem constricted. Helpers can never be seen as personal if they offer knowledge or skills instead of themselves. Murphy (1987) resented the trade: "What I needed was not a new instrument, but an old fashioned clinician with plenty of intuition" (p. 14). Patients argue that their helpers routinely neglect their feelings, that they have bought the argument in favor of impersonality.

But whenever anyone mentions using either selves or intuitive traits therapeutically, practitioners stir uneasily. They have a problem with being intuitive or personal. Some actually call caring *feminine*. Lear (1980) claimed that her husband felt care from women, distance from men: "They were with him constantly, those woman figures. They were gentle and good.... The male figures were with him for ten minutes a day, They were marginal figures, shadowy and cold. They touched him with instruments—stethoscopes, blood-pressure gadgets" (pp. 40–

41). It seems that here too helpers try to split the inseparable; they say that men will offer cures and skills, women service and caring. But patients argue that this and all other separations are unthinkable; all helpers must care.

Hodgins (1964) argued that encounters felt as personal are often what patients need most: "[The patient] will draw courage as he perceives human understanding underlying the professional techniques of those into whose care he has been given. Human understanding, however, is not to be found in the rituals of anything called medical science" (p. 841). Unhappily, concern for more personal issues seems to matter little in this formulaic belief: Correct procedures produce the superior results that serve the patient's best interests.

Occupational therapists are among those who must admit that techniques and protocols can preempt caring. Yerxa (1980) argued that "*technique*, once employed in the service of human needs, is rapidly moving us toward a society of total technology in which our ways of thinking and being themselves become so technical that we lose sight of other ways of thinking and being" (p. 530).

King (1980) concurred, claiming that "therapists have ignored their instinct for caring" (p. 525). Heller and Vogel (1986) described Heller's experience with the tight formula in his occupational therapy treatment for Guillain-Barré syndrome.

> As soon as I could sand a block of wood (with a need to rest both arms, it was written, after seven repetitions), a change was made to a coarser grade of sandpaper, increasing the amount of force required, and it was just as punishing for me to have to execute them as it had been in the beginning. (pp. 166–67)

Although Heller wanted to savor his gain and determine his next move in therapy, a protocol forbade his doing so.

Parham (1987) discussed the case of Longmore, a former faculty member at the University of Southern California Program in Disability and Society:

> He was subjected to long hours of occupational therapy training for self-care skills although he had no intention of performing these time-consuming tasks independently at home. He planned to hire an attendant who would expedite the process, freeing him to use his time and energy to pursue more stimulating and productive activities. (p. 556)

Neither Heller's nor Longmore's treatments heeded Baum's (1980) reminder that interventions notwithstanding, "we are nothing more than a bystander in the life of that individual until a relationship is formed" (p. 514).

A Health Care System Driven by Business, Efficiency, and Profit

Francis Peabody (1930), a physician, articulated the problem well when he argued that "hospitals, like other

---

institutions, founded with the highest human ideals, are apt to deteriorate into dehumanized machines" (p. 33). Many narratives suggest that this dehumanization stems from a system of providing health care that builds on business, efficiency, and profit.

The business of health care. Any business that aims to offer individual service to large numbers of people may suffer from criticisms such as Sarton's (1988):

> A small incident at the hairdresser's has given me something to try to understand … While Donna was securing my hair into curlers, an old lady was waiting to be picked up came and stood beside us and talked cheerfully about herself and her daughters and Donna responded. It was though I did not exsist, was an animal being groomed. (p. 255)

The number of patients who seek treatment can compromise caring expressions in hospitals. As Sarason (1985) wrote, "The clinician becomes a rationer of time, and that obviously sets drastic limits on the degree to which the ever-present client need for caring and compassion can be met" (p. 170). The result of that rationing is the feeling articulated by Peter Peabody during his visits to a busy clinic: "I just feel like they don't give a damn…. I feel like I'm always being ignored, they don't care" (1986), p. 172). Additional complications associate with the business of hospitals, however, by virtue of their lifesaving function. Hodgins (1964) discussed the personal estrangement that occurs with the rapid interventions warranted by life-threatening illness:

> Speaking as a patient, I think this point is important: that the stroke victim is most likely to encounter, as his first medical ministrant, a physician to whom he is a total stranger. Since speedy hospitalization is usually a first goal in stroke, treatment by strangers is likely to continue. (p. 839)

Peabody (1930) explained one consequence of the lifesaving business:

> When a patient enters a hospital, the first thing that commonly happens to him is that he loses his personal identity. He is generally referred to, not as Henry Jones, but as "that case of mitral stenosis in the second bed on the left"…. It leads, more or less directly, to the patient being treated as a case of mitral stenosis, and not a sick man. (p. 31)

The problem is a matter of focus; the institutional eye sees the relevance of saving Henry's life and so does not capture the wider clinical picture—that although "Henry happens to have heart disease, he is not disturbed so much by dyspnea as he is by anxiety for the future" (Peabody, 1930, p. 34).

The efficiency of the health care system. Murphy (1987) has spoken to the kind of ordering that occurs in institutions, renaming the hospital an island invaded by a rationalized system of schedules and shifts: "The hospital has all the features of a bureaucracy, and, like bureaucracies everywhere, it both breeds and feeds on impersonality" (p. 21)

The impersonality is well illustrated in Saxton's (1987) account:

> The scariest part of the hospitalization for me was not the surgery but the doctor rounds. On the mornings when these rituals were scheduled, the nurses and aides awakened us much earlier than usual. Meals and wash-ups were rushed…. Then they would come, the surgeons, the residents, the interns…. They entered our ward, about fifteen adults…. Strange long words were uttered; bandages were opened and quickly closed. (p. 53)

Gebolys (1990) recalled that only on the fourth day of her hospital stay did a nurse's aide wash her hair, which was bloody and dirty from an automobile accident. The aide did so after her shift was over because the highly regulated day precluded this helping task. Sacks (1983) concluded that "the hospital, in short, is a singular mixture, where freedom and bondage, warmth and coldness, human and mechanical, life and death, are locked together in perpetual combat" (p. 24).

The battle sometimes seems insane, Murphy (1987) explained, because like most bureaucracies, the hospital has turned "capricious, arbitrary, and irresponsible as Wonderland's Red Queen" (p. 44). One feels the capriciousness in Beisser's (1989) experience with heartless caretakers:

> In one hospital, the first hour of the nurses' shift was spent in a detailed discussion of who would take coffee breaks when. Medications, patient needs, all other things paled in comparison. Sometimes people would literally leave you in midair in a lift to go on a coffee break, or leave you in some other awkward position, and just say, "It's my break time." (p. 35)

Brice (1987) recalled a nurse in the recovery room whom she asked for a blanket. The nurse, seeming much like the Red Queen, "barked 'I just brought you one; I'm not going to bring you another' and disappeared" (p. 31). People are a hospital's only possible conveyors of personal care; there can be no social life there if helpers are capricious and irresponsible. Sarton (1988) wearied of her treatment that was "bland at best, cold and inhuman at worst" (p. 103).

The profit of health care provision. Hodgins (1964) thought that helpers produced mostly problems with the profit-driven business of health care:

> We have heard much sentimental lamentation over the disappearance of the old "family physician"—dear, lovable old Dr. Peatmoss, who delivered all the babies, saw them through diphtheria, whooping cough and scarlet fever, sat at the deathbeds of the elderly, and never sent anyone a bill. This last lovable quality is, I suppose, why he disap-

peared. I felt no sense of personal loss at his passing because I never knew him. I should have liked to. The physicians in my life all had very efficient accounting systems—if not actual departments. (p. 840)

Longcope (1962), a physician, had argued even earlier that a business orientation causes "the 'quantification, mechanization and standardization' which are said to characterize this country" (p. 547). Within a business orientation to health care, knowledge takes coin value, cure becomes a high-priced commodity, and ill persons are transformed into buyers. Success and solvency turn into treatment goals, productivity and efficiency into the means to achieve them. In this scheme, more accrues from procedures that cure than from manners that care. Rabin (1982), a physician with amyotrophic lateral sclerosis, remembered that his physician gave him a pamphlet outlining the course of a disease that he already knew too well. He regretted that this physician gave him no suggestions about "how to muster the emotional strength to cope with a progressive degenerative disease" (p. 307).

Practitioners face a major quandary when their patients' needs for time and compassion compete with the institution's need to prosper. When high regard falls to those who treat the most patients or accumulate the most billable units of time, moments spent noticing, listening, or communicating are harder to justify. Sarason (1985) explained: "Whose agent I was became a pressing, daily, moral problem. I know what it is to have divided loyalties, to want to give up the fight, to rationalize away the internalized conflict' (pp. 170–171). And although few helpers buy the idea that patients are mere customers, many budget their caring actions. Patients experience the cuts as hurtful. Lear (1980) wrote of her husband's regret that he had never attended to his patients' experiences. He thought: "Damn it, doctors *should* know. They should care. Say how're they treating you? How's the food? Accommodations comfortable? Staff courteous?.... He himself would never even have thought to ask. Didn't that make him negligent too? Ah. Bingo" (p. 43).

Occupational Therapists Within the System

According to Sacks (1983), occupational therapists are among those who struggle more successfully against the impersonality within the health care provision system: "There are, of course, gaps in this totalitarian structure, when real care and affection still maintain a foothold; many of the 'lower' staff nurses, aides, orderlies, physiotherapists, speech therapists, etc. give themselves unstintingly, and with love, to their patients" (p. 24). But occupational therapists speak openly about the frustrations of clinical practice; as Howard (1991) (see Chapter

64) wrote, "occupational therapy does not exist in a vacuum" (p. 878). Growing numbers of patients are a concern. Departments must handle more patients with fewer staff members because "productivity and efficiency are becoming high-priority goals" (p. 878). Howard argued that technological approaches are thus "valued more than the holistic use of a variety of methods" (p. 880).

The climate in hospitals seems one of "cost containment" rather than caring (Howard, 1991, p. 878 [see Chapter 64]. Kari and Michels (1991) (see Chapter 21) wrote of their regret that "daily life for those living within the institution can become compartmentalized and focused on receiving services to alleviate dysfunction" (p. 721). Trahey (1991) saw the combat to which Sacks (1983) referred as a "struggle to integrate quality care with a businesslike approach to fiscal soundness" (p. 397). Burke and Cassidy (1991) (see Chapter 65) called it the "disparity between reimbursement-driven practice and the humanistic values of occupational therapy" (p. 173). Boyle (1990) questioned one aspect of the dilemma:

> Are occupational therapists today meeting the needs of the rehabilitation population and considering their social, political, and economic status? Or are we compartmentalizing our services on the basis of our own need for neat, tidy treatment plans that fit our expertise and the selective mission of our institution? (p. 941)

The enormity of the challenge pressed Grady (1992) to ask a more fundamental question: "Is there still enjoyment in occupational therapy, or have we become so controlled with the realities of productivity, reimbursement, and modalities that we are failing to see the process as part of the outcome?" (p. 1063) A number of therapists have spoken to the powers essential for the struggle. Knowledge is one:

> All occupational therapists should have the knowledge, skills, and attitudes to position themselves to gain influence, power, and control of the systems in which they operate. To move upward in the power hierarchy, we must have knowledge (i.e., expertise), knowing (i.e., process skills), competencies, and credentials. (Nielson, 1991, p. 854)

But that competence, wrote Dickerson (1990), must be tempered by another concern: "Care must also be exercised so that therapists never sacrifice quality of care for increased profits" (p. 137).

The quality of care central to occupational therapy has traditionally included the assumption that "if therapists are to create individually designed, personally meaningful treatment programs, then they must spend considerable time and energy getting to know each patient as a person" (Burke & Cassidy, 1991, p. 173) (see Chapter 65). More and more, according to Burke and Cassidy, occupational therapists "must use a technical, protocol-driven approach to treatment" (p. 174). "Like physicians," they wrote, "we have had to amend our traditional allegiance to the patient due to increased fiscal restraint, which requires that we now consider the economic realities of the hospitals in which we work" (p. 174).

Conclusion

Caregivers such as Vanderwoude (1988) have paused after the course of their own illness to explain: "My illness was beneficial in helping me to be more reflective, in teaching me an element of patience, and in heightening my understanding of the person facing possible terminal illness" (p. 125). Sacks (1984) was similarly convinced: "I saw that one must be a patient, and a patient among patients, that one must enter both the solitude and the community of patienthood, to have any idea of what 'being a patient' means" (p. 172). Although such an experience offers a profound form of knowing, first-person narratives can also inspire helpers to consider the manner in which they care.

Occupational therapists who choose how they will be among their patients do so within a context shaped by an intermingling of personal, professional, and societal beliefs. Occupational therapists have traditionally endorsed a practice based on competence and caring (Peloquin, 1990). Therapists who act as either technicians or authoritarian parents disappoint patients with their over-valuation of competence. Several societal beliefs can be seen to connect with such overly competent enactments: an emphasis on the rational fixing of problems, an overreliance on method and protocol, and a health care system that thrives on business, efficiency, and profit.

A focus on fixing bodily parts and functional problems leads to a tendency to disregard a patient's understanding or feelings about illness. To a patient, the disregard feels technical rather than personal. A reliance on protocols that have success, authority, and reliability leads to a tendency to deny a patient's control, to dismiss a helper's intuition about what is right. To a patient, this preeminence of protocol feels impersonal and authoritarian. The routinization and rationalization of health care institutions lead to discourteous behaviors. The actions feel efficient but uncaring. Therapists who act as technicians or authoritarian parents reflect society's preference for the rational fixing of problems, the implementing of successful strategies, and the management of solvent businesses. And although each of these orientations is important and worthy of affirmation in any health care practice, overvaluation of any one of these can compromise the actions and words that mean care. Practice that values the person must build on both competence and caring.

Toward the end of his personal litany of complaints, Hodgins (1964) remembered the need that helpers also have for courage in the face of illness. He ended his address to the Academy of Physicians by suggesting that practitioners consider a picture of practice that might replenish their commitment: "Reclothe yourselves in humanity" (p. 843). It is hoped that occupational therapists will be among those who will hold fast to this image of personal caring as they practice competent care.

Acknowledgement

The research on which this article is based constitutes a portion of a dissertation that partially fulfilled requirements for a doctoral degree conferred by the Institute for the Medical Humanities, the University of Texas Medical Branch, Galveston, Texas. The dissertation is entitled *Art in Practice: When Art Becomes Caring*.

References

Baum, C. M. (1980). Eleanor Clarke Slagle lecture—Occupational therapists put care in the health system. *American Journal of Occupational Therapy, 34*, 505–516.

Bailey, D. M. (1990). Reasons for attrition from occupational therapy. *American Journal of Occupational Therapy, 44*, 23–29.

Beisser, A. (1989). Flying without wings: Personal reflections on becoming disabled. New York: Doubleday.

Benziger, B. F. (1969). *The prison of my mind.* New York: Walker.

Boyle, M. A. (1990). The Issue Is—The changing face of the rehabilitation population: A challenge for therapists. *American Journal of Occupational Therapy, 44*, 941–945.

Brice, J. (1987). Empathy lost. *Harvard Medical Letter, 60*, 28–32.

Burke, J. P., & Cassidy, J. C. (1991). Disparity between reimbursement-driven practice and humanistic values of occupational therapy. *American Journal of Occupational Therapy, 45*, 173–176. (Reprinted as Chapter 65.)

Cassell, E. J. (1985). *Talking with patients: Volume 1. The theory of doctor–patient communication.* Cambridge: MIT Press.

Dickerson, A. (1990). Evaluating productivity and profitability in occupational therapy contractual work. *American Journal of Occupational Therapy, 44*, 133–137.

Flagg, P. (1923). *The patient's viewpoint.* Milwaukee: Bruce Publishing.

Gebolys, E. (1990). Inadequacies, inequities and inanities in modern medicine—A personal experience. *Occupational Therapy Forum, 12*, 6–7, 13–18.

Grady, A. P. (1992). Nationally Speaking—Occupation as vision. *American Journal of Occupational Therapy, 46*, 1062–1065.

Heller, J., & Vogel, S. (1986). *No laughing matter.* New York: Avon.

Hodgins, E. (1964). Whatever became of the healing art? *Annals of the New York Academy of Sciences, 164*, 838–846.

Howard, B. S. (1991). How high do we jump? The effect of reimbursement on occupational therapy. *American Journal of Occupational Therapy, 45*, 875–881. (Reprinted as Chapter 64).

Jourard, S. (1964). *The transparent self: Self-disclosure and well being. New York:* Van Nostrand Reinhold.

Kari, N., & Michels, P. (1991). The Lazarus project: The politics of empowerment. *American Journal of Occupational Therapy, 44,* 719–725. (Reprinted as Chapter 21).

King, L. J. (1980). Creative caring. *American Journal of Occupational Therapy, 34,* 522–528.

Lear, M. (1980). *Heartsounds.* New York: Simon & Schuster.

Leder, D. (1984). Medicine and paradigms of embodiment. *Journal of Medicine and Philosophy, 9*(1). 29–43.

Lee, L. (1987). Transcendence. In M. Saxton & F. Howe (Eds.), *With wings: An anthology of literature by and about women with disabilities* (pp. 109–116). New York: Feminist Press.

Longcope, W. (1962). Methods and medicine. In W. H. Davenport (Ed.), *The good physician: A treasury of medicine* (pp. 546–559). New York: Macmillan.

Mattingly, C. (1991). The narrative nature of clinical reasoning. *American Journal of Occupational Therapy, 45,* 998–1005. (Reprinted as Chapter 36).

McClay, E. (1977). *Green winter: Celebrations of old age.* New York: Reader's Digest Press.

Moore, A. R. (1978). *The missing medical text: Humane patient care.* Melbourne, Australia: Melbourne University Press.

Murphy, R. F. (1987). *The body silent.* New York: Henry Holt.

Nielson, C. (1991). The Issue Is—Positioning for power. *American Journal of Occupational Therapy, 45,* 853–854.

Parham, D. (1987). Nationally Speaking—Toward professionalism: The reflective therapist. *American Journal of Occupational Therapy, 41,* 555–561.

Peabody, B. (1986). *The screaming room: A mother's journal of her son's struggle with AIDS.* New York: Avon.

Peabody, F. W. (1930). *Doctor and patient papers on the relationship of the physician to men and institutions.* New York: Macmillan.

Pekkanen, J. (1988). *M.D.: Doctors talk about themselves.* New York: Del Publishing.

Pellegrino, E. (1979). *Humanism and the physician.* Knoxville: University of Tennessee Press.

Peloquin, S. M. (1989). Sustaining the art of practice in occupational therapy. *American Journal of Occupational Therapy, 43,* 219–226. (Reprinted as Chapter 67).

Peloquin, S. M. (1990). The patient–therapist relationship in occupational therapy: Understanding visions and images. *American Journal of Occupational Therapy, 44*(1), 13–21.

Peloquin, S.M. (1993). The depersonalization of patients: A profile gleaned from narratives. *American Journal of Occupational Therapy, 47,* 830–837.

Rabin, D., Rabin, P., & Rabin, R. (1982). Compounding the ordeal of ALS. *New England Journal of Medicine, 307,* 506–509.

Reiser, D., & Schroder, A. K. (1980). *Patient interviewing: The human dimension.* Baltimore: Williams & Wilkins.

Sacks, O. (1983). *Awakenings.* New York: Dutton.

Sacks, O. (1984). *A leg to stand on.* New York: Harper & Row.

Sarason, S.B. (1985). *Caring and compassion in clinical practice.* San Francisco: Jossey-Bass.

Sarton, M. (1988). *After the stroke: A journal.* New York: Norton.

Saxton, M. (1987). In M. Saxton & F. Howe (Eds.), *With wings: An anthology of literature by and about women with disabilities* (pp. 51–57). New York: Feminist Press.

Schultz, S., & Schkade, J. K. (1992). Occupational adaptation: Toward a holistic approach for contemporary practice, Part 2. *American Journal of Occupational Therapy, 46,* 917–925.

Taylor, R. (1972). *The practical art of medicine.* New York: Harper & Row.

Trahey, P. (1991). A comparison of the cost-effectiveness of two types of occupational therapy services. *American Journal of Occupational Therapy, 45,* 397–400.

Van Eys, J. & McGovern, J. P., Eds. (1988). *The doctor as a person.* Illinois: Charles C Thomas.

Vanderwoude, J. (1988). The caregiver as a patient. In J. Van Eys & J. P. McGovern (Eds.), *The doctor as a person* (pp. 172–184). Illinois: Charles C Thomas.

Yerxa, E. J. (1980). Occupational therapy's role in creating a future climate of caring. *American Journal of Occupational Therapy, 34,* 529–534.

Section V

Tools of Practice: Media, Methods, and Strategies for Clinical Interventions

Introduction

The competent ethical use of a profession's legitimate tools enables practitioners to meet the needs of society (Mosey, 1986). Occupational therapists use a diversity of tools to effectively attain the goals of our profession. Purposeful activity is widely recognized as the fundamental tool of occupational therapy (OT) practice (Hopkins & Smith, 1993; Mosey, 1986), and for that reason it is the primary focus of this text. Additional legitimate tools of OT are the nonhuman environment, activity groups, conscious use of self, the teaching–learning process, and activity analysis and synthesis (Mosey, 1986). Clinical reasoning, technology, and a broad range of media and methods are also considered to be legitimate tools of OT practice (Hopkins & Smith, 1993). Many of these tools have been discussed in several chapters of this text, particularly, environmental contexts and modifications in Section II, activity groups in Section III, and therapeutic relationships and clinical reasoning in Section IV. This next section will further explore OT's tools of practice with emphasis placed on strategies and guidelines for the appropriate selection and competent use of these tools.

The profession of OT and the tools we, as occupational therapists, use in our daily practice are strongly influenced by sociopolitical forces and changes in the health care system. Chapter 39 by Reed critically examines the multitude of factors that determine whether a tool of practice is adopted, maintained, or discarded by the profession. Occupational therapists have used many media and methods for intervention over the years, yet the reasons for embracing or abandoning numerous media or methods are often unclear. Reed postulates that the lack of a rationale for the use of a medium or method may lead to limited understanding of its therapeutic value, for both the therapist and patient. This lack of awareness can compromise the therapeutic potential of the selected tool of practice. She suggests that eight factors—cultural, social, economic, political, technological, theoretical, historical, and research—influence the selection or abandonment of tools of practice in OT. Reed explores the nature of these influences, providing clear and relevant examples to highlight her points. She summarizes the effects of these eight factors by proposing 14 assumptions and providing three relevant, yet diverse, examples to illustrate how these factors and assumptions operate to affect the use of specific tools in OT practice. Reed emphasizes that the media, methods, and objectives of an activity must be consistent with each other for the activity to be purposeful and meaningful. She asserts that careful consideration of cultural, social, individual, and professional interests and values will ensure that the tools used in OT practice will have therapeutic value and be meaningful and purposeful to the individual. Reed's call for occupational therapists to increase their awareness of the "why" of practice to ensure their interventions are consistent with OT philosophy is a timely one.

A fundamental premise of our professional philosophy is that to achieve therapeutic goals there must be a "match" between a patient who has been holistically assessed and an activity that has been thoroughly analyzed and synthesized (McGarry, 1990; Mosey, 1986). Activity analysis and synthesis have been major tools of OT practice from the inception of the profession, and they have maintained their relevance and importance throughout the years. Chapter 40 by Creighton explores the origin of activity analysis from the early 1900s and the evolution of activity analysis up to the present. She examines the initial development of structural activity analysis based on motion studies. The first systematic application of activity analysis in an OT clinic is presented. These early analyses emphasized the study of movement required by each activity and the subsequent adaptations of the activities to improve physical function or compensate for a movement deficit. Creighton describes the evolution of activity analysis between World War I and World War II and the expansion of activity analysis to include psychosocial characteristics of activities. However, she states these analyses continued to perpetuate a physical and psychosocial split that was reflective of the dichotomy between psychiatric and physical disabilities practices. Creighton examines the refinement of activity analysis into an integrated, holistic approach in the 1970s and 1980s as frames of reference were further developed. The current view of activity analysis as a multifaceted process that also considers environmental contexts according to a frame of reference is emphasized.

Nelson, in Chapter 41, provides a useful and comprehensive model for activity analysis based on his challenging in-depth discussion of the multifaceted concepts of occupational form and occupational performance. He defines occupation as a relationship between occupational form and occupational performance. The multidimensional nature of occupational form and its relationship with occupational performance is presented, providing a systematic way to analyze occupation. The meaningfulness and purposefulness of occupational form to the individual and the influence of the individual's developmental structure on this meaning and purpose is examined. Nelson explores the dynamics of occupation and the impact of occupational performance on the environment, the individual, and his or her adaptation and occupation. The diverse multiple levels of occupation throughout different points in time are also considered. A series of figures graphically depict the interrelationships between occupational form, occupational performance, development, purpose, and meaning. A comprehensive outline of a sample activity analysis clearly illustrates the practical application of these concepts and supports the relevance of this framework to OT practice.

The exploration of the relationships among occupation, adaptation, development, and occupational performance follow in Chapter 43 by Levy. She also presents a comprehensive framework for activity analysis, expanding her discussion to consider activity adaptations and environmental modifications that enable an individual to successfully participate in desired activities and valued roles. The link between a functional assessment of an individual and activity analysis and synthesis is explored. Specifics on a number of functional deficits and clear suggestions, and practical guidelines for adapting activities and modifying the environment to enhance performance, given these functional deficits, are provided. Levy reviews basic principles of Allen's cognitive disabilities frame of reference and uses this as a basis for identifying adaptations to facilitate functional performance for different cognitive levels. The challenges of

adapting activities for an individual with a dual diagnosis of cognitive and physical disabilities are thoughtfully explored. Although Levy focuses on elderly individuals in this chapter, many strategies she identifies are applicable to persons of all ages with physical or cognitive disabilities. Her critique that there is often a lack of a match between activity participation and the strengths and capacities of the aged and her concerns over the dearth of role opportunities that use and maintain these strengths are clearly relevant to all populations with disabilities, regardless of age or diagnosis. Levy emphasizes that altering the demands and structure of activities and modifying the environment to maximize remaining capacities can facilitate successful performance in desired life activities and support the adaptation and development of valued social roles.

Although Levy's approach to disabilities is largely compensatory, Chapter 44 by Toglia presents a multicontext treatment approach for cognitive perceptual impairments that can enhance generalization of learning. Toglia reviews literature on learning and generalization, presenting an organizational framework of learning that considers the environmental context, nature of the task, learning criteria, metacognition processing strategies, and learners' characteristics. Based on this organizational framework she presents the multicontext treatment approach. The five components of this approach include the use of multiple environments, identification of criteria for transfer, metacognitive training, emphasis on processing strategies, and use of meaningful activities. Each treatment component is discussed with its relevance to function and its application to OT intervention clearly described and substantiated by a strong review of pertinent literature. Numerous practical examples and a comprehensive case report illustrate how the components of this treatment approach can be used in an integrated manner during cognitive–perceptual rehabilitation. Toglia addresses the realistic limitations of this approach given the diversity of brain injuries. Her call for increased research in this challenging area is a valid one. Fortunately, Tolgia's work here provides a solid theoretical foundation to guide this research and enhance the efficacy of clinical practice.

Chapter 42 by Dutton examines another topic of importance to occupational therapists that is worthy of further study through formal research and in clinical practice. The use of exercise versus activity has been a controversial topic that has often separated occupational therapists into two opposing factions with divergent views on what comprises a legitimate tool of OT and what defines OT's role on the health care team. Dutton reviews this divisive topic, identifying current issues affecting OT practice in acute care and rehabilitation settings that have resulted in an increased demand for the use of exercise instead of activity in OT intervention. She presents a thought-provoking and balanced discussion that recognizes the advantages and limitations of using exercise and activity in treatment, given the diversity of clinical problems and realities of current practice. She proposes a resolution of this exercise versus activity conflict that would use exercise as preparation and purposeful activity as application in a treatment plan. In her proposal, exercise and activity are not mutually exclusive or philosophically opposed treatment approaches; rather, they are two ends of a treatment continuum with preparation (exercise) at one end and application (activity) at the other. Dutton presents several specific continua from two OT frames of reference, the biomechanical and sensorimotor, that can be used to provide specific guidelines for treatment beginning with the use of exercise as preparation, then moving along each continuum to use purposeful activity as application. The value of integrating preparation through exercise with the application of purposeful activity is supported by clear, relevant clinical examples. Dutton emphasizes that movement along these continua must be planned according to a frame of reference to ensure functional improvement and satisfying role performance.

The question as to what constitutes the legitimate tools of OT and the press to integrate a diversity of potentially controversial approaches into current OT practice is further explored in Chapter 45, which reproduces three *Occupational Therapy Week* articles that addressed these vital issues. (The reader is referred to Appendix H, which contains the official AOTA Position Paper on Physical Agent Modalities for further information on this topic.) Pedretti begins this discussion by providing a frame of reference for the use of adjunctive modalities. She reviews OT's philosophical base, emphasizing the primary role purposeful activity plays in OT practice. Current health care issues and trends that have resulted in the use of adjunctive modalities are also presented. Pedretti proposes a four-stage treatment continuum according to the occupational performance frame of reference that takes the client from dependence to life role resumption by using a diversity of methods and modalities along this continuum. She emphasizes that all methods must consider the context of a client's occupational performance to be OT. This vital link between technique and functional performance is further supported by the review of the use of technology in OT presented in this chapter's next section. The historical relationship between technology and OT is discussed, and the cultural, social, individual, and historical relevance of technology is explored. The practice implications and the potential consequences of using technology in OT are examined with a caution voiced against using technology in an isolated manner. The ethical responsibilities of occupational therapists who use technology in their practice are emphasized because these ethical considerations are essential to ensure competent use of technology to enhance functional perfor-

mance. This discussion of competence and ethics is continued in the last section of this chapter, which examines the realistic limits of entry-level education and the need for continuing professional education to develop and maintain competence in accordance with AOTA's Code of Ethics and to ensure mastery in specialized areas. The need for occupational therapists to critically examine and reevaluate the expanding scope of OT practice, the growth of specialization, and the congruence between OT's philosophical base and media and methods used in practice is emphasized. This affirmation of the fundamental principles of OT and the call for individuation of treatment using purposeful activities in environmental contexts is reflected in each of the three sections of this chapter as they all appropriately reflect on OT's philosophical base.

This emphasis on integrating the fundamental principles of OT's philosophical base into daily OT treatment is continued in Chapter 46, which explores the integration of play (a most relevant purposeful activity for a child) into neurodevelopmental treatment (NDT). The authors, Anderson, Hinojosa, and Strauch, review the literature on play and the importance of play to a child with a disability, providing a conceptual foundation for their discussion. The ability of play to motivate a child to interact with his or her environment in an enjoyable and satisfying manner is clearly beneficial to treatment, adding a motivational dimension that isolated methods or modalities cannot. Issues related to combining play activities with neurodevelopmental principles are examined, and the challenges faced by therapists as they attempt to use play in NDT are realistically discussed. Selected suggestions for integrating and adapting activities to help solve some of the difficulties inherent in the introduction of activities to neurodevelopmental treatment with children with disabilities are provided. Concrete recommendations regarding the use of age-appropriate toys and play activities in treatment using NDT approaches provide a basis for creative individuation of treatment. This holistic approach to treatment using purposeful activities can fulfill a variety of therapeutic goals to help the child with a disability develop needed skills for current and future mastery of his or her environment.

The need for occupational therapists to work on environmental mastery is further explored in the next two chapters that examine the use of technological aids to enhance functional performance and increase independence. Many persons with disabilities cannot effectively master their environment, particularly if they have a severe disability or multiple disabilities; therefore, the use of technology to develop skills is often essential. Well-designed interdisciplinary programs that provide technological evaluations and interventions by using collaborative processes among occupational therapists, rehabilitation engineers, consumers, their families, and other team members are presented in these two chapters. The referral process, evaluation methods, various clinical problems, and potential solutions are described. In Chapter 47, Gordon and Kozole discuss and contrast benefits and limits of commercial aids, modified equipment, and custom devices; Pendleton, Somerville, Magdalena, and Bowman, in Chapter 48, discuss the alternatives of having a client learn a new technique for performing an activity or adapting behavior to eliminate the need for equipment. The benefits of a strong team approach in offering the most comprehensive services to individuals with disabilities are clearly presented in both chapters. The vital role occupational therapists perform on this team is emphasized by Pendleton et al.; they view occupational therapists as the experts in functional assessment, activity analysis, and the teaching of activities. Realistic considerations concerning cost containment, reimbursement limits, functional status, and prognosis are reviewed by Gordon and Kozole. Both chapters include two case studies that demonstrate the application of interdisciplinary principles to evaluation and intervention, resulting in increased functional levels and enhanced independent living through technology. A strong emphasis on considering the client's stated needs and goals relevant to his or her role environment and life activities is also reflected in both chapters, providing a humanistic perspective on technological approaches.

In Chapter 49, Friedland moves the exploration of OT tools of practice from a focus on high technology to the "low-tech" use of diversional activity. She presents a historical review of the concept of diversion, its philosophical foundations, and its relationship to the origins and development of the profession of OT. The psychological benefits of diversional activity, particularly as a way to decrease stress and increase morale, as evident in its use during the two world wars, are discussed. The impact of the adoption of the medical model on OT and the role that diversional activity played in OT treatment is explored. Friedland states that, as a result of reductionism, the entire concept of diversion was dismissed, along with much of the profession's focus on occupation. She finds the recent return to an emphasis on functioning and occupational performance to be heartening and offers a thoughtful exploration of current treatment rationales supportive of the therapeutic benefits of diversional activity. Three current and relevant treatment approaches—stress models, cognitive therapy, and logotherapy—that effectively use diversional activity in a purposeful manner to achieve treatment goals and increase quality of life are discussed. Friedland questions the total abandonment of diversional activity in OT practice and makes a strong case for the selective use of diversional activity for those patients who need assistance in coping with their illness or disability and who need guidance in selecting activities that can maintain health and prevent a secondary psychosocial disability.

A common diversional activity that many people use to relieve stress and maintain health is listening to music. Chapter 50 by MacRae examines the healing power of music and the potential for music to serve as a therapeutic modality. A literature review on how music is used in treatment for pain management, sensorimotor dysfunction, and cognitive disabilities is provided. MacRae discusses the therapeutic effects of music and its present and potential application in OT for a diversity of populations. Her view that the inherently motivating and pleasurable aspects of music, and the ability of musical activities to be easily graded to promote health, supports the use of music as a tool of practice that is consistent with OT's philosophical base. Although many occupational therapists use music in their practice, there is limited documentation on these clinical applications of music; therefore, MacRae calls for increased research on the use of music in OT to explore its effectiveness as a therapeutic modality.

The next chapter in this section also considers a therapeutic modality that has little documented research on its application in OT practice but is (hopefully) commonly used by many occupational therapists. This modality is the conscious use of humor. Tooper explores the purposeful use of humor as a therapeutic technique, reviewing the health benefits of humor and laughter as identified in the literature and presented at several seminars and workshops. She discusses commonly held viewpoints about humor and provides ideas on the use of humor as a planned activity in health and educational settings. Concrete suggestions and practical guidelines for the development and use of humor are provided and supplemented with case examples. She concludes that the use of humor by professionals can lighten the daily stresses of clinical practice and benefit clients' physical and mental health.

The broad range of OT tools of practice is evident in this section—from humor and music to computers and adjunct modalities—a diversity of treatment techniques are used in daily OT practice. However, these treatment approaches are not purposeful if they are not related to a goal that is meaningful to the client. Therefore, in Chapter 52, the last in this section, Peloquin presents an outstanding discussion on linking purpose to procedures during each therapeutic interaction we have with our clients. She explores the effectiveness of a collaborative approach that involves patients in their treatment and examines the increased efficacy of treatment when clients know the purpose of each given treatment session. Peloquin presents a clear rationale for discussing with patients the relevance and purpose of any and all procedures. Her stand, that each treatment session is an opportunity to link goals through patient–therapist collaboration with a structured activity in a manner relevant to clients' daily life, is a strong one. The critical importance of consistently integrating goal statements with

OT treatment is based on three realities that influence daily OT practice. These realities include current health care trends, traditional OT assumptions and the often ambiguous nature of activity that is OT's primary modality. Current health care emphasis on informed consent, treatment accountability, and patient rights provide strong justification for incorporating a collaborative approach into each OT session.

The collaborative approach is highly congruent with OT's philosophical assumptions and the traditional views of linking purpose to activity for all clients, regardless of functional level. Given the often limited knowledge the public has of OT and the often ambiguous nature of activity, the ability to consistently articulate the purpose of an OT treatment method is paramount. Peloquin provides concrete examples and realistic suggestions for developing a collaborative approach. Providing the purpose of each activity can increase patients' knowledge about the reasons for the treatment, thereby increasing the level of active participation in the session. Considering the decreases in treatment lengths of stays, the importance of occupational therapists recommitting themselves to developing meaningful relationships with their patients cannot be ignored, no matter what tools of practice are used in treatment.

Sadly, many therapists seem to forget the vital importance of the collaborative relationship in treatment because they limit their interactions with clients to the physical set-up of treatment methods. I've personally observed this many times and have had students express their concerns about the lack of individuation of OT treatment as they see therapists move from treatment set-up to treatment set-up with no personalization of goals provided to them or the clients. Although some clients will protest and demand explanations for their treatment activities, others will simply refuse to engage in the selected activity or will complete the activity in a superficial manner, thereby limiting the activity's therapeutic potential. To illustrate this point, a student told of a patient who was set up with a peg board and told to first remove all of the pegs from the board and then return them to their original position. The patient politely asked the therapist for a bottle of glue. When the therapist inquired as to why the patient needed glue, the patient adamantly replied "So I can glue these *!#?! pegs in permanently and not be forced to do this *!#?! again!" Fortunately for the patient, this therapist was a COTA, Daniel Ngowe, who recognized the lack of meaning in this treatment activity and who sought to introduce more purposeful activities with relevant therapeutic rationales into this client's treatment program. Daniel was also the OTR student who shared this story with his classmates as we discussed strategies for re-introducing purpose into OT treatment settings that have become dominated by techniques and modalities.

Although some therapists will argue that constraints within the current care system force them to use treatment techniques and modalities in an isolated, reductionist manner (as they scurry from patient set-up to patient set-up with little interaction with their clients), others will maintain a holistic approach in spite of system limitations and the use of adjunctive modalities (West and Wiemer, 1991). Ahlschwede (1992) describes an approach to treatment that is realistic in the current health care system and congruent with OT's philosophical base. She states that the time "during which a patient's hand is sandwiched between hot packs is spent discussing occupational performance or daily living components, collaborative goal setting, and patient education...or addressing psychosocial concerns or issues that the patient may have. The remainder (and majority) of each session is then spent in traditional, graded functional activities" (p. 650). It is hoped that the chapters in this section, and throughout the book, will provide the reader with invaluable information to facilitate the use of traditional and nontraditional OT tools of practice in a collaborative manner that is purposeful and meaningful to the patient, for this is the art and science of OT.

Questions to Consider

1. Identify major tools of OT practice. Describe the main therapeutic purposes of these tools. How would you explain these purposes to a client to increase their understanding of your therapeutic rationale and to enhance their participation in these treatment activities?

2. Pair up with a colleague to debate the pros and cons of using adjunctive modalities and physical agent modalities (PAMs) in OT treatment. Use the references provided here, at the end of each chapter, and in Appendix M to support your viewpoints.

3. Review the following case entitled "Helen and the disappearing pegs." Identify the tools of practice and principles of treatment that were used and those that were not used in the described treatment session. Explain how the missing tools of practice could be used to increase the relevance of Helen's OT treatment. Identify a diversity of purposeful activities that could have been used in this case to facilitate Helen's crossing of the midline with her upper extremity in a functional manner. Describe how you would have explained the purposes of these activities to this client to facilitate her active participation in this treatment session.

Helen and the Disappearing Pegs

Helen was an elderly woman with multiple physical disabilities including diabetes, double lower extremity amputations, expressive aphasia, upper extremity (UE) weakness, and decreased UE range of motion. She had a feeding tube and was dependent in all activities of daily living. She was also perceived by many to have a major cognitive deficit, for her interactions with her environment were limited to moans and attempts to remove her feeding tube and slide out of her wheelchair. One day, while waiting with my brother in the OT clinic, we observed a therapist place numerous pegs on the right side of Helen's lapboard and a basket on the floor to the left of her wheelchair. The therapist told Helen her activity for the day was to pick up each peg and drop it into the basket. She demonstrated the desired movement and then asked Helen to begin the activity. Helen dutifully picked up a peg, crossed her midline and dropped the peg into the basket. The therapist praised Helen and told her to continue this activity until all of the pegs were placed in the basket. She then walked away to set up another patient with a "treatment activity." Helen watched her walk away and as the therapist began to talk to another client, Helen placed her forearm on her lapboard and by moving her forearm across the surface she placed all of the pegs in the basket in one fell swoop. A gasp of breath and then laughter came from both my brother and I as we witnessed her cleverness in completing her assigned task. Helen instantly turned her gaze to us, giving us a stern look and placing her index finger to her lips, she nonverbally commanded us to "Shh!" We complied and Helen serenely waited for the therapist to return. After about 20 minutes,

the therapist returned to shower Helen with profuse praise for doing the activity so well. A transporter was then summoned to take Helen back to her room. As she was wheeled past us, Helen gave us a profound wink and a smile. Thereafter, each time Helen saw my brother and I, she would wink and put her finger to her lips. This supposedly cognitively disabled woman turned out to be one sharp lady with a great sense of humor. It was tragic that so few ever got to know her and that the potential of OT was never realized for her.

References

Ahlschwede, K. (1992). The issue is: Views on physical agent modalities and specialization within occupational therapy: A rebuttal. *American Journal of Occupational Therapy, 46,* 650–652.

Hopkins, H. L., & Smith, H. D. (Eds.) (1993). *Willard and Spackman's Occupational Therapy.* Philadelphia, PA: J.B. Lippincott.

McGarry, J. (1990). National perspective: Our special skill—Is it lost? *Canadian Journal of Occupational Therapy, 57,* 258–259.

Mosey, A. C. (1986). *Psychosocial Components of Occupational Therapy.* New York, NY: Raven Press.

West, N. L., & Wiemer, R. B. (1991). The issue is: Should the Representative Assembly have voted as it did, when it did, on occupational therapists' use of physical agent modalities? *American Journal of Occupational Therapy, 45,* 1143–1147.

Chapter 39

Tools of Practice: Heritage or Baggage?

1986 Eleanor Clarke Slagle Lecture

Kathlyn L. Reed

This chapter was previously published in the *American Journal of Occupational Therapy, 40*, 597–605. Copyright © 1986, American Occupational Therapy Association.

Over the years, occupational therapists have adopted or adapted numerous media and methods. The list is so long it staggers the imagination. Yet explanations for the changing practice scene are rare. Few therapists seem to know *why* media come and go or even *when* or *how* various media or methods became part of the occupational therapy tool kit. Why do occupational therapists drop some media or methods like so much excess baggage? Is occupational therapy losing its heritage or keeping up with the times?

The question of heritage first occurred to me during Mary Fiorentino's Slagle Lecture (Fiorentino, 1975). She said she used no arts and crafts in her clinic, implying that such media were no longer useful in the treatment tool kit of occupational therapists. Many people applauded her pronouncement as if occupational therapy finally had shed its 19th century image and joined the 20th century. Her denunciation of arts and crafts set me thinking. Why did arts and crafts become a medium of occupational therapy in the first place? What about other media and methods, such as sanding blocks or work-related programs? Discussions with colleagues produced few answers except that arts and crafts had always been taught since the days of the founders. Therefore, I decided to investigate the literature, historical documents, and old photographs to find some answers.

The objective of this article is to suggest reasons why certain media and methods have evolved as the treatment of choice in occupational therapy in a particular period of time. Likewise, a discussion of why certain media and methods fall into disfavor is relevant.

Definition of Media and Methods

A *medium* is an intervening mechanism through which a force acts or an effect is produced (Morris, 1981). In therapy the medium is the means by which the therapeutic effect is transmitted. A sanding block, a weaving loom, a vestibular board, and a large plastic ball are all media or means by which the therapeutic effect of occupational therapy is activated. Of course, the same objects can be used for other purposes not related to the therapeutic effect of occupational therapy.

Methods are the manner of performing an act or operation: a procedure or technique (*Dorland's*, 1985). In therapy the methods constitute the steps, sequence, or approach used to activate the therapeutic effect of a medium. Examples include one-handed techniques, joint protection, work simplification, and activity configuration. Thus, media and methods are two sides of the same coin. Media provide the means, and methods provide the manner through which the therapeutic effect of occupational therapy is achieved.

Definitions describe but do not determine what will become a therapeutic medium or method. To discover how an object or approach becomes identified as having therapeutic potential, one must look outside a dictionary. Analysis of media and methods over several years has suggested to me that there are eight primary factors that account for which media and methods are selected or discarded from the occupational therapy tool kit. These factors are cultural, social, economic, political, technological, theoretical, historical, and research (Christiansen, 1981; Cynkin, 1979; Di Sante, 1978; English, 1975; Jantzen, 1964; Johnson, 1983; Kielhofner, 1985; Kielhofner & Burke, 1983).

Factors in Selecting and Discarding Media and Methods

Culture is the most pervasive but hidden factor in the selection of media and methods in occupational therapy practice (Cynkin, 1979; Kielhofner, 1985). Occupational therapy was organized around the concept of improving people's abilities to deal with their daily lives. Therefore, it is logical that activities, occupations, or daily living tasks would be selected and used as media and methods. The activities, occupations, and daily living tasks are determined by the culture in which a person lives. A simple example is eating utensils. In Western culture the knife, fork, and spoon are used, but in Eastern culture chopsticks are used to get food from the serving vessel to the mouth. Thus, an occupational therapy clinic in America likely will contain eating utensils that resemble knives, forks, and spoons, but an occupational therapy clinic in Japan likely will contain chopsticks or adaptations of chopsticks.

The social factor is more conspicuous than the cultural (Cynkin, 1979; Kielhofner, 1985). Media and methods are subject to social acceptance or nonacceptance, which often is influenced by marketing and advertising strategies and changing values. The marketing strategies and changing values in turn create fads or trends that influence purchasing decisions. An example is the ongoing issue of whether handmade or machine-made products are superior in quality and value. Is there a difference in the warmth provided by a sweater made of the same yarn when one is handmade and the other made by machine? Probably not. Why then would a person pay

more for one than the other? Because social factors, such as perceived value, enter the picture.

The economic factor affects the selection or discarding of media because some media cost more to use and may or may not be reimbursable by third-party insurance. Building a 16-foot boat could be a very therapeutic occupational activity, but the cost is a little high for many therapists' budgets and probably not reimbursable through most health insurance plans.

The impact of political factors on media and methods has been well documented. Diversional methods of occupational therapy have been ruled out of reimbursable services for many years. More recently there have been disputes over the use of occupational therapy for people with hip replacements or sensory integrative dysfunction.

Technological factors can have a dramatic impact on the media and methods of occupational therapy. Perhaps the best example is the change that has occurred in splinting with the advent of plastics. Originally splints were made from plaster reinforced with wire. The process was tedious, and the product subject to frequent breakdown. Then came plastics, but they had to be heated at high temperatures and tended to become brittle with age. The advent of low temperature plastics allowed a splint to be made in a few minutes in a small frying pan. Splints from this material last for many months without noticeable change in molecular structure.

Some media and methods develop directly from a given theoretical model. An example is the use of vestibular boards, which is a direct application of the sensory integration model. When a medium or method is associated only with one theoretical model, it is easy to determine the origin. However, some media and methods can be used within a variety of theoretical models, and thus identification becomes more difficult. Cooking, for example, can be viewed as essential to nutrition, a pleasurable reward, a social activity, a paid vocation, a leisure skill, or an educational task. How many theoretical models encompass cooking as a medium and method?

The historical factor influences media and methods because some media and methods have been associated with occupational therapy from the earliest records and their origin is now obscure. For example, the use of the bicycle jigsaw can be traced back to occupational therapy clinics in 1918, but the trail is difficult to follow beyond that point. Who built the first bicycle jigsaw, and what was the original therapeutic objective?

Finally, research influences the selection and discarding of media and methods. For example, the research on building muscle strength led to the concept of progressive resistive exercise, which in turn led to the development or adaptation of media that can be modified to provide increased resistance. Many floor looms were modified in the 1950s and 1960s to provide increased resistance to shoulder, arm, hand, and leg muscles.

These factors can be explained further in a set of assumptions about their effect on the selection and discarding of media and methods in occupational therapy. The 14 assumptions can be stated as follows:

1. Media and methods become tools of occupational therapy through one or more of the eight factors.
2. Media and methods disappear from the tool kit of occupational therapy because of one or more of the eight factors.
3. The factors may operate to change the selection or discarding of media and methods singly or, more often, in combination.
4. Occupational therapists should understand the effects of the eight factors on the media and methods used in occupational therapy practice. (See Table 1 for a list of subfactors under the factors.)
5. Media and methods are selected from the dominant existing culture.
6. The sociocultural meaning of a medium and its methods may change over time and be used for a different reason or be discarded.
7. When the sociocultural rationale for a medium or method is lost or changed, the medium may be used in therapy in ways that make little sense to patients or other health professionals.
8. Economic considerations affect the selection and discarding of media and methods and thus restrict their use if the price is too high or if the cost is not reimbursable.
9. Changes in political issues may restrict or facilitate both the selection and use of various media and methods in occupational therapy based on decisions to cover them under or to exclude them from health care programs.
10. Technology introduces new possibilities or modifies existing ones, allowing new media or methods to emerge.
11. Media and methods may be selected because they operationalize an existing theoretical model recognized by the profession.
12. A medium or method may be used in more than one model. Therefore, the therapist must know why a medium or method is being used and change the explanation when a new model is adopted.
13. Historical precedent is the least desirable justification for the existence and continued use of a medium or method but the easiest to explain.
14. Selection and use of media and methods based on research and study is the most professionally responsible approach to justifying the use of a medium or method but the most difficult to obtain.

To illustrate how the eight factors and 14 assumptions operate, I have selected three media and their methods from among the many possible choices. The three are arts and crafts, sanding blocks, and work-related programs. Arts and crafts will illustrate the cultural, social, technological, and historical factors; the sanding blocks will illustrate the theoretical and research factors; and work-related programs will illustrate the political and economic factors.

Arts and Crafts

The use of arts and crafts as media and methods in occupational therapy is directly attributable to the arts and crafts movement that was in full swing during the formative years of occupational therapy early in this century (Levine, in press-a, in press-b [see Chapter 3]). The movement was designed as a cure for the social ills of a society struggling to deal with the impact of the Industrial Revolution. During the 1800s, Western civilization changed from an agrarian to a manufacturing economy; from a cottage industry to a mass production society; from a consumer-driven marketplace to a producer-driven marketplace; from a patronage system to an industrial wealth system; from pride in workmanship to concern for profit; and from an ordered society of similar cultural backgrounds to a disordered society of many cultures and customs. These factors all played a role in the demise of moral treatment. The arts and crafts movement provided a means of revitalizing the ideas of

---

Table 1
Factors in the Selection and Use of Media and Methods

1. Cultural factor	5. Technological factor
Dominant culture	New invention
Subdominant culture	Modification of
2. Social factor	known invention
Upper, middle or	6. Theoretical factor
lower class custom	Organismic philoso-
Fad or tradition	phy
3. Political factor	Mechanistic philoso-
Family or extended	phy
family politics	7. Historical factor
Local community	Significant
politics	Incidental
State or national	8. Research factor
politics	Supports statements
4. Economic factor	Refutes statements
Budget of department	
or hospital	
Reimbursement policies	

---

moral treatment in a new rationale, which the founders and early leaders of occupational therapy were quick to understand. Thus, the arts and crafts movement is the missing link between moral treatment, which dominated the practice of medicine in the 1800s, and the treatment models to follow.

The arts and crafts movement began in England. The original philosophy was based on the "conviction that industrialization had brought with it the total destruction of 'purpose, sense and life'" (Naylor, 1971). Mechanical progress had been gained at the expense of human misery and the destruction of fundamental human values. Thus, the arts and crafts movement "was inspired by a crisis of conscience" (Naylor, 1971). Its motivations were social and moral, and its aesthetic values derived from the conviction that a society produces the art and architecture it deserves (Naylor, 1971). To that idea could be added the thought that society produces the life-style it deserves.

Many people contributed ideas and thoughts to the arts and crafts movement, and not all agreed as to their importance. Therefore, a summary of concepts must be general. The arts and crafts movement did the following:

- Advocated the simplification of life and ordering of daily activity as opposed to the overcomplicated or idle life (Borris, 1986; Kornwolf, 1972; Lears, 1981; Shi, 1985; Wagner, 1904);
- Valued the "craftsman" ideal, in which occupation was pursued at its own pace and not on a production schedule (Borris, 1986; Kornwolf, 1972; Lears, 1981);
- Valued the standard of craftsmanship that gave an honest day's work for an honest day's pay, rather than exploitation of the worker or cheating by the employee (Borris, 1986; Kornwolf, 1972; Naylor, 1971);
- Favored returning to the land and the home as a means of escaping the crowded, unhealthy, unnatural conditions of the city and factory (Lears, 1981; Shi, 1985);
- Ennobled the power of handwork as useful, important, a joy, and a pleasure, as opposed to mindless, repetitive activity on an assembly line, which was viewed as drudgery (Borris, 1986; Lears, 1981);
- Promoted an appreciation of performing the process and the inherent satisfaction or pride in doing or making a product, as opposed to concern only for sale and profit (Naylor, 1971);
- Encouraged respect for the inherent properties of materials and opposed any deception designed to make a material look like something it was not (Kornwolf, 1972);
- Considered functionalism and fitness of purpose the best guide to decoration, as opposed to

ornamentation that served no purpose (Borris, 1986; Kornwolf, 1972);
- Believed that manual training of children would increase knowledge of moral aesthetics and improve work skills, as opposed to intellectual learning only (Borris, 1986; Lears, 1981);
- Valued the creative spirit in the artist and abhorred the mindless copying of designs (Borris, 1986);
- Attempted to improve the standards of taste and aesthetics, as opposed to allowing moral decay (Borris, 1986; Shi, 1985); and
- Viewed people as more than mere machines; human beings as having morals, values, and a sense of purpose (Kornwolf, 1972; Shi, 1985).

One early influence of the arts and crafts movement on occupational therapy came from Jane Addams. In 1900 she started the Hull House Labor Museum, because she wanted young people to see that the complicated machinery of the factory had evolved from the simple tools that their parents had used in the old country before immigrating to America. She wanted to interest young people in the older forms of industry so they would see "a dramatic representation of the inherited resources of their daily occupation" (Addams, 1945). The Labor Museum not only showed how spinning, weaving, pottery, and many other crafts were done, but also provided classes to teach people how to do the crafts. Addams admonished educators, saying that "educators have failed to adjust themselves to the fact that cities have become great centers of production and manufacture, and manual labor has been left without historic interpretation or imaginative uplift" (Addams, 1900, p. 236). Thus, when the training courses for attendants were started in 1907, in conjunction with the Chicago School of Civics and Philanthropy, there was a stress on the idea that occupation should be used as a means of education and that education was to substitute for custodial care of the mentally ill(20th *Biennial Report*, 1909).

In 1914, Eleanor Clarke Slagle started the Community Workshop under the auspices of the Illinois Society of Mental Hygiene. Its purpose was to serve as a clearinghouse for cases of doubtful insanity whom the courts considered as showing promise of a return to usefulness if given a proper environment and trade (Favill, 1917). The environment was the Hull House Labor Museum. In 1917 the Community Workshop became the Henry B. Favill School of Occupations. The following year, the first course in curative occupations and recreation was offered (*Special Courses*, 1917). Again the Labor Museum at Hull House served as the laboratory until the school was moved to the headquarters of the Illinois Society of Mental Hygiene in late 1919.

Another person to incorporate the ideas of the arts and crafts movement into treatment was Herbert J. Hall.

In 1904 Hall began his studies of alternate treatments to the "rest cure" for neurasthenia. He was assisted by Jessie Luther, OTR, the first curator of the Hull House Labor Museum (Luther, 1902). Hall states that the "modern Arts and Crafts idea appealed very strongly, because of the growing interest in the movement and because of the clean, wholesome atmosphere which surrounds such work, and because of the many-sided appeal which such a work as the making of pottery, for instance, has to most educated minds" (Hall, 1905). Hall believed that faulty living was the cause of neurasthenia and that what was needed was a change in occupation and habits. Manual work based on the life of the artisan (craftsman ideal) was recommended itself because it was simple. The "simple life," he felt, was best for neurasthenics because it offered the least food for the nourishment of neurasthenia and provided a structure of normality. Today the person with neurasthenia would be classified as suffering from stress or burnout. The "simple life" would be called stress reduction, and the "craftsman ideal" would be called time management.

In 1906 Hall received a grant from the Procter Fund of Harvard University for $1,000 to "assist in the study of the treatment of neurasthenia by progressive and graded manual occupation." His study at Marblehead, Massachusetts, probably was the first grant-funded research project on the use of occupation as a means of treating patients. He reported that 59 of 100 patients improved, 27 were much improved, and 14 received no relief (Hall, 1910).

The arts and crafts philosophy was summarized in the "Philosophy of Occupation Therapy" by Adolf Meyer (1922) (see Chapter 2). He said, "Our industrialism has created the false idea of success in *production* to the point of overproduction, bringing with it a kind of nausea to the worker and a delirium of the trader..."—in other words, loss of the craftsman ideal. Meyer said, "The man of today has lost the capacity and pride of workmanship and has substituted for it a measure in terms of money." In other words, there was a loss of respect for hand work. And he said that there is "a real pleasure in the use and activity of one's hands and muscles." In other words, one can find pride and satisfaction in performing and doing. Furthermore, "Our body is not merely so many pounds of flesh and bone figuring as a machine."

A final example of the influence of the arts and crafts movement on occupational therapy is the regional location of the arts and crafts societies that developed to organize the work of the arts and crafts movement. The three major areas of the country that responded to the arts and crafts movement were New England, Chicago and the Midwest, and the Pacific area (Clark, 1972). There is a strong correspondence between these three areas and the areas where there are large numbers of occupational therapists today.

The specific location of the societies also influenced occupational therapy. Thirteen states had at least one known arts and crafts society in 1904 (West, 1904). Of the 13, nine (69%) developed early programs in occupational therapy before 1920. All 13 states have occupational therapy programs today (West, 1904).

Considering its influence, what happened to the arts and crafts movement? It was overtaken by World War I. The rules of the game changed for many people. The war effort provided its own sense of purpose. Some industries did hire craftsmen to improve designs, and machine-made products did improve in quality. City life improved as sanitation efforts made inroads against the piles of garbage. The expanding population meant that machine manufacture was the only means of providing products for everyone. Hand production was just too slow and too expensive.

How did the changes influence occupational therapy? What factors were changing the role of the arts and crafts in practice? The cultural scene had shifted: Society was no longer struggling to adapt to city life, and the factory system had been integrated in the fabric of American life. The number of people living on the land would continue to decrease over the coming years. People had become used to the technological changes the factory had produced. Machine-made goods were acceptable and could be made in quantities unknown under the handmade system. Young therapists did not remember the arts and crafts movement and did not know what it represented. They only knew that arts and crafts always had been a part of occupational therapy's tool kit. Finally, a new philosophy was overtaking the profession. The humanistic ideas of the founding years were being challenged as unscientific and unmeasurable. The profession was being reformulated in such a manner that the arts and crafts philosophy made little sense. Not until the 1960s would the founding ideas resurface. Figure 1 illustrates the changing theory and philosophy of the arts and crafts ideology.

Sanding Blocks

Sanding blocks, or sandblocks, are a common sight in many occupational therapy clinics. Nearly all occupational therapists become acquainted with them during their education, and many have made sanding blocks. Yet, few can describe the origin and original purpose of the sanding block or trace the changes in thinking about their use over the years.

Woodworking and sanding can be traced to the beginning of occupational therapy history. The initial use of sanding blocks, however, is unclear. The first mention of them appears in 1934 in an article by Henrietta McNary. In the same article, the first description of an adapted sanding block also appears. Its purpose was to improve opposition. The last article in our literature on a sanding block, a reciprocal sanding device, appears in 1965 (Mathews, 1965). In all, 14 different types of sanding blocks are presented. These are listed in Table 2.

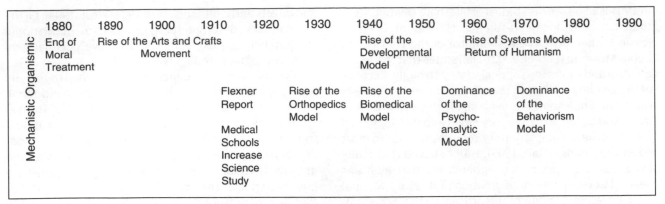

Figure 1. Relative influence of organismic and mechanistic models on occupational therapy practice.

Table 2
Types of Sanding Blocks

1. Proximal sanding blocks (Abbott, 1957; *Photographs,* 1947)
2. Proximal interphalangeal sanding block (Abbott, 1957; *Photographs,* 1947)
3. Metacarpal phalangeal sanding blocks (Abbott, 1957; *Photographs,* 1947)
4. Distal sanding block (Abbott, 1957)
5. Opponens sanding block (Abbott, 1957)
6. Shoulder abduction sanding block ("Adapted," 1957; Bennett & Driver, 1957)
7. Spring squeeze sanding block (Gurney, 1959)
8. Grip sanding block (Hightower et al., 1963)
9. Reciprocal sanding device (Mathews, 1965)
10. Weighted sander or progressive resistive exercise sander (Svensson & Brennan, 1954)
11. Bilateral sander, horizontal or vertical handles (*Photographs,* 1947)
12. Wrist exercise sander (Blodgett, 1947)
13. Hemiplegia sander (Forbes, 1951)
14. Graduated sanding blocks—graduated straight handles or graduated round knob handles (*Photographs,* 1947)

Table 3
Purposes or Objectives of Sanding Blocks

Sanding blocks were adapted to provide the following:

1. Different hand grip position for active or passive stretching:
   a. Handles were added and enlarged.
   b. Holes or grooves were drilled or carved for finger and thumb placement.
   c. Straps were added to hold the hand in place.
   d. Gloves were used to position the hand.
   e. Construction was altered to provide a different grip than that normally used.
2. Dynamic exercise of wrist, elbow, or shoulder—usually range of motion
3. Increased grip strength of hand and fingers
4. Bilateral activity of the upper extremities
5. Reciprocal activity of the upper extremities
6. Improved trunk stability
7. Standing and physical tolerance

The dates of the articles on sanding blocks coincide with the rise and fall of the orthopedic and kinesthetic treatment models of occupational therapy. The orthopedic model followed the arts and crafts model. It was concerned with muscle strengthening and range of motion. Stretching contractures, exercise, and physical tolerance also were included. These concepts form the basis of the objectives for which the sanding block was used. A summary of these purposes or objectives is found in Table 3.

The use of sanding blocks has not disappeared, but the theories underpinning their development and use have been superseded by the sensorimotor and sensory integration models. As a result some unusual uses of sanding blocks have surfaced. For example, one therapist was observed giving a patient a sanding block with no sandpaper and an incline plane made of formica. Because the patient did not want to make anything, the therapist explained that the purpose of the activity was bilateral exercise. In this example, the fundamental concepts of occupational therapy, performance through doing and the use of occupation toward some purpose, were overlooked or separated from the application. The medium of sanding blocks and the methods of setting up the activity to obtain selected objectives had been separated from the original concepts so the meaning and purpose of the activity were lost. The *motion* of sanding is a necessary but not sufficient part of the *activity* of sanding. The media, the methods, and the objective of an occupation must be consistent with each other. Three out of three—medium, method, and objective—must be the rule, not the exception.

Sanding blocks illustrate the factors of theory and research. The many adaptations of the sanding block are based on the theoretical concepts of the orthopedic and kinesthetic treatment models, which stress positioning the body part in the desired pattern of motion and then encouraging that motion to stretch, strengthen, or increase the motion of a particular body part or parts. Research supported the concept that increased amounts of resistance applied to a given muscle group would strengthen the muscle group involved. This concept became known as progressive resistive exercise.

Work-Related Programs

Work-related programs were a part of the early ideology of occupational therapy. The term *work-related programs* is used to represent all efforts to enable people to engage in productive occupations through occupational therapy, whether the effort is aimed at vocational education, vocational guidance, prevocational evaluation and training, vocational training or retraining, vocational readiness, work hardening, work adjustment, or career education.

Hall was very interested in helping patients find an alternate occupation that would be less stressful and more suitable to the person's needs. The "work cure" was based on the assumption that by substituting or bringing about "by a gradual process the conditions of a normal life, a life of pleasant and progressive occupations, as different as possible from the previous life, a person could overcome the mental and nervous problems in his life" (Hall, 1905).

George E. Barton said he was going to "try to prove that the hours of idleness in convalescence could be filled with pastimes which would be useful not only to pass the time, but to prepare the person for remunerative labor later on to get a job, a better Job, or to do a job better than it was before" (Barton, 1914). Consolation House was created to serve the needs of people who were learning to put their lives back together and who needed assistance to find an occupation suitable to their abilities but not limited by their disabilities.

Slagle had experience in assessing people's fitness for a job at the Community Workshop at Hull House. At the founding conference of occupational therapy in Clifton Springs, New York, she spoke of a family of five who had been supported by charities for many years. After one year at the Community Workshop, the family was self-sufficient (Dunton, 1917).

Thomas B. Kidner, Vocational Secretary to the Military Hospitals Commission in Ottawa, Canada, was well acquainted with the vocational side of occupational therapy. In June 1918, he was loaned by the Canadian government to the United States as a special adviser on rehabilitation to the Federal Board for Vocational Education (FBVE). The FBVE had been created the previous year to establish a federal-state program in vocational education. In 1918 it had been given the authority and responsibility for the vocational rehabilitation of veterans ("Editorial," 1922). Elizabeth G. Upham (later Davis), who had been instrumental in starting the occupational therapy course at Milwaukee Downer College, also joined the FBVE in 1918. She wrote two documents illustrating the role of occupational therapy with the disabled veteran (Upham, 1918a, 1918b) and recommended that the FBVE be given control of military patients as soon as possible in order to prepare them for adjustment to normal life (Davis, no date). Had her recommendation been accepted, occupational therapy's role in vocational preparation would have been larger than it has been. Both Kidner and Upham left the FBVE in 1919.

The medical department of the army also had a plan for the rehabilitation of disabled soldiers. It had created a system of orthopedic reconstruction hospitals that included vocational workshops and employment bureaus (Gritzer & Arluke, 1985). The dispute over who would do what came to the floor of the U.S. Senate in July 1918. The medical department of the Army was granted the exclusive right to all aspects of functional restoration and medical control over curative work. This action bound occupational therapy to medicine's domain. The FBVE on the other hand was given responsibility for vocational rehabilitation. The separation became more divided in 1920 when the Industrial Rehabilitation Act was passed without any coverage for medical services. Bulletin #57 of the FBVE makes it quite clear than any occupational work not related to the vocation for which the injured person is being trained is evidently given for its therapeutic value. Therapeutic use of work was viewed as part of the injured person's physical rehabilitation rather than vocational rehabilitation and therefore was not covered under the act ("Industrial rehabilitation," 1920). Thus, occupational therapy was cut off from many of its work-related programs by a political compromise over which it ultimately had little control. Work-related programs were not reestablished until 1943 when the Vocational Rehabilitation Act was changed to include coverage for medical services (Lassiter, 1972). In 1954, the Vocational Rehabilitation Act was further modified to include coverage for the training of rehabilitation personnel, including occupational therapists. In addition there were monies for research and demonstration projects (Lassiter, 1972). Among the demonstration projects were prevocational evaluation and training centers in which occupational therapists played a significant role. However, by the 1960s these projects became too expensive to continue, and the role of occupational therapy in work-related programs again went into a period of decline. Finally in the 1980s the interest returned. A position paper was written and a grant was funded to increase occupational therapists' awareness of the role of occupational therapy in work-related programs. Some of the current interests are assessment of work potential and aptitude skills, physical capacities assessment and work hardening, job evaluation, work experience, career exploration and job seeking skills, independent living, and industrial consultation.

The level of occupational therapists' interest and opportunities in work-related programs has waxed and waned over the past 80 years. The fluctuations can be traced to politics and economics. When both were favorable or neutral, occupational therapists provided many examples of programs designed to help a person to gain or regain productive skills. However, when the politics and economics made it difficult for occupational therapists to provide such skill assessment and skill training, their activity in work-related programs decreased. The challenge will be to shape the political and economic factors in favor of occupational therapy if therapists want to maintain their role in helping people attain or regain productive skills.

Occupational Analysis

As illustrated thus far, the selection and discarding of media and methods in occupational therapy has not been accidental. Factors converge and diverge to increase or decrease the likelihood that a particular medium and its methods will be selected or discarded in the practice of occupational therapy. Culture sets the major parameters, but changes in society frequently alter the cultural set. Political and economic factors often work in combination. Political factors can be influenced by occupational therapists, but some events may occur over which therapists have little control. The results may be felt most keenly economically when reimbursement patterns result in changes in coverage of occupational therapy services. Technology may lead to dramatic changes in media or methods. Theoretical factors often introduce new media and methods into the treatment setting. Sometimes the new theory or model brings new media and methods with it; at other times just the explanation and the use of an existing medium or method changes. History often is used to explain the existence of media or methods when the origin has been lost through time. Research offers a better explanation for the use of media and methods but is more difficult to obtain.

All of these factors need to be considered when examining why certain media and methods appear in a clinic or practice setting. Can practicing occupational therapists explain why each medium or method is used in their practice setting? Is the explanation the best one, or is the explanation of history used by default? Perhaps a more systematic use of occupational or activity analysis should be promoted which includes the selection and discarding of factors as well as considerations such as range of motion, sensory stimulation, or amount of social interaction obtained.

Central to each of the factors are the concepts of interests and values. A culture, individuals, and profes-

sionals have interests and values. An interest is defined as a set that guides behavior in a certain direction or toward certain goals (Chaplin, 1975). A value is a social end or goal that is considered desirable to achieve (Chaplin, 1975).

In occupational therapy there seem to be three major areas to consider in interest and values. These are culture and society, the individual, and the profession. The eight factors that affect selection and discarding of media and methods can be organized under the cultural and social interest and values and professional interests and values. Under the *cultural and social* area are the cultural, social, economic, political, and technological factors. Under the *professional* are the theoretical, historical, and research factors. Under the *individual* are factors that must be determined by assessment of each individual. These are the roles performed by the individual and the functional abilities, skills, and capacities of the individual. When the three areas of cultural-social, individual, and professional interests and values are considered, there should be less chance of using media and methods that are out-of-date in society, not meaningful to the individual, and of questionable use to the profession.

Summary

This article presents and illustrates the major factors that influence the selection and discarding of media and methods in occupational therapy. The eight factors are the cultural, social, economic, political, technological, theoretical, historical, and research factors. The factors may operate in various combinations or alone to influence the use of a specific medium or method in practice. Therapists are encouraged to know these eight factors and in particular to be familiar with (a) what media and methods occupational therapists use, (b) why occupational therapists use those media and methods, (c) from where the media and methods come, (d) with whom the media and methods should be used in treatment, (e) how the media and methods are used, (f) when the media and methods are used, and (g) how much of the medium or method should be used. Educators, in particular, need to teach why a medium or method is used as well as how. Researchers need to provide more information as to why certain media and methods became part of our tool kit. Practitioners would be wise to follow the statement, If you know how, be sure you know why and be sure the why is consistent with the philosophy of occupational therapy.

References

Abbott, M. (1957). *A syllabus of occupational therapy procedures and techniques as applied to orthopedic and neurological conditions.* New York: American Occupational Therapy Association.

Adapted sand block. Part I. (1957). *American Journal of Occupational Therapy, 11,* 198.

Addams, J. (1900). Social education of the industrial democracy. *Commons, 5,* 17–28.

Addams, J. (1945). *Twenty years at Hull House, with autobiographical notes.* New York: Macmillan.

Barton, G. E. (1914). A view of invalid occupation. *Trained Nurse & Hospital Review, 52,* 327–330.

Bennett, R. L., & Driver, M. (1957). The aims and methods of occupational therapy in the treatment of the after-effects of poliomyelitis. *American Journal of Occupational Therapy, 11,* 145–153.

Blodgett, M. L. (1947). Sanding for exercise. *American Journal of Occupational Therapy, 1,* 6.

Borris, E. (1986). *Art and labor: Ruskin, Morris, and the craftsman ideal in America.* Philadelphia, PA: Temple University Press.

Chaplin, J. P. (1975). *Dictionary of psychology* (2nd ed.). New York: Dell.

Christiansen, C. H. (1981). Editorial: Toward resolution of crisis: Research requisites in occupational therapy. *Occupational Therapy Journal of Research, 1,* 115–124.

Clark, R. J. (1972). *The arts and crafts movement in America: 1876-1916.* Princeton, NJ: Princeton University Press.

Cynkin, S. (1979). *Occupational therapy: Toward health through activities.* Boston: Little, Brown.

Davis, E. U. (no date). *Just another biography.* Unpublished manuscript.

Di Sante, E. (1978). Technology transfer: From space exploration to occupational therapy. *American Journal of Occupational Therapy, 32,* 171–174.

Dorland's illustrated medical dictionary (26th ed.). Philadelphia, PA: W. B. Saunders, p. 809.

Dunton, W. R. (1917). *The growing necessity for occupational therapy.* New York: Teachers College. (In AOTA Archives, Moody Library, Galveston, TX).

Editorial: The sixth annual meeting. *Archives of Occupational Therapy, 1,* 419–427.

English, C. B. (1975). Computers and occupational therapy. *American Journal of Occupational Therapy, 29,* 43–47.

Favill, J. (1917). *Henry Baird Favill: 1960-1916.* Chicago: Rand McNally, p. 87.

Fiorentino, M. R. (1975). Occupational therapy: Realization to activation—1974 Eleanor Clarke Slagle lecture. *American Journal of Occupational Therapy, 29,* 15–21.

Forbes, E. S. (1951). Two devices for use in treating hemiplegics. *American Journal of Occupational Therapy, 5,* 49–51.

Gritzer, G., & Arluke, A. (1985). The making of rehabilitation: A political economy of medical specialization, 1890-1980. Berkeley, CA: University of California Press.

Gurney, G. W. (1959). Spring-squeeze sandblock. *American Journal of Occupational Therapy, 13,* 278.

Hall, H. J. (1905). The systematic use of work as a remedy in neurasthenia and allied conditions. *Boston Medical & Surgical Journal, 112,* 29–32.

Hall, H. J. (1910). Work-cure: A report of five years' experience at an institution devoted to the therapeutic application of manual work. *Journal of the American Medical Association, 54,* 12–14.

Hightower, M. D., et al. (1963). Grip sander. *American Journal of Occupational Therapy, 17,* 62–63.

Industrial rehabilitation—A statement of policies to be observed in the administration of the Industrial Rehabilitation Act. (1920). *FBVE Bulletin, 57*

Jantzen, A. C. (1964). The role of research in occupational therapy. *Proceedings of the 1964 Annual Conference* (pp. 2–9). New York: American Occupational Therapy Association.

Johnson, J. A. (1983). The changing medical marketplace as a context for the practice of occupational therapy. In G. Kielhofner (Ed.), *Health through occupation: Theory and practice in occupational therapy* (pp. 163-177). Philadelphia, PA: F. A. Davis.

Kielhofner, G. (Ed.). (1985). *A model of human occupation: Theory and application.* Baltimore, MD: Williams & Wilkins.

Kielhofner, G., & Burke, J. P. (1983). The evolution of knowledge and practice in occupational therapy: Past, present and future (pp. 3–54). In G. Kielhofner (Ed.), *Health through occupation: Theory and practice in occupational therapy.* Philadelphia, PA: F. A. Davis.

Kornwolf, J. D. (1972). *M. H. Baillie Scott and the arts and crafts movement.* Baltimore, MD: Johns Hopkins Press.

Lassiter, R. A. (1972). History of the rehabilitation movement in America. In J. G. Cull & R. E. Hardy (Eds.), *Vocational rehabilitation: Profession and process* (pp. 5–58). Springfield, IL: Charles C Thomas.

Lears, T. J. J. (1981). *No place of grace: Antimodernism and the transformation of American culture: 1880-1920.* New York: Pantheon.

Levine, R. E. (in press-a). Guest editorial: Historical research: Ordering the past to chart our future. *Occupational Therapy Journal of Research.*

Levine, R. E. (in press-b). The influence of the arts and crafts movement on the professional status of occupational therapy. In W. Coleman (Ed.), *Written history monograph.* Rockville, MD: American Occupational Therapy Association.

Luther, J. (1902). The labor museum at Hull House. *Commons, 7,* 1–13.

Mathews, T. (1965). Reciprocal sanding device. *American Journal of Occupational Therapy, 19,* 354–355.

McNary, H. (1934). Anatomical considerations and technique in using occupations as exercise for orthopedic disabilities: III. Wrist and fingers. *Occupational Therapy Rehabilitation, 13,* 24–29.

Meyer, A. (1922). Philosophy of occupational therapy. *Archives of Occupational Therapy, 1,* 1–10. (Reprinted as Chapter 2).

Morris, W. (Ed.). (1981). *American heritage dictionary of the English language.* Boston: Houghton Mifflin, p. 815.

Naylor, G. (1971). *The arts and crafts movement: A study of its sources, ideals and influence on design theory.* Cambridge, MA: MIT Press.

Photographs of occupational therapy adapted equipment as developed in Veterans Administration and Army hospitals. (1947). Washington, DC: Department of Medicine & Surgery, Veterans Administration.

Shi, D. E. (1985). *The simple life: Plain living and high thinking in American culture.* New York: Oxford University Press.

Special courses in curative occupations and recreation. (1917, December). Chicago: Chicago School of Civics and Philanthropy Special Bulletin.

Svensson, V. W., & Brennan, M. C. (1954). Adapted weighted resistive apparatus. *American Journal of Occupational Therapy, 8,* 13.

20th biennial report of the board of public charities of the state of Illinois, July 1, 1906-June 30, 1908. Springfield, IL: Illinois State Journal Co., p. 58.

Upham, E. G. (1918a). Training of teachers for occupational therapy for the rehabilitation of disabled soldiers and sailors. *Federal Board for Vocational Education Bulletin, 6,* 1–76.

Upham, E. G. (1918b). Ward occupations in hospitals. *Federal Board for Vocational Education Bulletin, 25,* 1–57.

Wagner, C. (1904). *The simple life.* New York: Grosset & Dunlap.

West, M. (1904). The revival of handicrafts in America. *Bureau of Labor Bulletin, 55,* 1573–1622.

Chapter 40

The Origin and Evolution of Activity Analysis

Cynthia Creighton

In 1911, industrialization had resulted in unprecedented economic growth for the United States. The average employee worked a 9-hr to 12-hr shift, 6 days per week, for a wage of approximately $2 a day. The automobile assembly line had not yet been invented.

Two books that would revolutionize industry were published that year: *The Principles of Scientific Management* (Taylor, 1911) and *Motion Study* (Gilbreth, 1911). Taylor, past president of the American Society of Mechanical Engineers, proposed in his text that management in business and industry be approached as a true science with clearly defined rules and principles. An important element of Taylor's new system of management was the study and standardization of jobs to increase productivity. Soon, efficiency experts were observing and timing workers in shops and factories nationwide. As a laborer shoveled ore or cut metal, the consultant identified the fundamental operations, the most efficient tools, and the optimum speed for the task.

Gilbreth (1911), 10 years younger than Taylor and also an engineer, was the first to use the term *analysis* when discussing the systematic study of jobs. He believed that the worker's movements should be the focus of such studies. Gilbreth outlined the steps in analyzing a task as follows: "1. Reduce ... practice to writing. 2. Enumerate motions used. 3. Enumerate variables which affect each motion" (p. 5). Three categories of variables were considered in a motion study: characteristics of the worker (e.g., physical build, experience, temperament), characteristics of the surroundings (e.g., lighting, tools), and characteristics of the motion (e.g., direction, length, speed). Gilbreth documented these in chart form and in photographs. The purpose of analyzing a job was to identify and teach the "definite best" (most productive and least fatiguing) method of performance (p. 93).

Gilbreth (1911) also discussed adapting activity to make it more efficient:

> A careful study of the worker will enable one to adapt his work, surroundings, equipment and tools to him. "This will decrease the number of motions he must make, and make the necessary motions shorter and less fatiguing. (p. 10)

In his own bricklaying business, he made adaptations such as reversing the position of materials for left-handed workers and placing stock on a scaffold so the bricklayer no longer had to stoop when picking it up. In 1913, he began founding small museums of devices designed to simplify work and prevent fatigue (Gilbreth & Gilbreth, 1920).

Gilbreth and his wife, Lillian,[1] became well known both at home and abroad as consultants to the business community (Yost, 1949). In 1914 and 1915, Gilbreth visited hospitals in Europe to analyze surgeons' work. World War I had begun, and he met disabled veterans and learned about the groundbreaking research of Jules Amar.

Amar (1918) was a French physiologist appointed by his government to investigate scientific management and apply its principles to the training and reemploying of wounded soldiers. At that time, France led the world in the study of human physiology and the development of instruments to measure physiological functions; Amar began analyzing jobs in terms of their physiological requirements. He described the planes of motion in which work was performed and measured movements with simple goniometers. To document strength requirements, Amar attached spring dynamometers to tools such as a file, a plane, and a spade. He measured energy expenditure during work, using oxygen consumption, pulse rate and blood pressure, and urine and blood by-products as indicators. The results of the analyses were applied in a three-part program to reeducate soldiers (many of them with amputations). At the beginning of the convalescent period, exercise and crafts were used to strengthen stump muscles and build endurance. The patient was then fitted with a prosthesis or splint and taught to use it in vocational tasks.

Occupational Therapy and Motion Study

When Gilbreth returned from his travels, he and his wife presented papers to several professional groups about the application of motion study to "re-education of the crippled soldier" (Gilbreth & Gilbreth, 1920). The theme of the papers was as follows:

In considering any type of activity to which it is proposed to introduce the cripple, we first analyze this activity from the motion study standpoint, in order to find exactly what motions are required to perform the activity and in what way these motions may be adapted to the available, or remaining, capable members of the cripple's working anatomy or eliminated by altering the device or machine itself. (pp. 45–46)

One in this series of papers was presented in March 1917 at the founding conference of the National Society for the Promotion of Occupational Therapy (NSPOT) at Consolation House in Clifton Springs, New York (NSPOT, 1918). Titled "The Conservation of the World's Teeth," it recommended that disabled veterans be retrained as dental assistants (Gilbreth & Gilbreth, 1920). During the meeting, Frank Gilbreth and Jules Amar were elected honorary members of the Society (NSPOT, 1918).

The Gilbreths clearly believed that engineers were best qualified to analyze and adapt jobs for people with disabilities (Gilbreth & Gilbreth, 1920). Still, in their presentations after the Consolation House conference, they began acknowledging the contributions of George Barton and William Rush Dunton, Jr. (first and second presidents of the National Society). Barton and Dunton, in turn, began incorporating motion study into their work and their writings. A paper about Barton's practice with convalescents at Consolation House stated that he

considers what motions are possible or impossible, desirable or undesirable; then he finds some occupation which involves those possible and desired motions.... Failing to find such an occupation in his own knowledge, the "Director" turns to his "materia medica"—a huge fifteen-hundred page catalog of tools and machines—from which, by a visualization of each tool, how it is used and what motions are necessary for its use, he "compounds" his "prescription." (Newton, 1919, pp. 4–5)

Dunton (1919) discussed the work of both Amar and the Gilbreths in his second occupational therapy textbook and provided a bibliography of the Gilbreths's publications on motion study.

When the United States entered World War I, activity analysis was included in the new occupational therapy programs and in training courses that were developed to serve returning American soldiers. In early 1918, Elizabeth Upham wrote a curriculum plan for a proposed government course to train teachers of occupational therapy.[2] The plan, presented to the U.S. Senate and the Federal Board for Vocational Education, stated that students should study "1. Analysis of industrial, commercial and agricultural occupations in terms of therapeutic values. 2. Modification of processes, special devices and tools for special needs and fatigue prevention" (Dunton, 1918, p. 89). Upham's required reading list included selections from Amar's research.[3] Later that year, Upham became director of the first university-based occupational therapy school, at Milwaukee Downer College, Milwaukee (Reed & Sanderson, 1980).

The first systematic application of activity analysis in an occupational therapy clinic may also have been in 1918, at Walter Reed General Hospital in Washington, DC. Bird Baldwin (1919a), director of the new occupational therapy department, described the selection of therapeutic activities for patients as follows:

First, the work must be one which involves as an essential part the movements required by the prescription, or in which these movements recur from time to time as the work is performed by the normal individual. In order to discover the activities in which certain specific movements were thus involved, a survey was made of all the shop and ward activities, and insofar as it was possible by observation and practice, each activity was analyzed into its constituent movements. (p. 449)

Baldwin's activity analyses were detailed but addressed primarily joint position and action. For example, his analysis of engraving described the position of each body part: Fingers flexed at all joints, thumb extended at the interphalangeal and metacarpophalangeal joints to guide the tool, shoulders rigid and slightly abducted. Other important requirements, such as muscle strength and vision, were not delineated, although they were clearly considered when patients' programs were planned (Baldwin, 1919b). Activities were also adapted by changing the tools or methods used when this was indicated to improve the patient's physical function or compensate for deficits.

Between the Wars

In the 1920s, after the NSPOT had become the American Occupational Therapy Association (AOTA), a standing committee of the organization began publishing a series of papers designed to help therapists establish new departments in curative workshops and state psychiatric hospitals (AOTA, 1924). Dunton and Association president Thomas Kidner were among the influential members of the committee. Their reports included guidelines for analyzing crafts[4] in terms of joint motion and muscle strength (AOTA, 1928). Crafts requiring active motion with strength were listed for each body joint, and actions of the two sides of the body were differentiated. No attempt was made to quantify the requirements (e.g., in degrees of range or grades of strength). These craft analyses remained a standard reference for occupational therapists working with physically disabled patients for many years.

In psychiatric occupational therapy, activity analysis took the form of classification of crafts according to their characteristics or applications. Louis Haas, another member of AOTA's standing committee, developed an early system of classification that was widely accepted (Haas, 1922). He analyzed and rated activities in terms of the types of tools and materials used, the noise involved, the potential for modifying methods, the appeal to various ages and sexes, and the simplicity or complexity of processes. As was typical in psychiatry, he was most interested in the characteristics of activities that would address patients' emotional and social needs (e.g., channel aggression, promote self-esteem).

World War II stimulated renewed interest in motion study, now sometimes called *work simplification*. Frank Gilbreth had died, but Lillian Gilbreth published a paper in an occupational therapy journal recommending that engineers and rehabilitation professionals work closely together to help handicapped soldiers (Gilbreth, 1943). The army's War Department (1944) printed a technical manual on occupational therapy that contained the most detailed activity analyses to date. In addition to the traditional breakdown of joint motions, this manual listed activities for strengthening individual upper-extremity and lower-extremity muscles. Charts rating the intensity of motion at each joint during the performance of various tasks were also included.

Activity Analysis Comes of Age

In 1947, Sidney Licht, a physician who had been chief of physical medicine in an army hospital during the war, wrote a paper calling for more precise analysis of activities used in occupational therapy for physical dysfunction. He suggested the name *kinetic analysis* for the study of specific motions required in an occupation. Licht stated that a kinetic analysis should be based on actual observation of an experienced worker using proper body mechanics. It should describe the starting position and cycle of motion for the activity. The type of muscle contraction and degrees of joint range should be specified, as should the size and shape of tools used. Although Licht's terminology was not generally adopted, the elements of such an analysis are addressed today.

Through the 1960s, occupational therapists continued to analyze activities either in terms of physical requirements or in terms of emotional and social properties. In the 1970s and 1980s, however, a new way of thinking about the theory base of the profession led to major changes in activity analysis. Theorists began to delineate frames of reference within which occupational therapy intervention occurred (e.g., developmental biomechanical, behavioral). Because each frame of reference included a unique perspective on the selection and uses of activity, each required a different type of activity analysis. Llorens's (1973) analysis of activities for treatment of cognitive-perceptual-motor dysfunction focused on the sensory systems stimulated and the motor responses produced. Trombly and Scott (1977) differentiated biomechanical analysis (emphasizing range of motion and strength) from neurodevelopmental analysis (emphasizing postures and patterns of movement). Cubie (1985) discussed volitional, habituation, and performance analysis within the Model of Human Occupation. The cognitive requirements of tasks were Allen's focus (1985).

Conclusion

Today, activity analysis is viewed as a multifaceted process (Cynkin & Robinson, 1990; Hopkins & Smith, 1988; Lamport, Coffey, & Hersch, 1989; Mosey, 1986). A comprehensive analysis first places the activity within a cultural and environmental context. Then both its generic properties (e.g., steps, tools used, cost, safety considerations) and its characteristics related to a specific frame of reference are described. The activity is discussed as it is normally performed and as modified for remedial or compensatory applications with patients.

Okoye (1988) provided an example of activity analysis as it is currently applied in occupational therapy. She discussed the importance of the computer as a medium for skill development, education, and prevocational training in our computer age. She presents a form for analyzing a computer-based treatment activity in which the therapist lists the hardware and software needed and answers a series of questions about the characteristics of the activity. The form delineates the neuromotor requirements for accessing the computer (posture, alignment, coordination) and the basic cognitive and sensory integrative functions necessary (visual discrimination, attention, problem solving), because the persons most likely to have difficulty are those with severe physical or multiple handicaps. For each requirement identified, the therapist lists alternative positioning, equipment, or methods for access (e.g., breakaway keyboard, audio reinforcement, software with slower speed options).

Although the original link with industrial engineering and other fields doing time and motion studies in the pursuit of productivity has been severed, occupational therapists continue to use activity analysis essentially as the founders did: to improve the functioning and quality of the lives of persons with disabilities.

Acknowledgment

This work was supported in part by Grant #H133G00139 from the National Institute on Disability and Rehabilitation Research.

References

Allen, C. K. (1985). *Occupational therapy for psychiatric diseases.* Boston: Little, Brown.

Amar, J. (1918). *The physiology of industrial organization and the re-employment of the disabled.* London: Library Press Limited.

American Occupational Therapy Association. (1924). Report of Committee on Installations and Advice. *Archives of Occupational Therapy, 3,* 299–318.

American Occupational Therapy Association. (1928). Report of Committee on Installations and Advice. *Occupational Therapy and Rehabilitation, 7,* 29–43, 131–136, 211–216, 417–421.

Baldwin, B. T. (1919a). Occupational therapy. *American Journal of Care for Cripples, 8,* 447–451.

Baldwin, B. T. (1919b). *Occupational therapy applied to restoration of function of disabled joints.* Washington, DC: Walter Reed General Hospital.

Cubie, S. H. (1985). Occupational analysis. In G. Kielhofner (Ed.), *A Model of Human Occupation: Theory and application.* Baltimore: Williams & Wilkins.

Cynkin, S., & Robinson, A. M. (1990). *Occupational therapy and activities health: Toward health through activities.* Boston: Little, Brown.

Dunton, W. R. (1918). Rehabilitation of crippled soldiers and sailors: A review. *Maryland Psychiatric Quarterly, 7,* 85–101.

Dunton, W. R. (1919). *Reconstruction therapy.* Philadelphia: Saunders.

Gilbreth, F. B. (1911). *Motion study.* New York: Van Nostrand.

Gilbreth, F. B., & Gilbreth, L. M. (1920). *Motion study for the handicapped.* London: Routledge.

Gilbreth, L. M. (1943). The place of motion study in rehabilitation work. *Occupational Therapy and Rehabilitation, 22,* 61–64.

Haas, L. J. (1922). Crafts adaptable to occupational needs: Their relative importance. *Archives of Occupational Therapy, 1,* 443–445.

Hopkins, H. L., & Smith, H. D. (Eds.). (1988). *Willard and Spackman's occupational therapy* (7th ed.). Philadelphia, Lippincott.

Lamport, N. K., Coffey, M. S., & Hersch, G. I. (1989). *Activity analysis handbook.* Thorofare, NJ: Slack.

Licht, S. (1947). Kinetic analysis of crafts and occupations. *Occupational Therapy and Rehabilitation, 26,* 75–78.

Llorens, L. A. (1973). Activity analysis for cognitive-perceptual-motor dysfunction. *American Journal of Occupational Therapy, 27,* 453–456.

Mosey, A. C. (1986). *Psychosocial components of occupational therapy.* New York: Rover.

National Society for the Promotion of Occupational Therapy. (1918). *Proceedings of the first annual meeting of the National Society for the Promotion of Occupational Therapy.* Towson, MD: Author.

Newton, I. G. (1919). *Consolation House.* Clifton Springs, NY: Consolation House.

Okoye, R. L. (1988). Computer technology in occupational therapy. In H. L. Hopkins & H. D. Smith (Eds.), *Willard and Spackman's occupational therapy* (pp. 340–345). Philadelphia: Lippincott.

Reed, K. L., & Sanderson, S. R. (1980). *Concepts of occupational therapy.* Baltimore: Williams & Wilkins.

Taylor, F. W. (1911). *The principles of scientific management.* New York: Harper & Brothers.

Trombly, C. A., & Scott, A. D. (1977). *Occupational therapy for physical dysfunction.* Baltimore: Williams & Wilkins.

War Department. (1944). *Occupational therapy.* Washington, DC: U.S. Government Printing Office.

Yost, E. (1949). *Frank and Lillian Gilbreth.* New Brunswick, NJ: Rutgers University Press.

Notes

[1] Lillian Gilbreth also applied motion study methodology to organizing the Gilbreth's home and raising 12 children while earning her doctorate at Brown University. The American public came to

know the family through the books *Cheaper by the Dozen* and *Belles on Their Toes,* written by two of the children.

[2]The term *occupational therapist* was not yet in use. Practitioners in the new discipline were called *teachers of occupation* or *reconstruction aides.*

[3]An English translation of Amar's most recent text had been published in 1918, making his ideas more accessible to American students.

[4]During this period, the term *crafts* was used more broadly than it is today. Early craft analyses included work-related and recreational activities such as tennis, typing, gardening, and bookbinding.

Chapter 41

Occupation: Form and Performance

David L. Nelson, PhD, OTR, FAOTA

As used in everyday language, *occupation* and its verb root *occupy* are ambiguous terms. The same ambiguity marks other terms of key significance to the profession of occupational therapy, including *activity*, *play*, and *work*. On one hand, each of these terms refers to actual performance, or doing. On the other hand, each of the terms also refers to a preexisting format that guides the human performance. For example, on one hand we can speak of the *occupation* or *activity* of baseball as an established format of rules, procedures, locus, and equipment that preexists and is independent of the actual doing of any specific person. In contrast, we can also speak of a person *being occupied* as a way of describing the actual doing of a series of *activities* over a 2-hour period (e.g., the person throws a ball, hits a ball, runs, talks with teammates, etc.). Is *occupation* the format of the game (the structure) or is it the playing of the game (the doing)?

The ambiguous use of these terms appears in the language of occupational therapists also. We speak of work in the abstract as an *occupation*, and we also speak of a particular worker's behavior as *occupation*. We speak of art forms and crafts as *activities*, and we also speak of the specific actions taken by a particular person as his or her *activity*. This type of ambiguity is common in the everyday usage of words and is documented in dictionaries, such as *Webster's Third New International Dictionary* (s.v. "occupation" and "occupy"). However, such ambiguity can inhibit the development of a profession. One of the first steps in any logical inquiry is to ensure that everyone knows exactly what is being discussed.

Figure 1 eliminates the ambiguity in the term *occupation*. *Occupational form* is the preexisting structure that elicits, guides, or structures subsequent human performance; *occupational performance* consists of the human actions taken in response to an occupational form. The

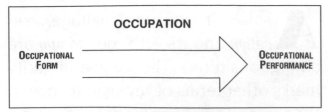

OCCUPATION

OCCUPATIONAL
FORM

OCCUPATIONAL
PERFORMANCE

Figure 1. Occupation defined as a relationship between occupational form and occupational performance, with occupational form as the objective preexisting structure eliciting and/or guiding occupational performance.

term *occupation*, then, need no longer be used ambiguously (to refer to either form or performance); *occupation* can be thought of as the relationship between occupational form and occupational performance. As used in the framework presented here, the term *occupation* always refers to the occupational performance of an occupational form (i.e., the doing of something or the engaging in something).

Occupational Forms

An *occupational form* is an objective set of circumstances, independent of and external to a person. The individual's occupational performance (the doing) can be understood only in terms of the environmental context in which the performance takes place (that is, only in terms of the occupational form). Almost all human contexts are full of richness and variety—the typical occupational form is multidimensional. An occupational form not only tends to have many facets, but also frequently has a preestablished order in the arrangement of its many facets.

Broadly, each occupational form has two types of dimensions.[1] First, each occupational form can be described objectively in terms of physical stimuli present in the immediate environment of the individual at any given point in time. These stimuli include (a) the materials, including the number of objects, their spatial interrelationships, and the physical characteristics of each object; (b) the environmental surround, including the location, the features that separate the immediate environment from the "outside," and potentially competing materials on the fringes of the immediate environment; (c) the human context, including the movement, speech, and appearance of all those in the immediate environment; and (d) the temporal context, including the occupational form's relationships to prior and future events, and the step-by-step changes in the physical environment over the course of the occupation.

Second, each occupational form has a sociocultural reality that exists independently of any specific individual but that depends on social or cultural consensus. Each level of society has its own values, norms, sanctions, symbols, roles, and practical guidelines for interpreting the physical aspects of occupational forms. For example, at the cultural level, there are definite rules governing the symbolic interpretation of speech utterances. Or, at a community level, a specific building may symbolize something recognized by all who see it. Or, at a much more basic level of society, the family, there may be specific norms governing household objects. Other levels of society include the universal (cross-cultural) level, subcultures, political units, regions, institutions, organizations, and friendship circles.

The sociocultural reality of an occupational form might be highly prescribed (ritualistic) or might be loosely organized with much sanctioned opportunity for typical variations or individual interpretations. In addition, though the sociocultural reality of an occupational form might include norms for a typical performance, the actual occupational performance of an individual at a particular time might or might not conform to those norms. The sociocultural reality of an occupational form depends on group consensus, but the consensus is seldom unanimous. Furthermore, the individual encountering an occupational form may or may not be familiar with its socioculturally defined norms and processes (this is a matter of acculturation).

As presented in this paper, an occupational form is a specific environmental context as opposed to a *medium*. A *medium* is a hypothetical set of occupational forms that vary from circumstance to circumstance. For example, weaving is a socioculturally defined medium that can vary considerably from situation to situation depending on the materials (the type of thread and loom); the environmental surround (the nature of the setting, whether one is in one's own home, at school, or at work); the human context (the type of instructions given and the presence or absence of other weavers); and the temporal context (the occupations preceding and following the weaving as well as the step-by-step physical changes occurring during the weaving).

Occupational Performance

The term *performance* means to go through or to carry out something, and *occupational performance* means to go through or carry out the occupational form. Occupational performance is the doing, the action, the active behavior, or the active responses exhibited within the context of an occupational form. Usually, occupational performance is observable to others in the environment (because the response by the doer typically involves behaviorally observable movement). Such responses include gross as well as fine patterns of movement, speech and related vocalizations, ocular movements, facial expressions, and all other voluntary (nonreflexive) movements and postures made possible by motor control. Occasionally, occupational performance may be covert (e.g., an individual may mentally solve a puzzle not requiring any observable response).

As is implied by the arrow in Figure 1, occupational form precedes occupational performance in time. This does not mean that all of the occupational form always precedes all of the performance; on the contrary, as will be seen later, performance at one point in time frequently alters the occupational form guiding subsequent performance. What it does mean is that, at any point in time, occupational performance is guided by a preexisting occupational form, even if the preexisting occupational form is not entirely complete.

Although the arrow in Figure 1 implies temporal precedence, it leaves open the possibility of different types of relationships between occupational form and occupational performance. Changes in occupational forms frequently cause changes in occupational performances. For example, seemingly small changes in the form's materials or instructions can cause large changes in performance. The identification of possible relationships between occupational forms and occupational performances is a matter for empirical research as well as theoretical inquiry. A science of occupation would include research investigating the relationships between the degree of structure in typical occupational forms and the degree of predictability in the occupational performances. Also, the relationship between occupational form and occupational performance could be studied as a "match" or a "mismatch" to the requirements of the preexisting occupational form. Furthermore, performance could be investigated as a function of "press," a term used by Barris, Kielhofner, Levine, and Neville (1985, p. 45) to describe novelty, challenge, or arousal-eliciting properties.[2]

Meaning and Occupational Forms

Occupational form can be said to predict or have an effect on occupational performance, but it cannot be said to determine or control occupational performance. Determinism is a false position for several reasons, and one of the primary reasons is that the effect of the occupational form on the occupational performance depends on the individual's interpretation of the form. The concern for the individual's interpretation of the environment has been a major theme in the profession from Slagle (1914, p. 19) to Kielhofner (1985, p. 19). This interpretation is an active process on the part of the individual, and potentially the individual's entire developmental history can be brought to bear on that interpretation. The same occupational form may be interpreted differently by different individuals depending on all the factors that have contributed to each individual's current state of development (Cynkin, 1979, p. 123).

Meaning or *meaningfulness* is the term to be used in labeling the individual's interpretation of the occupational form.[3] Here the *meaningfulness* of an occupational form refers both to the perceptual sense it makes to the individual as well as to the cognitive associations elicited in the individual. We can describe an occupational form in terms of the presence or absence of meaningful-

ness (is an interpretation made?), in terms of its degree of meaningfulness, and in terms of the types of meanings assigned to it by an individual. The meaning of the occupational form to an individual may or may not conform to sociocultural norms. For example, a cultural symbol such as a Thanksgiving Day turkey may have no meaning or only an idiosyncratic meaning to a particular person.[4]

Developmental Structure

The meaningfulness of an occupational form depends on the individual's developmental structure. The structure that an individual brings to bear on the interpretation of an occupational form is complex, yet the multitudinous attributes are integrated into a working whole that is greater than the sum of its parts. These attributes may be classified in terms of an individual's (a) sensory, (b) motor, (c) perceptual, (d) cognitive, (e) emotional, and (f) interpersonal structural characteristics.[5] Within each of the six structural characteristics are many identifiable attributes. These include abilities, attitudes, beliefs, predispositions, memories, and other qualities (such as the individual's current state of arousal) enabling the individual's responses to occupational forms. Although it is generally easy to classify certain attributes into one of the six categories of structural characteristics, this is not always the case. Certain complex attributes, such as language, love, values, or creativity, are interactions among several of the six identified structural characteristics.

An individual's structure at any given point in time is a function of his or her development. Genetic, maturational, and experiential factors contribute to this development. Furthermore, as Huss (1981) pointed out, each attribute has a physiological basis in the human being; however, little is known at the present time about the physiology of many of the structural characteristics of the human being. Figure 2 shows how the occupational form takes on meaning as a function of the individual's developmental structure.

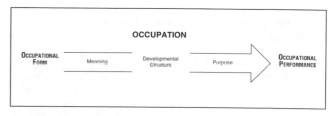

Figure 2. Occupation defined further, with the relationship between occupational form and occupational performance depending on the meaningfulness of the occupational form to the individual and the purposefulness of the occupational performance to the individual. (Both meaning and purpose depend on the individual's developmental structure.)

Purposefulness

All occupation includes a sense of purposefulness. This is true for the specific terminology proposed in this paper and for the everyday usage of the term (*Webster's Third New International Dictionary*, s.v. "occupation"). Figure 2 clarifies the relationship between purposefulness and other aspects of occupation. *Purpose* is the goal orientation of the individual and the link between the individual's developmental structure and occupational performance. As Breines (1984) (see Chapter 12) pointed out, purposefulness varies from individual to individual. Depending on the meanings assigned to the occupational form by the individual, the individual purposefully organizes his or her structural characteristics in such a way as to achieve a goal through occupational performance. Whereas meaning is constituted by the interaction between occupational form and the individual's developmental history (a "looking back"), purpose is constituted by the interaction between the individual's developmental structure and his or her future occupational performance (a "looking forward"). Meaning involves reflection; purpose involves prediction.

As used in this paper, the purpose of an occupational performance is always from the point of view of the actor. In other words, the term *purpose* is restricted to the goal orientation of the individual and does not refer to the goals of others, whether in the immediate environment or not. Another aspect of purposefulness is that the individual may be seeking more than one goal when engaged in a single occupational performance. For example, in performing a particular occupation, an individual may simultaneously be seeking (a) specific changes in the occupational form's materials (a "product"), (b) the praise of a supervisor, (c) money, (d) the tactile sensations of handling the materials, and (e) satisfaction of the need to be productive, leading to confirmation of personal efficacy.[6] Just as all occupational forms are not equally meaningful to an individual, all occupational performances are not equal in terms of purposefulness. Although the goal orientation of an individual is not always perceptible to an outsider, observation of the occupational performance is usually a means of inferring the individual's purposes.

The Impact of Occupational Performance

Frequently, occupational performance leaves an observable effect on the environment. Materials are transformed; others in the environment are influenced; and the sequence of events is altered. As Cubie (1985, p. 148) pointed out, occupation not only depends on the environment, but also serves to create the environment. Therefore, occupation can be said to be dynamic, in that occupational performance tends to affect subsequent occupational forms, which, in turn, tend to affect subse-

quent occupational performance. The impact of an individual's performance on the environment is another factor refuting the proposition that individual behavior is controlled or determined by external forces.

Figure 3 depicts occupational dynamics. The occupational form at one point in time is interpreted in terms of the individual's developmental structure; upon this interpretation the individual organizes himself or herself for performance designed to achieve specific purposes; and the performance, in turn, contributes to the occupational form at the next point in time. This is depicted in Figure 3 as the "impact" arrow. Of course, other events occurring in the environment, such as the actions of other individuals, also influence the occupational form. Just as the individual is not totally determined by the environment, so the environment, especially if shared with others, is not totally determined by the individual. Occupational performance that orders and sequences subsequent occupational forms in a balanced way was important to Meyer (1922) (see Chapter 2) and is part of what Kielhofner (1977) (see Chapter 17) has termed *temporal adaptation*.

Adaptation and Occupation

As Fidler and Fidler (1978) (see Chapter 7) stated, purposeful action is the means by which human beings become themselves. Meyer (1922) (see Chapter 2) stated that "It is the use that we make of ourselves that gives the ultimate stamp to our every organ" (p. 5). Meyer used the term *adaptation* to describe the change process facilitated by occupation; King (1978) (see Chapter 8) also recommended that the term *adaptation* be used to describe this process.[8]

As depicted in Figure 3, adaptation includes any effect on the individual's developmental structure that is not exclusively due to purely physical means (i.e., physiological maturation or disease). Figure 3 depicts two possible kinds of adaptation. The section of the arrow originating over "Purpose" in Figure 3 depicts a type of adaptation that occurs once the individual has a sense of purpose in relation to the occupational form but before the occupational performance is actually emitted. Gil-

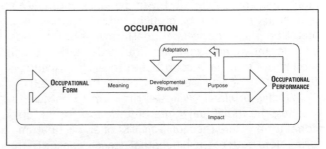

Figure 3. The dynamics of occupation: Occupational performance influences subsequent occupational forms, and purposefulness and/or performance results in adaptations in the individual's developmental structure.

foyle, Grady, and Moore (1981, p. 48) cited the accommodation of the individual's own resources to the requirements of the task as one of the major types of adaptation. The exact nature of adaptation may vary depending upon which structural characteristic is challenged (e.g., cognitive structures may adapt somewhat differently from motor structures).

The other possible route of adaptation as displayed in Figure 3 is the effect of the performance itself on the performer's developmental structure. Once the performance is carried out, the individual frequently stores in memory the action and the context of purposefulness in which the action took place. Gilfoyle, Grady, and Moore (1981, p. 48) described the types of associations that can be generated by performance. This memory is incorporated within the individual's structure for possible use in assimilating and differentiating future situations.

There are different types of adaptation. Structural characteristics may be strengthened, weakened, added, eliminated, restored, or simply maintained (the effect of maintenance can be thought of as a change from the weakening that would have otherwise occurred without the occupation). Although all occupation has the potential to foster adaptation, the quality and magnitude of adaptation varies from occupation to occupation and from person to person. As Slagle (1914, p. 20) stated, "little common things" from everyday life can become "powerful levers" fostering human development.

Levels of Occupation

The relationships presented in Figure 3 depend on the concept *point in time*; an arrow connects one point in time to a subsequent point in time. Point in time can be conceptualized at different levels. A point in time may be at an immediate level; for example, the occupational form may be the "catchability" of a baseball flying through the air, with the individual's sensory, perceptual, emotional, and motor structures organized around the purpose of catching the ball. Or, a point in time may be at a somewhat enhanced level; for example, the occupational form may involve a nine-inning baseball game, with the individual's developmental structure organized around the purpose of effective competition. To extend the analogy of the baseball player, a third level of occupation can be thought of as taking place at the level of the baseball season, and a fourth as taking place at the career level. Finally, Figure 3 can describe an entire life of occupation, with socioculturally available occupational forms interacting with an individual's developmental structure to promote purposeful performance and subsequent development throughout the life span. This idea that there are different levels of occupation is consistent with the view of Meyer (1922) (see Chapter 2), who used the term *occupation* both to describe that which could be performed in a single sitting and to describe

long-term patterns. A related concept is the *adaptation continuum*, developed by Kleinman and Bulkley (1982).

Of course, the user of the ideas in Figure 3 must be clear about the level of discourse. Empirical research conducted at the immediate level should not be automatically generalized to levels employing larger points in time. On the other hand, longer term occupations have identifiable relationships to shorter term occupations. Some of the individual's purposes in an immediate occupation often relate to higher levels of occupation (for example, the baseball player might want to catch the ball not only for its own sake but also to win the game, contribute to a winning season, enjoy a successful career, and so forth). Higher levels of occupational performance are actually made up of lower levels of occupation, and the relationships between occupational performance at the various levels are important areas for empirical inquiry. The reader can imagine a multidimensional version of Figure 3 in which any given occupation is actually made up of lower levels of occupation, and, together with others at its own level, makes up higher levels of occupation.

Although examples of ascending levels of occupation can be given, there appears to be no universally effective way of labeling them.[9] Whereas five levels may work well for baseball playing, different numbers of levels appear useful for other types of occupation. However, one distinction that might be useful in differentiating levels of occupation is between the occupation that typically has an uninterrupted beginning, middle, and end, and the occupation that is seldom completed in one continuous session.

An Abbreviated Example of Occupational Analysis

The details of Table 1 are not novel; most of them can be found in the formats for activity analysis presented by Cynkin (1979, pp. 121–124). What is novel about Table 1 is the categorization of the details. It happens that Tiffany (1983, pp. 299–300) has also analyzed the planting of a garden from an occupational therapy point of view; the reader is urged to compare the two analyses, particularly in regard to the separation of the objective physical and sociocultural features of the occupation from the developmental structure and occupational performance of the individual.

Conclusions

1. Thinking of occupation as a relationship between occupational form and occupational performance enables a systematic analysis of the nature of that relationship. The intent is to begin to raise what Slagle (1922, p. 16) termed *occupational analysis* (often called *activity analysis*) from its status as a set of techniques within the profession of occupa-

Table 1
Planting a Small Garden (by a 40-Year-Old Man With His 7-Year-Old Daughter): An Abbreviated Example of the Relationship Between Occupational Form and Occupational Performance

OCCUPATIONAL FORM	**Physical Aspects.** *Materials*—Packages of various types of seeds; a gardening book; tools, including trowels, hoes, and rakes (weight, size of parts, sturdiness, color, etc); plot of prepared soil; spatial relationships between objects. *Surround*-Sunny spring day; fenced-in backyard with toys and sandbox; nearby house with typical supports and distractions (telephone, etc.); residential neighborhood sounds (children, slamming screen doors, etc.). *Human aspects*—Seven-year-old daughter's presence and the absence of others; the girl's speech (frequency, duration, volume, pitch, phonetic qualities, and responsiveness); the girl's movements (garden- or toy-related). *Temporal aspects*—Events that occur after tilling and shopping and before cleaning up (daily level) and garden care (seasonal level); the moment-by-moment physical changes during the two hours of planting. **Sociocultural Aspects.** *Universal*—Crosscultural and historical significance of growing things with regard to self-sufficiency and physical survival, nurturance and the father-daughter relationship; rejuvenation of spring. *Cultural Context*—Industrialized society's view of gardening as leisure, particularly among upper socioeconomic classes; society's norms and values concerning leisure and father-daughter interaction; the culture's storehouse of knowledge concerning plants, gardening, and tool use; the culture's linguistic rules for interpreting speech and written instructions; appropriateness of occupation for both genders. *Family*—Backyard as shared space and family norms regarding child care and scarce leisure time; man's grandparents' dependence on, but his parents' avoidance of, farming/gardening.
INDIVIDUAL MEANINGS	His sensory and perceptual abilities (listed below) allow him to make sense out of the shapes, sizes, colors, and spatial interrelationships of the seed packages, the seeds, the tools, and the soil, and also enable him to see potential matches between his body parts and the objects (he sees the trowel as a graspable object). He focuses attention on small features of the environment while not being distracted by events on the periphery (in contrast, the daughter is frequently distracted). Comprehension of the daughter's speech depends on a complex of sensory, perceptual, cognitive, affective, and interpersonal abilities (including auditory temporal processing and symbol interpretation). Many objective aspects in the occupational form do not take on meaning (some of his daughter's speech); other aspects elicit thoughts and memories about helping his grandmother garden (when he was about his daughter's age), interacting with his father, and observing his daughter's birth.
DEVELOPMENTAL STRUCTURE	*Sensory*—Vision; audition; touch; proprioception; vestibular sensation; smell; general state of arousal (beginning the occupation in a generally under aroused state). *Motor*—Muscle stiffness; stamina; coordinative structures (these underlying abilities are conceptually separate from the observable performances they make possible—see "Occupational Performance," below). *Perceptual*—Processing of raw sensory input, including depth, shape, weight, texture, figure-ground, rhythm, body scheme, and spatiotemporal relations of the body scheme to objects (praxia). *Cognitive*—Memory, associational ability, comprehension of symbols, symbol creation, sequencing and ordering, imagination, evaluation of alternatives, plan making, inductive and deductive reasoning. *Emotional*—Capacity for various positive and negative feelings, including a temperamental proclivity for certain moods; the capacity to give affective coloring to meanings and purposes. *Interpersonal*—Inherent social nature (distinguishing between the human and the nonhuman); his developed proclivities (e.g., dependence/independence, empathy); his way of assuming roles (father, son, grandson, husband).

Table 1 (continued)

Planting a Small Garden (by a 40-Year-Old Man With His 7-Year-Old Daughter): An Abbreviated Example of the Relationship Between Occupational Form and Occupational Performance

INDIVIDUAL PURPOSES	The focal goal sought is a properly planted vegetable garden (he repeatedly imagines the outcome). He seeks to explore this new experience and also to demonstrate a beginning level of mastery. His levels of purposefulness match his levels of occupation: Each movement (e.g., dropping a seed) is goal oriented, and each phase of the occupation is goal oriented (e.g., completing the measurements of the layout). The occupation also is motivated by future goals (the anticipated sprouting, growing, harvesting, and eating of the vegetables). In the long term, he explores gardening as a possibly enduring hobby. A strong purpose is the desire to spend time and communicate with his daughter. Other purposes are relatively weak (e.g., the yard's aesthetics).
OCCUPATIONAL PERFORMANCE	Manipulation of the various tools (sometimes against resistance, as in digging), grasping/releasing, reaching, the assumption of various postures (kneeling, squatting), maintenance of postures, joint stabilization, walking, head orientation (to look at the materials or the daughter), laughing, gesturing, and speech. Some speech related to gardening, and some meant to pass along information about his daughter's grandparents and great-grandparents. An example of a cognitively based, covert operation: measuring and dividing up the plot (though not directly observable, this performance could be inferred through subsequent movements). Notable is the fact that the man's occupational performance is not the only method that could have been used to accomplish many of his purposes (e.g., some movements could have been performed in reverse order, or the left hand could have been used instead of the right).
OCCUPATIONAL DYNAMICS	*Impact*—Concretely, physical changes from the beginning of the occupation to end include: seeds in the ground, seed packages impaled on sticks marking rows, water sprinkler on, soil level and loosely packed, tools back in the garage (tools tend not to be affected much by occupation, whereas other materials are transformed), and daughter in the house, cleaning. Less concrete are the cognitive/affective impacts on the man's daughter: She now knows something about planting and has memories of doing things with her father (she probably remembers only what she saw as particularly meaningful). *Adaptation*—Minor accommodations to the man's developmental structure result from assuming novel postures in order to plant seeds without stepping on vulnerable areas, and from applying book knowledge about planting seeds to an actual (and partly unanticipated) situation. In future seasons, the man will be prepared in terms of tool use, guidelines concerning various seeds, and movement in a garden. Another adaptation is relaxation (creating readiness for future leisure and work). More deeply, the occupation provides a context for moving toward resolution in mourning for his father and grandparents, and in sensing his own development as a father and as a contributor within a series of human generations. Although the more significant adaptations of this occupation are in the affective/cognitive realms, the significant adaptations resulting from other occupations may be motoric/perceptual.
LEVEL OF OCCUPATION	This planting occupation has an uninterrupted beginning, middle, and end. Within it are many lower level occupations (e.g., covering a seed with dirt), but the 2-hour occupation cannot be reduced into the simple sum of lower level occupations (because of the man's unity of purpose in wanting to plant a vegetable garden). The planting occupation also helps make up higher levels of occupation (e.g., gardening at the seasonal level, and parenthood at the lifelong level).

tional therapy to a scientific status with its own theoretical structure and empirical possibilities. Writings on occupational analysis, whether from Tracy (1907–08), Dunton (1931), Fidler (1948), Llorens (1973), Cynkin (1979), or Tiffany (1983) can be readily interpreted in terms of the model presented in Figure 3 and in terms of the example presented in Table 1.

2. The relationships between occupational form and occupational performance (the nature of occupation) is dynamic, not deterministic. The dynamics of occupation are such that (a) the effects of the occupational form depend on the meanings assigned to the form by the individual; (b) occupational performance is furthermore influenced by the individual's multi-level sense of purposefulness; (c) prior occupational performance affects subsequent occupational forms; and (d) the individual's purposefulness and performance promote adaptations in his or her own developmental structure.

3. Occupations can be analyzed at different conceptual levels depending on the unit of time used by the occupational analyst. These levels range from the most immediate level of a particular act; to the level of a multistep occupation with an uninterrupted beginning, middle, and end; to higher levels descriptive of long-term roles and entire life spans.

Recommendations for Future Inquiry

1. Given the description of occupation presented in this paper, the next logical step is to define *therapeutic* occupation. What are the relationships between the occupational therapist and the occupational dynamics depicted in Figure 3?

2. The framework for thinking about occupation presented in this paper readily prompts empirically answerable questions, and the science of occupation requires research. What types of research methodologies are suited to answer the questions raised within this framework for thinking about occupation?

3. Past research, conducted both within the profession of occupational therapy and by other professions, can be classified in terms of the framework presented in this paper. Which past research has spoken to which aspects of Figure 3?

4. Because the intent of this paper is to provide an overall framework for thinking about occupation, much of the richness of many aspects of occupation has necessarily been excluded. Historical inquiry as well as further theoretical work could examine and expand on each of the concepts presented in Figure 3.

5. The description of occupation presented here is not the only way to conceptualize occupation. Other frameworks include those by Barris et al. (1985), Clark (1979), Katz (1985), Kielhofner (1985), Llorens (1976), Mosey (1981, chap. 8), and Reed (1984, chap. 16). There is a need to compare and contrast the various frameworks in terms of completeness, clarity, internal logic, adherence to historical conceptions of the profession, generation of frames of reference to guide clinical practice, and promotion of research.

Acknowledgments

I thank the following colleagues for their helpful suggestions made on an earlier draft of this paper: Yuen Hon Keung, BOT, OTR; Doris A. Smith, MEd, OTR, FAOTA; Barbara Baker, BS, OTR; Sandra Edwards, MA, OTR; Claire Callan, EdS, OTR; Gary Kielhofner, DrPH, OTR, FAOTA; Lela Llorens, PhD, OTR, FAOTA; and Anne Mosey, PhD, OTR, FAOTA.

References

Allen, C. K. (1987). Activity: Occupational therapy's treatment method. *American Journal of Occupational Therapy, 41*, 563–575.

American Occupational Therapy Association. (1972). *Project to delineate the roles and functions of occupational therapy personnel.* Rockville, MD: Author.

Barris, R., Kielhofner, G., Levine, R. E., & Neville, A. M. (1985). Occupation as interaction with the environment. In G. Kielhofner (Ed.), *A model of human occupation: Theory and application* (pp. 42–62). Baltimore: Williams & Wilkins.

Breines, E. (1984). The issue is—An attempt to define purposeful activity. *American Journal of Occupational Therapy, 38*, 543–544. (Reprinted as Chapter 12).

Clark, P. N. (1979). Human development through occupation: A philosophy and conceptual model for practice, part 2. *American Journal of Occupational Therapy, 33*, 577–585.

Cubie, S. H. (1985). Occupational analysis. In G. Kielhofner (Ed.), *A model of human occupation: Theory and application* (pp. 147–155). Baltimore: Williams & Wilkins.

Cynkin, S. (1979). *Occupational therapy: Toward health through activities.* Boston: Little, Brown.

Dunton, W. R. (1931). Occupational therapy. *Occupational Therapy and Rehabilitation, 10*, 113–121.

Fidler, G. S. (1948). Psychological evaluation of occupational therapy activities. *American Journal of Occupational Therapy, 2*, 284–287.

Fidler, G. S., & Fidler, J. W. (1978). Doing and becoming: Purposeful action and self-actualization. *American Journal of Occupational Therapy, 32,* 305–310. (Reprinted as Chapter 7).

Gilfoyle, E. M., Grady, A. P., & Moore, J. C. (1981). *Children adapt.* Thorofare, NJ: Slack.

Huss, A. J. (1981). From kinesiology to adaptation. *American Journal of Occupational Therapy, 35,* 574–580.

Katz, N. (1985). Occupational therapy's domain of concern: Reconsidered. *American Journal of Occupational Therapy, 39,* 518–524.

Kielhofner, G. (1977). Temporal adaptation: A conceptual framework for occupational therapy. *American Journal of Occupational Therapy, 31,* 235–242. (Reprinted as Chapter 17).

Kielhofner, G. (1983). Occupation. In H. L. Hopkins & H. D. Smith (Eds.), *Willard and Spackman's occupational therapy* (6th ed.) (pp. 31–41). Philadelphia: Lippincott.

Kielhofner, G. (Ed.). (1985). *A model of human occupation: Theory and application.* Baltimore: Williams & Wilkins.

King, L. J. (1978). Toward a science of adaptive responses. *American Journal of Occupational Therapy, 32,* 429–437. (Reprinted as Chapter 8).

Kleinman, B. L., & Bulkley, B. L. (1982). Some implications of a science of adaptive responses *American Journal of Occupational Therapy, 36,* 15–19.

Leont'ev, A. N. (1978). *Activity, consciousness, and personality* (M. J. Hall, Trans.). Englewood Cliffs, NJ: Prentice-Hall.

Llorens, L. A. (1973). Activity analysis for cognitive-perceptual-motor dysfunction. *American Journal of Occupational Therapy, 27,* 453–456.

Llorens, L. A. (1976). *Application of a developmental theory for health and rehabilitation.* Rockville, MD: American Occupational Therapy Association.

Llorens, L. A. (1986). Activity analysis: Agreement among factors in a sensory processing model. *American Journal of Occupational Therapy, 40,* 103–110.

Lyons, B. G. (1983). Purposeful versus human activity. *American Journal of Occupational Therapy. 37,* 493–495.

Meyer, A. (1922). The philosophy of occupation therapy. *Archives of Occupational Therapy, 1,* 1–10. (Reprinted as Chapter 2).

Mosey, A. C. (1981). *Occupational therapy: Configuration of a profession.* New York: Raven.

Mosey, A. C. (1986). *Psychosocial components of occupational therapy.* New York: Raven.

Nelson, D. L. (1984). *Children with autism and other pervasive disorders of development and behavior: Therapy through activities.* Thorofare, NJ: Slack.

Reed, K. L. (1984). *Models of practice in occupational therapy.* Baltimore: Williams & Wilkins.

Reilly, M. (1962). Occupational therapy can be one of the great ideas of 20th century medicine. *American Journal of Occupational Therapy, 16,* 1–9. (Reprinted as Chapter 6).

Sharrott, G. W. (1983). Occupational therapy's role in the client's creation and affirmation of meaning. In G. Kielhofner (Ed.), *Health through occupation: Theory and practice in occupational therapy* (pp. 213–235). Philadelphia: F. A. Davis.

Slagle, E. C. (1914). History of the development of occupation for the insane. *Maryland Psychiatric Quarterly, 4,* 14–21.

Slagle, E. C. (1922). Training aides for mental patients. *Archives of Occupational Therapy, 1,* 11–17.

Tiffany, E. G. (1983). Psychiatry and mental health. In H. L. Hopkins & H. D. Smith (Eds.), *Willard and Spackman's occupational therapy* (6th ed.) (pp. 267–334). Philadelphia: Lippincott.

Tracy, S.E. (1907–08). Some profitable occupations for invalids. *American Journal of Nursing, 8,* 172–177.

[1]This discussion builds on many of the concepts I presented in an earlier work (Nelson, 1984. pp. 119–121). In that book, as in most of the occupational therapy literature, the terms *activity* and *occupation* are used ambiguously without a clear distinction between *occupational form* and *occupational performance* as defined in this paper. Other corrections of that earlier work are that this paper treats the sociocultural reality of an occupational form as a separate dimension from its physical characteristics and that the meaningfulness of an occupation refers only to an individual's interpretation of an occupational form, not to the socioculturally defined attributes of the form.

[2]The chapter by Barris et al. (1985) is entitled "Occupation as Interaction With the Environment," a phrase that in some ways parallels the title of this paper. A specific quotation in that chapter reads, ". . . it is not enough for therapists to know only about the person. The therapist must also understand the process of person/environment interaction...." (p. 61). This quotation is also consistent with the spirit of the present paper. Some ideas in the present paper that may be somewhat different from those in the chapter by Barris et al. are the following: (a) in this paper, the immediate environment of the person (the inner layer) may be made up of other persons and an environmental surround, all in a temporal context, as well as objects (materials); (b) the immediate presence or absence of others is considered to be at a different level of discourse (a different layer) from the expectations of social entities not immediately present; (c) in this paper, a *task* is one type of occupation (usually work oriented as pointed out by Llorens, 1986, p. 104), and as such it is the relationship between an occupational form and an occupational performance (it is not considered to be once removed from the person in a hierarchy between objects and sociocultural features); and (d) in this paper, each occupational form has an objective reality that is external to the person (the meanings found in the form by an individual may be entirely different from sociocultural expectations, depending on the individual's developmental structure). Although *occupation-*

al form as presented in this paper cannot be described graphically by the rings of concentric circles as presented by Barris et al. (p. 43), the concepts presented by Barris et al. are indeed relevant to the concepts in this paper. In this paper, the same phenomena would be classified and arranged in a different fashion.

[3]This usage of *meaning* is different from the term *meaningful activity* as presented by Sharrott (1983, p. 213). From the point of view of this paper, Sharrott's interesting discussion refers to the creation of future meaning *through* occupation, not to the meaningfulness *of* an occupational form. From the point of view of this paper, Sharrott presents an example of adaptation, not meaning.

[4]Mosey's discussion of cultural and idiosyncratic symbols (Mosey, 1981, pp. 104–105) is relevant here. One difference between the idea of idiosyncratic meaning as presented in this paper and Mosey's notion of idiosyncratic symbols can be seen in her charming example of the family who could not conceive of Thanksgiving without "squash, peanuts, and sour cream." In this paper, the symbolic values assigned to these foods by the family would be considered part of the occupational form external to any individual. In this paper, the idiosyncratic meaning of an occupational form is always an individual matter. One of the implications of this is that a family member may not yet know how others interpret these foods, or may lose the ability to find meanings in them.

[5]I defined these six attributes of developmental structure in detail in an earlier work (Nelson, 1984, chap. 3). They refer to essentially the same phenomena that have been labeled *performance components* by a 1972 project of the American Occupational Therapy Association and by Mosey (1986). Within the conceptual framework presented in this paper, the term *performance components* would be misleading in that this label implies that the attributes referred to are components of, or make up, performance. Within the framework of this paper, they are performance *enablers,* not performance *components.* The rationale for using the label *structural characteristics* is to emphasize that the individual encountering an occupational form has a preexisting *structure* (that the individual is not a blank slate upon which the environment writes its messages).

[6]Reilly (1962) stated that occupation involves a particular sense of purposefulness not present in all activity. In like manner Kielhofner (1983, pp. 31–32) specified that the purposefulness of occupation involves the satisfaction of the need to explore and master the environment whereas nonoccupational activities are motivated by other kinds of purposes. [Note: The more recent work of Kielhofner (1985, p. 7) does not make the same distinction.] The position taken in this paper is somewhat different from Reilly's (1962) (see Chapter 6) and the 1983 work of Kielhofner. Here it is proposed that extrinsic motivation also plays a role in many types of occupation. From its inception, the profession has recognized the importance of extrinsic motivation; for example, Slagle (1914, p. 19) described the importance of others' appreciation in motivating the occupational efforts of the individual. The very desire to survive is often an extrinsic motivator for work and activities of daily living. Hence, although doing for its own sake may be the most important

(even sublime) form of purposefulness, the richness of occupation is in part due to its many dimensions of purposefulness.

[7]Meyer (cited in Slagle, 1922, p. 11) differentiated activity characterized by "nervous fickleness" from health-producing activity, and, in like vein, Fidler and Fidler (1978) (see Chapter 7) and Mosey (1981, p. 99) maintained that some activities are purposeful in that they are goal oriented, whereas others are not. in this paper, however, it is maintained that all voluntary human action (this excludes reflexive activity) necessarily involves a minimum of purposefulness on the actor's part (otherwise the action would not take place). In other words, this paper recommends that purposefulness be thought of in terms of degrees instead of in terms of absolute presence or absence. Therefore, although all occupation involves purposefulness, some occupations (so-called busywork) are characterized by a minimal sense of purposefulness whereas others are full of the health-producing energy described so aptly by Meyer.

[8]The restriction of the term *adaptation* to the human change process is at variance with the use of the term by Mosey (1986, p. xvi), who described adaptation "as having two interrelated parts": one involving self-modification and the other involving environmental modification. In this paper, self-modification would indeed be termed *adaptation,* but environmental modification would be termed *impact.*

[9]This thorny problem of smaller units of occupation within larger units of occupation, all with their own levels of purposefulness, may explain the difficulty that occupational therapists have had in defining *occupation.* Understandably, a would-be definer wants to be able to give an example of what one unit of the thing being defined is like. Where does one unit of the thing begin and end? The problem with occupation is that an immediate occupation, such as steering the wheel of a car, is nested within the intermediate occupation of a trip, which is nested within higher and higher levels of occupation. The proposed solution within this article is to use the same term *occupation* for each level, but this proposal is different from that advanced by the Russian psychologist Leont'ev (1978) and discussed by the occupational therapy authors Lyons (1983) and Allen (1987). In analyzing "the general structure of activity," Leont'ev (pp. 62–74) proposed three levels: *activities* (linked to *motives*); *actions* (linked to *purposes* and the achievement of *goals*); and *operations* (linked to the modification of *conditions*). In this article, the phenomena Leont'ev calls *activities, actions,* and *operations* can all be termed *occupations,* albeit at different levels, and the phenomena Leont'ev calls *motives, purposes,* and the goal-oriented modification of *conditions* can all be termed *purposes,* albeit at different levels. The justification for this paper's economy of terms is that the model presented in Figure 3 works as well with lower levels of occupation as it does with higher levels. Therefore, why should the same term not be used? Regardless of terminology, Allen (1987) makes the excellent observation that occupational therapy authors tend to focus only on one level. For example, she suggests that authors in the area of occupational behavior/human occupation tend to focus on higher levels, whereas many writers within the area of physical disabilities have tended to focus on lower levels.

Chapter 42

Guidelines for Using Both Activity and Exercise

Rebecca Dutton, MS, OTR/L

O ccupational therapy is based on the belief that the active participation of a client is facilitated by the performance of purposeful activity (Hopkins, 1988a). Occupational therapists believe that purposeful activity enhances effort by (a) tapping cognitive, social, and emotional sources of motivation and (b) showing the patient the immediate application of treatment procedures to daily function. The emergence of exercise as an occupational therapy modality has created a controversy regarding our legitimate tools and our true role as part of the health care team (Bing, 1981 [see Chapter 5]; English, Kasch, Silverman, & Walker, 1982; Huss, 1981; Reed, 1986 [see Chapter 39]; West, 1984). Historically, occupational therapists have been called the "activity specialists" because they teach patients how to use their new mobility (Hopkins, 1988b). Physical therapists have been called the "exercise specialists" because they restore mobility to body structures. However, this simplistic view of role delineation ignores some basic facts about changes in the health care system.

Occupational therapists used to treat patients only after they were medically stable and ready for purposeful activity. Today, occupational therapists are treating some patients in acute stages, which imposes new role responsibilities (Affleck, Lieberman, Polon, & Rohrkemper, 1986). The occupational therapist in an acute care setting must put homeostasic (life-threatening) issues first and restoration of function second. Repeated medical tests and procedures take priority over functional goals such as self-feeding. The occupational therapist must initially restrict treatment to simple, isolated movements that can be completed in 5- to 10-min windows.

Even certain activity materials may be prohibited in an acute care setting. Additionally, during acute stages, the patient's cognition is often temporarily impaired by pain, fear, medication, fever, metabolic imbalances, the inability to communicate orally, and sensory deprivation (Affleck et al., 1986). Even patients who appear lucid during the acute stage can later exhibit large memory gaps and distortions about what actually happened.

The acutely ill patient with a spinal cord injury, who must be ventilated because of compromised respiration illustrates the problems that can arise from the treatment of patients in acute care settings. The therapist may have to interrupt a treatment session to perform an assisted cough to clear the airway or to accommodate a respiratory therapy procedure. In doing so, the therapist must also use an activity that does not overstress the patient's current vital capacity. If this patient experiences respiratory distress during an activity, the activity must be stopped. Although the occupational therapist can break a purposeful activity down into 5-min segments, the patient may feel frustrated. This frustration may be due to the delayed completion of even a simple project, to a restricted selection of activities, to repeated interruptions for life-preserving procedures or medical tests, or to temporarily impaired cognition. Therefore, a few simple, short exercises might be more desirable in this temporary acute phase.

The rehabilitation phase of treatment is also changing. Occupational therapists could once concentrate on purposeful activity in this phase, but changes in the provision of health care services have forced therapists to reconsider their role. Although traditional inpatient programs permit a team approach, today's rehabilitation efforts are being diverted to more cost-effective outpatient programs and home health care (Levy, 1988). Independently functioning health care professionals in these new service provision systems cannot ensure a cohesive, logical sequence of treatment on the basis of traditionally defined roles (Taira, 1985). There is often little interaction between team members, which further fragments care. This fragmentation has forced each member of the long-term care team to reconsider how to ensure a smooth transition from preparation to application.

The diagnosis-related-group guidelines have also changed the provision of both acute care and rehabilitation services. Shortened lengths of stay in both settings have put a premium on time management. Time constraints often interfere with patient education. Compliance is jeopardized when a patient does not understand his or her medical condition and treatment.

Although our profession has acknowledged these changes in the health care system (Levy, 1988; West, 1984), the fear persists that if an occupational therapist starts a treatment session with a preparatory exercise, then purposeful activity will be forgotten or devalued.

The controversy over the role of occupational therapists has persisted because activity and exercise have been seen as mutually exclusive, philosophically opposed treatment approaches. Activity and exercise are actually at complementary ends of the same continuum.

The literature defines purposeful activity in several ways. Nelson (1984) identified two types of purposeful activity. The first type is directly related to the facilitation of occupational performance. This includes the practice of specific skills used in work, leisure, and self-care. Some skills, like brushing one's teeth, are generic cultural expectations. Other skills, like the use of a baton by a symphony conductor, are role specific. Nelson called the second type of purposeful activity dual-purpose activity. Dual-purpose activities seek to remediate foundation skills such as strength or attention, which support occupational performance. A modality can be a direct or dual-purpose activity. A client may play wheelchair basketball to assess it as a future leisure interest. Wheelchair basketball can also be used as a dual-purpose activity to increase cardiovascular conditioning in a client who has no intention of continuing this activity after discharge.

Both types of purposeful activity differ from what Huss (1981) called *pure exercise*, which she defined as a person's ability to consciously control a body part without having to think about anything else. Even simple activities require at least some subcortical control of movement, which enables the patient to divide his or her attention. For example, a patient racing to put clothespins on a line must monitor his or her competitor's actions, deal with his or her own emotional response to performance, and control his or her pinch and release movements.

This paper explores how the biomechanical and sensorimotor frames of reference provide specific guidelines for movement along the continuum from exercise (preparation) to purposeful activity (application). These guidelines are not hard-and-fast rules. They describe when it is easier for the therapist to adapt an activity or an exercise to achieve a specific goal. Ease of a treatment plan, characterized by good time management, safe treatment, and better patient education, is directly related to how well the inherent characteristics of an activity or an exercise match the patient's current level of performance. The closer the match, the less time the therapist has to spend modifying the modality to make it appropriate and safe. A closer match also has better face validity, so it takes less time to explain the purpose of the treatment to the patient and family.

Biomechanical Frame of Reference

The biomechanical frame of reference provides six continua that suggest criteria for when to use both activity and exercise. The continua are (a) isolated versus coordinated movements, (b) rhythmical versus arrhythmical movements, (c) linear versus diagonal movements,

(d) reciprocal versus asymmetrical movements, (e) movements to increase versus movements to maintain range of motion, and (f) movements against excessive resistance versus maximal repetitions.

Isolated versus coordinated movements. Isolated movements are easy to achieve with exercises. A good example of this is an isolated finger extension exercise for a flexor tendon injury (Van Strien, 1987). Active finger extension to the limit of the dressing is followed by passive finger flexion achieved with rubber bands that have been attached to each fingernail. These isolated finger movements, which can be prescribed as early as 1 week after surgery, prevent adhesions from forming by making the flexor tendons glide inside the tendon sheath. Functional grasp, which requires active finger flexion and wrist extension, is prohibited at this early stage, to keep all tension off the sutured flexor tendons. The modification of a purposeful activity that meets these severe restrictions may be difficult, because the patient is still wearing a bulky, compressive dressing. In addition, the patient could become so engrossed in an activity that he or she might actively flex the fingers instead of letting the rubber bands passively perform this motion. This is an example of what the occupational therapist faces when ordered to immediately start isolated remobilization. It is therefore easier and safer to facilitate isolated movements with exercises during this temporary phase of acute care.

Normal movements, however, are rarely isolated. Most movements involve the coordinated action of several muscle groups (Bobath, 1970; Voss, Ionta, & Myers, 1985). Yet the transition from simple, isolated movements to complex, coordinated movements is not always automatic. This is especially true for patients with central nervous system deficits, but even patients with no brain damage may have abnormal sensory feedback. Distorted feedback can be created by peripheral conditions such as pain, edema, impaired circulation, changes in the skin, peripheral nerve injury, or stabilization devices. Patients with either abnormal sensory feedback or abnormal sensory throughput often have to relearn how to execute coordinated movements. Purposeful activities, which have this inherent characteristic, make such relearning easy. For example, writing requires the coordinated action of the long finger flexors and extensors, the interossei and lumbrical muscles, several thumb extrinsic and intrinsic muscles, and the wrist and forearm muscles. Although the occupational therapist could have a patient perform complex nonsense movements in an exercise format that uses all of these muscles, it would be easier to use a purposeful activity that shows the patient how to move.

Rhythmical versus arrhythmical movements. Rhythmical movements performed at constant speeds are easy to achieve with exercise. For example, by using free weights or exercise pulleys, the patient can concentrate on per-

fecting one smooth, slow motion executed through a full range of motion without having to respond to unexpected changes. The therapist could use a purposeful activity, such as a ceramics project, to practice rhythmical movements, but it may be difficult for a patient to remember to reach for the glue and move each tile at the same speed each time. It is easier to reinforce rhythmical movement performed at a constant speed with exercises that already have these inherent characteristics.

Many human movements are, however, arrhythmical and performed at irregular speeds. For example, to ambulate around the kitchen in order to prepare a meal, a person must make frequent small turning motions. The person must pivot to turn on the stove and then pivot and lean forward to turn on the water faucet and fill a pot. Such a task becomes even more variable when obstacles such as table legs, open cabinet doors, and other people are present. The therapist could use exercises to practice arrhythmical movements performed at irregular speeds, but these exercises require the patient to visualize complexly timed nonsense sequences. Arrhythmical movements are reinforced more easily with purposeful activities like cooking, which already have these inherent characteristics and which remind the patient of the unpredictability of an unprotected environment.

Linear versus diagonal movements. Linear movements performed in anatomical planes are easy to achieve with exercise. Skateboard exercises, for example, require only horizontal shoulder abduction and adduction and elbow flexion and extension. Anyone who has watched a patient struggle with just these two simple movements knows that linear movements are sometimes the only movements a patient can perform initially. Some activities can be adapted to require only linear movement, but the selection is limited and the activity must be simplistic. Some patients may not be any more motivated by a repetitive bilateral sanding activity than by a repetitive skateboard exercise. It is therefore easier to design a linear exercise for this brief period of early mobilization.

Normal human movement, however, is not linear. Joint structures produce diagonal movements performed in irregular parabolic curves (Voss et al., 1985). Diagonal movement is more easily facilitated with purposeful activities that are intrinsically diagonal. For example, the shoulder and elbow joints travel through one set of parabolic curves during self-feeding and travel through a different set of parabolic curves during hair combing. Although the therapist could have a patient trace a number of imaginary parabolic curves in the air, a purposeful activity such as pushing a toy truck would more easily show the patient where to move.

This particular continuum, which was first described by sensorimotor theorists (Voss et al., 1985), is discussed here to emphasize the fact that all human movement is diagonal. These theorists would counsel against the therapist beginning with linear movements during initial treatment sessions. They believe that assisted diagonal movements are easier, more natural, and less painful to perform than linear movements, even for acutely ill or debilitated patients.

Reciprocal versus asymmetrical movements. Reciprocal movements are easy to achieve with exercise. Exercise pulleys, free weights, exercise bicycles, and ergometers facilitate reciprocal movements. Few purposeful activities require only reciprocal movements (e.g., walking). Reciprocal exercises are easy to design, so why not use them?

Although reciprocal exercises are an easy way for patients to achieve early remobilization, they are more readily generalized to gait training than to upper extremity function. Upper extremity movements are more typically asymmetrical. The nondominant hand stabilizes the object while the dominant hand manipulates the object. Although some patients can generalize from reciprocal to asymmetrical movements, the occupational therapist cannot always predict which patients can make this transition unaided. Because purposeful activities such as opening a bottle often have the inherent characteristic of asymmetry, it is easy to use purposeful activities to achieve this goal.

Increasing versus maintaining range of motion. Movements to increase joint motion beyond a patient's currently available range are easy to achieve with exercise. For example, manual or static stretching can reverse a shoulder flexion contracture. Although the occupational therapist can design many activities that require increasing amounts of shoulder flexion, it is difficult for the patient to actively move beyond his or her own currently available range. Even normal muscles become actively insufficient at the extreme end of range, which decreases their power. In addition, the frequent presence of pain, disuse atrophy, and loss of endurance makes it difficult for a patient to actively stretch beyond his or her current performance ceiling. Exercise techniques such as a manual or static stretch allows the therapist to prevent substitutions and to assist the patient to the maximal range long after the patient's current strength and endurance have been exhausted.

However, one cannot assume that once the therapist has increased the patient's passive range of motion with exercise, the patient will automatically use that range of motion daily. For example, a woman with a shoulder injury may diligently perform her shoulder exercises at home, but end up with a refrozen shoulder because she constantly holds the injured arm against her body. Even well-educated patients may believe that doing a few daily exercises will maintain their increased range of motion despite constant disuse. The therapist must prescribe purposeful activities that require full range of motion in order to generalize the gains achieved by exercise in the hospital to occupational roles at home and work.

Excessive strength versus endurance. Movements against excessive resistance to develop above-average strength are easy to achieve with exercise. For example, a patient with C_6 quadriplegia needs excessive strength in the wrist extensors to achieve functional pinch strength through tenodesis. It is easy to use free-weight exercises to strengthen these wrist muscles. Technically, it is also possible to put a 10-lb weight on a patient's wrist during self-feeding, but that is not very practical. First, failure to lift, which is required to increase strength, permits few repetitions. This can frustrate a patient who is trying to eat an entire meal in an allotted amount of time. Second, excessive weight can significantly interfere with the smooth, coordinated movements required to get the food to the mouth. Although above-average strength can be achieved with activities, it is more easily achieved with exercise.

Above-average strength alone does not ensure role performance. Strength is not functional without endurance, which is the ability to sustain effort. Exercises that increase endurance require the use of maximal repetitions, but such exercises can be boring. Instead, a meaningful activity can facilitate the compliance that is needed to ensure these maximal repetitions. Some patients would be more motivated to increase upper extremity endurance by playing basketball than by doing wheelchair laps up and down the hospital corridors.

Summary. In the biomechanical frame of reference, there are at least six continua that provide guidelines for the use of both exercise and activity. When considering whether to use an exercise (preparation) or a purposeful activity (application) for treatment, the occupational therapist should consider the patient's current status (see Table 1). Exercise is easier to use if the patient is capable of only isolated, rhythmical, linear, or reciprocal movements. Purposeful activities are easier to use once the patient is ready to advance to more complex skills, such as coordinated, arrhythmical, diagonal, or asym-

---

Table 1
Exercise-Purposeful Activity Continuum for the Biomechanical Frame of Reference

Movements More Easily Achieved Through Exercise	Movements More Easily Achieved Through Purposeful Activity
Isolated movement	Coordinated movement
Rhythmical movement	Arrhythmical movement
Linear movement	Diagonal movement
Reciprocal movement	Asymmetrical movement
Increase in range of motion	Maintenance of range of motion
Excessive resistance for strength	Maximal repetitions for endurance

metrical movements. Exercise is also easier to use if the therapist's biomechanical goals are to increase range of motion beyond the currently available range and to develop above-normal strength. When the therapist's biomechanical goals eventually shift, it is easier to use purposeful activity to maintain the new gains in range of motion and to develop the endurance needed to make strength functional.

Sensorimotor Frames of Reference

The sensorimotor frames of reference provide five continua that suggest specific criteria for the use of both activity and exercise. These continua are (a) therapist-controlled versus patient-controlled muscle tone, (b) tracking versus initiating normal movement, (c) initial versus repetitive weight shifts, (d) conscious versus automatic monitoring, and (e) routine movements versus motor planning.

Control of tone. Spasticity must be controlled initially by the therapist, who gives the sensation of what normal tone feels like (Bobath, 1970). Therapists are taught to give this normal sensation by using handling techniques, which are a form of preparation (exercise). One handling technique for a patient who has tight scapular retractors is to slowly roll the patient onto the hemiplegic side with the hemiplegic shoulder flexed and the scapula protracted. An activity cannot always be used at this early stage of giving the sensation of elongated refractors because active effort of spastic muscles increases their tone. This would give the patient the wrong sensation.

Before going home, however, the patient must take responsibility for his or her own muscle tone. The therapist must risk active movement even though it will increase tone. For example, the therapist might teach a patient to inhibit scapular refractors while putting on a button-down shirt by leaning forward with the hemiplegic arm dangling between abducted thighs. Because the patient's use of the sound arm to manipulate the shirt will initially increase tone in the hemiplegic arm, the therapist must initially use his or her hands to keep the patient's scapula protracted and elbow extended. Gradually, the therapist must remove his or her hands or at least fade to more distal key points of control to make the patient more responsible for controlling the tone. The therapist could have the patient perform a number of nonsense movements with the sound arm while trying to inhibit tone in the hemiplegic arm, but a purposeful activity like dressing would more accurately replicate the on-going problems that the patient will encounter with high tone after discharge.

Tracking versus initiating normal movement. Brain-damaged patients initially relearn normal movement patterns by "tracking" a therapist's normal movement (Becker et al., 1985). The patient imitates this normal movement by maintaining physical contact with the therapist's moving body part and by learning not to resist the therapist's

movements. The therapist might want a patient with a tightly retracted scapula to learn to roll. In such a situation, the patient lies on his or her side and remains passive while the therapist slowly rolls the patient back and forth in tiny midranges. Gradually, the patient is asked to actively follow the therapist's movement (Becker et al., 1985; Bobath, 1970). At this early stage, a purposeful activity is too stressful because it divides the patient's attention between tracking the therapist's motions and watching and thinking about the activity.

Eventually, the patient must stop tracking the therapist's normal movement and start initiating his or her own movement. At this stage, it is easy to use activity to teach initiation of movement. For example, the patient described above could roll in bed to reach for the bedside telephone or the nurses' call button. As the patient learns to initiate movement with graded control, the therapist gradually withdraws his or her control of the patient's movement. Although the patient could instead perform repetitive rolling exercises, it is easier for the patient to understand the purpose for performing a movement in his or her daily life if the movement is already incorporated into a purposeful activity.

Initial versus repetitive weight shifts. When brain-damaged patients first get motor return, they may expend all of their effort maintaining themselves in a fixed position (Adams & Dieterich, 1982). The therapist must discourage fixing immediately by teaching the patient to move within a posture. For example, stroke patients often have excessive extensor tone in the lower extremity, which inhibits weight shifts. A common handling technique for this problem is to place the patient in a sitting position, which has strong flexor characteristics, and then to passively shift the patient's trunk forward and backward in tiny ranges. Although the therapist could introduce an activity at this point, patients with moderate to severe extensor spasticity often cannot tolerate activity at this early stage. Initially, this weight shift can be a very frightening experience. The patient is so used to fixing the trunk behind the vertical position while sitting that he or she experiences an exaggerated sense of falling forward during any weight shift.

The patient usually accepts weight shift quickly and becomes less dependent on fixing for stability. At this point, the patient is able to perform repeated weight shifts. An activity such as opening a refrigerator door without falling forward while leaning forward to reach for an object and then stepping back to close the door is an excellent way to achieve repetitive weight shifts. An exercise could be used instead, but movements such as leaning forward and stepping backward are inherently boring and often have poor face validity. Many patients and family members do not understand the purpose of moving between and within postures until they see it incorporated in a functional activity.

Conscious versus automatic monitoring. Once patients can initiate a few normal movements, they can begin to teach themselves other normal movements by paying conscious attention to their own somatic sensation. This is called a *feedback loop* (Stockmeyer, 1978). For example, once a hemiplegic patient learns how to roll and how to put the hemiplegic arm on a tabletop without retracting the scapula, he or she can learn to consciously inhibit scapular retraction in other movement situations. It is easy to use handling techniques to reinforce this conscious monitoring. By lightly touching the patient's scapula, the therapist can remind the patient to generalize scapular protraction to new situations. An activity could be used at this point, but the patient might regress when asked to generalize a newly learned movement while also being cognitively challenged.

Eventually, however, the patient must stop consciously attending to somatic feedback. The cerebellum must assume the job of automatically monitoring somatic feedback and coordinating habitually performed movement so that the cortex can deal with cognitive challenges. This process of automatic monitoring by the cerebellum is called *feed forward* (Stockmeyer, 1978). For example, a normal college student does not walk up the steps to get to class by looking intently at his or her feet. Instead, the cerebellum monitors the walking while the student attends to cognitive challenges such as conversing with a friend as they walk up the steps together. If patients don't develop this kind of automatic monitoring of movement, they will regress to primitive movement patterns whenever they are cognitively challenged. Although a patient could practice automatic monitoring by reciting the names of the presidents of the United States while walking up and down the hallway, a purposeful activity such as walking through a cafeteria line while choosing from the menu inherently requires automatic monitoring of limb movements.

Routine movements versus motor planning. Some brain-damaged patients have dyspraxia in addition to spasticity. Dyspraxia is the inability to generalize familiar, routine movement schema to new, unfamiliar movement situations. An explanation or demonstration of the component parts of new movements is not always successful with the dyspraxic patient. Handling techniques, however, can be very useful, especially when the dyspraxic patient perseverates during familiar routine movements instead of trying new patterns.

Eventually, the patient must be able to move about in an environment that offers a variety of subtly changing demands. These subtle variations do not impede normal persons, but dyspraxic patients find them to be exasperating. It is therefore not sufficient for the dyspraxic ambulatory patient to repeatedly practice navigating an uncrowded, fire-regulation width hospital corridor. This patient will not be able to shop in a crowded store if he or she cannot motor-plan while in a crowd. The therapist could have the patient practice a sequence of subtly changing nonsense movements, but it is more effective to use purposeful activity such as walking around different obstacles. This helps the dyspraxic patient understand the functional value of quick changes in motor output. Any therapist that has seen a dyspraxic patient trying to sit on an unfamiliar surface can understand the suffering that new, unfamiliar movements create for these patients.

Summary. When using the sensorimotor frames of reference, the occupational therapist should consider the patient's current status when choosing a handling technique or an activity (see Table 2). The therapist more easily ensures quality movement by using handling techniques alone when the patient is functioning at a primitive level. This includes when the patient is (a) unable to control his or her own muscle tone, (b) dependent on tracking normal movements, (c) resistant to initial attempts at weight shift, (d) dependent on conscious monitoring, and (e) capable of learning only a few routine movements.

When the patient progresses to a more advanced level, handling techniques can be faded gradually while purposeful activity is added. The advanced patient is ready to (a) learn to control his or her own muscle tone, (b) initiate his or her own normal movement, (c) perform repetitive weight shifts, (d) progress to automatic monitoring, and (e) practice motor planning.

Conclusion

Some occupational therapists feel strongly that our activity base must be maintained at all costs. I believe, however, that purposeful activities are not always practical or safe for every phase of a patient's treatment. I do not believe that occupational therapists are going to stop using splints, massage, Reflex Inhibiting Patterns,

---

Table 2
Exercise-Purposeful Activity Continuum for the Sensorimotor Frames of Reference

Conditions in Which Exercise is Desirable	Conditions in Which Purposeful Activity is Desirable
Patient unable to control tone tone	Patient ready to control tone
Patient dependent on tracking	Patient ready to initiate movement
Patient resists initial weight shift	Patient ready to perform repetitive weight shifts
Patient uses conscious monitoring	Patient ready to practice automatic monitoring
Patient must relearn routine movements	Patient ready to relearn motor planning

and many other "nonpurposeful" modalities. These modalities are too closely matched to the primitive needs of acutely ill and seriously debilitated patients to be abandoned. Exercises and handling techniques are also advantageous because they have no clear end product. These techniques can be abruptly terminated without frustrating the patient by failing to complete a project. These modalities are especially helpful during the brief period of early remobilization.

Some occupational therapists believe that the only way that we can establish our efficacy in this age of accountability is to use exercise. I believe that the use of only exercise and handling techniques is not valid. Many patients cannot or will not make the transition from simple to complex movements independently. Many patients need to practice complex movements in a purposeful activity before they go home or return to work. Purposeful activity implicitly tells the patient which complex movements to make, makes the patient less dependent on the therapist's physical contact, and embeds complex movements in a functional context. The more closely the activity in the hospital resembles the activity at home or work, the more likely the patient is to retain what was learned and apply it in daily life.

Although some patients find exercise more intrinsically motivating than craft activities, this misses the point. Movement occurs in an environment that does not permit undivided attention to what various parts of the body are doing. There is always an object, another person, or an internal cognitive or emotional process that demands attention. Exercise alone does not prepare a patient to reenter this jungle of competing stimuli. Ironically, because shortened stays have prompted third-party payers to reimburse for functional goals, some occupational therapists are eliminating functional activities from their treatment plans.

I advocate the use of both activity and exercise within a single treatment plan. This can be an emotional issue, but the following example illustrates how these two approaches blend together in a more neutral context. A football coach knows that players who scrimmage (application) without first warming up (preparation) are at a greater risk of injury. The coach also knows that running laps around the field (preparation) does not fully prepare a player for running downfield with 1,000 pounds of crazed linemen coming at him from three directions (application). The coach therefore combines preparation and application without questioning the validity of these legitimate tools.

Changes in the health care system have forced the allied health professions to look at how they use both preparation and application. Occupational therapists have had to look at how safely acutely ill or seriously debilitated patients are handled. Preparation is also an issue for home health care patients and outpatients who

are treated by individual contractors. These health care systems lack the sequencing and overlapping techniques of several disciplines, which are typical of inpatient programs. Changes in the health care system have simultaneously triggered an increased focus on application with its persuasive cost-benefit ratio. It is no longer a question of preparation or of application. Occupational therapists must be prepared to do both.

Because patients progress at different rates, the timing of the transition from preparation to application depends on clinical experience and observation. As a stimulus for dialogue, I would like to briefly describe my own experience with this transition. When I begin treatment, I use both preparation and application. Although the first few treatment sessions may focus on preparation, I usually bring a purposeful activity to these early sessions. I may ask the patient to try one or two purposeful movements, such as taking two bites of food, knowing that the patient may initially fail. This brief application experience helps the patient see the long-term benefits of his or her effort from the beginning of the therapeutic program.

I sometimes find it difficult to accurately predict when to make the transition from preparation to application without actually trying it. This is another reason to bring materials for both to treatment sessions from the beginning. The patient's progress can surprise even the experienced therapist. Conversely, if the patient initially performs well on an activity, he or she might still regress in the middle of the activity. When I begin an activity very early and the patient gets into trouble, I implement a brief return to preparation and then try the activity again later in the session. I find that moving freely back and forth between preparation and application is effective and practical. I gradually spend less time on preparation and more time on application as the patient improves.

I believe clinicians are already using both preparation and application. However, this makes marketing our services difficult. Gilfoyle (1988) suggested that our inability to define our product impairs our ability to control our destiny in the marketplace. This article has attempted to explain why our product changes as the patient's condition improves.

I hope this article has stimulated some constructive thought about the question, Are both exercise and activity part of an occupational therapist's repertoire? If the reader finds merit in this continuum approach to the prolonged debate about our legitimate tools, perhaps additional frames of reference would be analyzed from this perspective. Whatever the profession of occupational therapy does to resolve this conflict about activity versus exercise, it will have to be a constructive and creative solution. To remain viable, the profession must be able to respond to the changing needs of both the individual and the health care system.

Acknowledgments

I would like to thank Linda Levy, MA, OTR/L, and my students for challenging my old schema and constantly making occupational therapy new for me. I would also like to thank Judie Perinchief, MS, OTR/L, for her many hours of thoughtful feedback. This article could not have been written without their influence and support.

References

Adams, M., & Dieterich, G. (1982). *Neurodevelopmental treatment certification course.* Memphis: Les Passees Rehabilitation Center.

Affleck, A. T., Lieberman, S., Polon, J., & Rohrkemper, K. (1986). Providing occupational therapy in an intensive care unit. *American Journal of Occupational Therapy, 40,* 323–332.

Becker, P., Myers, B. J., & Mukoyama, S. (Chairs). (1985). Meeting of the Rehabilitation Institute of Chicago, Chicago.

Bing, R. B. (1981). Eleanor Clarke Slagle Lectureship—Occupational therapy revisited: A paraphrastic journey. *American Journal of Occupational Therapy, 35,* 499–518. (Reprinted as Chapter 5.)

Bobath, B. (1970). *Adult hemiplegia: Evaluation and treatment* (2nd ed.). London: Heinemann.

English, C., Kasch, M., Silverman, P., & Walker, S. (1982). The Issue Is—On the role of the occupational therapist in physical disabilities. *American Journal of Occupational Therapy, 36,* 199–202.

Gilfoyle, E. M. (1988). Nationally Speaking—Partnerships for the future. *American Journal of Occupational Therapy, 42,* 485–488.

Hopkins, H. L. (1988a). Current basis for theory and philosophy of occupational therapy. In H. L. Hopkins & H. D. Smith (Eds.), *Willard and Spackman's occupational therapy* (7th ed.) (pp. 38–42). Philadelphia: J. B. Lippincott.

Hopkins, H. L. (1988b). An historical perspective on occupational therapy. In H. L. Hopkins & H. D. Smith (Eds.), *Willard and Spackman's occupational therapy* (7th ed.) (pp. 16–37). Philadelphia: J. B. Lippincott.

Huss, A. J. (1981). From kinesiology to adaptation. *American Journal of Occupational Therapy, 35,* 574–580.

Levy, L. L. (1988). Occupational therapy's place in the health care system. In H. L. Hopkins & H. D. Smith (Eds.), *Willard and Spackman's occupational therapy* (7th ed.). (pp. 153–164). Philadelphia: J. B. Lippincott.

Nelson, D. L. (1984). *Children with autism and other pervasive disorders of development and behavior: Therapy through activities.* Thorofare, NJ: Slack.

Reed, K. L. (1986). 1986 Eleanor Clarke Slagle Lecture—Tools of practice: Heritage or baggage? *American Journal of Occupational Therapy, 40,* 597–605. (Reprinted as Chapter 39).

Stockmeyer, S. (1978). [Foundations of motor control]. Unpublished lecture notes.

Taira, E. D. (1985). After treatment what? New roles for occupational therapists in the community. *Occupational Therapy in Health Care, 2*(1), 13–24.

Van Strien, G. (1987, March). *Post-operative care of primary tendon repair.* Paper presented at the 11th Annual Surgery and Rehabilitation of the Hand '87 Symposium and Workshop, Philadelphia.

Voss, D. E., Ionta, M. K., & Myers, B. J. (1985). *Proprioceptive neuromuscular facilitation* (3rd ed.). Philadelphia: Harper & Row.

West, W. L. (1984). A reaffirmed philosophy and practice of occupational therapy for the 1980s. *American Journal of Occupational Therapy, 38,* 15–23.

Chapter 43

Activity, Social Role Retention, and the Multiply Disabled Aged: Strategies for Intervention

Linda L. Levy, MA, OTR

This chapter was previously published in *Evaluation and Treatment of the Psychogeriatric Patient*, (1990), p. 1–30. Copyright © The Haworth Press, Inc.

A well established tenet in the gerontological literature is that maintaining activity is important to adaptation, life satisfaction, and retention of social roles in the later years (Atchley, 1980; Burrus-Bammel & Bammel, 1985; Havinghurst, 1963; Havinghurst & Feigenbaum, 1968). And yet, in the face of the all too common physical and cognitive disabilities that occur, the capacity to maintain active participation in preferred activities and social roles is compromised (Gordon, Gaitz, & Scott, 1976; Harris & Associates, 1975). One critical question is how best to enable disabled older adults to participate in desired life activities, to maximize their independence, life satisfaction, and quality of life. An equally critical question is how therapeutic regimens whose goal is to assist older adults to restore their lives to fullest use and satisfaction can be adapted to meet the needs of the multiply disabled aged.

This chapter will provide an overview of concepts that can be used by therapists and caregivers in rehabilitation of the physically and cognitively disabled elderly individual to facilitate his or her participation in therapeutic regimens and preferred life activities. It will describe intervention strategies that are responsive to a central dilemma in the gerontological literature, as it applies to the multiply disabled aged: the mismatch between the strengths and capacities of the aged on the one hand and the inadequate social role opportunities to utilize and sustain those strengths on the other (Riley & Riley, 1989). It is intended as a reference point in initiating activity adaptation responsive to the strengths, capacities, and limitations experienced by physically and cognitively disabled older adults.

Activity Analysis

The influence of disabilities on activity participation and role retention is assessed first by means of a comprehensive process known as activity analysis. Simply stated, activity analysis is the examination of an activity to determine its multifaceted components and the effects of those components on the activity participant (Cynkin, 1979; Llorens, 1986; Mosey, 1981). A number of characteristics are considered, including the intrinsic properties of the activity (e.g., necessary tools, materials, and motor patterns) and the demands of the activity on affective, cognitive, and neuromuscular capacities. Activity analysis serves as the necessary precursor to the design of activity adaptations required to optimize capacities and to compensate for the limitations presented by disability. It is only after the essential components of a desired activity are identified that strategies can be considered for adapting those components of the activity causing difficulties for the disabled older adult.

Analyzing an activity to match the capacities and limitations of older adults who have physical and cognitive disabilities is a complex process. The factors involved must be considered at three different levels: operations, results, and meaning (Allen, 1987). These levels are hierarchical in nature and will be briefly examined starting with the most concrete level, that of operations.

Operations

The term operations refers to the required technical processes of engaging in an activity to produce an end result. Considerations include the materials, tools, strength, endurance, attention, memory, problem solving capacities, procedures, and neuromuscular patterns required to complete the activity. These considerations must then be juxtaposed to the comprehensive assessment of the functional capacity of the disabled older adult to conceptualize required activity adaptations. The functional assessment identifies operations that are limited by the disability. Compensatory strategies for accomplishing the activity can then be developed.

Two major types of compensatory strategies are used: adaptations that capitalize on remaining neuromuscular and cognitive capabilities and adaptations that use environmental modification. When the therapist's assessment of the individual's functional capacities reveals that a specific motor pattern necessary to do the activity is not available to the individual, the therapist can capitalize on the individual's remaining motor and cognitive capacities to compensate for the motor function deficit by adapting the procedures required by the activity. To illustrate: Although two hands are ordinarily required to fasten buttons, if the individual has lost the use of one hand, it is possible to learn to fasten buttons with one hand. The other type of compensation involves modification of elements of the physical and social environment to compensate for motor, sensory, or cognitive limitations. For example, button closures can be replaced with velcro fastenings which can be secured one-handed; safety treads and grab bars can be added to bathtubs and showers to promote the safety of those experiencing balance and coordination limitations; or, the living environment can be modified to provide the most effective kind of visual, auditory, and tactile stimulation to compensate for specific sensory limitations (Levy, 1986).

Results

The therapist next considers the goals or results that are produced by the requisite operations. A key assumption within this level of activity analysis is that activities are performed with goals in mind, and ultimately the success of any activity is measured in relationship to its goal. The problem here is that although activities are carried out with specific intent, the reasons for pursuing an activity may not always be those inferred by an observer. In fact, there are varying reasons that nondisabled individuals pursue activities, ranging, for example, from the simple pleasure of moving, to an interest in the effects of actions, to an investment in producing a high quality end product. Results are a particularly problematic area for the cognitively disabled, because the range of reasons for pursuing an activity that are available to the cognitively disabled elder is limited by the specific nature of his or her disability (Allen, 1985). All too often, the seemingly simple intent of producing a satisfactory end product exceeds the individual's cognitive capacities. Consequently results that are unsatisfactory by traditional standards are common. It is especially important to provide the cognitively disabled individual with opportunities to pursue activities that are adapted to ensure success because without this intervention, opportunities to pursue activities with successful results are limited.

Meaning

The third hierarchical level in activity analysis considers the implicit or explicit meaning of the activity to the individual. The meaning of an activity is related to diverse factors such as the individual's sense of self as competent rather than incompetent as well as the his or her interests and values. It is also related to the individual's perception of meaningful social roles and the expectations of significant others for role performance. To be meaningful, then, activities must not only be consistent with one's expectations for success, interests, and values, but must also have some relationship to one's desired and expected social roles.

There are several issues to be considered at this level of activity analysis. First, at its most basic level, the intent of intervention in occupational therapy is to enable the individual to maintain a sense of competence despite his or her disability through successful participation in valued life activities and social roles. Concepts of competence and success are central to the profession's philosophy and approach to rehabilitation. At the same time, research amply demonstrates that these concepts are inextricably linked to survival. Seligman (1975), Langer and Rodin (1976), and others (Banziger & Roush, 1983; Langer, Rodin, Beck et al., 1979; Mercer & Kane, 1979; Rodin, 1989; Rodin & Langer, 1977) provide data that supports the notion that individuals who are unconnected to their world and who expect consistent failure are especially prone to depression, accelerated deterioration, and even death. Surely there can be no more convincing argument of the critical need to enable disabled individuals to participate successfully in valued activities and social roles.

And yet, in the face of disability, the older individual or his or her caregiver is forced to reexamine the requirements and expectations of desired social roles. Ultimately it is the ability to carry out the activities that maintain those roles that determines the roles that can be pursued successfully. Often, disabled older adults need assistance in objectively assessing their capacities and limitations in performing desired activities to become aware of their functional potentials and to determine realistic, desirable, and perhaps new social roles. In addition it is vital to appreciate the extent to which severe disability imposes significant limits on the range of desirable activities that the individual can engage in successfully. In these instances therapists intervene by making available opportunities to engage in as wide a range of activities adapted to capitalize the individual's strengths and capacities as possible, including activities in the areas of self-care, work, and leisure. The intent is to provide the individual with the opportunity to choose those activities that are most desirable and to offer assistance in retaining a sense of connection and role investment within one's social world.

This approach to intervention with multiply disabled older adults has much in common with the "Excess Disabilities" approach that is, well documented in the gerontological literature (Brody, Kleban, Lawton et al., 1974) The key to the excess disability approach is to identify and to target treatment toward each individual's "excess disabilities," that is, the discrepancies between the individual's actual functioning in any sphere (physical, psychological, and social) and one's potential functioning. What occupational therapy shares with this approach is the comprehensive assessment of the individual's capabilities and disabilities to determine those specific factors that promote or hinder activity participation. However, the excess disability approach is more generic than that used within rehabilitation, and must be operationalized by the by use of activity analysis to determine those components of an activity that can best be adapted given the capacities and limitations presented by the disability, in order that the individual can participate in desired activities and roles successfully.

Functional Considerations

The functional assessment of the older individual is coupled with activity analysis to design intervention strategies to facilitate the participation of disabled elders in desired activities and social roles. The functional assessment identifies motor, sensory, cognitive, and affective capacities as well as the specific nature of the limitations imposed by the disability which may limit activity participation.

The chronic conditions causing functional limitations in the older population are broad ranging, diverse, and all too common. Four out of five persons over the age of 65 have at least one chronic condition; and, with increasing age, multiple disabling conditions are commonplace (U.S. Senate, 1986). The leading chronic conditions causing activity limitations for the elderly are arthritis, hypertensive disease (including hemiplegias), hearing impairments, heart conditions (U.S. Senate, 1986), and dementia (Katzman, 1976). Each of these conditions impose varying limitations in activity participation which are specific to factors such as the severity of the condition, the presence of additional conditions, and the adaptive capacity of the individual involved. However, the most common limitations imposed by these conditions include decreased strength, endurance, and range of motion as well as deficits in memory, learning, and problem solving. Activity adaptations that are responsive to these limitations will be highlighted shortly.

Notwithstanding, even in the absence of specifically diagnosed conditions, there are a number of functional limitations which occur as a natural consequence of the aging process that confound the limitations imposed by diagnosable conditions. These age-related functional limitations include:

Visual Limitations

For most people, the aging process leads to a slow but steady decrease in visual efficiency. It produces reduced visual acuity, a steadily decreasing ability to focus (accommodation), a reduced capacity to adjust to changes in illumination, a decreased resistance to glare, and a shift in color vision. Compensatory strategies for these limitations are discussed in detail elsewhere (Levy, 1986), but involve environmental modifications that control contrast, glare, and lighting in order to aid acuity, visual field accommodation, and dark adaptation, and to compensate for sensitivity to glare. Generally, these interventions involve the use of increased illumination of the activity environment, magnifiers, large print lettering for written words, supplemental tactile cues, and strong color cueing.

Hearing Limitations

As aging advances, the ability to hear progressively lower frequencies declines. Specifically, age-related losses result in a decreased ability to discriminate speech and increased difficulty in hearing high frequency sounds, especially soft consonants (e.g., c, ch, f, s, sh, th, and z). Hence, many messages sound garbled and are frequently misunderstood, and it becomes increasingly difficult to discriminate speech from background noises. Compensatory strategies for these limitations are also discussed in detail elsewhere (Levy, 1986), but generally involve lowering the pitch of one's voice, the pace of one's speech, amplification, the elimination of background noise (such as radio or television), and the use of supplementary visual and tactile cues.

Cardiovascular Limitations

Age related changes in the arteries and the heart contribute to a decline in cardiac output, losses in the capacity of the heart to respond and recover from extra work, a progressive increase in resistance to blood flow, and a consequent increase in systolic blood pressure (Menks, 1986). These changes result in a diminished supply of oxygenated blood which becomes a major cause of decreased stamina and endurance. Compensatory strategies require that the individual learn principles of work simplification and energy conservation, such as breaking down desired activities in terms of duration and severity of effort; organizing work and leisure space to minimize the need for lifting, bending, and walking; sitting in lieu of standing whenever possible; and storing supplies in close proximity to their place of use.

Muscular System Limitations

Muscle weight and strength tend to decline with age which compounds the problem of diminished strength and endurance induced by the cardiovascular system, especially in those activities requiring major muscle groups. Here, too, compensatory strategies require the individual to learn principles of work simplification and energy conservation.

Respiratory System Limitations

The aging process leads to decreases in expiration and inspiration due to factors such as atrophy of intercostal muscles, thickening of pulmonary walls, and thinning of alveolar walls (Menks, 1986). This further contributes to a decrease in oxygen content of the blood, and consequent limitations in stamina and endurance. Basic principles of work simplification and energy conservation are no less essential to compensate for these limitations.

Skeletal System Limitations

Bone mass tends to decrease with age and become more vulnerable to fracture, which requires increased vigilance to potential safety hazards within the environment to avoid accidental falls. The vertebral column becomes more compressed, is less flexible, and shorter, which can be compensated for by modifications in the height of work surfaces and by optimal placement of supplies. Decreases in cartilage mass also causes the head and neck to flex forward, and flexion in the elbows, hips, and knees such that increased energy is required merely to maintain balance (Jacobs, 1981). Eighty percent of the population experience degeneration of synovium in joints resulting in joint stiffness and pain (Kane, Kane, & Arnold, 1985). Compensation for joint limitations to reduce joint stress and preserve joint structures requires the individual to learn principles of joint protection that will be introduced shortly.

Activity Adaptation with Physical Disabilities

Activity adaptations are derived from the analysis of the essential components of the activity that may be modified to compensate for the individual's functional limitations. For physically disabled individuals there, is particular emphasis on the analysis of the "operations" level of activities. An activity analyzed at this level most often reveals that compensatory strategies should be introduced that modify four major activity components:

1. position of the individual performing the activity
2. the amount of resistance in the activity
3. the properties of materials and tools used, and
4. the procedures for performing the activity (Trombly & Scott, 1984).

Before proceeding it is important to recognize that whenever an activity adaptation requires new learning (e.g., learning to use a modified tool or adaptive device to carry out a desired activity, or learning new procedures for carrying out a highly familiar activity), the cognitive demands of an activity markedly increase. This demand limits the use of such adaptation strategies when, as often occurs, a physical disability is complicated by a cognitive disability. In these instances, therapists must rely on compensatory strategies using modification of environmental elements rather than those which capitalize on the individual's remaining neuromuscular and cognitive capacities. The components that are most often modified by therapists in response to the limitations presented by a physical disability are described here.

Changing the Position of the Individual

The position of the individual relative to the activity can be adapted to compensate for limitations such as poor sitting posture, decreased endurance, and lack of upper extremity strength. Poor posture (induced by disabilities including hemiplegia, arthritis, and osteoporosis) serves to decrease vital capacity, reduce oxygen intake, decrease mental alertness, and increase fatigue.

Activity adaptations designed to compensate for postural limitations might include the use of environmental supports (e.g., a wheelchair cushion with a supporting seat board or modification of the height of the work surface to accommodate reduced sitting height). Individuals with generalized weakness and low endurance should be encouraged to sit rather than stand whenever possible (e.g., use a high stool for meal preparation or laundry tasks), and materials should be stored to minimize the need to bend, reach, or walk.

In addition, limitations in upper extremity strength can contribute to dysfunctional positioning. In the case of hemiplegia, these limitations can be compensated for by the provision of a lap tray or an arm sling to support the arm from excess gravitational pull and by the use of a splint to support the wrist and encourage functional grasp positioning during activity. Functional hand splints are also used to align dislocated joints and muscles and to reduce pain for individuals with arthritis (Shah, Avidan, & Sine, 1981; Spencer, 1988; Trombly, 1984; Trombly & Scott, 1984).

Changing Resistance

Another environmental modification strategy involves the addition or deletion of resistance within an activity to compensate for limitations such as incoordination, decreased range of motion, lack of upper extremity strength, and joint deterioration. For example, a weighted cuff can be placed directly on the wrist to reduce hand tremors. The movement of a weakened hemiparetic extremity can be facilitated by the provision of a mobile arm support or suspension sling that eliminates gravitational resistance. Because excess resistance increases joint destruction and pain, individuals with arthritis must select objects for use in their activities that are as light in weight as possible, i.e., an aluminum pan can substitute for a cast iron pan. Similarly, individuals with decreased strength or endurance induced by cardiopulmonary conditions should avoid lifting or carrying materials that weigh more than two to three pounds and should select clothing that avoids excess weight, e.g., a down coat can substitute for a heavy wool coat (Shah, Avidan, & Sine, 1981; Spencer, 1988; Trombly, 1984; Trombly & Scott, 1984).

Changing Property of Materials and Tools

Environmental modifications can also be made in materials selected for desired activities. Materials are most often adapted in relationship to their pliability, resistance, size, and texture as well as in relationship to the intensity of tactile, visual, and auditory stimulation that they provide. For example, limitations in muscle strength can often be compensated for by selecting materials that are more pliable and that offer less resistance (e.g., thin aluminum can be selected in lieu of

heavy copper when metal tooling, thin muffin batters are more easily mixed than biscuit batters, paper back books can be selected rather than hard-backed books). Coordination or visual limitations can be compensated for by enlarging sizes of recreational materials, such as puzzle pieces and chessmen, or craft materials, such as yarn and tiles. Tactile limitations can be compensated for by selecting materials that are highly textured.

In addition, limitations such as decreased muscle strength, range of motion, and coordination can be compensated for by adaptations in the size and shape of tools. For example, limitations in pinch and grip strength can be compensated for by enlarging handles on tools of daily living such as pencils, combs, toothbrushes, eating utensils, doorknobs, and faucet handles. Limitations in reach can be compensated for by means of extended handles on tools such as combs, bathing sponges, and eating utensils as well as by the use of long handled reacher tongs. Coordination limitations can be compensated for by weighted utensils as well as by the selection of heavier tools rather than lighter ones, e.g., a claw hammer instead of a tack hammer, a cast iron frying pan instead of an aluminum one, or the heaviest electric shaver rather than the lightest (Shah, Avidan, & Sine, 1981; Spencer, 1988; Trombly, 1984; Trombly & Scott, 1984).

Changing Method of Performance

Limitations can also be compensated for by capitalizing on cognitive capacities to teach the individual alternative methods to carry out desired tasks. For example, individuals with hemiplegia can compensate for decreased range of motion and strength in the involved upper extremity by learning to use adaptive equipment for one-handed cooking or dressing. Individuals with arthritis can compensate for joint deterioration by learning how to avoid actions that contribute to joint stress and deformity. Individuals with low stamina and endurance can learn ways of organizing routines, materials, and work areas to make maximal use of available energy. And, because fluctuating energy expenditures are detrimental for those with cardiopulmonary conditions, individuals must learn to carry out activities at a moderate and consistent pace. To reiterate, however, strategies involving new learning have limited use when the individual is experiencing concomitant cognitive limitations.

Clinical Application of Activity Adaptation: Physical Disabilities

The two most commonly experienced chronic physical conditions in the older population are hemiplegias and arthritis (U. S. Senate, 1986). The most frequently used activity adaptations designed to compensate for the limitations imposed by these disabilities are introduced here.

Hemiplegia

The individual who has experienced hemiplegia exhibits a complex pattern of limitations. These include paralysis or muscle weakness on one side of the body, absent or reduced sensation on the affected side, spasticity or flaccidity on the affected side, loss of the visual field on the affected side or unilateral neglect of objects, persons, and sounds on the affected side, and loss of bilateral coordination and balance. In some cases, these neuromuscular limitations are compounded by communication limitations including difficulty in speaking or understanding speech and written words, or by cognitive limitations in learning, memory, judgment, and concentration (Spencer, 1988). The following will provide examples of activity components that are frequently adapted to compensate for the neuromuscular dimensions of these limitations.

Changing the Position of the Individual

The backs, arm rests, foot rests, and seats of wheelchairs can be adapted to compensate for limitations in trunk stability. Trunk stability can also be encouraged by appropriate placement of seat cushions. Tools and materials should be placed within normal reach of the unaffected side to compensate for one-handedness as well as balance limitations. Arm troughs and lapboards can be added to wheelchairs to position and support the paralyzed arm and to eliminate gravitational pull on weak muscles. Hand splints also encourage functional positioning, and grasp.

Changing Resistance

Suspension slings and mobile arm supports support and facilitate movement of the affected extremity by eliminating gravitational resistance. Lighter weight tools and supplies compensate for limitations in strength and endurance.

Changing Properties of Materials and Tools

Tools are frequently adapted to compensate for limitations in range of motion, decreased strength, and incoordination. As indicated earlier, limited range of motion is often compensated for by using extended handles on utensils and tools, such as a long handled spoon to reach the mouth. Limited range is also compensated for by reaching tongs that are used, for example, to remove clothes from shelves, to initiate pulling clothes over parts of the body, or to pick up objects from the floor. Limitations in grasp strength and prehension are compensated for by enlarging handles of the variety of tools and utensils used in daily activities by, for example, wrapping handles or writing utensils with foam secured with a rubber band for temporary use, or by purchasing commercially available utensils with built-up handles for permanent use. When grasp is not possible, a "universal cuff," or utensil holder, can be used that fits around the palm and has a pocket for the insertion of the utensil handle. Bilateral coordination limitations can be compensated for by the use of loafer style shoes or elastic shoelaces which avoid the need to tie shoelaces with two hands. Lack of a stabilizing hand to perform activities can be compensated for adaptations including: the use of masking tape, a clipboard, or weights to stabilize paper when writing longhand; the use of clamps to hold craft objects, such as an embroidery hoop, on a tabletop; the use of a suction cup to secure a nail brush to the side of the sink to clean fingernails of the unaffected hand; or, the use of a spiked cutting board to hold meat, vegetables, and fruit while cutting and peeling.

Materials can also be adapted to compensate for limited range, decreased strength, and incoordination. For example, self dressing is facilitated by selecting loose fitting clothing, converting buttons to Velcro, using waistbands for skirts, having dresses open in the front, and changing zippers in pants to Velcro (Shah, Avidan, & Sine, 1981; Spencer, 1988; Trombly, 1984).

Changing Method of Performance

With sensory and motor loss on the affected side of the body, the individual functionally becomes one-sided. And yet, a number of procedures for performing bilateral activities can be adapted so that they can be done unilaterally. For example, numerous one handed cooking procedures can be learned, as can one-handed dressing procedures. The individual can learn how to cut meat with the use of a rocker knife (a knife with a sharp curved blade that cuts when rocked over meat); one can learn how to spread bread by trapping it in the corner of a spikeboard, and spreading it toward the corner; or, one can learn to manage a one-handed can-opener. And, one can learn one-handed dressing routines such as putting clothing on the affected side of the body first, and taking clothes off the unaffected side of the body first. Procedures can also be learned to conserve limited strength and energy. These involve such routines such as organizing storage to eliminate wasted trips, eliminating all but essential steps of a task, and incorporating regular rest periods into the day's work plan (Shah, Avidan, & Sine, 1981; Trombly, 1984).

Arthritis

The older adult with rheumatoid or osteoarthritis experiences pain and stiffness in joints, where there may be subluxation (when the bones slip out of their normal position), dislocation, swelling, and deformity. The result is functional limitations in joint range of motion affecting reach, grasp, and coordination as well as limitations in strength due to the disuse that is caused by pain and limited range of motion (Spencer, 1988). Components of activities that are adapted to compensate for these limitations include the following.

Changing the Position of the Individual

Positioning is an essential adaptation for the individual with arthritis because poor positioning encourages pain, poor functional alignment, joint stiffening, and deformity. High straight backed chairs with firm cushions are necessary to provide trunk and head support while sitting, and a firm mattress is necessary for support while sleeping. And yet, static positioning encourages stiffness and muscle imbalance. Hence, any prolonged position (e.g., sitting) should be avoided, and activities should be designed to accommodate change of position at 20 minute intervals.

With limited joint function, joints can assume dysfunctional and painful positions. If the wrist is unstable, wrist splints are fabricated to position the wrist in a more functional position and to reduce pain. Dislocated joints and muscles in the hand can also be properly aligned, and pain reduced, with a functional hand splint (Spencer, 1988).

Changing Resistance

Activities requiring strength must be carefully considered for the individual with arthritis, because too much resistance can increase joint destruction and pain. Any object used within activities should be as light in weight as possible, e.g., an aluminum frying pan rather than a cast iron one, and heavy objects should either be slid across flat surfaces or transported in a wheeled cart, rather than lifted or carried (Spencer, 1988).

Changing Properties of Materials and Tools

Adapted tools and materials similar to those used by the individual with hemiplegia are used, with differences due to the fact that in arthritis, the major limitations to be compensated for are decreased range of motion and strength, whereas with hemiplegia these same limitations are compounded by the limitations imposed by one-handedness. Hence, for the individual with arthritis, long handled tools and special holders are used to compensate for limitations in range and strength, as well as to conserve energy and reduce stress on joints. For example, long-handled lightweight utensils compensate for limited range of the shoulder and elbow; i.e., a long handled bath sponge facilitates self-bathing if the individual cannot reach his feet, and lipstick can be mounted on aluminum tubing and independently applied if the individual cannot reach her mouth. A swivel spoon may prevent spillage and assist self-feeding if the individual experiences limitations in range of motion in rotation of the forearm. Built-up handles or universal cuffs also compensate for limited range of motion and weakness of the hand. Built-up handles minimize the joint stress that results when objects are tightly grasped. Other strategies to reduce the joint stress caused by tight grasp include: cleaning fingernails with a brush that fits over the palmar part of the hand, or using a nail brush secured to the sink with suction cups; using equipment such as jar openers or electric can openers; and, using a book holder to hold books for an extended period of time. In addition, the clothing adaptations that were suggested to compensate for limited range and strength for individuals with hemiplegia are also suitable for those with arthritis; for example, selecting clothing that opens in the front compensates for limitations in range and strength, and replacing fastenings with large buttons or velcro closures compensates for limitations in range and strength while reducing the joint stress imposed by buttoning small buttons or pinching small zippers (Shah, Avidan, & Sine, 1981; Spencer, 1988; Trombly, 1984).

Changing Method of Performance

The individual with arthritis must learn principles of joint protection, energy conservation, and work simplification to reduce joint stress and pain and to preserve joint structures. Often, life-long habits in performing routine activities serve to exacerbate symptoms and increase joint destruction, and must be changed. Consequently, the cognitive demands involved are high.

For example, individuals must learn to remember to change positions or activities frequently, to stretch tight muscles and relieve pressure on the joints. Or, they must learn how to avoid positions that increase deformity by, for example, turning door knobs with one hand rather than two, and dialing phones with pencils rather than fingers. They must also learn to use proper body mechanics when sitting, standing, walking, climbing stairs, pulling, lifting, or pushing weight to minimize stress on other joints; and, they must learn to avoid lifting, pulling, or carrying *any* heavy objects. Carts or wheeled tables should be substituted to transport heavy items. Routine activities must also be simplified, and frequent rest periods need to be balanced with periods of activity in one's daily schedule. For example, the individual needs to plan to complete components of the evening meal in periodic sessions that are balanced with rest periods throughout the day rather than attempting to prepare the entire meal within one prolonged activity period prior to serving it (Spencer, 1988).

Activity Adaptation in Cognitive and Physical Disabilities

Theoretical Formulations

Just as a physical disability imposes limitations on the individual's ability to pursue desired life activities, so does a cognitive disability. A cognitive disability presents different challenges to the adaptation of activities because the limitations that must be compensated for involve the thought patterns that are prerequisite to participation in normal life activities (Allen, 1985; Levy,

---

1986). Similar to activity analysis in light of physical disabilities, activity analysis here is used to determine which components in the desired activity the individual can and cannot do, and activities are adapted to maximize use of carefully assessed capabilities and to compensate for limitations. Given the nature of limitations imposed by a cognitive disability, however, therapists place particular emphasis on the "results" level of activity analysis, in contrast to emphasis placed on the "operations" level for the physically disabled.

The analysis of activities for those with cognitive disabilities involves the identification and assessment of thought patterns that are by their very nature abstract. It is important therefore to gain some familiarity with concepts and assumptions of Allen's (1985) cognitive disability theory as a basis for understanding activity adaptations specific to the thought patterns that impose limits on successful activity and role participation. The following provides a brief overview of concepts and assumptions used in functional assessment, activity analysis, and activity adaptation for the cognitively disabled elder.

A primary intent of cognitive disability theory is to identify the thought patterns that need to be assessed to determine whether an individual can perform a desired activity successfully. To this end, Allen (1985) has proposed a hierarchy of six cognitive levels that identify those dimensions of thought that differentiate and explain functional limitations in day to day activities. Three dimensions of thought are considered at each of the six cognitive levels. These are:

1. Sensory cues. These cues capture and sustain attention. Allen identifies two sources of sensory cues that serve as precursors to motor action: those that arise from the individual's inner world, including subliminal and proprioceptive cues and those that arise from the environment, including tactile, visual, auditory, and, finally, complex symbolic cues. At lower cognitive levels, individuals can attend only to internal cues, such as musculoskeletal sensations. At higher cognitive levels, individuals can respond to progressively wider ranges of cues, including internal cues as well as those from the environment.

2. Sensorimotor associations. This term refers to the reasons why an individual performs an action. The implicit goal of the individual performing an activity may not be consistent with the explicit goals of a given activity. For example, a cognitively disabled individual who chooses to vacuum a rug may well be more invested in the *action* of pushing the vacuum back and forth, than the *result* that would be intended by a less disabled individual (i.e., a clean rug). Consequently, at lower cognitive levels, unintentional results become commonplace.

3. Motor actions. Motor actions are elicited by sensory cues and are guided by sensorimotor associations. There are two types: spontaneous (self initiated) and imitated (copied from another person). At lower cognitive levels, individuals are only able to initiate or imitate motor actions that are already very familiar behavioral patterns. At higher cognitive levels, self initiated motor actions are more diverse and individuals are able to imitate motor actions not already mastered.

The principle contribution of cognitive disability theory to activity adaptation is that it provides means for analyzing the relative difficulty of any activity in terms of requisite dimensions of thought. From this analysis, environmental factors are identified that are associated with deficient dimensions of thought. Activity adaptations are derived from an understanding of how the cognitive elements of the environment might best be modified to compensate for cognitive limitations and to place desired activities within an individual's range of comprehension. Therapists modify the structure of a desired activity to capitalize on (1) the sensory cues that are attended to in the process of doing an activity at any given cognitive level; (2) the quality of sensorimotor association, or the reason why the individual performs the activity at any given level; and (3) the amount of assistance required to enable the individual to complete the activity at any given level (i.e., whether the desired motor action must be imitated from the therapist or can be self initiated by the individual).

Clinical Application

The identification of environmental factors associated with the dimensions of thought required for activity and role participation provides the conceptual basis for activity adaptation. The discussion that follows will identify dimensions of thought, associated environmental factors, and guidelines for the design of activity adaptations required at each of the cognitive levels. In addition, guidelines for the adaptation of activity for older individuals experiencing both cognitive and physical disabilities will be emphasized, given the reality that single disabilities rarely occur in the aging population and that multiple disabilities are common (U.S. Senate, 1986).

Therapists will find it useful to note that cognitive levels 1 and 2 are most often associated with conditions such as severe hemiplegia, severe dementia, and acute head injuries. Levels 3, 4, and 5, are associated with moderate hemiplegia, moderate and mild dementia, and major mental disorders.

Cognitive Level 1

At this level, *attention* is directed to subliminal internal cues, such as hunger, taste, and smell, and individuals are largely unresponsive to external stimuli. Few motor actions are being performed because there is no reason for performing motor actions. *Motor actions* are limited to the potential to follow near-reflexive one-word directives, such as "sip" or "turn." With little, if any, purpose and few, if any, motor actions available, there are few cognitive capabilities to capitalize on, and it is unrealistic to conceptualize activity adaptations.

Therapists and caregivers find that the individual either actively resists or is at best uncooperative in efforts to provide required maximal assistance in grooming, bathing, and feeding. The individual may need to be fed or allowed to eat with the fingers. Walking and transfers from bed to wheelchair may be achieved with physical guidance. An orienting response can be elicited by familiar gustatory and olfactory stimuli (e.g., favorite foods and spices, fragrant plants, hand lotion, aftershave), gentle touch, massage, or a family pet. (Allen, 1985; Allen, 1988; Levy, 1986; Levy, 1987).

Cognitive Level 2

At this level, *attention* is directed to proprioceptive cues from muscles and joints that are elicited by one's own highly familiar body movements. The *goal* in performing a motor action is to repeat the one-step motor action component of the activity for the pleasure of its effect on the body alone (i.e., on one's sense of position and balance, or on sensory input to muscles and joints). *Motor actions* are limited to the ability to imitate, albeit inexactly, a one step direction only if it involves the use of a highly familiar near reflexive gross motor pattern. New learning is not possible.

Activities that can be successfully accomplished at this level are those that are adapted to capitalize on the capacity to imitate one step familiar repetitive gross motor actions. Therapists and caregivers will find that providing opportunities to imitate simple movement, calisthenics, and modified sports activities are most often useful, but one step activities such as folding laundry, chopping vegetables, and polishing furniture can be imitated if these activities were near habitual prior to the onset of the disability. Spontaneous behaviors are largely unproductive or bizarre (e.g., sitting backward on the toilet and "driving" it like a car—flushing to "shift gears," constantly disrobing and redressing, reapplying the same lipstick over and over again). It appears as though individuals are searching for opportunities to apply very familiar gross motor patterns to the environment regardless of the context. Hence it is critical that therapists and caregivers provide individuals with opportunities to imitate activities specifically adapted to their cognitive capacities to optimize functional performance and to enable the retention of some sense of dignity, connection to the external environment, and role investment within their social world.

Therapists and caregivers find that individuals at this level may cooperate by moving body parts to assist in activities such as grooming, dressing, and feeding but that maximal assistance and direct supervision are still essential. With supervision individuals may be able to eat unassisted with spoons and non-slip scoop-edged plates, although other utensils are used incorrectly. Aimless pacing is common, but the individual will walk in directions guided by companions. To avoid voiding in unacceptable locations, individuals should be escorted to the bathroom. Individuals at this level are easily confused when objects are hidden by doors, drawers, or closets. Whenever possible it is helpful to leave bathroom and bedroom doors open and to place frequently used objects or treasured possessions on furniture surfaces or hangers where they can be seen easily.

Individuals in wheelchairs can often manage the repetitive movement required to propel the chair; however, they are unable to initiate the planning required to direct that motion and frequently run into objects or walls. In addition, they may not recognize their motor limitations and may attempt to get up to walk. In these instances wheelchair restraints may be indicated. Notwithstanding, therapists and caregivers need to be alert to the need to design environmental strategies and to provide continuous supervision to protect individuals functioning at this level from safety hazards (Allen, 1985; Allen, 1988; Levy, 1986; Levy, 1987).

Cognitive Level 3

At this level, *attention* is directed to tactile cues and to familiar objects that can be manipulated. The *goal* in performing a motor action is limited to the process of discovering the kinds of effects one's actions have on the environment. These actions are typically repeated to verify that similar results occur. *Motor actions* are limited to the ability to follow a one step highly familiar action-oriented direction which has been demonstrated for the individual to follow. It is unrealistic to expect the individual to learn new behavior.

Activities that can be successfully accomplished at this level are those that are adapted to capitalize on the capacity to imitate one step familiar, repetitive, and tactile actions. The intent is to provide opportunities to participate in adapted activities to reinforce the relationship between one's actions and predictable effects on the environment. Possibilities include sports activities, such as swimming, biking, and playing "catch"; household maintenance activities, such as washing the car, mowing lawns, cultivating gardens, hand washing laundry; and kitchen activities, such as washing and drying the dishes, peeling and chopping vegetables, and cleaning counter tops. As in the previous level, functional performance can be maximized by teaching the caregiver how to present activities to the individual in a manner that will elicit productive motor actions.

Spontaneous motor actions include such unproductive behaviors as clicking dials on and off, using keys indiscriminately in locks, and pouring soup in the coffee maker. It is no less critical at this level to provide the individual with opportunities for more productive "face saving" use of familiar movement patterns to enable a sense of competence and role investment within his or her social environment. At this level the goal of the activity is *not* related to a specific outcome or end product but rather to the relationship between actions and their predictable effects. Consequently therapists and caregivers need to appreciate the need for the individual to do the same thing over and over again, even though by traditional standards this behavior might appear to be unnecessary. Allowance should be made for behaviors such as vacuuming the same spot over and over again and polishing the same spot on the car door.

Caregivers find that individuals are able to brush teeth, wash hands and face, and use familiar table utensils independently, although they need to be reminded to do these activities. In the absence of a concomitant physical disability, they are also able to manage dressing. However, if the caregiver does not select clothing and hand items to the individual one at a time, errors are frequent. For example, underwear may be placed over trousers, clothes may be donned inside out or backwards, and nightclothes may be selected for daytime wear. Most self-maintenance activities must be broken down into one step motor actions, and supplies for activities such as tooth brushing, shaving, bathing, and hair washing should be presented one at a time. Note that physically disabled individuals at this level will still require assistance in self-care activities such as dressing because the routines required to perform adapted self care techniques often entail procedures that are not highly familiar.

For the individual with concomitant physical disabilities, the repetitive actions required to manage a wheelchair or a walker can be initiated, but individuals will not be able to attend to safety concerns which entail two or three steps, such as applying wheelchair brakes or the manipulating foot plates, nor will they without an escort be able to arrive at proper locations at proper times. To follow through on an activity mastered in therapy (e.g., wheeling one's chair to the dining room), caregiving staff need to be instructed about the individual's need to be cued to each successive step of the activity. Individuals may benefit from adapted equipment that requires the use of familiar motor actions (e.g., traditional eating utensils with extended or built up handles to compensate for limited range of motion or grasp), but will not be able to make use of adapted equipment requiring the use of unfamiliar motor patterns (e.g., reaching tongs to initiate pulling clothes over parts of the body). Therapists will also find that individuals at this level require one to one supervision to sustain attention to therapeu-

tic exercises (Allen, 1985; Allen, 1988; Levy, 1986; Levy, 1987).

Cognitive Level 4

Attention at this level is directed to tactile as well as visible cues, and it is sustained throughout short-term activities to their completion. The *goal* in performing a motor action is to perceive cause and effect relationships between a tangible cue and a desired outcome. *Motor actions* are limited to the ability to follow a two to three step, highly familiar motor process that leads to the accomplishment of familiar goals. It is now possible to learn two to three step procedures that have visible and predictable results.

Activities that can be accomplished successfully at this level are those that are adapted to capitalize on the capacity to use two to three step familiar motor actions that have predictable visible results. Because mistakes at this level are not noticed, the challenge is to provide opportunities to engage in simple, relatively error proof activities that support desired social roles. This goal is best accomplished by incorporating into the individual's daily routine yard work, household chores (e.g., laundry, simple meal preparation, shopping for a few familiar purchases), familiar sports and dance activities, simple board games and puzzles, letter writing or typing, and walks to familiar destinations.

Despite significant cognitive impairment, the individual appears to be less confused at this level because activities are pursued with specific outcomes in mind. Caregivers and therapists should encourage individuals to engage in comprehensible concrete activities to protect personal dignity and enable social role retention, but should not expect the individual to notice mistakes or solve problems when they occur, to retain directions out of context, to plan beyond the immediate situation, to generalize learning to new situations, or to anticipate safety hazards. At this level individuals are more easily engaged in activities and therapeutic regimens than at previous levels because the goal is to achieve a desired outcome (e.g., "to get the job done"). Desired outcomes, however, are restricted to those that are concrete and predictable, and that entail no more than a three step process.

Caregivers find that individuals can complete familiar grooming activities, although they frequently neglect areas that are not clearly visible. For example, the back of the body may remain unwashed, shampoo may not be rinsed from the back of the head, and the individual may neglect to shave under the chin. Dressing can be accomplished relatively independently, although the appearance of the backs of garments may be ignored. The individual can eat independently but may require assistance to season foods, share a limited quantity of food, open unfamiliar containers, or avoid burns. Individuals should be protected from invisible hazards from sources such as heat, chemicals, and electricity.

Therapists find that physically disabled individuals at this level can learn to follow an exercise program and wheelchair safety precautions but will require weeks of practice to master their skills. Adaptive equipment can be successfully introduced if the actions required are highly familiar, if they involve no more than three steps, and if the intended effect is highly visible. For example, the individual with hemiparesis can learn how to cut meat unilaterally with the use of a rocker knife or an individual with arthritis can learn to use an electric can opener to reduce the joint stress caused by tight grasp. In addition, modified procedures such as those required in one-handed dressing (e.g., putting clothing on the hemiparetic side first and taking clothes off the unaffected side first) can be mastered after weeks of practice (Allen, 1985; Allen, 1988; Levy, 1986; Levy, 1987).

Cognitive Level 5

At this level, *attention* is captured and sustained by the interesting properties of objects. The *goal* of action is to explore the effects of self initiated motor actions on physical objects and to investigate these effects through the use of overt trial-and-error problem solving. *Motor actions* are exploratory to produce interesting effects on material objects, and they extend to the ability to follow through on a four or five step concrete process. The individual is now able to learn through doing. Hence, in the event of a concomitant physical disability, teaching new procedures for carrying out desired activities becomes an appropriate rehabilitation objective.

Numerous activities can be accomplished successfully at this level because in concrete activities (i.e., those involving familiar four to five step motor actions with visibly perceivable results), individuals function relatively independently. However, the cognitive limitations experienced by elders at this level become apparent when individuals are engaged in activities that require attention to abstract and symbolic cues, such as those that involve spoken and written instructions, diagrams, or drawings. Activities requiring attention to these cues will accentuate the disability and should be avoided.

Caregivers find that individuals can complete grooming, dressing, and eating activities without assistance. Household activities are carried out relatively independently, although the individual may require assistance in the abstract reasoning required to establish safety procedures and to anticipate hazardous situations. Difficulties in cooking may be reflected in the inability to anticipate burning of food or to anticipate the need to coordinate the timing of several dishes.

Because individuals with physical disabilities are now able to follow a series of demonstrated instructions containing new information, they can now follow a ther-

apeutic exercise program and learn requirements within two to four sessions. In addition, most adaptive equipment can be successfully introduced, although attention to safety precautions that must be anticipated may be neglected (e.g., the chaffing of a splint strap). The cognitive demands of activity adaptations such as work simplification and energy conservation techniques may be beyond the cognitive capabilities of individuals at this level. These techniques often require the individual to use abstract reasoning in, for example, prioritizing activities and organizing future routines; the individual at this level is limited to reasoning that is concrete. When involved in daily routines, however, the individual can be cued by others to make use of such strategies (Allen, 1985; Allen, 1988; Levy, 1986; Levy, 1987).

Cognitive Level 6

Attention at this level is captured by abstract and symbolic cues. The *goal* is to use abstract reasoning to reflect about the range of possible actions, including reconsideration of old plans and creation of new ones. Spontaneous *motor actions* are those that have been planned in advance and on which there are no restrictions on performance. Learning uses symbolic thought and deductive reasoning, and can be generalized to new situations. Theoretically, this level represents the absence of cognitive disability. Activity adaptations to compensate for cognitive limitations are not required (Allen, 1985).

For the individual with a physical disability, activity adaptations can now be introduced that compensate for physical limitations by learning complex alternative procedures for carrying out activities, or that require the individual to change life long patterns in performing routine activities. For instance, individuals with arthritis can learn to remember to change positions frequently and to avoid highly-habituated positioning that increase joint deterioration, such as turning door knobs with two hands rather than one, or using improper body mechanics when sitting, standing, walking, or climbing stairs. Now that the individual is able to organize the home environment and can plan a schedule for completing chores in light of priorities and energy constraints, more abstract activity adaptations such as those that involve work simplification and energy conservation techniques can be learned and incorporated into daily routines.

In conclusion, the process of activity adaptation for the cognitively disabled elder requires familiarity with concepts of cognitive disability theory. Environmental elements associated with the dimensions of thought that affect activity and role participation have been identified at each of the cognitive levels and include (1) the cues that should be provided by the therapist or caregiver, (2) an appreciation of what is perceived based on those cues, and (3) the type and complexity of assistance and directions to be given to elicit productive motor actions. Adapted activities for the cognitively disabled individual maximize remaining cognitive capabilities of the individual by modifying both the cognitive demands and the structure of the activity to enable best performance in activities that support desired social roles.

Concepts that are considered in adapting activities for the cognitively disabled individual are critical to the design of activity adaptations for the elder who is both physically and cognitively disabled. The presence of a cognitive disability places limits on the use of those strategies for adapting activities to compensate for neuromuscular limitations that require unfamiliar tools, modified procedures, or new learning; in these instances emphasis is placed on compensatory strategies that involve environmental modifications. Hence, concepts used to adapt activities for the cognitively disabled elder assume high priority when therapists consider how best to design activity adaptations to compensate for the limitations experienced by the individual who is both physically and cognitively disabled.

Conclusion

Activity adaptation presents an approach to rehabilitation that helps the disabled older adult maintain active participation in as many preferred activities and social roles as possible, given the disability that exists. The primary purpose of activity adaptation is to enable a sense of competence by facilitating the best performance of activities that the individual needs and wants to do. Activity adaptation entails the knowledgeable modification of the multifaceted components of activities to allow the elder with limitations to still meet activity demands. Appropriately adapted activities optimize remaining strengths and capacities to provide ongoing success experiences that enable the disabled individual to retain a sense of competence, dignity, and social role involvement. In this way, adapted activities contribute significantly to enhanced functional independence, life satisfaction, and quality of life in the later years.

References

Allen, C.A. (1985). *Occupational therapy for psychiatric diseases: Measurement and management of cognitive disabilities.* Boston: Little, Brown.

Allen, C.A. (1987). Activity: Occupational therapy's treatment method. *American Journal of Occupational Therapy, 41,* 563–575.

Allen, C.A. (1988). Cognitive disabilities. In S. Robertson (Ed.). *Focus: Skills for assessment and treatment.* Rockville, Md.: American Occupational Therapy Association.

Atchley, R. (1980). *The social forces in later life: An introduction to social gerontology,* 3rd Ed. Belmont, CA.: Wadsworth Publishing Co.

Banziger, G., & Roush, S. (1983). Nursing homes for the birds: A control-relevant intervention with bird feeders. *Gerontologist, 23,* 527–531.

Brody, E., Kleban, M., Lawton, M., & Moss, M. (1974). A longitudinal look at excess disabilities in the mentally impaired aged. *Journal of Gerontology, 29,* 79–84.

Burrus-Bammel, L., & Bammel, G.(1985). Leisure and recreation. In J.E. Birren & K.W. Schaie (Eds.). *Handbook of the psychology of aging,* 2nd Ed. New York: Van Nostrand Reinhold.

Cynkin, S. (1979). *Occupational therapy: Toward health through activities.* Boston: Little, Brown.

Gordon, C., Gaitz, C.M., & Scott, J. (1976). Leisure and lives. In R.H. Binstock & E. Shanas E (Eds.). *Handbook of aging and the social sciences.* New York: Van Nostrand Reinhold.

Harris, L., & Associates (1975). *The myth and reality of aging in America.* Washington DC: National Council on the Aging.

Havinghurst, R.J., & Feigenbaum, K. (1968). Leisure and lifestyle. In B. Neugarten (Ed.). *Middle age and aging.* Chicago: University of Chicago Press.

Havinghurst, R.J. (1963). Successful aging. In R.H. Williams, C. Tibbitts, and W. Donahue (Eds.). *Processes of aging.* New York: Atherton Press.

Jacobs, R. (1981). Physical changes in the aged. In M. Devereaux (Ed.). *Elder care: A guide to clinical geriatrics.* New York: Grune and Stratton, Inc.

Kane, R.L., Kane, R.A., & Arnold, S.B. (1985). Prevention and the elderly: Risk factors. *Health Services Research, 19*(6, pt.II), 945–1005.

Katzman, R. (1976). Prevalence and malignancy of Alzheimer's disease. *Archives of Neurology, 33,* 217–218.

Langer, E. J., & Rodin, J. (1976). The effects of choice and enhanced personal responsibility for the aged: A field experiment in an institutional setting. *Journal of Personality and Social Psychology, 34,* 191–198.

Langer, E.J., Rodin, J., Beck, C. et al. (1979). Environmental determinants of memory improvement in late adulthood. *Journal of Personality and Social Psychology, 27,* 2000–2013.

Levy, L.L. (1986). Sensory change and compensation. In L.J. Davis and M. Kirkland (Eds.), *Role of occupational therapy with the elderly.* Rockville, Md.: American Occupational Therapy Association.

Levy, L.L. (1986). A practical guide to the care of the Alzheimer's disease victim. *Topics in Geriatric Rehabilitation, 1,* 16–26.

Levy, L.L. (1987). Psychosocial intervention and dementia, part 2. *Occupational Therapy in Mental Health, 7,* 13–36.

Llorens, L. (1986). Activity analysis: Agreement among factors in a sensory processing model. *American Journal of Occupational Therapy, 40,* 103–110.

Menks, F. (1986). Anatomical and physiological changes in late adulthood. In L.J. Davis and M. Kirkland (Eds.), *Role of occupational therapy with the elderly.* Rockville, Md.: American Occupational Therapy Association.

Mercer, S., & Kane, R. (1979). Helplessness and hopelessness among the institutionalized aged: An experiment. *Health and Social Work, 4,* 90–116.

Mosey, A.C. (1981). *Occupational therapy: Configuration of a profession.* New York: Raven Press.

Riley, M.W., & Riley, J.W. Jr. (1989). The lives of older people and changing social roles. *Annals of the American Academy of Political and Social Science, 503,* 14–28.

Rodin, J. (1989). Sense of control: Potentials for intervention. *Annals of the American Academy of Political and Social Science, 503,* 29–42.

Rodin, J. & Langer E.J. (1977). Long-term effects of a control-relevant intervention with the institutionalized aged. *Journal of Personality and Social Psychology, 35,* 897–902.

Seligman, M. (1975). *Helplessness: On depression, development, and death.* San Francisco: W.H. Freeman.

Shah, M., Avidan, R., & Sine, R. (1981). Self care training for patients with hemiplegia, Parkinsonism, and arthritis. In R.D. Sine, J.D. Holcomb, R.E. Roush et al.(Eds.). *Basic rehabilitation techniques.* Rockville, Md.: Aspen.

Spencer, E.A. (1988). Functional restoration: Neurologic, orthopedic, and arthritic conditions. In H.L. Hopkins & H. Smith (Eds). *Willard and Spackman's occupational therapy, 7th Ed.* (Philadelphia: Lippencott.

Trombly, C.A. (1984). Activities of daily living. In C.A. Trombly (Ed.). *Occupational therapy for physical dysfunction,* 2nd Ed. Baltimore: Williams and Wilkins.

Trombly, C.A. & Scott, A.D. (1984). Activity adaptation. In C.A. Trombly (Ed.). *Occupational therapy for physical dysfunction,* 2nd Ed. Baltimore: Williams and Wilkins.

U.S. Senate, Special Committee on Aging (1986). *Aging America, Trends and projections, 1985-1986.* Washington DC: U.S. Government Printing Office 498-116-814/42395.

Chapter 44

Generalization of Treatment: A Multicontext Approach to Cognitive Perceptual Impairment in Adults with Brain Injury

Joan Pascale Toglia, MA, OTR

The ability to apply what has been learned in therapy to a variety of new situations and environments is termed *generalization* (Sufrin, 1984). Transfer of learning is included within the concept of generalization but is narrower in scope and refers only to the ability to apply specific strategies to a related task (Parente & Anderson-Parente, 1989). Both transfer and generalization refer to the use of skills in contexts other than those of their initial use.

Approaches used by occupational therapists in the treatment of perceptual deficits have been categorized by Neistadt (1988) as either remedial or adaptive. Adaptive, functional approaches capitalize on the patient's assets and are used to provide direct training in activities of daily living. Remedial approaches focus on the impaired area and are used to improve abilities through the retraining of specific perceptual components of behavior with the use of tabletop activities or sensorimotor exercises. These two approaches contain different assumptions regarding generalization. In the remedial approach, generalization of learning is a process that is assumed to occur automatically. For example, retraining specific perceptual cognitive skills with tabletop drills, computer activities, or sensorimotor exercises assumes that observed improvements in specific skill areas will affect performance on other tasks requiring the same underlying skill. In contrast, an adaptive, functional treatment approach uses techniques that minimize requirements for generalization (Neistadt, 1990). In this approach, the patient with brain injury is bound by context and is unable to generalize new information to different contexts. This, repetitive practice with specific functional activities is emphasized rather than transfer of learning to a variety of situations (Davis & Radomski, 1989).

These two opposing treatment approaches are reminiscent of arguments regarding transfer of learning that occurred at the turn of the century. In that era, one group of theorists argued that transfer of learning was rare and occurred only when cued by physical similarities (Thorndike & Woodworth, 1901). Other theorists believed that transfer occurred automatically when a task or piece of information learned in one context was relevant to the second context. The more general the skill, the greater the likelihood of transfer (Ferguson, 1956; Hebb, 1949; Judd, 1908).

Recently, a number of studies in the psychology literature have identified conditions that maximize the probability of transfer of learning in nondysfunctional children and adults (Belmont, Butterfield, & Ferretti, 1982; Brown & Kane, 1988; Gick & Holyoak, 1983, 1987). The findings support the contention that transfer of learning does not occur automatically. "One must teach for transfer rather than merely hoping or even praying that it will occur" (Sternberg, 1987, p. 258). These more recent theorists argued that transfer occurs during learning, not after. Transfer is part of the learning process and must be directly addressed throughout the treatment process (Brown, Bransford, Ferrara, & Campione, 1983). These findings contain implications for the promotion of transfer of learning with brain-injured adults where difficulty in learning has been identified as a major barrier in rehabilitation (Ben-Yishay & Diller, 1983a).

Current treatment approaches used by occupational therapists contain few guidelines for addressing generalization. In the present paper, I propose a multicontext treatment approach based on a cognitive psychology framework for learning. Literature on learning and generalization is reviewed, and direct applications to treatment with the adult with brain injury are discussed.

Learning: An Organizational Framework

In contemporary cognitive psychology, learning is conceptualized as knowledge acquisition through an interaction of internal and external factors that influence the ability to process information (Brown et al., 1983; Glaser, 1990). Six basic factors have been identified as being critical to the process of learning and generalization. The first three factors—environmental context, nature of the task, and learning criteria—are external to the learner. The last three factors—metacognition, processing strategies, and learner's characteristics—are internal to the learner (Bransford, 1979; Jenkins, 1979). Internal and external factors are interrelated in their effect on learning and generalization. Performance is a result of interaction between the total set of variables. In essence, learning is a function of the relationship between the learner and the task to be learned (Bransford, 1979; Brown et al., 1983; Jenkins, 1979).

Environmental context. The familiarity of the environment as well as the type of environment (physical, social, or cultural) can influence learning (Abreu & Toglia, 1987). For example, a crowded, unfamiliar environment filled with auditory and visual distractions can alter the learner's attitude and ability to process and monitor information.

Nature of the task. The numbers, spatial arrangement, and familiarity of stimuli as well as the rate of response, task directions, type of materials, and movement and postural requirements can influence the learner's attitude, choice of strategies, and self-monitoring skills

(Abreu & Toglia, 1987; Bransford, 1979). For example, as the number of items in a task increases, more demands are placed on the ability to select relevant stimuli, prioritize, screen out irrelevant details, and plan. If the amount of information presented exceeds the patient's processing capacity, the patient will have difficulty developing effective responses and may become frustrated or overwhelmed and withdraw from the task. In addition, the body alignment, positioning, and active movement patterns used during an activity can require different types of information processing and self-monitoring strategies (Abreu & Toglia, 1987).

Learning criteria. These are the kinds of tasks used to evaluate the degree of learning or performance outcome. Many different tasks can be used to measure learning. These measures can yield quite different results and conclusions regarding the person's learning capacity (Bransford, 1979).

Metacognition. Metacognition includes two aspects that are interrelated: knowledge concerning one's own cognitive processes and capacities and the ability to monitor one's own performance. Inaccurate perception of the nature of the task and its level of difficulty can lead to inability to initiate or choose appropriate task strategies (Brown et al., 1983).

Processing strategies. The kinds of strategies that learners use when presented with material (e.g., selecting relevant information, prioritizing, rehearsing, categorizing information, associating, elaborating) depend on the nature of the task (e.g., stimuli parameters, environmental context, movement requirements) as well as the familiarity and perceived difficulty of the task (Brown et al., 1983).

Learner's characteristics. These characteristics include previous knowledge, existing skills, attitudes, emotions, and experiences. Information that can be easily related to previous knowledge, experience, and skills will be more easily learned and remembered (Bransford, 1979; Gagne, 1985). The patient's motivation and attitude toward a task can influence the extent to which information is processed and monitored (Bransford, Sherwood, Vye, & Rieser, 1986; Brown, 1988).

The Multicontext Treatment Approach

The multicontext treatment approach is based on the organizational framework of learning described above. It involves the practicing of a targeted strategy in multiple environments with varied tasks and movement demands (Toglia, 1989b). Task parameters are analyzed and graded to place increasing demands on the ability to transfer learning. Direct training of metacognitive skills and self-awareness is incorporated throughout treatment. Treatment begins at the level at which the patient is functioning. Level of difficulty is not increased until the patient is able to demonstrate the ability to apply the targeted strategy to a variety of tasks. The treatment components of the multicontext approach are (a) use of multiple environments, (b) task analysis and establishment of criteria for transfer, (c) metacognitive training, (d) processing strategies, and (e) relation of new information to previously learned knowledge or skills.

Use of Multiple Environments

Generalization involves the differentiation of the strategy or skill from the environment in which it was learned (Gagne, 1985). Several studies on nondysfunctional children and adults have demonstrated that transfer of information is facilitated when the person is required to apply the newly learned skill or strategy to multiple situations or environments (Brown et al., 1983; Brown & Kane, 1988; Fried & Holyoak, 1984; Gick & Holyoak, 1983; Palincsar & Brown, 1984). This has been shown to decrease the likelihood that a particular piece of information will be associated with a particular context. For example, Nitsch (as cited by Bransford, 1979) found that a combination of single-context and varied-context examples facilitated the ability of adults to learn new concepts. When learning was restricted to single-context conditions, the range and flexibility of transfer was reduced. Gick and Holyoak (1983) reported that transfer of problem solving by analogy in adults increased with the number of examples and situations provided. Brown and Kane (1988) also found that exposing preschool children to a variety of transfer experiences involving problem solving taught them to search for the underlying commonalities. It has been demonstrated that many of the difficulties in transfer involve recognition that a new situation is similar to one previously encountered (Brown & Campione, 1984; Gick & Holyoak, 1980). Studies have shown that telling subjects that a new situation is similar to an old one results in dramatic increases in transfer in both adults and children (Gagne, 1985; Gick & Holyoak, 1983).

Several authors have observed that some adults with brain injury, particularly those with frontal lobe dysfunction and diffuse brain damage, have a strong tendency to be bound by the effects of context (Goldstein & Ruthven, 1983; Gross, 1982; Trexler, 1982; Wilson, 1987), that is, they have difficulty differentiating the task from the environment in which it occurs. Goldstein and Scheerer (1941) devised numerous sorting tasks that demonstrated this concrete, stimulus-bound behavior in populations with neurological impairment. Learning involves moving from a context-dependent state to a context-independent state (Brown et al., 1983). Patients with brain injury appear to need help with this process (Cicerone & Wood, 1987). Treatment approaches that grade only the difficulty of the task while maintaining a set context may reinforce context-dependent learning. The benefit of exposure to multiple situations, although demonstrated in the literature on normal learning, has only recently started to be examined in the literature on brain injury. For example, Cicerone and Wood found that generalization of training occurred in one case only after direct and extended training was used in a variety of situations. In addition, Diller, Goodgold, and Kay (1988) compared two conditions of treatment in 37 brain-injured adults with right-hemisphere lesions. In one condition, table-top training materials were used daily. In the other condition, the emphasis of treatment was on optimization of consistent performance across a variety of activities and contexts. Although gains had resulted from both treatment conditions, they were better maintained by the multicontext training condition.

The therapist may facilitate transfer of learning by asking the patient to apply the same strategy to different contexts during treatment. Brown et al. (1983) stated that "seeing the strategy applied in several contexts allows the learner to understand its significance and infer some of the properties of situations in which it is applicable" (p. 145). Transfer is part of learning and should be required during treatment rather than at the end of treatment. Probability of transfer in nondysfunctional persons has been shown to increase with exposure to situations that vary widely on irrelevant attributes (Gagne, 1985; Gick & Holyoak, 1987). For example, if a left-to-right scanning strategy is emphasized with practice on cancellation tasks, the patient should gradually be required to apply the strategy to other tasks and environments, such as locating an item in a medicine cabinet, counting paintings on the wall or books on a shelf, or identifying a row of items on a store shelf. The situations in which application of the strategy will be practiced need to be carefully selected through detailed task analysis. The learner also needs to practice identifying the situations in which the strategy does not apply (Gagne, 1985). For example, the left-to-right scanning strategy is most efficient in the location of targets when stimuli are arranged in horizontal lines. When stimuli are scattered and nonlinear, the left to right scanning strategy may be an inefficient method to use to locate targets.

Task Analysis and Establishment of Criteria for Transfer

Transfer of learning is not an all-or-none phenomenon. It occurs in different degrees along a continuum (Campione & Brown, 1987; Gordon, 1987; Perkins, 1987).

In therapy, establishment of criteria is appropriate for the determination of when and to what extent transfer of learning has taken place. These criteria enable the therapist to define what is being trained and to objectively evaluate progress of transfer separately from that of task training (Brown & Campione, 1982). One can establish transfer criteria by identifying a graded series of tasks that display decreasing degrees of physical and conceptual similarity to the original learning situation. It has been demonstrated that the more two tasks or situations are perceived as similar, the easier it is for transfer of learning to occur (Gagne, 1970; Gick & Holyoak, 1983). For example, Gick and Holyoak examined mechanisms that promoted transfer in nondysfunctional adults and found that any manipulation that stressed the similarity of the original problem and transfer situation led to enhanced transfer. Establishment of transfer criteria requires a detailed analysis of the surface characteristics of the task as well as the conceptual characteristics. The task characteristics outlined in Table 1 can be used to establish criteria for transfer distance.

Near transfer. In near transfer tasks, only one or two surface task characteristics are changed. The task is physically similar to the previous one and can be described as an alternate form of the original task (Toglia, 1990). An example of near transfer is the ability to spontaneously apply one-handed techniques originally learned in donning a pullover T-shirt to the task of donning a pullover sweater. The task is easily recognizable as being like the initial task; only one surface characteristic—variable attributes of color and texture—is changed.

Intermediate transfer. Intermediate transfer tasks share some physical similarities with the original task but are less readily identified. Three to six surface task characteristics are changed (Toglia, 1990). The ability to spontaneously apply one-handed principles learned in donning a pullover sweater in the therapy area to putting on a button-down silk blouse in the patient's room is an example of an intermediate transfer task. In this case, four surface characteristics are changed—type of clothing, color and texture of material, movement requirements, and environment.

Far transfer. Far transfer tasks are conceptually similar to the initial task, but the surface characteristics of the task are either completely different or share only one surface similarity. The task is physically different from the original learning task (Toglia, 1990). The ability to spontaneously apply one-handed principles learned in putting on a blouse (e.g., dress the affected limb first) to putting on pants or socks is an example of far transfer. In this case, the underlying strategy of dressing the affected side first remains the same, while almost all the surface characteristics are changed.

Very far transfer. Very far transfer is generalization, or the spontaneous application of what has been learned in treatment to everyday functioning. Very far transfer may include use of an external aid within everyday activities, for example, reading a checklist or a list of cues placed on the closet door prior to dressing.

Once some evidence of transfer is observed, the ability to independently maintain the skill over time must be monitored. For example, a patient may demonstrate intermediate transfer learning but may not be able to maintain the newly learned skill over time.

Table 2 illustrates how the surface characteristics of a letter cancellation task, which is a task typically used in the treatment of unilateral inattention, can be gradually changed so that eventually the task is completely different in physical appearance from the initial task. In all tasks, the amount of stimuli and complexity are generally held constant while the patient learns to apply the same strategy in every task.

Once the patient demonstrates the ability to initiate and successfully use a targeted strategy in a variety of situations with 90% accuracy, the complexity and number of stimuli are increased. It should be noted that there are wide gaps between the various levels of transfer described in Table 2. Task grading and practice in multiple situations need to be combined with other aspects of the multicontext approach. For example, training in

Table 1
Analysis of Surface Task and Underlying Task Characteristics

Task Characteristic	Examples
SURFACE TASK	
Type of stimuli	Objects, shapes, numbers, letters, words, sentences, symbols.
Presentation mode	Three-dimensional, two-dimensional, photographs, drawings, written form, auditory mode, tactile mode.
Variable attributes	Color, texture, size, thickness.
Stimuli arrangement	Scattered, horizontal, rotated, overlapping.
Movement	Body alignment, positioning, active requirements movement pattern.
Environmental	Physical surroundings, familiarity, context number of people.
Rules or directions	Number of steps required.
UNDERLYING TASK	
Underlying skills	Eye-hand coordination, selective attention, memory, visual discrimination, categorization.
Nonsituational	Planning, self-questioning, pacing strategies speed, checking outcomes, anticipating results.
Situational strategies	Grouping, association, left-to-right scanning, rehearsal, elaboration, visual imagery.

Table 2
Surface Characteristic Changes for a Letter Cancellation Task[a]

Transfer Distance	Task
Near	Patient is instructed to cross out the number 5 (number cancellation task).
Intermediate	Four horizontal rows of various coins are presented. Patient is instructed to place a marker over all the nickels (tabletop task).
Far	Patient is presented with a spice rack and is asked to pick out all of the jars that need to be refilled (standing and reaching at kitchen cabinets).
Very far	Patient is evaluated on the ability to spontaneously initiate left-to-right scanning in the context of simple, everyday life tasks, such as when reading four lines in a large-print magazine or locating an item in the medicine cabinet or on a shelf.

[a]For the initial task of letter cancellation, the patient was instructed to cross out the letter A on a page of four horizontal rows of random letters (paper-and-pencil task, tabletop task).

awareness and self-monitoring techniques, described below, is critical in the moving of a patient from a cued to an uncued condition.

The tasks used to measure the success of treatment must be identified in terms of transfer distance. Near transfer has been shown to occur effortlessly and spontaneously in the nondysfunctional population (Campione, Brown, & Bryant, 1985; Perkins, 1987). Evidence of near transfer has also been demonstrated in persons with mental retardation (Campione & Brown, 1977) as well as in adults with brain injury (Carter, Howard, & O'Neil, 1983). In the examination of the outcome of remediation, near transfer is not a sufficient criterion by which to determine effectiveness. Intermediate transfer tasks have been used most commonly to evaluate outcome of cognitive remediation, but there are problems in relating the changes to everyday function. Use of very far transfer tasks to evaluate outcome is most desirable, but examples in the literature are sparse (Gordon, 1987).

Awareness of the patient's capacity for generalization can be used as a guide to treatment planning and appropriate goal setting (Cicerone & Tupper, 1986). Near-transfer learning may be the maximum level of success that a patient can achieve and, if so, then this information can be used to plan treatment. For example,

domain-specific training, or the learning of task-specific skills, requires only near transfer skills. Domain-specific training involves extensive repetition of a specific task. For example, when teaching a patient to operate a computer through the use of the method of vanishing cues, the patient initially may require more than 100 cues to perform the task. Gradually, these cues are withdrawn.

Glisky and Schacter (1988) studied domain-specific training with adults with brain injury who had severe memory impairments and found that although learning occurred, many more training trials were required, and the knowledge acquired was described as hyperspecific. The researchers described a patient with severe memory problems who was able to apply the skills learned in operating a microcomputer to a data-entry job. In this case, however, the training situation closely resembled the actual work tasks, so the requirements for transfer were minimal and did not extend beyond near transfer.

Metacognitive Training

As noted earlier, metacognition refers to awareness and control of one's own thinking skills (Flavell, 1985). It includes two interrelated aspects: (a) knowledge concerning one's own cognitive processes and capacities and (b) the ability to monitor one's own performance. Metacognitive skills include the ability to evaluate the difficulty of a task, predict the consequences of action, formulate goals, plan, self-monitor performance, and demonstrate self-control (Brown et al., 1983). These skills have been identified by several authors as critical components in the learning and generalization processes. Belmont et al. (1982) argued that meaningful transfer can be attained only if such metacognitive skills as strategy planning and self-monitoring are addressed in addition to training for specific skills. They reviewed 114 published studies on the use of cognitive instruction with nondysfunctional, learning-disabled, and retarded persons and found that the 6 out of 7 studies that achieved generalization included training in metacognitive skills, whereas the other 107 studies did not.

Insight, or the degree of awareness one has regarding one's cognitive or physical capacities, is often impaired in adults with brain injury. Studies have shown that a large number of adults with brain injury underestimate the severity of their deficits (Anderson, DaMasio, Damasio, & Tranel, 1989; Anderson & Tranel, 1989; Rimel, Giordani, Barth, Boll, & Jane, 1985). Anderson and Tranel used a standardized interview to measure unawareness and found that 72% of patients with stroke and 68% of patients with head trauma demonstrated poor insight concerning their cognitive deficits. It has been demonstrated that there is a greater incidence of unawareness in patients with frontal lobe injury or right-hemisphere damage, but this phenomenon is still poorly understood

(Anderson et al., 1989; Anderson & Tranel, 1989; McGlynn & Schacter, 1989; Stuss & Benson, 1986).

McGlynn and Schacter (1989) stated that it is crucial to differentiate between defensive denial, which can be observed after nonneurological disease, and neurologically based unawareness. In neurologically based unawareness, the patient is not consciously aware that a once-intact function is impaired. Defensive denial signifies a motivated reaction by a patient who is aware of but unwilling to confront his or her problem. Although firm criteria for separating these two types of phenomena are not available, the clinician should be aware that there may be different mechanisms involved in unawareness. A multidisciplinary team approach involving psychological consultation is needed to gain a complete understanding of the patient's behavior.

Decreased awareness results in an inability to effectively use compensatory strategies. Compensation for disability assumes that a patient recognizes the need to compensate. Patients with brain injury often do not possess this prerequisite skill (Crossan et al., 1989; Diller, 1987). Their concept of what they can and cannot do is based on their cognitive performance before the injury. A person who does not understand his or her true cognitive capacity and limitations may be unwilling or unable to employ various strategies (Cicerone & Tupper, 1986; Wheatley & Rein, 1989). If the person perceives a task as easy, he or she will be less likely to exert effort, use special strategies, or monitor and verify performance outcome. In addition, the inability to accurately evaluate task difficulty in relation to oneself and to predict performance outcomes can create a perceived loss of control that can increase anxiety, decrease motivation, and further impede the learning process (Toglia, 1989b). Several authors have observed a positive relationship between awareness and treatment outcome (Ben-Yishay, Silver, Piasetsky, & Rattok, 1987; Klonoff, O'Brien, Prigatano, Chiapello, & Cunningham, 1989; Prigatano, 1986).

Therapists often complain that the patient's lack of insight interferes with treatment. Instead of attempting to teach the patient compensatory strategies, it is suggested that treatment directly address the problem of awareness. Modification of a patient's perception concerning his or her own problems may "significantly affect the subsequent course of treatment and modifiability of more specific cognitive processes" (Cicerone & Tupper, 1986, p.78). The literature contains little information, however, that can be used to guide the clinician in awareness training. Feedback has typically been used to help patients gain awareness of their performance (Carter et al., 1983; Craine, 1982), but feedback that provides information about results may be ineffective in improving performance unless the patient understands why the error occurred. The patient must learn how to monitor and evaluate his or her own performance (Bransford, 1979).

With the exception of a few small studies, this area has been unexplored in the adult with brain injury. Fordyce and Roueche (1986) attempted to increase head-injured patients' awareness of their deficits through a patient education program, videotape feedback, group discussions, and consistent reinforcement for behaviors that reflected increased awareness. Nine of the 17 patients who initially greatly underestimated their level of dysfunction showed increased awareness at the end of training. The authors concluded that only some patients with head injury benefit from attempts to increase awareness.

McGlynn and Schacter (1989) described an awareness training program with a severely involved brain-injured patient with memory problems. The program required the patient to predict his recall performance before performing recall tasks. Extensive feedback and discussion concerning the discrepancies between prediction and performance were incorporated into treatment. With training, the patient's predictions became more realistic, and his responses on a questionnaire reflected increased awareness of his current state of memory function. He was not, however, able to apply his knowledge to other situations. Training did not include practice with a variety of tasks.

The use of self-instruction techniques with adults with brain injury has been documented in a number of single case studies. Self-instruction techniques require a patient to verbalize strategies or a plan before and during the execution of a task. The goal is to help patients focus their attention on the task, organize their thoughts, and monitor the speed and accuracy of their performance (Cicerone & Wood, 1987; Fetherlin & Kurland, 1989; Lawson & Rice, 1989; Webster & Scott, 1983).

Treatment techniques that aim to help the patient detect errors, predict outcomes, estimate task difficulty, and evaluate performance outcome are suggested to increase insight and self-monitoring skills (Ben-Yishay & Diller, 1983b; Cicerone & Wood, 1987; Lawson & Rice, 1989; McGlynn & Schacter, 1989; Pollens, McBratnie, & Burton, 1988). Examples of awareness training techniques that can be integrated into daily treatment activities are self-estimation, role reversal, self-questioning, and self-evaluation.

Self-estimation. The patient estimates one or more of the following parameters before, during, or after completing a task: (a) task difficulty (e.g., the patient is asked to rate task difficulty on a scale of *very easy and unchallenging, it will not require any extra concentration or effort* [1] to *very difficult and beyond my abilities, I will not be able to complete the task even if I try hard* [5]); (b) time to complete the task; (c) number correct (or amount of errors); and (d) amount of assistance needed (number of cues). Initially, the patient is asked to estimate his or her performance during or immediately after performing a task. The patient's self-assessment is compared with the actual results to help the patient evaluate his or her performance. If necessary, a scoring system is used in which the patient is assisted in keeping track of his or her score or time. When the patient can accurately assess his or her performance, he or she is then asked to predict his or her performance before performing a task. The patient's original prediction is compared with his or her actual performance. The objective is to increase the accuracy of predictions so that they become more realistic; the emphasis is not on improving accuracy of performance. Self-estimation can be incorporated into functional activities, such as dressing or cooking, as well as in computer games or tabletop activities (McGlynn & Schacter, 1989; Toglia & Golisz, 1990). Research on normal populations has shown that adults are remarkably reliable in their predictions of their cognitive abilities (Flavell, 1985).

Role reversal. The patient observes a therapist performing a task. The therapist makes errors and the patient must identify the therapist's errors and hypothesize why the errors occurred (e.g., the therapist went too fast or did not pay attention to details). The goal is to increase error detection and analysis skills (Ben-Yishay & Diller, 1983b).

Self-questioning. At specific times during a task, the patient is asked to stop and answer the same two or three questions, such as "How am I doing?" "Am I looking all the way to the left?" "Have I followed the directions accurately?"; The goal is to help the patient monitor performance during a task (Fertherlin & Kurland, 1989).

Self-evaluation. After performing an activity, the patient fills out a self-evaluation form to help him or her accurately assess outcome. Questions include, "Have I checked over all my work carefully?" "Have I paid attention to all the details?" "Have I crossed out or removed all of the unnecessary information?" "How confident do I feel with my results?" (e.g., "I feel 100% confident that my results are accurate").

Processing Strategies

Processing strategies are organized approaches, tactics, or rules that operate either unconsciously or consciously. These strategies help the patient select relevant information from the environment and guide the organization of incoming material for information processing (Abreu & Toglia, 1987). Information processing involves the way information is collected, organized, modified, assimilated, interpreted, and used. Although the amount of information that can be processed at any one time is limited, the quality and amount of information processing is also partially influenced by the kinds of strategies used by the learner (Brown et al., 1983). Examples of strategies are the ability to prioritize, to cluster related information together, or to eliminate irrelevant details. The learner's strategies can determine the depth at which information is processed. Informa-

tion that is processed at deep levels has been shown to be more readily retained than information processed at shallow or superficial levels (Anderson, 1985).

Brain injury not only reduces the capacity to process information but also decreases the ability to use strategies to order and structure incoming information (Bolger, 1982; Melamed, Rahamani, Greenstein, Groswasser, & Najenson, 1985). The patient either fails to automatically initiate use of strategies or uses strategies ineffectively (Toglia & Golisz, 1990). Processing strategies can be divided into two groups: situational and nonsituational.

Situational strategies. Situational strategies are effective in specific tasks and environments. Examples of such strategies are grouping, rehearsal, association, visual imagery, and left-to-right scanning. Each of these strategies may result in deeper information processing when used in certain situations and may be less effective in other situations. For example, the strategy of rehearsal is best suited to tasks where the amount of information to be remembered is small and where exact reproduction is required (Campione & Brown, 1977). When the strategy of rehearsal is used with large amounts of information, the system becomes overloaded, and information processing is inhibited. The adult with brain injury often chooses strategies that are inefficient for the task (Abreu & Toglia, 1987; Bolger, 1982; Rao & Bieliauskas, 1983).

Nonsituational strategies. Nonsituational strategies are effective in a wide range of tasks and environments. Examples of such strategies are planning ahead, removing or blocking out irrelevant information, prioritizing information before beginning a task, using time-management techniques, and using self-monitoring strategies such as self-questioning.

Both situational and nonsituational strategies involve the elaboration or reorganization of information to allow for deeper processing of the material to be learned. Learning situations that address a combination of strategies have been shown to be most effective in promoting transfer in children (Brown et al., 1983). The emphasis in treatment of the adult with brain injury may therefore be shifted from specific skills, such as form constancy, figure-ground perception, categorization, memory, or problem solving, to the processing strategies that underlie these skills. Improved use of processing strategies should influence performance on a variety of tasks (Toglia, 1989a).

Relation of New Information to Previously Learned Knowledge or Skills

Knowledge and familiarity with a task affects both processing speed and strategy selection (Brown & Campione, 1982). Information is better learned and better retained when the person can relate new information to previously learned skills or knowledge. Information that cannot be connected to experience is devoid of meaning. The learner usually makes attempts to elaborate new information and associate it with experiences to make it more meaningful (Bransford, 1979).

The adult with brain injury may have difficulty elaborating new information or associating it with experience (Rahmani, 1982). In addition, he or she may not be able to automatically access previous knowledge and experiences when needed. For example, in a memory recall experiment, patients with brain injury demonstrated no spontaneous attempt to cluster related words together to help them remember, even though they were able to do so when specifically requested. In contrast, nondysfunctional adults immediately used their knowledge of object and event categories to reorganize the material and help them remember (Mattis & Kovner, 1984). An important prerequisite for learning is the ability to activate knowledge and skills when needed (Bransford et al., 1986).

The nature of the material as well as the way in which the task is presented have been shown to have powerful effects on the degree to which relevant knowledge is accessed in nondysfunctional persons (Bransford et al., 1986). Abstract materials, such as dot matrices and abstract line drawing, were originally used in perceptual remediation and education because they were content-free and conceptually neutral. It was therefore thought that the skills involved were equally generalizable to all applicable situations. These programs, however, failed to show impressive results (Adams, 1989; Sternberg & Bhana, 1986). It has since been argued that if what is taught is abstract and removed from the context and conditions of its application, it will be unrelated to previous experience and learned as an isolated, meaningless structure (Adams, 1989). Conversely, if what is taught is embedded in only one context, such as a dressing task, the skills learned may be accessible only in relation to that specific context (Adams, 1989). The implication is that exclusive use of either abstract tasks or functional tasks results in a decreased ability to transfer the skills learned in therapy to other situations.

Patients must be able to deal with both familiar and novel situations to be independent in the community. At the same time, the patient needs to be able to understand the relevance of a treatment activity and be able to connect it to other experiences. In the field of education, it has been shown that a few words or questions that show the student how the new materials relate to previous experiences or knowledge can substantially increase learning and recall (Gagne, 1985). If the therapist cannot help the patient understand the relevance of an activity, then the activity should be discarded. Many different tasks can be used to work on cognitive skills. The task itself is unimportant: The critical component of treatment is the way in which the task is structured, manipulated, and presented to elicit the proper response.

Case Study

The purpose of the following case study is to demonstrate the application of theory to practice. The intent is not to demonstrate efficacy of this approach, but rather, to illustrate how the treatment components of the multicontext approach can be used in an integrated manner during cognitive perceptual rehabilitation. The person studied is a 38-year-old man with a closed head injury resulting from a fall.

On cognitive perceptual testing 5 weeks after the injury, the patient, Mr. R., demonstrated difficulty on a variety of tasks (e.g., memory, visual discrimination, categorization). Use of the dynamic investigative assessment procedure, however, revealed that a factor underlying performance on the majority of tasks was difficulty in switching attention to new tasks or task components. Mr. R. had particular difficulty with tasks that involved moving from one step to the next or tasks that required altering his course of action. Perseveration of thoughts between tasks was observed. Performance improved with cues that assisted the patient in shifting his focus of attention. The initial emphasis of treatment, therefore, was on helping the patient become aware of his tendency to become stuck on parts of a task and on helping him deal with activities that involved shifting attention to accommodate to changing circumstances.

Treatment Program

Treatment encompassed all aspects of the multicontext approach.

Metacognitive training. Self-monitoring techniques (described previously) were used to increase self-awareness. For example, the patient was initially asked to estimate his score during and after the performance of tasks. Eventually, he was required to predict his performance before beginning a task. In addition, at 10-min intervals, the patient was required to answer questions written on a card, such as "Am I following changes in rules?" "Am I remembering to talk out loud when there is a change in the rules?" "Am I doing as I thought I would do or should I change my prediction?" "Am I stopping to take a time-out when I feel stuck?"

Processing strategies. Both situational and nonsituational strategies were emphasized consistently in a variety of activities. An example of a situational strategy was for the patient to shift his attention back and forth with changes in rules. An example of a nonsituational strategy was for the patient to verbalize the plan, goal, or rule to help shift or maintain attention. Another nonsituational strategy used was for the patient to initiate time-out when errors began to increase or when he felt stuck.

Use of multiple environments. Treatment took place in the patient's room, the occupational therapy clinic, quiet rooms, and hospital corridors. Different movement positions and patterns were required in various tasks. Table-top as well as gross motor, computer, and functional tasks were used.

Task analysis and criteria for transfer. The tasks used to observe levels of transfer learning were divided into task components and were clearly defined (see treatment tasks below).

Relation of new information to previously learned knowledge. Each task was related to previous treatment tasks and to functional tasks during every session. For example, the patient was told the following: "Just as that tendency to get stuck in one thought makes it difficult to think of other ways of making 45¢, the same thing happened when we looked at the map yesterday and when you tried to call your sister and kept dialing the same number (even though it was wrong). If you see you are making the same mistake over and over, stop and tell me. Right now that is our major goal." Problems and behaviors interfering with successful completion of treatment tasks need to be related to difficulties experienced in functional activities so that the patient can understand the connection between them.

Sample Treatment Activities or Tasks

Initial treatment activity. The patient sits on the edge of a mat and throws red shapes into a blue hoop on the floor and blue shapes into a red hoop on the floor until the therapist says "Change." At this point, the patient throws the red shapes into the red hoop and the blue shapes into the blue hoop. A scoring system by which to calculate the number of correct responses after each change is used and the scores are charted. The patient initially made three to four errors after each change.

Near transfer. The same activity as described above is used, except that the patient throws odd numbers into the blue hoop and even numbers into the red hoop until the therapist says "Change."

Intermediate transfer. The patient places pennies on all of the red beanbags and nickels on all of the blue beanbags until the therapist says "Change." At this point, the patient must place each penny on a blue beanbag and each nickel on a red beanbag. The beanbags are spread around a mat, and the patient has to shift weight and reach in different directions to place the coins on the beanbags.

Far transfer. First, the patient is shown 10 objects that are assigned various prices. The patient is asked to find three objects he could buy with 98¢. Then he is told that two of the objects are out of stock. He is asked to find three other objects to buy for the same amount of money. Second, the patient is presented with assorted coins and is asked to make as many different combinations of 45¢ as

he can think of. Third, the patient is asked to find a route from one point to another on a simple map. Once the patient draws the route, he is asked to find another route that could be used to get to the same point.

In near transfer, intermediate transfer, and far transfer, the emphasis is on comparison of performance before a change is requested with performance after a change is requested.

Very far transfer. Very far transfer is not addressed directly during treatment. It involves observation of performance within the context of everyday function. Evidence of very far transfer is obtained through repeated observations of patterns of behavior. Mr. R. initially demonstrated difficulty whenever he was confronted with an unexpected problem. His tendency to become stuck in one thought or course of action overshadowed his performance in both treatment and functional activities. For example, one day he repeatedly looked in the same drawer for his comb. He did not think to look in any other place, even though it was obvious that the item was not in the drawer. On another occasion, he wanted to get soda from a soda machine. The machine had a sign on it saying "Quarters only." Mr R. concluded he could not get soda because he had only dimes and nickels. He did not initiate alternative solutions, such as going to the cashier, who was located a short distance away. On another occasion, he wanted to speak to a relative but could not recall the person's telephone number. His solution was to wait for his relative to call him. Shortly before discharge, patterns of behavior observed in the context of everyday function suggested that Mr. R. had become better at dealing with simple problems. For example, Mr. R. went to the gift shop to buy a thank-you card. He looked carefully in different sections, and when he found that the thank-you card section was empty, he looked in the all-occasion card section and chose a blank card instead. On another occasion, Mr. R. came into the therapy area looking for a telephone book because he wanted to speak to his business partner but did not have his phone number. On another occasion, Mr. R. put on a shirt and realized that it had a large spot on the front. He spontaneously picked out an alternative shirt without difficulty. All of the above observations suggest very far transfer, but the evidence is inconclusive. It is difficult to determine when very far transfer has occurred. Because everyday situations cannot be simulated or contrived, the opportunity to observe the same situation twice may not occur. Additionally, if the same functional situation is repeated, any changes in performance would reflect near transfer skills, not very far transfer skills. Evidence for very far transfer is provided with changes in behavioral patterns across situations rather than in a specific task. Improvements that are observed during treatment sessions, even if related to spontaneous recovery, should be looked for within the context of everyday function.

Once very far transfer is observed, treatment activities are increased in complexity.

On discharge to an outpatient facility after 4 weeks of daily occupational therapy sessions of 30- to 45-min duration, the patient demonstrated all levels of transfer with basic-level tasks involving switching attention and was able to identify errors as they occurred. Although he no longer demonstrated perseveration and could alternate his attention back and forth between two or three stimuli, cope with changes between tasks, and generate alternative solutions to simple problems with limited stimuli, he still had difficulty functioning with more complex tasks. In these more complex tasks, the patient often overattended to unimportant details within a task, while at the same time omitting essential details. Although he still had problems with attention, such problems were no longer apparent in basic-level tasks, that is, in tasks with fewer than 12 stimuli and with gross discriminations of objects or shapes. Instead, the problems were expressed with complex tasks, that is, in those tasks with large amounts of stimuli (e.g., 20) and subtle discrimination of detail. When strategies that emphasized the ability to identify and remove irrelevant task information were introduced, near transfer skills were readily observed.

Summary. Although cognitive deficits interfered with the patient's ability to perform community living skills and ability to work, he appeared to have learning potential at discharge. These improvements, however, may have been related to many other factors, such as spontaneous recovery and treatments provided through other disciplines. The case example illustrates how the multicontext approach guides the selection and progression of cognitive rehabilitation treatment techniques and activities.

Summary

Remedial treatment approaches that emphasize tools and techniques to facilitate cognitive skills have been criticized, because the results are not generalizable. Functional treatment approaches also have been criticized for training skills that are too narrow in scope and that can be used only in the training context. Remedial treatment is based on the belief that generalization occurs automatically, whereas functional treatment appears to be based on the concept that patients with brain injury do not have the capacity to generalize. The dissatisfaction with these cognitive perceptual treatment approaches suggests that information is lacking to assist the clinician in examining and addressing the issue of generalization. The educational and cognitive psychology literature proposes that in nondysfunctional persons, transfer of learning does not happen automatically. Instead, learning relies on certain conditions that increase the probability that transfer will occur. Practical guidelines for teaching of transfer skills were extrapolated from this literature, and their use in the treatment of the adult

with brain injury was discussed. The result is termed the *multicontext treatment approach.*

In the multicontext treatment approach, learning is conceptualized as a dynamic interaction between the learner's processing strategies, metacognitive skills, and experiences and the nature of the task, environment, and learning criteria. Treatment based on this approach addresses all of these components. The same strategy is practiced with a variety of carefully selected tasks, movement patterns, and environments. Learning criteria for near, intermediate, and far transfer are identified. The surface similarities of treatment tasks are gradually changed, whereas the underlying skills and strategies required for performance of the task remain consistent across varied conditions. Simultaneously, metacognitive training techniques that emphasize the ability to anticipate and detect errors are employed to assist the patient in developing the self-monitoring skills necessary to move from a cued to an uncued condition.

Advocacy for this treatment approach does not presume that all patients with brain injury have the ability to generalize learning. Instead, this approach asserts that the ability to transfer learning occurs at different levels. Certain conditions increase the probability that some degree of transfer will occur. Patients with brain injury may need more help in transferring the effects of learning. Facilitation of the transfer process may help some patients to gain a higher level of transfer of learning than that which could happen spontaneously. If the patient does not show any ability to transfer learning after a trial period, then this knowledge could be used to plan an intervention program that does not require transfer.

The efficacy of the multicontext treatment approach requires examination with different patient populations and comparison with other approaches used in the management of cognitive perceptual problems. The multicontext approach, particularly, the awareness training techniques that require verbal mediation, probably would not benefit patients with language deficits or severe global cognitive impairments. The level of severity and stage of recovery influence the type of intervention that is most effective.

Many of the topics discussed in this paper, although important to cognitive perceptual rehabilitation, have not been well explored with the adult with brain injury. Strategy use, training in multiple contexts, metacognitive skills, awareness training, and effects of the nature of material on learning are just a few of the topics that need such exploration with the brain-injured population. Additionally, the extent to which models of normal learning are relevant to persons with impaired cognition has not yet been determined. Research examining the parameters that influence learning in adults with brain injury is only in its infancy, yet the issue of generalization is critical to rehabilitation. Third-party payers will not continue to reimburse treatments that have not been demonstrated to influence everyday function. In this paper, I have proposed a theoretical foundation for the guidance of clinical practice and research, in the hope that this would stimulate thinking and exploration in a challenging area that is in need of further development and research.

Acknowledgments

This paper was partially based on a presentation made at the Cognitive Rehabilitation: Principles and Practices Conference in New York, June 1990, sponsored by the Department of Rehabilitation Medicine, New York Hospital, Cornell Medical Center, New York, New York. This paper was supported by the C. S. Scribner Fund.

References

Abreu, B. C., & Toglia, J. P. (1987). Cognitive rehabilitation: A model for occupational therapy. *American journal of Occupational Therapy, 41*, 439–448.

Adams, M. J. (1989). Thinking skills curricula: Their promise and progress. *Educational Psychologist, 24*, 25–77.

Anderson, J. (1985). *Cognitive psychology and its implications.* New York: Freeman.

Anderson, S. W., Damasio, A. R., Damasio, H., & Tranel, D. (1989). Impaired awareness of disease states following right hemisphere damage. *Neurology, 39* (Suppl. 1), 232.

Anderson, S. W., & Tranel, D. (1989). Awareness of disease states following cerebral infarction, dementia and head trauma: Standardized assessment. *Clinical Neuropsychologist, 3*, 327–339.

Belmont, J. M., Butterfield, E. C., & Ferretti, R. P. (1982). To secure transfer of training: Instruct self-management skills. In D. K. Detterman & R. J. Sternberg (Eds.), *How and how much can intelligence be increased* (pp. 147–154). Norwood, NJ: Ablex.

Ben-Yishay, Y., & Diller, L. (1983a). Cognitive deficits. In M. Rosenthal, E. Griffith, M. Bond, & J. Miller (Eds.), *Rehabilitation of the head injured adult* (pp. 167–182). Philadelphia: F. A. Davis.

Ben-Yishay, Y., & Diller, L. (1983b). Cognitive remediation. In M. Rosenthal, E. Griffith, M. Bond, & J. Miller (Eds.), *Rehabilitation of the head injured adult* (pp. 367–391). Philadelphia: F. A. Davis.

Ben-Yishay, Y., Silver, S. M., Piasetsky, E., & Rattok, J. (1987). Relationship between employability and vocational outcome after intensive holistic cognitive rehabilitation. *Journal of Head Trauma Rehabilitation, 2*, 35–48.

Bolger, J. P. (1982). Cognitive retraining: A developmental approach. *Clinical Neuropsychology, 4*, 66–70.

Bransford, J. (1979). *Human cognition: Learning, understanding and remembering.* Belmont, CA: Wadsworth.

Bransford, J., Sherwood, R., Vye, N., & Rieser, J. (1986). Teaching thinking and problem solving: Research foundations. *American Psychologist, 41*, 1078–1089.

Brown, A. (1988). Motivation to learn and understand: On taking charge of one's own learning. *Cognition and Instruction, 5*, 311–321.

Brown, A., Bransford, J., Ferrara, R., & Campione, J. (1983). Learning, remembering and understanding. In J. Flavell & E. Markman (Eds.), *Handbook of child psychology* (Vol. 3, pp. 77–158). New York: Wiley.

Brown. A. L., & Campione, J. C. (1982). Modifying intelligence or modifying cognitive skills: More than a semantic quibble? In D.K. Detterman & R. J. Sternberg (Eds.), *How and how much can intelligence be increased?* (pp. 215–230). Norwood, NJ: Ablex.

Brown, A. L, & Campione, J. C. (1984). Three faces of transfer: Implications for early competence, individual differences, and instruction. In M. Lamb, A. Brown, & B. Rogoff (Eds.), *Advances in developmental psychology* (Vol. 3, pp. 143–192). Hillsdale, NJ: Erlbaum.

Brown, A. L., & Kane, M. J. (1988). Preschool children can learn to transfer: Learning to learn and learning from example. *Cognitive Psychology, 20*, 493–523.

Campione, J. C., & Brown, A. L. (1977). Memory and metamemory development in educable retarded children. In R. V. Kail, Jr., & J. W. Hagen (Eds.), *Perspectives on the development of memory and cognition* (pp. 367–406). Hillsdale, NJ: Erlbaum.

Campione, J. C., & Brown, A. L. (1987). Linking dynamic assessment with school achievement. In C. Lidz (Ed.), *Dynamic assessment* (pp. 83–109). New York: Guilford.

Campione, J. C., Brown, A. L., & Bryant, N. R. (1985). Individual differences in learning and memory. In R. J. Sternberg (Ed.), *Human abilities: An information processing approach* (pp. 103–126). New York: Freeman.

Carter, L. T., Howard, B. E., & O'Neil, W. A. (1983). Effectiveness of cognitive skill remediation in acute stroke patients. *American Journal of Occupational Therapy, 37*, 320–326.

Cicerone, K. D., & Tupper, D. E. (1986). Cognitive assessment in the neuropsychological rehabilitation of head injured adults. In B. P. Uzzell & Y. Gross (Eds.), *Clinical neuropsychology of intervention* (pp. 59–83). Boston: Martinus-Nijhoff.

Cicerone, K D., & Wood, J. C. (1987). Planning disorder after closed head injury: A case study. *Archives of Physical Medicine and Rehabilitation, 68*, 111–115.

Craine, J. F. (1982). Principles of cognitive rehabilitation. In L. Trexler (Ed.), *Cognitive rehabilitation conceptualization and intervention* (pp. 83–97). New York: Plenum.

Crossan, C., Barco, P. P., Velozo, C., Bolesta, M. M., Cooper, P. V., Werts, D., & Brobeck, T. C. (1989). Awareness and compensation in postacute head injury rehabilitation. *Journal of Head Trauma Rehabilitation, 4*, 46–54.

Davis, E. S., & Radomski, M. V. (1989). Domain-specific training to reinstate habit sequences. *Occupational Therapy Practice, 1,* 79–88.

Diller, L. (1987). Neuropsychological rehabilitation. In M. Meier, A. Benton, & L. Diller (Eds.), *Neuropsychological rehabilitation* (pp. 3–17). New York: Guilford.

Diller, L., Goodgold, J., & Kay, T. (1988). *Project: R7 innovative intervention programs to rehabilitate perceptual, cognitive, and affective deficits of stroke patients* (NIDRR Grant No. G008300039). New York: New York University Medical Center, Institute of Rehabilitation Medicine.

Ferguson, G. A. (1956). On transfer and abilities of man. *Canadian Journal of Psychology, 10,* 121–131.

Fertherlin, J. M., & Kurland, L. (1989). Self-instruction: A compensatory strategy to increase functional independence with brain injured adults. *Occupational Therapy Practice, 1,* 75–88.

Flavell, J. H. (1985). *Cognitive development.* Englewood Cliffs, NJ: Prentice-Hall.

Fordyce, D. J., & Roueche, J. R. (1986). Changes in perspectives of disability among patients, staff, and relatives during rehabilitation of brain injury. *Rehabilitation Psychology, 31,* 217–229.

Fried, L. S., & Holyoak, K. J. (1984). Induction of category distributions: A framework for classification learning. *Journal of Experimental Psychology: Learning, Memory, and Cognition, 10,* 234–257.

Gagne, E. (1985). *The cognitive psychology of school learning.* Boston: Little, Brown.

Gagne, R. M. (1970). *The conditions of learning* (2nd ed.) New York: Holt, Rinehart & Winston.

Gick, M. L., & Holyoak, K. J. (1980). Analogical problem solving. *Cognitive Psychology, 12,* 306–355.

Gick, M. L., & Holyoak, K. J. (1983). Schema induction and analogical transfer. *Cognitive Psychology, 15,* 1–38.

Gick, M. L., & Holyoak, K. J. (1987). The cognitive basis of knowledge transfer. In S. Cormier & J. D. Hagman (Eds.), *Transfer of learning: Contemporary research and applications* (pp. 9–42). San Diego: Academic Press.

Glaser, R. (1990). The reemergence of learning theory within instructional research. *American Psychologist, 45,* 29–39.

Glisky, E. L., & Schacter, D. L. (1988). Acquisition of domain-specific knowledge in patients with organic memory disorders. *Journal of Learning Disabilities, 21,* 333–339.

Goldstein, G., & Ruthven, L. (1983). *Rehabilitation of the brain damaged adult.* New York: Plenum.

Goldstein, K. H., & Scheerer, M. (1941). Abstract and concrete behavior: An experimental study with special tests. *Psychological Monographs, 53*(2) (Whole No. 239).

Gordon, W. A. (1987). Methodological considerations in cognitive remediation. In M. Meier, A. Benton, & L. Diller (Eds.), *Neuropsychological rehabilitation* (pp. 111–131). New York: Guilford.

Gross, H. (1982). A conceptual framework for interventive cognitive neuropsychology. In L. Trexler (Ed.), *Cognitive rehabilitation conceptualization and intervention* (pp. 99–114). New York: Plenum.

Hebb, D. O. (1949). *The organization of behavior.* New York: Wiley.

Jenkins, J. J. (1979). Four points to remember: A tetrahedral model and memory experiments. In L. S. Cermak & F. I. M. Craik (Eds.), *Levels of processing in human memory.* Hillsdale, NJ: Erlbaum.

Judd, C. H. (1908). The relation of special training to general intelligence. *Educational Review, 36,* 28–42.

Klonoff, P. S., O'Brien, K. P., Prigatano, G. P., Chiapello, D.A., & Cunningham, M. (1989). Cognitive retraining after traumatic brain injury and its role in facilitating awareness. *Journal of Head Trauma Rehabilitation, 4,* 37–45.

Lawson,M. J., & Rice, D. N. (1989). Effects of training in use of executive strategies on a verbal memory problem resulting from closed head injury. *Journal of Clinical and Experimental Neuropsychology, 11,* 842–854.

Mattis, S., & Kovner, R. (1984). Amnesia is as amnesia does: Toward another definition of the anterograde amnesias. In L. R. Squire & N. Butters (Eds.), *Neuropsychology of memory* (pp. 115–121). New York: Guilford.

McGlynn, S., & Schacter, D. (1989). Unawareness of deficits in neuropsychological syndromes. *Journal of Clinical and Experimental Neuropsychology, 11,* 143–205.

Melamed, L., Rahamani, L., Greenstein, Y., Groswasser, Z., & Najenson, T. (1985). Divided attention in brain-injured patients. *Scandinavian Journal of Rehabilitation Medicine, 12*(Suppl.), 16–20.

Neistadt, M. E. (1988). Occupational therapy for adults with perceptual deficits. *American Journal of Occupational Therapy, 42,* 434–440.

Neistadt, M. E. (1990). A critical analysis of occupational therapy approaches for perceptual deficits in adults with brain injury. *American Journal of Occupational Therapy, 44,* 299–304.

Palincsar, A. S., & Brown, A. L. (1984). Reciprocal teaching of comprehension-fostering and comprehension-monitoring activities. *Cognition and Instruction, 1,* 117–175.

Parente, R., & Anderson-Parente, J. K. (1989). Retraining memory: Theory and application. *Journal of Head Trauma Rehabilitation, 4,* 55–65.

Perkins, D. N. (1987). Thinking frames: An integrative perspective on teaching cognitive skills. In J. B. Baron & R. J. Sternberg (Eds.), *Teaching thinking skills: Theory and practice* (pp. 41–59). New York: Freeman.

Pollens, R., McBratnie, B., & Burton, P. (1988). Beyond cognition: Executive functions in closed head injury. *Cognitive Rehabilitation, 6,* 26–31.

Prigatano, G. (1986). *Neuropsychological rehabilitation after brain injury.* Baltimore: Johns Hopkins University Press.

Rahmani, L. (1982). The intellectual rehabilitation of brain damaged patients. *Clinical Neuropsychology, 4,* 44–45.

Rao, S. M., & Bieliauskas, L. A. (1983). Cognitive rehabilitation two and one-half years post right temporal lobectomy. *Journal of Clinical Neuropsychology, 5,* 313–320.

Rimel, R. W., Giordani, B., Barth, J. T., Boll, T. J., & Jane, J. A. (1985). Disability caused by minor head injury. *Neurosurgery, 9,* 221–228.

Sternberg, R. J. (1987). Questions and answers about the nature of teaching thinking skills. In J. B. Baron & R. J. Sternberg (Eds.), *Teaching thinking skills: Theory and practice* (pp. 251–259). New York: Freeman.

Sternberg, R. J., & Bhana, K. (1986). Synthesis of research on the effectiveness of intellectual skills programs: Snake-oil remedies or miracle cures? *Educational Leadership, 42* (2), 60–67.

Stuss, D., & Benson, F. (1986). *The frontal lobes.* New York: Raven.

Sufrin, E. M. (1984). The physical rehabilitation of the brain injured elderly. In B. A. Edelstein & E. T. Couture (Eds.), *Behavioral assessment and rehabilitation of the traumatically brain-damaged* (pp. 191–221). New York: Plenum.

Thorndike, E. L., & Woodworth, R. S. (1901). The influence of improvement in one mental function upon the efficiency of other functions. *Psychological Review, 8,* 247–261.

Toglia, J. P. (1989a). Approaches to cognitive assessment of the brain-injured adult: Traditional methods and dynamic investigation. *Occupational Therapy Practice, 1,* 36–57.

Toglia, J. P. (1989b). Visual perception of objects: An approach to assessment and intervention. *American Journal of Occupational Therapy, 43,* 587–595.

Toglia, J. P. (1990, June). *Cognitive rehabilitation: Principles and practices* [Supplemental manual]. Workshop conducted at New York Hospital, New York.

Toglia, J. P., & Golisz, K. (1990). *Cognitive rehabilitation: Group games and activities.* Tucson: Therapy Skill Builders.

Trexler, L. (1982). Cognitive and neuropsychological aspects of affective change following traumatic brain injury. In L. Trexler (Ed.), *Cognitive rehabilitation conceptualization and intervention* (pp. 173–197). New York: Plenum.

Webster, J. S., & Scott, R. R. (1983). The effects of self-instructional training on attentional deficits following head injury. *Clinical Neuropsychology, 5,* 69–74.

Wheatley, C. J., & Rein, J. J. (1989). Intervention in traumatic head injury: Learning style assessment. In S. Hertfelder & C. Gwin (Eds.), *Work in progress: Occupational therapy in work programs* (pp. 197–212). Rockville, MD: American Occupational Therapy Association.

Wilson, B. (1987). *Rehabilitation of memory.* New York: Guilford.

Chapter 45

Use of Adjunctive Modalities in Occupational Therapy

Section 1
Lorraine Pedretti, MS, OTR

Section 2
Roger Smith, PhD, OTR, FAOTA
Joy Hammel, PhD, OTR, FAOTA
Judy Rein, MS, OTR
Denis Anson

Section 3
Mary Jo McGuire

This chapter reproduces a series of three OT *Week* articles that were developed to frame the issues around the use of treatment modalities that may or may not include the use of physical agent modalities. Each author was asked to write a short paper that addressed a particular issue related to the use of adjunctive modalities. The first section, written by Lorraine W. Pedretti, provides a frame of reference for using modalities. The second section, written by the Technology Special Interest Section Standing Committee (Roger O. Smith, Joy Hammel, Judy Rein, and Denis Anson), reviews technology as an occupational therapy treatment modality. The final section, written by Mary Jo McGuire, presents issues of competency and ethics when using modalities. All three sections are based on the central theme of the profession's philosophical base and the engagement in purposeful activity.

Section 1: A Frame of Reference for Occupational Therapy

The occupational performance frame of reference identified the areas of concern for occupational therapy (American Occupational Therapy Association [AOTA], 1974). These are the performance areas of activities of daily living, work activities, and play or leisure activities and the performance components of sensorimotor components, cognitive integration and cognitive components, and psychosocial skills and psychological components (AOTA, 1989). Using this framework, the occupational therapy treatment program addresses remediation of the performance areas and the performance components. Its primary concern is with the client's achievement of maximal independence in the performance areas from the acute stage of illness or injury through extended rehabilitation (Pedretti & Pasquinelli, 1990).

The philosophical base states that participation in purposeful activity can improve or influence health. Purposeful activity is the central theme of the philosophical base and characterizes the primary tools of occupational therapy. Affirmations accompanying the philosophical base placed facilitating procedures in perspective as preparatory to purposeful activity and stated that they are not acceptable as occupational therapy if they are used as ends unto themselves ("Highlights of Actions," 1979).

Although occupational therapy practitioners continue to be committed to the original beliefs and values of the profession and to purposeful activity as the core of practice, many consider their competence and expertise to encompass treatment methods and approaches that are preliminary to or support the client's ability to perform purposeful activity (English, Kasch, Silverman, & Walker, 1982; Kasch, 1982; Pedretti, 1982).

In response to the changing needs of a dynamic health care system, occupational therapy practitioners have developed new skills and practices that precede, support, and enable the ability to perform purposeful activity (Pedretti, 1982). They have become increasingly skillful in the use of sensorimotor and neurophysiological approaches to treatment, therapeutic exercise, and, in some segments of practice, physical agent modalities. There is evidence that occupational therapy practitioners are practicing these treatment techniques with increasing frequency and using purposeful activity less frequently (Bissell & Mailloux, 1981; Cynkin, 1979; Shannon, 1977). Although these treatment techniques are practiced or shared in practice by other disciplines, they can be justified for use in an occupational therapy treatment program because they may be necessary to the development of the client's ability to perform skills essential to occupational roles.

Trombly (1982) proposed that these methods may be considered adjunctive to purposeful activity in the occupational therapy treatment program. The word *adjunctive* implies that they are added to and complement (McKechnie, 1979) the primary methods and modalities used in treatment, that is, purposeful activity.

A four-stage treatment continuum can be conceptualized that addresses the performance components and performance areas in the occupational performance frame of reference and takes the client through a logical progression from dependence to resumption of life roles. It accommodates methods and modalities used in current practice. The stages in this continuum overlap and are concurrent in any comprehensive treatment program. When one works on the remediation of the performance areas, purposeful activity is likely to constitute the more significant portion of the treatment program. For example, when the treatment goal is self-care independence, the treatment method is training in hygiene and dressing skills. When one works on remediation of performance

components, adjunctive and enabling activities are likely to constitute a greater share of the treatment program. For example, if trunk balance is inadequate for independent hygiene and dressing skills, stimulation of balance reactions on mat table or bedside might be used in the treatment program before hygiene or dressing training is initiated. It is essential that adjunctive methods be directed to the mastery of performance areas in occupational therapy practice. Exclusive use of adjunctive and enabling methods out of the context of the client's occupational performance cannot be considered occupational therapy (Pedretti & Pasquinelli, 1990). The treatment continuum is described below.

Stage 1: Adjunctive methods. These methods or modalities are preliminary to the use of purposeful activity and are meant to prepare the client for occupational performance. Examples are exercise, facilitation and inhibition techniques, splinting, sensory stimulation, and selected physical agent modalities (Pedretti & Pasquinelli, 1990).

Stage 2: Enabling activities. Activities that simulate purposeful activities, such as stacking blocks or cones, using activities of daily living practice boards, sanding boards, and performing tabletop activities to train perceptual skills are examples of enabling activities. Such activities may not be considered purposeful because they do not have an autonomous goal (Ayres, 1960) and may not engage the coordination of the physical, emotional, and cognitive systems (Hinojosa, Sabari, & Rosenfeld, 1983). However, they constitute a necessary preparatory step to the performance of purposeful activity in the treatment program because they are used to train the subskills of purposeful activity, such as particular movement patterns, strength, or shape discrimination.

Stage 3: Purposeful activity. These activities have an autonomous purpose; are relevant and meaningful to the client; engage the client's physical, emotional, and cognitive systems; and address the performance areas in the occupational performance frame of reference. Examples are feeding, dressing, arts and crafts, mobility, and simulated work activities.

Stage 4. Occupational performance. Appropriate real life tasks essential to independent living are used in treatment. Activities of daily living, mobility, work, education, and play or leisure tasks are performed to the client's maximal level of independence. The client begins to assume or resume occupational roles in his or her living environment and in the community. Occupational therapy intervention decreases and is ultimately discontinued in this stage. Performance at this level is the ultimate goal and desired outcome of occupational therapy intervention (Pedretti & Pasquinelli, 1990).

Many years ago, Ayres (1958) stated that "the use of purposeful activities ... constitutes the common element and distinguishing feature of occupational therapy" (p. 301). She added that procedures associated with purposeful activity and essential to its maximal therapeutic utilization are also the concern of occupational therapy. Examples given were testing eye–hand coordination, cutaneous stimulation, and the use of reflex-inhibiting postures preceding purposeful activity. Thus, the notion of the need to use adjunctive methods has been developing for more than 30 years.

Occupational therapy practitioners are skillful in the application of treatment approaches unknown to the profession a few years ago. If adjunctive methods are to be considered "only acceptable as occupational therapy when used to prepare the patient/client for better performance and prevention of disability through self-participation in occupation" ("Highlights of Actions," 1979, p. 1), their continuity with and relationship to purposeful activity and the extent to which they duplicate the services of other disciplines demand further study.

Section 2: Technology as an Occupational Therapy Treatment Modality

Historical Relationship Between Technology and Occupational Therapy

Technology and occupational therapy have been closely associated for decades. In fact, technology has been an integral part of occupational therapy since the early 1900s, when occupational therapy began defining itself as a profession. Occupational therapy and a branch of engineering even crossed professional paths in the first decades of the century. The Gilbreths, who later were responsible for the story *Cheaper by the Dozen* (Gilbreth & Carey, 1948), were promoters of the science of activity analysis. They attended and presented at occupational therapy meetings and are now known to have founded many concepts in industrial engineering (Creighton, 1992). This relationship between technology and occupational therapy has had two dimensions. First, occupational therapy practitioners used technology as tools and media for therapeutic activities. Second, practitioners discovered early that these tools and the technological environment frequently needed to be adapted to accommodate impairments of persons with disabilities.

The early occupational therapy practitioners applied nonelectronic, but complex, technologies in craft activities. This was a key part of therapy. Human-powered saws and sanding equipment were used extensively in occupational therapy clinics for woodworking projects. Complex looms were used for weaving projects. Technology was not always in the form of large equipment; needles, hoops, brackets, hammers, clamps, and brushes were also tools of occupational therapy. These technologies as therapeutic media were not only commonplace in occupational therapy clinics, but also expected. Occupational therapy education required that therapy practitioners learn how to use these technologies and how to teach them to their clients. In 1918, Dunton described occupa-

tional therapy education as needing to teach the application and modification of special tools and devices.

Early occupational therapy practitioners also became adept at modifying equipment and the task environment so it best fit the particular needs of their clients. If a client were working on a project that required sanding but only had use of one hand, the practitioners needed to design a jig or a method for performing the functions of stabilizing the wood and using the sanding block unilaterally. If a client had an angry disposition and required a medium to express his or her feelings, the occupational therapy practitioners might try to adapt an activity to incorporate more gross motor involvement and physical expression. In the 1950s, equipment modifications were frequently discussed in the literature with article titles such as "Adapted Floor Loom for Strengthening Weak Ankle Dorsiflexors" (Geiss, Myers, & Bevill, 1954), "A Device to Supply a More Comprehensive Kinetic Therapy in Occupational Therapy" (Jackson, 1954), "Adaptations and Apparatus" (Parlin, 1948), and "Adapted Weight Resistant Apparatus" (Svensson & Brennan, 1954). This modification of the equipment and the tasks used in occupational therapy became a natural part of the therapeutic process.

Cultural, Social, and Individual Appropriateness of Technology

Occupational therapy practitioners have always needed to assess the cultural, social, and personal appropriateness of a therapeutic activity. The context in which technology is being used is as important as the intervention itself. Working with needlepoint, for example, may not be of interest to a specific person. A business executive may not want to work on a car engine. A modern farmer may not be interested in learning how to prepare the soil with a horse-driven plow. An older person may not want to join in a group calisthenic activity. Although the therapeutic value of any of these activities might be optimal in terms of developing needed motor, sensory or cognitive skills, the context and the preference of the participant direct the ultimate suitability of the activity. In occupational therapy, cultural, social, and personal preferences must drive the choice of a therapeutic activity. This concept is fundamental to occupational therapy and applies to the use of technology in occupational therapy as well.

Less often noted, however, is that the value of an activity is greatly affected by historical relevance. Therapeutic modalities change as the life activities of occupational therapy clients change. Our lives as occupational therapy practitioners, too, are changing, and the use of technology is one major area of change. Many therapeutic activities that are appropriate today were not even conceptualized 75, 20, or even 10 years ago. Activities that help clients develop the skills to use an automated banking machine, push buttons on a memory-dial telephone, use a remote control for television, hold and activate a hair dryer, monitor traffic on a busy highway, or use a digital microwave oven were not always part of occupational therapy. Technological progress has changed what we do in practice because it has changed the way people function in their daily lives. Along with these changes, the use of technology that physical agent modalites represent needs to be considered.

Technology as a Modern Occupational Therapy Modality

Philosophically, occupational therapy has not been changed by time. Today's occupational therapy clinics are not much different from those in the early days. If we could walk into an occupational therapy clinic of 50 or 75 years ago, we would see therapy practitioners working with technology and adapting it. Today, we would see the same picture, but the technologies being used would be more modern. In the 1990s, occupational therapy practitioners can be seen using new media. The interests and activities of our clients have expanded, so to make therapy relevant, purposeful, and functional, the intervention media of occupational therapy practitioners must expand in a parallel fashion. Modern therapeutic activities might include using video games, creating stories on a computer, cooking a microwave meal, driving through a wheelchair obstacle course, exercising for a more balanced lifestyle (to compensate for the sedentary technological life), or doing warm-up exercises to prepare for subsequent functional activity. Occupational therapy textbooks reflect these changes. Biofeedback modalities were included as occupational therapy topics in the sixth edition of *Willard and Spackman's Occupational Therapy* (Hopkins & Smith, 1983). A chapter on computer technology was entered into the text in the seventh edition (Hopkins & Smith, 1988).

Today's technology modalities can be categorized. Technologies used as modalities for direct intervention technology can be rehabilitative and educational or assistive and adaptive (Smith, 1991). The rehabilitative and educational technologies assume that a person has some deficits that can be resolved or improved through treatment. Technology provides one medium for bringing this about. Examples of rehabilitative and educational technologies are cognitive rehabilitative software and the computer on which it runs; biofeedback in all of its forms, ranging from sophisticated electromyographic screen-based feedback to simple single-switch toys used in pediatrics with students with a low cognitive level; exercise or drill systems for clients who are involved in fitness regimens; pressure systems for reducing edema and increasing functional motion during activity; and computer games controlled by fine- or gross-motor-activated transducers for motor skill development. Assistive and adaptive technologies include those devices that are not targeted to improve skills, but those that assume a static level of

function and therefore aim to supplement a person's intrinsic function. Examples of assistive and adaptive technologies are seating and positioning systems, static positioning splints and other orthoses, limb prostheses, robotics, computer access equipment, functional electrical stimulation used as an orthotic device, architectural barrier assessment and modification, and wheelchairs.

Physical agent modalities are often thought of as new technologies. A brief mention of how they fit into this conceptual model is helpful, because in many respects they are a type of technology unto themselves. In other respects, however, they are just like the other technologies. Physical agent modalities tend to be adjunctive. Some of them are used in preparation for functional activity. Some are used in conjunction with functional activity. The properties of physical agent modalities, "of light, water, temperature, sound, and electricity [aim] to produce a response in soft tissue" (AOTA, 1991c, p. 6). They are intended to facilitate functional performance. Examples of these physical agent technologies may include, but are not limited to, "paraffin baths, hot and cold packs, fluidotherapy, contrast baths, ultrasound, whirlpool, and electrical stimulation units (FES—Functional Electrical Stimulation/NMES—Neuromuscular Electrical Stimulation devices, TENS—Transcutaneous Electrical Nerve Stimulator)" (AOTA, 1991c, p. 6). Applied examples of these adjunctive interventions as a rehabilitative and educational technology might be the use of hot or cold to prepare an orthopedic client for a manual activity and the use of tools or functional electrical stimulation for neuromuscular reeducation so that a person can increase specific movements necessary for dressing activities. In the area of assistive and adaptive technologies, functional electrical stimulation might be used as an electronic splint, that is, an orthotic device allowing a person to engage in functional activity such as self-feeding.

Consequences of Using Technology as an Occupational Therapy Modality

Although technology is an answer for many people who have disabilities and enables them to enjoy a better quality of life, technology can be harmful through misuse or neglect. It can be purchased and remain in a closet or it can be put to use building homes and communities. Owning a tool also means owning the responsibility for its proper and safe use. If we own a hammer or saw, we must be careful in how we use it. Using assistive and rehabilitation technology requires responsible ownership, as true of any tool. In using technology, occupational therapy practitioners have a fourfold responsibility. Occupational therapy practitioners must (a) use technology when it can be of benefit, (b) not use technology when it will not be of benefit, (c) be competent with the technology when it is used, and (d) use technology in the context of meaningful activity. The fourth responsibility implies that there is a difference between an occupational therapy practitioner who uses technology (or becomes a technologist) and a technologist from another professional base. All of these responsibilities carry an ethical burden. Occupational therapy practitioners should apply the technology needed and should acquire the skills that they need to do so.

We as occupational therapy practitioners bring a tradition of using technology to provide a positive effect on the health and functional performance of the clients we serve. This tradition implies that we as occupational therapy practitioners use technology in the context of the specific environments of our clientele. Cultural, social, and personal preferences are incorporated in the technology-consideration process to select meaningful therapeutic activities. This also suggests that technology can never be considered alone. It must always be evaluated for use with full cognizance of the client's current and future intrinsic abilities.

Technology provides yet another challenge for occupational therapy practitioners to be competent. It is easy to become so enamored of technology that the context of occupational therapy is lost. Practitioners might, for example, focus so intently on identifying the exact dimensions of a seating system, calibrating the correct continuous passive range of motion machine settings, following the proper edema reduction machine protocol, or adjusting the optimal electronic delay in a computer keyboard that they forget the reason they are using the technology. They may focus so carefully on the details of the technology that the functional reasons that initially set the directions of the interventions were forgotten. The nature of technology is particularly conducive to this phenomenon. Occupational therapy practitioners must, therefore, be vigilant in monitoring their use of modalities to ensure that the modalities are a means to function.

The appropriate selection and application of assistive or rehabilitative technology can be the precise solution to help persons with a disability become so fully functional that they eliminate their disability. As occupational therapy practitioners, we need to provide these interventions. This can only happen, however, if we retain our use of technology in the context of occupational therapy tradition. This should not be too hard. As the occupational therapy profession reaches its 75th birthday, we review our roots and can see that assistive and rehabilitative technology and occupational therapy have a lot of experience working together.

Technology as a Future Occupational Therapy Modality

The future of occupational therapy and technology is full of suspense. Many science fiction stories, like *The Time Machine* (Wells, 1964) depict technology as a tool eventually leading us to the end of civilization. "Star Trek," however, portrays technology as a tool leading to the survival of civilization. Whichever the case, technolo-gy is here now, and occupational therapy practitioners must deal with it. Technology is changing our lives every day as we communicate with each other, travel, work, perform household tasks, and prepare for our daily activities. Although we can only guess what effect the role of robotics, pictorial telephones, virtual telecommunication and computing environments, prosthetic body parts, world economies, and artificial intelligence will have on occupational therapy, one thing is certain— occupational therapy practitioners will always be updating their treatment modalities and tools for the benefit of the clientele for whom they work.

Section 3: Methods and Media in a Growing Profession

The articles in the special 75th anniversary issue of the *American Journal of Occupational Therapy* (Schwartz, 1992) provide new perspectives for understanding the founding of occupational therapy. Reading the articles confirms the fact that controversy and disagreement are not new (or bygone) phenomena in AOTA. The profession's valuing of occupation has withstood the storms and struggles of the past 75 years and, I hope, will continue to be the central purpose and plan of occupational therapists for the next 75 years.

The foundation of knowledge on which the profession stands has greatly expanded in the past seven and a half decades. The expansion of clinical services has reached the point that the needs of persons at every developmental stage after birth are served in a wide variety of health care provision systems. This has resulted in many changes in the needs of and demands placed on occupational therapy practitioners in the 1990s. Debates, such as those over the inclusion or exclusion of specific methods and media, touch on important issues that must continually be examined and reevaluated as the profession grows.

In her Eleanor Clarke Slagle Lecture, Kitty Reed, PhD, MLIS, OTR/L, FAOTA, provided interesting guidelines for analyzing the evolution of methods and media. She described eight primary factors that influence media change: cultural, social, economic, political, technological, theoretical, historical, and research (Reed, 1986) (see Chapter 39). As growth occurs, occupational therapy practitioners are challenged to continually examine and reevaluate the scope of practice, the congruence of the basic philosophy of occupation with methods and media used, specialization, limits of entry-level education, competence issues, and ethical dilemmas created by internal and external demands and conflicts.

Scope of Practice

The scope of occupational therapy practice has increased dramatically in the past 75 years, taking practitioners into places such as prisons, school systems, hospices, private practices, well-baby clinics, and patients' homes.

The occupational therapy community has worked hard to educate itself as well as society about the far-reaching applications of the paradigm of occupation. The increase in the types of populations served has placed increasing demands for growth on the discipline. The knowledge and technology explosion associated with each specialty area continually provides occupational therapy practitioners with a new array of information, problems, answers, methods, and media for evaluation and treatment. Occupational therapy practitioners have had to accept the responsibility to discern what is and what is not within the scope of occupational therapy practice.

Specialization

Specialization is a process that occurs naturally within our profession. Educational and workplace choices directly and indirectly affect the direction and speed of growth for persons. If the specialist has received the proper education and training, specialized media and methods may be integrated into the occupational therapy treatment program. Practitioners who have been certified by more than one organization or who have acquired the necessary education and training to use specific methods or media may be able to provide specialized occupational therapy to specific populations. The expertise of the experienced occupational therapy practitioners should not be under-estimated or devalued by defining the specialized competencies (which have been acquired through years of practice and education) as generalist or entry-level skills. It is important, however, to emphasize the importance of staying true to our basic paradigm, regardless of specialty, if we are to continue to call what we do *occupational therapy*. The generalist skills of the entry-level practitioners, on the basis of the paradigm of occupation, are a foundation that must never be denied or forgotten. If they are, then, unfortunately for the patient, occupational therapy may not truly be provided. Occupation must be at the core of our purpose and of our plan.

Education

As the scope of occupational therapy has expanded and the technology and information explosion of our times has occurred, the educational system has been challenged and strained to its limits. The entry-level education of the occupational therapist and the occupational therapy assistant is limited by many factors, including time, space, and economic restraints. Currently, it is inappropriate and impossible to expect entry-level professionals to possess the knowledge and skills that would make them experts in all the areas in which occupational therapy serves. Continuing education is not a luxury; it is essential for mastering the methods and media used in any specialty area.

As growth occurs in the discipline, the appropriateness and effectiveness of the educational objectives must be evaluated. The Association's Commission on Education continually monitors and modifies the "Essentials and Guidelines of an Accredited Educational Program for the Occupational Therapist" (AOTA, 1991a) and the "Essentials and Guidelines of an Accredited Educational Program for the Occupational Therapy Assistant" (AOTA, 1991b), upon which curricula are based. Moreover, the vision and hopes of *Directions for the Future* (AOTA, 1987) may greatly alter the occupational therapy educational system of tomorrow.

Competence and Ethics

The issue of competence is usually associated with two major concerns related to the use of media and methods: the identification of professionals who possess special competencies and the protection of the consumer from those professionals who are not practicing competently. The American Occupational Therapy Certification Board has been established as the entry gate into the profession. It is designed to evaluate entry-level skills. There is no national system designed to programmatically evaluate the maintenance or development of competence in the experienced professional. However, a variety of systems exist that encourage professional development: States have written continuing education requirements into their regulatory laws, specialty courses offer certification in specific methods of media, and AOTA has recently begun to organize systems for acknowledging the advanced qualifications of its experienced members. In addition, some practitioners choose to join related professional organizations or to become certified or licensed by other organizations to have their special expertise acknowledged.

Beyond certification, the evaluation of the competence of certified occupational therapists and occupational therapy assistants is basically left to the individual professional, the consumer, and the state regulatory boards. Regardless of the methods or media a therapist chooses to use, the occupational therapy code of ethics (AOTA, 1988) must be respected. In particular, practitioners must "demonstrate competency by meeting competency-based standards" (AOTA, 1988, p. 795) and maintain competency by involvement in continuing education" (AOTA, 1988, p. 795). Competencies that were not acquired in entry-level education should be gained through appropriate continuing education or in-service education. The Association does not have extensive documentation on competency standards against which individual practitioners can assess their competence; however, such standards may provide a catalyst for professional growth for experienced practitioners. It is particularly important that high standards of competence be established for the application of methods and the use of media that our Association considers to be advanced. Practitioners who pioneered the integration of new techniques or media into occupational therapy practice must also take the responsibility to initiate or at least stay abreast of research that investigates the effectiveness of the selected treatment approach.

Methods and media in occupational therapy change as a result of many factors. Issues related to the scope of practice, specialization, education, competence, and ethics must be considered as important factors that shape and guide the growth of the profession. As the profession changes, it must continually examine these issues and work to preserve the essence of our profession that society needs: the opportunity to actively select and engage in occupation to promote one's health.

Summary

This chapter reminds us that as practice evolves, we must revisit and reaffirm the fundamental philosophy and precepts in which our profession is grounded. The face of practice is fluid. Its superficial appearance is molded by external forces and stresses. These include the changes in the needs of the persons we serve, the emergence of new and different treatment modalities, and the realities of the socioeconomic environment in which we work. Beneath the surface, however, are the basic structures that all of us hold in common. These are our philosophical beliefs that are articulated both in the professional literature and in the ethical principles that we espouse.

References

American Occupational Therapy Association. (1974). *A curriculum guide for occupational therapy educators.* Rockville, MD: Author.

American Occupational Therapy Association. (1987). *Directions for the future.* Rockville, MD: Author.

American Occupational Therapy Association. (1988). Occupational therapy code of ethics. *American Journal of Occupational Therapy, 42,* 795–796.

American Occupational Therapy Association. (1989). Uniform terminology for occupational therapy—Second edition. *American Journal of Occupational Therapy, 43,* 808–815.

American Occupational Therapy Association. (1991a). Essentials and guidelines of an accredited educational program for the occupational therapist. *American Journal of Occupational Therapy, 45,* 1077–1084.

American Occupational Therapy Association. (1991b). Essentials and guidelines of an accredited educational program for the occupational therapy assistant. *American Journal of Occupational Therapy, 45,* 1085–1092.

American Occupational Therapy Association (1991c). *Physical agent modality task force report.* Rockville, MD: Author.

Ayres, A. J. (1958). Basic concepts of clinical practice in physical disabilities. *American Journal of Occupational Therapy, 12,* 300–302.

Ayres, A. J. (1960). Occupational therapy for motor disorders resulting from impairment of the central nervous system. *Rehabilitation Literature, 21,* 302–310.

Bissell, J. C., & Mailloux, Z. (1981). The use of crafts in occupational therapy for the physically disabled. *American Journal of Occupational Therapy, 35,* 369–374.

Creighton, C. (1992). The origin and evolution of activity analysis. *American Journal of Occupational Therapy, 46,* 45–48. (Reprinted as Chapter 43.)

Cynkin, S. (1979). *Occupational therapy: Toward health through activities.* Boston: Little, Brown.

Dunton, W. R. (1918). Rehabilitation of crippled soldiers and sailors: A review. *Maryland Psychiatric Quarterly, 7,* 85–101.

English, C., Kasch, M., Silverman, P., & Walker, S. (1982). The Issue Is—On the role of the occupational therapist in physical disabilities. *American Journal of Occupational Therapy, 36,* 199–202.

Geiss, G. W., Myers, C., & Bevill, H. (1954). Adapted floor loom for strengthening weak ankle dorsiflexors. *American Journal of Occupational Therapy, 8,* 11–12.

Gilbreth, F. B., & Carey, E. M. (1948). *Cheaper by the dozen.* New York: Crowell.

Highlights of actions taken by the Representative Assembly during its recent meeting. (1979, June). *Occupational Therapy Newspaper,* p. 1.

Hinojosa, J., Sabari, J., & Rosenfeld, M. S. (1983). Purposeful activities. *American Journal of Occupational Therapy, 37,* 805–806.

Hopkins, H. L., & Smith, H. D. (Eds.). (1983). *Willard and Spackman's occupational therapy* (6th ed.). Philadelphia: Lippincott.

Hopkins, H. L., & Smith, H. D. (Eds.). (1988). *Willard and Spackman's occupational therapy* (7th ed.). Philadelphia: Lippincott.

Jackson, F. W. (1954). A device to supply a more comprehensive kinetic therapy in occupational therapy. *American Journal of Occupational Therapy, 8,* 158–161.

Kasch, M. (1982, March). Professional relationships [Guest editorial]. *Occupational Therapy Association of California Newsletter,* pp. 1, 6.

McKechnie, J. L. (Ed.) (1979). *Webster's new universal unabridged dictionary.* (2nd ed). New York: Dorset & Baber, New World Dictionaries/Simon & Shuster.

Parlin, F. W. (1948). Adaptations and apparatus. *American Journal of Occupational Therapy, 2,* 206.

Pedretti, L. W. (1982, May). *The compatibility of treatment methods in physical disabilities with the philosophical base of occupational therapy.* Paper presented at the 62nd Annual Conference of the American Occupational Therapy Association, Philadelphia.

Pedretti, L. W., & Pasquinelli, S. (1990). A frame of reference for occupational therapy in physical dysfunction. In L. W. Pedretti & B. Zoltan (Eds.), *Occupational therapy practice skills for physical dysfunction* (pp. 1–17). St. Louis: Mosby.

Reed, K. L. (1986). 1986 Eleanor Clarke Slagle Lecture—Tools of practice: Heritage or baggage? *American Journal of Occupational Therapy, 40,* 597–605. (Reprinted as Chapter 39).

Schwartz, K. B. (Ed.). (1992). Special 75th anniversary issue [Special issue]. *American Journal of Occupational Therapy,*

Shannon, P. D. (1977). The derailment of occupational therapy. *American Journal of Occupational Therapy, 31,* 229–234.

Smith, R. O. (1991). Technology applications to enhance human performance. In C. Christiansen & C. Baum (Eds.), *Human performance deficits* (pp. 746–786.) Thorofare, NJ: Slack.

Svensson, V. W., & Brennan, M. C. (1954). Adapted weight resistant apparatus. *American Journal of Occupational Therapy, 8,* 13.

Trombly, C. A. (1982). Include exercise in "purposeful activity" [Letter to the editor]. *American Journal of Occupational Therapy, 36,* 467–468.

Wells, H. G. (1964). *The time machine.* New York: Airmont.

Chapter 46

Integrating Play in Neuro-developmental Treatment

Jill Anderson
Jim Hinojosa, PhD, OTR, FAOTA
Carrie Strauch

This chapter was previously published in the *American Journal of Occupational Therapy*, *41*, 421–426. Copyright © 1987, American Occupational Therapy Association.

The integration of play activities with neurodevelopmental treatment (NDT) can be a challenge even for the experienced occupational therapist. A primary goal of occupational therapy in treating children with cerebral palsy is to promote normal patterns of movement and prevent abnormal postural reactions of movement and prevent abnormal postural reactions while the child is engaged in functional, purposeful activities.

Treating a child with cerebral palsy often involves a variety of treatment techniques and methodologies from several theoretical frames of reference. Occupational therapists in pediatrics commonly use the neurodevelopmental therapy frame of reference, which involves the use of specific handling techniques to facilitate normal muscle tone, patterns of movement, and automatic responses. When NDT principles are integrated into occupational therapy intervention, the therapist must have a basic understanding of the tonal and movement characteristics of each type of cerebral palsy, specific handling techniques, and the performance components of developmentally appropriate activities.

Integrating play activities with NDT can be difficult. It is a complex task to try to elicit specific responses through handling while simultaneously engaging the child in purposeful play activities. Unsuccessful attempts to integrate play with NDT may be frustrating and may result in a limited use of activities during occupational therapy intervention.

This article discusses some of the issues involved in combining play with NDT and offers selected activity solutions. The authors believe that play interaction with children with cerebral palsy is generally compatible with the application of NDT principles. However, we recognize that the integration of activities involving specific play materials, objects, and manipulative or motor skills may not always be possible.

Review of the Literature

The occupational therapist's unique use of play as a therapeutic activity involves the reconceptualization of play as a purposeful activity (Hinojosa, Sabari, & Rosenfeld, 1983). Play is an action on human and nonhuman objects that is engaged in for its own sake. Florey (1981) has identified six principles of play common to many theories: Play is a complex set of behaviors characterized by fun and spontaneity; play is sensory, neuromuscular, mental, or a combination of these three; play involves repetition of experience, exploration, experimentation, and imitation of one's surroundings; play integrates the child's internal and external world; play permits the child to rehearse his or her interpretation of reality and fantasy; and play follows a sequential, developmental progression. Thus, play activities develop the skills that will allow the child to interact with the demands of his or her environment.

There is agreement in the psychoanalytical literature on two points—that play has a central role in a child's development and that the inhibition of play in childhood has severe pathological implications (Erikson, 1950; Pellar, 1954; Winnicott, 1971). When the natural drive to play is thwarted during therapy, the young child may become distressed. Older children may lose concentration and repeatedly ask when therapy will be finished or may become less cooperative, more resistant, and manipulative.

From a psychoanalytic perspective, play helps children achieve instinctual satisfaction by creating substitutes that permit emotional expression (Plaut, 1979). A bright, socially interactive, 15-month-old infant with spastic diplegia appeared to have a "psychological need" to constantly manipulate objects and exercise control over the play materials during therapy. This upper extremity play may be a substitute for gross motor exploration and independent ambulation. The play also provided her with control over her environment and possibly fulfilled her needs for autonomy—needs that are characteristic of the separation–individuation process.

Play facilitates mastery over anxiety by active rather than passive means. When this same 15-month-old child was first positioned in a supported standing position in inhibitory casts, she appeared distressed and fearful. She tolerated the lower extremity weight bearing and calmed when her favorite play materials were presented.

Handicapped children follow a developmental play sequence similar to the sequence followed by normal children, but sometimes at a delayed rate (Field, Roseman, De-Stefano, & Koewler, 1982). An 8-year-old developmentally delayed child required the use of dramatic interactive play typical of the preschool period to meet her developmental play needs during therapy. Imaginative play progressed from symbolic play with animals to role play with human figures during the course of 1 year. The primary goal for this child was to facilitate normal motor development and the acquisition of fine motor skills.

The NDT frame of reference, an interdisciplinary therapy approach, focuses on the normalization of tone and the integration of primitive postural patterns into the development of normal postural responses and movement patterns (Smith, 1984). Therapists evaluate the quality of the child's movement, developmental milestones, skills, movement sequences, and postures (Stengel, Attermeier, Bly, & Heriza, 1984). To establish an appropriate goal for the child, occupational therapists identify movement components required to achieve a functional goal (Boehmme, 1985). Through handling and movement, appropriate automatic reactions are elicited to achieve functional goals (Scherzer & Tscharnuter, 1982).

One goal of NDT is to produce automatic movement patterns without placing conscious attention on the process. Historically, occupational therapists have selected, used, adapted, and synthesized activities in their treatment. A child absorbed in play is not focused on the motor demands inherent in the activity. Through motor analysis, activity (play) integration, problem solving, and facilitation of normal tone and movement, occupational therapists address the specific developmental needs of the child (Smith, 1984).

Issues in Play and NDT

A primary objective of the NDT certification course is to refine observation skills while developing handling techniques through facilitation labs and hands-on clinical practice. The course does not tend to focus on play activity integration, possibly because of time constraints. Participants are expected to synthesize NDT concepts in their particular domain of concern and into future clinical practice. Because the emphasis in the NDT course is on handling and normal motor development, potential conflicts may arise when occupational therapists try to integrate purposeful goal-directed activities into NDT.

Traditionally, occupational therapists are expected to effectively use activities in treatment. Many therapists who complete the NDT certification course may experience role conflict if they perceive NDT strategies as inconsistent with occupational therapy treatment approaches. Aside from perfecting handling skills, occupation therapists may feel that they must also master the integration of activities with NDT. To develop and perfect handling methods with a specific child while providing relevant play experiences may create additional challenges. These complex practice issues may be resolved in a variety of ways. Therapists who specialize in NDT may disregard the notion of combining play activities as a "personal philosophy of practice" and concentrate primarily on handling techniques. Others may limit handling and focus more on positioning while facilitating the development of specific skills through activities. Therapists may also alter the activity and NDT emphasis with different children or during treatment sessions depending on the child's specific needs.

Occasionally therapists have difficulty integrating play activities and may feel they have compromised their occupational therapy roles. However, because of the sophistication of skills required to integrate play with NDT, certain difficulties may be inherent in the treatment process. Positioning the play activity while simultaneously handling the child can be a difficult, almost impossible, task with some children. Handling techniques are modified according to the child's responses during movement sequences, and therapists constantly analyze the child's reactions to determine the effectiveness of handling methods. The addition of a play activity creates another component for the occupational therapist to plan, integrate, and monitor in an already demanding treatment situation.

During the child's treatment, the therapist may need periods of time to select, organize, and change activities. Unfortunately, the child's attention or normalized muscle tone and posture may be lost during these periods. The efforts of a child with cerebral palsy to participate in activities may also cause associated reactions and abnormal postures that conflict with the NDT approach. Thus, highly developed observation and handling skills are essential to coordinate all aspects of treatment. The sophistication and complexity of this intervention process is often not recognized by occupational therapists and other professionals.

Intervention

Because of their motor impairment, most children with cerebral palsy cannot fully participate in many play activities. Incorporating play within NDT has many benefits and can fulfill a variety of therapeutic goals: (a) to develop specific cognitive and perceptual skills, (b) to provide appropriate activity experiences as stimuli for normal movement patterns, and (c) to motivate the child for intervention that supports normal developmental needs. Play activities may satisfy both the goal of the child to participate with his or her world and the therapeutic goals of the therapist. There are a number of ways of adapting and integrating activities with NDT.

Activity Adaptation

Activity adaptation is inherent in the effective use of play activities and involves (a) adapting the size, shape, or consistency of the equipment or materials used, (b) modifying the rules and procedures, (c) adjusting the position of the child, materials, and/or environment, and (d) controlling the nature and degree of interpersonal interaction. Thus, play activities are continually modified to meet the changing needs of the child. Using play activities while handling a child involves continuous analysis and adaptation of the activity. If the motor demands placed on the child are high, the cognitive demands of the activity may have to be lowered accordingly. Behavioral changes and the child's emotional responses to activities and treatment influence activity choice, adaptation, and integration. Activities must be

meaningful and purposefully incorporated into treatment sessions.

The occupational therapist draws from the knowledge of activity analysis and grading to adapt activities. By using activity analysis, the therapist identifies the critical aspects of the activity related to the individual child and NDT goals. The two processes involved in this analysis are an assessment of the motor, cognitive, perceptual, and psychosocial needs of the child and an evaluation of the components of the activity. The specific NDT equipment needs of the child are also considered. A mobile (therapist lap, ball, or roll) or nonmobile surface is selected to meet the therapeutic goals. Having analyzed both aspects, the therapist is challenged to provide the appropriate play activity while incorporating NDT techniques. Each element or characteristic (size, shape, etc) of the activity and the type of play (dramatic, games with rules, etc.) may be modified to meet the specific needs of the particular child. For example, if a 5-year-old girl with severe spasticity in both her upper and lower extremities and normal intelligence and language wants to play with the doll house, the therapist first needs to analyze the various components involved in playing with the doll house. In this case, the activity analysis may lead to adapting the activity by changing the location of the doll house, the child's postural demands, or the manner in which the child will manipulate the objects.

Issues in Intervention

The successful integration of activities depends on an appropriately structured physical environment with the activity at the correct height and distance. Lack of equipment or environmental restrictions (e.g., home and school settings) can complicate integrating play activities in treatment.

Two factors that influence activity choices are the neurodevelopmental goals (i.e., techniques and sequences used with the specific child) and the therapist's own body mechanics and coordination. During treatment, the therapist must be prepared to move with the child in a dynamic interplay. Therapists must be mobile in their positioning and, therefore, use postures that facilitate their own movement as well as that of the child. Assisting a child onto a roll may be difficult for a therapist who is in a tailor sitting position. During dynamic movement sequences, less complicated play activities may be indicated.

Therapists adapt the degree of movement within a given activity and also the sequence of movements. Therapists may select static or dynamic positioning. For example, the child with severely involved, left hemiplegia may need to sit on a stable surface to perform a puzzle or other perceptual motor activity. When side-sitting and reaching with the affected arm this child experiences movement in a different way (i.e., subtle weight shifts and postural reactions). When using static positioning and weight shifting, elongation and the active use of these components may be facilitated through subtle handling or by adapting the activity. Thus, NDT principles are incorporated in a treatment session without the use of therapy tools (balls, rolls).

In a dynamic movement sequence, movement through space occurs with assisting the child from one position to another. For example, the therapist helps the child with mild, left hemiplegia down to the floor to grasp puzzle pieces, step over a roll, and then place pieces in the puzzle held in a high easel. Dynamic versus static positioning and movement sequences (i.e., child on floor, roll, ball, or activity on table, wall, or floor) are determined by the therapist.

Children with severe or complex physical limitations often require more hands-on treatment. Intervention demands by the therapist may increase with the child's motor, psychological, cognitive, and perceptual needs. It may at times be necessary during treatment for the therapist to find a balance between the child's ability to participate concurrently in movement sequences and play activities. Efforts to promote one aspect may lead to loss of control of another aspect.

Skill Development

Developing specific cognitive and perceptual skills in a child while actively handling the child can be a complex process. The child with delays in both motor and perceptual spheres may be unable to participate in treatment sequences that demand a combination of these skills. The therapist must prioritize goals both in treatment planning and during the treatment session. A previously planned activity may be abandoned or modified when the child is unable to successfully participate or when the treatment objectives cannot be achieved with the activity.

Occupational therapists may use a variety of theoretical frames of reference with the same child. For example, the child may benefit from the NDT frame of reference with regard to motor deficits but also require treatment for cognitive or perceptual deficits. A therapist may even use more than one frame of reference during a treatment session either simultaneously or sequentially. For example, the treatment of an 8-year-old child with mild spastic athetosis and visual perceptual deficits involved selected visual motor tasks during upper extremity activities to promote proximal shoulder girdle control. Because efforts to combine higher level visual motor tasks during movement caused excessive distress, this sequence was followed with a more sophisticated visual motor task on the table.

Motivational Use of Play

Creative and innovative use of play materials, the environment, and use of the self as a play agent are the critical aspects in the effective integration of motivational play with NDT. The child's play interests and capabilities have an extremely important role in activity selection. Although other disciplines use activities for motivation during NDT, occupational therapists educational background and clinical expertise with play provide a solid foundation for play intervention. One of the unique contributions of occupational therapy is the adaptation of developmentally appropriate activities to meet the specific neuromuscular needs of the child.

The use of current play materials and activities may have an impact on the success of play during therapy. Popular and contemporary activities and the broad spectrum of play interests (i.e., games, television shows, computers, technology, and humor) are important both in activity selection and in interaction with the child. Battery-operated toys may be adapted with various kinds of on/off switches for the severely impaired child with cerebral palsy. Less impaired children may respond to electronic toys and technological devices, including toys that speak, respond to touch, light up, or move, as well as academic learning toys and computers.

Movement is an important aspect of the child's developmental process and play repertoire from infancy onward; for example, the 8-month-old rocks on all four extremities in the quadruped position, the 18-month-old climbs on and off chairs, or the 8-year-old rolls down a hill. Developmentally appropriate movements may be considered play activities. Play can be used to encourage normal movement patterns when NDT is applied. By varying upper extremity actions on objects or toys (reaching, throwing, or placing objects), or the posture (sitting, quadruped or high kneeling), and/or the size of the objects, treatment objectives can be met. Upper extremity elongation, trunk rotation, head and trunk positioning, appropriate grasp, or a combination of these motor components may be developed by using play activities as stimuli for movement.

Activities which are simple, organized, and limited in scope allow the therapist to more effectively handle the child while involving the child in play activities. Less complicated activities with fewer positioning requirements are effective and interfere less with handling. With the young infant (birth to 3 months), the therapist's face and voice can be effective play objects to stimulate visual fixation and tracking, thereby facilitating side-to-side rolling while the child lies supine. With the preschool child, simple play materials can stimulate dramatic or imaginary play. For example, a variety of hats (baseball, fireman, or space helmet) were used with a 5-year-old boy with spastic diplegia. First he was seated on a therapy ball with his shoulders positioned behind his pelvis to develop abdominal control. Lateral weight shifting and rotation were encouraged when he reached out to grasp and switch hats with the therapist.

The repetitive use of an activity with variations during a treatment session can also simplify the activity component. A 2-year-old girl with spastic diplegia had graduated rings placed over her feet as she lay supine. She reached for and stacked the rings while side-sitting and wore them as bracelets when laterally shifting her weight on the roll. For a 5-year-old child with athetosis and normal intelligence, a pretend game of gardening using colored cubes was used throughout the therapy session. While sitting on a roll, the child planted the garden (colored cubes), emphasizing her trunk rotation and upper extremity weight bearing. Kneeling, she harvested the vegetable garden by placing the vegetables on a small table. Moving to stand, she prepared a vegetable soup, mixing the blocks while holding on to a large spoon with both hands.

Age-appropriate toys and activities are used to encourage participation in treatment. For example, when an 18-month-old toddler straddled a bolster to facilitate rotation and lateral weight shifting, three large dolls were strategically placed on each side of the roll. The child was encouraged to reach out an identify the doll's facial features. Stuffed animals, an effective alternative to bolsters and wedges for positioning, can also be used as a stimulating material for dramatic play. With a 5-year-old child, small stuffed animals were used to encourage pretend games while the child was standing. Animals were placed appropriately under the feet to facilitate weight shifting in the step position.

School-age children often create games involving rules and competition: the number of seconds a child can stand on the roll while laterally shifting weight can prompt interest and motivation. Playing baseball for a 6-year-old boy with spastic diplegia, while he was sitting on a therapeutic ball to promote lower extremity weight bearing, provided the opportunity to integrate basic motor skills in a developmentally appropriate manner. The ultimate long-term goal for children is to develop skills that will allow them to fulfill their life roles.

Summary

Occupational therapists' educational background in normal growth and development, therapeutic use of activities, and neurophysiological theory provide the basis for play intervention. Combining clinical experience with NDT and play activities with a willingness to experiment and learn from the child's responses may result in more creative and appropriate activities. Similar movements, actions, and thought processes during play may facilitate participation in activities of daily living; thus, play activities may support acquiring skills in other areas.

Although this paper has focused on the integration of NDT with play, the issues discussed may arise with other neurophysiological treatment approaches. Activities analysis and adaptation, positioning of the child, and handling methods are all equally important aspects of therapeutic intervention. While considering the realistic physical limitations of the child, therapists encourage the child's involvement in play activity to develop the child's physical, cognitive, and psychosocial abilities. Play involves the active participation of the child with his or her environment in a manner that is enjoyable, rewarding, and satisfying. Through play the child with cerebral palsy may explore and discover the world—learn, practice, and become an interactive human being.

References

Boehme R. (1985, November 1). Self-care assessment and treatment from an NDT perspective. *Neuro-Developmental Treatment Association Newsletter*, pp. 1, 5.

Erikson, E. H. (1950). *Childhood and society.* New York: Norton.

Field, T. M., Roseman, S., De-Stefano, L. J., & Koewler, J. (1982). The play of handicapped preschool children with handicapped and non-handicapped peers in integrated and non-integrated situations. *Topics in Early Childhood Special Education. 2,* 28–38.

Florey, L. L. (1981). Studies of play: Implications for growth, development and for clinical practice. *American Journal of Occupational Therapy, 35,* 519–528.

Hinojosa, J., Sabari, J., & Rosenfeld, M. S. (1983). Purposeful activities. *American Journal of Occupational Therapy, 37,* 805–806.

Peller, L. E. (1954). Libidinal phases, ego development, and play. *Psychoanalytic Study of the Child, 9,* 178–198.

Plaut, E. A. (1979). Play and adaptation. *Psychoanalytic Study of the Child, 34,* 217–232.

Scherzer, A. L., & Tscharnuter, I. (1982). *Early diagnosis and therapy in cerebral palsy.* New York: Marcel Dekker.

Smith, M. M. (1984, December). Applying the neurodevelopmental treatment approach to OT. *Developmental Disabilities Special Interest Section Newsletter.* pp. 1–2.

Stengel, T. J., Attermeier, S. M., Bly, L., & Heriza, C. B. (1984). Evaluation of sensorimotor dysfunction. In S. K. Campbell (Ed.), *Pediatric Neurological Physical Therapy* (pp. 13–87). New York: Churchill Livingstone.

Winnicott, D. W. (1971). *Playing and reality.* New York: Basic Books.

Related Readings

deRenne-Stephan, C. (1980). Imitation: A mechanism of play behavior. *American Journal of Occupational Therapy, 34,* 95–102.

Gunn, S. L. (1975). Play as occupation: Implications for the handicapped. *American Journal of Occupational Therapy, 29,* 222–225.

Hindmarsh, W. A. (1979). Play diagnosis and play therapy. *American Journal of Occupational Therapy, 33,* 770–775.

McEnvoy, J., McConkey, R. (1983). Play activities of mentally handicapped children at home and mothers' perception of play. *International Journal of Rehabilitation Research, 6,* 143–151.

Reilly, M. (Ed.). (1974). *Play as exploratory learning.* Beverly Hills, CA: Sage Publications.

Sparling, J. W., Walker, D. F., & Singdahlsen, J. (1984). Play techniques with neurologically impaired preschoolers. *American Journal of Occupational Therapy, 38,* 603–612.

Vanderburg, B., Kielhofner, G. K. (1985). Play in evolution, culture, and individual adaptation: Implications for therapy. *American Journal of Occupational Therapy, 36,* 20–28.

Chapter 47

Occupational Therapy and Rehabilitation Engineering: A Team Approach to Helping Persons with Severe Physical Disability to Upgrade Functional Independence

Ruth Ellen Gordon, OTR
Ken P. Kozole, BSME, OTR

This chapter was previously published jointly in *Occupational Therapy Strategies and Adaptations for Independent Daily Living* (Haworth Press, 1984) and in *Occupational Therapy in Health Care, 1,* (4), 117–129. Copyright © 1984, The Haworth Press, Inc.

Occupational therapists who work in clinical settings serving persons with severe disabilities often face difficult problems of selection and modification of aids to independence. At the Rehabilitation Institute of Chicago (RIC), Alan J. Brown Center for Communication and Environmental Control, many solutions to such needs are facilitated by the interaction and collaboration of occupational therapists, clinical rehabilitation engineers and speech/language pathologists. This paper will describe the occupational therapist/rehabilitation engineer collaboration in conjunction with the total team as various clinical problems and their solutions are presented.

Engineers available for both service and research at RIC come from one of two entities, the Rehabilitation Engineering Service Delivery Program (RESDP) which provides direct service to clients on a regular basis, and Northwestern University Rehabilitation Engineering Program, (NUREP) whose major focus is federally funded research and special problem solving. From their joint efforts, much up-to-date clinical and research information about special aids for disabled persons is made available for clients. Services include consultation, evaluation, fabrication of devices and re-evaluation as needed for both inpatients and outpatients at RIC.

As a way of offering the most comprehensive services possible to all patients at RIC, a strong team approach is practiced. Rehabilitation engineers, who combine in their education training in both engineering and rehabilitation principles, add a special dimension to the team solutions for patients seeking more independent function.

In the Alan J. Brown Center, services are offered to non-verbal and otherwise severely disabled persons who in general come wishing to increase their independence in communication and/or to gain control over their environments. The majority of individuals seen are from the diagnostic categories of spinal cord injury, brain-stem level cerebral vascular accident, cerebral palsy, amyotrophic lateral sclerosis, or other progressive neuromuscular disorders.

Communication equipment and environmental aids of many kinds are available in the Center for client evaluation through trial use, and for use as training activities. Services offered focus on the skills of team specialists consisting of the occupational therapist, rehabilitation engineer and speech/language pathologist. The services offered include: comprehensive evaluation and training of inpatients and outpatients in the use of alternative/augmentative communication and environmental control systems; education, training and counseling services for disabled individuals, their families and friends and for rehabilitation and educational professionals; site visits in home or work environments to set up assistive systems when required or requested; follow-up evaluations and counseling, as necessary.

Solving Problems

The Referral

The engineer works closely with the therapists beginning with the receipt of the doctor's referral (most often initiated by the occupational, speech or physical therapist who realizes a patient needs technical aid assistance). The therapists and engineer discuss the person's needs and an appointment is scheduled with the client and his family and other involved team members for the actual evaluation, a critical phase in the problem solving process.

To begin, the team considers the client's total living situation as well as his goals and objectives in seeking the staff's help. Focusing on only one need such as mobility or communication without reviewing other aspects of the person's life will undoubtedly result in recommendation of inadequate or inappropriate aids. Also, since most individuals must pay for second devices themselves if the first ones prove inadequate or inappropriate (third party payers rarely will *reconsider* technical aids purchased for clients), it is important that correct decisions be made the first time. Also, since the equipment a person receives will affect him and his life style for years to follow, it is imperative to listen and discuss alternatives carefully with him to increase his acceptance of equipment ultimately selected. In addition, at this stage the prognosis of the person's functional status should be considered to determine how the future course of events will affect his use of aids.

The Evaluation

A review of the medical record and conferences with other health professionals provide much of the necessary base-line information regarding functional expectations. However, a functional evaluation with careful observation and discussion with the client is conducted to get specific information needed. The evaluation then involves the disabled person trying to use various technical aids or modified aids as arranged by the evaluation team. This is the first step.

The most basic element in determining functional capacities and equipment solutions, however, is that the client be initially properly seated and positioned for optimum function. A stable base and appropriate body support is essential for comfort and cosmesis as well as function. The individual's posture and body position (balance and alignment) will define and affect his motor abilities. Often temporary seating adjustments are necessary and are provided *before* any trial use of equipment can be attempted. In addition to the occupational therapist and rehabilitation engineer, at RIC the physical therapist is a key team member involved in seating, positioning and mobility.

Also important to the decision making about equipment are the person's cognitive skills, such as orientation, concentration, attention span, memory, judgement, ability to follow directions, error recognition and problem solving skills. These abilities are appraised by the team through trials in structured activities.

Evidence of sensory awareness in both general and specific terms, so necessary in operation of equipment, is often determined both by review of formal testing results and by direct questioning. Perceptual abilities (visual perception, visual motor skill and body integration) are also verified in the same manner. As an example, visual motor abilities, so critical in one's potentials for operating an electric powered wheelchair, can be observed through his playing Pacman or other joystick operated video games.

A complete formal evaluation of motor skills is provided by physical and occupational therapy departments; however, motor skills necessary for performing specific functions are reevaluated. Head, neck, upper and lower extremity motions are all potentials for operation of switches to control a technical aid. Therefore, measures of active range of motion, strength, placement ability, coordination, dexterity and endurance of such body parts must be known. In addition, muscle tone (hyper and hypo), reflex and synergistic influences must be appraised because they too are significant in determining control potentials.

Finally, the person's general psychological status and adjustment to disability figure largely in making determinations about his potentials as an equipment user. This kind of information is acquired by various team members through their contacts with the client and by review of his record.

Identification of the client's functional (daily living) needs is next in the evaluation process. Needs may involve his mobility, ability to communicate (needs, wants, as well as emotions and general conversations), ways to control devices needed for him to function in his environment, the environment itself (where the person spends his time and what he does there), or work and leisure activities. The direction of this phase of the evaluation comes from the client's stated needs and goals as well as from the therapist's knowledge of the interrelationships among various life activities.

Team Problem Solving

Even before the evaluation is begun, the range of the client's financial resources is explored since various options exist as solutions to most problems. Costs can vary considerably depending on which devices are chosen. General information and cost constraints must be known before service can proceed and recommendations made.

Following the evaluation as described, the entire team gathers with the client (and family members if possible), for discussion. The client, or referring party, defines his needs; the occupational, physical and speech/language therapists present their assessments of the person's abilities and deficits, and possible methods of enhancing his function; the rehabilitation engineer offers suggestions for effective and efficient use and set-up of technical aids. The resultant conference is more of a joint problem solving session with each team member presenting his perspective and ideas for potentials for resolution of the difficulties. Compromise in the selection of the optimal technical aid is based upon the client skills and needs, his interests in the solution, financial resources and available solutions.

Solution Guidelines

When choosing equipment, it is important to reflect on a few basic principles. *Prognosis* of the client's condition is primary to consider since it determines operation potentials. For example, knowing the patterns of progressive motor loss characteristic of muscular dystrophy, one might choose a wheelchair system which can be changed as the person's ability to control diminishes. A powered wheelchair that allows for operation by both a light-touch joystick and sip and puff control without major electrical modification may be an appropriate system for this client. Communication aids must be such that they offer *growth potential* as the user's vocabulary grows. Can the electric communication aid be operated by more than one type of control? Does the simple communication board allow for adding more media easily? The environmental control system should be *flexible*. For instance, perhaps the client cannot now speak, but if in the near future he does talk, will the environmental control unit (ECU) operate a telephone without extensive electrical changes? The person may not be mobile now, but if he becomes independently mobile in the future, could he operate his ECU from his wheelchair? Can more devices be added to the system or is the unit capable of operating only a few devices? Is there a means for both family members or attendants and the client to operate the same devices?

An Option Approach

Correlation of all these factors inevitably results in a ranking of possible options. For example, if the client is a student who has achieved his maximum level of physical function and no change in his physical status is expected, his most immediate need may be control of his environment which would enable him to live independently, as in a room in a dormitory. With his good head and neck function, the occupational therapist may recommend that the optimal control interface for him is head or chin control; sip and puff control would be another alternative. The environmental control options are then presented based on the control method finally decided. The occupational therapist and rehabilitation engineer will present the pros and cons of the various systems and explore the best set up for each system. The client states his preference after trial use of all the options. The rehabilitation engineer often provides temporary modifications to the controls or devices to enhance independent access for the client and thus increase his effectiveness in using them. After the exploration process, a final list of options is compiled.

Commercially available aids are the usual first choice of the team. They often present a variety of potentials for application or modification of either simple or sophisticated electronic aids. The majority of client problems can be solved using commercial aids. One excellent source of information about what is available commercially is provided by a federally funded source called ABLEDATA. Based on one's request, ABLEDATA will send a list of commercially available equipment related to solving the client's needs. That list then offers additional alternatives for technical aids.

Environment/Home Devices
The Home Itself

Environment/home modifications are generally straightforward in providing solutions to client's problems. Installation of devices may include: ramps, elevators or lifts; replacement of door handles, special light switches, faucet handles, telephones; rearrangement of furniture, or commonly, redesign of a bathroom to assure wheelchair access. Much of the hardware that must be installed in such instances can be purchased in a neighborhood hardware store or lumber supply store. Also, many catalogues of equipment for disabled persons provide useful ideas and devices.

Work and Leisure

Aids for work and leisure activities tend to overlap in function depending on the client's daily responsibilities and interests. Regardless of why a person engages in an activity using a device, however, he must have *independent access* to the technical aid he needs to use if it is to be considered effective. This is generally assured by having a set 'work station,' which might be a large table of proper height, a bed table of adjustable height, possibly a turntable desk, or other work surface. In any case, devices which the user operates need to be both accessible and mounted securely where they are to be used.

If needed, page turning can be accomplished with books mounted on holders (or a rotating book holder) and the person flips the pages with a mouth stick if he is unable to use his hands. Use of an electric page turner is an alternative choice; however a good mouthstick user can easily out-perform the electric device. For recording or dictating, a conventional tape recorder, preferably with a one button 'record' feature or with variable speech control is recommended when hand use is limited. Other options or modifications which enhance independent operation of a recorder include the addition of projections to lengthen control levers, use of remote switches or control by an environmental control unit (ECU). Available portable and non-portable typewriters present a wide range of features helpful to clients with disability. Automatic correction features are necessary and effective. Use of paper in a roll or self-feeding perforated computer paper makes independence in typing possible for the severely handicapped because paper loading is eliminated.

Computers

With the advent of personal computers and the wide variety they offer in functions, costs and features available, more persons with physical disabilities are now able to engage in a diverse range of work and leisure activities. Now it is easier for the disabled person to undertake many activities because of widely varying software for such things as word processing, accounting, bookkeeping, graphics as well as for recreation in things like video games. Special computer programs are available which allow one to use many personal computers as communication aids. Television sets and stereo systems can be operated by their own 'remote controller' or through an ECU. Telephones with a wide variety of operational features also are now readily available. They offer such functions as wireless transmission, push-button memories, automatic re-dial and a choice of either hand held receivers or desktop speakers, all excellent aids to those needing special telephoning assistance.

Positioning for Use

Many aids to be effective must be positioned semi-permanently in a manner that is not only stable and accessible but also cosmetically appealing. Commercially available mounting systems can be purchased, but an occupational therapy department offers a variety of equipment and materials that can solve mounting problems. Goose neck extensions, lapboards, calculator stands, thermoplastic materials, plywood, aluminum stock and bars, and plastic strapping all might be used in devising mounting systems. In addition, a walk through the local hardware store often reveals a variety of solutions for the enterprising therapist.

Most of the technical aids previously mentioned require an interface, or method of control, compatible with the client's abilities. Since electronic technology presents many options for easily operated devices, there are, not surprisingly, many commercially available microswitches and low force switches which can be operated by limited hand force or movement, mouth stick or headpointer. Thus they prove appropriate for the person with limited motor function.

The Occupational Therapist/ Rehabilitation Engineer Problem Solving

In approaching any client's needs, the therapist and engineer pool their resources along with those of the client when problem solving to come up with the best man/machine combination. The occupational therapist contributes a broad knowledge of human function and of the effects of various degrees and kinds of disability on the performance of daily activities. The engineer brings rich resources in human factors engineering, design, materials and fabrication resulting in his knowing what is possible to devise. Their shared philosophies of problem solving approaches to difficult problems meld to bring about effective solutions which may evolve as devices for person, setting or activity depending on the goal.

Commercial Aid Solutions

As stated before, commercial aids are the first choice for solving most functional needs. Their cost advantages and greater availability are significant incentives for using them. Further, service and maintenance warranties are often available for major items, whereas with custom designed items, quick and accessible repair is not always possible and is inevitably costly. Many commercial aids also have replacement parts readily accessible so that 'down–time' in breakdown may be reduced. Finally, with use of commercial equipment loan equipment may be more readily available while the client is waiting for his personal device to be operable again.

Modifications

Even though the number and variety of commercial aids continue to expand, a large number of people have needs which cannot be met completely by such equipment. This is where the skills of both the occupational therapist and the rehabilitation engineer come into play again to develop modifications which either allow for independent operation by the user or satisfy other needs not found in the particular item which was available.

Care must be taken in making modifications however, so that the device is not damaged nor its warranty voided by changes made. A phone call to the manufacturer should be made to clear up modification/warranty questions before proceeding, especially on major items. For example, use of permanent adhesives or screw fasteners to attach plastic projections on operating buttons of a cassette recorder may void the manufacturer's warranty. However, since the projections enable the user to operate the device, many clients in such circumstances choose to have the modifications, regardless.

Commercially available materials and components also reduce time and cost in modifying devices and may permit home repair if a part becomes damaged or inoperable. The rehabilitation engineer uses such materials as much as possible to keep client costs down. For example, plastic pipe fittings are useful and durable as mounting fixtures or holders for ADL equipment, such as for a stand for a telephone headset or countertop positioning post for an electric shaver. Joystick controllers for electric wheelchairs can also be modified with plastic pipe fittings to provide 'custom' fitted hand tillers.

Custom Devices

The design and fabrication of custom devices is chosen as a last resort at RIC in solving client needs. In cases where it is the only viable option for RIC clients, the research group at NUREP is often contacted since they provide valuable research-related input. Other sources of ideas include other Rehabilitation Engineering Centers and vendors of durable medical equipment. Considerable care is taken in making these decisions using all possible relevant data along with the evaluation process previously described to choose the final device or system. Staff supervise both installation and trial of the custom devices to assure final 'fit' to the client's needs.

Case Studies

Case One: JD

JD, a 58 year old woman with post-polio quadriplegia, sought help from NUREP to explore recent technological developments which could enhance her functional abilities. Tired of being dependent upon her husband and daytime attendants for all activities of daily living, she was discouraged by being able to do so little for herself. With these needs in mind she was referred to the Brown Center for evaluation by the occupational therapist and rehabilitation engineer team. JD was evaluated while seated in her manually powered, reclining wheelchair even though she spent the majority of each day in a rocking bed (assisted breathing). She demonstrated fair head mobility if external support was provided, limited right arm placement and hand function (with armrest and mobile arm support) but she was unable to complete any of her activities of daily living independently. Following the assessment of her skills and needs, as well as discussion with her husband, primary goals were seen as giving her changes in her means of mobility and control of her immediate environment. However, since the client was a recipient of Medicare which disallows funding for such equipment, decisions had to be made with her and her husband to provide private funding for whatever system was finally chosen.

Problem solving by the team resulted in two suggestions: (1) An electric powered wheelchair with both light touch joystick and sip and puff controls was recommended to provide a means of independent mobility and pressure relief while sitting. An electric powered recliner system operated by head switches was also recommended as part of the wheelchair package to provide independent weight redistribution. (2) An environmental control system to be operated either from the rocking bed or wheelchair was recommended. After trial and training with recommended equipment at the Center, a home visit was made by the OT/RE team to set up the system and to identify additional needs. Training followed and periodic follow-up continues, initiated either by the client or the therapist as changing needs dictate. JD reports that use of her equipment does indeed allow her independent mobility and personal control of her telephone, rocking bed, positive ventilator unit, radio, home intercom unit, room lights, TV and an emergency call unit. Thus the ECU has reduced the need for constant attendant care because JD can now call for assistance if she needs it. Her independence in operating the devices not only enables her to be alone for longer periods of time, but also has given her considerable confidence and a significant boost psychologically. Equipment carefully selected and installed for use by the team resulted in markedly increased levels of independence for JD.

Case Two: JW

JW, a boy 12 years of age, is non-verbal and non ambulatory as a result of cerebral palsy. He was evaluated by teams at both RIC and NUREP to find a means for him to be independently mobile and to be able to communicate effectively. A custom wheelchair seating system was first provided. The postural insert was mounted in a variety of wheelchairs until the proper fit for JW was achieved. Staff of the physical and occupational therapy departments determined that JW's upper extremity motions were non-functional due to his severe athetosis. However, foot placement was functional, and further testing showed that JW could press tread switches mounted on the wheelchair footplate and thereby operate a wheelchair. Rehabilitation engineers designed and fabricated a footplate controller to match JW's ability so that he could drive his chair.

The footplate control also operated a laptray-mounted, electric powered, row-column/scanning communication aid. Staff from NUREP wired the control in a way so that JW would use the same footplate switches for both mobility and communication to eliminate the addition of more controls. Experience has shown that the fewer and less complicated the gadgets, the better.

JW has gained sufficient head control to enable him to use a head-pointer unit for doing desktop activities. The head-pointer has proven to be his 'physical link' to the immediate environment. Recently when he was reevaluated for upgrading his communication system, it was noted that he could select desired words on the communication board display more efficiently when using head motions to direct the optical head pointer (rather than with the foot control). Because the communication system is designed to accept a variety of controls, JW can immediately upgrade his level of communication by using the faster head-pointer direct selection method. He still, however, operates the wheelchair using the foot plate switches. Both the independent mobility and effective means of communication have helped JW significantly. He now can express his emotions, demonstrate control over his environment through commands and wishes, interact with his peers and show us an emerging personality which we all enjoy.

Summary

Persons who have severe physical disabilities can upgrade their levels of functional independence through the use of technical aids which are carefully selected to meet their needs. Many seek such solutions. The occupational therapist is often mainly responsible for solving functional problems by determining needs and possible answers, and ultimately for recommending particular devices that change either the environment or the way a person interacts with his surroundings. At the Rehabilitation Institute of Chicago, and in a growing number of other Centers, however, the occupational therapist now works with a clinical rehabilitation engineer for reaching solutions to such client needs. Combining the occupational therapist's knowledge of human function and needs in daily living activities with the rehabilitation engineer's resources in human factor engineering, design, materials and fabrication and their shared problem-solving approaches to difficult functional problems, they together develop effective solutions in the form of either commercial, readily available 'use' devices, custom modifications to such devices, or, as a last resort, custom-designed and built assistive equipment.

The results in two case studies presented and many others like them, bear testimony to the effectiveness and success of this combination of skills. Many persons so helped achieve marked levels of independence.

Chapter 48

Project Threshold: A Systematic Approach to Solving Functional Problems of Persons with Physical Disabilities Using Occupational Therapy and Rehabilitation Engineering Services

Heidi McHugh Pendleton, OTR
Nancy J. Somerville
Gail K. Magdalena, OTR
Kathryn L. Bowman, OTR

This chapter was previously published jointly in *Occupational Therapy Strategies and Adaptations for Independent Daily Living* (Haworth Press, 1984) and *Occupational Therapy in Health Care*, 1, (4), 131-142. Copyright © 1984, The Haworth Press, Inc.

Throughout people's lives circumstances change, opportunities arise and challenges result which require adaptation and growth. To ensure success in meeting these life challenges, many people seek the assistance of others, taking advantage of their experience and expertise. For the person with a physical disability, challenges might occur in school, vocational training, employment, or by assuming a more independent living situation. Project Threshold is a service delivery program designed to offer the practical assistance necessary to those who are encountering such challenges.

Evolution of the Program

Project Threshold began in a much needed attempt to deliver engineering services to disabled individuals in the community.[1] The Rehabilitation Engineering Center (REC) at Rancho Los Amigos Hospital (RLAH) had been involved for many years in research and development of treatment oriented equipment for severely disabled patients in this comprehensive rehabilitation center. As an offshoot to this in-house activity, the engineering group began to work with a small number of disabled individuals in the community as they attempted to solve specific problems encountered in performance of everyday activities at home, school, or work. In 1976, these services were made available to a larger number of individuals through an Innovation and Expansion Grant. Subsequent case service contracts from the California State Department of Rehabilitation provided the necessary funding to allow continued program development. During this period of development, the program became formally known as Project Threshold.

During the initial period of the program's development, clients were seen by a team of four to six people which included engineers, machinists, technicians and a coordinator. Evaluations were generally limited to investigating one problem area which usually resulted in each client receiving custom equipment to solve his or her specific problem. As more clients with a wider variety of problems were referred, changes in staff and procedures for providing services were required. These resulted in emphasis being placed on client involvement, functional assessment of each client and research of commercial products prior to recommending the more costly alternative of design and fabrication of custom equipment.

In making these changes, it was felt that an interdisciplinary team would be better equipped to solve the myriad of problems presented by severely disabled clients. The program however, could not support the wide variety of personnel that might be needed in providing services. A decision was made to employ occupational therapists as consultants and later as full-time employees; engineers and individuals from other disciplines, such as physical therapy were and continue to be used as consultants on an as-needed basis. The engineering consultants are readily available because of Project Threshold's link with the REC already existing at Rancho Los Amigos Hospital.

A key factor in the effectiveness of staff and consultants is the use of the case coordinator. While a variety of people may become involved at some point in providing services to any given client, one staff member assumes responsibility for the management of each case beginning with reviewing the referral and coordinating interventions until completion of the final recommendations. In this way, services are provided with only essential staff and consultants involved. Each staff member assumes responsibility for management of a caseload. Individual cases are assigned at random or, on occasion, to match disability-related problems with a staff member's specific areas of expertise.

Case coordinators are not always occupational therapists. However, with few exceptions, an occupational therapist participates in every evaluation conducted through Project Threshold. The expertise of the occupational therapist lends itself particularly to evaluating and solving the independent living and worksite problems characteristic of those presented by clients. Occupational therapists are educated to assess clients' functional capabilities, to analyze and teach activities of daily living and to recognize the characteristics of tools and equipment which will facilitate successful performance of an activity.[2] Further, the occupational therapy philosophy views clients within the context of their life roles and environments with concern for home, work, play and rest needs of each individual.[3] This awareness helps to ensure that solutions for one problem will not interfere with the client's performance of other activities.

Individuals with a wide variety of physical disabilities are referred to Project Threshold. The majority of referrals are made by counselors from the California State Department of Rehabilitation with other referral sources including allied health professionals, rehabilitation nurses, vocational counselors in private agencies as well as the clients themselves. Although clients generally have been discharged from rehabilitation settings for at least a year, some have never been involved in rehabilitation programs. While problems presented by clients typically involved difficulty with performance of activities in the home, school, or worksite, an evaluation may address problems encountered in more than one of these areas.

Evaluations are conducted in either home, school, or work environments, or in Project Threshold's Model Home. The Model Home is a building with a furnished living room, kitchen, bedroom, bathroom and office. In addition, the rooms are stocked with numerous assistive devices and equipment items available for trial use.

Another resource used during the evaluation process is an extensive file of information on commercially available equipment from over 1500 manufacturers. Much of this product information has been entered into a computerized information retrieval system called ABLEDATA. Using ABLEDATA and the file, Project Threshold staff can search for specific equipment items which are currently available, often avoiding the need for generally more expensive custom devices.

Process of Service Delivery

A systematic approach is used in providing services to severely disabled clients. This process provides for definition of clients' problems in the context of their daily activities, rather than as an isolated dysfunction. The client is continually involved throughout the process to ensure that the definitive solution will be useful and so that he or she learns problem solving skills which can be independently applied in the future.

Information Gathering

The first step is review of the referral information by the case coordinator to determine appropriateness for services. The information in the referral includes basic data regarding the client: age, diagnosis, medical history, statement of problem areas, and the referring party's or agency's expectations of the evaluation. To augment this information it is sometimes necessary for the coordinator to study further the nature of a disability, to clarify the reason for referral, or to consult with allied health professionals who have previously worked with the client.

As the next step, an in-depth telephone interview with the client follows using a comprehensive form which addresses all aspects of daily living.[4] During the interview, clients are asked to describe their functional abilities and limitations in performing activities of daily living, including use of adaptive behavior or equipment. In addition, information related to a client's personal care schedule, use of attendants, living situation, vocational and avocational activities is obtained. Often problems are identified during the course of the interview which were not included in the referral, but which may affect successfully solving the original problem. Obtaining detailed information from the client prior to the actual hands-on evaluation provides a total picture of the client's needs within the context of his or her daily lifestyle as well as a beginning plan that will facilitate the efficient use of time during the actual evaluation.

After reviewing these data, a team meeting is conducted when the case coordinator presents a tentative plan for service. The team members help the case coordinator to further define the plan and determine the goal for evaluation, where it should be conducted, what specialized equipment is needed and who should be included. A schedule is then established to accommodate the client, necessary consultants and the referral source. At times it may be appropriate to include the client's employer, family members or others who can contribute to, or benefit from the evaluation.

Client Evaluation

Although most evaluations take place in the Model Home, visits to the client's home or worksite are made when there is an identified need for assessment of specific environments. All evaluations include the assessment of the client's actual function which serves as the foundation for determining solutions. The functional assessment is a thorough evaluation of the client's problem areas, compensatory methods of performance and assets in terms of both physical and cognitive skills. The assessment may include traditional standardized tests, however, it focuses on observation of the client's function during performance of various tasks. Identification of specific problems is accomplished through observation of key activities beyond those listed in initial descriptions from the referral and interview. Demonstration of alternative methods of performing activities and trials with various equipment items are also part of the session. When needed equipment is not available in the Model Home, such items can often be obtained on a short-term loan basis from manufacturers. Persons with complex needs may require several problem solving sessions, as well as an extensive search for appropriate equipment resources.

Choosing Solutions

The intended outcome of the evaluation is to determine feasible solutions and to make recommendations. Solutions to problems may include learning adaptive behavior, or acquisition of commercial or custom equipment. Consideration is first given to the possibility of the client learning alternate techniques for performing activities or adapting behavior to eliminate the need for equipment. When problems cannot be resolved through adaptive behavior, commercially available equipment is next investigated and actually tried when possible. Although there are numerous equipment items manufactured specifically to meet the needs of persons with disabilities, frequently products designed for general use in homes and offices can be used.

Only after the preferred solutions of adaptive behavior or commercial equipment have proven unsuccessful, is design and fabrication of custom equipment considered. When such equipment is required, or adaptation of a commercial product is indicated, engineering personnel become extensively involved and remain so from evaluation to fabrication of the end product.

During the evaluation, the occupational therapist is responsible for teaching the client adaptive behavior techniques and methods of using both the commercial and custom equipment. For most clients this short training period, followed by practice at home, is sufficient for learning the particular skill. If, however, it becomes evident during the evaluation that more extensive and specialized training is necessary, the clients are referred to an outside resource or agency, such as an outpatient occupational therapy program in their community.

Reporting

Following the determination of solutions, a written report is prepared and sent to the referral source. The report summarizes the evaluation results and lists the recommendations, often including solution options. When commercially available equipment is recommended, exact model numbers, local sources and approximate costs are given. In the report, the client's potential for increased function as a result of using the recommended equipment is well documented. This is essential if financial assistance from third party payers is being sought. When recommendations include provision of custom equipment, sources for this work as well as time and cost estimates are given. At the end of the report the referral source is invited to contact the case coordinator for clarification or any assistance.

Follow-up

After the report is prepared and sent to the referral source, the Project's contract commitment is completed. Project Threshold does not conduct a formal follow-up on each individual case, however in order to determine the program's effectiveness and the extent to which recommendations are implemented, two formal studies have been conducted. One study surveyed the satisfaction of referral sources with the services provided[1] and the other assessed former clients' perceptions of the services and the benefits derived from their involvement with Project Threshold.[5] The results of both studies indicated a high level of satisfaction with services and implementation of recommendations.

Informal follow-up frequently occurs as many of the referral sources continue to use Project Threshold and provide information on the status of former clients. This repeat business is evidence of the counselors' satisfaction with services. In addition, a number of former clients contact the program relating the outcome of their involvement with the program.

Case Examples

Two case examples are presented to demonstrate application of the process.

Case 1: Shirley

The first example concerns Shirley, a 53-year-old woman four years following a stroke that resulted in right hemiplegia. She was referred by her vocational rehabilitation counselor to enable her to function as a homemaker in an independent setting in order to meet her vocational goal. At the time of referral, Shirley was residing in a board and care home where she was functioning at a high level of independence with minimal supervision. An evaluation was needed to determine her potential to meet her goal of living independently. Clarification of the referral revealed that the reason for evaluation was not only to identify equipment needs in relation to her one-hand function, but to determine if problems in behavior, such as mild confusion and memory loss, would affect her safety in performance in home activities. These problems were viewed by the counselor as the only potential obstacles preventing Shirley from achieving her goal.

During the telephone interview, Shirley revealed that she had had little opportunity to attempt homemaking activities since her stroke, but was independent in her personal care. She was managing her money independently, had a checking account and made small purchases at the local store. It was noted however, that her speech was rambling and ideas were often tangential causing the case coordinator to question her organizational abilities.

After discussion in a team meeting, a plan for evaluation in the Model Home by an occupational therapist was formulated. Emphasis was to be placed on her performance in cooking an actual meal and performing other home tasks to determine the feasibility of commercially available devices as aids. The client's ability to adapt to new methods of performing tasks would also be assessed. Of particular concern would be an evaluation of her judgement, problem solving skills, abilities to organize and her safety in the kitchen with environmental distractions present. The equipment thought to enhance her function was located, preparations were made for a cooking experience and homemaking evaluation. The time and location for the assessment were arranged with the staff, client and counselor.

Functional assessment showed that Shirley was left dominant with good dexterity, but non-functional in the right upper extremity. She was ambulatory for short distances, but sat frequently in a wheelchair to perform activities. The evaluation further revealed that Shirley's task performance was far better than her verbal skills.

She was observed to be organized, attentive and safe in home activities. Shirley proved to be an ideal candidate for commercial devices designed for one-handed use and for home convenience items such as a toaster oven, drawer and cupboard organizers. She learned quickly how to use these devices in the equipment trial. Overall problem solving and planning skills were noted to be adequate for independent living despite verbal distractibility. Once it was determined she was capable of making changes in her performance, adaptive behavior was introduced to her for methods of kitchen organization as well as for other household activities. Specific commercially available equipment was recommended for her use in a written report to the rehabilitation counselor.

The report also included recommendations for further professional assistance once Shirley obtained an apartment. After several months, she did move to an apartment and was re-referred to Project Threshold for an assessment of her ability to function in this new environment. An evaluation in her home revealed the need for equipment to assist her with toileting and bathing. The recommended equipment included a raised toilet seat and a tub safety rail for greater ease and safety in these activities. An additional report with description of performance in the apartment was made including specific equipment recommendations. From this point, purchase of the equipment and follow-up was the responsibility of the counselor. Contact with Shirley a few months later revealed she was using her equipment and performing well in her own environment.

This is an example of a relatively simple evaluation in terms of personnel, time, complexity and cost of solutions. Even so, the design and sequence of the problem solving process was valuable in determining evaluation needs early and in assuring a thorough, relevant assessment and subsequent reintervention once her living situation changed. To Shirley, this intervention was a major factor in her being able to change her lifestyle and achieve a reported happier, independent existence.

Although a majority of clients referred to Project Threshold are experiencing problems with performance of activities in the home, such as in the case previously described, there have been an increasing number of referrals requesting evaluation of problems encountered at work. In the majority of such cases, addressing the concerns of the employer is critical to ensure successful implementation of proposed solutions. Early communication with employers, therefore, can help to eliminate pre-conceived ideas or misconceptions they may have regarding the extent of changes needed to accommodate a worker who is disabled. This involvement also serves to increase employers' acceptance of solutions.

Case 2: Martha

An example of a referral concerning work-needs is Martha, a 28-year-old woman with a diagnosis of arthritis who was employed full-time as an invoice records clerk for a department store. She was experiencing fatigue and joint pain which seemed to increase with the performance of work duties. She experienced an acute flare-up of her arthritis and was hospitalized. During her hospitalization, an occupational therapist who provided Martha's inpatient treatment noted the need for assessment of her work duties in relation to her symptoms. She subsequently became a client of the Department of Rehabilitation and was referred to Project Threshold. She was seen for a worksite evaluation to assess the extent of her current physical complaints, their relationship to job requirements, and for recommendations to permit daily work performance with less discomfort.

Martha was interviewed by telephone for information concerning her perceptions of her physical abilities and limitations and her current difficulties at work. As an invoice records clerk, her job responsibilities included a great deal of writing, filing, using a stapler, and operating a calculator. She indicated that she was experiencing increasing pain in her back, neck and all extremities which seemed to be intensified by her job tasks. Because of these symptoms, she was concerned about her ability to maintain her job.

Martha's job-related problems were then presented in a team meeting where causes and potential solutions were identified. An evaluation at the worksite was subsequently scheduled with the client, employer and referral source present. The evaluation began with an assessment of Martha's physical status and progressed to observation of her performance of the various tasks involved in her job. It became evident during this observation that working from the horizontal surface of the desk was a major factor contributing to her problems. It forced her to position her neck in pronounced flexion while working resulting in pain and fatigue. Further, repeated stapling, as well as removing staples with a pinch-type remover resulted in hand and wrist pain. Retrieving fallen papers and objects from the floor also resulted in pain through her back and lower extremities. Her entire work space needed rethinking; desk, chair and arrangement of work area. Filing and operating the calculator posed additional problems resulting in joint pain.

Recommendations for solving this client's work-related problems included use of a portable somewhat angled drawing board which could be placed on the desk top to minimize the need for constant neck flexion. The angled surface also provided support to her arm while operating the calculator, resulting in less pain while performing this task. In addition, non-slip matting to prevent objects from slipping off this angled surface was suggested. An electric stapler and a light-weight reacher solved problems with stapling and accessing items.

In addition to these commercially available items, a custom modification was made to an ordinary staple remover to limit strain on her finger joints. A removable

custom file holder was designed to clamp on the desk edge positioning file folders at a convenient height. This alleviated neck pain previously caused by accessing file folders in her lap. These recommendations were described in a written report which was shared with the referral source and the employer. All of the suggestions were implemented and resulted in reduced pain for Martha and greater efficiency on the job.

Summary and Conclusions

Project Threshold located at Rancho Los Amigos Hospital, is a program which uses the skills of an interdisciplinary team to solve functional problems encountered at home or at work by persons with physical disabilities. The program evolved because there was a community need to provide rehabilitation engineering services in an efficient and cost-effective manner. The program, using a systematic process for delivering services, emphasizes functional assessment, client involvement, and research of solutions. Occupational therapists are involved in almost all cases because of their knowledge and skills in assessing and teaching activities of daily living. Solutions recommended include either teaching adaptive behaviors, using commercially available equipment or custom designing and fabricating equipment for unique situations. Two case examples were presented which demonstrated how this team process for solving home and worksite problems works.

Project Threshold is an example of a non-traditional rehabilitation program in which occupational therapists play an integral part. The program focuses on providing services to individuals who are encountering problems with activities of daily living in their own home and community settings. Generally, the clients have had adequate time and opportunity to experience these problems and the effects of their disability within their own environments.

Project Threshold has learned that as disabled individuals pursue the challenges of more active roles in the community, there is definitely a need for community-based helping services. In addition, with health trends leading toward shortened hospital stays, further increases in the need for assistance to clients on an outpatient basis will follow. Accordingly, the demand for occupational therapists to practice in such settings will increase and bring challenges to therapists to broaden their knowledge of community resources, commercial products used in everyday living and working, and application of specialized technology. Since the rehabilitation engineer is an ideal resource for assistance in the use of such technology, the link between occupational therapists and rehabilitation engineers is ideal for solving these daily living functional problems. The expansion of this role of the occupational therapist to the community, applicable in many areas of practice, is a current and growing challenge to the profession.

References

1. McNeal, D. and Bruno, G.: *Project Threshold—A Model System for Delivery of Rehabilitation Engineering Services.* Professional Staff Association of the Rancho Los Amigos Hospital, Downey, California, 1979.

2. American Occupational Therapy Association, Inc., Council on Education: Essentials of an Accredited Educational Program for the Occupational Therapist. *American Journal of Occupational Therapy 29* (8):485–496, 1975.

3. Revised Licensure Definition. American Occupational Therapy Association, 1981.

4. Somerville, N. and Pendleton, H.McH.: *Project Threshold—A Model System for Delivery of Rehabilitation Engineering Services.* Available from Project Threshold, Rancho Los Amigos Rehabilitation Engineering Center, Downey, California 90242, 1980.

5. Somerville, N.: *Client Perceptions of Project Threshold Services.* Unpublished manuscript, 1983. Available from Project Threshold, Rancho Los Amigos Rehabilitation Engineering Center, Downey, California 90242.

Chapter 49

Diversional Activity: Does It Deserve Its Bad Name?

Judith Friedland, PhD, OT(C)

No word in the English language is as upsetting to an occupational therapist's ears as the word *diversion*. It strikes at the core of the occupational therapist's being and threatens her or his very existence. The idea that some activities used in occupational therapy might be diversional is heretical to many in the profession; diversion is seen as unscientific and therefore dismissed as inappropriate for use by professionals as a means of treatment. In this chapter I reexamine the original concept of diversional activity so that we will be better able to decide whether it should have a place within the current context of treatment. To examine this issue in some breadth, I will make reference to both American and Canadian experience and I will assume that the profession has developed in a similar fashion in both countries.

Historical Review

The concept of diversion is deeply embedded in the origins of the profession. The direct lineage of the birth of occupational therapy from within the Moral Treatment movement of the 1800s makes this clear (Barris, Kielhofner, & Watts, 1983). In fact, throughout history, diversion has been a strong theme in the treatment of illness in general, and of mental illness in particular. Along with purposeful occupation and employment, diversion was given a prominent place by the Egyptians in 2000 B.C., the Hebrews in 1030 B.C., and during later periods in both Greece and Rome (Haas, 1946).

According to the account given by Haas (1946), it was not until around 1915 that the therapeutic value of diversional occupation was called into question. However within a few years, World War I had begun to take its toll, and therapists no longer had the luxury of pondering this question; instead they began to treat the thousands of sick and injured soldiers who returned home using the wide range of activities then at their disposal. In Burnette's (1923) words, it appeared that occupational therapy had been "transformed overnight by the exigencies of the war into an honoured if somewhat bewildered guest at the doctor's table" (p. 179).

In the early twenties, diversional activity was given an important place in Adolf Meyer's (1977 [see Chapter 2]) psychobiological approach to the treatment of mental illness. Meyer, a prominent psychiatrist and one of the founders of the profession of occupational therapy, saw occupation as helping to fulfill one of the necessary conditions for health, that is, in achieving a proper balance between work, play, rest, and sleep—the activities of life. And if a balance was necessary to maintain health in those who were well, then it was also good treatment for those who were ill. In fact, Meyer stated "the proper use of time in some helpful and gratifying activity appeared to me a fundamental issue in the treatment of any neuropsychiatric patient" (p. 639). It should be noted here, that Meyer believed in providing opportunities for activity and not prescriptions. Neither was he concerned about an activity's ability to simulate work; rather he suggested that the leading principle in selecting activities should be any form of helpful enjoyment.

The psychobiological theory that Meyer advocated saw mental illness as primarily stress induced. According to this theory, any one person could be more or less predisposed, biologically, to respond poorly to stress, but it was socioenvironmental forces that caused disequilibrium, and disequilibrium resulted in mental illness. To recover, the individual needed to be protected both physically and mentally from the stressors. Physically this could be accomplished with the help of a supportive family or by admission to a hospital; but mentally this protection could only be achieved—in the days before medication—by activity. Since the Moral Treatment era the view had prevailed that no two absorbing thoughts could occupy the mind at the same time (Bockhoven, 1972). Activity, it was thought, could not only divert one's attention from stressors, it could even preclude stressful thoughts from invading. Ultimately, activity would become habit, and in this way, the balance and rhythm of healthy life would be reestablished (Kaplan & Sadock, 1985).

The idea that attention should be diverted from stressful situations, and that activity could be used for this purpose, continued to be incorporated into treatment during World War II when it became obvious that socioenvironmental stress was a contributing factor to the conditions seen in soldiers. Canadian occupational therapists, sent abroad to treat their country's soldiers, were asked to give special consideration to the needs of these people who, being away from home, were seen as suffering an additional, specific stress. Howland, the first president of the Canadian Association of Occupational Therapists (CAOT), noted that Canadian soldiers would have fewer visitors than English soldiers, and hence less stimulation. Thus, activities were used in something of a preventive fashion, with the understanding that if morale were poor, recovery would be impeded (Howland, 1944). It is interesting here to recall that one of the meanings of the word *moral* in the Moral Treatment movement was expressed in terms of *morale*: It was considered important to instill in patients feelings of enthusiasm, hope, and confidence (Bockhoven, 1972). Thus it was not uncommon to see injured servicemen occupied in activities unrelated to their disorders, activities that had been provided solely for the purpose of maintaining or raising morale. The activities were relevant and therefore meaningful, and they were often product oriented and therefore purposeful, but they were, nonetheless, diversional; they were designed to divert the soldier's attention from the stressful situation.

At that time most conflict over the idea of diversional activities not being therapeutic probably stemmed from the fact that diversional activities could not be considered work or simulations of work. In the early years of the profession in Canada, work played a very central role and activities were often selected for their ability to assess vocational interests and aptitudes, particularly with war veterans (Robinson, 1981). It should be remembered, however, that work-like activities had initially been chosen because of their ability to divert attention, that is, for the explicit purpose of diverting the ill person's preoccupation with himself or herself and with his or her brooding and destructive thoughts. This was the case particularly for those suffering from mental illness, but it was also recognized as necessary for the physically ill. In an article written for the *Canadian Geographical Journal* in 1944, which was reprinted in the *Canadian Journal of Occupational Therapy* in 1986, Howland delineated five forms of occupational therapy, as follows:

1. *Diversional* treatment for the purpose of keeping the patient interested over a long period of time.
2. Physical treatment for restoring the activity of muscles, joints, and tendons.
3. Recreational treatment, a combination of *diversional* and physical activity associated with games and sports.
4. Psychological treatment for nervous and mental cases, to restore normal mental action by carefully selected *diversion*.
5. Preventive treatment, which is purely *diversional* or recreational, for the prevention of nervous and mental states and for the retention of morale in hospitals, and for troops in camp. [italics mine] (p.19)

It is clear from Howland's account that occupational therapy was considered an important form of treatment and that within occupational therapy, diversional activity played a significant role.

The next and perhaps the most serious challenge to the concept of diversion as part of the treatment process came in the forties and fifties when the impact of the medical model came to be felt in occupational therapy (Kielhofner & Burke, 1983). The reductionist paradigm of the medical model demanded that everyone on the team be engaged in treating the broken parts of the individual. Occupational therapy rose to the challenge, and activities soon became directed almost exclusively at attacking pathology. Dunton and Licht, writing in 1957, still alluded to the need for mental stimulation for those who were bedridden. They stated, somewhat begrudgingly, that "although it is not strictly therapeutic, it remains highly desirable for patients who wish to be occupied . . . to have that wish granted if it is consistent with their medical management" (p. 27). But the idea that occupation in itself could be health giving was no longer considered respectable.

The reductionist paradigm of the medical model first found its expression in psychiatric occupational therapy within a psychodynamic perspective. As psychiatrists began to see value in occupation, they began to prescribe the form it should take, thus placing occupational therapy even more squarely within the framework of the medical model. Diagnostic categories became very important, and patients who exhibited symptomatology x were now given activity y, with the firm conviction that this was a treatment that directly addressed the psychopathology (Dunton, 1945). Although there undoubtedly was some merit to this approach, it is important to note that studies which have examined the meaning of activity (Allard, 1964; Fox & Jirgal, 1967; Henry, Nelson, & Duncombe, 1984; Kremer, Nelson, & Duncombe, 1984; Smith, Barrows, & Whitney, 1959) have found striking discrepancies between the meanings attributed to activities both within and across various populations and under varying conditions (see McColl, Friedland, & Kerr, 1986, for a review and discussion of this literature).

Thus, the focus in occupational therapy which had hitherto been on the importance of occupation per se, and which had included diversion, receded into the background both in physical medicine and in psychiatry. This reductionist period was of enormous importance for the profession because it gave therapists a more clear-cut idea of what treatments to provide. The security was short-lived, however, and in the sixties and seventies, occupational therapists found themselves in a territorial struggle. In physical medicine they were often competing with physical therapists, while in psychiatry they competed with social workers, nurses, and psychologists. As treatment in psychiatry moved away from psychoanalytic models, it became apparent that the longed-for respectability and acceptance of occupational therapy within psychiatry would not be found within a reductionist approach. Meanwhile, activities no longer considered purposeful by occupational therapists, and therefore ignored, went by default to other groups—to music and drama specialists, to recreationists, to art therapists, to craft workers, and to volunteers.

It was difficult to fit diversional activity into a reductionist view because its purpose was very different; instead of focusing on the patient's identified problems diversional activity set out to take the patient's attention away from the identified problems. Although it had never claimed more than a small part within our treatment repertoire, the whole concept of diversion was now dismissed, along with much of the concept of occupation itself. To those who have analyzed the developmental history of the profession, the shift away from the focus on occupation as health giving and toward a direct attack on pathology signaled that a paradigm shift, that is, a change in our way of thinking about old concepts, had taken place (Gilfoyle, 1984).

In the last decade or so, there has again been discontent within the profession. Concern has grown that we have lost much as we have strayed from our original focus on occupation. This discontent, we now recognize, is not only normal but healthy in terms of the stages of scientific revolution through which we can expect to pass (Kielhofner & Burke, 1983). More recently, emphasis in occupational therapy has been on function and the model of occupational performance. At this moment in our history, it seems quite clear that occupational therapists are in the business of helping clients develop skills, restore function, and maintain abilities—all within the areas of self-care, productivity, and leisure.

Diversional Activity and Current Treatment Rationales

Central to the concept of diversion is the old idea from the Moral Treatment movement that the mind cannot think two thoughts at once. It was assumed then that there was a limited amount of space for thinking, and that if healthy thoughts—necessitated by the carrying out of an activity—were in place, then there would be no room for unhealthy thoughts, if only for that period of time during which the activity was taking place (Bockhoven, 1972). This phenomenon remains under study more than a century later within the field of cognitive science where time-sharing and multiple processors, serial and parallel processing, and conscious and unconscious processing are among the dual-task paradigms being explored (see Gardner, 1985, for a detailed discussion). Within the field of neuropsychology, the concept of intrahemispheric functional distance put forth by Kinsbourne and Hicks (1978) and the limited-capacity theory of interhemispheric processing advanced by Friedman and Polson (1981) are being put to empirical tests. The answer to the question, Can two different thoughts be processed in the brain at the same time? is still not clear, but it appears to depend on several factors. These include the position of the competing thoughts along the processing continuum, the modalities of both input and output, the complexity of the competing tasks, and the locations in terms of the actual brain space in which the thoughts are processed (Eysenck, 1982; Gardner, 1985; Parasuraman & Davies, 1984). Therefore, although we can no longer say unequivocally that two thoughts cannot be processed at the same time, we can say unequivocally that processing is affected when attention is distracted from one task or thought by another task or thought.

There are treatment approaches outside of the discipline of occupational therapy that capitalize on this ability of diversional activity to interfere with cognitive processing. Three treatment approaches that use diversional activity in a very purposeful manner are stress models, cognitive therapy, and logotherapy.

Stress Models

Selye's (1976) discovery that a variety of stressors could result in the same stress reaction brought with it the notion that generic stress-reducing activities could be used as treatment. Selye's general adaptation syndrome, which results in biochemical changes irrespective of the origin of the stressors, is composed of three stages: the alarm reaction, the stage of resistance, and, because our bodies have a finite amount of adaptation energy, the stage of exhaustion. When the body is trying to achieve general adaptation, it is trying to restore itself to its former state of homeostasis (Selye).

Although much research has been carried out in this field in recent years (e.g., on stressful life events, person-environment fit, and the notion of perceived stress), Selye's (1976) original concept of stress still appears to maintain a central position (Cooper, 1983), and his ideas on how to deal with stress are readily perceived in most stress management courses. Selye made it clear that stress was not only inevitable in human life but to some extent desirable. To have ways of dealing with stress, then, is necessary for maintaining health. Management techniques that focus on the alarm reaction stage of the general adaptation syndrome facilitate a return to homeostasis. Selye suggested four general ways of dealing with stress: removing unnecessary stressors from life, not allowing certain neutral events to become stressors, developing a proficiency in dealing with conditions that are not wanted but cannot be avoided, and seeking relaxation, or diversion, from stressful demands.

Central to Selye's treatment approach is the idea that people must learn to observe their own responses to stress and recognize when it is time to stop or change their activity, that is, when it is time to find a diversion. In reference to mental stress, he suggests that by highlighting some other problem through diversion, or by activating the whole body by exercise or relaxation, the source of worry automatically becomes less important in proportion. He said, "you must find something to put in the place of the worrying thoughts to chase them away" (p. 417). This simple idea is no different from that expressed during the Moral Treatment movement when

it was said that "no two absorbing thoughts or emotions can occupy the mind or heart at the same instant" (as cited by Barris et al., 1983, p. 177).

Cognitive Therapy

Interest in cognitive therapy has steadily increased since Beck (1976) first introduced this approach to the treatment of emotional disorders in the 1970s. Beck placed great importance on what an individual thinks about an event because it is this thinking which affects the response. The goal in cognitive therapy is to identify intervening thoughts, which tend to be automatic and generally negative in character, and then to contradict or refute them (Beck). Although the technique is verbal in nature, it depends in large measure on the activities in which the patient engages. In many instances, particularly with depressive disorders, therapy consists of scheduling activities designed to be pleasurable and successful, which can then be used as evidence for contradicting the patient's negative thoughts. In addition, these "structured exercises" as they are called, provide the patient with an opportunity to practice focusing or concentrating. However, all of this can be achieved only if the activity is capable of diverting the patient from perseverative negative thinking. Because the choice of activities is crucial, the therapist must know about the patient's strengths, understand his or her background, and appreciate his or her values. Not only does the activity have to be of sufficient interest to motivate the patient at the outset, it also must be carefully graded to ensure continued success and thus be capable of undermining the patient's belief that he or she cannot do it (Beck, Rush, Shaw, & Emery, 1979). These concepts are all very familiar to occupational therapists.

The techniques of diversion are obviously not solutions to the patient's problems; they are, however, tools for producing short-term attitudinal changes. The patient is then ready to work at finding more long-term, basic solutions. In addition, diversion per se is often taught to patients as a coping skill. It is suggested that simple activities such as taking a walk, talking on the telephone, or observing the environment may be used as a means of distraction. Humor may also be used for these purposes. Beck and his colleagues (Beck et al., 1979) think that when a patient has learned to use diversion as a coping skill, he or she has gained an important sense of control.

The Humanist School: Logotherapy

In the humanist school of thought, one of the essential goals of treatment is to help the patient find meaning in life (Goleman & Speeth, 1982). In the existential philosophy that pervades this body of work, life is viewed as an entity in itself; it is imbued with meaning only as the individual experiences it, that is, in a phenomenological context. Life must be viewed with detachment, yet it also must be experienced. Frankl (1967), a major contributor to this theoretical perspective, notes the specifically human capacity for self-detachment. He refers to this state of detachment as the *noetic* dimension, in contrast to the *somatic* and *psychic* dimensions. Man, he suggests, can leave the "plane" of the biological and psychological, to enter the "space" of the noological. This capacity for self-detachment can be used in different ways. For example, it may be used for the purpose of paradoxical intention, that is, to be able to do something that appears to be the opposite of what is needed; or it may be used to counteract a compulsive inclination for self-observation through what Frankl (1967) called "dereflection" (p. 156). Thus, patients can ignore their neuroses and focus their attention on something away from themselves. They are directed to a life full of potential meanings and values that have specific personal appeal. This is known as "right activity." Frankl also speaks of "right passivity," which is a ridiculing of symptoms rather than running away from them or fighting them. In both cases, the individual must gain distance to achieve perspective. To do so, Frankl suggests that the patient be "dereflected" from his or her anticipatory anxiety to something else. Therapists working within a humanist frame of reference are familiar with these approaches to helping a patient find meaning in life.

Diversional Activity and the Current Paradigm of Occupational Therapy

Are there patients/clients who would benefit from diversional activity? Are there people who need to be distracted or diverted, either to maintain health, as in the tradition established by Meyer (1977) (see Chapter 2), Howland (1944), and Selye (1976) or as a preparation for treatment, as outlined in the approach by Beck (1976) and Frankl (1967)? Should occupational therapists be the ones to provide such treatment?

Society is filled with people who suffer greatly from psychological and physical stress. In some cases, the stress is overwhelming, the individual decompensates, and hospitalization is required before any other form of treatment can begin. In other cases, people suffer in a more chronic fashion because they have not learned how to manage their stress. In either case, occupational therapists and other professionals try to teach these people to manage their stress. These programs all employ the techniques of relaxation and diversion. There is little doubt that more should be done in this area of stress management by occupational therapists both in terms of treatment and in the area of health promotion (King, 1978 [see Chapter 8]).

The stressful effects of hospitalization are basically no different today than they were in Meyer's day, or after the world wars when therapists saw the positive effects of diversional activity on their patients' morale. Both Gray (1972) and Parent (1978) pointed out that intervention is needed in this important area, which still tends to be ignored. It is rare, for example, to find occupational therapists on trauma and orthopedic floors unless there are upper extremity or head injuries to be treated. Who, then, is intervening to facilitate the patient's ability to cope with the stress of his or her illness or disability? Who is seeing to it that patients can occupy their time with activity that simulates and thus maintains health? Who is working to prevent secondary psychological complications and speed recovery by raising morale and facilitating the patient's sense of control?

Fortunately there are many people who, no matter how ill, are able to take control of their lives and maintain their mental health while progressing through the stages of recovery. They do not need diversional therapy. They find activities for themselves, they have good social support, they do not need to be made ready for rehabilitation, they achieve a healthy balance for their day. The others, the "difficult" patients, the ones with limited or severely strained emotional and physical resources, need all the help they can get. They do not form relationships with the staff so readily, they do not have good social support, they may not be highly motivated, and they do not seek out available services. Unfortunately and paradoxically, because they are so needy, they may not receive the help they need. The Matthew Effect (Link & Milcarek, 1980, p. 280), as it is sometimes called in health care, will ensure that those who most need help will receive it the least. Diverting these people from their preoccupation with themselves and their conditions is no easy task. And they will not be ready for rehabilitation until they have been able to gain this distance from their conditions. This intervention requires the services of a skilled occupational therapist.

Conclusion

We are told that a *paradigm* shift is occurring in occupational therapy, that there is again a shift in our way of thinking about old concepts (Gilfoyle, 1984). In recent years there has been a recognition that much of what we originally had was of value and should not have been tossed aside. Kielhofner (1982) suggested that three broad premises of early theory need to be restored: (a) human beings have an occupational nature; (b) when occupation is disrupted health can be threatened; (c) occupation can help restore health. Within that philosophy, diversional activity should maintain a small but important place. For some individuals, it will be a necessary first step, preparing them for treatment; for others, it may be a last step, preparing them to cope better on their own.

As has been recommended by West (1984), it is time to reaffirm the concept of occupation in occupational therapy and to implement it once again, in all its forms. We must not continue to reject it because of its apparent simplicity. For as Mary Reilly said in one of her less

---

familiar but no less profound statements: "The wide and gaping chasm which exists between the complexity of illness and the commonplaceness of our treatment tools is, and always will be, both the pride and the anguish of our profession" (Reilly, 1962, p. 1 [see Chapter 6]).

Diversional activity is a commonplace tool for treatment. It has existed for centuries and was recognized as important by the founders of the profession of occupational therapy. The concept deserves to be researched more thoroughly and put to empirical tests. We may find that it deserves to reclaim a small but important place among our treatment tools.

Acknowledgments

I thank former students Devora Basser, Cathy Laws, Elaine Jackson, and Lisa Rezler whose essays on this topic proved particularly helpful, and former teachers Isobel Robinson and Thelma Cardwell for the opportunity to discuss this material.

This paper is based on a presentation at the June 1987 Conference of the Canadian Occupational Therapists in St. John, New Brunswick.

References

Allard, I. (1964). Our professional judgement: Sound or haphazard? *American Journal of Occupational Therapy, 18,* 104–107.

Barris, R., Kielhofner, G, & Watts, J. (1983). *Psychosocial occupational therapy: Practice in a pluralistic arena.* Laurel, MD: RAMSCO.

Beck, A. (1976). *Cognitive therapy and the emotional disorders.* New York: New American Library.

Beck, A. T., Rush, J., Shaw, B., & Emery, G. (1979). *Cognitive therapy of depression.* New York: Guilford Press.

Bockhoven, J. S. (1972). *Moral treatment in community mental health.* New York: Springer.

Burnette, N. (1923). The status of occupational therapy in Canada. *Archives of Occupational Therapy, II* (3), 179–183.

Cooper, C. (Ed.). (1983). *Stress research.* New York: John Wiley & Sons.

Dunton, W. R. (1945). *Prescribing occupational therapy.* Springfield, IL: Charles C Thomas.

Duntohen, W. R., & Licht, S. H. (1957). *Occupational therapy principles and practices.* Springfield, IL: Charles C Thomas.

Eysenck, M. (1982). *Attention and arousal.* Heidelberg: Springer-Verlag.

Fox, F. V. D., & Jirgal, D. (1967). Therapeutic properties of activities as examined by the clinical council of the Wisconsin Schools of Occupational Therapy. *American Journal of Occupational Therapy, 21,* 29–33.

Frankl, V. (1967). *Psychotherapy and existentialism.* New York: Washington Square Press.

Friedman, A., & Polson, M. (1981). Hemispheres as independent resource systems: Limited capacity processing and cerebral specialization. *Journal of Experimental Psychology, Human Perception and Performance, 7,* 1031–1058.

Gardner, H. (1985). *The mind's new science.* New York: Basic Books.

Gilfoyle, E. M. (1984). Eleanor Clarke Slagle lectureship, 1984: Transformation of a profession. *American Journal of Occupational Therapy, 38,* 575–584.

Goleman, D., & Speeth, K. (Eds.). (1982). *The essential psychotherapies.* New York: New American Library.

Gray, M. (1972). Effects of hospitalization on work-play behavior. *American Journal of Occupational Therapy, 26,* 180–185.

Haas, L. J. *(1946). Practical occupational therapy.* Milwaukee: Bruce.

Henry, A. D., Nelson, D. L., & Duncombe, L. W. (1984). Choice making in group and individual activity. *American Journal of Occupational Therapy, 38,* 245–251.

Howland, G. (1986). Occupational therapy across Canada. *Canadian Journal of Occupational Therapy, 53,* 18–26. (Reprinted from *Canadian Geographical Journal,* Vol. 28).

Kaplan, H., & Sadock, B. (1985). *Modern synopsis of comprehensive textbook of psychiatry* (4th ed.). Baltimore: Williams & Wilkins.

Kielhofner, G. (1982). A heritage of activity: Development of theory. *American Journal of Occupational Therapy, 36,* 723–730.

Kielhofner, G., & Burke, J. (1983). The evolution of knowledge and practice in occupational therapy: Past, present and future. In G. Kielhofner (Ed.), *Health through occupation. Theory and application.* Philadelphia: F. A. Davis.

King, L. J. (1978). 1978 Eleanor Clarke Slagle lecture: Toward a science of adaptive responses. *American Journal of Occupational Therapy, 32,* 429–437. (Reprinted as Chapter 8).

Kinsbourne, M., & Hicks, R. (1978). Functional cerebral space: A model for overflow, transfer and interference effects in human performance: A tutorial review. In J. Requin (Ed.), *Attention and performance: Vol. VII.* Hillsdale, NJ.: Lawrence Ehrlbaum.

Kremer, E. R. H., Nelson, D. L., & Duncombe, L. W. (1984). Effects of selected activities on affective meaning in psychiatric patients. *American Journal of Occupational Therapy, 38,* 522–528.

Link, B., & Milcarek, B. (1980). Selection factors in the dispensation of therapy: The Matthew Effect in the dispensation of mental health resources. *Journal of Health and Social Behavior, 21,* 279–290.

McColl, M., Friedland, J., & Kerr, A. (1986). When doing is not enough: The relationship between activity and effectiveness in anorexia nervosa. *Occupational Therapy in Mental Health, 6*(1), 137–149.

Meyer, A. (1977). The philosophy of occupational therapy. *American Journal of Occupational Therapy, 31,* 639–642. (Reprinted as Chapter 2.)

Parasuraman, R., & Davies, D. (Eds.). (1984). *Varieties of attention.* Orlando, FL: Academic Press.

Parent, L. H. (1978). Effects of a low stimulus environment on behavior. *American Journal of Occupational Therapy, 32,* 19–25.

Reilly, M. (1962). Eleanor Clarke Slagle lecture: Occupational therapy can be one of the great ideas of 20th century medicine. *American Journal of Occupational Therapy, 16,* 1–9. (Reprinted as Chapter 6).

Robinson, I. (1981). The mists of time. *Canadian Journal of Occupational Therapy, 48,* 145–151.

Selye, H. (1976). *The stress of life* (rev. ed.). New York: McGraw-Hill.

Smith, P. A., Barrows, H. S., & Whitney, J. N. (1959). Psychological attributes of occupational therapy crafts. *American Journal of Occupational Therapy, 8,* 16–22.

West, W. L. (1984). A reaffirmed philosophy and practice of occupational therapy for the 1980s. *American Journal of Occupational Therapy, 38,* 15–23.

Chapter 50

Should Music Be Used Therapeutically in Occupational Therapy?

Anne MacRae, PhD, OTR

The healing power of music has been recognized by various cultures for many centuries. This power, however, was often attributed to magic, either of the performer, such as a shaman or medicine man, or of the music itself (Deschenes, 1989; Hamel, 1979). The past century has brought forth efforts to empirically understand the effects of music on the human mind and body. Belief in the healing value of music has spawned the development of new disciplines, such as music and dance therapy. Occupational therapists have not fully explored its potential as a therapeutic modality. Should music be included in the repertoire of occupational therapy? I believe that music is not only a legitimate healing tool, but also an appropriate expression of the philosophy of occupational therapy. Music is a vocational activity for some and an active or passive leisure pursuit for others. It is a pleasurable, intrinsically motivating activity that can be easily graded and used to promote overall health through relaxation and movement. Music is both versatile and powerful in that it has the potential to involve all of the components of occupational performance—motor, sensory, cognitive, social, and emotional. In this chapter, I describe the healing effects of music and discuss its present and potential uses in occupational therapy.

Therapeutic Effects of Music

The experience of music occurs "physiologically, psychologically, affectively, and aesthetically" (Rouget, 1985, p. 119). On the physiological level, music affects auditory perception. The sensorial manifestations, however, go far beyond audition. Music is also vibration, which is palpable (tactile) and, possibly, even visible (Rouget, 1985). In addition, music has somatic qualities in that it is essentially body movement. That is, we receive the vibrations and, in the case of participatory music, we can feel ourselves singing and interacting with the instruments.

Deschenes (1989) stated, "Music has much more than a simple physical impact on our body. In influencing the body kinetics and posture through the cerebellum and our emotions through the pneumo-gastric nerve, music happens to have a dynamogenic effect on humans.... When music reaches our ear, it also reaches our whole body and emotions imprinted in our muscles" (p.2). The effects of music on the human mind and body occur simultaneously, but it is perhaps in the emotional and affective spheres that music has its greatest therapeutic potential. "Nothing is more laden with emotional associations than music; nothing is more capable of recreating situations that engage one's entire sensibility" (Rouget, 1985, p. 123). Music can facilitate mood changes, alter states of awareness, modify one's consciousness, and increase affective response.

Considering the wide range of human response and ease of access, it is reasonable to assume that music has great healing potential. Heinze (1990) suggested that music can be used to uncover formerly buried memories and emotions. Also, music can be effectively used to shift a person's attention, to soothe agitation, and to aid with visualization techniques. Hamel (1979) stated that relaxing music can be used by healthy persons as well as by those with a wide variety of disorders, including active psychosis.

Application of Music in Occupational Therapy

Occupational therapy addresses the dysfunction found in a wide variety of psychiatric, developmental, and physical disorders. The motor, sensory, cognitive, social, and emotional components of a person's functional performance are all addressed. Considering the holistic philosophy of occupational therapy, its broad client base, and its traditional use of creative and purposeful activity, music would seem to be an ideal modality. Unfortunately, a search of the occupational therapy literature reveals that although music is being used in specific areas of practice, its full potential as a therapeutic tool has not been explored. Published accounts of the therapeutic use of music by occupational therapists appear to be limited to the practice areas of pain management, motor and sensory dysfunction, and certain forms of cognitive dysfunction.

Pain Management

Heck (1988) used an experimental design to determine the effectiveness of activity in prolonging tolerance to pain. He concluded that significant pain relief can be obtained through engagement in activity that is purposeful, that is intrinsically motivating, and that captures the attention and interest of the patient.

Unfortunately, there was minimal discussion of the specific activity used in this study, and activity involving sound or music was not mentioned. McCormack (1988) concurred with the conclusion of Heck's study and provided specific examples of music as purposeful activity for pain reduction. These examples include active listening (including motoric involvement), auditory distraction, the use of background music to promote muscle relaxation, and rhythmic breathing.

Motor and Sensory Dysfunction

Van Deusen and Harlowe (1987) described a study in which dance with accompanying music is used in an exercise program for persons with rheumatoid arthritis. An audiotape with the ROM [range of motion] Dance (1984) was used in a group format and then provided to each participant for home use. The experimental group in this study reported "significantly greater enjoyment of exercise and rest" as well as "better scores in range of motion then did the control subjects" (Van Deusen & Harlowe, 1987, p. 94).

Miller (1979) also supported the use of music and movement for increasing range of motion. In addition, she suggested specific musical techniques to be used with persons with limited muscle strength, abnormal gait, lack of proprioception, loss of sensation, speech and communication problems, and muscular tension. Unfortunately, there have been no efficacy studies on the use of these techniques.

Cognitive Dysfunction

Farber (1982) stated that auditory input is useful in the treatment of comatose patients. Although music is not specifically mentioned, it is suggested that a small radio, conversation, and tape recordings of family members be used. Farber cautioned against the continuous use of the radio, because adaptation may result, thereby rendering the treatment ineffective.

Miller (1979) stated that musical recordings can increase reality orientation to persons, places, and things. Time orientation is not specifically mentioned, but it is certainly plausible that music could enhance one's sense of time by increasing awareness of the environment and the relationship between timing and rhythm. However, it is also possible for the opposite effect to occur. Heinze (1990) reported that some persons lose time orientation while involved in a musical activity.

Silberzahn (1988) stated that there is a unique cell-firing rhythm in the brain that appears to be related to learning and memory. Therefore, rhythmic repetition may be an appropriate therapeutic modality. However, information on specific techniques or efficacy data is not available.

Music is used extensively with mentally retarded patients. Orff-Schulwerk techniques, originally developed for children, have been easily adapted for use with this population (Bitcon, 1969) and are employed by many rehabilitation specialists, including occupational recreation, and music therapists. These techniques do not specifically address the cognitive deficits of this population; rather, they are designed to facilitate self-expression in a nonjudgemental atmosphere.

Discussion

The therapeutic potential of music is multifaceted and profound. It legitimately belongs in the domain of occupational therapy because it can promote health through the use of activity that involves all of the occupational performance components. Yet the occupational therapy literature shows limited use of music as a modality.

It is especially surprising to find a lack of documentation regarding music as a facilitator of emotional health and social skills. A possible explanation for this deficit is that occupational therapists are indeed using music for such purposes but are not publishing their protocols or clinical results. It is interwoven into the fabric of our culture to believe that music, particularly with active involvement (song) and movement (dance), can heighten social involvement and can have an emotional effect. Because this knowledge is considered commonplace or intuitive, it may not be given sufficient consideration in formal studies. This is unfortunate, because the effectiveness of music as a therapeutic modality would have increased significance if its use were specifically applied and goal directed, as in clinical protocols and research.

I believe that the occupational therapy profession could enhance its repertoire of skills while simultaneously increasing the validity of its methods by undertaking the rigorous study of music as a therapeutic modality. The studies conducted by music therapists and psychologists provide important background information for the occupational therapist interested in the therapeutic application of music. We need research specifically grounded in an occupational therapy frame of reference.

This topic lends itself to a wide variety of research methods. Certainly, rich descriptive information could be culled with the use of ethnographic or phenomenological methods, and many aspects of this topic could be studied using quantifiable studies. In addition, it is possible to use existing research designs in occupational therapy settings and modify them to study the effects of music. For example, Llorens (1986) employed a laboratory model to study tasks and activities, with the goal of assessing the degree of agreement among participants "regarding the sensory stimuli, intersensory stimuli, sensory integrative processes, motor activity, and sensory feedback" (p. 106). None of the activities used in Llorens's study had a strong auditory component (i.e., drawing, spinning, buttoning), but the model could easily lend itself to the study of musically oriented activities such as dance.

Boyer, Colman, Levy, and Manoly (1989) also used an experimental design with 45 subjects. The purpose was to document variation in affective responses to several activities. As with the Llorens (1986) study, none of the chosen activities involved music. However, this design would also be an ideal vehicle for a study of the effects of music as a modality.

Summary

It has long been common knowledge that music profoundly affects human beings on a variety of levels. Occupational therapists have at their disposal a potentially powerful therapeutic tool, but the specific effects of this tool have not been documented.

Occupational therapists have a history of using music in their treatment probably to a greater extent than is documented in the literature. It would be advantageous for us to engage in research regarding the application of music to occupational therapy.

References

Bitcon, C. (1969). 1 AM! Orff-Schulwerk: Clinical application. In *Proceedings of the Fourth National Symposium on Creative Communication*. Bellflower, CA: Creative Practices Council.

Boyer, J., Colman, W., Levy, L., & Manoly, B. (1989). Affective responses to activities: A comparative study. *American Journal of Occupational Therapy, 43*, 81–88.

Deschenes. B. (1989). Healing beyond music: The application. In *Proceedings of the Sixth International Conference of the Study of Shamanism and Alternate Modes of Healing*. Berkeley, CA: Independent Scholars of Asia.

Farber, S. D. (1982). *Neurorehabilitation: A multisensory approach*. Philadelphia: Saunders.

Hamel, P. M. (1979). *Through music to self*. Boulder, CO: Shambhala.

Heck, S. A. (1988). The effect of purposeful activity on pain tolerance. *American Journal of Occupational Therapy, 42*, 577–581.

Heinze, R. (1990, January). *The effect of sound and music on the human mind and body*. Symposium conducted at the National Meeting of Saybrook Institute, Belmont, CA.

Llorens, L. A. (1986). Activity analysis: Agreement among factors in a sensory processing model. *American Journal of Occupational Therapy, 40*, 103–110.

McCormack, G. L. (1988). Pain management by occupational therapists. *American Journal of Occupational Therapy, 42,* 582–590.

Miller, K. J. (1979). *Treatment with music: A manual for allied health professionals.* Kalamazoo, MI: Western Michigan University.

ROM Dance [Audiocassettes]. (1984). Madison, WI: University of Wisconsin, St. Marys Hospital Medical Center.

Rouget, G. (1985). *Music and trance.* Chicago: University of Chicago Press.

Silberzahn, M. (1988). Integration in sensorimotor therapy. In H. L. Hopkins & H. D. Smith (Eds.), *Willard and Spackman's occupational therapy* (7th ed., pp. 127–141). Philadelphia: Lippincott.

Van Deusen, J., & Harlowe, D. (1987). The efficacy of the ROM dance program for adults with rheumatoid arthritis. *American Journal Of Occupational Therapy, 41,* 90–95.

Chapter 51

Humor as an Adjunct to Occupational Therapy Interactions

Virginia O. Tooper, EdD, OTR

This chapter was previously published in *The Changing Roles of Occupational Therapists* (Haworth Press, 1984). Copyright © 1984, The Haworth Press, Inc.

Wipe that smile off your face." "Settle down and get serious, now." "Don't laugh in church!"

These are just some of the expressions the adult members of our culture have used to begin to program the joy and fun out of our lives or at least make us feel guilty about expressing it, even if unintentionally. And though the Bible and Readers Digest are common references for the physical and emotional benefits of humor, individuals and groups in the health professions have been slow to accept the idea that a program for using fun and laughter as a therapeutic tool can be developed.

Humor and laughter have not only distinguished man from other species, they have been a natural part of human life in all cultures as far back as recorded history can determine. But there have been myths and associated anxieties that leave many of us unwilling to explore new directions and possibilities or to believe that anything of genuine value could come out of such a frivolous subject area.

One popularly held myth is that humor or a "sense-of-humor" is something you are either born with or without. If you are born with it, you are lucky. If not, then you are unfortunate. A second associated myth is that if you are born without a "sense-of-humor" there is little you can do to change your situation. The evidence disproves these and other commonly held ideas regarding the humor in the individual. A few weeks or months after birth, normal children begin to smile, laugh and enjoy play. Even children born deaf and blind will exhibit some of these qualities without seeing or hearing a role model. Furthermore, a "sense-of-humor" has been described by health professionals and educators as an "attitude" and attitudes can be learned or changed. Dr. O. Carl Simonton, a radiation oncologist and medical director of the Cancer Counseling and Research Center in Dallas, Texas has noted that

> "It is . . . essential for you to understand that you can influence your own attitudes. When you are convinced it is desirable to do so, you are capable of changing them." He further states that, "Simply by exposing yourself to these (positive) processes and ideas you will become sensitive to alternative ways of viewing life, and ultimately your beliefs may begin to change." [1]

Adults do a good job of encouraging spontaneity and joy in early childhood. Yet kindergarten and primary teachers know that frequently parents are struck with fear just before their child is to enter school. They worry that their child's behavior at that point may appear immature to others, and may abruptly change from emphasizing playful interaction to a "time to get very serious" approach.

Health professionals may find themselves in a similar paradoxical position. On one hand, we realize the value of positive attitudes and encouraging the patient's active participation in the therapeutic process, while on the other hand we fear being thought of as "lightweights" as we deal with individuals who may be concerned with life and death matters. Added to these fears are confusion related to our own personal experiences with humor.

Who among us does not recall the pain of being the butt of a joke? Or who can not remember telling a funny story that no one laughed at? We wonder what is wrong when others laugh at something we don't think is funny at all. It's so difficult to sort out these experiences that many of us just decide it's safer to say, "I enjoy a good laugh as much as anyone, but I'm not good at using humor, so I'll just forget it."

Though there are those who have quickly accepted the myths, there are many others in health and education who are coming out of the closet with ideas they have been developing and successfully using for sometimes. The turning point seems to be the publication of Norman Cousins' 1976 article in the New England Journal of Medicine[2] that was expanded into a book in 1979 entitled, Anatomy of an Illness.[3] In this work, Cousins, formerly editor of the Saturday Review, tells of his bout with a serious collagen disease, a condition that affects the connective tissue. Given only one chance in 500 to survive, he devised his own therapeutic program with his physician's assistance. The major emphasis of the program included up to a half-hour or more of sustained laughter using old Candid Camera and Marx brothers films. Cousins worked on the premise that if negative emotions can lead to disturbances in body chemistry producing ulcers, cardiovascular problems, migraine headaches and other illnesses, might not positive emotions, particularly laughter, produce an opposite reaction. He found that laughter did release endorphins, the body's own natural pain killer and that ten minutes of genuine belly laughter had an anesthetic effect and would give him at least two hours of pain-free sleep.

In 1978, about a year after Norman Cousins' article appeared in the medical journal, Dr. Raymond Moody, a Virginia physician, published Laugh After Laugh[4] in which he discussed the history of humor and health, the pathology of laughter and the socio-cultural aspects of humor. Dr. Moody notes that in medical school, students are taught to find out everything about a patient from his/her blood pressure and respiration to language peculiarities and sexual functioning, but never to probe for sense-of-humor or willingness to laugh. In his work with patients, he has devised a set of questions that he uses to expand medical histories. Among them are: What sort of role did humor play in the person's family as he was growing up? Was he teased excessively as a child? What kinds of jokes, humor, etc. does he like best?

How often does he laugh? Moody's ideas are in keeping with a psychologist who is reported to have said, "Tell me what you laugh at and I will know more about you than through any other means."

Others who have reported on the health benefits of laughter are Dr. William F. Fry, Jr.,[5] an associate clinical professor at Stanford University Medical School and Dr. Wayne Dyer who points out in his book, The Sky's the Limit,[6] that laughter is the first of "Seven Paths to the Fountain." Dyer is referring to the "Fountain of Youth" and is describing how individuals can recapture "childlike" not "childish" qualities of their earlier years.

Finally, Dr. Vera Robinson, a California State University professor of nursing education, must not be overlooked. It is interesting to observe that although she did not get the attention of the previously mentioned authors, her research in Colorado hospitals and other facilities appears to predate that of other writers and led to her very comprehensive book, Humor and the Health Professions.[7] In it, she deals with (1) humor in our society, (2) importance for health professionals, (3) humor as a planned tool, (4) current uses of humor and questions (5) variables to be considered in the conscious use of humor and (6) methods and procedures for the conscious use of humor.

State of the Art

A look at several seminars and workshops in addition to the literature on the positive uses of humor reveals that work is being done by individuals in over a half-dozen states who represent a variety of professional disciplines including occupational therapy, education, psychiatry, social work, nursing and speech communication. Although individuals from different professions naturally place emphasis on different aspects of a subject area, there seem to be some common elements.

1. It is necessary to understand your own attitudes toward humor and its values in order to use it with others.

2. It is important to recognize that humor is individual. What is funny to one, may not be to another. Careful observation of others using humor gives you clues for your own approaches to individuals and groups and helps in establishing rapport.

3. There are many kinds of humor, but they fall in two basic categories: laughing AT others and laughing WITH others. The former includes acid-wit of the "put-down" variety and is not favored as a tool for therapy or education. Laughing with others involves putting pain in perspective and playfully choosing to see humorous options.

4. It is just as important to know when NOT to use humor as when TO use it. Humor can be the appetizer or dessert, sometimes the main course, but not the whole meal or steady diet.

5. Everyone has a "sense-of-humor." Just try to get anyone to admit that he does not. It is just that some seem to have it buried deeper inside due to environmental and cultural programming than others do and they will have to work harder to recapture it. However, the individual must want to work on his humor development. One cannot develop humor in another person who does not want to go along with the idea.

6. In order to develop and use humor with yourself and others, observation is the first key and practice, practice, practice are the next three. Humor does not come easily and for this reason, people tend to give up too fast. Training programs generally emphasize experimenting in small steps and in safe surroundings. After all, one does not learn to speak French, play the guitar, or tap dance overnight.

7. With practice, individuals can learn to produce their own humor and develop unique ways of using it, just as they may begin to put together their own humor modalities.

Seminar and Workshop Presentations

Due to the fact that people delivering and receiving humor in an educational or therapeutic setting have many different preconceived ideas of what they want to present or get out of it, some ideas to help avoid some of the pitfalls are offered. These seminars and workshops are designed for health and education professionals who plan to use the methods with their own patients, clients, or students.

Seminar/Workshop Suggestions

I. Evaluation of seminar/workshop attendees
A. Initially, attention must be given to the particular audience present and members' reasons for interest in humor as a tool in the therapeutic/educational process. Those who attend for the purpose of doubting or challenging the ideas can be encouraged to listen with an open mind and begin to determine which of the suggestions or approaches they might be willing to try.
B. In many humor classes, a larger than average number of workshop attendees will identify themselves as lacking humor in their lives. If such individuals feel their attitudes or backgrounds make the use of humor difficult for them, they may form another group that could be encouraged to take in ideas slowly and try them out in small steps.
C. There are persons who actually think they can bring humor and laughter to others without experiencing the emotion themselves. They may say, "I didn't come to a class to learn to laugh, I came to learn how to get others to laugh." Until

a person feels comfortable with humor himself he will have about as much luck as a physician trying to get someone to stop smoking as he sits and puffs away.
D. Whether the therapist is teaching a workshop or dealing with patients, it is important to first be a careful observer and questioner. When humor fails, it quite often does so because the individual using the humor delivers it with little regard to the receiver's preferences.

II. Identifying one's own humor style
A. Prior to the use of humor in treatment, it is of value to look at one's own attitudes, background, and previous uses of humor. Identifying what one likes and doesn't like as well as what one feels comfortable with or wants to work toward will be important building blocks in determining and establishing a humor style.
Example #1: Robert L., an occupational therapist, did not feel comfortable telling jokes or spontaneously observing the humor in a communication event with his elderly patients in a gerontology facility. He did, however, develop warm relationships with the people he served by asking them to tell him (or the patient group) short humorous stories from their life experiences. He listened and laughed with them and encouraged other group members to do the same.
Example #2: Susan J., a nurse, was able to help patients feel less apprehensive in receiving shots by kidding herself out loud as if she were the patient speaking. "Oh, no! Here's the nurse again. Well, I'll just roll over, think of a sunny beach in Hawaii and it'll be done with."
B. In classes and in individual treatment, the leader or therapist emphasizes the importance of choosing to look at daily problems, irritations and annoyances from many different angles in an effort to see the humor in the situation. Frequently there is humor in the realization that we are responsible for the problem and that our control does not end there.
Example: In one group situation, Karl P., looked at his fellow group members "irritations" that had been written on the chalkboard. He raised his hand and said, "I'm sitting here looking at what really bothers people in this class and thinking how ridiculous they all are!" The group broke out in laughter as they pointed out that HIS irritation was not on the list.
C. Specialists who work in the area of stress reduction strongly suggest that it is the little petty, everyday incidents that constantly grind on us that produce illness. Humor has been found to be a very effective tool in dealing with these seemingly unrelenting annoyances. And since

---

humor has a foundation in truth, it helps us see some of these problems for what they really are and to do something about them. When one has tried to look at a problem from the side, the top and the bottom with humor and still has difficulty, it may be an indication that this is a problem where a bit of "straight-talk" is indicated instead of humor.

Example: A group of humor problem solvers were stuck on a matter that other groups had worked on unsuccessfully. How do you use humor with one employee in an office who has body odor? Suggestions such as "Give him/her a bar of soap and a washrag gift wrapped, " or "Spray his/her work area with deodorant," are not in the spirit of positive humor. The group concluded that this was a problem for straight-talk, one-on-one by an immediate supervisor of the same sex.

III. Some humor applications

A. Humor participants identify the stresses of life as fast as they can list them. They may run from "long lines at the grocery store" to "people who ask personal questions," or even "people who say you look tired!" Then groups of 3-6 persons take one or two of these irritants or "bugs" as they are sometimes called and quickly brainstorm all the funny ways they can look at them or possibly solve them. Usually a group will come up with many silly suggestions, have some fun, and find among them one or two that can be put to practical use.

Examples: A group working on the "bugs" above came up with: Long lines at the grocery store: "That's how I get the National Enquirer read without paying for it. This week, it took me four trips to the store to finish it. I sometimes find myself getting into longer lines to give myself more time." People who ask personal questions: "Since they usually have to do with my age or weight, I answer them in stones, liters, minutes or seconds. If they're that nosey, let them do their own multiplication or division." People who say you look tired: "When people tell me that, I will say, "You should've seen him!'"

B. Some of the new ways of looking at the irritants of life can now be translated into appropriate responses that leave both parties laughing and feeling good.

Example: A seventh grade student who didn't like the math assignment his substitute teacher gave him went all over the school saying she was a centerfold in Playboy Magazine. Initially upset, the teacher found herself getting angry and tense in the neck and jaw area when she remembered to practice looking at things humorously. Then,

at recess, when two regular teachers sidled up and asked her if what everyone was saying were true, she replied, "No, it's a filthy, dirty lie and I certainly hope no one gets ahold of August of '59." Everyone had a good laugh, no one was put down and the subject was dropped.

C. Other resources can include a variety of activities a therapist can offer her patients for fun along with the tasks that may be necessary, but not as enjoyable.

Examples: "When I see you tomorrow, Mr. Jones, I want you to be ready to tell me your best joke." Or, "Here is a book of cartoons. When I see you next week, I want to know which one you thought was the funniest and why." Or, "Look at these photos in the newspaper. Can you come up with a funny caption to one or more of them?"

Summary

Both empirical and scientific studies are revealing the benefits of humor and laughter in physical and mental health. As work progresses in this field, occupational therapists and other allied health professionals may become more aware of the benefits of humor techniques when they are selectively applied in treatment programs.

Professionals experimenting with newer methods for health motivation may begin to find some of the suggestions in this paper can lead to further applications and study that will assist them in their own attitude changes as they seek to lighten the realities of the day-to-day burdens derived from illness and disability.

References

1. Simonton, OC: *Getting Well Again*, New York: Bantam Books, 1978.

2. Cousins, N: "Anatomy of an Illness (as Perceived by the Patient)," *New England Journal of Medicine, 295* (1976), 1458–63.

3. Cousins, N: *Anatomy of an Illness*, New York: Bantam Books, 1979.

4. Moody, RA: *Laugh After Laugh*, Jacksonville, FL: Headwaters Press, 1978.

5. Fry, WF: *Sweet Madness: A Study of Humor*, Palo Alto, CA: Pacific Books, 1968.

6. Dyer, WW: *The Sky's the Limit*, New York: Simon and Schuster Pocket Books, 1980.

7. Robinson, V: *Humor in the Health Professions*, Thorofare, NJ: Charles B. Slack, 1977.

Related Readings

Peter, LJ: *The Laughter Prescription,* New York: Ballantine Books, 1982.

Andrus Gerontology Center: *Humor: The Tonic You Can Afford,* Los Angeles, CA: Andrus Volunteers, University of Southern California, 1983.

Goodman, J: *Laughing Matters,* 110 Spring St., Saratoga Springs, NY 12866: Sagamore Institute, 1982–3.

Tooper, VO: *Laugh Lovers News,* P.O. Box 1495, Pleasanton, CA, 94566 1981–83.

Chapter 52

Linking Purpose to Procedure During Interactions with Patients

Suzanne M. Peloquin, PhD, OTR

This chapter describes a rationale and some methods for incorporating statements of purpose, or goal statements, into the daily practice of occupational therapy. Given the clinical pressures generated by brief lengths of stays in care facilities, occupational therapists need to recommit themselves to meaningful relationships with their patients. The need for this renewed commitment sharpens when one considers three realities basic to practice: current trends in health care, traditional occupational therapy assumptions, and the often ambiguous nature of activity, occupational therapy's primary modality. Each of these realities provides a context within which the process of discussing goal statements with patients will be explored.

Rosen (1974, p. 292) used the term *therapy set* to refer to statements or directives that inform patients about a therapeutic procedure, motivate them to cooperate, and heighten their expectations of the benefits to be derived from treatment. When this treatment approach is used, patients (a) understand what they are doing and why they are doing it and (b) feel encouraged to engage in the process.

As applied to occupational therapy, a communication in psychiatric practice that encourages informed patient involvement might be the following:

> We'd like to have you join us in the 9 AM craft group today. You will probably experience this as a pleasant hour since you enjoy working with your hands. Our main interest in having you attend this group, however, is that your participation will give you an opportunity to use several skills, such as your ability to concentrate, to solve problems, and to organize your thoughts.

Effectiveness of the Collaborative Approach

Although the purpose of this article is not to investigate the effectiveness of enlightening patients about and involving them in their therapy, but to explore a rationale for the use of such a collaborative approach in occupational therapy practice, some brief discussion of the effectiveness of the approach seems indicated. Rosen (1974) cited several studies involving subjects receiving desensitization therapy procedures accompanied by different forms of "therapy set." He indicated that two primary approaches dominated the research on the effectiveness of informing and involving the patient. The first group of studies investigated the extent to which varied instructions might alter subjects' expectations for a therapeutic outcome. The second group of studies explored the effects of changing subjects' knowledge of the procedure through instructions. In the first approach, control groups were given a general therapeutic orientation, whereas experimental groups were given instructions that might influence their expectations of the treatment outcome positively. Small between-group differences that failed to achieve statistical significance were reported in these studies (Lomont & Brock, 1971; McGlynn, 1971; McGlynn & Mapp, 1970; McGlynn, Mealiea, & Nawas, 1969; McGlynn, Reynolds, & Linder, 1971; McGlynn & Williams, 1970; Woy & Efran, 1972). In the second approach, groups given therapeutic orientation were compared with groups who believed they were being studied for physiological reactions only. In this approach, subjects' knowledge of the purpose of the procedure was being manipulated. Most studies of this type demonstrated significant effects attributable to the type of instruction given (Borkovec, 1972; Leitenberg, Agras, Barlow, & Oliveau, 1969; Miller, 1972; Oliveau, Agras, Leitenberg, Moore, & Wright, 1969; Rappaport, 1972). Subjects who knew that the purpose of the treatment was therapeutic had better therapeutic outcomes.

In his own study, Rosen (1974) concluded that subjects aware of the purpose of procedures designed to make them less afraid of snakes demonstrated significantly higher mean behavioral changes, that is, became more desensitized to the offending stimulus, than subjects unaware of the purpose. Those informed that test procedures were therapeutic demonstrated more confident behavior in approaching snakes than those told that the procedures were simply experimental.

The collaborative approach's focus on patients' expectations resembles a construct called "expectancy of therapeutic gain." Historically, this construct emerged from research on the placebo effect described in the medical literature (Wilkins, 1973). Cartwright and Cartwright (1958) explained that in the 1950s the concepts of anticipation, belief, confidence, and conviction emerged in psychotherapy, giving rise to the concept of the placebo effect. Frank (1959) said that a patient's expectancy of benefit from treatment may in itself have enduring and profound effects on his or her physical and mental health. Krause, in 1967, wrote that the client's beliefs about treatment determine his or her valuation of the

process, and that this valuation determines his or her motivation to participate. Kielhofner (1985) echoed this conviction in his conceptualization of volition as the human subsystem that provides the energy and desire for choosing an action, that energy being generated by what a person believes to be interesting and valuable.

Wilkins (1973) proposed that an individual's expectancy of therapeutic gain may be treated as either (a) an attitude that the individual brings to a situation concerning how much benefit he or she will receive or (b) a state that can be induced by instructions delivered about the effectiveness of procedures to which he or she will be exposed. The idea of the collaborative approach is predicated on the assumptions that instructions can induce an expectancy of therapeutic gain and that creating a state of expectancy potentiates the therapeutic procedure.

There is justification for the use of the collaborative approach in occupational therapy when one considers its efficacy; there is additional justification for its use when one reflects on current demands in health care practice.

Current Demands in Health Care

In light of the current emphasis on bioethical issues such as informed consent and patients' rights, there is sound reasoning for incorporating a collaborative approach into each occupational therapy procedure. Engelhardt (1986) described the patient's status as that of a stranger in a strange land:

> Patients, when they come to see a health care professional, are in unfamiliar territory. They enter a terrain of issues that has been carefully defined through the long history of the health care professions. A patient is unlikely to present for care with as well-analyzed and considered judgments as those possessed by health care professionals. . . . The patient in this context is a stranger, an individual in unfamiliar territory who does not fully know what to expect or how to control the environment. . . . Things no longer happen as usual; they no longer take place in their taken for granted ways. As an outsider in a strange culture, the patient always runs the risk of being a marginal person. (pp. 256–257)

The care giver must explain this new and strange land to the patient, thereby reducing the patient's sense of being a marginal person. The care giver must augment the patient's sense of belonging by providing him or her with access to information and by giving him or her control in the form of consent over the treatment process (Engelhardt, 1986).

Current emphasis on patients' rights reminds those in positions of power that the ultimate power is changing hands. Patients have the right to know the precise relevance and nature of their treatment and to choose it or reject it on the basis of their understanding of its value to them (Bloomer, 1978). This patient/consumer right gives the practitioner a powerful incentive for explaining procedures and for collaborating with patients throughout treatment.

Clinicians face a demand from agencies, both accrediting and reimbursing, to be accountable for the treatment they provide. They face requests from patients and their families to prove the utility of their service and to clarify the expected outcome of their treatments. Current trends to exact statements of purpose from therapists can be perceived as the public's validation of a professional and ethical response that is their due.

Traditional Occupational Therapy Thinking

Even before the emergence of current trends, traditional occupational therapy assumptions supportive of the collaborative approach were well represented in the literature. The assumptions can be summarized as follows: The patient is rational. The patient is a collaborator with the therapist. The patient is free to choose or reject therapeutic services. The therapist, in turn, is a teacher and a motivator in the therapy process.

Excerpts from *Willard and Spackman's Occupational Therapy* highlight these assumptions. McNary (1947) wrote: "An activity entered into without a purpose is not occupational therapy" (p. 10). If the patient is the one entering into the activity, it is he or she who must understand the purpose. It then becomes the therapist's responsibility to share that information. Edgerton (1947) said that "the ability to relate an activity to the need of the individual is one of the characteristics that distinguishes the occupational therapist from the . . . crafts instructor" (p. 42). Here is clear endorsement of any procedure that communicates the relevance of a therapeutic activity. If occupational therapists resent having their role minimized by others, they must take measures to ensure that they are not sabotaging themselves by failing to define their work so that others will recognize it unmistakably as therapy.

Wade (1947) said that "if the patient is unable to participate actively in the plan, its existence should be kept in his consciousness as a justification for the task" (p. 90). When meaningful collaboration with the patient is not possible, the therapist still retains responsibility for explaining the plan on some level. When the patient is elderly, psychotic, young, or cognitively impaired, it may seem easier to abandon explanations in favor of expediting the procedure. Therapists are encouraged to do otherwise. At whatever level of comprehension is possible, care givers need to inform. The information may be brief, simple, and even reductionistic. The information is nonetheless "placed in the patient's consciousness." When in doubt about the potential for awareness, one communicates.

An anecdotal contribution to *Reader's Digest* ("Speedy Recovery," 1987) illustrates a response that even patients assumed to be minimally aware can furnish. A nurse's aide described her patient as a 96-year-old woman immobilized after a stroke. The aide's task was to get the patient out of bed. She communicated her plan to her assistant as follows: "I'll take an arm and a leg on this side, you take an arm and a leg on that side and then...." The explanation was interrupted by the patient's saying in a weary voice: "Oh, God, she's not even going to make a wish!" (p. 53).

This anecdote clearly reminds therapists that the presence of a significant disability does not justify excluding the patient from an active understanding of any procedure. Exclusion constitutes treatment of the patient as a marginal person. The publication of this anecdote as a humorous short in a popular magazine reflects perhaps the universality of the situation. The treatment is all too familiar. The poignancy of the story lies in the fact that the patient's best defense was that of taking the offensive by being more humane and personable than the care giver.

Current literature supports these examples taken from the past. Reed and Sanderson (1983) described several attitudes and assumptions about the occupational therapy process consistent with those underlying the idea of the collaborative approach. They emphasized salient points made more subtly 40 years ago by encouraging therapists to regard the client as a *valuable, worthwhile person, even if the client does not respond readily to the program*" (p. 153). Here stands a declaration of the patient's right to challenge services offered on the basis of his or her understanding of them. A consequent responsibility for the therapist is to maintain the patient in high regard and to respond to the challenge with information. "The client has a right to be informed, but also the information should be in a manner that is comprehensive and at a rate that can be absorbed by the client" (p. 154).

Reed and Sanderson (1983) drew up a list of patient's rights that included the following:

1. A person has the right to decide whether to seek and accept health care services within legal limitations.
2. A person has the right to determine the state of health and level of wellness that person will seek to attain and maintain, as long as the decision does not threaten or endanger the health and wellness of other persons.
3. A person has the right to be consulted regarding the objectives, goals and methods to be used in individual health care plans. (p. 71)

These three rights merit observance during daily sessions when specific treatments are being proposed. The patient's right to be consulted and to decide needs to be reinforced daily. Providing the patient with the necessary information at each session can operationally reaffirm his or her rights.

Motivating the patient becomes an inevitable therapist responsibility if one endorses the patient's right to choose. Reed and Sanderson (1983) identified the last step of the occupational therapy process as being "to facilitate and influence client participation and investment" (p. 81). This step constitutes a directive to communicate the rationale, the importance, and the relevance of the therapy process in such a manner as to facilitate the patient's investment in a successful outcome.

Traditional occupational therapy has been a process of teaching, motivating, and collaborating with the patient during therapeutic activity. More recently, proponents of a psychoeducational approach to occupational therapy have contrasted it with traditional occupational therapy. Fine and Schwimmer (1987) described the psychoeducational approach to occupational therapy as a derivation from social learning theory:

> The life skills curriculum (LSC) is further differentiated from its traditional counterpart by structuring the educational format and techniques, emphasizing the patient's active participation in setting and evaluating treatment goals, identifying learning needs and influencing the teaching-learning process, planning the integration and continuity of problem-solving and communication skills among all groups, providing multiple opportunities to practice skills through graded repetition and homework assignments, and matching treatment tasks to patient's problems and priorities. (p. 3)

Excerpts from traditional and more current literature, cited earlier, support the premise that traditional occupational therapy (a) has incorporated the tenets of social learning theory to a considerable extent and (b) has promoted active involvement in goal formulation all along.

The Public's Knowledge of Occupational Therapy

The rationale for using the collaborative approach sharpens considerably when we reflect on the profession's unclear image. "Occupational therapy is not understood well by the average client because it is not a common profession, such as medicine, nursing, engineering, law, teaching or the ministry" (Reed & Sanderson, 1983, p. 161). Practitioners often find themselves explaining the word *occupational*, differentiating occupational therapy functions from those of other therapies, and otherwise clarifying their professional roles. If the public expects physicians, nurses, and engineers, whose professions are better understood, to clarify their procedures, the expectation increases for those representing less well understood professions.

Occupational therapy is often not understood; it can, in fact, often be misunderstood. A particularly noteworthy example of that misunderstanding appears in Joyce Rebeta-Burditt's novel *The Cracker Factory* (1977). In the story a young female patient, a self-described alcoholic, writes from the psychiatric hospital to a friend:

> I should write to you every day. I could not only unravel the Gordian knot in my psyche, but appear to be busy and involved when Brunhilde, the misplaced Viking lady, comes tapping on my door every afternoon in an effort to intimidate me into going to Occupational Therapy. She marches around the seventh floor telling all the patients that their doctor has "ordered" Occupational Therapy and they must come IMMEDIATELY. She herds them out in the hall where they mill around until she lines them up in two columns and goose steps them out the door ...
>
> Patients are forever trying to hide by taking a shower or even [having] a fit, but she doesn't care. Wet or screaming, it makes no difference. She drags them along anyway.
> . . .
> I go sometimes and hate myself for it. I sit and dab grout on a metal shell and try to decide what color ashtray I'm going to mess up that day. I listen to the conversations around me, and the tape recorder in my head jots down snatches and fragments and I smile and pretend that I am not listening in. (pp. 114–115)

Fiction will often exaggerate or satirize those aspects of our functioning that create interesting reading material, such as the domineering qualities of Brunhilde and the perceived irrelevance of occupational therapy. Fiction also mirrors reality. In this case the reality is that occupational therapy is sometimes misunderstood.

The consequence of this misunderstanding can be significant. Patients uninformed of the purpose of occupational therapy are free to infer its meaning based on their observations. The result may well be compliance with the procedure. It might as easily be noncompliance accompanied by hostility. One probability is that patients who are uninformed or misinformed will be less able to generalize to their life situations those concepts the therapist had hoped might be learned in therapy.

The Ambiguous Nature of Activity

Because occupational therapists use activity as a primary modality, they increase the risk of being misunderstood. Any single activity can have many therapeutic possibilities. Proficiency in activity analysis enables clinicians to recognize the multiple goals that can be attached to any one activity. Therapists need to apply that theoretical concept clinically and consider its practical consequences. Therapeutic methods can easily confuse patients. A patient can be given leather stamping as a task to achieve a wide range of goals, including (a) the enhancement of grip strength, (b) the redirection of nervous energy through gross motor release, or (c) the use of organizational and problem-solving skills in the planning of a balanced design. If the only focus patients have is the one they can infer while doing the task, the relationship between the leather-stamping activity and the treatment plan may elude them. Because they do not clearly understand the therapeutic concepts supporting the activity, they may be less apt to apply them to their personal life situations.

A pleasant staff development exercise that illustrates the multifaceted aspect of any activity is the following: Divide the total group into five working subgroups. Provide each small group with a bowl of sliced oranges. The primary activity will be to eat the oranges. From the list given in the appendix to this paper, provide each group with a different set of written directions. Allow each group to complete the activity as directed. Following the group activity, ask a representative from each group to share both the directions given and the results of their activity. Reports from the representatives will reflect the different end points that one task with different directions can have. The exercise can stimulate reflection on the importance of clarifying the specific focus of a planned activity.

Methods of Providing a Collaborative Approach

A collaborative approach can be used creatively. Therapists can provide feedback formally or informally, use the printed or the spoken word, and communicate the purpose of occupational therapy procedures at various phases in the treatment process. Any method used that communicates the purpose of or the expectations for the treatment can qualify.

In an earlier article (Peloquin, 1983), I endorsed integrating information about the expectations and relevance of the occupational therapy program into the structure of an initial interview format in an acute care psychiatric setting. The three-part interview stresses the continuous provision of feedback to the patient. My conviction remains that, if nothing else, we give patients methods of self-help when we provide them with informative goal statements that they can readily apply to their personal environments after discharge.

One way to enlighten patients is to give them printed materials. A general description of the occupational therapy program might be a suitable accompaniment to the initial contact between a patient and a therapist. The descriptive introduction might include a statement of the various purposes of the occupational therapy program. Next, a brief, goal-oriented paragraph at the top of an occupational therapy schedule might serve as a motivational reinforcement. Posters listing typical occupational therapy goals for various groups can be displayed in both residential and treatment areas. In more financially comfortable settings, pamphlets or video messages discussing the programmatic goals of occupational therapy might be used as part of a general hospital orientation.

Feedback can be provided in formal groups and individual orientations. On a daily basis, a brief discussion can either precede or follow each activity group. More articulate patients can be asked to help clarify the purposes and expectations of various groups for new patients. Less organized patients can be reminded informally on the way to and from groups about the specific purpose of each group. Brief personal contacts reminding patients about individualized goals can occur during large parallel groups.

It might be helpful to include here a few illustrations of how the collaborative approach can be incorporated into occupational therapy. Each illustration includes vocabulary that can be adjusted upward or downward to match the intellectual level of the patient population being addressed. Any verbal delivery of the feedback needs to reflect, in its tone, rate, and inflection, the therapist's perception of the patient as intelligent. A singsong or overly didactic delivery, suggesting condescension, could vitiate or at least compromise the purpose of the feedback. A respectful intent requires respectful delivery.

An introductory explanation of a psychiatric occupational therapy program might read, in part, as follows:

Occupational therapy adds to your total treatment by encouraging you to use activities and occupy your time in a therapeutic way. Purposeful activity has an organizing and beneficial effect on an individual. Because it involves the total person, activity meets several mental health needs.

Occupational therapy offerings here include crafts, exercise, greenhouse, relaxation, communication, and life skills groups. By participating in these activities you help ready yourself to return to your community. During group and individual sessions, you can set goals and practice skills essential to your coping more effectively outside of the hospital.

You will have daily opportunities to plan and organize tasks, to solve problems, to improve your physical condition, to interact effectively with others, to make decisions, to boost your self-confidence, to learn new ways of relaxing and coping with different life situations. Activity becomes therapy because of the adaptive skills you practice when you are active.

A poster mounted in the clinical area to provide information about a typical occupational therapy craft group might list some of the following goal statements:

Why Crafts?

to improve your concentration
to organize your thoughts
to have you solve problems
to help you make decisions
to exercise your work skills
to boost your self-confidence

---

to increase your independence
to help you interact with others
to increase your sense of control
to keep you alert and involved

A poster describing the purposes of a communication group might read as follows:

Why Communication Group?

to improve your listening skills
to help you share and interact
to increase your self-awareness
to help you identify your feelings
to help you express yourself
to help you better deal with anger
to increase your assertiveness
to help you clarify your thoughts
to help you make or keep friends

A discussion at the end of a particular group might follow a basic outline such as the following, addressing a different goal from day to day. The following format has been used with groups of adults having cognitive problems:

1. Explain the purpose of the group: "One of the goals for this particular group is to have you use your cognitive or thinking skills. During the course of this hour each of you has had some opportunity to use a number of thinking skills, such as concentrating, problem solving, decision making, comprehending instructions, or organizing your activity."

2. Set the stage for a discussion: "Take a minute to think about the thinking skills you used while working on your project. I'll be asking a few of you to share with the rest of us how you used your skills during the past hour."

3. Facilitate a brief discussion of skills used, making sure to clearly link for patients the various task steps they completed with the cognitive skills they used. Examples of therapist responses might be:

   a. "That's right, Jim. You had to follow several complex verbal instructions today. I also noticed that you were doing a lot of planning and organizing for the design you want to put on your belt tomorrow."

   b. "Lorene, you're feeling that you didn't use your thinking skills today, but I noticed that you had to make several color choices when you were painting. That's decision making. You also had to pay attention to the shapes you were painting. That required you to concentrate on what you were doing. You really were using thinking skills for the better part of the hour."

4. Summarize what was accomplished and encourage patients to return to the next session.

Formulating and providing a set of goals in collaboration with the patient can be a creative process evolving from the basic premise that patients have rights, capabilities, and a vested interest in knowing the relevance of therapy. Using the collaborative approach can potentiate our therapeutic activities by communicating their value to patients in the real world outside the treatment setting. An old proverb says, "Give a man a fish and you have fed him for a day; teach a man to fish and you have fed him for a lifetime." Sharing goal statements with patients can give them an understanding of a process that can provide a link to improved functioning.

Summary

There is a rationale for a collaborative approach with patients in the daily practice of occupational therapy. Effective collaborative procedure provides patients with (a) knowledge about what they are doing and why they are doing it and (b) encourages them to engage in the process.

The effectiveness of this approach has not been established conclusively, but studies suggest that subjects exposed to the therapeutic purpose of desensitization procedures tend to have better therapeutic outcomes than those unaware of the purpose. Current emphasis on the patient's right to be informed and on the therapist's responsibility to inform reflects the public's growing insistence that practitioners explain the utility of the treatments they provide to the patient.

Excerpts from past and present literature indicate that assumptions underlying the practice of traditional occupational therapy reflect similar assumptions underpinning the use of a collaborative approach. These assumptions describe the patient as rational, as having rights, and as a collaborator in therapy. The therapist is assumed to be a teacher and a motivator in the therapeutic process, the person who articulates the relevance of therapy and encourages the patient's participation.

The general public often lacks understanding of the occupational therapy process. Additionally, the versatility and multiple possibilities associated with any activity can confuse the patient about its purpose. The uninformed patient might be less inclined to participate in therapy and less able to generalize helpful concepts from the experience.

Feedback to patients can be provided in a number of creative ways throughout treatment. Providing such feedback need not require a major time investment, but can represent the therapist's renewed commitment to the therapeutic alliance and to the goal directedness of occupational therapy practice.

Acknowledgments

I thank Lillian Hoyle Parent, MA, OTR, FAOTA, for her support and encouragement in the preparation of this paper.

The topic of this paper featured in a workshop entitled "Goal Formulation: Clinical Leverage in Challenging Times," which I copresented with Debora Davidson, MS, OTR. The workshop was sponsored by the Department of Occupational Therapy at the University of Texas Medical Branch Hospitals, L. Randy Strickland, EdD, OTR, FAOTA, Director.

Appendix

1. You have been given orange sections as a help in your discussion. The tangible and sensual experience of the orange will enable you to complete your task. As you are eating the sections, discuss as a group the various memories you have that are associated with eating oranges. Appoint a spokesperson who will later present a 30–60 second summary of your discussion.

2. You have been given orange sections as a help in your discussion. The actual taste of the orange will help you to better focus on your task. As you are eating the sections, discuss as a group as many dishes or recipes as you can think of that use oranges. Appoint a spokesperson who will later present a 30–60 second summary of your discussion.

3. You have been given orange sections as a help in your discussion. The visual and tactile experience of the orange will help you in your task. As you are eating the sections, discuss as a group as many functions as you can think of that an orange might have aside from its function as a food item. Appoint a spokesperson who will later present a 30–60 second summary of your discussion.

4. You have been given orange sections as a help in your discussion. The sight of the orange will help you in your task. As you are eating the sections, discuss as a group as many other natural items as you can think of that share a similar color. Appoint a spokesperson who will later present a 30–60 second summary of your discussion.

5. You have been given orange sections as a help in your discussion. The smell of the orange will help you in your task. As you are eating the sections, discuss as a group as many other items as you can think of that share a similar odor, or that have the orange scent. Appoint a spokesperson who will later present a 30–60 second summary of your discussion.

References

Bloomer, J. S. (1978). The consumer of therapy in mental health. *American Journal of Occupational Therapy, 32,* 621–627.

Borkovec, T.D. (1972). Effects of expectancy on the outcome of systematic desensitization and implosive treatments for analogue anxiety. *Behavior Therapy, 3,* 29–40.

Cartwright, D. S., & Cartwright, R. D. (1958). Faith and improvement in psychotherapy. *Journal of Counseling Psychology, 5,* 174–177.

Edgerton, W. B. (1947). Activities in occupational therapy. In H. Willard & C. Spackman (Eds.), *Occupational therapy* (pp. 40–59). Philadelphia: Lippincott.

Engelhardt, H. T., Jr. (1986). *The foundations of bioethics.* New York: Oxford University Press.

Fine, S. B., & Schwimmer, P. (1986, December). The effects of occupational therapy on independent living skills. *Mental Health Special Interest Section Newsletter,* pp. 2–3.

Frank, J. D. (1959). The dynamics of the psychotherapeutic relationship. *Psychiatry, 22,* 17–39.

Kielhofner, G. (1985). The human being as an open system. In G. Kielhofner (Ed.), *A model of human occupation: Theory and application* (pp. 2–11). Baltimore: Williams & Wilkins.

Krause, M. S. (1967). Clients' expectations of the value of treatment. *Mental Hygiene, 51,* 359–365.

Leitenbheerg, H., Agras, W. S., Barlow, D. H., & Oliveau, D.C. (1969). Contributions of selective positive reinforcement and therapeutic instructions to systematic desensitization therapy. *Journal of Abnormal Psychology, 74,* 113–118.

Lomont, J. F., & Brock, L. (1971). Cognitive factors in systematic desensitization. *Behavior Research and Therapy, 9,* 187–195.

McGlynn, F. D. (1971). Experimental desensitization following three types of instructions. *Behavior Research and Therapy, 9,* 367–369.

McGlynn, F. D., & Mapp, R. H. (1970). Systematic desensitization of snake-avoidance following three types of suggestion. *Behavior Research and Therapy, 8,* 197–201.

McGlynn, F. D., Mealiea, E. L., & Nawas, M. M. (1969). Systematic desensitization of snake-avoidance under two conditions of suggestion. *Psychological Reports, 25,* 220–222.

McGlynn, F. D., Reynolds, E. J., & Linder, L. H. (1971). Systematic desensitization with pre-treatment and intra-treatment therapeutic instructions. *Behavior Research and Therapy, 9,* 57–63.

McGlynn, F. D., & Williams, C. W. (1970). Systematic desensitization of snake-avoidance under three conditions of suggestion. *Journal of Behavior Therapy and Experimental Psychiatry, 1,* 97–101.

McNary, H. (1947). The scope of occupational therapy. In H. Willard & C. Spackman (Eds.), *Occupational therapy* (pp. 10–22). Philadelphia: Lippincott.

Miller, S. B. (1972). The contribution of therapeutic instructions to systematic desensitization. *Behavior Research and Therapy,* 159–169.

Oliveau, D. C. (1969). Systematic desensitization in an experimental setting: A follow–up study. *Behavior Research and Therapy, 7,* 377–380.

Oliveau, D. C., Agras, W. S., Leitenberg, H., Moore, R. C., & Wright, D. E. (1969). Systematic desensitization, therapeutically oriented instructions and selective positive reinforcement. *Behavior Research and Therapy, 7,* 27–33.

Peloquin, S. M. (1983). The development of an occupational therapy interview/therapy set procedure. *American Journal of Occupational Therapy, 37,* 457–461.

Rappaport, H. (1972). Modification of avoidance behavior: Expectancy, autonomic reactivity, and verbal report. *Journal of Consulting and Clinical Psychology, 39,* 404–414.

Rebeta-Burditt, J. (1977). *The Cracker Factory.* New York: Macmillan.

Reed, K. L., & Sanderson, S. R. (1983). *Concepts of occupational therapy.* Baltimore: Williams & Wilkins.

Rosen, G. M. (1974). Therapy set: its effects on subjects' involvement in systematic desensitization and treatment outcome. *Journal of Abnormal Psychology, 83,* 291–300.

Speedy recovery. (1987, July). *Reader's Digest,* p. 53.

Wade, B. D. (1947). Occupational therapy for patients with mental disease. In H. Willard & C. Spackman (Eds.), *Occupational therapy* (pp. 81–117). Philadelphia: Lippincott.

Woy, J. R., & Efran, J. S. (1972). Systematic desensitization and expectancy in the treatment of speaking anxiety. *Behavior Research and Therapy, 10,* 33–49.

Wilkins, W. (1973). Expectancy of therapeutic gain: An empirical and conceptual critique. *Journal of Consulting and Clinical Psychology, 40,* 69–77.

Section VI

Research: Applied Scientific Inquiry on Purposeful Activity and Occupational Therapy

Introduction

The selection and use of purposeful activity, media, and methods based on research can increase the efficacy of Occupational Therapy intervention. As Reed emphasized in Chapter 39, using research to justify the use of a tool of practice is the most professional and responsible approach; however, it is also the most difficult to obtain. Given current health care system demands for professional accountability and proven functional outcomes, it is essential for occupational therapist to engage in clinical research to establish the efficacy of our tools of practice and to provide objective, persuasive evidence of the effectiveness of occupational therapy for the various patient populations we serve (Rogers and Holm, 1994). Professions and professionals who are able to provide documented, data-based research will have important roles in health care and service provision in the future (Royeen, 1995).

Occupational therapists know their interventions make a difference, we see qualitative changes every day. Now we have to provide the documentation to back up our observations. Fortunately, many leaders in our profession have recognized this need with a significant increase in resources being devoted to research during the last several years (AOTA, 1995). As a result of this research emphasis, a number of excellent studies and texts have been published; thereby, strengthening our profession's body of knowledge (See chapter reference lists and Appendix L for these resources). This section includes a number of previously published research studies representing several broad areas of concern regarding the use of purposeful activity in occupational therapy. These studies were selected based upon their relevance to the field, demonstrated outcomes, and use of replicable designs. Obviously, there are limitations in the scope of the research presented here as there are

several gaps in our professional literature itself. However, these studies are generally well designed with clear implications for the use of purposeful activity in occupational therapy, and while they have their limitations, they do make solid contributions to our professional research literature.

Steinbeck begins this section with a description of a controlled study designed to measure the effect of purposeful versus non-purposeful activity on activity performance. The definitions and characteristics of purposeful versus non-purposeful activity are reviewed and their effect on motivation and activity performance are explored. Relationships between purpose, motivation, and activity performance are analyzed. The study's objectives, subjects, apparatus, instruments, procedures, and results are identified. Results are analyzed with implications for future research provided. These results demonstrated that adding purpose to an activity increases the amount of time an individual will engage in an activity and enhances the person's level of expressed interest in the activity. While the study has its limitations, its findings affirm the intrinsically motivating qualities of purposeful activity, substantiating the therapeutic value of the process of engaging in purposeful activity. The premise that individuals will be more motivated to perform an activity when it is purposeful was clearly supported by this study, validating a fundamental principle of OT intervention.

The next chapter by Miller and Nelson also explores the effect of purposefulness on activity performance as measured by task duration, exertion level, and affect. They first explore the controversial question as to whether exercise is to be included in the definition of purposeful activity. They discuss a number of different definitions of purposeful activity and review the concept of "single purpose" activity (i.e., activity for exercise alone), versus "dual-purpose" activity (i.e., activity for exercise and an added goal). Miller and Nelson then present their study which compared the performance of a single purpose activity to the performance of a dual purpose activity. Specifics regarding subjects, apparatus, instruments, and procedures are provided. Results are presented and analyzed with questions for further study outlined. This study found positive correlations between performance of a dual purpose activity and exertion, duration, and the person's value of the activity. Although this study cannot be generalized to other populations, its findings support the assumption that having an additional goal beyond exercise will be more motivating to an individual than exercise alone, reaffirming the use of purposeful activity in treatment.

As Steinbeck, Miller, and Nelson demonstrated in these first two chapters, purposefulness can be added to an activity by physically adding materials for task performance. Providing concrete materials to use during an activity is often the most common and realistic method for adding purposefulness to an OT session, and the documented increased efficacy of dual purpose activity versus single purpose activity make these efforts clearly worthwhile. However, many therapists continue to use single purpose exercise activities in treatment, citing a lack of supplies, space constraints and/or limited time for activity set-up and clean-up as reasons for not developing meaningful dual-purpose treatment activities. While these reasons may be rationalizations at times for a lack of creativity, there can be clinical setting realities that challenge the resources and imagination of even the best of therapists. Therefore, some therapists add imagery to exercise to make it a "dual purpose" treatment activity. The addition of imagery as a alternative to adding an activity to exercise to make it purposeful is explored in this section's next chapter. The authors, Riccio, Nelson, and Bush, examine the use of imagery in therapeutic clinical practice and provide an overview of the literature on the relationship between imagery and movement. The therapeutic use of imagery and its link to the theoretical construct and philosophical principles of occupational therapy are explored. A study which examined the effects of verbally elicited imagery on the performance of two exercises as compared to rote exercise, that is, repetitive exercise done without any added purpose is presented. Details on study's subjects, method, procedures, and results are provided. This study found that the addition of imagery to an exercise increased the duration and frequency of the exercise performance and increased participants spontaneous favorable verbalizations about the activity performance. The authors conclude that in the absence of suitable materials for an activity, imagery-based instruction during exercise can increase the purposefulness of the exercises. They offer

a number of clear, concrete suggestions as to how imagery can be used in day-to-day OT practice to enhance activity performance and they urge therapists to further explore the advantages and disadvantages of using imagery during activities in OT intervention.

While imagery can add purpose to exercise, its use is limited when one is concerned with non-physical goals. A purposeful activity with materials, directions, and a final product is more useful than imagery when treatment is aimed a attaining psychosocial and/or cognitive goals. Project completion is often an inherent part of many OT treatment plans, but policies regarding clients keeping, or not keeping, their products vary among programs, The following chapter by Rocker and Nelson explores the psychosocial implications of keeping, or not keeping a product produced in OT treatment. The potential reactions and affective responses of clients to not being allowed to keep a product are reviewed. A controlled study which explores these issues is presented. Subjects, instruments, procedures, data reduction, and results are described. The results show that not being allowed to keep an activity product significantly effects certain moods of participants. Implications of keeping, and not keeping, an activity product for OT clinical practice are examined. Although this is a limited study, these findings warrant thoughtful consideration, given the potential emotional reactions of a client to keeping, or not keeping, a product produced during a treatment session.

The next chapter also examines the implications of keeping, or not keeping a product but the focus here is on the altruistic act of purposefully giving an activity product to others. Hatter and Nelson investigate altruism as an influential factor in task participation among the elderly. The intrinsic value of purposeful activity to the quality of life of the elderly and the relationship of participation in occupation to life satisfaction is explored. Emphasis is place on the enhanced value of altruistic activities. Study's subjects, procedures, and results are described. The authors found a significant relationship between altruism and task participation and concluded that incorporating altruism into a purposeful activity may increase motivation and participation. While this study was limited to elderly persons residing in an institutionalized setting, I have observed, in my practice, similar outcomes with clients on an acute, inpatient psychiatric unit and with members of a day treatment program for persons with chronic mental illnesses. From baking cookies and making wooden toys for a pediatric unit, to knitting hats and scarves for a homeless shelter, these clients universally express a great deal of satisfaction with altruistic activities, As one client commented,"It feels so good to finally give. I feel I've been useless and taking from everyone since I got sick. It's great to be able to give again and make a difference to someone." Many individuals with physical and mental illnesses have few opportunities "to give" to others, limiting their ability to be contributing members of society. Occupational therapists can plan and structure activities that enable persons with disabilities to use their abilities in an altruistic manner, enhancing the therapeutic value of purposeful activities and increasing their contributions to society.

The ability of occupational therapists to structure activities for therapeutic purposes is further explored in the following chapter by Nelson, Peterson, Smith, Boughten, and Whalen, which examines the effect of group structure on social interaction and affect. Nelson, et al, describe the characteristics and purposes of group structure, reviewing literature relevant to activity group structure and the creative use of purposeful activities in OT practice. Their study compared subjects working in a parallel group with participants having their own task to subjects working in a project group with all participants sharing a common task. Results indicated that group structure and the sharing of a task may have a significant effect on group members' social interaction and their affective responses to the group's activity. Limitations of the study are identified and implications for OT evaluation and intervention are thoughtfully considered. The authors concluded that the results of this study, although limited, are supportive of OT's activity heritage and can serve as a base for future activity analysis research.

The next chapter, by Klyczek and Mann, also studies group structure but in a broader sense, for their research focused on the overall structure of two psychiatric day treatment programs, comparing a verbally-oriented program to an activity-oriented program. Literature on day treatment program effectiveness with respect to symptom reduction, relapse, and community tenure is reviewed. Types of day treatment program groups are defined with goals and methods discussed. Their research methods including subjects, treatment approaches, variables, and outcome measures are identified. A program that offered twice as much activity based treatment as verbal-oriented treatment was compared to a day treatment program offering the exact opposite, that is, twice as much verbal-oriented treatment than activity-oriented treatment to determine if there were differences in the outcome measures of symptom reduction, community tenure, and relapse for participants in each of the described programs. Their results indicate that these different approaches do influence clients' functioning within their community. Although these results cannot be generalized to other populations, the differences in outcomes between the two treatment approaches supports the value of activities based treatment in mental health, for it is an effective approach to increase functioning within the community.

Community programming is also the focus of the following chapter by Kirchman, Reichenbach, and Giambalvo. They studied the effects of adding a purposeful activity program to a community-based preventative service for the well-elderly. A literature review on the value of activity to the elderly and on quality of life is provided. The rationale for this model project's development, program structure, and activities are clearly described. The research component, using pre and post intervention interviews, was designed to examine the effect of purposeful activity and support services on the ability of elderly to remain in their communities are an enhanced quality of life. They found that the addition of a structured activity program to a senior nutritional site did result in increased social resources and networks, enhanced life satisfaction, and improved affect for the well elderly. The authors conclude that these results validate the efficacy of purposeful activities and support systems in keeping the elderly in their home communities.

The final chapter in this section also presents research conducted on an activity program for elders living in the community; however, this program is a home-based one for persons with chronic disabilities. The authors, Levine, and Gitlin, identify the incidence of chronic disability in the elderly and discuss the functional effects of these chronic disabilities on daily life. Models for service provision and treatment approaches for chronic illness and the elderly are analyzed. The need for collaboration and individuation of treatment through the use of relevant and meaningful purposeful activity is emphasized, serving as a foundation for the program developed for this research project. This model program's four phases of intervention—exploration, competence, achievement, and termination—are described with comprehensive case data and purposeful activity examples substantiating the use of purposeful activity to promote competence and adaptation in the study's subjects. A clear description of the program, including therapist training, client characteristics, visit patterns, and documentation guidelines is provided. This collaborative approach to intervention emphasized using treatment strategies that evolved from an understanding of the clients' ascribed meaning to activities and unique daily life issues. Many areas of treatment focus are identified and implications for OT practice are explored. Although the interventions identified may seem to have resulted in small functional gains, the meaning of these accomplishments to the clients and the corresponding qualitative changes in their daily life were great. This research supports the efficacy of a collaborative, client-driven, activity-based approach for increasing clients' competence and quality of life in the community, even with the presence of a chronic illness.

The increased effectiveness of OT intervention which includes the use of purposeful activity has been demonstrated in this section for a diversity of populations in a variety of clinical and community-based settings. While these studies all have their limitations, which were realistically identified and openly discussed by the authors, they can provide the reader with a number of excellent ideas for increasing the efficacy of OT treatment. In addition, several of the authors have made viable suggestions for future research on the therapeutic use of purposeful activity and many of the research designs presented can be replicated with improvements made to eliminate the cited limitations of the original designs. This increase in research can further substantiate the therapeutic value of our professions's tools of practice. Understandably, some OT practitioners may view this call for clinical research as unrealistic, given the complex and multiple demands on a clinician's time or others may fear research, questioning their skills and supports for competing a research study (Bailey,1994; Oakley, 1993). However, research can be viewed as a natural extension of the orderly, sequential process used by OTs to provide clinical care (Oakley, 1993). There are also numerous alternatives to solo research which can counter these concerns. Collaboration with a colleague and/or academician, membership in study groups, research networks, and research symposia and replication of well-designed studies are all effective methods for conducting clinical research (Baily, 1993; DePoy and Gallagher, 1993; and Oakley, 1993). The reader is referred to the reference lists in Appendix L for resources on research principles and designs and for additional published research studies relevant to the use of purposeful activity in occupational therapy.

Questions to Consider

1. Select a research study from the reference list in Appendix L. Critically review the study. Was the study well-designed? What were it's major shortcomings? How could the research design or procedures be improved to eliminate these flaws? What were the major contributions of this study to occupational therapy's body of knowledge? Can this study's findings be used to provided justification for OT services?

2. Identify a relevant purposeful activity that can use altruism as a motivating factor for a client population. Using Chapter 57 as a guide, set up a small research study to determine if the addition of altruism to an activity has an effect on activity performance. Suggested populations for this pilot study are a.) adolescent teens with developmental disabilities in an after school program, b.) young adults with quadriplegia in a long term rehabilitation center, c.) adults with multiple sclerosis attending an outpatient support group, d.) well elderly persons attending a senior citizen center.

3. What are the resources available from the American Occupational Therapy Foundation (AOTF), AOTA and your state and local OT associations to support research? Contact these organizations to obtain this information and attend available research symposia, networks, and presentations to further develop research skills and expand your resources.

References

American Occupational Therapy Association (1995). National speaking-American Occupational Therapy Association and American Occupational Therapy Foundation Outcomes-Related Activities. *American Journal of Occupational Therapy, 49,* 759-762.

Bailey, D.M. (1993). The challenge of conducting research in a clinic. In R.P. Cottrell (Ed.). *Psychosocial Occupational Therapy: Proactive Approaches* (pp. 505-507). Bethesda, MD: American Occupational Therapy Association.

DePoy, E. and Gallagher, C. (1993). Steps in collaborative research between clinicians and faculty. In R.P. Cottrell (Ed.). *Psychosocial Occupational Therapy: Proactive Approaches* (pp. 509-513). Bethesda, MD: American occupational Therapy Association.

Mosey, A.C., (1986). *Psychosocial Components of Occupational Therapy.* New York , NY: Raven Press.

Oakley, F, (1993). Research and professional growth in a clinical setting. In R.P. Cottrell (Ed.). *Psychosocial Occupational Therapy: Proactive Approaches* (pp 501-503). Bethesda, MD: American Occupational Therapy Association.

Rogers, J.C. And Holm, M. (1994). Nationally speaking-Accepting the challenge of outcome research: Examining the effectiveness of Occupational Therapy Practice. *American Journal of Occupational Therapy, 48,* 871-876.

Yasuda, L. And Royeen, C.B. (1995). Considering environmental context: Thinking about functional outcomes. In C.B. Royeen (Ed.). *The Practice of the Future: Putting Occupation Back into Therapy* (pp 9-11). Bethesda Md: American Occupational Therapy Association.

Chapter 53

Purposeful Activity and Performance

Thomas M. Steinbeck, MOT, OTR

In formulating the first principles of occupational therapy in 1918, Dunton wrote that occupation must have some useful end to be an effective tool in the treatment of mental and physical disabilities. Today, purposeful activity remains a cornerstone of occupational therapy, and its importance to the field is cited throughout the professional literature. Numerous authors have taken a variety of approaches in attempting to advance an understanding of the concept of purposeful activity. King (1978) (see Chapter 8) views it as part of an adaptive process that characterizes individual development and mastery of the environment. Fidler and Fidler (1978) (see Chapter 7) speak of purposeful action, of "doing," as a means of self-actualization. DiJoseph (1982) identified purposeful activity in terms of a triad of mind, body, and the environment. These authors and others (Breines, 1984 [see Chapter 12]; Kleinman & Bulkey, 1982) articulate support for the view that purposeful activity is a legitimate tool in the evaluation and treatment of physical and mental dysfunction.

However, despite apparent support for this view among occupational therapists, the concept and value of purposeful activity appears to have been accepted largely through a qualitative process with relatively little evidence of an empirical nature. With debate continuing over the definition and efficacy of purposeful activity (Breines, 1984 [see Chapter 12]; West, 1984), the need for controlled studies to measure its effectiveness or value is necessary since it is a basic premise in occupational therapy.

In identifying what sets purposeful activity apart from activity per se, one can begin by defining purposeful activity as "tasks or experiences in which the person actively participates" (Hinojosa, Sabari, & Rosenfeld,

1983, p. 805). By selecting activities in which the patient has an interest, the therapist assumes the patient will experience enough satisfaction to sustain performance (Fidler, 1981). According to King (1978[see Chapter 8]), each successful effort elicited by the occupational therapist serves as an incentive for greater effort by the patient. In other words, purposeful activity is thought to provide an intrinsic motivation to act.

Trombly (1983) refers to motivation as the determination or persistence with which one pursues a goal. She reasoned that a patient provided with interest-sustaining activities is likely to pursue those activities longer than would be expected with less interesting activities or exercises. In a recent study, Kircher (1984) compared exertion, as perceived by the subject, during purposeful and nonpurposeful activity and found that, in normal subjects, heart rate at a predefined level of perceived exertion was significantly higher in the performance of a purposeful activity than in the performance of a nonpurposeful activity. The implication is that an individual may not perceive fatigue as readily when the focus of attention is on the end product or purpose of the activity rather than on the act itself. However, Kircher's conclusions may have been somewhat compromised by her methodology.

Occupational therapists have long believed that purposeful activity would motivate the patient to perform longer. If this is true, then a greater number of repetitions or a longer duration of performance should be obtained during purposeful activity than during nonpurposeful activity before a point of fatigue is reached.

Purpose of Study

This study examined the hypothesis that the presence of a purpose or a goal would have an effect on the number of times an individual would repeat a desired motion before reaching a point of perceived exertion. For the scope of this study, purposeful activity was defined as an activity, task, or process in which the individual actively focuses on the achievement of a goal inherent in the activity. Nonpurposeful activity was defined as the absence of an inherent goal other than the specific muscle or extremity function.

Two activities designated as purposeful were matched with two designated as nonpurposeful. An Oliver Rehabilitation Woodworking Machine requiring reciprocal pedaling to operate an integral drill press was chosen for the purposeful lower extremity activity (see Figure 1), and a Fiton Cycle Ergometer, adapted to duplicate the physical requirements of the drill press, was chosen for the nonpurposeful lower extremity activity (see Figure 2). In preparing the cycle ergometer to duplicate the motions of the drill press, the handlebars were removed and replaced with a platform of the same height which served as the drill press worktable. A spring-loaded lever was installed on the platform to reproduce the motion used in operating the drill press.

The speedometer on the cycle was covered to eliminate that particular incentive.

A game requiring the rapid unilateral squeezing of a rubber bulb to produce a steady jet of air necessary to maintain a Ping–Pong ball at a particular level of suspension on an inclined track was developed and designated the purposeful hand activity (see Figure 3). The same rubber bulb, detached from the game, was designated for the nonpurposeful hand activity.

The activities designated as purposeful had goals inherent in their performance whereas the nonpurposeful activities did not. In operating the drill press, the subject's attention was focused on drilling holes to produce a solitaire strategy game. Keeping the Ping–Pong ball suspended on a specific color–coded section of the inclined track was the focus of the purposeful hand activity.

In addition to the number of repetitions performed for each activity, heart rate and electromyogram (EMG) measures were recorded to establish comparable levels of activity in the subjects.

Method

Subjects

Thirty undergraduate students not studying occupational therapy or physical therapy (15 males, 15 females) with a mean age of 19.0 years participated in the study.

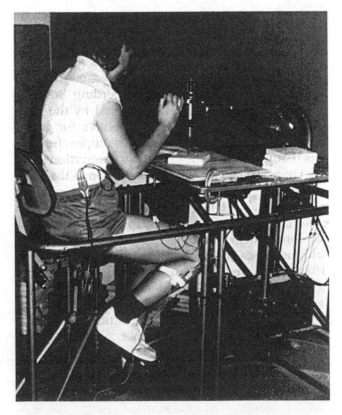

Figure 1. Subject performing puposeful lower extremity activity.

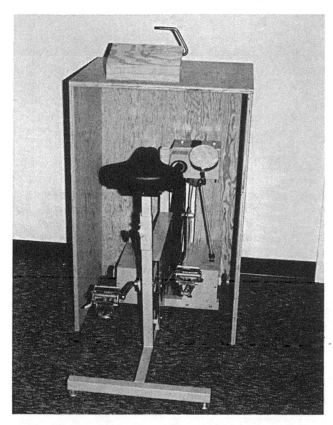

Figure 2. Cycle ergometer adapted to serve as nonpurposeful lower extremity activity.

The selection was based on results of an eight-item assessment of activity and health factors. Volunteers were considered for selection if they reported performing fewer than 3 hours of aerobic activity per week, did not participate in regular weight lifting, and had no physical conditions that might have been aggravated by a performance of the activities required in the study.

Apparatus

Range of motion on the drill press and Fitron was set ar 33 cm diameter, and the seats were set at equal positions. The Fitron was adjusted to require the same

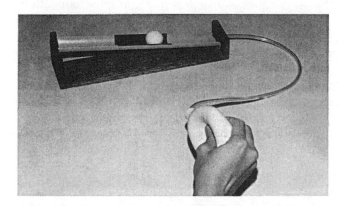

Figure 3. Ping–pong ball game for purposeful hand activity.

pedaling resistance as the drill press by recording EMG activity in the right rectus femoris muscle of a single control subject who performed both activities. The statistical analysis following this method of calibration indicated no significant difference between EMG readings taken on the two activities ($t = .12$, $p > .05$). Since EMG registers muscle action potentials evoked by the discharge of motor neurons which increases with the level of muscle contraction (Kimura, 1983), it could be reasonably assumed that the similar EMG readings generated by the control subject on the two activities were an indication that the physical demands of the activities were essentially the same.

Repetitions of the pedaling activities were recorded by mechanical revolution counters attached to the machines, and an observer took a back-up count. Repetitions of the hand activities, were counted by an observer using a hand-held counter.

Instrumentation

A Cyborg Biolab was used to monitor and record surface EMG activity in the right forearm flexors and the right rectus femoris muscle of each subject during the respective performance of the upper and lower extremity activities.

Heart rate was monitored at 1-minute intervals 'with a Quinton 650 Heart-rate Meter, which utilized a 3-lead chest pick-up to display an updated heart rate every 10 seconds. Accuracy is reported at ±4 beats per minute.

The Borg Scale of Ratings of Perceived Exertion (Borg, 1970) was used to establish levels of exertion at which the subjects would stop each activity (see Table 1). The validity ($r = .79$) and reliability ($r = .80$) of this instrument have been reported in the literature (Skinner, Hutsler, Bergsteinova, & Buskirk, 1973).

The subject's opinion of the activity in terms of interest and physical requirements was assessed with the aid of a three-item interest questionnaire. Scaled answers were assigned values ranging from 3 to 12 with a higher value indicating greater interest. After completing all four activities, the subjects ranked the activities in order of preference and were given an opportunity to make additional comments.

Table 1
Borg Scale of Perceived Exertion

6	14
7 very, very light	15 hard
8	16
9 very light	17 very hard
10	18
11 fairly light	19 very, very hard
12	20
13 somewhat hard	

Procedure

Subjects were not informed about the primary purpose of the experiment; they were told that the purpose was to study the effect of various activities on heart rate. After giving informed consent, subjects were randomly assigned to one of eight possible sequences of activities that controlled for order effects as well as for the effects of fatigue by alternating upper and lower extremity activities. Once a sequence had been established and resting heart rate taken, the subject was given an explanation of the Borg Scale. Subjects were told to stop performance of each activity when they felt they were working *somewhat hard*, which is at midpoint on the scale. With heart rate and EMG monitors in place, subjects were given a demonstration of the activity, heart rate was recorded, and they were told to begin. A pendulum metronome, placed outside the subject's view, was used to regulate the rate of pedaling in the lower extremity activities. The purposeful lower extremity activity involved drilling a series of 32 holes in a 13.5 cm square pine board to construct the game, which the subjects were told they could keep upon completion. No limit was placed on the number of games each subject could produce. On the nonpurposeful lower extremity activity, subjects pedaled at the same rate while depressing the nonpurposeful lever at a rate of approximately once every 10 seconds.

Subjects performed the hand activities in a seated position with the arm in slight abduction, elbow flexed to 90 degrees, and forearm in the neutral position. The proper grasp was demonstrated, and the subjects were instructed to squeeze the bulb all the way at a rate sufficient to keep the Ping–Pong ball suspended on the color-coded section of the track. Subjects who performed the nonpurposeful hand activity before the purposeful hand activity were instructed to squeeze at a demonstrated rate of approximately twice per second.

Immediately following each activity, the interest questionnaire was administered. Subjects then rested for a minimum of 5 minutes to allow their heart rate to return to its resting level before they resumed activity (Lunsford, 1978).

Results

Table 2 shows means and standard deviations for the dependent variable of repetitions. Dependent t tests indicated that the mean number of repetitions for the purposeful lower extremity activity was significantly greater than for the nonpurposeful lower extremity activity ($p < .001$), and purposeful hand activity repetitions were significantly greater than nonpurposeful hand activity repetitions ($p = .05$).

Table 3 shows the means and standard deviations for the control variables of heart rate and EMG. For heart rate, significantly higher levels were recorded on ending heart rates for the nonpurposeful lower extremity activity ($p = .05$) and the purposeful hand activity ($p = .05$).

For the control variable EMG, there was no significant difference between the purposeful and nonpurposeful lower extremity activities. EMG, however, was significantly higher for the purposeful hand activity than for the nonpurposeful hand activity ($p = .01$).

Subjects' responses on the interest questionnaire indicated that interest was significantly greater in the purposeful than in the nonpurposeful activities for both the lower extremity ($p = .005$) and the hand ($p < .001$). No significant differences were found between male and female responses on the questionnaire; however, males preferred the purposeful activities over the nonpurposeful ones, whereas females indicated no significant preference.

Discussion

The hypothesis that purposeful activity will have a positive effect on performance, as measured by the number of repetitions, was supported empirically. For the field of occupational therapy, this clearly supports a basic premise of the profession. If one views purposeful activity as a process engaged in by patients rather than as the tools of the profession (Breines, 1984) the value of this study becomes apparent. The results substantiate the philosophy of occupational therapy—the therapeutic value of the process of purposeful activity—and the modalities utilized in that process. When therapists choose a purposeful activity for a patient, that decision is based on the assumption that the patient will find sufficient satisfaction in the activity to sustain performance. This satisfaction is a key property of intrinsic motivation leading to the performance of an activity that can lay the foundation upon which competent behavior can be built (Florey, 1969). Results of this study strongly support the intrinsic motivational qualities of purposeful activities. Comments

Table 2
Means and Standard Deviations for Dependent Variable of Repetitions

Repetitions	Purposeful Activity		Nonpurposeful Activity			
	Mean	SD	Mean	SD	t	p
Lower extremity	677.80	489.15	323.30	185.67	4.32	<.001
Hand	105.67	33.55	95.50	32.45	2.26	.05

Table 3
Means and Standard Deviations for Control Variables of Heart Rate and EMG

Control Variables	Purposeful Activity		Nonpurposeful Activity		t	p
	Mean	SD	Mean	SD		
Heart rate						
Lower extremity	141.27	23.68	144.90	24.33	−2.17	.05
Hand	101.50	17.44	98.27	16.35	−2.60	.05
EMG						
Lower extremity	42.86	13.16	43.01	13.27	-.23	—
Hand	81.36	9.95	77.04	11.18	2.89	.05

Note. EMG = Electromyogram

from subjects also endorse this view. One wrote, "Certainly physical activity seems easier when my mind is kept busy." Another commented that it is "easier to do activities where there is a goal to achieve."

Although this study attempted to designate two activities as purposeful, it is true, as Lyons (1983) has stated, that "there are no generic purposeful activities (p. 493). Therefore the study may have been somewhat limited by the fact that the subjects were not able to choose the activities they performed. This, however, raises the question of whether or not a patient's choice is, in fact, a necessary prerequisite in determining a purposeful activity or whether the presence of an inherent goal provides sufficient motivation regardless of choice. Of the 6 subjects in the study who reported a preference for the nonpurposeful lower extremity activity over the purposeful lower extremity activity, only 2 actually performed longer on the nonpurposeful lower extremity activity. Among females, there was no significant difference in expression of interest between the purposeful lower extremity activity and the nonpurposeful lower extremity activity although females performed a significantly greater number of repetitions on the purposeful activity. This indicates that the particular motivational properties of a goal-directed activity may be capable of sustaining interest when none has been expressed. An examination of how the presence or absence of choice affects motivation could be the focus of future research. It is important to determine the extent to which choice defines the purposefulness of an activity and how it affects performance.

With regard to heart rate and perceived exertion, results failed to totally support Kircher's (1984) findings that a given level of exertion is perceived at a higher heart rate in the performance of a purposeful activity than in the performance of a nonpurposeful one. Kircher found that mean ending heart rate for the purposeful activity of jumping rope was 11.15 BPM greater than for the nonpurposeful activity of jumping in place without a rope. It has been established elsewhere that heart rate can be used effectively to classify exercise in terms of relative intensity

with a higher heart rate indicating a greater work load (McArdle, Katch, & Katch, 1981; Astrand & Rodal, 1977). Consequently, the heart rates recorded in Kircher's study indicate that her subjects performed two dissimilar activities in terms of work load and, therefore, her conclusion that the differences in performance were due to purposefulness is compromised by her procedure.

In this study, the differences in heart rate were in both directions: Heart rate was higher in the nonpurposeful lower extremity activity (p = .05) and in the purposeful hand activity (p = .05). In contrast to the 11.15 BPM difference found in Kircher's (1984) study, the differences recorded in this study were less than the ±4 BPM margin of error reported for the recording instrument. Therefore, one can consider these differences to be of statistical rather than of clinical significance. The similarity in heart rates between the two activities is, in fact, a strong indication that work loads were essentially the same for the matched activities. Therefore, one can conclude that the differences in performance, in this case, can be attributed directly to the purposefulness of the activities.

Future research in this area might examine physiologic factors and levels of perceived exertion in subjects following performance of matching purposeful and nonpurposeful activities of controlled duration rather than exertion levels.

Finally, in considering results of the EMG readings, the absence of a significant difference between the purposeful lower extremity activity and nonpurposeful lower extremity activity indicates that the differences in repetitions were recorded at equal levels of activity. In the performance of the hand activities, however, the force exerted for each activity could not be regulated and this may have contributed to significantly higher readings on the purposeful hand activity. Despite this limitation, the results demonstrate that the subjects worked longer and harder at the purposeful hand activity than at the nonpurposeful hand activity, which ultimately supports the original hypothesis.

Because of the uniformity of the work loads between the purposeful and nonpurposeful activities, as measured by heart rate and EMG, one must examine the cognitive and emotional aspects of the activity to account for the differences in performance. DiJoseph (1982) collectively labeled these emotive and cognitive processes the "mind" and emphasized the therapeutic importance of considering these processes as intimately linked to the other dimensions of body and environment. Results of this study support that contention and demonstrate that purposeful activity involves the mind as well as the body in a process that can lead to greater performance. The facilitation of that process, through the utilization of appropriate modalities, is the fundamental challenge to be met by occupational therapists in all areas of practice.

Summary

In examining the effect of purpose on performance, it was found that, when working to a given level of perceived exertion, 15 male and 15 female subjects performed a significantly greater number of repetitions during a purposeful pedaling activity than during a nonpurposeful activity. Similar results were obtained for purposeful and nonpurposeful hand function activities. An assessment of the subjects' interest in the activities showed a significantly greater interest in the purposeful activities. These results support occupational therapy's basic premise that purposeful activity is a motivating factor in performance. Implications were discussed in general terms for the practice of occupational therapy and the process of purposeful activity.

Acknowledgments

The author thanks Margo Holm, PhD, OTR, Steve Morelan, PhD, OTR, and Roberta Wilson, MS, for contributing time, energy, and insight to the preparation of this study; Watson Wade, COTA, for helping construct and adapt the activities used in the study; and Debra Steinbeck, RN, for assisting in collecting the data.

This article is based on materials submitted in partial fulfillment of the requirements for the degree of master of occupational therapy from the School of Occupational Therapy at the University of Puget Sound, Tacoma, Washington.

References

Astrand, P. O., & Rodahl, K. (1977). *Textbook of work physiology: Physiological bases of exercise.* New York: McGraw–Hill.

Borg, G. (1970). Perceived exertion as an indicator of somatic stress. *Scandinavian Journal of Rehabilitation Medicine, 2–3,* 92–98.

Breines, E. (1984). An attempt to define purposeful activity. *American Journal of Occupational Therapy, 38,* 543–544. (Reprinted as Chapter 12).

DiJoseph, L. M. (1982). Independence through activity: Mind, body, and environment interaction in therapy. *American Journal of Occupational Therapy, 36,* 740–744.

Dunton, W. R. (1918). The principles of occupational therapy. *Public Health Nurse, 10,* 320.

Fidler, G. S. (1981). From crafts to competence. *American Journal of Occupational Therapy, 35,* 567–573.

Fidler, G., & Fidler, J. (1978). Doing and becoming: Purposeful action and self-actualization. *American Journal of Occupational Therapy, 32,* 305–310. (Reprinted as Chapter 7).

Florey, L. L. (1969). Intrinsic motivation: The dynamics of occupational therapy theory. *American Journal of Occupational Therapy, 23,* 319–322.

Hinojosa, J., Sabari, J., & Rosenfeld, M. S. (1983). Purposeful activities. *American Journal of Occupational Therapy, 37,* 805–806.

Kimura J. (1983). *Electrodiagnosis in diseases of nerve and muscle: Principles and practice.* Philadelphia: F. A. Davis.

King, L. J. (1978). Toward a science of adaptive responses. *American Journal of Occupational Therapy, 32,* 429–437. (Reprinted as Chapter 8).

Kircher, M. A. (1984). Motivation as a factor of perceived exertion in purposeful versus nonpurposeful activity. *American Journal of Occupational Therapy 38,* 165–170.

Kleinman, B. L., & Bulkey, B. L. (1982). Some implications of a science of adaptive responses. *American Journal of Occupational Therapy, 36,* 15–19.

Lunsford, B. R. (1978). Clinical indicators of endurance. *Physical Therapy, 58,* 704–709.

Lyons, B. G. (1983). Purposeful versus human activity. *American Journal of Occupational Therapy, 37,* 493–495.

McArdle, W. D., Katch, F. I., & Katch, V. L. (1981). *Exercise physiology: Energy, nutrition, and human performance.* Philadelphia: Lea and Febiger.

Skinner, J., Hutsler, R., Bergsteinova, V., & Buskirk, E. (1973). The validity and reliability of the rating scale of perceived exertion. *Medicine and Science in Sports, 5,* 94–96.

Trombly, C. A. (1983). *Occupational therapy for physical dysfunction.* Baltimore: Williams & Wilkins.

West, W. L. (1984). A reaffirmed philosophy and practice of occupational therapy for the 1980s. *American Journal of Occupational Therapy, 38,* 15–23.

Chapter 54

Dual-Purpose Activity versus Single-Purpose Activity in Terms of Duration on Task, Exertion Level, and Affect

Lynette Miller, MS, OTR

David L. Nelson, PhD, OTR

This chapter was previously published in *Occupational Therapy in Mental Health*, 7, (1), 55–67. Copyright © 1987.

Historically, occupational therapy has been involved in a broad spectrum of therapeutic activities (Barris & Kielhofner, 1983). The strength of the occupational therapy profession lies in the integrative functions of activities that unite the mind, will, and body in doing (Cynkin, 1979). Occupational therapists use the term "purposeful activities" to describe activities that have an integrative function.

However, occupational therapists have different views of a working definition of purposeful activity. Reed (1984) defined purposeful activity as "the goal-directed use of a person's resources, time, energy, interest and attention" (p. 118). According to another source, "Activity becomes purposeful when the nature of and participation with the activity/event facilitates meaningful responses for the nervous system" (Gilfoyle, Grady & Moore, 1981, p. 135). Many other definitions exist of purposeful activities, but controversy arises when exercise is proposed to be included in the definition of purposeful activity.

Those occupational therapists who exclude exercise from the definition for purposeful activity do so on the basis that exercise tends not to produce adaptation as well as purposeful activity. King (1978) (see Chapter 8) believed that activities can produce adaptive responses that exercise cannot. Huss (1981) also expressed concern for the loss of adaptation when exercise is used for a treatment modality.

On the other hand, Trombly (1983a) and Yerxa (1967) have supported the inclusion of exercise in the definition of purposeful activities. Trombly (1982a, p. 467) argued three main points for the inclusion of exercise in purposeful activities.

1. Motor output that reflects any goal to move involves an internally organized plan to move and results in automatic activation of lower level circuits.
2. Most movement is consciously attended to (only postural changes which are reflex adjustments are unconscious and not attended to).
3. Voluntary movement is learned and therefore reflects purposefulness.

Yerxa (1967) also stated that exercise may be maximally productive for some individuals. Moreover, Trombly and Yerxa argued that exercise fulfills a need in the practice of occupational therapy.

The concept of dual-purpose activity proposed by Nelson (1984, p. 147) provides another context for discussing exercise and purposeful activity. Nelson stated that an activity often has two goals. For example, a client may mix cookies as part of therapy. In addition, the client may also seek a final product that can be eaten. Here there are two purposes or goals. The first is the exercise of the arm. The second is to make cookies. According to this analysis, pure exercise is indeed purposeful; however, single-purpose activity (exercise) can be distinguished from dual-purpose activity. Historically, occupational therapists have often used dual-purpose activities in their therapy. However, it is not clear that occupational therapists are necessarily involved in dual-purpose activity.

In choosing between dual-purpose and single-purpose activity, occupational therapists need data that dictate the relative benefits of the two approaches in different situations. However, little research has been done to prove the benefits of activities. As early as 1960, Reilly noted the need for research of activities. She stated, "For us, in occupational therapy, the most fundamental area of research is, and probably always will be, the nature and meaning of activity" (p. 208) (see Chapter 6). However, Fidler and Fidler (1978) (see Chapter 7) expressed the concern that our understanding of activities has remained limited. Trombly (1982a) also expressed concern for the need of research in the area of activities and exercise.

Concerning exercise, research studies have been done in respect to perceived exertion in the field of psychology (Ekblom & Goldberg, 1971; Pandolf, 1978). However, these studies do not compare exercise to the use of activities. In the occupational therapy literature, one study (Kircher, 1984) was done comparing exercise and exercise combined with an additional goal. Exercise alone was simulated by having the subject jump in place. Exercise with activity was simulated by having the subject jump rope. Kircher's guiding question was "whether purposeful activity provided intrinsic motivation to exercise performance" (p. 166). Kircher measured perceived exertion in terms of maximal heart rate, total exertion, and total exercise time. Kircher's results indicated that heart rate was significantly higher for individuals who participated in exercise combined with activity. Kircher discussed the possibility that exertion level was perceived to be less when activity was used in combination with exercise, and Kircher emphasized the importance of adaptive responses.

A postulate of occupational therapy is that the meanings of different types of activities vary according to the inherent characteristics of activity (Weston, 1960). Determining the meaning of the activity is a problem in using both single-purpose and dual-purpose activity. One way of measuring the meaningfulness of an activity for an individual is the use of Osgood's small-case semantic differential (Osgood, 1952). Several recent studies have used this set of scales to measure how individuals perceive different activities (Henry, Nelson & Duncombe, 1984; Shih, Nelson & Duncombe, 1983; Carter, Nelson & Duncombe, 1983). This instrument measures the affective meanings of evaluation, power, and action.

> *Evaluation* is defined as the factor of affective meaning that summarizes the degree to which a person feels positively or negatively about something. *Power* is the factor of affective meaning that summarizes the person's feelings in terms of the magnitude of the effect something potentially has on its environment. *Action* is the factor of affective meaning that represents the person's feelings about the degree of movement or volatility associated with something. (Nelson, Thompson & Moore, 1982, p. 382)

The present study compared dual-purpose activity to exercise. Often in a clinical setting, occupational therapists use cooking as a treatment modality. The process of mixing batter in a cooking activity may have two goals: exercise and a final edible product. Does this dual-purposefulness affect the exertion level, affect, and duration of the task in normal college students as compared to exercise alone? In other words, does the act of stirring cookie batter for the purpose of making cookies have benefits over stirring for the sake of exercise alone?

The following hypotheses are stated as expected outcomes:

1. Dual-purpose activity will be engaged in longer than exercise alone.
2. Dual-purpose activity will have a higher exertion level than exercise alone.
3. Dual-purpose activity will be perceived as higher on each factor of the Osgood semantic differential than exercise.

Method

Subjects

An available sample of 30 female Western Michigan University undergraduates was used. Males were not studied for two reasons. First, it seemed theoretically likely that men would respond differently to a cooking-related activity; and the study of this difference would have required a sample size that was impractical for the principal investigator. Second, the exercise involved might have been insufficiently challenging to some males, and they might not have believed that cookies needed as much stirring as they were able to give. There were 15 undergraduate occupational therapy students and fifteen undergraduate non-occupational therapy students used as subjects. Information concerning age and major in college was recorded at the time of the experiment.

Apparatus

A special mixing apparatus was constructed for this experiment. An aluminum 9.46 L cooking pot with lid was the container used. A shaft ran down the center of the pot and through the lid. The lid was secured during the experiment by a nut, and a wooden ball was placed at the top of the shaft. The purpose of the lid was to prevent the subject from viewing the contents of the container while stirring. In the lid was a 2.54 cm hole that was 5.04 cm from the edge of the lid. The hole allowed a metal spoon to fit through the lid for the purpose of stirring. Thus all revolutions made while stirring were comparable.

Instruments

These were the dependent variables: evaluation, power, action, duration, and exertion. The Osgood's short-form semantic differential (Osgood, May & Miron, 1975, p. 172) was used to assess the feelings of the subjects in relationship to exercise and exercise with a dual-purpose. Each subject was given the scale at the completion of the experimental procedure and was asked to fill out the form by placing an "X" on the continuum drawn as a line. The line was equally divided into seven sections. Each section could be scored by a corresponding number ranging from one to six. Each of the three factors of affective meaning results in scores with a possible range from 0 to 24.

In order not to distract the subject, the researcher sat off to the side and slightly behind the subject. The researcher used a stopwatch to determine the duration of time the subjects engaged in the activity. The researcher also counted the number of revolutions the subject made with the spoon during the experiment (this is the operational definition of exertion) by hand-scoring each revolution on a sheet of paper. Since the number of revolutions and duration of time were functions of strength, grasp strength was planned as a covariate for this study. A grasp dynamometer was used to assess grasp strength.

Procedure

The subjects were randomly divided into two groups, A or B. Each subject individually participated in the experimental procedure. The experimental procedure was conducted in an activity of daily living room of an occupational therapy teaching clinic. Every subject was given the grasp strength test upon entering the testing room. The subject was given two separate trials with a three minute rest period between each trial. The higher score was recorded (Trombly, 1982b).

Group A subjects stirred a substance for the purpose of exercise and making cookies. Group B subjects stirred the same substance for the purpose of exercise alone.

Neither group was allowed to see the contents of the mixing pot. The contents of the pot for both Group A and Group B consisted of the following: 145 ml shortening, 145 ml sugar, 1 egg, 280 ml flour, 5 ml soda, and 2.5 ml salt. However, the contents of Group A's pot contained 5 ml vanilla whereas Group B's pot contained 5 ml water. The vanilla was added to Group A's contents to make the substance smell like cookie batter. The purpose for having the same amount of liquid for both groups was to equalize the physiological resistance placed on both groups.

Group A was given added environmental stimuli to convince each subject that she was making cookies. Before the subject began to stir, a batch of fresh cookies was placed into the oven to bake. Homemade cookies were placed on the table in front of the subject, and the subject was allowed to eat the cookies. Group A subjects were told:

Activities are part of the practice of occupational therapy and are often used for rehabilitation purposes. Incorporated into this activity is an element of exercise, but you will also be participating in the process of making cookies by stirring the cookie batter. I am trying to determine the length of time and how hard a person will stir a substance for the therapeutic value of exercise and cookie making.

Group B did not receive any additional environmental stimulus. Only a verbal explanation of the purpose of this experiment was given. The subjects were told:

Exercise is part of the practice of occupational therapy and is often used for rehabilitation purposes. In this research project, I am trying to determine the length of time and how hard a person will stir a substance for the therapeutic value of exercise.

After telling the subjects the purpose of the experiment, the researcher gave specific instructions. The subjects were told to stir the contents of the pot with the dominant hand for as long as possible with a constant motion and without changing hands. The researcher demonstrated how to hold the mixing pot (on the lap stabilized by the non-dominant arm). Subjects were timed from the onset of stirring. Revolutions were counted as the spoon made a complete rotation. At the completion of the stirring process, the subjects were given instructions for filling out the Osgood's short-form semantic differential. The researcher then recorded duration and exertion data on a prepared form. The subject was instructed not to discuss the experimental procedure with other students who might be in the study.

Results

A two-way analysis of variance (type of exercise X type of student major) was done on each dependent variable. Since grip strength did not correlate significantly with any of the dependent variables, it was not needed as a covariate.

Osgood's Factors of Affective Meaning

The dual-purpose activity was evaluated significantly higher than exercise, $F(1,26) = 14.3$, $p < .001$. There was also a main effect for student majors on this variable. Non-occupational therapy students generally rated both the dual-purpose activity and the exercise higher than occupational therapy students, $F(1,26) = 5.2, p < .05$. This difference between subject groups does not detract from the meaningfulness of the difference between dual-purpose activity and exercise. Occupational therapy students evaluated dual-purpose higher than exercise and so did non-occupational therapy students. See Table 1.

Exertion and Duration

The difference between dual-purpose activity and exercise in terms of exertion approached significance at the .05 level, $F(1,26) = 4.1, p = .052$. There was no significant difference on duration. See Table 2.

There were positive significant correlations between duration and exertion on the one hand and the affective meanings of evaluation, power, and action on the other hand. This was true across all subjects, regardless of group.

Discussion

This study supported the hypothesis that dual-purpose activity was perceived greater on the evaluation scale of the Osgood's short-form semantic differential scale than exercise. Exertion level differences approached significance. These results support the finding by Kircher (1984) that activity with an added purpose may be more motivating to a patient/client than exercise alone. However, further research is needed to determine all the implications of dual-purpose activities for various tasks in different populations. Though this study's results

Table 1
Perceived Evaluation, Power, and Action By Group Across Majors of Students (the Possible Range is from 0 to 24)

Variable		Dual-Purpose (Group A)	Exercise (Group B)
Evaluation	M	16.2*	11.1
	SD	3.9	4.4
	n	15	15
Power	M	12.9	13.3
	SD	2.8	3.4
	n	15	15
Action	M	13.4	12.6
	SD	3.7	2.2
	n	15	15

Note.   *Significantly greater than the exercise group at the .001 level.

Table 2
Duration and Exertion Level Across Student Majors

Variable		Dual-Purpose (Group A)	Exercise (Group B)
Exertion	M	103.3*	77.07
	SD	67.3	54.2
	n	15	15
Duration	M	233.4	141.07
	SD	169.3	87.4
	n	15	15

Note.   *$p = .052$ that the two means are equal

cannot be automatically generalized to clinical populations, this study and that of Kircher provide a starting point for theory-building and for research with clinical populations.

The findings provide theoretical support for the importance placed on dual-purpose activities in occupational therapy practice. The cookie group felt more positively toward the activity than the exercise group. If an individual perceives an activity more positively he/she may participate more vigorously in the treatment process.

Another finding in this study was that the higher the value placed on the activity, the more work was done and the more active the individual was during the activity. This was true for both the exercise group and the cookie group. This statement is supported by the positive correlations between exertion, duration, evaluation, power, and action. The value one places on an activity may determine in part the benefits one may gain from that activity. Other factors also should be considered in the analysis of an activity, such as the individual meaning held by the activity. Further research is needed to determine how the value of an activity affects the treatment process in occupational therapy.

The finding that the non-occupational therapy students evaluated both activities higher than the occupational therapy students was not expected. The reason for this phenomenon is unclear, and it may be due to chance alone. The presence of non-occupational therapy students is a methodological improvement over studies involving occupational therapy students alone. Regardless of the reasons for the difference between student groups, the important thing is that both groups preferred the dual-purpose activity to the single-purpose exercise. This enhances the generalizability of the findings.

It is difficult to interpret statistics that closely approach the designated alpha level. As Ottenbacher (1984) has discussed, those adhering to the decision-making school of statistics do not reject the null hypothesis if

$p = .052$ (as in this study) but would reject the null if $p = .049$. Other statisticians find this categorical approach overly rigid. The approach taken in this study is to alert the reader that a p of .052 is *approaching* statistical significance at the .05 level. Such a finding should be interpreted with caution but should not be ignored. Further studies with more subjects may well confirm the difference.

Despite the importance of dual-purpose activity, it is important to recognize that certain highly motivating dual-purpose exercise activities may in some instances be contraindicated. For a client with a cardiac condition the physiological stress of a dual-purpose exercise activity may be too strenuous. While mixing of cookie batter places relatively little physiological stress on an individual, gross motor games may be too stressful for certain individuals. It is also acknowledged that single-purpose exercise can and does have beneficial qualities. Some individuals may prefer a single-purpose activity.

The main limitation of this study was that the principal investigator was present during the experiment. The optimum experimental procedure would have used a naive individual to gather the data and conduct the experimental procedures. However, this was not practical. Standardized procedures were used in both groups to prevent experimental bias.

The same instrument (the mixing pot) was used for both experimental groups to provide equal physiological stress for all subjects. This relates to a criticism of Kircher's research study. As Kasch (1985) stated, the difference between jumping in place and jumping rope may not be due to internal motivation as much as to the fact that jumping rope is a more strenuous activity involving the upper extremities as well as the lower extremities. The present study controlled for this by making both activities identical in terms of motor requirements.

This study has also shown that dual-purpose activity is not restricted to the task studied by Kircher (1984). As occupational therapists, we must be careful not to generalize findings from one task context to another. The appropriate way to deal with this is to conduct parallel experiments on different tasks. Future research might also examine the following questions:

1. Do other dual-purpose activities have an increased benefit over single-purpose activities, and if so, for which populations?
2. When is exercise the optimal treatment technique?
3. How does affective meaning change with different populations and different tasks?
4. How do different environmental factors influence affective meaning?
5. Are there identifiable differences between sexes in terms of purposefulness?

Conclusion

Dual-purpose activity has a long and central place in occupational therapy history, but little systematic research has been done on this basic phenomenon. The practice of occupational therapy should be based on theory that is well-grounded by research. Group research deals with generalities. But each client is unique, and the dual-purpose activity should be tailored for individual needs. The individualized incorporation of dual-purpose activities is left up to the creativity of the occupational therapist.

References

American Psychological Association. (1983). *Publication Manual of the American Psychological Association* (3rd ed.). Washington, DC: Author.

Barris. R., Keilhofner. F., & Waits. J. H. (1983). *Psychological occupational therapy: Practice in a pluralistic area.* Laurel, MD: RAMSCO Publishing Co.

Carter. B. A., Nelson, D. L., & Duncombe, L. W. (1983). The effect of psychological type on the mood and meaning of two college activities. *The American Journal of Occupational Therapy, 37,* 688–693.

Cynkin. S. (1979). *Occupational therapy: Towards health through activities.* Boston: Little, Brown & Co.

Ekblom, B., & Goldberg, A. N. (1971). The influence of physical training and other factors on the subjective rating of perceived exertion. *Acta Physiology Scandanavia, 83,* 399–406.

Fidler, G. S., & Fidler, J. W. (1978). Doing and becoming: Purposeful action and self-actualization. *The American Journal of Occupational Therapy, 32,* 305–310. (Reprinted as Chapter 7).

Gilfoyle, E. M., Grady, A. P., & Moore, J. C. (1981). *Children adapt.* Thorofare, New Jersey: Charles B. Slack. Inc.

Henry, A. D., Nelson, D. L. & Duncombe, L. W. (1984). Choice making in group and individual activity. *The American Journal of Occupational Therapy. 38,* 245–251.

Huss, J. (1981). From kinesiology to adaptation. *The American Journal of Occupational Therapy, 35,* 574–580.

Kasch, M. C. (1985). Motivation and activity. *The American Journal of Occupational Therapy, 39,* 114–115.

King, L. J. (1978). Toward a science of adaptive responses. *The American Journal of Occupational Therapy, 32,* 429–437. (Reprinted as Chapter 8).

Kircher, M. A. (1984). Motivation as a factor of perceived exertion in purposeful versus nonpurposeful activity. *The American Journal of Occupational Therapy, 38,* 165 –170,

Nelson, D. L. (1984). *Children with autism and other pervasive disorders of development and behavior: Therapy through activities.* Thorofare, New Jersey: Charles B. Slack.

Nelson, D. L., Thompson, G., & Moore, J. (1982). Identification of factors of affective meaning in four selective activities. *The American Journal of Occupational Therapy, 36,* 381–387.

Osgood, C. E. (1952). The nature and measurement of meaning. *Psychological Bulletin, 49*(3), 197–237.

Osgood, C. E., May, W. H., & Miron, M. J. (1975). *Cross-cultural universe of affective meaning.* Chicago: University of Illinois Press.

Ottenbacher, K. & York, J. (1984). Strategies for evaluating clinical change: Implications for practice and research. *The American Journal of Occupational Therapy. 38,* 647–659.

Pandolf, K. B. (1980). Influences of local and central factors in domination rated perceived exertion during physical work. *Perceptual Motor Skills, 46,* 683–689.

Reilly, M. (1960). Occupational therapy can be one of the great ideas of 20th century medicine. *American Journal of Occupational Therapy, 16,* 2–9. (Reprinted as Chapter 6).

Shing-Ru Shih, L., Nelson, D. L. & Duncombe, L. W. (1984). Mood and affect following success and failure in two cultural groups. *Occupational Therapy Journal of Research, 4,* 213–230.

Trombly, C. A. (1982a). Include exercise in "purposeful activity". *The American Journal of Occupational Therapy, 36,* 467–468.

Trombly, C. A. (1982b). *Occupational therapy for physical dysfunction* (2nd ed.) Baltimore: Waverly Press. Inc.

Weston, D. L. (1960). Therapeutic crafts. *The American Journal of Occupational Therapy, 14,* 121–123.

Yerxa, E. (1967). Authentic occupational therapy. *The American Journal of Occupational Therapy, 21,* 2.

Chapter 55

Adding Purpose to the Repetitive Exercise of Elderly Women through Imagery

Christine M. Riccio
David L. Nelson, PhD, OTR
Mary Ann Bush

This chapter was previously published in the *American Journal of Occupational Therapy*, *44*, 714–719. Copyright © 1990, American Occupational Therapy Association

Imagery is an internal psychological process involving the evocation of the physical characteristics of objects or events that are absent from the perceptual field (Denis, 1985). A person can form a mental image of an object, such as a flower, for example, even when no flower is physically present. Likewise, a person can form a mental image of an event, such as picking a flower, even though no movement is actually taking place. Paivio (1985, p. 26) stated that imagery depends either on "memory for a specific performance episode" or on "general knowledge of performance skills in appropriate situations." It is important to recognize that a person can have an image of an event without actually having experienced or witnessed that specific event. One can imagine picking up a snake, for example, without ever having actually done so. In the construction of this image, general knowledge of snakes is integrated with general knowledge of the act of picking things up.

The relationship between imagery and human movement has been the topic of many studies in the disciplines of physical education, sports psychology, and movement. In these studies, imagery is elicited through protocols encouraging mental practice (i.e., symbolic rehearsal or introspective visualization) to enhance a motor skill or strength. A typical experimental design involves a comparison of three conditions: imagery-based mental practice, actual physical practice, and a control condition. Examples of motor skills that have been enhanced experimentally through mental practice include ring tossing (Twining, 1949), basketball shots (Clark, 1960), gymnastic moves (Jones, 1965), dart throwing (Wichman & Lizotte, 1983), and golf putting (Woolfolk, Parrish, & Murphy, 1985). An example of a study that used imagery to test strength was performed by Tynes and McFatter (1987). A meta-analysis of 60 studies (Feltz & Landers, 1982) has indicated that the use of imagery is particularly efficacious in the promotion of skills requiring cognition but is also somewhat effective in promoting strength.

Physical therapists Fansler, Poff, and Shepard (1985) investigated mental practice by studying a basic component of normal movement: equilibrium. Elderly women in their study were assigned to three experimental conditions: mental practice involving vivid images, progressive relaxation, and a control condition involving nonsensical instructions requiring the subject's attention. The results tended in the direction of improvement after mental practice, but the statistical comparison of the three conditions' improvement scores was nonsignificant (perhaps because of high subject-to-subject variance). The authors urged the future study and use of mental practice in the rehabilitation of elderly persons and other populations.

According to wide-ranging literature reviewed by Bortz (1982), elderly persons have special needs for physical exercise because physical inactivity tends to results in the deterioration of several of the body's biological systems. Mobily (1982) showed that a lack of exercise among elderly persons also tends to be associated with psychosocial problems. Cantu (1980) is among those who have described specific exercises for the elderly that promote flexibility, coordination and agility, balance, muscular strength, and endurance. As Mobily pointed out, however, elderly people are frequently unmotivated to exercise.

Clinicians have often employed imagery to motivate repetitive exercise patterns in elderly patients. Caplow-Linder, Harpaz, and Samberg (1979) stated that many geriatric groups respond well to suggestions such as, "Stretch your arms up as if you're touching the stars." Ross and Burdick (1981) encouraged group members to act out images related to gardening (e.g., spading the ground, raking, pulling weeds) or winter actions (e.g., shoveling snow, throwing snowballs, ice skating) while exercising. Lewis (1987) elicited exercise by urging her elderly, immobile clients to "push the water away" or to pretend to be various animals with characteristic movements. The use of this type of imagery-based instruction in the absence of materials is also a common feature of exercise groups for well persons of various ages.

But how does this use of imagery relate to the theoretical constructs of the profession of occupational therapy? Nelson and Peterson (1989) suggested that occupation can be categorized as (a) naturalistic, (b) simulated, or (c) imagery-based. Occupational therapists frequently employ simulated environments (e.g., hospital-based therapeutic kitchens) to enhance future performance in naturalistic environments (e.g., the patient's home kitchen). The distinction between imagery-based occupation and simulated occupation is that verbal or pictorial cues referring to absent materials are used to elicit imagery-based occupation, whereas props are used in simulated occupation.

In imagery-based occupation, the occupational form is the verbalization or picture within the environmental context. The person finds meaning in the occupational form depending on memories of past occupations. Given meaning and the development of purpose, occupational performance occurs (see Figure 1).

In the present study, for example, one of the occupational forms was the verbalization, "Stretch your arms up one at a time as if you're picking apples." We predicted that this form would then to be meaningful to the research subjects. Meaning, however, is an individual matter dependent on a particular person's developmental structure. A person could conceivably come to this occupation with the loathing of apple picking on the basis of experience (i.e., negative adaptations due to past occupations). We predicted that, generally speaking, most research subjects would be favorably disposed to the apple-picking imagery. We further predicted that this verbalization would have the type of meaning that would add purpose to the subjects' performance.

To test this prediction, we compared the subjects' occupational performance (exercise repetitions) in the imagery-eliciting condition to their occupational performance in a suitable control condition. The control condition was called rote exercise, a term used by Nelson and Peterson (1989) to describe repetitive exercise done without any special added purpose. We reasoned that if statistically significant differences could be documented between these two conditions, then the apple-picking prompt probably had meaning and added purpose. We also predicted that exercise repetitions would be increased in a different, subsequent occupation, in which the subjects were instructed to reach down as if picking up dropped coins, compared with a rote exercise of reaching down.

Methods

Subjects

The Parachek Geriatric Rating Scale (Parachek & King, 1976) was administered as a screening device to

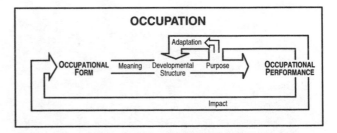

Figure 1. The dynamics of occupation. From "Occupation: Form and Performance" by D. L. Nelson, 1988, *American Journal of Occupational Therapy, 42,* p. 637 (see Chapter 41).

female volunteers residing in a nursing home, a residential retirement home, and foster care home. The Parachek scale determines the overall functional level of potential subjects in three categories: (a) physical capabilities, (b) self-care skills, and (c) social interaction skills (Parachek & King, 1976). Those persons who demonstrated sufficient physical and communication skills by obtaining a score of 25 or more on the Parachek scale were eligible for the study. Persons scoring 25 to 39 points show awareness of their surrounding, recognition of staff members, some concern for their own care, and increased awareness and capability in group activities organized by an occupational therapist. Persons scoring 40 to 50 points are generally independent in self-care, are self-motivating, and benefit well from an occupational therapy program consisting of various activities.

On the basis of this screening tool, 30 female subjects were selected; 2 subjects, however, did not participate in both conditions of the study because of conflicting appointments, and another subject refused to participate in both conditions. These 3 were excluded from the study, leaving 27 subjects. The subjects' ages ranged from 62 to 96 years, with a mean age of 80.9 years (SD = 9.2). The mean Parachek scale score of the sample was 44.70 points (SD = 4.85).

Procedure

The subjects were randomly assigned to different orders in accordance with a counterbalanced design. In Order 1 (n = 12), the subject received the control condition first and the imaging condition second. These conditions were reversed for the subjects in Order 2 (n = 15).

In the rote exercise condition, the subjects were told that the researcher (the first author) was interested in the kinds of exercises women over 62 years of age like to do and that they would be asked to do two exercises. They were then given the following instructions for the reaching-up exercise:

Today we are going to exercise our arms. Listen to all of the directions first. I will demonstrate the exercise and give you a chance to try a few. First, stretch your arms up one at a time. Reach all the way up with your right arm, then place it in your lap. When your right arm touches your lap, reach all he way up with your left arm, then put it in your lap. Repeat with your right arm. Watch me. Now you try a few. When I tell you to begin, do as many as you can without becoming too tired. Stop when you are too tired. Ready? Begin.

When the subjects stopped, they were told to rest for a few minutes and take some deep breaths. Next the researcher continued with instructions for the reaching-down exercise:

Now we are going to do another exercise. Listen to all of the directions first. Reach all the way down with both of your hands. Bring both hands back up and touch your lap. Watch me. Now you try a few. When I tell you to begin, do as many as you can without becoming too tired. Stop when you are too tired. Ready? Begin.

As in the rote-exercise condition, in the added-purpose (imagery-based) condition the subjects were told that the researcher was interested in the kinds of exercises women over 62 years of age like to do and that they would be asked to do two exercises. They were then given the following instructions for the reaching-up exercise:

Today we are going to exercise our arms. Listen to all of the directions first. I will demonstrate the exercise and give you a chance to try a few. First, stretch your arms up one at a time as if you are picking apples. Reach all the way up with your right arm, pick an apple, then place it in a basket on your lap. When your right arm puts the apple in the basket, reach all the way up with your left arm, pick another apple, then place it in the basket. Repeat with your right arm. Watch me. Now you try a few. When I tell you to begin, pick as many apples as you can without becoming too tired. Stop when you are too tired. Ready? Begin.

When the subjects stopped, they were told to rest for a few minutes and to take some deep breaths. Then the researcher continued:

Now we are going to do another exercise. Reach all the way down with both of your hands as if you are picking up some coins you have dropped. Bring both hands back up and put the coins in your lap. Watch me. Now you try a few. When I tell you to begin, pick up as many coins as you can without becoming too tired. Stop when you are too tired. Ready? Begin.

The researcher remained in a chair approximately 1.7 m away from and facing the subjects throughout the proceedings. If a subject asked when she could stop or how many exercises she should do, the instruction of "Stop when you are tired" was repeated. For both conditions, the procedure took place in the dayroom of the premises or in the residents' rooms (each subject's setting was the same for both conditions).

The researcher measured the frequency and duration or exercise repetitions. A repetition in the reaching-up exercise was defined as the raising of a hand over the top of the head and the placing of that hand in the lap. A repetition in the reaching-down exercise was defined as the movement of both hands to ankle length or lower and the placing of both hands in the lap. Interobserver reliability was confirmed by an independent observer, who observed 11 subjects. The independent observer sat to the side of the researcher and approximately 1.7 m from the subject. The researcher and the independent observer kept their stopwatches out of each other's sight, and the operation of the stopwatches was inaudible. The silent count of repetitions (frequency) was necessarily independent. We determined reliability by dividing the smaller number by the larger number for each subject, by multiplying the result by 100, and by taking the mean across the 11 subjects dually observed. In the reaching-up exercise, interobserver reliability was 98.5% (frequency) and 97.3% (duration). In the reaching-down exercise, interobserver reliability was 99.4% (frequency) and 97.6% (duration).

Results

As is often the case when the dependent variable involves a frequency count (Neter, Wasserman, & Kutner, 1985), the data were positively skewed. Therefore, nonparametric statistics were used. Additionally, as expected, within each type of exercise, frequency was highly correlated with duration. Because frequency and duration cannot be assumed to be independent, only frequency was analyzed through inferential statistics (see Table 1).

Reaching-up exercise. Preliminary Mann Whitney U tests were done to test for possible order effects in terms of frequency; none was found (for the imaging condition, $U = 57$, $p = .11$; for the rote exercise condition, $U = 77$, $p = .52$). The Wilcoxon matched-pairs signed rank tests confirmed our hypothesis that the subjects would exercise more in the imaging condition than in the rote exercise condition [$z = 2.25$, p (one-tailed) = .012].

Reaching-down exercise. Preliminary Mann Whitney U tests computed to test for possible order effects revealed that the 12 subjects randomly assigned to Order 1 scored higher than the 15 subjects randomly assigned to Order 2 for both the imagining condition ($U = 40.5$, $p = .016$) and the rote exercise condition ($U = 46.5$, $p = .033$). Possibly, subjects in Order 1 did not tire as quickly as those in Order 2. Given this qualification, the Wilcoxon matched-pairs signed rank test of the hypothesis resulted in $z = 1.60$, p (one-tailed) = .055.

Discussion

The results for the reaching-up exercise are clear and support the study's hypothesis. The results for the reaching-down exercise are not so clear due to (a) differences between randomly assigned order groups and (b) the difficulty in interpreting a probability level that closely approaches but does not pierce the traditional .05 level. As shown in Table 1, however, the mean levels of performance tended to be in the direction of favoring the imaging condition in both the reaching-down and reaching-up exercises. Future research that replicates the reaching-down design, independent of the reaching-up design, would be desirable.

Table 1
Differences in Frequency and Duration Between the Imaging and Control Conditions for Two Exercises (N = 27)

Outcome Measures	Condition	
	Imaging	Rote Exercise
Reaching-up Exercise		
Frequency (no. of repetitions)		
M	38.44	20.67
SD	42.94	38.85
Median	19.00	15.00
Mean rank	14.90	11.90
($z = 2.25$, $p = .012$)		
Duration (sec)		
M	84.78	60.93
SD	85.46	84.96
Median	59.00	35.00
Reaching-down Exercise		
Frequency (no. of repetitions)		
M	20.11	15.89
SD	17.16	16.11
Median	15.00	10.00
Mean rank	12.70	10.70
($z = 1.60$, $p = .055$)		
Duration (sec)		
M	66.15	53.30
SD	53.35	46.34
Median	48.00	36.00

Note. The nonparametric Wilcoxon matched-pairs signed rank test was used to compute one-tailed z scores.

The subjects' spontaneous verbalizations after the exercise were generally consistent with the statistical findings. They responded to the imaging conditions with statements such as "My apple tree is plentiful," "I will have to go to another tree when I finish here," and "I used to pick apples" for the reaching-up exercise and "I have enough coins to go to Detroit now" and "I will be rich pretty soon" for the reaching-down exercise. In the control condition, the subjects replied with comments such as "This is silly" or "I'm not tired, but I want to stop."

The unambiguous results for the reaching-up exercise and, to a lesser extent, the results for the reaching-down exercise suggest important implications for occupational therapy theory. First, this study documents another approach by which the therapist can add purpose to needed exercise. The use of occupation to encourage therapeutic exercise is one of the oldest traditions within the profession of occupational therapy. For example, Baldwin (1919) postulated that therapeutic exercise is especially beneficial when done within the context of everyday occupations and descried this idea as a basic principle of occupational therapy. Fidler and Fidler (1978) (see Chapter 7) provided a theoretical link between imagery and purpose. They wrote how action leading to achievement can be thought of as "the *product* of a mental image that sets an objective" (p. 307), In other words, mental imagery adds purpose to occupation.

Eight recent research articles (Bloch, Smith, & Nelson, 1989; Heck, 1988; Kircher, 1984, Miller & Nelson, 1987 |see Chapter 54|; Mullins, Nelson & Smith, 1987, Steinbeck, 1986 |see Chapter 53|; Thibodeaux & Ludwig, 1988; Yoder, Nelson & Smith, 1989) have investigated how purpose can be added to encourage movement. The present study is similar to these projects in that an occupational form is used to add purpose to therapeutic exercise. It differs, however, in that, whereas the occupational forms in the previous studies relied on materials as well as verbal instruction to simulate an occupational situation, the present study relied on verbal instruction only. We showed in the present study that physical materials (e.g., the apples described in the instructions) are not always necessary in order to create an occupational form eliciting added purpose. As Paivio (1985) stated, language is an efficient and accurate way of eliciting imagery, which, in turn can guide human movement.

To what extent is imagery involved even when materials are physically present in the occupational form? To explore this question, let us consider the hypothetical example of an occupational form consisting of some modeling clay, and let us further assume that this occupational form elicited occupational performance resulting in a sculpture in the shape of a cat. Here we have no verbal instructions, but almost certainly the person who encountered the clay experienced mental images of cats or remembered pictures o cats before completing the sculpture. We can thus theorize that imagery may well have been involved in all eight of the studies cited above. The occupations examined n these studies were rope jumping (Bloch, et al., 1989, Kircher, 1984), a table tennis game and the drilling of holes to make a game board (Steinbeck, 1986),(see Chapter 53), the sanding of a cutting board (Thibodeaux & Ludwig, 1988), the drawn reproduction of a design (Heck, 1988), the stenciling of a design (Mullins et al., 1987), and the stirring of cookie dough (Miller & Nelson, 1987 (see Chapter 54), Yoder et al., 1989) Mental images on the part of the research subjects may have been involved in all of these studies. The subjects imagery was not ruled out in any of the studies. Although all occupation does not necessarily involve imagery, we believe that imagery is involved in much developmentally advance complex occupation, particular occupation that depends on subjects' memories of occupation.

These theoretical ideas have substantial implications for future occupational therapy research. Self-reports of imagery could serve as dependent variables in studies of occupation. As Fidler and Fidler (1978) (see Chapter 7) asserted, imagery not only adds purpose to action but also is the result of action. The characteristics of self-reported imagery could be studied in relationship to the characteristics of motor performance. Furthermore, it seems reasonable to expect differences across populations and individuals in terms of imagery Other suggestions for future research related to the present study are (a) a comparison of verbally elicited imagery to materials-elicited imagery to a control condition of rote exercise in terms of exercise repetitions and (b) a study of the effect of imagery on additional dependent variables, such as the development or regaining of motor skills or other qualities of movement. Future research might also attempt to overcome a limitation in the present study, namely, that the first author of the study also served as the administrator of the independent variable.

The literature on imagery also has implications for occupational therapy practice. Descriptive phrases that begin with "Try it as if ..." or "Imagine that ..." could be used to guide movement and enhance performance. When using therapeutic exercise to improve a client's coordination, for example, the therapist could introduce rhythmic images, such as a see-saw, rocking horse, or cross-country skier. Additionally, the therapist could use such images as the swinging of a golf club or the imitating of the sun's pattern across the sky to promote full range of motion. Imagery could also be use din sensory integrative therapy to help children or psychiatric patients explore different movement qualities. By encouraging patients to imagine or act out stories, vocations, the functions of inanimate objects, or the behavioral patterns of animals, the therapist can elicit varied qualities of speed, shape, directions, or range of movement and promote relaxation, postural flexibility, and coordination,. The therapist may also employ imagery for the development and practice of self-care, work, or leisure skills. Imaging actual occupations such as shaving may facilitate strength and endurance as well as the learning of this specific movement pattern.

Vivid images of well-remembered events are considered the best for eliciting skilled movement, according to Paivio (1985). The use of imagery has several advantages in clinical use. First , the therapist is not restricted by materials that are difficult to obtain. Second, verbally elicited imagery may be more gradeable (e.g., in terms of range) than physical materials when the therapist tires to elicit specific movements. Third, imagery may be used in combination with standard equipment associated with rote exercise (e.g., the rowing machine). Finally, imagery has the power to communicate complex events. The therapist's saying "Imagine picking up a robin's egg" is a more efficient communication than an attempt to describe the complex finger and hand movements involved in performing that action.

The use of imagery outside of the context of physical materials, however, can have disadvantages in certain situations. The patient's image, memory, or both, on which imagery is based, may be incorrect. Even if the image is correct, the movement might still be faulty because of an inability to match intention to performance. For example, the person might believe that a particle movement would be effective in holding an egg, whereas a real egg would be crushed or dropped.. In other words, imagery does not provide knowledge of results, one of the frequent advantages of naturalistic, malleable occupational forms. Additionally, some populations might have special difficulties in experiencing mental images. Future research will help clinicians choose between the use of physical materials, imagined materials, and rote exercise.

Conclusion

This study presents a beginning stp in the consideration of the potential uses of imagery in occupational therapy. We have introduced a way to enhance purposefulness and occupational performance without the use of physical materials. The verbal and nonverbal forms that elicit imagery have important theoretical, research, and clinical implications, specifically regarding therapeutic exercise.

Acknowledgements

We thank Jackie Knapp, activity director and social work designee of Brookhaven Care Facility, Kalamazoo, Michigan; Donna Jones, Administrative assistant of Park Place Manor, Kalamazoo, Michigan; and Jean VanderSteen, activity director of Park Village Pines, Kalamazoo, Michigan, for their interest and cooperation. We also thank Karen Palmer Milbourne, OTR, and Anne Rogers, OTR, for their assistance with data collection.

References

Baldwin, B.T. (1919). Occupational therapy applied to restoration of function of disabled joints. *Walter Reed Hospital Monograph* (pp. 5-6). Washington, DC.

Bloch, M.W., Smith, D.A. & Nelson, D.L. (1989). Hearty rate, activity, duration, and affect in added-purpose versus single-purpose jumping activities. *American Journal of Occupational Therapy, 43*, 25-30.

Biortz, W.M. (1982). Disuse and aging. *Journal of the American Medical Association, 248*, 1203-1208.

Cantu, R.C. (1980). *Toward fitness: Guided exercise for those with health problems.* New York: Human Sciences.

Caplow-Linder, E., Harpaz, L., & Samberg, S. (1979). *Therapeutic dance/movement: Expressive activities for older adults.* New York: Human Sciences.

Clark, L.V. (1980). Effect of mental practice on the development of certain motor skill. *Research Quarterly, 31*, 560-569.

Danis, M. (1985). Visual imagery and the use of mental practice in the development of motor skills. *Canadian Journal of Applied Sports Sciences, 10*, 4S-16S.

Fansler, C., Poff, C., & Shepard, K. (1985). Effects of mental practice on balance in elderly women. *Physical Therapy, 65*, 1332-1337.

Feltz, D.L., & Landers, D.M. (1982). The effects of mental practice on motor skill learning and performance: A meta-analysis. *Journal of Sport Psychology, 5*, 25-67.

Fidler, G.S., & Fidler, J.W. (1978). Doing and becoming Purposeful action and self-actualization. *American Journal of Occupational Therapy, 32*, 305-310.

Heck. S.A. (1988). The effect of purposeful activity on pain tolerance. *American Journal of Occupational Therapy, 42*, 577-581.

Jones, J.G. (1985). Motor learning without demonstration of physical practice, under two conditions of mental practice. *Research Quarterly, 36*, 270-276.

Kircher, M.A. (1984). Motivations as a factor of perceived exertion in purposeful versus nonpurposeful activity. *American Journal of Occupational Therapy, 38*, 165-170.

Lewis, C.B. (1987, December 15). *Dysmobility of the elderly: Evaluation and treatment* [Video conference]. Pittsburgh: American Rehabilitation Education Network.

Miller, L. & Nelson, D.L. (1987). Dual-purpose activity versus single-purpose activity in terms of duration on tasks, exertion level and affect. *Occupational Therapy in Mental Health, 7*, 55-67 (Reprinted as Chapter 54).

Mobly, K. (1982). Motivational aspects of exercise for the elderly: Barriers and solutions. *Physical and Occupational Therapy in Geriatrics, 1* (4), 43-53.

Mullins, C.S., Nelson, D.L., & Smith, D.A., (1987). Exercise through dual-purpose activity in the institutionalized elderly. *Physical and Occupational Therapy in Geriatrics, 5* (3) 29-38.

Nelson, D.L., (1988). Occupational: Form and performance. *American Journal of Occupational Therapy, 42*, 633-641. (Reprinted as Chapter 41).

Nelson, D.L., & Peterson, C.Q. (1989). Enhancing therapeutic exercise through purposeful activity: A theoretic analysis. *Topics in Geriatric Rehabilitation, 4* (4), 12-22.

Nieter, J., Wasserman, W., & Kutner, M.H. (1985). *Applied linear statistical models* (2nd ed.). Homewood, IL: Richard D. Irwin.

Paivio, A. (1985). Cognitive and motivational functions of imagery in human performance. *Canadian Journal of Applied Sports Sciences, 10,* 22S-28S.

Parachek, J.F., & King, L.J. (1976). *Parachek Geriatric-Rating Scale* (2nd ed.). Scottsdale, AZ: Greenroom.

Ross, M., & Burdock, D. (1981). *Sensory integration: a training manual for therapists and teachers for regressed, psychiatric and geriatric patient groups.* Thorofare, NJ: Slack.

Steinbeck, T.M. (1986). Purposeful activity and performance. *American Journal of Occupational Therapy, 40,* 529-534. (Reprinted as Chapter 53).

Thibodeaux, C.S., & Ludwig, Ferol M. (1988). Intrinsic motivation in product-oriented and non-product oriented activities. *American Journal of Occupational Therapy, 42,* 169-175.

Twining, W.E. (1949). Mental practice and physical practice in learning a motor skill. *Research Quarterly, 20,* 432-435.

Tynes, L.L. & McFatter, R.M. (1987). The efficacy of "psyching" strategies on a weight-lifting task. *Cognitive Therapy and Research, 11,* 327-336.

Wichman, H., & Lizotta, P. (1983). Effects of mental practice and locus of control on performance of dart throwing. *Perceptual and Motor Skills, 56,* 807-812.

Woolfolk, R.L., Parrish, M.W., & Murphy, S.M. (1985). The affects of positive and negative imagery on motor skill performance. *Cognitive Therapy and Research, 9,* 335-341.

Yoder, R.M., Nelson, D.L., & Smith, D.A. (1989). Added-purpose versus rote exercise in female nursing home residents. *American Journal of Occupational Therapy, 43,* 581-586.

Chapter 56

Affective Responses to Keeping and Not Keeping an Activity Product

Janice Dale Rocker, MS, OTR, CHT
David L. Nelson, PhD, OTR

Activity, or what Fidler and Fidler (1978) (see Chapter 7) called "doing," is a primary concern in occupational therapy. Cynkin (1979) stated that craft activities, which are adaptable and versatile, have played an important role in occupational therapy programs because they simulate situations encountered in the real world.

Sometimes occupational therapists may overlook the whole person if they concentrate more on the necessity that an activity meet certain treatment requirements than on the activity's meaningfulness and purposefulness to the patient (Allard, 1964). In 1981, Bissell and Mailloux explored the role crafts have played both in the history of the profession and in current practice by sampling 250 U.S. occupational therapists specializing in physical disabilities. The authors concluded that "overall, the occupational therapists surveyed seemed to stress the physical aspects of therapy with less emphasis on the psychological and social domains of treatment" (p. 374). Cynkin (1979) pointed out that whereas technical excellence improves physical rehabilitation, an excessively technical focus "negates what is essentially the strength of occupational therapy: the integrative function of activities that unite the mind, will, and body in doing" (p. 8).

In some clinics, therapeutic activity involves the creation of a product which the patient is not always allowed to keep. For example, it is common practice to recycle materials. In addition, clinics serving chronically disabled patients often have their patients create products to be sold at bazaars for institutional benefit. Other institutions place formal or informal restrictions on patient property. What effect does keeping or not keeping an activity product have on the person who created the product? Although the variable of "keeping" has not been directly studied, this issue relates to several principles of normal human development and occupational therapy.

The occupational behavior model (Kielhofner, Burke, & Igi, 1980) stresses that a disabled person tends to experience imbalances among volition, habituation, and performance subsystems. If a patient cannot do what is valued because of physical or mental limitations, he or she probably senses a loss of independence. The occupational therapist must counteract this.

A sense of independence develops, in part, from being able to make and carry out decisions. Kielhofner and Burke (1980) noted the importance of a sense of personal causation. If a patient expects to keep a hand-crafted product and is persuaded not to (or denied this opportunity), he or she might sense a loss of control over the environment, which might reinforce dependence and feelings of powerlessness. In contrast, if able to keep the activity product, the patient receives concrete, ongoing feedback on mastery. In adapting to a disability, a patient must reexplore and remaster the world (Kielhofner, 1980). Craft activities provide opportunities to do this.

Denying patients their activity products has additional possible negative effects. Patients might become hostile if the products have potential utility in everyday life. Also, not being able to keep a product violates expectations: People have learned that they are able to keep whatever they make in most situations outside of formal work. A person who has lost mental or physical functions might need to be able to count on fulfillment of expectations. A fourth possibility is that a patient might feel that the object made has personal symbolic meanings. If so, discarding or dismantling the object is a personal affront or loss.

Mosey (1973) outlined the interaction skills necessary at five developmental levels. Perhaps patients functioning at egocentric levels of development are especially distraught when they cannot keep their craft products. Their needs for mastery are particularly acute, and they might be especially vulnerable to situations in which expectations are not fulfilled. Persons with weak ego skills might confuse the value placed on their work in a particular situation with their inherent value as individuals.

Many occupational therapists have long recognized the psychological effects of crafts on patients, but research in this area is limited. The first controlled quantitative and replicable study examining the psychological effects on crafts was published in 1959 by Smith, Barrows, and Whitney. These researchers used Osgood's semantic differential to study how subjects respond emotionally to selected arts and crafts. Three groups of subjects were asked to rank nine activities on scales of paired opposites. Smith et al. found that affective responses to the names of various crafts differed in terms of three factors: appeal, potency, and difficulty.

In a study that built on the work of Smith et al., subjects ranked four activities, three of which were crafts, on Osgood's semantic differential after participating in the activities (Nelson, Thompson, & Moore, 1982). In this study, the semantic differential included only those three factors of affective meaning identified by Osgood as having the most universal significance. The quantitative evidence showed that the four activities did elicit different affective responses in terms of the three factors of evaluation (which summarizes the degree to which a person feels positively or negatively about something), power (which summarizes a person's feelings in terms of the magnitude of effect something potentially has on its

environment), and action (which represents a person's feelings about the degree of movement or volatility associated with something).

Another study (Carter, Nelson, & Duncombe, 1983) investigated how different types of people respond differently to activities. The authors suggested that personality types should be considered in planning occupational therapy activities. They also argued that a distinction should be made between creativity and imitation when activities are planned to suit a patient's personality.

These studies, then, established a foundation for quantifying the affective meanings of activities and the effects of activities on mood. The present study took a further step by addressing how keeping or not keeping the product of one's activity influences affective responses and mood. Making stationery was thought to be a generally meaningful and purposeful activity that would motivate the subjects to create attractive, useful products. Subjects would have the opportunity to personalize the products if they wished.

Methods

Subjects

Forty-three occupational therapy students volunteered to participate in the study. Of these, 20 were first-year professional master's students and 23 were junior undergraduates. The undergraduates were approached in their lab sessions on their first day of class. The principal investigator asked the potential subjects to be available for the study during class time, but also told them they could leave if they wished and would not suffer any detrimental consequences. All students chose to participate. The study was conducted during class time without a time lapse between request and participation.

The master's students were initially approached during their second class lecture in a required course. The principal investigator requested that they set aside time to participate after lab the next week and made a second request the following week during lab. About half of the students stayed after class to participate in the study.

All subjects were female except for one male master's student who could not keep his product and another who could.

Instruments

The instruments used to measure the subjects' responses to keeping or not keeping their products were the Bipolar Profile of Mood States (POMS-BI) and the Osgood 12-scale short-form semantic differential. The measurement procedure was similar to that of Carter et al. (1983).

The 12-scale short-form semantic differential consists of 7-point scales of paired opposites: nice–awful, fast–slow, quiet–noisy, sour–sweet, powerful–powerless, young–old, good–bad, weak–strong, alive–dead, deep–

shallow, big–little, and helpful–unhelpful. Scoring produces three factors: evaluation, power, and action. Research supports the use of the semantic differential as a valid and reliable method of comparing different concepts in terms of their affective meanings (Bentler, 1969; Green & Goldfried, 1965; Osgood, 1952).

POMS-BI lists 72 adjectives describing positive and negative moods and feelings. Each adjective has a set of four possible responses, and subjects choose one response for each adjective based on their feelings "right now." Possible responses are *much unlike this* (0), *slightly unlike this* (1), *slightly like this* (2), and *much like this* (3). Scoring produces six factors that have been identified through extensive factor analysis (Lorr & McNair, 1982; Lorr, McNair & Fisher, 1982; Lorr & Shea, 1979): elated–depressed, agreeable–hostile, composed–anxious, energetic–tired, clearheaded–confused, and confident–unsure.

Procedure

The first tested group, 11 undergraduates who could not keep their stationery, met in the morning. The second group, 12 undergraduates who could keep their stationery, met in the afternoon on the same day and in the same room. The third group, 9 master's students who could not keep their products, met in the afternoon the following week, in a different room. The final group, 11 master's students who could keep their stationery, met in the same room as the other master's students, at the same time on the following day.

Subjects in all four groups read and signed consent forms and then completed the POMS-BI. Next, the researcher demonstrated printing techniques by pointing out the various ink colors available: blue, red, and brown. Choices of stationery colors were light blue and light brown.

Predesigned blocks were available for printing, but potatoes were also available so that subjects could design their own prints if desired. Thus, the activity would be more meaningful to subjects who would rather not use precut blocks, but would prefer to create unique designs. Two charts and examples of block-printed stationery were displayed. One chart described printing procedures; the other chart explained how to cut a potato design. Subjects practiced on newsprint before finally block-printing on high-quality textured stationery.

After they finished the activity, subjects assigned to the "not keeping" groups were told that they could not keep their stationery. The investigator collected it and placed it in a brown grocery bag. The subjects then completed the semantic differential (recording their feelings about the activity) and the POMS-BI. The first three groups were told not to discuss the experiment with other students. The total procedure took 1 hour.

The "keeping" groups followed an identical protocol, except before completing the forms subjects in these groups were told they could keep their stationery.

In a critique of the semantic differential, Green and Goldfried (1965) observed that the subject might think that marking the continuum of paired opposites in the middle indicates that the subject views both sides of the scale as appropriate. Therefore, in this study, the researcher explicitly explained to subjects that a mark in the middle of the form means that the concept is neutral on the scale, not that the subject believes both sides of the scale are appropriate. This point was also prominently written on the forms.

Data Reduction

The 12 scales of the semantic differential are reduced to three dependent variables, each of which consists of the sum of four scales. The lowest rating on each scale is 0, and the highest is 6. Therefore, the score for each dependent variable can range from 0 to 24. The six mood scores are calculations of the difference between pretests and posttest (for each mood, the pretest score is subtracted from the posttest score). The possible range of scores for each mood change is from +36 to -36, but it is rare for an individual to score at either extreme.

Results

Preliminary analysis revealed some differences between graduate and undergraduate groups. Therefore, two-way analyses of variance were computed on each dependent variable. The two independent variables were condition (keeping vs. not keeping) and student group (graduate vs. undergraduate). See Table 1 for a summary of all results.

There was a significant mood difference between conditions on the agreeable–hostile factor. Subjects who could not keep their stationery (particularly the master's students) displayed more hostile moods than subjects who could keep their stationery, $F(1, 39) = 6.66$, $p<.05$.

There was also a significant mood difference on the energetic–tired factor. Subjects who could not keep their stationery became more energetic than subjects who could keep it, $F(1, 39) = 4.17$, $p<.05$.

For both of these factors, differences between student groups and interactions were not significant. Also, there were no statistically significant differences on the remaining four factors of mood states: composed–anxious, elated–depressed, clearheaded–confused, and confident–unsure.

There were no significant differences between keeping and not keeping for any of the affective factors, and only one significant difference between student groups. Graduate students scored higher on the Evaluation factor than undergraduates (regardless of whether they kept the product or not), $F(1, 39) = 7.35$, $p < .05$.

Discussion

The results indicate that not keeping a product of activity can elicit hostile feelings in normal subjects. In

Table 1
Affective Meaning and Change in Mood as a Function of Keeping or Not Keeping a Craft Project

Dependent variable	Kept Project		Could Not Keep Project		Significant Effects
	M	SD	M	SD	
Agreeable–Hostile					
Jr. UG	-0.1	3.9	-2.7	6.2	Keeping vs. not keeping*
MS in OT	1.6	5.8	-5.3	8.3	
Energetic–Tired					
Jr. UG	2.5	6.1	6.6	6.7	Keeping vs. not keeping*
MS in OT	0.7	7.2	5.0	6.8	
Composed–Anxious					
Jr. UG	-2.2	3.9	-2.2	2.9	—
MS in OT	0.8	6.1	-1.8	6.5	
Elated–Depressed					
Jr. UG	-0.6	4.5	3.4	6.2	—
MS in OT	1.9	4.7	0.1	6.4	
Clearheaded–Confused					
Jr. UG	-3.1	4.7	-0.4	4.3	—
MS in OT	0.6	7.5	0.3	5.0	
Confident–Unsure					
Jr. UG	-1.3	6.5	0.8	3.8	—
MS in OT	2.4	7.5	1.1	4.9	
Evaluation					
Jr. UG	14.2	5.3	14.2	5.7	Jr. UG vs. MS in OT*
MS in OT	17.6	3.6	18.3	2.4	
Power					
Jr. UG	11.1	4.8	9.9	3.3	—
MS in OT	11.4	4.2	12.3	1.7	
Action					
Jr. UG	12.8	2.9	15.3	3.6	
MS in OT	15.0	2.5	15.0	2.8	

Note. ns = no significant effect. Jr. UG = junior undergraduates (*n* = 23). MS in OT = master's students in occupational therapy (*n* = 20). * *p* < .05.

fact, one master's student who could not keep her stationery was not satisfied with merely indicating her displeasure on a standardized form. Her face turned red as she loudly and repeatedly argued about this condition with the tester. Another student tried to calm her down, but frowns on other subjects' faces further indicated their distress.

It is surprising that subjects who could not keep their stationery rated themselves more energetic than subjects who could keep their products. Did keeping the stationery reduce subjects' energy levels? No. A close look at the data shows that although subjects who kept their stationery felt more energetic after the activity than before, subjects who did not keep their products became even more energetic. Perhaps this energy directly relates to their hostile feelings. In other words, either they became energetically more hostile or their hostility energized them. They did not passively accept the fact that

they could not keep their products, and their moods became charged.

Perhaps not keeping a product violates a learned expectation that starts in early childhood—that people usually may keep their products. Violations of learned expectations could have particularly detrimental effects in therapy. If a patient molds clay into a useful bowl and then must reshape it into a ball (to be stored away and used for other patients), the patient might well feel that he or she is in an insensitive and uncaring environment and has wasted time. The patient might perceive that the therapist thought the product was poorly done.

Developmentally, the patient may be able to focus only on his or her own egocentric needs, and therefore may have difficulty accepting the fact that the product cannot be kept. Egocentric people especially need positive feedback about their productive efforts, whether from self-assessment or from the assessment of other persons in the environment.

Kielhofner et al. (1980) suggested that feedback on handiwork guides skill building and, in part, determines future interests. If the therapist urges the patient to donate his or her craft to the annual bazaar, if the product is dismantled in front of the patient, or if the product is dismantled by the patient in order to recycle materials, the patient receives feedback that does not guide skill building or stimulate interest in future occupational therapy activities.

No attempt was made in this study to assess the relationship between the individual's personal investment in the stationery and his or her feelings about the experience. It is possible that subjects who invested a great deal of personal symbolic meaning in their stationery felt especially upset when told that they could not keep it. This possibility would provide an interesting area for future research, but it would be difficult to measure the degree of a subject's personal investment in his or her activity.

Strictly speaking, this study investigated only the effects of not being able to keep one's activity product. Donating or dismantling a product might have different effects, depending on the type of subject. Another limiting factor is that subjects were told whether they could keep the product after they had completed their work to ensure that all groups had equivalent experiences and comparable products up to the point at which the independent variable was administered. Subjects told in advance might respond differently than these subjects did, and future research could investigate this point. A necessary limitation of this study is the possibility that subjects in earlier groups told subjects in later groups what to expect (even though they were told not to). However, this possibility cannot explain the differences found in the study.

Despite the fact that subjects became hostile and energetic when told they could not keep their work, they still evaluated the activity highly (a score of 12 on the evaluation factor is a neutral score). And all subjects liked the activity regardless of whether or not they could keep their work. When subjects filled out the Osgood semantic differential, they were told that the scale measured their feelings about the block-printing activity. Perhaps they did not even consider the fact that they could not keep the stationery when they evaluated the *activity* but did consider it when asked how they felt *right now*. If in a future study subjects realize that they should rate the entire session on the semantic differential, significant differences on the evaluation factor might appear.

Both groups of master's students evaluated the activity significantly higher than both undergraduate groups. This effect might have been due to the testing situation. The undergraduates volunteered to partici-

pate during class time. The graduate students, however, stayed after class, thereby forfeiting their own free time.

Although the students showed no significant differences between conditions on seven of nine factors (evaluation, power, action, elated–depressed, composed–anxious, clearheaded–confused, and confident–unsure), perhaps people with disabilities might be more vulnerable to negative effects of losing their products. These seven factors should not be discarded in further research. They might be important in other activities and under different conditions. For example, anxiety might reflect conditions of performance more than conditions of outcome (i.e., process rather than product). Also, whether a craft product may be kept might affect different personality or diagnostic groups in different ways. Occupational therapists must therefore examine these variables to determine the importance of keeping an activity product.

Conclusions

The results show that not keeping an activity product can significantly affect certain moods of subjects. This study contributes to the profession's theoretical underpinnings in regarding the impact of activity situations. Clinicians should not automatically generalize the results of this study to everyday practice, but they can make use of its theoretical implications. Therapists should consider the meanings of activity products to patients when developing treatment plans. Because activities and crafts are basic to occupational therapy, the study of the importance of activity products will enhance occupational therapy theory and clinical decision making.

Acknowledgments

We thank Suzanne Poirier, MS, OTR, for her support and assistance during data collection. This study is based on Janice Dale Rocker's master's thesis, conducted in partial fulfillment of the master of science in occupational therapy degree at Sargent College of Allied Health Professions, Boston University.

References

Allard, I. (1964). Our professional judgment. *American Journal of Occupational Therapy, 18,* 104–107.

Bentler, P. (1969). Semantic space is (approximately) bipolar. *Journal of Psychology, 71,* 33–40.

Bissell, J., & Mailloux, Z. (1981). The use of crafts in occupational therapy for the physically disabled. *American Journal of Occupational Therapy, 35,* 369–374.

Carter, B. A., Nelson, D. L., & Duncombe, L. W. (1983). The effect of psychological type on the mood and meaning of two collage activities. *American Journal of Occupational Therapy, 37,* 688–693.

Cynkin, S. (1979). *Occupational therapy: Toward health through activities.* Boston: Little, Brown.

Fidler, G., & Fidler, J. (1978). Doing and becoming: Purposeful action and self-actualization. *American Journal of Occupational Therapy, 32,* 305–310. (Reprinted as Chapter 7).

Green, R., & Goldfried, M. (1965). On the bipolarity of semantic space. *Psychological Monographs: General and Applied, 79,* 599.

Kielhofner, G. (1980). A model of human occupation: Part 2. Ontogenesis from the perspective of temporal adaptation. *American Journal of Occupational Therapy, 34,* 657–663.

Kielhofner, G., & Burke, J. P. (1980). A model of human occupation: Part 1. Structure and content. *American Journal of Occupational Therapy, 34,* 572–581.

Kielhofner, G., Burke, J. P., & Igi, C. H. (1980). A model of human occupation: Part 4. Assessment and intervention. *American Journal of Occupational Therapy, 34,* 777–781.

Lorr, M., & McNair, D. (1982). *Profile of mood states, bipolar form.* San Diego: Educational and Industrial Testing Service.

Lorr, M., McNair, D., & Fisher, S. (1982). Evidence for bipolar mood states. *Journal of Personality Assessment, 46,* 432–436.

Lorr, M., & Shea, T. M. (1979). Are mood states bipolar? *Journal of Personality Assessment, 43,* 468–472.

Mosey, A. C. (1973). *Activities therapy.* New York City: Raven Press.

Nelson, D., Thompson, G., & Moore, J. (1982). Identification of factors of affective meaning in four selected activities. *American Journal of Occupational Therapy, 36,* 381–387.

Osgood, C. E. (1952). The nature and measurement of meaning. *Psychological Bulletin, 49,* 197–237.

Smith, P., Barrows, H., & Whitney J. (1959). Psychological attributes of occupational therapy crafts. *American Journal of Occupational Therapy, 13,* 16–21, 25–26.

Chapter 57

Altruism and Task Participation in the Elderly

Jan K. Hatter, MS, OTR/L

David L. Nelson, PhD, OTR, FAOTA

Occupation, as the word is used in occupational therapy, refers to activities and tasks that engage a person's time, energy, and resources. Kielhofner (1980) suggested that the absence or disruption of occupation may produce a threat to health. He proposed that occupation could be an effective means for reorganizing behavior in the event of a biological or a psychological disturbance in health.

It is common for the elderly to experience disruption of occupation because of health problems or institutionalization. Winston (1981) noted a high incidence of reports of isolation, boredom, and lack of activity in institutions for the aged. She pointed out that although many institutions have activity programs, they are seldom tailored to individual physical, psychological, social, and economic needs. Reviewing studies of the elderly residing in nursing homes, Lieberman (1969) suggested that these residents share such characteristics as poor adjustment, depression and unhappiness, intellectual ineffectiveness, negative self-image, and feelings of personal insignificance. They tend to be docile and submissive, to show a small range of interests and activities, and to live in the past rather than in the future.

Numerous investigators have attempted to determine how participation in occupations is related to life satisfaction in the elderly. Havighurst, Neugarten, and Tobin (1968) noted a positive correlation between life satisfaction and activity level with increasing age. Similarly, Anantharaman (1979) found that the greater number of activities persons engaged in, the better adjustment they had in old age. A study by Graney (1975) confirmed research indicating that happiness is positively related to social participation in old age. Tobin and Neugarten (1961) conducted a study that demonstrated that social interaction is positively associated with life satisfaction in advanced age. Their findings suggested that with advancing age, engagement is more closely related to psychological well-being than is disengagement. These studies seem to indicate that continued occupational involvement is positively correlated with various measures of life satisfaction in the elderly. Kielhofner (1983) suggested that opportunities to pursue valued occupations should restore the morale of elderly persons, as well as exercise their physical capabilities.

It seems important to consider the intrinsic value a particular activity has for the individual as well as the number of activities he or she is engaged in. Gregory (1983) asserted that the meaning of the activity is of primary importance in producing satisfaction and helping individuals adapt to their environments. In a study of retirees, Gregory found a significant relationship between being occupied in purposeful activity and life satisfaction. Winston (1981) also said that activities for the elderly must be tailored to their interests and needs. Stafford and Bringle (1980) suggested that engaging in activities that are defined and acknowledged as worthwhile should increase self-esteem in the elderly.

Of the activities having meaning or value for the elderly, altruistic activities may have especially high reward value. In a review of the literature related to altruism, Krebs (1970) noted that researchers have generally employed everyday definitions in their studies of the concept. These definitions most frequently suggest that altruistic acts are ends in themselves (i.e., are not directed at gain), are emitted voluntarily, and do good of some type.

In a survey on which activities elderly citizens feel contribute to their general happiness and facilitate their positive adjustment to growing older, Reid and Ziegler (1977) found a high degree of emphasis on the importance of helping other people in maintaining happiness. For example, many respondents said it made them happy to run errands for others.

A review of the recent literature revealed few studies focusing on altruistic behavior and the elderly. Trimakas and Nicolay (1974) investigated the altruistic behavior of elderly women in relation to self-concept and social influence. They found that both self-concept and social influence had significant impacts on altruistic behavior. Subjects with high self-concept scores were more altruistic than those with low self-concept scores. Subjects under negative social influence were less altruistic than those under positive or no influence. Volunteer work could often be considered an altruistic act, and Perry (1983) noted the existence of a significantly large group of older persons willing to do volunteer work if asked. In a discussion of elderly volunteerism, Hunter and Linn (1980–1981) noted that volunteerism offers the participants the opportunity to increase their feelings of usefulness and self-respect. Hunter and Linn found volunteers over 65 years old to have significantly higher degrees of life satisfaction, stronger wills to live, and fewer symptoms of depression, anxiety, and somatization than elderly persons who did not engage in volunteer work.

The purpose of the present study was to examine whether elderly persons would be more likely to participate in an activity if it was designed to help or benefit other people than if it was not.

Method

Subjects. The 130 residents of a retirement home in Kalamazoo, Michigan, served as subjects. They ranged in age from 63 years to 104 years, with the average age being 83.2 years. Twenty-four of the residents were men and 106 were women. The average length of stay at the retirement home was 2.6 years. All residents were conscious, ambulatory, and capable of independently participating in a craft activity.

Procedure. Subjects were individually invited to participate in a holiday cookie-decorating activity. Written invitations were distributed 2 days before the activity date, and a verbal announcement was made immediately before the activity time. Activity groups were scheduled at times when few competing activities were offered.

In the altruism condition, subjects were asked to decorate cookies that would be given to a local preschool. In the nonaltruism condition, subjects were asked simply to participate in a cookie-decorating activity. The cookie-decorating activity was selected for its appeal and familiarity to elderly individuals and because it required no special skills or extraordinary physical exertion. The retirement home has two wings, each made up of two floors. This physical division was the basis for the formation of four activity groups, two of which incorporated altruism and two of which did not. All residents from two randomly chosen floors were assigned to the altruism condition, and all residents of the other two floors were assigned to the nonaltruisim condition. This method was chosen so that next-door neighbors would not be concerned about receiving different types of invitations. The use of four groups also enabled the two conditions to be balanced for time of day. Because residents were assigned to rooms in an essentially random manner on initial admittance to the home, all floors were comparable in terms of the physical and mental status of the residents who lived there.

The following invitation was extended to each subject in the altruism groups:

> I am a graduate student in occupational therapy at Western Michigan University. I'm doing a project which involves decorating Valentine cookies. The cookies will be a surprise for the children at a preschool in Kalamazoo. I could sure use your help. Hope you can come.

This invitation made an appeal to altruism in two ways. The subjects were asked to create a gift for a group of children and were also asked to help the researcher by agreeing to participate.

The invitations distributed to the subjects in the non-altruism groups read as follows:

> I am a graduate student in occupational therapy at Western Michigan University. I'm getting together a group of people to decorate Valentine cookies. Won't you join us at the date and time above?

Invitations for the altruism and nonaltruism groups were identical except in wording. For each group, the number of subjects participating was recorded.

Data Analysis. The chi-square statistic was calculated to test the relationship of altruism to task participation. Statistical significance was set at the .05 level.

Results

See Table 1 for a summary of the results. Computation of the chi-square statistic revealed a significant relationship between the altruism condition and activity participation, $x2(1) = 3.96$, $p<.05$. Of the 39 subjects choosing to participate in the activity, 25 were in the altruism groups. No significant relationship was found between time of day and activity participation.

Discussion

This study demonstrates a significant relationship between altruism and task participation in a group of institutionalized elderly persons. The findings suggest that participation in altruistic activities is meaningful to older persons and that incorporating altruism in an activity may motivate some elderly individuals to participate. The results support previous work (Reid & Ziegler, 1977) that indicated elderly persons want the opportunity to help other people.

When working with the institutionalized elderly, occupational therapists are faced with the dual challenge of designing meaningful activities and motivating individuals to participate in them. The results of this study suggest that activity participation may be increased by incorporating altruism into the activity. The elderly desire responsible roles in society and feel the need to be depended on. It seems important, then, that these needs be considered in occupational therapy planning.

Although the majority of persons invited to participate in the activity groups in this study did not choose to participate, attendance in the altruism groups was higher than would normally be expected at the comparable activities regularly offered at this nursing home. Residents lead relatively independent lives and are busy with a wide variety of individual interests. The intent of the study was not to cause a majority to participate, but to demonstrate the existence of a factor that may serve as a motivator for activity participation.

This is the first study on altruism as a motivating factor in activity participation. It is a very short-term study of participation rates only. No consideration was made of the effect of altruism on length of participation or quality of the product of the activity. These and other factors remain to be examined. Such variables as who benefits from the altruistic act and the activity involved in the altruistic act could also be manipulated and studied. Finally, altruism should also be studied as an element of activity analysis in other populations treated by occupational therapists.

Acknowledgments

We thank the staff and residents of Park Village Pines Retirement Home for their participation and help, Barbara J. Hemphill, MS, OTR, FAOTA, for her advice, and students Ellen Siegel and Susan Juchartz for their assistance in the data collection.

This study is based on a research project submitted in partial fulfillment of the requirements for a master of science degree from the Department of Occupational Therapy, Western Michigan University, Kalamazoo.

References

Anantharaman, R. N. (1979). Activity vs. disengagement for successful ageing in old age. *Journal of Psychological Researches, 23*, 110–112.

Graney, M. J. (1975). Happiness and social participation in aging. *Journal of Gerontology, 30*, 701–706.

Gregory, M. D. (1983). Occupational behavior and life satisfaction among retirees. *American Journal of Occupational Therapy, 37*, 548–553.

Havighurst, R. J., Neugarten, B. L., & Tobin, S. S. (1968). Disengagement and patterns of aging. In B. Neugarten (Ed.),. *Middle age and aging* (pp. 173–177). Chicago: University of Chicago Press.

Hunter, K. I., & Linn, M. W. (1980–1981). Psychosocial differences between elderly volunteers and non–volunteers. *International Journal of Aging and Human Development, 12*, 205–213.

Kielhofner, G. (1980). A model of human occupation, Part 2. Ontogenesis from the perspective of temporal adaptation. *American Journal of Occupational Therapy, 34*, 657–663.

Kielhofner, G. (1983). Occupation. In H. L. Hopkins & H. D. Smith (Eds.), *Willard and Spackman's occupational therapy,* (pp. 31–39). Philadelphia: J. B. Lippincott.

Krebs, D. L. (1970). Altruism—An examination of the concept and a review of the literature. *Psychological Bulletin, 73*, 258–302.

Lieberman, M. A. (1969). Institutionalization of the aged: Effects on behavior. *Journal of Gerontology, 24*, 330–340.

Table 1
Task Participation as a Function of Altruistic Quality of the Activity

Condition	No. of Persons Participating	No. of Persons Not Participating
Altruism	25	41
Nonaltruism	14	50

Note. $x^2(1) = 3.96$, $p < .05$

Perry, W. H. (1983). The willingness of persons 60 or over to volunteer: Implications for the social services. *Journal of Gerontological Social Work, 5*, 107–118.

Reid, D. W., & Ziegler, M. (1977). A survey of the reinforcements and activities elderly citizens feel are important for their general happiness. *Essence, 2*, 5–24.

Stafford, J. L., & Bringle, R. G. (1980). The influence of task success on elderly women's interest in new activities. *Gerontologist, 20*, 642–648.

Tobin, S. S., & Neugarten, B. L. (1961). Life satisfaction and social interaction in the aging. *Journal of Gerontology, 16*, 344–346.

Trimakas, K. A., & Nicolay, R. C. (1974). Self–concept and altruism in old age. *Journal of Gerontology, 29*, 434–439.

Winston, E. B. (1981). An older population: Meeting major needs through occupational therapy. *American Journal of Occupational Therapy, 35*, 635–637.

Chapter 58

Effects of Project Versus Parallel Groups on Social Interaction and Affective Responses in Senior Citizens

David L. Nelson, PhD, OTR
Cindee Peterson
Doris A. Smith
Judith A. Boughto
Gail M. Whalen

This chapter was previously published in the *American Journal of Occupational Therapy, 42,* 23–29. Copyright © 1988, American Occupational Therapy Association.

Through activity analysis and synthesis, occupational therapists structure occupation to meet the needs and goals of their patients. Groups have provided an important context for occupational therapy since the early days of the profession (Howe & Schwartzberg, 1986, p. 39), and the special characteristics of groups make group activity analysis a complex but rich task. The occupational therapist using group activities must determine (a) the degree of sharing required by the task among group members and (b) the degree of creativity allowed by the predetermined structure in the task. These variables within the group activity may be used to foster or inhibit different types of social interaction or affect, depending on the needs of group members.

The concept of the *project group* as a therapeutic tool has been credited to Anderson (1936). According to this author, in a project group all group members share the responsibility for the end product. This is seen in contrast to a situation where the individual is solely responsible for the end product whether working alone or in a group. In 1937 Dunton analyzed the activity of quilt making in terms of its potential effects on socialization and affect. He described how the specialization of group members and the alternation of roles within the project could increase the "social idea" and lead to increased verbal and nonverbal interaction. Mosey (1970) theorized that the project group can be thought of as the next developmental step beyond the minimal sharing seen in parallel groups.

Occupational therapy research into the nature of group task structure is limited, as is research in other areas of activity analysis. Hyde, York, and Wood (1948) compared the effects of different group games on social responses in institutionalized psychiatric patients. Efron, Marks, and Hall (1959) compared group-centered activity (making lawn chairs for use on hospital grounds) with individual activity in terms of rated psychiatric improvement. It should be noted that these authors mistakenly labeled individual activity as "occupational therapy" and group projects as "industrial therapy."

More recently, DeCarlo and Mann (1985) confirmed a key principle of occupational therapy groups by finding that an activity-based group enhanced self-perception of interpersonal communication skills more than a verbally oriented group. In a similar vein, Schwartzberg, Howe, and McDermott (1982) compared three different types of groups: a community group meeting, a self-expression group combining task- and process-oriented occupational therapy, and an open occupational therapy group oriented to individual activities. The acute psychiatric inpatients were found to communicate more in the individually oriented group than in the other two group contexts.

Two recent studies conducted with nondisabled populations (normal college students) investigated task-structured sharing as a variable of significance to activity analysis. Adelstein and Nelson (1985) studied two types of sharing within the context of collage activity: the sharing of materials and the sharing of end products. Affective meanings of the different activity experiences were measured by Osgood's shortform semantic differential (OSD), which measures evaluation (the affective value placed on the activity), power (the potency held by the activity), and action (the liveliness of the activity). No differences were found due to sharing on these dependent variables. Steffan and Nelson (1987) compared three levels of sharing brought about by the presence or absence of tool scarcity within the context of a stenciling activity. In addition to using the OSD, these authors used the Group Climate Questionnaire (GCQ). This instrument measures engagement, avoidance, and conflict in groups at various stages of development. It was found that subjects in groups experiencing a moderate level of sharing reported significantly more engagement than subjects experiencing either a high level of sharing or no required sharing.

The present study extended this line of inquiry into task-structured sharing through activity analysis. A project group in which subjects worked together to make the same shared end product was compared with a parallel group in which subjects engaged in the same types of activity to make individual products. Group task structure (project vs. parallel) was compared both under the relatively less structured conditions of a creative collage activity and under the relatively more structured conditions of imitating a previously constructed collage from a photograph.

The study of creative vis-a-vis imitative activity is of theoretical significance to the profession of occupational therapy in its own right. Tiffany (1983, p. 300) and Cynkin (1979, p. 122) specified creativity, as a factor occupational therapists should consider in conducting activity analyses. Fidler and Fidler (1978) (see Chapter 7) reasoned that creative activity has an important role in

the development of a sense of self-worth. On the other hand, imitative activity of the type considered in this study requires problem solving to fulfill external criteria. Since creative activity and imitative activity involve different kinds of challenges, the provision of both in this study extended the generalizability of the comparison between project and parallel groups.

Another feature of the present study was the measurement of directly observable social behavior in addition to the use of the OSD and the GCQ. Carlsmith, Ellsworth, and Aronson (1976, p. 197) have argued that research of small group situations has relied too much on self-report rating scales. Needed are behavioral studies to supplement rating scales such as the OSD and the GCQ. The present study included the measurement through time-sampled direct observation of four variables: talking, looking at another person, laughing, and on-task behavior. Ottenbacher (1986, pp. 71–74) is among those who have described the time-sampling of prespecified behaviors.

Previous study (Froehlich & Nelson, 1986) indicated that collage making is a highly rated activity among healthy older women. The study of older people, for many reasons, including the demographic distribution of seniors, the prevalence of seniors' activity programs, and the special needs of seniors for leisure activities, is important to the profession. However, Johnson (1983) stated that occupational therapy research with the elderly is rare and that occupational therapists are "scarcely recognized in the broad field of gerontology" (p. 729). Although the study of disabled groups should be a high priority, the study of normal populations at various levels of the developmental span is also important for several reasons: (a) basic principles of occupational therapy depend on an understanding of normal function and occupation; (b) an understanding of normal function is directly relevant to the role of occupational therapy in the prevention of disability; and (c) a logical progression of research is from studies of normal function to studies of abnormal function (for example, many of the procedures used in this study to measure social interaction are directly transferable to studies of clinical populations).

This study tries to determine (a) whether the effects of project and parallel group structure on healthy seniors differ in terms of affective responses, group climate, or directly observed measures of social interaction and (b) whether there are differences between creative and imitative activity.

Method

Subjects. Forty-one subjects (32 women and 9 men) living in a small Midwestern city participated in the study. Research assistants asked staff at a variety of senior citizen activity and educational centers for their assistance in identifying healthy seniors who might be interested in participating in a research project involving collage making. They were told of the following selection criteria: independent mobility, adequate vision and hearing for reading and following instructions, ability to fill out forms, and ability to engage in a fine motor activity for 2 half-hour periods. Activities center staff allowed the research assistants to post signs advertising the project and encouraged individuals meeting the criteria to call the research assistants for appointments. All subjects attending the research sessions had the basic abilities required by the study's procedure.

The mean age of those participating was 68.9 years, with a standard deviation of 5.1 and a range from 62 to 83. Socioeconomic status was measured by the Four Factor Index of Social Status (Hollingshead, 1975). This instrument has a possible range from 8 to 66. The mean score of subjects on this index was 40.0, with a standard deviation of 11.1. This score indicates a sample broadly reflective of the community, with family educational and occupational backgrounds varying considerably.

Measurements. The OSD (Osgood, May, & Miron, 1975, p. 172) consists of twelve 7-point scales of paired opposites. Each of the three factors of affective meaning (evaluation, power, and action) are calculated by adding together four of the scales. Osgood et al. have identified the OSD's construct validity and internal reliability through extensive factor-analytic studies.

The GCQ (MacKenzie, 1983) is based on several other group dimension scales and the factor analysis and refactoring of items. It has 12 items on 7-point Likert scales, each ranging from *not at all* to *extremely*. Scoring involves the calculation of a weighted *t* score for each item; in addition to that, the mean of the *t* scores for each factor is calculated (five scales make up the engaging factor; three, the avoiding factor; and four, the conflict factor) (MacKenzie, 1984).

Four of the 41 subjects left missing data on scales of the OSD and GCQ. For the OSD, averaging of the remaining scales of the factor was used (Nie, Hull, Jenkins, Steinbrenner, & Bent, 1975, pp. 119–120). Missing data on the GCQ were handled in accordance with the calculations recommended by MacKenzie (1984).

Directly observed behaviors were measured in accordance with a protocol established through extensive pilot testing. Three observers sat behind a one-way vision window with a full view of the subjects. Generally the observer on the left observed 2 or 3 subjects on that side, and the observer on the right observed the 2 or 3 remaining subjects on the right. Except for one session in which the middle observer substituted for the observer on the left, the middle observer checked for interobserver reliability by independently scoring behaviors of observed subjects.

Each of the observers had a Radio Shack TRS-80 Model 100 portable computer. The middle observer's computer was programmed to signal 10-second observation and 5-second recording intervals through beeps audible only to the observers. A single high-pitched beep indicated that each observer should start observing a designated subject; a single low-pitched beep indicated that 5 seconds were available for recording the 1st subject's behaviors before the double high-pitched beeps indicating the beginning of another subject's observation. The progression continued until after the 3rd subject's behaviors were recorded, at which time the program signaled the return to observing the 1st subject. This continued for 16 cycles, at which time the computer signaled a 4½-minute break for the observers. After the break, 16 more cycles were signaled.

The middle computer was programmed both to signal with beeps and to accept recorded data, whereas the other two computers were programmed only to accept recorded data. During each recording interval each observer had to choose among four left-hand keys to press (which represented no talking or laughing, laughing but no talking, talking but no laughing, or both talking and laughing) and among four right-hand keys to press (no looking at any other person or at task, looking at another person but not at task, looking at task but not at another person, and both looking at another person and at task). Laughing was operationally defined as any audible nonverbal exhalation accompanied by smiling (smiling without making a sound did not count). Talking included any audible vocalization with communicative intent and excluded laughing or coughing. Looking at another person included any orientation of the eyes in the direction of any part of another person. On-task behavior was any orientation of the eyes to the collage materials or tools.

After each session, the data were uploaded to a mainframe computer programmed to recode the variables, add up the intervals so that each of the four variables had a possible range from 0 to 32, and compute interobserver reliability. Computed as the percentage of interobserver agreements divided by the total number of intervals, the mean interobserver reliability across sessions and across observers was (a) talking—90%; (b) looking at another person—85%; (c) laughing—95%; and (d) on-task—98%.

Procedure. As soon as each subject contacted the recruiting research assistants, he or she was randomly assigned to either the project condition or the parallel condition. Next each subject signed up for one of the scheduled sessions. Men were much harder to recruit than women, and they were scheduled in such a way that there would always be at least one man per group but no more than two. The recruiter used Reiss's Interpersonal Contacts Categories scale (Reiss, 1959) to ensure that good friends, close associates, and kin were not scheduled for the same session. Six persons were scheduled for each session; if fewer than four appeared, the session was rescheduled.

A 4 by 6.4 m room equipped with a one-way vision window and located in a university building was the site. On entering the room each subject was greeted by the group leader and was asked to choose one of six colored cards that randomly determined initial seating position along one side of a 1 by 3 m table.

The group leader carefully followed a written protocol. After the group leader welcomed and oriented the group, each subject filled out a short form eliciting demographic information. As a warm-up exercise, subjects were encouraged to pair up for approximately 5 minutes and to share some background information with each other; each then shared one or two pieces of information about the other person with the group.

For the four sessions designated as parallel groups ($n = 22$), subjects were told to use a 45.7 by 61 cm sheet of railroad board as the background for each person's collage. In two of these sessions subjects were first told to create their own collage: "What you make is up to you." In the other two sessions the imitative collage came first; these subjects were asked to "copy one of the collages on these photographs." Two identical sets of nine mounted 10 by 15 cm color photographs of different collages were then distributed. Subjects were told that they would have about a half-hour to make the collage, and the computer program behind the one-way mirror was not started until subjects actually began the collage. Every 5 minutes the group leader told the group that all was going well but did not otherwise interact with the subjects unless asked a direct question. At the end of the half hour, subjects were asked to finish up, and then subjects filled out the OSD and GCQ before taking a refreshments break outside the room. After the break and without another warm-up exercise, the group that had made a creative collage received the instructions for the imitative collage, and vice versa. All other procedures were the same as before the break.

The four groups ($n = 19$) assigned to the project group condition experienced exactly the same protocol except that subjects were asked to work together as a group in making a single collage. They were given background railroad board that was six times as large as that provided for the parallel group collages.

At the start of each collage experience, the same types of tools and materials were available: glue, scissors, varieties of dried flowers, grains, macaroni, peas, felt and other patterned and nonpatterned materials and trims, ribbons, yarn, feathers, construction paper, and other small patterned objects made of plastic, metal, Styrofoam, or paper. Magazines and newspapers were not used because it was impossible to copy many types of photographs, and thus the imitative condition could not have been compared with the creative condition.

Results

Table 1 summarizes the results. Three of the variables—observed laughing, observed on-task behavior, and GCQ conflict—were not normally distributed and did not meet the assumptions for analysis of variance. Laughing was an infrequent behavior for most subjects, and all subjects remained on task for most of the intervals observed. Most subjects reported very little conflict.

Each of the other dependent variables was submitted to a two-way analysis of variance with one repeated measure (Group Structure x Type of Activity) via the SPSS MANOVA repeated measures (default model) facility.

Observed Talking and Looking at Other Persons

The project group structure elicited significantly more talking than the parallel group structure, $F(1,39) = 62.4$, $p < .001$. As can be seen by the mean scores in Table 1, there were more than twice as many talking intervals in the project group than in the parallel group. There was no significant difference between the creative task structure and the imitative task structure in terms of talking, $F(1,39) = 0.9$, and the interaction between the two factors was not significant, $F(1,39) = 2.2$.

The ANOVA for observed looking at another person revealed a significant main effect for group structure, $F(1,39) = 25.2$, $p < .001$, and a significant interaction between group structure and type of activity, $F(1,39) = 13.3$, $p < .001$. As Table 1 shows, the difference between the project and parallel means is greater in the imitative condition than in the creative condition. F tests for simple effects demonstrated that subjects looked at each other more when they were in the project groups than when they were in the parallel groups both while being engaged in the creative collage, $F(1,39) = 4.8$, $p < .05$, and in the imitative collage, $F(1,39) = 40.1$, $p < .001$.

Affective Meanings and Group Climate

For the OSD factors of evaluation and power and for the GCQ factors, there were no significant main effects or interactions. However, for the OSD factor action, there was a significant difference between project group structure and parallel group structure, $F(1,39) = 7.4$, $p < .01$. Project groups were experienced as more active than parallel groups.

Discussion

The data demonstrate that task group structure may have a significant effect on social interaction. Specifically, groups structured in a project fashion elicited much more verbal and nonverbal (visual regard) interaction than groups structured in a parallel fashion. This was true both under the relatively unstructured conditions

Table 1
Effects of Task Group Structure and Activity Type on Directly Observed Variables, Factors of the OSD, and Factors of the GCQ ($n = 41$)

Dependent Variable	Possible Range	Group Structure	Type of Activity			
			Creative Collage		Imitative Collage	
			M	SD	M	SD
Observed talking	0–32	Project*	18.1	4.7	18.7	5.2
		Parallel	9.0	6.6	6.6	4.7
Observed looking at other person	0–32	Project*	16.2	5.9	18.2	6.4
		Parallel	12.4	5.1	7.7	4.1
Observed laughing	0–32	Project	2.6	3.3	2.9	3.3
		Parallel	1.8	2.0	0.7	0.9
Observed on task	0–32	Project	31.9	0.2	31.8	0.4
		Parallel	31.2	1.6	31.9	0.5
OSD evaluation	0–24	Project	18.2	4.9	19.4	4.3
		Parallel	18.0	5.3	19.6	3.8
OSD power	0–24	Project	13.8	5.2	14.8	5.0
		Parallel	13.6	6.9	14.0	6.1
OSD action	0–24	Project*	14.8	3.9	16.0	3.1
		Parallel	12.9	3.3	13.1	3.0
GCQ engaging	23–68	Project	50.7	6.8	53.7	8.4
		Parallel	49.2	8.1	48.0	10.0
GCQ avoiding	34–75	Project	58.2	6.1	60.4	–.6
		Parallel	55.0	5.9	57.4	10.8
GCQ conflict	37–82	Project	39.2	5.3	39.7	6.9
		Parallel	38.0	3.4	40.2	4.0

Note. OSD = Osgood semantic differential. GCQ = Group Climate Questionnaire.
*Project scores greater than parallel scores, $p < .01$ for main effect on this factor.

provided by the creative collage activity and under the relatively high degree of structure provided by the imitative collage.

As pointed out by Howe and Schwartzberg (1986, p. 205), a major role for the occupational therapist group leader is to adapt the group's structure in a way that will help group members achieve their therapeutic goals. For example, the occupational therapist may want to encourage social interaction among socially isolated individuals, or may want to increase the rate of interaction so that individuals have more opportunities to become aware of self-defeating interpersonal patterns. On the other hand, the occupational therapist may want to decrease the rate of social interaction in a particular group. For example, the members of a group might not

yet be ready to deal with a high level of interpersonal demands, or they might need a temporary retreat from interpersonal stresses. Another possibility is that the members of a group might be more in need of individual task achievement than enhanced interpersonal skills.

The other significant difference found to be due to group task structure was in the affective dimension of action. In factor-analytic studies conducted by Osgood et al. (1975), the scales making up this factor (fast–slow, noisy–quiet, young–old, and alive–dead) were found to be independent of the scales making up the evaluation and power factors. In the present study the subjects may have found the project group to be faster moving and livelier than the parallel group because of the added stimulation brought about by working together on a project.

Task group structure is not only one of the most important variables in group work, it is also a variable that is highly specific to the profession of occupational therapy. Whereas a verbally oriented group therapist would be unlikely to consider the presence or absence of a shared end product as a source of affective meaning and increased or decreased social interaction, the occupational therapist using activity groups has this added tool in fostering behavioral change. This is part of our heritage of activity.

It is improper to extrapolate research findings with a healthy population to clinical practice with patients in convalescent hospitals and nursing homes. The study reported here is theoretically oriented rather than oriented to the efficacy of intervention. However, the present study is relevant to the clinician insofar as it strengthens occupational theory in the area of group work. The practitioner makes clinical judgments based on theoretical considerations, situational matters, and other factors. This study has confirmed a theoretically based relationship in a healthy population; it is up to the clinician to apply the theory to actual clinical situations.

Although the present study does document the importance of group task structure, there were few differences between creative and imitative activities as defined in this study. This is in contrast to the findings of Carter, Nelson, and Duncombe (1983) who showed that college students asked to create a collage expressing their own image rated this activity significantly higher both in evaluation and power than the activity of imitating a magazine picture with the same collage materials. In the present study elders' mean ratings of the four experimental conditions ranged from 18.0 to 19.6 on the evaluation factor; these scores were high given the fact that a score of 12 can be considered a neutral rating. In contrast, the mean evaluation scores of the college students in the Carter et al. study were 14 for the imitative condition and 16.8 for the creative personal collage condition. This suggests the possibility that there may be age-related differences both in how collage activities are perceived and in how creativity and imitation are perceived. There is a need to study this possibility under controlled conditions within the same investigation using a factorial model.

The main limitation to this study in terms of research design is the fact that any competent group leader would be aware of the differences between groups and therefore could deduce the independent variables under study. It is important to acknowledge the possibility that such a group leader could bias the study's results. To mitigate this problem, the group leader in this study followed a carefully established protocol and interacted minimally with the subjects. The nature of the variables observed from behind the one-way mirror was not discussed with the group leader until after the study was over.

Methodologically, the present study advances activity analysis research by documenting the reliable use of direct observation technology to measure the effects of occupation on activity participants. Although more time-consuming and costly than the use of self-report forms, direct observation technology can provide valid, sensitive measures of a wide variety of clinically relevant behaviors. This is especially important for future activity analysis research with clinical populations who do not have the cognitive abilities required by self-report measures. For example, many seniors living in nursing homes would be hard-pressed to fill out the OSD or the GCQ; however, most people in nursing homes are capable of engaging in a wide variety of occupations. Future research should explore those occupations, including the differences between project and parallel activities, through the use of direct observation technology.

Conclusion

With healthy seniors as its sample, this study has demonstrated that task group structure can have a significant effect on verbal interaction, nonverbal interaction, and the perception of action in the group. This was true within the contexts both of a creative activity and of an imitative activity. Further activity analysis research should be done to extend the methodologies used in this study to investigations of clinical populations.

Acknowledgments

We wish to acknowledge the assistance of Ellen Winter, MA, OTR, in the design of the activity under study; Jean Steffan, MS, OTR, for contributions to instrumentation; and students Jeanne Burns and Chris Cummings for recruiting subjects.

Work was supported by a fellowship from the Western Michigan University Faculty Research and Creative Activities Fund, by a grant from the American Occupational Therapy Foundation, and by a grant from the Western Michigan University Center for Human Services of the College of Health and Human Services.

References

Adelstein, L. A., & Nelson, D. L. (1985). Effects of sharing versus non-sharing on affective meaning in collage activities. *Occupational Therapy in Mental Health, 5,* 29–45.

Anderson, C. L. (1936). Project work—An individualized group therapy. *Occupational Therapy and Rehabilitation, 15,* 265–269.

Carlsmith, J. M., Ellsworth, P. C., & Aronson, E. (1976). *Methods of research in social psychology.* Reading, MA: Addison-Wesley.

Carter, B. A., Nelson, D. L., & Duncombe, L. W. (1983). The effect of psychological type on the mood and meaning of two collage activities. *American Journal of Occupational Therapy, 37,* 688–693.

Cynkin, S. (1979). *Occupational Therapy: Toward health through activities.* Boston: Little, Brown.

DeCarlo, J. J., & Mann, W. C. (1985). The effectiveness of verbal versus activity groups in improving self-perceptions of interpersonal communication skills. *American Journal of Occupational Therapy, 39,* 20–27.

Dunton, W. R., Jr. (1937). Quilt making as a socializing measure. *Occupational Therapy and Rehabilitation, 15,* 265–269.

Efron, H. Y., Marks, H. K., & Hall, R. (1959). A comparison of group-centered and individual-centered activity programs. *Archives of General Psychiatry, 1,* 120/552–123/555.

Fidler, G. S., & Fidler J. W. (1978). Doing and becoming: Purposeful action and self-actualization. *American Journal of Occupational Therapy, 32,* 305–310. (Reprinted as Chapter 7).

Froehlich. J., & Nelson, D. L. (1986). Affective meanings of life review through activities and discussion. *American Journal of Occupational Therapy, 40,* 27–33.

Hollingshead, A. B. (1975, June). *Four Factor Index of Social Status.* (Available from August B. Hollingshead, PO Box 1965, Yale Station, New Haven, CT 06520).

Howe, M. C., & Schwartzberg, S. L. (1986). *A functional approach to group work in occupational therapy.* Philadelphia: Lippincott.

Hyde, R. W., York, R., & Wood, A. C. (1948). Effectiveness of games in a mental hospital. *Occupational Therapy and Rehabilitation, 27,* 304–308.

Johnson, L. A. (1983). Gerontology. In H. L. Hopkins & H. D. Smith (Eds.). *Willard and Spackman's occupational therapy* (6th ed.) (pp. 721–736). Philadelphia: Lippincott.

MacKenzie, K. R. (1983). The clinical application of a group climate measure. In R. K. Dies & K. R. MacKenzie (Eds.), *Advances in group psychotherapy: Integrating research and practice* (pp. 159–179). New York: International University Press.

MacKenzie, K. R. (1984, April). Group climate questionnaire. *Information Bulletin No. 1.* (Available from K. R. MacKenzie, Foothills Hospital, Calgary, Alberta, Canada).

Mosey, A. C. (1970). The concept and use of developmental groups. *American Journal of Occupational Therapy, 24,* 272–275.

Nie, N. H., Hull, C. H., Jenkins, J. G., Steinbrenner, K., & Bent, D. H. (1975) *Statistical package for the social sciences* (2nd ed.). New York: McGraw-Hill.

Osgood, C. E., May, W. H., & Miron, M. S. (1975). *Cross-cultural universals of affective meaning.* Urbana, IL: University of Illinois Press.

Ottenbacher, K. J. (1986). *Evaluating clinical change: Strategies for occupational and physical therapists.* Baltimore: Williams & Wilkins.

Reiss, A. J. (1959). Rural-urban and status differences in interpersonal contacts. *American Journal of Sociology, 65,* 182–195.

Schwartzberg, S. L., Howe, M. C., & McDermott, A. (1982). A comparison of three treatment group formats for facilitating social interaction. *Occupational Therapy in Mental Health, 2* (4), 1–16.

Steffan, J. A., & Nelson, D. L. (1987). The effects of tool scarcity on group climate and affective meaning within the context of a stenciling activity. *American Journal of Occupational Therapy, 41,* 449–453.

Tiffany, E. G. (1983). Psychiatry and mental health. In H. L. Hopkins & H. D. Smith (Eds.). *Willard and Spackman's occupational therapy* (6th ed.) (pp. 265–333). Philadelphia: Lippincott.

Chapter 59

Therapeutic Modality Comparisons in Day Treatment

James P. Klyczek, PhD, OTR
William C. Mann, PhD, OTR, FAOTA

Psychiatric day treatment is a community mental health service that provides patients with intensive treatment as frequently as 5 days per week and up to 6 hours per day, depending on the individual patient's needs. Several different approaches to treatment can be found among day treatment programs. Some programs employ concepts from occupational therapy, with patients working directly on skill development through a task or activity approach (Angel, 1981; Howe, Weaver & Dulay, 1981; Lilly & Armstrong, 1982; Mauras–Corsino, Daniewicz & Swan, 1985). Other centers rely more on a verbal approach, with individual and group psychotherapy and an emphasis on the development of insight into the basis of the psychiatric problems (Sappington & Michaux, 1975). The relative effectiveness of the various approaches remains largely untested.

The purpose of this study was to compare the effectiveness of two different approaches to day treatment programs using a verbally oriented approach versus a program using an activity-oriented approach. Two day treatment programs were compared, one offering twice as much verbal therapy as activity therapy, the other offering twice as much activity therapy as verbal therapy.

The authors viewed day treatment effectiveness within the framework of the occupational behavior paradigm which posits that people have a vital need to master their environment in the areas of self-care, work, and play/leisure (Reilly, 1966). This drive for mastery is thought to be innate, and the resulting feeling of efficacy is intrinsically motivating (Fidler, 1981; White, 1971). Day treatment is perceived as an intervention designed to increase the patient's level of functioning in these areas through a variety of therapeutic modalities. Therefore this study looked at concrete indicators of functioning such as the reduction of symptomatology in the areas of vocational adjustment, decision-making skills, and the use of leisure time, in addition to the less tangible measure of self-esteem, the patient's community tenure or ability to remain in the community for extended periods of time, and the recidivism or readmission rate. This study did not attempt to measure change in insight development. While the occupational behavior paradigm as a framework focuses effectiveness on changes in environmental mastery, it is believed that approaches such as verbal therapy which focus on less tangible change such as insight, also assume that patients increase their ability to function in areas of self-care, work, and play/leisure.

Review of the Literature

A number of studies support the effectiveness of day treatment in symptom reduction (Fink, Longabough & Stout, 1978; Guy, Gross, Hogarty & Dennis, 1969; Herz, Endicott, Spitzer & Mesnikoff, 1971; Kris, 1965; Linn, Caffey, Klett, Hogarty & Lamb, 1979; Michaux, Chelst, Foster & Pruim, 1972; Washburn, Vannicelli, Longabough & Scheff, 1976). A number of studies found that day treatment reduces rehospitalizations or relapse rates (Edwards, Yarvis & Mueller, 1979; Ettlinger, Beigl & Feder, 1972; Guy et al., 1969; Herz et al., 1971; Linn et al., 1979; Meltzoff & Blumenthal, 1966; Michaux, Chelst, Foster, Pruim & Dasinger, 1973; Sappington & Michaux, 1975; Wilder, Levin & Zwerling, 1966). And a number of studies found that day treatment increases community tenure (Ettlinger et al., 1972; Guy et al., 1969; Herz et al., 1971; Kris, 1965; Linn et al., 1979; Meltzoff & Blumenthal, 1966; Michaux et al., 1973; Washburn et al., 1976; Wilder et al., 1966). Most of these studies compare day treatment with other forms of aftercare, whereas other studies compare day treatment with hospitalization. There is evidence suggesting that day treatment is more effective with symptom reduction than are other modes of treatment. However, until now most studies have examined only single centers, and it is questionable whether these data can be generalized to larger populations.

One study compared different approaches within day treatment. When other methods of treatment were similar, Linn et al. (1979) found the following:

> Poor result centers more often used group psychotherapy and more family counseling at a highly significant level statistically. Good result centers used more occupational therapy ($p < .05$). (p. 1064)

Since studies evaluating the effectiveness of treatment approaches in day treatment settings do not exist, we studied the literature on treatment approaches in general, including approaches used in institutional and other community-based settings.

Symptom Reduction

Five studies found day treatment to be more effective in symptom reduction than the mode of treatment being contrasted (Guy et al., 1969; Herz et al., 1971; Kris, 1965; Linn et al., 1979; Washburn et al. 1976). Michaux et al. (1972), however, found full-time hospitalization to be more effective than day treatment in symptom reduction on seven cognitive and affective scales. Yet at a 1-year follow-up the groups were essentially the same. One study (Fink et al., 1978) found little difference in symptom reduction comparisons, another (Michaux et al., 1973) found that day treatment patients were more intrapunitive and that hospitalization seemed to provide symptomatic relief more quickly than day treatment.

Relapse

Of nine studies examining relapse data, only one (Sappington & Michaux, 1975) provided significant evidence that day treatment patients relapse less often. This study compared one group of patients receiving day treatment as an aftercare treatment with a group of patients receiving conventional aftercare treatment, including individual counseling, medication, and psychotherapy, but not day treatment. The study findings showed that the day treatment group relapsed half as often as the groups receiving conventional aftercare. Two studies (Herz et al., 1971; Edwards et al., 1979) provide evidence that relapse rates were lower for day treatment clients, but these studies did not treat the data statistically. Five studies found no statistically significant difference in relapse between day treatment patients and patients receiving other forms of treatment (Guy et al., 1969; Linn et al., 1979; Michaux et al., 1972; Sappington & Michaux, 1975; Wilder et al., 1966). Ettlinger et al. (1972) found no significant differences in the number of rehospitalizations but did find evidence that the greatest effect of partial hospitalization may be in preventing rehospitalization during the 2-month period immediately following discharge from the hospital.

Community Tenure

In contrast to relapse data, which are simply a measure of the number of rehospitalizations, the community tenure measure relates to the number of days during a specified period of time that the patient was not an inpatient in a psychiatric hospital. Relapse data are less indicative of success since lower rates of relapse may in fact reflect lengthy hospitalizations and fewer days in the community. A treatment that increases a patient's community tenure, however, would suggest a more successful treatment. It can be argued that day treatment reduces the likelihood of chronic social breakdown and subsequent institutionalization and should therefore result in lower rates of relapse. However, this argument has been contradicted by two studies, which found no significant difference in relapse data, but did find increased community tenure for day treatment patients (Guy et al., 1979; Wilder et al., 1966).

Several studies examined community tenure. One found that remission in day treatment lasted as long as remission achieved with hospitalized patients but did not take as long to achieve (Kris, 1965). Another found that day treatment patients spent only half as many days in the hospital as those patients receiving conventional aftercare (Sappington & Michaux, 1975). Several studies reported day treatment patients to have spent more days in the community than patients receiving other forms of aftercare treatment (Guy et al., 1969; Herz et al., 1971; Michaux et al., 1973; Washburn et al., 1976; Wilder et al., 1966). One study with Veterans Administration (VA) patients found no statistically significant difference between groups (Linn et al., 1979).

Methods

The purpose of this study was to test the hypothesis that there are differences in patient outcome measures between a day treatment center using primarily an activity-oriented approach and a day treatment center using primarily a verbally oriented treatment approach.

Subjects

Data were gathered on patients in two adult psychiatric day treatment programs in western New York. Both centers were administered by the same not-for-profit community mental health agency, although each center was under the direction of its own program director. Both centers received county, state, federal, and private funds. Both centers were functioning under approved operating certificates granted by the New York State Office of Mental Health.

Subjects included 122 patients who were admitted to either of the two day treatment centers during the 29-month study period, or who were already on the rolls of one of the centers at the start of the study. This total did not include subjects who did not receive at least 10 full days of treatment or who were not on the rolls for at least 30 days. It was thought that patients unable to meet these criteria would not accurately represent the population being studied. Table 1 summarizes the demographic data collected.

The average age of patients in the activity center was 37.8 years, 44% of the patients were male, and 56% female (n = 89). Patients with chronic illness made up 51 %, and patients with an acute illness made up 49% of the activity center sample. Only 26% of the patients in this group were married or living with an intimate other; 74% were single, widowed, or divorced. The primary diagnosis for individuals in both centers was chronic schizophrenia, and all patients were Caucasian.

The average age of patients in the verbal center was 40 years; 67% of the patients were male, and 33% female (n = 33). Patients with chronic illness made up 54% of the sample in this group, whereas patients with an acute illness made up 46%. Only 15% of the patients in this group were married or living with an intimate other, whereas 85% were single, widowed, or divorced. There

Table 1
Demographic Variables

| | Treatment Approach | | | |
| | Activity | | Verbal | |
Variable	N	%	N	%
Sex				
Male	39	44	22	67
Female	50	56	11	33
Age (years)				
18 to 29	34	38	9	27
30 to 39	21	24	11	33
40 to 49	15	17	5	15
50 to 59	10	11	5	15
60 or older	9	10	3	10
Marital Status				
Single	51	57	23	70
Widowed	5	6	1	3
Divorced	10	11	4	12
Married	21	24	4	12
Living together	2	2	1	3
Type of Illness				
Chronic	45	51	18	54
Acute	44	49	15	46

Note.   All subjects were Caucasian.

were no statistically significant differences in the groups on any of the demographic variables.

Treatment Approach

The independent variable, the treatment approach, was determined by examining treatment schedules for each of the centers for a 29-month period. Treatment groups were categorized on the basis of the goals and objectives of the treatment group, and the format with which it was carried out. All treatment groups on the schedules were assigned to one of the following five categories: *activities*, *verbal*, *social/leisure*, *social skills/activities of daily living*, and *other*. The intent and method of each of the categories are listed in Table 2.

Total average treatment time per week per category was calculated. The center using primarily activity-oriented therapy scheduled an average of 4.21 direct treatment hours per week in activity groups and 2.17 direct treatment hours per week in verbal groups. The center using primarily verbally oriented therapy scheduled only 1.75 direct treatment hours per week in activity groups and 3.16 direct treatment hours per week in verbal groups. Both centers provided virtually equal amounts of treatment in the other three treatment group categories. In summary, patients receiving treatment from the activity-oriented day treatment center received twice as much activity therapy as verbal therapy, whereas the verbally oriented day treatment center provided

Table 2
Treatment Group Classification

Group	Intent	Method
Activity	Increase skills in decision making, attention span, time management, and other areas	Use traditional craft media, including leather, woodworking, ceramics, photography, and weaving
Verbal	Increase awareness of issues related to illness and the development of insight	Use discussion and paper-and-pencil tasks
Social/ leisure	Increase social interaction and leisure skills	Use parties, dinners, games, craft hobbies, bowling, and cultural/ educational trips
Social skills/ ADLs	Increase communication, assertiveness, and other social skills	Use combination of discussion, role-playing, and paper and pencil tasks
Other	Groups that provide a sense of community and help integrate the various components of the program with the use of any or all of the above listed methods	

Note.   ADL = activities of daily living.

patients with twice as much verbal therapy as activity therapy.

Control Variables

Two control variables were included in this study: attendance rate and length of stay in the treatment program. Attendance rate was included because it was thought that the patient's actual participation in the program, represented by the number of days he or she attended treatment, would influence the study outcome measures. The patient's length of stay in the treatment program was also included as a control variable because it was thought that patients treated for longer periods could be expected to demonstrate higher levels of functioning and have a longer community tenure than those treated for shorter periods.

Outcome Measures

The dependent variables in this study included symptom reduction, relapse, and community tenure. Symptom reduction was defined as the difference between the level of psychiatric symptomatology present at the end of treatment and the level present at the beginning of the study or the beginning of treatment as measured by the Comprehensive Mental Health Assessment (CMHA), a

quarterly assessment used at both centers. The CMHA was administered by the patient's primary day treatment therapist rather than by an outside investigator. It was thought that the continuity and integrity of the total assessment process would be better maintained by not introducing a new variable, that is, an individual foreign to the patient. The assessment reports current functioning in 16 life areas and uses a 5-point rating scale to derive a score for each area evaluated. A score of 1 indicated the lowest level of symptomatology in that area, a score of 5 reflected the highest level of symptomatology. A narrative report summarized the patient's progress since the last assessment. Ratings from six life areas were used to derive symptom scores for this study. The areas included were vocational/occupational adjustment, decision making, leisure time use, lethality to the self, lethality to other, and self-esteem. The initial symptom scores were obtained from the CMHA completed at admission to day treatment, or from the CMHA completed nearest to the start of the study.

Relapse was the number of times an individual was hospitalized in a psychiatric facility during the course of the study. Community tenure was the number of days during the 29-month period that the patient remained in the community. It was calculated by subtracting the number of days the individual was an inpatient from the total number of calendar days in the time period studied for each patient.

Data were analyzed using descriptive statistics. Since this was a two-center study, generalizations cannot be made, and thus inferential statistics are not appropriate. This study was meant to be suggestive rather than definitive.

Results

The hypothesis of this study was that there would be meaningful differences in outcome measures between a day treatment center offering primarily an activity-oriented treatment approach and a center offering primarily a verbally oriented approach.

Table 3 presents the group means for the outcome measures of symptom reduction, community tenure, and relapse. Patients receiving activity therapy experienced greater gains in symptom reduction, which translates to one or more of the following: increased self-esteem, better decision-making skills, clearer cognitive processing, improved use of leisure time, greater awareness of feeling states and their impact on functioning, and decreased potential for self-injurious behaviors and/ or harm to others. Patients receiving verbal therapy showed more symptomatology, indicating that during the treatment period studied, patients receiving this therapy showed lower functioning in the areas listed.

Community tenure means were essentially the same for both groups. Relapse rates were three and a half times greater for patients receiving activity therapy, although the mean length of stay per hospitalization was only one third of that for patients receiving verbal therapy. These data may suggest that through the use of activities patients achieve treatment goals via their alterations of the environment. These experiences in therapy allow patients to demonstrate some level of competence and mastery of the environment that over time reduces the feelings of helplessness and hopelessness characteristic of patients with chronic mental illness. It is a fairly well accepted notion that patients approaching recovery and/or wellness experience fears related to the increased responsibility they need to assume to return to independent functioning in the community, and this may result in increased hospitalizations. However, through the use of activities, the patients' motivation to return to the community may be higher because of their previous successful interactions with the environment through therapy, and this may lead to shorter hospitalizations.

Summary and Conclusions

Since the results of the study may have been influenced by uncontrolled variables, the outcomes cannot be generalized to other populations. However, the following statements can be made about the relationship between therapeutic approach and the outcome measures of symptom reduction, community tenure, and relapse, found for the two centers in this study.

1. Overall, patients receiving activity therapy achieved a much greater reduction in symptomatology, and this symptomatology translates to increased levels of independent functioning in community living skills.
2. There was little overall difference in length of community tenure between patients receiving activity therapy and patients receiving verbal therapy.
3. Patients receiving activity therapy were rehospitalized significantly more often than those receiving verbal therapy, but these hospitalizations were for shorter durations than for verbal therapy patients.

Acknowledgment

The authors thank Professor Phillip Shannon, MPH, OTR, Associate Dean, School of Health Related Professions, State University of New York at Buffalo, for his editorial contributions.

References

Angel, S. L. (1981). The emotion identification group. *American Journal of Occupational Therapy, 35,* 256–262.

Edwards, D. W., Yarvis, R. M., & Mueller, D. P. (1979). Evidence for efficacy of partial hospitalization: Data from two studies. *Hospital and Community Psychiatry, 30,* 97.

Ettlinger, R. A., Beigl, A., & Feder, S. L. (1972). The partial hospital as a transition from inpatient treatment: A controlled follow-up study. *Mount Sinai Journal of Medicine (New York), 39,* 251–257.

Fidler, G. (1981). From crafts to competence. *American Journal of Occupational Therapy, 35,* 567–573.

Fink, E. B., Longabough, R., & Stout R. (1978). The paradoxical under-utilization of partial hospitalization. *American Journal of Psychiatry, 135,* 713–716.

Guy, W., Gross, M., Hogarty, G. E., & Dennis, H. (1969). A controlled evaluation of hospital effectiveness. *Archives of General Psychiatry, 20,* 329–338.

Herz, M. I., Endicott, J., Spitzer, R. L., & Mesnikoff, A. (1971). Day vs. inpatient hospitalization: A controlled study. *American Journal of Psychiatry, 127,* 1272–1382.

Howe, M. C., Weaver, C. T., & Dulay, J. (1981). The development of a work-oriented day center program. *American Journal of Occupational Therapy, 35,* 711–718.

Kris, E. B. (1965). Day hospitals. *Current Therapeutic Research, 7,* 320–323.

Lillie, M. D., & Armstrong, Jr., H. E. (1982). Contributions to the development of psychoeducational approaches to mental health service. *American Journal of Occupational Therapy, 36,* 438–443.

Linn, M. W., Caffey, E. M., Klett, D. J., Hogarty, G. E., & Lamb, H. R. (1979). Day treatment and psychotropic drugs in the aftercare of schizophrenic patients. *Archives of General Psychiatry, 36,* 1055–1066.

Mauras-Corsino, E., Daniewicz, C. V., & Swan, L. C. (1985). The use of community networks for chronic psychiatric patients. *American Journal of Occupational Therapy, 39,* 374–378.

Meltzoff, J., & Blumenthal, R. L. (1966). The day treatment center: Principles, applications, and evaluation. Springfield, IL: Charles C. Thomas.

Michaux, M. H., Chelst, M. R., Foster, S. A., & Pruim, R. J. (1972). Day and full time psychiatric treatment: A controlled comparison. *Current Therapeutic Research, 14,* 179–292.

Michaux, M. H., Chelst, M. R., Foster, S. A., Pruim, R. J., & Dasinger, E. M. (1973). Post release adjustment of day and full time psychiatric patients. *Archives of General Psychiatry, 29,* 647–651.

Reilly, M. (1966). A psychiatric occupational therapy program as a teaching model. *American Journal of Occupational Therapy, 20,* 61–67.

Sappington, A. A., & Michaux, M. H. (1975). Prognostic patterns in self report, relative report, and professional evaluation measures for hospitalized and day care patients. *Journal of Consulting and Clinical Psychology, 43,* 904–910.

Washburn, S., Vannicelli, M., Longabough, R., & Scheff, B. J. (1976). A controlled comparison of psychiatric day treatment and inpa-tient hospitalization. *Journal of Consulting and Clinical Psychology, 44,* 665–675.

White, R. W. (1971). The urge towards competence. *American Journal of Occupational Therapy, 25,* 271–274.

Wilder, J. F., Levin G., & Zwerling, I. (1966). A two year follow-up evaluation of acute psychotic patients treated in a day hospital. *American Journal of Psychiatry, 122,* 1095–1101.

Chapter 60

Preventive Activities and Services for the Well Elderly

Margaret M. Kirchman, PhD, OTR, FAOTA

Velma Reichenbach, MS, OTR/L

Barbara Giambalvo, MS, OTR/L

A growing movement in the United States encourages the development of support systems to help the elderly remain in their communities. Program efforts have ranged from Federal to grass roots levels. Exploring the possible role of the occupational therapist in such a movement led to a search for identifying the value of purposeful activity and components that constitute quality life.

Value of Activity. The value of activity for the elderly has been well documented in the literature. Pikunas (1) described the theory of activity as stressing the need to maintain vocational interests and to augment recreational activities in order to occupy one's time fully and to make the later years gratifying and productive. Maddox (2) suggested that individuals whose activity levels are high or low generally maintain that ranking throughout life. Spelbring and Rhee (unpublished paper, 1972) found this to be true in an aging population in Michigan: the activity level of people during adulthood continued into their later years.

In contrast, Cumming and Henry (3) in 1961 introduced the disengagement theory, suggesting that gradual disengagement from social roles and withdrawal from social interaction in order to accept death more easily benefits both the individual and society. Havighurst's study in 1961 found that both social and psychological engagement decreased with age (4). Further study of these data by Neugarten, Havighurst, and Tobin showed that social engagement, not disengagement, is generally related to psychological well-being. They found that people who remained relatively active in the various social roles of family member, citizen, club member, or friend showed the greatest satisfaction with their lives (5). Smith and Lipman (6) studied satisfaction in the elderly relative to the constraints of their environment. They found that people constrained in performance of self-care, moving about, and gainful employment were less likely to be satisfied.

Purposeful activity is claimed to be the trademark of the occupational therapy profession. King (7) (see Chapter 8) drew an analogy between occupational therapy and corresponding elements of adaptation: that it is an active response; that it is evoked by environmental demands of needs, tasks, and goals; that it is organized below the level of consciousness, with conscious attention directed to objects or tasks; and that it is self-reinforcing, with each success serving as a stimulus for the next, more complex environmental challenge.

The 1974 Task Force on Target Populations specified the elderly in its identification of populations needing occupational therapy. The report targeted the well elderly as being at risk by virtue of living in environments that failed to support health (8).

Nontraditional examples of occupational therapy include one by Menks et al. who, in collaboration with a community health center, implemented a successful outreach activity group for psychogeriatric clients in the community (9). Another use of activity was reported by Kales-Rogoff (10), who arranged community outings for patients for purposes of evaluating functional abilities and providing an opportunity for patients to practice activities outside the center. Therapists assessed problem-solving skills in conjunction with the outings.

Warren (11) and Nystrom (12), in separate studies, interviewed the elderly in the community about their perceptions of independence and leisure activities and found that most interviewees participated in both active and passive activities. In another unique setting, Hasselkus and Kiernat studied an independent living project for the elderly in the community and delineated the contributions of the occupational therapist in helping the elderly maintain their independent living status. Activity was inherent in independent living (13).

From the perspective of occupational therapy, no problem is found in interpreting these studies that correlate high activity with high satisfaction as likely preventives of isolation, boredom, and preoccupation with problems.

Quality Life Components. Many studies were reviewed to determine how to assess quality in a person's life. George and Bearon suggested that the components of a quality life are life satisfaction, self-esteem, general health and functional status, and socioeconomic conditions (14). Campbell, Converse, and Rodgers defined the quality of life experience mainly in terms of satisfaction of needs (15). They concentrated on the experiences of life, rather than on the conditions of life, using the latter only to help account for the differences in the quality of experience that subjects report. Cantril used a Self-Anchoring Striving Scale to measure self-rated health and life satisfaction in an attempt to measure psychological well-being (16).

As early as 1972, Palmore and Luikart found self-rated health to bear the strongest relationship to life satisfaction (17). Six years later, Larson, in reviewing the literature of the previous 30 years, found that studies of life satisfaction, morale, and related constructs yielded a consistent body of findings. He was able to identify a single summary construct on subjective well-being (18). His research on Americans more than 60 years of age shows well-being to be most strongly related to health, followed by socioeconomic factors and degree of inter-action with others. Maddox and Douglas found that a patient's self-assessment of health tended to be more congruent with well-being than the physician's rating of the patient's health (19), and supported the theory that how people feel about themselves assumes the greatest importance in an overall feeling of well-being. Returning to the focus of the study of activity and well-being, Mancini suggested that satisfaction with one's use of time and leisure activities may have an impact upon well-being, regardless of monetary resources or health level (20).

Although all these studies show some relationship to each other, researchers generally agree that perfect criteria have not been developed to predict and validate subjective well-being (21–23). Our study most closely approximates Campbell's viewpoint—that personal interpretation of life experiences most often determines quality of life.

Description of the Service Project

The Preventive Activities and Service Project was a joint service and research project established for a well elderly population that attended a nutrition site at the University of Illinois at the Medical Center. The object of the service program was to offer a support system to maintain the elderly in their own communities while attempting to improve the quality of their lives. The purposes of the program were to build on the participants' meaningful former relationships, to generate new opportunities for socialization, education, and purposeful activity, and to enrich their problem-solving abilities.

The need for intervention became apparent when a few of the seniors were observed arriving for lunch as early as 8:00 in the morning and sitting around the periphery of the room without interacting, much like the scene in a physician's waiting room. Something was needed to dispel the isolation so apparent there.

The program was initiated with one therapist working 2 days a week for a total of 10 hours. The time period between 9 and 1 o'clock appeared to be the most beneficial for client contact.

The therapist met with the principal investigator once a week (2 or 3 times per week during the orientation phase) to discuss the progress of the project, the growth of individual clients, and the effect of therapist behavior upon individuals and groups.

The occupational therapy intervention used avocational and recreational activities, physical exercise, and educational sessions to achieve the stated program goals. Initially, music (either records or piano playing), as well as dancing and singing, were used to encourage interaction. Then crafts and exercise sessions were introduced. Crafts were used to help rebuild the esteem diminished through loss of income when employment ceased. The exercise sessions included general exercises appropriate for seniors, and specific exercises for individual physical problems.

Bingo, a medium that requires a minimum of interaction, was used to help some of the seniors who were not able to interact or develop friendships easily. This activity also provided the therapist with an opportunity to evaluate and intervene in individual problem areas such as reversal of letters, inability to read, varied handicaps caused by arthritis, and decreased dexterity. The crafts and bingo activities helped some seniors regain confidence in their ability to be productive and enjoy activities, despite severely diminished vision, the result of cataracts or glaucoma.

As trusting relationships developed and participation increased, the therapist used more active listening in order to be informed of their clients' problems and needs. It became clear that the seniors needed suggestions or referrals to appropriate agencies for help with their individual problems. A second therapist, working 6 hours a week, was added to the program, making more one-to-one interactions possible. Because of the cold and deep snows that winter, information was provided on emergency services, danger of exposure, and proper nutrition. The development of spontaneous activities both at home and at the nutrition site was encouraged to help dispel the isolation caused by the long winter and by personal losses, such as the ability to get around, that altered each person's life space.

An intergenerational aspect, involvement with handicapped children at a nearby hospital school, was also added to the program. The seniors regularly visited the school and personally interacted with the children, giving gifts they made during the craft sessions. The visits helped the seniors put their ailments in perspective in relation to the children's severe physical limitations and provided opportunities for personal friendships to develop and grow. These visits were very popular with both the children and the seniors.

The goals of the project were met within the time constraints of its operation. Participants assumed increased responsibility for all aspects of the program. They became more tolerant of each other's idiosyncrasies. Peer pressure and peer support helped seniors accept each other. Racial discrimination noticeably decreased as interaction increased. Therapeutic intervention in individual needs provided the support necessary to meet the project's objective of maintaining the elderly in their communities, while working to improve the quality of their lives.

Description of the Research Component

The research component of this project used pre- and post-interviews to measure change in self-care independence, and other aspects of the quality of the subjects' lives after a period of 6 to 8 months of occupational therapy intervention. The following areas were measured: Activities of Daily Living, Social Resources, Economic Resources, Performance of Household Activities, Health, Life Satisfaction, and General Affect.

Subjects. Forty-five senior citizens were interviewed at the beginning of the project and 31 of this group still in attendance and willing to participate were reinterviewed 6 to 8 months later. Attrition was caused by death, moving, or attendance at other nutrition sites. The demographic characteristics appear in Table 1. Most participants' attendance averaged 4 days per 5-day week.

Interviewers. The interviews were conducted by the occupational therapists who worked in the service program and by volunteers from the occupational therapy faculty. These therapists were selected because of their interest and/or experience with the elderly and because it was felt that occupational therapists, more than other professionals, could add an in-depth perception to the interviews and could intervene therapeutically as needed. All interviewers attended instructional sessions with the principal investigator.

Instrument. The main part of the instrument in this study was adapted from a questionnaire developed by Spelbring (24) because it covered many of the components defined by the quality of life: functional independence, socioeconomic resources, health, and life satisfaction. Spelbring's instrument reflects Katz's Activities of Daily Living instrument (25), Darsky's instrument from the Detroit Survey of the Aged (unpublished, 1964), and Cantril's Ladder (16). Another measurement of quality, or how persons feel about their life in general, was taken from Campbell (15) and used to tap General Affect.

Our adapted instrument consisted of 38 questions divided into 4 areas: 8 questions on Activities of Daily Living, including performance on bathing, dressing, transfer, toileting, continence, feeding, walking, and home confinement; 12 questions of Social Resources, including living arrangements, marital status, transportation, amount of contact with relatives and friends, and amount of participation in clubs and organizations, as well as specific questions on leisure time activities; 3 questions on Economic Resources concerning major source of funds for food, clothing, shelter and medical care; employment status, interest in finding a part-time job, and 15 questions on Household Activities including car repairs, disposing of trash, driving (for errands), taking care of children, grocery shopping, household repairs, laundry, clothing care, paying bills, yard care, planning and preparing meals, and light or heavy cleaning.

The Cantril Ladder (Figure 1) was used to measure Health and Life Satisfaction. People were asked to suppose that the top of the ladder represented the best possible health, and the bottom, the worst possible health, and to show where they stood on the ladder at that time. A similar question was related to their perception of life satisfaction.

Table 1
Demographic Characteristics of 31 Subjects on PAS Project

	No. Subjects	Percent
Age:		
60–79	17	55
70–79	12	39
80–89	2	6
Sex:		
Male	10	32
Female	21	68
Race:		
White	28	90
Black	1	3
Other	2	7
Place of Birth:		
Illinois	18	58
Other U.S. town	6	19
Foreign born	7	23
Marital Status:		
Married	13	42
Single	5	16
Widow, Widower	11	35
Divorced	2	7
Education:		
Grade School – Grades Completed		
3 years	1	3
5 years	2	6
8 years	15	48
High School – Grades Completed		
1 year	2	7
2 years	6	19
3 years	2	7
4 years	3	10
Nature of Residence:		
Single Home	11	36
Apartment	19	61
Boarding House	1	3
Living Arrangements:		
Alone	10	32
With spouse	14	45
With son, daughter	4	13
With sibling	2	7
Other	1	3

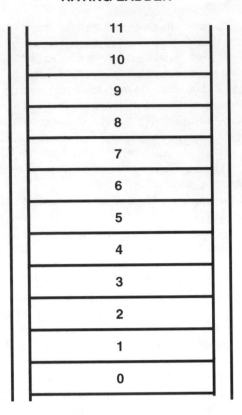

RATING LADDER

Figure 1. Cantril Ladder used for measuring Perception of Health and Life Satisfaction.

General Affect was measured on a 7-point scale, rating ten semantic variables (Figure 2) that described how persons feel about their present life.

Indexes were constructed for Activities of Daily Living, Social Resources, Economic Resources and Performance of Household Activities by submitting answers on a 6-point scale. Measurable criteria in each area made it possible to arrive at a single figure that summarized an overall performance for each Index.

In constructing the Index of General Affect, the decision to include eight items in the Index (eliminating easy-hard and dependent-independent) was based on intercorrelations and factor analysis from an earlier study (26). A single additive score was then made available on each individual.

Pre- and post-mean-scores on the five Indexes—Activities of Daily Living, Social Resources, Economic Resources, Performance of Household Activities, and General Affect—and the two measures of Perception of Health and Life Satisfaction were submitted to statistical analysis by means of the t-test.

Results and Discussion

Table 2 shows the mean scores on interviews before and after occupational therapy intervention. Significance was achieved on Social Resources, Economic Resourc-

Here are some words we would like you to use to describe how you feel about your present life. If you think your present life is very boring, put an X in space next to Boring. If you think it's very interesting, put an X in space next to Interesting. If it's somewhere in between, put it where you think it belongs.

	1	2	3	4	5	6	7	
Boring	❑	❑	❑	❑	❑	❑	❑	Interesting
• Enjoyable	❑	❑	❑	❑	❑	❑	❑	Miserable
Easy	❑	❑	❑	❑	❑	❑	❑	Hard
Useless	❑	❑	❑	❑	❑	❑	❑	Worthwhile
• Friendly	❑	❑	❑	❑	❑	❑	❑	Lonely
• Full	❑	❑	❑	❑	❑	❑	❑	Empty
Discouraging	❑	❑	❑	❑	❑	❑	❑	Hopeful
Disappointing	❑	❑	❑	❑	❑	❑	❑	Rewarding
• Brings out the best in me	❑	❑	❑	❑	❑	❑	❑	Doesn't give me much chance
Independent	❑	❑	❑	❑	❑	❑	❑	Dependent on others

• Items reversed to avoid making all answers in one column.

Figure 2. Questions measuring General Affect (taken from Campbell, Ref. 15).

Table 2
Mean Scores Pre- and Post-Occupational Therapy Intervention on the PAS Project

Indexes	Pre-OT Mean Scores	Post-OT Mean Scores	t	Significance
ADL	5.6	5.8	1.68	N.S.
Social Resources	4.7	5.0	2.79	.01
Economic Resources	4.7	4.5	−2.52	.02
Household Activities	5.2	5.4	1.65	N.S.
Perception of Health	7.13	7.06	− .17	N.S.
Life Satisfaction	8.0	8.7	2.38	.05
General Affect	5.9	6.2	2.42	.05

Note. $n = 31$; $p < .05$ (set as acceptable level of significance); $df = 30$.

es, Life Satisfaction, and General Affect. The greatest significance ($p < .01$) was shown in Social Resources, reflecting the increase in socialization, both within the group and within social networks that developed outside the group setting. The Index on Economic Resources was significant at the .02 level in a negative direction. Many seniors' only income was a Social Security check, which made their economic future bleak in the face of inflation. The measurements on Life Satisfaction and General Affect were both significant at the .05 level, demonstrating increases that could not happen by chance alone. Since the occupational therapy took place between the pre- and post-measurements, the positive changes on Social Resources, Life Satisfaction, and General Affect suggest that they may be related to the occupational therapy intervention.

The ADL Index was not significant. The subjects' ADL level was higher than expected, a condition explained by the fact that they were "well elderly." At times serious illness or disability prevented them from attending the program, eliminating them temporarily or permanently from the group. The level of performance on Household Activities also did not change significantly. It paralleled the ADL level of "mostly independent," with the number of activities reflecting independent living for the most part during both measurements. The negative t of −.17 on the Perception of Health measurement did reflect the serious illnesses within this group and a natural concern for chronic illness.

The second interview was conducted just as the seniors were able to return to the nutrition site after a severe snowstorm had paralyzed the city. The storm seemed to affect their health and morale, and those who had experienced bouts of illness were concerned about what they perceived as deteriorating health.

The significant findings on Self-Satisfaction and General Affect were a positive corroboration of the improvement in the seniors' affective level, as demonstrated in the program.

Summary

A project that combined research and an ongoing service program as the intervention was described. The goals were to maintain a well elderly population in the community and to improve life satisfaction. The program included avocational and recreational activities, physical exercises, and educational sessions to help improve the overall quality of life.

Of the seven areas measured to assess the quality of the subjects' lives, four were found to have significant results between pre- and post-measurement: Economic Resources, Social Resources, Life Satisfaction, and General Affect.

The findings in the three areas of Social Resources, Life Satisfaction, and General Affect validate the existence of a support system to help maintain these elderly in the community.

Acknowledgments

This project was funded by a grant from the College of Associated Health Professions. Thanks are extended to all who helped with this project.

Parts of this paper were presented at the AOTA Conference in Denver, Colorado, 1980.

References

1. Pikunas J: *Human Development: An Emergent Science,* New York: McGraw Hill (3rd Edition), 1969.

2. Maddox GL: Persistence of life style among the elderly: A longitudinal study of patterns of social activity in relation to life satisfaction. In *Middle Age and Aging: A Reader in Social Psychology,* BL Neugarten, Editor. Chicago: University of Chicago Press, 1975, pp 181–183.

3. Cumming E, Henry WE: *Growing Old: the process of disengagement,* New York: Basic Books, 1961.

4. Havighurst RJ: Successful aging. *Gerontologist 1:* 8–13, 1961.

5. Havighurst RJ, Neugarten B, Tobin SS: Disengagement and patterns of aging. *In Middle Age and Aging,* B Neugarten, Editor. Chicago: University of Chicago Press, 1975.

6. Smith JJ, Lipman A: Constraint and life satisfaction. *J Gerontolo 27:* 77–82, 1972.

7. King LJ: Toward a science of adaptive responses. *Am J Occup Ther 32:* 429–437, 1978 (Reprinted as Chapter 8).

8. Task Force on Target Populations. *Am J Occup Ther 28:* 231–236, 1974.

9. Menks F, Sittler S, Weaver D. Yarnow B: A Psychogeriatric activity group in a rural community. *Am J Occup Ther 31:* 376, 381–384, 1977.

10. Kales-Rogoff L: Community skills experience for rheumatic disease patients. *Am J Occup Ther 33:* 394–395, 1979.

11. Warren HH: Self-perception of independence among urban elderly. *Am J Occup Ther 31:* 71–74, 1977.

12. Nystrom EP: Activity patterns and leisure concepts among the elderly. *Am J Occup Ther 28:* 337–345, 1974.

13. Hasselkus RR, Kiernat JM: Independent living for the elderly. *Am J Occup Ther 27:* 181–188, 1973.

14. George LK, Bearon LB: *Quality of Life in Older Persons: Meaning and Measurements,* New York: Human Sciences Press, 1980.

15. Campbell A, Converse PE, Rodgers WL: *The Quality of American Life: Perceptions, Evaluations and Satisfactions,* New York: Russell Sage Foundation, 1976.

16. Cantril H: *The Pattern of Human Concerns,* New Brunswick, NJ: Rutgers University Press, 1965.

17. Palmore E, Luikart C: Health and social factors related to life satisfaction. *J Health Soc Behav 13:* 68–80, 1972.

18. Larson R: Thirty years of research on the subjective well-being of older Americans. *J Gerontol 33:* 109–129, 1978.

19. Maddox GL, Douglas EB: Aging and individual differences: a longitudinal analysis of social, psychological, and physiological indicators. *J Gerontol 29:* 555–563, 1974.

20. Mancini JA: Leisure satisfaction and psychologic well-being in old age: effects of health and income. *J Am Geriat Soc 12:* 550–552, 1978.

21. Wan TH. Livieratos B: Interpreting a general index of subjective well-being. *Milbank Memorial Fund Quarterly/Health Soc 56:* 531–556, 1981.

22. Kaplan RM, Bush JW, Berry CC: Health Status: types of validity and the index of well-being. *Health Serv Res 11:* 478–507, 1976.

23. Ware JE: Scales for measuring general health perceptions. *Health Serv Res 11:* 396–415, 1976.

24. Spelbring LM: *Loss and resumption of role activities following stroke.* Doctoral dissertation: Ann Arbor, Michigan: University Microfilms, 1981.

25. Katz S, Ford AB, Moskowitz RW, Jackson BH, Jaffee WW: Studies of illness in the aged. *J Am Med Assoc 185:* 914–919, 1963.

26. Kirchman MM, Loomis B: A longitudinal study assessing the quality of occupational therapy. *Am J Occup Ther 34:* 582–586, 1980.

Chapter 61

A Model to Promote Activity Competence in Elders

Ruth Levine Schemm, EdD, OTR/L, FAOTA
Laura N. Gitlin

Today, 1 in every 10 Americans is chronically disabled, and this number is expected to rise dramatically by the 21st century as the population ages. Estimates from national health surveys indicate that close to 13% of community-living elders aged 65 years or older report difficulty with walking or with at least one self-care task, whereas 17.5% report difficulty with at least one instrumental daily life activity, such as meal preparation, housekeeping, or shopping. Although most elders function independently, the proportion of those who do so diminishes with age. The percentage of those unable to function without some type of assistance rises dramatically to 34.5% for those aged 85 years and older (Leon & Lair, 1990).

As advances in technology prolong life, it is anticipated that the number of elderly persons with chronic illness and disability will steadily increase. Chronic illness presents unique social, psychological, and physical issues that are distinct from those presented in acute illness (Corbin & Strauss, 1988). It necessitates long-term care over time where prognosis is often uncertain, function and dysfunction are episodic, progressive deterioration in physical well-being occurs, and quality of life is "intrusively" affected for both caregivers and chronically ill persons (Strauss, 1975, p. 35). Professionals who assist persons in accommodating and adapting to their disabilities will be important participants in the effort to provide quality care and contain rising health care costs.

This chapter describes an occupational therapy home-based intervention in which purposeful activities were used to promote adaptation and competence in older adults with chronic disabilities. The intervention is based on an application of Reilly's (1974) concept of an activity continuum in which the specific concerns and issues identified by older adults as affecting the quality of their daily lives form the basis of therapeutic actions. The intervention was developed and evaluated as part of a research project that examined home-based strategies for older home-bound elders. Seven home care occupational therapists visited 17 community-living elders who were chronically disabled. The subjects were randomly selected and volunteered to participate in the program.

Background and Significance of Approach

Current service provision and treatment approaches to chronic illness continue to be based on an acute care, medical model focus. This focus emphasizes therapist-driven intervention strategies to promote independence in functional abilities and a symptom-based and time-limited approach to treatment. However, an emerging body of literature has identified unique conditions confronted by older adults with multiple chronic illnesses that challenge the acute care model. Research studies varying widely in methodological approaches have identified the need for health professionals to develop a care perspective that extends beyond current temporal boundaries of service, one that incorporates the specific goals and issues of persons and their caregivers in the management of daily activities and complex life changes presented by chronicity and aging (Becker & Kaufman, 1988; Chiou & Burnett, 1985; Hasselkus, 1988; Kaufman, 1983; Ory & Williams, 1989). Ory and Williams (1989) suggested that, although the goals of older adults often seem qualitative to a therapist, basing treatment on small goals may encourage and maintain interest in the older patient who is working through the disability recovery process. By focusing on small goals that are important to the person, a therapist provides a series of successful experiences that are immediately relevant to the person's life. The identification and incorporation of patient and caregiver goals in the treatment process challenges therapists to assume a collaboration-based approach in the development of intervention strategies.

The concept of collaboration has emerged in the health care literature as a pivotal factor in treatment effectiveness (Gitlin & Corcoran, 1991; Peloquin, 1990; Shelton, Jeppson, & Johnson, 1989). Identification of patient goals in occupational therapy is important to assure a successful therapeutic process. Therapists often use therapeutic activities to motivate a person through the occupational therapy process (Barris, 1982; Barris et al., 1985; Dunning, 1972; Meyer, 1922 [see Chapter 2]). Activities or goal-directed occupations are the interface between the person and his or her environment. Activity participation offers feedback and behavioral evidence of the person's effect on the environment (Barris, 1982, 1986; Kielhofner & Burke, 1980). Barris (1986) described occupational therapy as a "created environment" (p. 48) where the therapist offers options for the person to engage in activities. Feelings of mastery and satisfaction, which are derived from participation, then become a positive influence on future behavior. Persons become motivated and gain a positive sense of self when an activity matches their own goals for recovery and their interests and needs. In this approach, the choice of activity and its fit with the person's sense of self are critical to successful treatment. A series of studies by Nelson and colleagues showed that episodic involvement in an exercise activity was enhanced when a meaning was attached to that activity (Nelson, 1988; Nelson & Peterson, 1989). In these studies, meaning seemed to stimulate further investment, self-fulfillment and pleasure, and, hence, positive treatment outcomes. The literature on activity and aging provides further evidence that older adults participate more readily in activities that are important to them and that provide or reinforce a sense of identity and self (Barris, 1986; Heppe & Ray, 1986).

The development of a meaningful activity for patient participation is the most complex aspect of therapeutic intervention. This therapeutic process can be seen as a hierarchy of occupational performance (Christiansen & Baum, 1991; Levine & Brayley, 1991; Llorens, 1986) in which occupation refers to engagement in activities (Nelson, 1988). The most basic component of the hierarchy is the introduction of an activity or specific action or pursuit designed to capture the client's interest quickly. The next layer of the hierarchy is the performance of a series of interrelated activities or tasks that have a common purpose and are mutually understood and recognized by persons (Levine & Brayley, 1991). Barris et al. (1985) maintained that persons participate in these actions "to satisfy either external societal requirements or internal motives to explore and be competent" (p. 49). The highest level of the occupational performance hierarchy contains activities that contribute to or reflect the doer's participation in a role. Such activities fulfill role or social expectations or requirements and are personally satisfying (Levine & Brayley, 1991, p. 621).

When developing activities, tasks, and roles for a client, the therapist must consider the influence of the environment or the "composite of all external forces and influences affecting the competence and maintenance of an individual" (Hopkins & Smith, 1983, p. 920). White (1959, 1964, 1971) defined competence as efficacy in meeting environmental demands. To enhance competence, occupational therapists adjust the level of press of the environment during an activity by using carefully selected activity choices, adapting the materials or process, grading the activity upward or downward, designing parallel choices, using repetition, and assisting the patient with verbal and nonverbal cues. Murray developed the concept of *press*, which refers to the demands or forces in the environment that activate the physical, interpersonal, or social needs of a person and thus affect behavior in that environment (Murray, Barrett, & Hamburger, 1938). Competence develops as the person explores, manipulates, and learns to adjust behaviors to meet external demands (Christiansen, 1991).

Description of Intervention Program

As part of a study to evaluate home-based occupational therapy strategies, seven therapists from across the Unites States volunteered to participate as home visitors to elderly persons with chronic disabilities living in their communities. Therapists participated in a 5-day training program, sponsored by the funding source, in which they were oriented to the conceptual basis of the intervention. Through lecture, group discussion, and case presentations, therapists were instructed in the collaboratively driven, activity-based approach of the intervention. Therapists were instructed not to *treat* the person, but to listen and build a trusting relationship from which to identify the daily problems for which clients expressed interest in receiving assistance. Participatory observation techniques were introduced to the therapists to enhance their ability to enter the client's social and cultural system (Gitlin & Corcoran, 1991; Levine & Gitlin, 1990; Spradley, 1979). Therapists were also taught to use assessment instruments that included closed-ended and open-ended questions to establish a collaborative relationship and gain insight into the client's interests and needs.

Description of Clients

After training, therapists returned to their respective work place and contacted a supervisor or director of a home care agency, public or subsidized housing, or retirement or rehabilitation center to request a pool of clients who might benefit from a home-based activity program. Clients had to be 65 years of age or older with a chronic illness that had been medically stable for one year. Each therapist randomly selected up to 10 clients from this pool. Therapists then randomly selected up to 5 clients to participate in the intervention. Seventeen clients agreed to be visited and evaluated for their living situation, social network and time use, and their ability to perform self-care and instrumental activities of daily living. Fifty-nine percent were women and 41% were men. Seventy-seven percent lived alone: 59% were widowed, 12% divorced, and 6% never married. The remaining 23% were married and lived with their spouses. Eighty-eight percent of the clients were white, 6% were black and 6% represented a wide range of ethnic backgrounds. More than half (59%) of the clients lived in either an apartment building or an apartment in a house, whereas 24% lived in housing for the elderly. Although chronically disabled, 53% classified their health as good to excellent, whereas only 18% rated their health as poor. Clients reported a wide range of disabilities: 53% indicated arthritis as a primary, secondary, or tertiary diagnosis, and 18% indicated polio as a primary diagnosis. Other primary diagnoses included Parkinson disease, diabetes, brain injury, and high blood pressure.

Visit Pattern

Each occupational therapist visited from one to five clients. Every client received an evaluation and an average of 7 visits, each of which lasted an average of 45 min.

The number of visits ranged from 3 to 10 with a mode of 6. Therapists were not bound by fiscal constraints, made visits on their own time according to the needs and wishes of the client, and determined with the client the appropriate number of visits. The average number of days between visits was 14, the range was from 5 to 40 days and the mode and median between visits was 7. Except for four clients, all had at least 1 or more visits scheduled with more than 20 days between visits. This scheduling pattern was based on client need and indicates the importance of flexibility in timing service provision to this population. Also, administrative time was not wasted on closing and opening cases even if service was interrupted by several weeks.

Documentation

Therapists completed a fieldnote form for each visit that documented the following: time, visit number and date, place, adverse conditions, observations of client, observations of environment, activities, personal themes, and preparation for next visit (see Table 1). This documentation served two purposes: it provided a mechanism for therapists to reflect about their own interactions and activity choices, and it assisted the investigators in evaluating the components of the intervention and its outcomes as reported by the therapists.

The investigators reviewed 112 fieldnote forms to identify three aspects of the intervention process: activities that clients engaged in, a description of the activity that was introduced or pursued during each visit, and the outcome of the visit.

Intervention Process

Four phases of intervention parallel the occupational performance hierarchy (Kielhofner, 1985; Reilly, 1974). Each phase is described here with examples from the therapists' fieldnotes.

Phase I: Exploration —Activity as a means to learn about the client. During Visits 1–3, exploratory activities were used to evaluate the client, attempt to understand client concerns, and generate interest by the client. Visit 1, an evaluation tool that involved both structured and unstructured questions, was used to structure activity. These questions probed the client's daily activities and the meaning of objects and tasks. A functional assessment of self-care was obtained using the Functional Independence Measure (FIM), which rates level of independence on a 7-point scale (FIM, 1987). This rating scale was also used to evaluate performance of 15 instrumental activities of daily living.

During Visit 2, therapists raised questions and formulated hypotheses about the client and caregivers. This questioning process indicated that therapists were actively working to understand the client, the environment, and the client's interests. Some examples from therapists' notes are as follows:

Table 1
Items Included In Therapist Fieldnotes

Items	Description
Time	Time when therapist arrived and left.
Visit number	Visits numbered consecutively.
Place	Place of visit.
Adverse conditions	Notation of environmental forces that may have impinged on client's performance.
Observations of client	Included physical status, affect, or mood of care-giver or family.
Observation of environment	Objects and how they were used, tasks and social groups client was involved in, and cultural aspects of the environment.
Activities	Activities used during session, description of any new activities client engaged in during therapist's absence, client's reaction to activities introduced during the session, description of therapist's reflections on activity choice and use of self.
Personal themes	Description of themes, statements and concerns that provide insight as to the therapist's understanding of the client's self-identity, values, and interests.
Preparation for next visit	Ideas for next visit and list of questions therapist wanted to explore.

She told stories that I had a hard time understanding [in terms of] their relevance to the evaluation questions.

She was more animated in conversation about family members than about herself.

[After he expressed interest in indoor gardening] He is going to be an interesting person to get to know.

During Visit 3, therapists began to test initial hypotheses and to further explore client interests through the introduction of therapist-generated or client-generated activity ideas. Throughout these initial activities, therapists and clients searched for role boundaries. Therapists who joined in the client's activity tended to develop rapport more readily and were able to amend their own activity ideas to assure client success. Examples of activities introduced by therapists included dressing the upper extremity, planning exercise groups, arranging flowers, playing card games, looking through an equipment catalog, gardening indoors, playing an electric organ that the therapist brought, reminiscing, making bread dough, sharing family photographs, and sharing food. Therapists continued to question their understanding of the client, the level of rapport achieved, and how to work more effectively and collaboratively. One therapist wondered, "Why is he discussing [the] Depression era and World War II in all three of my visits?" and later wrote "He is a challenge and I'm not sure I'll be able to do anything." Another indicated, "I am still building rapport with her. I think she is somewhat suspicious yet. Needs to trust me more." "How comfortable will she become with me? I her? She surprises me already with things she discusses with me."

A clear example of rapport building is illustrated by the following therapist's description. The therapist had noted the client's past interest in music during the evaluation interview and encouraged the client to discuss this interest and her previous role as a pianist. In the next visit, the therapist brought her own electronic organ so the client could exercise this old skill. "We experimented with her religious music used for notes and chords. She chose a country music base [sic] chord and beat while I played 'Amazing Grace' to it. We laughed and enjoyed ourselves. Rapport building."

Phase II. Competence—Creating Tasks. By Visit 4, the focus of the interventions tended to be clearer to the therapist and the fieldnotes indicated their growing sense of confidence. As one therapist explained,

> The importance of the opportunity to try our activity in the home setting, whether an adaptation or a renewed skill, has been reinforced with each client. Talking about proposed change generally produces a negative response. The *key* is therapist creating a cognitive bridge between old habits and roles and accommodation to new physical or emotional needs.

Another therapist exclaimed, "I feel I hit this one on the head."

Throughout visits 4 through 6, the fieldnotes reveal that therapists were able to incorporate the client's culture and environment into treatment. Whereas rapport building and achieving an understanding of the client's goals and values were concerns in visits 1 through 3, the issue in this phase of the intervention was control. *Control* can be defined as taking charge and guiding and directing the process and outcome of the intervention. In working with chronically ill clients, it may be advantageous to share control and ultimately relinquish it so that clients become empowered to take more responsibility for the management of their care. In this phase, a shift in control was evident as therapists and clients continued to collaborate. The following passage indicates how one therapist guided the therapeutic process but was flexible enough to share control and foster increased client participation in decision making: "I offered suggestions when needed, but let him have control for organizing, combining, and categorizing his items....I would like to be more structured with an activity next time or we'll never get anywhere."

Once trust was established, therapists could focus on adaptations and physical accommodations, at times assuming a more directive role and offering suggestions or displaying samples or pictures to better explain their ideas. One therapist commented, "The surprising thing this time was that she asked me to help her see if she could go up a step or two. This was something I was curious about and prepared to help her with." The client had serious problems and the therapist talked with her about "scooting up and down the stairs." The client thought this would be a good idea.

An evaluation of the fieldnotes revealed that, when therapists were unable to collaborate and relinquish control, therapeutic outcomes did not appear to be as positive and meaningful to the client or to be perceived as effective by the therapist. In 5 of the 17 cases, therapists allowed the clients to direct the activities throughout the intervention. In the other 12 cases, the therapists used the client's activities during the first two visits to gain trust and rapport. These therapists allowed the clients to direct the activities and become participants in choices such as card playing, reorganizing a closet, talking about the client's family, or having coffee and cake and socializing. Therapists introduced their own ideas after they felt that they had gained some rapport. At times, therapists expressed feelings of guilt because they were not directing and controlling the provision process. Integrating the client's ideas with the therapist's often seemed to be mutually beneficial. However, it also created anxiety in some therapists because responsibility for decision making was being shared.

Examples of activities that were introduced once rapport and trust had been established included buying incontinence pants, adjusting the volume knob of the television, raising the height of the client's bed, and demonstrating Kegel exercises to improve incontinence. Each of these activities reflected an increased level of comfort and trust that had been gained through the activities pursued by the therapist and client.

Visit 6 was primarily devoted to teaching and reinforcing previously introduced ideas. Activities were used to skillfully link the client's daily tasks and interests. Therapists emphasized feelings of competence to develop activities into habits. The theme that emerged during this visit was the increase in positive results based on the therapist's understanding of the client's preferred way of doing things. One therapist said, "I appear to be a motivator for him to take charge in doing self-care activity." A former gardener with left hemiplegia took the therapist to see his sprouting indoor herb garden, and the client who had not played the organ in years shared her playing with another friend.

Phase III: Achievement—Establishing Roles. The theme that emerged from visits 7 through 10 was "tucking in loose ends." One therapist stated: "I saw myself as agent of change and facilitator for client and family."

In two cases, the clients were eager to receive life review tapes that the therapist used during reminiscence activity. Therapists also reviewed adaptive equipment use and reinforced the link between activity interests and roles. "I wasn't sure how the volunteer suggestions would go so I brought other things also. Glad those worked."

One therapist took a client to the mall and taught her to use the automatic teller machine. For some clients, the role of church attendee, exercise group organizer, organ player, Bible group participant, photographer, and independent dresser were restored. Other clients developed new interests such as making string art and socializing with neighbors.

Phase IV: Final Visit: Saying Goodbye. Therapists reviewed their accomplishments during this visit. Contacts with appropriate referral sources were arranged and some therapists arranged for further, less intense communication. One therapist wrote, "I think he has been thinking more about things he can't do ... than the things he can." This statement captures the therapist's investment in maximizing the client's competence and suggests that occupational therapy raised new issues that might be addressed later once these ideas were further integrated into the client's life.

Summary of Intervention Outcomes

An evaluation of the fieldnotes revealed that the clients who participated in the intervention engaged in a range of activities such as making wine, visiting relatives, attending church, making bread, doing craft work, socializing, reading, playing bingo, cleaning, doing arm chair exercise, and reading. The great variety of interests and abilities among the members of this group of chronically impaired persons suggests that a treatment focus on functional status provides a limited framework for occupational therapy.

Therapists reported a variety of positive outcomes that were critical for what Ory and Williams (1989) called "small standards of measurement" (p. 68). Examples of these qualitative gains include a client who agreed to volunteer his time, one who renewed socializing with neighbors, and another who organized and directed an exercise group. One woman resumed church attendance, another agreed to make aprons for the occupational therapy department, one man made a series of tapes about his life for family members, and several used adaptive equipment more skillfully, thus enhancing their self-care performance.

There were 10 areas of concern on which therapists tended to focus:

1. Mobility (e.g., getting to church on Sundays)
2. Activities of daily living (e.g., installing and operating shower hose)
3. Instrumental activities of daily living (e.g., using an automatic teller machine)
4. Equipment selection and purchase (e.g., buying incontinence pants, finding an appropriate magnifier and purchasing it for the client)
5. Updating of previously prescribed adaptive equipment (e.g., placing a basket on the front of a walker)
6. Repair of equipment (e.g., repairing reacher and wheelchair, replacing cushion of wheelchair)
7. Expansion of present participation in activities (e.g., encouraging client to use ceramics class to make Christmas presents for family, introducing windowsill herb garden to gardener, encouraging exerciser to organize a group)
8. Introduction of new activities (e.g., tape recording reminiscence activity for family members, making a string art picture)
9. Upgrading or downgrading of previous interests (e.g., introducing electronic keyboard to someone who played the organ, encouraging a photographer to purchase an automatic 35mm camera so he could resume taking pictures)
10. Using activities as the basis for building a new area of competence or achievement (e.g., earning money for sewing aprons previously made as gifts).

Conclusion

This paper presents an intervention approach that involves extended contact and involvement with an older client with chronic illness. The purpose of extended contact is to derive an insider's perspective, or what is referred to in anthropology as an *emic* viewpoint, on the issues and concerns of caring for oneself or a family member with chronic illness. In this intervention approach, treatment strategies evolve from an understanding of the meaning of activities and issues of daily life as identified and defined by the client. The fieldnotes revealed that therapists come to understand a client's needs and concerns differently when treatment is not time bound by present-day service provision and fiscal constraints. A client's feelings and story of how he or she is managing unfold within each therapist visit and through the introduction, presentation, reformulation and upgrading of an activity program over time. The visit patterns that emerged indicate the necessity of obtaining optimal flexibility in reimbursement from fiscal intermediaries for such services to the chronically ill. The intervention strategies may appear to have resulted in small qualitative outcomes or accomplishments. However,

understood in the context of what is meaningful to these persons, each adaptation, activity introduction, and equipment choice resulted in advancing a client's personal need or goal for achieving a self-care activity, a socialization experience, or a reintegration of their compromised competencies with their former personal identities. These outcomes are important to the person's quality of life.

This client-driven intervention has three major consequences for therapists and traditional therapeutic practice. The first involves that of trust and control. Development of trust generally took two to three visits. Although therapists continued to build rapport over time, they often belittled or minimized their skills and expressed concern with visits that were totally devoted to client needs. Some therapists expressed a loss of control and said they were not "doing anything." Others were initially nondirective and unsure when to assume control and direct the intervention while still preserving the client's role as an active participant. Obtaining the right balance is perhaps the most difficult aspect of a collaborative approach to treatment. In one case, the therapist was not able to obtain the right balance of control until the final visit. Once a collaborative and focused relationship was achieved, therapists tended to report success.

The second issue concerns the accuracy of therapists' interpretations of client concerns. Therapists often felt equivocal regarding their perceptions and understandings of a client's life-style and personal values. It was evident from the fieldnotes that clients rarely expressed their real concerns in direct ways and these concerns often unfolded over time. For example, one therapist discovered a client's problem of incontinence while they were looking at assistive devices in a catalogue. The case illustrated the complex ways in which clients perceive their health problems and share intimate concerns with formal health providers. It is up to a skilled professional to read the many cues in the home environment and in a client's presentation of self to discover the client's story.

The third issue raised by this service approach is the potential for conflict because of differences in the therapist's and client's vision of how to frame a problem. This issue can only be resolved if rapport and trust have been achieved and a collaborative relationship has been developed.

One final consideration is that this approach may expose clients to a range of issues and areas in their life that they may not want to have examined by therapists. For example, one therapist who bought incontinence pants for a client on one visit discovered a new feeling of distance after the next visit when she gently inquired about the success of the adaptation.

In conclusion, the intervention is based on the premise that chronic illness presents a set of complex issues that affect the person's personal identity and sense of self as well as issues of daily functioning and self-care. Strict adherence to medical diagnosis and medical functional independence in activities of daily living ignores the multiple needs and concerns that older clients confront in managing their illness over time. The unique skills of occupational therapists as collaborators and listeners who can incorporate client values and interests in therapy provide a critical approach from which to develop innovative and meaningful interventions that promote quality of life for this growing client population. Evaluation of extensive fieldnotes that documented each step of the intervention process from the therapists' perspectives indicated that clients derived positive benefits. Further systematic research is necessary to test the efficacy of the intervention for chronically disabled, medically stable older adults living in the community.

Acknowledgments

We thank Laura A. Schluter, OTR, Ronald A. Stone, MS, OTR/L, Karen F. Barney, MS. OTR/L, Jan Stube, OTR, M. Jean Stolzenberg, OTR, Barbara N. Jackson, MS, OTR/L, and Anne Long Morris, MPA, OTR, for their assistance.

A version of this paper was presented at the Pennsylvania Occupational Therapy Association Meeting, October 1991, Pittsburgh, Pennsylvania, and at the 72nd Annual Conference of the American Occupational Therapy Association, April 1992, Houston, Texas.

The research on which this paper is based was supported in part by funds from the American Occupational Therapy Foundation. The opinions expressed in this paper are those of the authors and do not represent the funding agency.

References

Barris, R. (1982). Environmental interactions: An extension of the Model of Occupation. *American Journal of Occupational Therapy, 36*, 637–644.

Barris, R. (1986). Activity: The interface between person and environment. *Physical & Occupational Therapy in Geriatrics, 5*(2), 39–49.

Barris, R., Kielhofner, G., Levine, R. E., Neville, A. M. (1985). Occupation as interaction with the environment. In G. Kielhofner (Ed.), *A Model of Human Occupation: Theory and application* (pp. 42–62). Baltimore: Williams & Wilkins.

Becker, G., & Kaufman, S. (1988). Old age rehabilitation and research: A review of the issues. *Gerontologist, 28*, 459–468.

Chiou, I. L, & Burnett, C. N. (1985). A survey of stroke patients and their home therapists. *Physical Therapy, 65*, 901–906.

Christiansen, C. (1991). Occupational therapy: Intervention for life performance. In C. Christiansen & C. Baum (Eds.), *Occupational therapy: Overcoming human performance deficits.* Thorofare, NJ: Slack.

Christiansen, C., & Baum, C. (Eds.), (1991). *Occupational therapy: Overcoming human performance deficits.* Thorofare, NJ: Slack.

Corbin, J.M., & Strauss, A. (1988). *Unending work and care: Managing chronic illness at home.* San Francisco: Jossey–Bass.

Dunning, H. (1972). Environmental occupational therapy. *American Journal of Occupational Therapy, 26*, 292–298.

Functional Independence Measure (1987). *Guide for use of the Uniform Data Set for Medical Rehabilitation.* Buffalo, NY: Data Management Service of the Uniform Data system for Medical Rehabilitation, Research Foundation, State University of New York.

Gitlin, L., & Corcoran, M. (1991, September/October). Training occupational therapists in the care of the elderly with dementia and their caregivers: Focus on collaboration. *Educational Gerontology, 17*(5), 591–605.

Hasselkus, B. (1988). Meaning in family caregiving. *Gerontologist, 28*, 686–691.

Heppe, G., & Ray, R. O. (1986). Older adult happiness, the contribution of activity: Breadth of intensity. *Occupational and Physical Therapy in Gerontology, 4*(4), 31–43.

Hopkins, H. L., & Smith, H. D. (Eds.), (1983). *Willard & Spackman's occupational therapy* (6th ed.). Philadelphia: Lippincott.

Kaufman, S. (1983). Cultural components of identity in old age: *Ethos, 9*, 51–87.

Kielhofner, G. (1985). Occupational function and dysfunction. In G. Kielhofner, *A model of Human Occupation: Theory and application* (pp. 63–75). Baltimore: Williams & Wilkins.

Kielhofner, G., & Burke, J. P. (1980). A Model of Human Occupation, Part 1. Conceptual framework and content. *American Journal of Occupational Therapy, 34*, 572–581.

Leon, J., & Lair, T. (1990). Functional status of the noninstitutionalized/elderly: Estimates of ADL and IADL difficulties. (DHHS Publication No. PHS 90–3462). National Medical Expenditure Survey Research Findings IV, Agency for Health Care Policy and Research. Rockville, MD: Public Health Service.

Levine, R. E., & Brayley, C. R. (1991). Occupation as a therapeutic medium. In C. Christiansen & C. Baum (Eds.), *Occupational therapy: Overcoming human performance deficits* (pp. 591–631). Thorofare, NJ: Slack.

Levine, R. E., & Gitlin, L N. (1990). Home adaptations for persons with chronic disabilities: An educational model. *American Journal of Occupational Therapy, 44*, 923–929.

Llorens, L. (1986). Activity analysis: Agreement among factors in a sensory processing model. *American Journal of Occupational Therapy, 40*, 103–110.

Meyer, A. (1922). The philosophy of occupational therapy. *Archives of Occupational Therapy, 1* (1), 1–10. (Reprinted as Chapter 2).

Murray, H. A., Barrett, W. G., & Hamburger, E. (1938). *Explorations in personality.* New York: Oxford University Press.

Nelson, D. L (1988). Occupation: Form and performance. *American Journal of Occupational Therapy, 42,* 633–641.

Nelson, D. L, & Peterson, C. Q. (1989). Enhancing therapeutic exercise through purposeful activity: A theoretical analysis. *Topics in Geriatric Rehabilitation, 4*(4), 12–22.

Ory, M., & Williams, T. F. (1989, May). Rehabilitation: Small goals, sustained interventions. *Annals of the American Academy of Political and Social Science,* 60–71.

Peloquin, S. M. (1990). The patient-therapist relationship in occupational therapy: Understanding visions and images. *American Journal of Occupational Therapy, 44,* 13–21.

Reilly, M. (1974). An explanation of play. In M. Reilly (Ed.), *Play as exploratory learning* (pp. 117–149). Beverly Hills: Sage.

Shelton, T., Jeppson, E., & Johnson, B. (1989). Facilitation of parents/professional collaboration at all levels of health care. In B. E. Hanft (Ed.), *Family centered care* (pp. 63–66). Rockville, MD: American Occupational Therapy Association.

Spradley, J. P. (1979). *The ethnographic interview.* Fort Worth, TX: Holt, Rinehart & Winston.

Strauss, A. L. (1975). *Chronic illness and the quality of life.* St. Louis: Mosby.

White, R. W. (1959). Motivation reconsidered: The concept of competence. *Psychological Review, 66,* 297–333.

White, R. W. (1964). Sense of interpersonal competence. In R. White (Ed.), *The study of lives.* New York: Atherton Press.

White, R. W. (1971). The urge toward competence. *American Journal of Occupational Therapy, 25,* 271–274.

Section VII

Current Realities and Future Directions for Purposeful Activity in Occupational Therapy

Introduction

The influence of historical movements, sociopolitical forces, and health care system trends on occupational therapy has been comprehensively discussed in many of the chapters in this text. From the profession's early struggle to define practice to the recent debate on PAMs, occupational therapy has faced a number of challenges and changes throughout its first century of growth (Schemm, 1994; West, 1984). We have a strong history of divergent viewpoints as occupational therapists have always strove to balance the art and science of patient care (Schemm, 1994). However, there is growing concern that current challenges faced by occupational therapy may result in the future loss of the heart and soul of our profession if we do not actively work to sustain this balance between the art and science of practice. In 1984, West expressed concern that the term, activity, while clearly a core principle of our philosophical base, has become "narrow and impoverished, bearing little resemblance to its rich, original connotations" (p.22). This concern was clearly valid, as now, many OT practices appear to be clones of their physical therapy or social work counterparts, emphasizing physical modalities or verbal therapies (Haase, 1995; Joe, 1995). The infrequent use of meaningful occupation and purposeful activity in treatment results in the loss of the uniqueness and distinctive benefits of occupational therapy. The need for occupational therapists to integrate our fundamental theoretical principles with client information to collaborate and design natural, real-life occupations and meaningful, purposeful activities is vital if patients, caregivers, reimbursing agencies, and the public are to view occupational therapy as a viable and distinct profession, separate from physical therapy and social work (Haase, 1995; Joe, 1995). Grady asks "have occupational therapists become so controlled by the realities of productivity, reimbursement, and modalities that we

are failing to see the process as part of the outcome and therefor (also) measurable, reimbursable, and valuable?" (1992, 1013). The chapters in this section explore this question, examining the current realities influencing our profession while sustaining a commitment to our founding beliefs which emphasize the value of the therapeutic process and the use of purposeful activity in occupational therapy. While this section may become quickly dated, give the rapidly changing health care system and the absence of a crystal ball in which to foresee the future resolution of the current debate, many of the issues raised by the authors in this section will likely remain pertinent as we enter the next millennium and the next century of OT practice.

Wilma West begins this section be reviewing the fundamental beliefs and basic principles of our profession as articulated by the founders of occupational therapy, which, as she emphasizes, are still relevant today. She shares her vision of the potential of occupational therapy in a changing world by examining the profession's history of adaptation over 2 1/2 generations. A review of the challenges faced by first and second generation occupational therapists and a description of the accomplishments of these earlier generations of professionals is provided. West explores the changes and pressures confronting today's third generation of occupational therapists and declares that ongoing allegiance to occupational therapy's basic beliefs and the continued application of these beliefs in practice has enabled OTs to historically and successfully adjust to change. Continuance of this unified vision of occupational therapy will enable current and future generations of occupational therapists to accommodate to change as needed without losing the essence of occupational therapy. West calls for focusing and defining the core of our service as the use of occupation in therapy; thereby, reunifying OT practice. she gives a number of thoughtful and realistic short and long-term imperatives for practice, education, and research. According to West, a unified professional commitment to meeting these imperatives will enable occupational therapists to meet the serious and challenging changes that are facing our profession today.

The value of our professional history to current and future OT practice is further explored in the next chapter by Johnson, who examines the "old" values of humanism, caring, and the therapeutic relationship and the "new" directions of science, logic and depersonalization. She examines the conflict between being humanistic and caring while striving to meet demands to be scientific and objective, expressing concern that the profession is moving toward reductionism and away from holism. An historical review of the characteristics of the founders of OT and the evolution of the profession up to the present is provided. While there has been growth in the profession with respect to the types of clients served, settings in which we provide service, and our repertoire of tools of practice; Johnson cautions that this growth may have sacrificed depth for breadth. She challenges occupational therapists to question their work so that they can maintain holistic values while developing knowledge and skills in a scientific sense. Johnson calls for increased professional support for entry-level therapists, administrators, researchers and educators to ensure they are able to meet the challenges of their roles. Increased research is also needed to substantiate the value of occupational therapy by developing a solid unifying theoretical foundation. Personal poignant examples highlight Johnson's presentation, emphasizing the depth of meaning inherent in these professional values, considering the complexities of OT practice. She concludes that the combination of old values of humanism and holism with new values of science, research, and knowledge will enable OTs to acquire new competence and attain professional unity.

Maintaining this balance between our old values and new competencies to meet current practice demands is increasingly complex as the societal values of the current health care system sharply contrast with our professional philosophy. One of the biggest challenges to occupational therapy's maintenance of a holistic and humanistic approach to treatment are the demands of reimbursement agencies. The following chapter by Howard explores the effect of reimbursement on occupational therapy, examining the extent to which third party reimbursement dictates day-to-day practice. The history and meaning of reimbursement with respect to OT practice is explored through a thoughtful and comprehensive analysis of the literature. According to this review, OT's definition, scope of practice, professional roles, management of OT departments, and profession-

al ethics have been modified over the years in response to changes in reimbursement. Howard thoroughly explores each of these impacts on occupational therapy, analyzing the profession's response to changes in reimbursement including licensure, public relations, and political actions. Societal forces which influence reimbursement policies and subsequently affect OT practice are examined. Howard contends that third party payers currently control the definitions of occupational therapy, rewarding the use of the medical model which leads to changes in our professional language and how we define ourselves to accommodate these pressures. Implications of reimbursement driven practice and the resulting values conflict experienced by many OTs working in the current health system are explored. Howard concludes that occupational therapists who understand the causes of reimbursement imposed on OT practice will be able to be proactive with respect to issues of health care policy, maintaining viable professional roles, now and in the future, that are grounded in OT's humanistic base.

This conflict between the values of reimbursement-driven practice and the humanistic values of occupational therapy are further explored in the next chapter by Burke and Cassidy. They consider the opposing forces faced by therapists today whose practices are fundamentally based on OT's humanistic philosophy, yet these practices are located in a health care environment that is determined by economics. The philosophical foundations of our profession are reviewed and the question as to how these individually oriented, humanistic values can survive within the current health care system with numerous economic, political, and social factors impacting on this philosophy of care is analyzed. The impact of economically driven practice on OT treatment approaches and service provision models and the conflicts between evaluation and intervention based on individual needs versus evaluation and intervention based on reimbursement for service are explored. The need for occupational therapists to shift their allegiance from being solely focused on the patient to also include concern for employers' economic viability and the fiscal constraints of reimbursement, is emphasized by the authors, as being a reality in current practice. Burke and Cassidy analyze the expansion of the "consumer" of OT services to include the government, HMOs, third party payers, health corporations and school administrations, resulting in increased pressures for accountability and leading to the development of a number of vested interests that can lead to ethical conflicts and practice dilemmas. A number of relevant practice dilemmas which result from these ethical conflicts and a series of though provoking questions for OTs to consider as they attempt to manage these dilemmas are presented. A series of directives that will lead to occupational therapy's inclusion in the health care marketplace are provided. The challenge to OT practitioners is to effectively implement these directives while maintaining a humanistic and holistic philosophy of practice.

The next chapter, by Schwartz, offers a way to deal effectively with the challenges, demands, and frustrations of reimbursement-driven practice. She presents the excellence perspective as a way to ensure quality of care, as well as efficient care. The excellence perspective is contrasted with the efficiency perspective, which emphasizes productivity. The history of the efficiency perspective is presented and its introduction to health care management is examined. The adoption of the efficiency perspective in health care resulted in a change from a humanistic emphasis to a business administration focus. The incongruence between a business mode and the provision of humanistic health care presents a dilemma as to how to achieve quality as well as efficiency. Schwartz proposes the excellence perspective as an alternative to the efficiency perspective, stating that if one stresses excellence as their primary goal, productivity will also be enhanced. Since leadership is a critical factor in successful implementation of the excellence perspective, she identifies way leaders can shape organizations in which members strive for excellence. A case study of a hospital program that exemplifies many of the characteristics of the excellence perspective with leaders that epitomize the leadership qualities fundamental for success is provided. The excellence perspective can be used as a guide for program innovation as it is congruent with OT's concern for quality patient care and with the health care system's concern for productivity. Occupational therapists need to develop leadership skills and knowledge of management to be able to articulate consumer needs, and design and implement programs based on excellence.

Peloquin further explores methods for maintaining excellence in practice in the following chapter which focuses on sustaining the art of practice in occupational therapy. She thoughtfully reviews the literature on the art and science of occupational therapy, examining fundamental principles and assumptions of our profession. While mastering the art of practice has always been challenging, current demands from a changing health care system limits the ability of therapists to develop and engage in meaningful relationships with their patients. Decreased lengths of stay, increased documentation requirements, and heightened emphasis on productivity take time and energy away from caring; thereby, constraining therapeutic relationships. According to Peloquin, the health care system focuses on the science of practice and does not value, nurture, or reward the art of practice. Therefore, occupational therapists must obtain sustenance and nurturance of their art from other sources. She suggests therapists use literature to affirm the value of the art of practice as it can provide sustaining images to support their commit-

ment to the therapeutic relationship and in using occupation as therapy. Providing a number of poignant examples from fiction, Peloquin accentuates the power of images and the written word to occupational therapist reflecting on the art of practice. Insightful reading of literature containing both positive and negative images of the profession of OT and its practitioners can increase the reader's awareness of the type of therapist he, or she, would like to emulate. Self reflection on character strengths and weaknesses is vital to maintaining the art and soul of occupational therapy. Peloquin's unique suggestion to use literature to increase self awareness is an effective tool for it can be used individually at one's own convenience. Given the multiple demands on therapists' time, this can be an efficient method of sustaining the art of practice in a challenging health care system.

Sustaining the art of practice in Occupational therapy will be critical if our profession is to successfully meet the demands of the next millennium. This text concludes with two thought provoking chapters which eloquently present the authors' viewpoints on OT practice in the next millennium. Yerxa presents an American perspective and Polatjko presents a Canadian perspective on dreams, dilemmas and decisions for OT practice in the 21st century. Yerxa puts forth the assumption that the next century will have a number of unique characteristics that will be important to occupational therapists and the consumers of our services. These characteristics-increase in chronicity, knowledge of human purpose, complexity of daily living, awareness of demands from the environments in which people live and work, emphasis on personal power, autonomy, self directions and self responsibility, and a new conceptualization of health as persons' capacities to achieve goals through a repertoire of skills-are briefly described. A clear link between each of these characteristics and the philosophy and unique body of knowledge of the profession of occupational therapy is provided. Based upon the congruence between these characteristics and occupational therapy, Yerxa asserts that the 21st century will begin a millennium of occupation, for occupational therapists can effectively meet the needs reflected in each of the identified characteristics. Yerxa strongly emphasizes the value of authentic occupational therapy and reflects on the potential of occupational science to enrich and broaden OT practice. Implications for the future of occupational therapy are discussed and the need for occupational therapists to establish their priorities in the "millennium of occupation" is examined. She calls for OT practice to emphasize the potential of person with disabilities, with OTs serving as advocates and allies for individuals and their families. Yerxa concludes that the knowledge, skills, and values of occupational therapists, as founded in our early philosophical base, will enable us to ensure that persons with chronic illnesses and disabilities will develop the skills they need to achieve their goals of competency. Social barriers to this self definition will be removed, enabling them to thrive in their environments throughout the next century.

Polatajko continues this theme of viewing persons with disabilities in a "new light" in the 21st century, thereby, requiring occupational therapy to shift its emphasis as enter the next millennium. She proposes that in the future, the world will eliminate the concept of handicap by creating an environment where individuals with different abilities and disabilities can live meaningful lives with dignity. In this new world, the focus of occupational therapy will change from reducing impairments to preventing handicaps through empowerment. The definitions of handicap, impairment, and disability are provided and contrasted. The relationship of occupation to these concepts is examined and a review of the basic assumptions and core values of OT are reviewed. Polatajko realistically discusses the limits of current OT practice which is heavily influenced by the medical model and puts forth her vision that an OT profession which emphasizes the full potential of occupation can assume a leadership position in the 21st century. Adopting occupation as the core concept of our profession and entrenching occupation into our professional value system is essential to achieve the ultimate goal of practice which is the empowerment of occupational competence. Clear figures illustrate what OT is in a medical model and what it can become in an occupational competence model. Polatajko concludes that occupational therapists are uniquely positioned to eliminate handicaps and enable all to achieve occupational competence during the next millennium.

The tremendous future potential of occupational therapy, as envisioned by Yerxa and Polatajko, is exciting and heartening, given the current debate on the future of health care, While many authors in this section realistically recognized present constraints on OT practice, it is interesting to note that they also emphasized the need to reaffirm the core values of occupational therapy to successfully counter these limitations. The fundamental principles and rich heritage of occupational therapy has made the profession strong, sustaining it through many decades of change (Grady, 1992). However, the environments in which we apply these principles and the activities, methods, media, and modalities we use have changed greatly over the years and we now are faced with an era that is promising even greater changes which will affect the day-to-day practice of occupational therapy (Grady, 1992; Van Deusen, 1995). While some may view these changes as a threat to our profession, questioning occupational therapy's ability to survive in this new health care system; others view these changes as an opportunity for occupational therapists to thrive and assume leadership positions to develop these new practice arenas and service delivery systems. Occupational therapists are the professionals best suited to take on the role of the primary health care professional in managed care, for we have traditionally been directly concerned with evaluating a client's functioning to determine what components need to be addressed to restore the ability to maintain a productive lifestyle (Van Deusen, 1995). In addition, our professional philosophy of having persons do for themselves and be actively involved in this process is completely congruent with the growing consumer movement (Grady, 1992). New models of community-based practice that improve the health and life opportunities for persons with disabilities have already been developed, and visible alternatives to hospitalization and nursing home care will continue to be sought in the future (Yerxa, 1995). Many professionals and consumers are also recognizing the limitations of scientific medicine and calling for a return to the art of patient care. Occupational therapist who have historically struggled to balance the art and science of practice can be leaders and guide other professionals to develop more integrative health care services (Schemm, 1994). "These present and future needs require an army of occupational therapist" (p.296), committed to holism and our profession's founding beliefs (Yerxa, 199). Since the early 20th century our profession has focused on people's ability to engage in meaningful occupations and purposeful activities in a need satisfying manner. Along the way some OTs have lost this relatively clear vision of our profession, leading to an overemphasis on specific techniques, modalities, and specialties. Therefore, as we enter the 21st century, "we need to be constantly vigilant to build, rather than divide our core of practice. We need to make decisions that support our core values about meaningful activity and active involvement by persons themselves, rather than an emphasis on what we do to people" (Grady, 1992, 1065). Grady's articulate call for a reaffirmation of our profession's fundamental beliefs brings this last section on current realities and future directions full circle back to the text's first section on historical and philosophical foundations. It is hoped that the chapters selected for this text will sustain the readers' commitment to our profession's founding principles as they face the inevitable challenges of practice today, and in the 21st century. Occupational therapists upholding this professional heritage by holistically using purposeful activity in a manner meaningful to a person's daily occupations and relevant to their environment will contribute greatly to society in the next millennium, enabling persons with disabilities and chronic illnesses to be self directed, engage in worthwhile pursuits, and achieve a satisfying quality of life. This was the vision of the founders of occupational therapy in the early 20th century, and it is the ongoing promise of our profession as we enter the 21st century.

Questions to Consider

1. Reflect on your personality, your assets, and limitations. What are your character strengths that will assist you in maintaining the art of practice in a changing health care system? What are your character weaknesses that may make it difficult to maintain this art of practice? What resources are available to help you work on your limitations, and strengthen your assets to meet the demands of current and future practice, while sustaining a commitment to the fundamental, holistic beliefs of occupational therapy?

2. What is your vision of OT in the next millennium? How can occupational therapy work to sustain the art and science of practice in the 21st century? How will recent and impending federal and state legislation impact on current and future OT practice? How can current societal movements and sociopolitical trends serve as a foundation for the enhancement of holistic health care?

3. Review the following case entitled "The Student Who Dared To Care." What were the major value conflicts experienced by Carina? What are the potential ethical dilemmas exhibited in this case? How can an OT balance the psychosocial and physical needs of a client in a health care system that does not recognize the need for holism? What are practice models and alternative delivery systems supportive of holistic OT intervention?

The Student Who Dared To Care

Carina Pavarini was an Occupational Therapy student who had just finished her first Level II Fieldwork experience at a physical disabilities setting and was now completing her final six weeks of academic course work. Carina spoke to me of her experience during this fieldwork placement and of her struggle to maintain the art of practice in today's health care system. She has generously agreed to share her story in this text.

Carina had been assigned to evaluate and formulate a treatment plan for a forty year old woman, Charlotte, diagnosed with late stage cancer. The patient was cooperative with the evaluation, but felt she did not need therapy, as she was very sick, and weak, and in a lot of pain. Carina consulted with her supervisor, who suggested she work on endurance and ADLs with this patient, 2 times per week for thirty-minute sessions. The first time Carina met with Charlotte, she asked her about her interests and learned that Charlotte liked to read and listen to music. Carina then attempted to get Charlotte to sit up to do basic grooming activities. Charlotte was unable to sit up to brush her hair due to low endurance. Carina encouraged her to try to just sit up for a short period of time without performing an activity. The client agreed to try, and, during the next few sessions, Carina read several paragraphs from a collection of short stories, while Charlotte maintained a sitting position. Carina also loaned her walkman to Charlotte so she would be able to listen to music in between treatment sessions. During each session, Carina encouraged Charlotte to try to sit longer and do basic grooming tasks such as combing her hair and brushing her teeth. At this point, Carina experienced mixed feelings about her role in helping this patient.

The physical disabilities setting emphasized increased endurance and ADL performance, as the only appropriate goals for this client, yet Carina saw Charlotte had other needs to be met. Charlotte needed someone to listen to her as she spoke of her pain, her concern for her daughters, about giving up hope and the reality of dying. Carina sought to help this client by listening and validating her feelings.

Sadly, this was not supported in this setting as psychosocial issues were not considered an appropriate focus of OT treatment for persons with physical disabilities. Throughout her affiliation, Carina struggled to treat this person holistically, addressing Charlotte's feelings, as well as her physical symptoms. She met with Charlotte two or three times per week for a few minutes at a time, just to talk. This was not scheduled treatment time, but it provided Charlotte with an opportunity to reflect on her battle with cancer and her impending death, and enabled Carina to develop her ability to meet a client's psychosocial needs, as well as their physical. Carina's fieldwork supervisor continued to emphasize the need to only work on ADLs and endurance while Carina recognized that Charlotte was dying and her immediate need was for someone to listen to her concerns and not give her false hope. Charlotte died during this hospitalization.

Carina's ability to treat Charlotte in a holistic manner in a health care system which did not encourage, reward, or nurture holism, is a tribute to her humanism and her developing skill as an occupational therapist. Her commitment to the fundamental beliefs of occupational therapy, and her willingness to focus on the art of practice, in addition to the science of practice, certainly enabled Charlotte to receive greater benefits from her OT interventions and, as Carina hoped, helped make her last days of life easier and more meaningful.

References

Grady, A.P. (1992). Nationally Speaking—Occupation as a vision. *American Journal of Occupational Therapy, 46,* 1062-1065.

Haase, B. (1995). Clinical interpretation of "Occupationally embedded exercise versus rote exercise: A choice between occupational forms by elderly nursing home residents." *American Journal of Occupational Therapy,* 403-404.

Joe, B.E. (1995, August 24). 50 years an OT and still going strong—Gail Fidler. *OT Week,* 22-23

Schemm, R.L. (1994). Looking back: Bridging conflicting ideologies: The origins of American and British Occupational Therapy. *American Journal of Occupational Therapy, 48,* 1082-1088.

Van Deusen, J. (1995). The issue is: What is the role of Occupational Therapy in Managed Care? *American Journal of Occupational Therapy, 49,* 833-834.

West, W.L. (1984). A reaffirmed philosophy and practice of Occupational Therapy for the 1980s. *American Journal of Occupational Therapy, 38,* 15-23.

Yerxa, E.J. (1995). Nationally speaking: Who is the keeper of Occupational Therapy practice and knowledge? *American Journal of Occupational Therapy, 49,* 295-298.

Chapter 62

Perspectives on the Past and Future

Wilma L. West, MA, OTR, FAOTA

In support of the American Occupational Therapy Association's (AOTA's) Commitment to the implementation of the Directions for the Future initiatives, I intended for this chapter to reinforce a vision of the potential of occupational therapy in a changing world and to emphasize the practice–education–research linkage and its dynamic influence on professional growth.

A Vision of Potential

The word *vision* expresses far more than its ethereal quality first implies. My vision of occupational therapy's potential embodies concepts and beliefs embraced by our founders that are as viable today as when they were proposed initially. The philosophical importance and practical value of these beliefs have enabled them to endure over the 70-plus years of our profession and far longer as an early treatment for physical and mental disabilities.

The clinical reasoning study conducted by Gillette and Mattingly (1987) yielded a list of beliefs held by today's occupational therapists that reaffirm many of the beliefs of our founders. In synthesizing my own professional beliefs, I developed a more generic list, but one which contains most of the same abiding principles of both early and modern practitioners. I precede this statement with a disclaimer to authorship: I am echoing that which I have heard, read, and thought.

As occupational therapists, we hold these truths to be the reason for our being:

1. The individual has an inherent and compelling need for activity.
2. Such activity must stimulate the individual's intellect and emotions as well as his or her sensory and motor systems.
3. Self-fulfillment is best realized through engagement in activity that meets the individual's inner drives and the requirements the outer world places on his or her behavior and performance.
4. When disease or disability interrupts either the will or the ability to engage in activity, the individual needs special help through the medium of restoration, adaptation, or, at a minimum, maintenance of independent function and performance.

These tenets of our profession originated in the writings of our founders, who conceived and promoted them as the fundamental bases of our calling. They have been preserved in our literature by our modern colleagues, who have perceptively and expressively elaborated their meaning. They have been instilled in our practitioners by educators, who have professed our heritage and shared its valued principles. They have been reconfirmed by our practice through demonstration of apparent improvement in patients of all ages and with a broad range of disabilities. They are now being validated through research to support our claim that there is a science as well as an art of therapy through occupation.

I have thus far expressed a collective vision of the potential of occupational therapy. I believe most of us would agree that sound concepts underlie our efforts—concepts that include the occupational nature of human beings; the role of activity in human development, adaptation, and self-actualization; and the worth of the goal of social reintegration of the individual for physical and psychosocial function. Thus, many of us see the effect of activity or its absence on health as the most easily identified, readily understood, and generally compelling concept that makes our service unique and distinguishable among the health professions.

Why, then, do society in general and medicine in particular not value our service? Reilly (1962) (see Chapter 6) suggested, "The wide and gaping chasm which exists between the complexity of illness and the commonplaceness of our tools is, and always will be, both the pride and the anguish of our profession" (p. 1). Our anguish stems from the lack of mystery and magic in what we do, the lack of scientifically enhanced equipment to aid our evaluation and treatment, and the absence of a laying on of hands or the administration of cures that, if not fully understood, appear to have ameliorating and positive effects. Conversely, we take pride in the commonsense principles of enlisting the patient's own effort in his or her recovery and of engaging the patient in everyday, interest-motivating activities of play, work, leisure, and self-maintenance, which are essential to a healthy and satisfying life. Because I cannot accept that these principles are flawed and that our mode of intervention is therefore inappropriate; because I have neither heard nor read a serious challenge to either; and because we have not only continued to exist but also have grown and developed on an upward curve over the past 70 years, I can only reaffirm my vision of our potential.

Potential in a Changing World

To consider the potential of occupational therapy in a changing world, we must first look back at some early changes.

We are told that a new generation is born about every 30 years. Using that measure against our organized origins, I count the first generation of occupational therapists in the years 1917 to 1947 and the second in the years 1947 to 1977. Because the next 30-year period takes us to 2007, a date not clearly visible to a person of my age,

I have opted to think of our third-generation therapists as approaching, in 1992, the midpoint of their time span.

Is the world faced by this generation the only one characterized by change? Far from it! Our founders and their early successors contended with the dramatic challenges of the Great Depression and two world wars, yet they expanded practice from the single specialty of psychiatry to a broad range of disabilities and increased the profession's course of study from a mere few weeks to 4 or more years. Some of the accomplishments of the first generation of our profession include (a) the accreditation of schools, (b) the national registration examination, (c) the first master's degree program, (d) the first textbook by and for occupational therapists, and (e) our own journal.

One of the earliest and most threatening challenges for the second generation of occupational therapists was the near loss of control of our practice and education to physical medicine and rehabilitation. Only by the wise counsel of a leading educator and the strong support of our other medical friends did we win the case for the availability of our clinical services to all medical specialties and the self-direction of our educational programs (AOTA, 1960; Kahmann, 1950; Willard, 1950). Another controversial and potentially divisive issue was the education, certification, and recognition of the occupational therapy assistant. Only recently has that development been credited as a partial solution to the personnel shortage, thereby freeing registered occupational therapists for more professional roles and furthering the professional educational ladder. The deinstitutionalization of mentally disabled patients, the mainstreaming of disabled children, and the emerging health mode of practice required new roles in health promotion and disability prevention; new, nonhospital commmunity-based settings; and diversifications in practice, for which this generation had not been prepared. These changes, plus the chronic problems of personnel shortages, recognition for reimbursement, and galloping health legislation in which we were not initially represented, pervaded the years 1947 to 1977 and, to some extent, persist today. This period also saw the profession's move from a long-standing negative stance, through a brief neutrality, and then to a positive stance on the state regulation of practice. Therapists nationwide paid a high price to secure the enactment of laws that would prohibit practice by unqualified personnel, to say nothing of the cost to the national association for legislative and legal staff. A later development experienced by second-generation therapists was the government's effort to impose regulations on education, certification, and practice. The most visible and near-tragic effect of this trend was the proposed substitution of competency-based education and proficiency testing as alternative methods of professional entry that would have bypassed our long-standing educational standards and requirements. Finally, our intraprofessional debate about specialization and appropriate media and intervention strategies have threatened the cohesion and unity so needed in a group's movement toward mutual goals.

Not all changes are negative, however. In fact, the changes that have confronted third-generation therapists over their tenure to date may be grouped into three major categories: (a) benefits, (b) pressures, and (c) conflicts. Among benefits, there might be listed the broadened definition of the Developmental Disabilities Amendments of 1984 (Public Law 98–527), which makes many more diagnostic groupings than mental retardation eligible for health services; the Education of the Handicapped Act Amendments of 1986 (Public Law 99–457), which created two new programs for children from birth to age 5; enactment of the Medicare Part B Amendments (omnibus Budget Reconciliation Act of 1986), which cover occupational therapy services in skilled nursing facilities, rehabilitation agencies, clinics, and independent practice; and lastly, new roles in hospice care and the treatment of patients with AIDS or Alzheimer disease. These new frontiers required adaptation to new patient populations in diverse new settings, plus new applications of basic principles in treatment. Perhaps the ultimate challenge has been in meeting all of the needs brought about by these changes in the face of the profession's chronic personnel shortage.

The pressures on individual therapists include the emphasis on continued competence to practice and increased participation in research. The pressure on occupational therapy programs and departments includes quality assurance and program evaluation, the reduced length of hospital stays, and the expanding use of computer technology in both program administration and patient treatment.

The conflicts within the profession include the continuing debate about media and the appropriate form of intervention strategies: problems in the use of sensory integration techniques in the schools and in teachers' versus therapists' use of computers as educational tools or as treatment tools; the emerging patient-client issue; and the prospective payment system (PPS) and the diagnosis-related groups (DRGs), which replaced retrospective reimbursement based on treatment costs. The PPS-DRG model resulted in shorter hospital stays and treatment of more acutely ill patients, for whom occupational therapists were expected to increase productivity, facilitate early discharge, and maintain quality of care—certainly competing if not conflicting goals. For educators, who are already struggling with the most functional mix of courses to prepare therapists for changes in practice, there is the ultimate conflict of making the field an academic discipline to counter the mounting threat to the survival of professional schools at the university undergraduate level.

A changing world? No doubt about it. But as Burke (1984) pointed out, "Occupational therapists are used to change. It is very much a part of our everyday practice when we work with people who are experiencing disruption and dysfunction in their lives" (p. 24). To the aspect of change that we have always faced, there must now be added the external forces that have caused multiple changes in the health care provision system of which we are a part. The form of change that challenges our third generation is admittedly different from the changes that confronted the earlier generations of therapists, and such changes will undoubtedly differ for those who follow. If we are not, as Burke said, used to change, we should think about becoming so, because as Heraclitus, a fifth century B.C. Greek philosopher noted, "There is nothing permanent except change" (Bartlett, 1955, p. 12a).

Even those who accept the inevitability and permanence of change despite the opposing connotations of those words, may still find change uncomfortable—a natural reaction to the unfamiliar and unknown. If, however, we consider the alternatives to change—stagnation and obsolescence—we can see the logic of accommodation. Mindful that change is not a synonym for progress, we must expend extra effort to ensure that change will not pass us by.

This brief review of our history shows that we have, indeed, adapted to many changes over two and a half generations. I believe that the factor enabling us to adjust to those changes has been our allegiance to our basic beliefs in the interrelationships between occupation and health and our continuing application of those beliefs in the occupations we use to maintain or restore health and to prevent disability. I also believe that the vision we hold of our potential in a changing world will facilitate whatever other accommodations may be required of future generations.

The Practice–Education–Research Linkage

The interrelatedness of practice, education, and research—the three essentials of any enterprise—has been well established in the scientific literature and in our own literature as well. I did not feel it necessary to review the scientific literature for two reasons. First, in nearly all instances, our colleagues have used the scientific references in their respective reviews of the literature. Second, our colleagues have applied and related the rationale for linkages directly to our own field, thus sparing us the task of translations from the biological, behavioral, and social sciences.

I have therefore compiled the following brief statements on the subject of linkages and recommend that the reader review not only the statements but the total papers from which they were taken. With the exception of Flexner, all of the authors cited below are occupational therapists with both commitment to and expertise in research.

First, from Flexner (1910):

Professions are learned in nature and their members are constantly resorting to the laboratory and seminar for a fresh supply of facts. (p. 49)

And from our own ranks:

Yerxa (1964) said. "The development of the research attitude in every student and every clinician is the beginning of the development of professionalism in occupational therapy. Once critical thinking becomes a habit, research activity inevitably follows." (p. 22)

Ethridge and McSweeney (1971), authors of the first textbook on research in occupational therapy, noted that "through practice, questions are raised to be studied through research, the results of which . . . modify and improve practice." (p. 1)

Writing about education for research functions, Rogers (1982) said, "The proposed goals for professional education are to educate therapists who are inquisitive about their practice, use research findings to improve it, and participate in the conduct of research." (p. 10)

Gillette (1983), writing of Kielhofner's Health Through Occupation, said the book was devoted to "an examination of the full range of knowledge that has accrued through practice and research." (p. xii)

Reed (1984) stated that the purpose of her book was "to suggest some directions for research on theoretical and practice models in occupational therapy." (p. v)

Ottenbacher, Barris, and van Deusen (1986) advocated proceeding "from technical research literature to theory and from theory to practice to enhance the knowledge base of occupational therapy practice." (p. 111)

The American Occupational Therapy Foundation's (AOTF's) Research Advisory Council stated, "The national commitment to . . . research that is related to occupational therapy theory, practice, education, and philosophy has been established." (Llorens & Snyder, 1987)

Research is probably the least accepted component of the practice–education–research linkage. Why, then, is research in occupational therapy so important to our future? Perhaps the most cogent reason is that the value of occupational therapy is more evident to ourselves than to others. The truth of this observation is best seen in our profession's belief that no age or disability is beyond the potential benefits of our services. Although we have always been motivated by these high ideals, and although many have realized them in resourceful ways, few among us would contest the need for greatly increased efforts to transform solid conviction and partial demonstration into the scientific documentation that is required to merit professionalism.

In this concluding section, I have outlined short-and long-term imperatives by which we can strengthen the components of and the linkages between occupational therapy practice, education, and research. The achievement of these imperatives will lend credibility to our professional vision.

Short-Term Imperatives

Practice

My overarching short-term imperative for practice is that we focus and define with a single voice the core of our service, which is the use of occupation as therapy. Professional books and journal articles of the 1980's have elaborated on the rationale for this imperative. Yet external forces that have emphasized outcome measurability seem to have persuaded some of our colleagues to use more tangible techniques such as physical agents of treatment and a concomitant devaluation of self-help through activity. This, in turn, has led to such diversification of practice that we can no longer identify our uniqueness and thereby jeopardized our legitimate claim for reimbursement. Age-appropriate, interest-motivating, and self-actualizing occupations abound in everyday play and work environments. These occupations are infinitely better suited to meeting human need to be accepted, to be useful, and to know the dignity of independence than are all the heat, light, water, electricity, and other physical agents in the world. Let us stop borrowing modalities from other disciplines while selling short our own. Let us apply sound critical thinking and creative problem-solving skills to the task of reunifying our practice.

Education

The first short-term imperative for occupational therapy education, I believe, is the use of other university faculty to buttress our program. One obvious but important reason for this lies in our shortage of qualified educators, but another is the richness of knowledge available from other fields. Several of our schools are currently using such resources, but I urge the significant expansion of both the number of schools doing so and the range of fields from which faculty are drawn.

The second short-term imperative for education is that we teach principles rather than techniques, and knowledge rather than skills. In the past, we have taught skills at the expense of content and developed our curricula in scope but not in depth. Some teachers seem to have catered to their students' low tolerance for ambiguity and preference for concrete over analytical or abstract material. Such a curriculum, however, does not produce therapists who can meet challenging clinical problems with creative and alternative solutions. One of our most limiting professional traits is our propensity to seek solutions before gaining a fundamental understanding of the reason for the problem. A chronic nightmare of such pioneers as Ayres and Rood was the number of their disciples who sought only the techniques and not the theory upon which they rested.

The third short-term imperative for education is increased support of graduate education, consistent with the American Occupational Therapy Association's policy of expanding graduate-level education for professional entry. The American Occupational Therapy Foundation's Board of Directors, at its meeting in June of 1989, passed a motion to allocate at least 50% of its annual scholarships to graduate-level students.

Research

A primary short-term imperative in research, in my opinion, is the greater use of specific requests for proposals that will result in studies specifically responsive to established priorities. Because there is never enough money to support all we would like to do, this shift will require a corresponding decrease in the number of small research grants for separate and unrelated research and on funding education for research. Although such aspects of the research program supported by the Association and Foundation since 1978 represent a sound investment in new researchers, I suggest that we give more support to research that holds promise of meeting our identified needs, for example, the standardization of measurement instruments developed through requests for proposals.

A second imperative for research is the need for outcome studies to document the efficacy of interventions. I feel strongly that our best hope for such documentation, with numbers that will have significance, lies in collaborative studies that link together therapists using the same treatment strategies for patients with the same conditions. Potentials for these studies previously existed in caseloads of cerebrovascular accident patients in acute hospitals. Do these or other patient populations still exist in other settings where time is not a restriction and colleagues could be motivated to standardize their strategies for common benefit?

The third imperative for occupational therapy research is the greater use of qualitative methodology, which seems eminently suited to the study of the psychosocial and behavioral problems that pervade occupational therapy caseloads. Qualitative research methods employ the use of recorded observations of human behavior and performance in natural contexts such as at home, at work, and during leisure time. What a natural form of study for our field!

Long-Term Imperatives

I believe that education is the most important focus in the long term; practice and research follow from education. I applaud and commend the Entry Level Study Committee for their report entitled *Occupational Therapy: Directions for the Future* (American Occupational Therapy Association, 1987). I am such a fan of this report

that I believe it should be required reading for every occupational therapist. I wish to emphasize the importance of three key imperatives for the future of education as identified in that report:

1. We must move from our current linear/vocational/allied health model to a hierarchial/academic/professional model of education.
2. We must accept the necessity of a liberal arts baccalaureate degree as a prerequisite for entry to professional education at the graduate level.
3. To accomplish the first and second imperatives, we must develop an academic discipline based on an abstract body of knowledge and on applied sciences that translate that body of knowledge into solutions for the problems we confront in practice.

Although I believe that these encapsulated imperatives reflect the major recommendations of the report, we do the authors and ourselves an injustice if we do not study the full report in considerable depth. This scholarly and comprehensive report is clear, logical, and well documented. We must do more, however, than simply accept the serious and challenging changes that we are to implement in the next several years; we must comprehend the rationales for all of them. This requires a full understanding and internalization of the entire report.

The outcomes of our commitment will, indeed, be worth our efforts. These outcomes are the survival of our educational programs in the university, the achievement of recognition as a profession, and the proof of our right to practice. Who among us would ask for anything less?

References

American Occupational Therapy Association. (1960). Annual meeting, Board of Management. *American Journal of Occupational Therapy, 14,* 100–105.

American Occupational Therapy Association (1987). *Occupational therapy: Directions for the future.* Rockville, MD: Author.

Bartlett, J. (1955). *Bartlett's familiar quotations* (13th ed.). Boston; Little, Brown.

Burke, J. P. (1984). Occupational therapy: A focus for roles in practice. *American Journal Of Occupational Therapy, 38,* 24–28.

Developmental Disabilities Amendments of 1984 (Public Law 98–527).

Education of the Handicapped Act Amendments of 1986 (Public Law 99–457), 20 U.S.C. § 1400.

Ethridge, D. A., & McSweeney, M. (1971). *Research in occupational therapy.* Dubuque, IA: Kendall/Hunt.

Flexner, A. (1910). *Medical education in The United States and Canada: A report to the Carnegie Foundation for the Advancement of Teaching* (Bulletin No. 4). Boston: Updyke.

Gillette, N. P. (1983). Foreword. In G. Kielhofner, *Health through occupation; Theory and practice in occupational therapy* (pp. xi-xiii). Philadelphia: F. A. Davis.

Gillette, N. P., & Mattingly, C. (1987). The Foundation—Clinical reasoning in occupational therapy. *American Journal of Occupational Therapy, 41,* 399–400.

Kahmann, W. C. (1950). Nationally Speaking—From the president. *American Journal of Occupational Therapy, 4,* 111–112.

Kielhofner, G. (1983). *Health through occupation: Theory and practice in occupational therapy.* Philadelphia: F. A. Davis.

Llorens, L. A., & Snyder, N. V. (1987). Nationally Speaking—Research initiatives for occupational therapy. *American Journal of Occupational therapy, 41,* 491–493.

Omnibus Budget Reconciliation Act of 1986: Medicare Part B Amendments.

Ottenbacher, K. J., Barris, R,, & Van Deusen, J. (1986). Some issues related to research utilization in occupational therapy. *American Journal of Occupational Therapy, 40,* 111–116.

Reed, K. L. (1984). *Models of practice in occupational therapy.* Baltimore: Williams & Wilkins.

Reilly M. (1962). Eleanor Clarke Slagle Lecture—Occupational therapy can be one of the great ideas of 20th century medicine. *American Journal of Occupational Therapy, 16,* 1–9. (Reprinted as Chapter 6).

Rogers, J. C. (1982). Guest Editorial—Educating the inquisitive practitioner. *Occupational Therapy Journal of Research, 2,* 3-11.

Willard, H. S. (1950). Committee Reports—Report of the Education Committee. *American Journal of Occupational Therapy, 4,* 35–37.

Yerxa, E. J. (1964). Observe—theorize-relate: Our professional responsibility. In the American Occupational Therapy Association's *Proceedings of the 1964 Annual Conference* (pp. 15–22). Rockville, MD: American Occupational Therapy Association.

Chapter 63

Old Values–New Directions: Competence, Adaptation, Integration

Jerry A. Johnson, EdD, OTR/L, FAOTA

One of the truly exciting and stimulating benefits that derives from being president of an organization like the American Occupational Therapy Association is the opportunity to be exposed to the problems and concerns of 20,000–25,000 people and to be involved in the resolution of some of those issues. It is an incredible experience, and one can never be quite so provincial or so quick to render judgment after having held such a position.

One of the privileges of no longer serving as president is the opportunity to reflect upon the experience and its meaning for my life. For me, that has meant devoting a considerable amount of time exploring the values of our profession, the directions in which the profession seems to be headed, my values, and the way that I want to spend the remainder of my life.

So, when invited to make this presentation, I accepted immediately. The topic seemed so natural in relation to my thoughts about our profession and about me, and it offered an opportunity to address issues of personal concern and professional interest. When it was time to write, however, the process was slow and arduous. Concepts that seemed clear were, upon examination, ambiguous. Connections between and among competence, adaptation, and integration were more tenuous than I had assumed. Concepts were supported by beliefs and anecdotal experience, rather than by hard scientific evidence.

In the final analysis, it was my own internal conflict that made writing difficult. The title of this presentation, "Old Values–New Directions," epitomized a conflict between the old, enduring values of humanism, caring, belief in the individual, and concern for the client, and the new values and new directions pointing toward science, rigor, objectification, logic, analysis, dehumanization, and depersonalization. This conflict seems to represent a decision: a choice between being humanistic and caring, or being scientific and objective.

Thus my challenge today is to discuss this conflict, not because I have answers, but in the hope that clarification of the issues surrounding the conflict may help us find a satisfactory means of resolving it. I believe that the conflict is serious, that it has the potential to divide our profession, with one group opting for the old values and the comfortable, traditional approaches to practice, and the other seeking to move in the direction of scientific advancement. Intuitively, I feel that the creativity and sensitivity that are generally characteristic of occupational therapists offer hope for resolution of the conflict. However, we must be consciously aware of our fears as well as of our aspirations if we are to succeed in our endeavors.

To address this complex matter of conflict, I will first give you my interpretations of the concepts to be addressed. Then I will discuss values and their meaning for us as professionals. Next, I will review the "discovery" and evolution of occupational therapy as it occurred factually and conceptually. Finally, I will describe the nature of the conflicts, as I understand them, and offer some general thoughts about their resolution.

Definition of Terms

I will explain my interpretations of each of the words contained in the title of my presentation so that there will be a common understanding of the context within which I use each concept.

For the terms *old* and *values*, I have opted for the interpretation that suggests our values have been in existence for a long time and are familiar or known from the past. As such they have intrinsic worth, exist as social principles, and are held in high esteem.

New directions, when contrasted with *old values*, suggests that we are dealing with a phenomenon that has not existed before or has only recently been observed, experienced, and made manifest. *Direction* is defined as the way a person or thing faces or points, or a line or point toward which a moving person or thing goes. Thus the term *new directions* suggests that we are facing a particular way, a way that is new and unfamiliar and that may change our course by replacing the more comfortable and enduring values that we esteem.

Definitions of *competence*, *adaptation*, and *integration* offer interesting possibilities for interpretation within the context of a potential shift in our direction. *Competence* is defined as being fit or able, or as having capacities equal to expectations or requirements. When expectations or requirements shift, *adaptation*, or change, is necessary if we are to conform to new or revised circumstances, and if we are to achieve a better adjustment to a different environment. *Integration* suggests that the parts can be brought together and made whole, or renewed.

In summary, we confront the possibility of a change in our directions, a change that is currently perceived in our literature as moving toward science and reductionism and away from humanism and holism. However, competence, adaptation, and integration suggest that there may be hope for satisfactory resolution of the conflict between old values and new directions. This is the context from which I will speak today.

The Meaning of Values

The literature about professions and professionalization suggests that professionals conceptualize certain problems, or perplexing questions, that are of primary concern to members of their profession. Resolution of these problems becomes the focus of the profession's attention and energy and determines actions to be taken by its members in every sphere of practice, education, research, political activity, decision making, and other endeavors. These problems, or questions, significantly affect the standards for content of educational programs, as well as the organization, location, and structure of the profession's services. They are influential in attracting and recruiting prospective students and may influence the degree to which there is high attrition or "burn-out" at certain levels of professional achievement or practices. These problems, or perplexing questions, frequently reflect the values of the profession's members and may heavily influence the directions of the profession.

The directions that our profession has taken seem to be predicated on values, rather than on the basis of problems or perplexing questions. Our literature consistently reflects some of our values:

1. the value of the individual as a total person (1);
2. the value of purposeful activity (2), the value of occupation (3) in producing change and recovery;
3. the value of goal-oriented activity designed for a given individual's skills and abilities (3);
4. the value of permitting patients to choose meaningful activities (1)—activities that might, as Susan Tracy suggested, run parallel to the activity or occupation in which they would have been normally engaged (4);
5. the value of seeing the individual interacting within the framework of the environment (5); and
6. the value we place upon ourselves, our feelings, and our interactions with the patient/client as vital, integral, and caring components of the therapeutic process.

Rarely do occupational therapists do things *to* clients; rather, we engage in a collaborative process *with* them. Each party assumes responsibility and understands that the ultimate goal is for clients to achieve the degree of full responsibility for their lives of which they are capable.

These values appear throughout our literature. Although the language has changed, their meaning to us as occupational therapists has not. These are our espoused values (6), and the assumptions upon which they rest are that life is more than mere existence and that health is more than the absence of disease. For us, as therapists, health is a dynamic state of being that is reflected in the behaviors of people who have optimized their resources and who are living their lives fully, creatively, and expressively.

In my experience it seems that people are attracted to a profession because that profession, in its practice, demonstrates actions and behaviors that reflect its values, values that probably are common to and shared by both individuals in the profession and the profession itself.

As I considered this, I reflected on the experiences that brought me into occupational therapy as well as the experiences that reinforced my values and belief in the inherent and potential powers of our profession.

I was the older of two children; my father was a lawyer; my mother, a school teacher. About the time I was four or five, my father became an active alcoholic. His addiction rapidly worsened, and within a very short time span, our lives seemed to shift dramatically while many of our resources went into alcohol. It finally became necessary for my mother to seek employment. Divorce was out of the question both because of the prejudices of the time and because alimony was not permitted under state laws.

As his drinking patterns increased in severity, so did violence. Many nights I ran to town—barefooted, in my pajamas—to get the police to come stop the threats or the fighting—hoping that no one would be killed or seriously injured before I could return home with help. The police would attempt to reason with my father and to calm him; if that failed, he was sometimes whipped soundly. If that approach, too, failed, he would be taken to jail to sober up. It then became my responsibility to go to his cell to bargain with him: If we would let him come home, would he stay sober?

During one of these visits I saw a woman in a cell who was very psychotic. She had been jailed because there was no place to restrain her, no drugs to sedate her, and she had to be declared insane by the court before she could be transferred to a distant state hospital for treatment.

Later, during my college years, I spent two summers with the American Friends Service Committee in institutional service units. The purpose of these units was twofold:

1. to promote understanding among people by having representatives of varied races and religions work for a common goal, which was
2. to improve treatment of the mentally ill in state hospitals.

I spent one summer in a Texas hospital and another summer in a hospital in Ohio. In both hospitals I was assigned to wards with the most disturbed, paranoid, suicidal, or homicidal patients. Most of them had been hospitalized for a long time; few had any contacts with family or friends.

Treatment consisted of insulin or electric shock, isolation in empty cells, restraints—which usually meant being chained to a bench—or occasional beatings. There were no occupational therapists to come to the wards, and generally, the patients could not leave the wards.

We used games, discussion, and behavior modeling to bring about change, and I realized our effectiveness only after returning to visit later. During that visit one of the patients described to me, in exquisite detail, what it meant to her when I took a crayon and paper in for her to use while I talked with her when she was disturbed and shackled to a bench.

As I thought about these and other experiences, I realized how strongly developed was my sense of value about humane treatment and concern for the individual patient. So, as I reviewed the literature in preparing this presentation, it was not surprising to find these and similar values occurring repeatedly. This led me to believe that others had had similar experiences. In retrospect, many of the values we have that relate to caring may well come from experiences in state hospitals and other long-term care facilities where there was only the staff to care about patients and in which sometimes caring was the only treatment medium available.

I suspect that many of you selected occupational therapy as your career choice because you, too, found that your values could be reinforced and channeled in satisfying ways through the therapist/client relationship. We care—and we believe in what we do. This I know from personal experience as well as from visits with so many of you during my terms as president.

To summarize this discussion of values and their meaning for us, I believe that competent, thoughtful, caring people are drawn to a profession like occupational therapy for several reasons:

1. Commitment to the conceptual, perplexing questions that the profession addresses (which in my earlier experience related primarily to humane care of the ill and disabled);
2. Shared concern for the values espoused by and seen in a profession's practice, particularly as that practice reflects attempts to resolve specific questions; and
3. Opportunity to commit one's creativity, energies, and life to resolution of problems that matter—that make a difference in the quality of life and the quality of the environment.

The commitment to our values is deep and strong, but there may be pitfalls for us as professionals if values are not expressed within a context of scientific thought. So let us move to a discussion of the "discovery" and evolution of occupational therapy and see how our values fit into a larger scheme.

The "Discovery" and Evolution of Occupational Therapy

The concepts and observations upon which our profession was founded were formulated when medicine and related sciences lacked knowledge and tools to understand or eliminate the causes of many illnesses, diseases, and social problems. Many illnesses, such as tuberculosis or mental illness, required prolonged hospitalization, or institutionalization. Problems such as abject poverty resulted in placements in poor farms. These conditions resulted in decreased or impaired activity and often necessitated removal of the "sick" or impoverished individual from home and family.

Physicians, having limited knowledge and without the technology available today, had to develop and systematically use their powers of observation and judgment. In the absence of diagnostic tests, they relied upon intuition to connect scientific or systematic observations and empirical evidence with limited knowledge to make a diagnosis. (The term *empirical evidence* as used herein refers to reliance on practical experience without reference to scientific principles; empiricism is the dependence of a person on his or her own experience and observation, disregarding theory, reasoning, and science. At times it may be necessary to rely upon one's experience and observations because there are no scientific principles to explain the phenomenon.) It was necessary to diagnose and treat within a broad context and to look for external (to the body) or environmental causes and cures. It was acknowledged that microbes or germs produced illness or disease, but many physicians believed that external stress, produced perhaps by work or other environmental conditions, created the conditions in which germs or microbes were triggered into action.

Consequently, focus on a broad spectrum of interrelationships led to the following conclusions:

1. a relation existed between the environment and a person's state of health;
2. recovery from illness or depression was influenced by activity; and
3. more specifically, when certain conditions were present, improvement occurred following engagement in activity or occupation.

It was thus hypothesized that activity, or occupation, and improvement in one's medical condition were related. Most members of society, lacking disciplined skill in observation and trust in their intuitive powers, would likely describe the same phenomenon as "busy work."

Our founders were physicians, architects, social workers, secretaries, teachers of arts and crafts, nurses, and of course, the first occupational therapists. Each brought a different perspective and came from a unique background and orientation, yet each observed the effects of occupation in their individual environments and believed in its curative powers. In some ways, this gathering of "specialists" represented the context in which systems theory has been most effective—that is, in situations when a group of specialists representing different perspectives and backgrounds meet to consider the resolution of complex problems.

The individuals who gave life to our profession were visionaries, persons with strong convictions and the courage to uphold and support their convictions. The men who participated in our "discovery" were humanists as well as scientists, exerting leadership to change the course of illness and medical care. Female founders were also unique: educated and dedicated professionals, exerting leadership to change social conditions and to promote healing—people who opted for a life that did not conform to the expectations of women as held by society at that time. These pioneers had competence, discipline, and the determination to succeed.

They seemed to share similar characteristics: the ability to define problems broadly and to organize an effective response to such problems; the ability to act and to reflect upon what they learned from their actions, thereby modifying their behaviors as necessary; the ability to transmit their goals and the rationale underlying these goals to others. They also had power—power granted not by the sanction of society but power that comes from within: intuitive power; power created by belief and conviction, as they are honed by knowledge and observation; the power of disciplined minds and compassionate spirits. These qualities are demonstrated in their writing, their decisions, their interactions with others, and, most importantly, in their legacy to us. Their lives were devoted to bringing about change in the human condition. Their experience convinced them that occupation was the vehicle by which such change could be made possible.

Rene Dubos, whose life has been devoted to study of the interrelationships between living organisms and their environment, suggests that great discoveries are often intuitive and occur when surprising outcomes result from an observed phenomenon (7).

Robert Merton, the noted sociologist of science from Columbia University, "has shown in his writings that almost all major ideas arise more than once, independently, and often virtually at the same time." (8) Our professional literature reflects the concepts expressed by Dubos and Merton.

In this sense, our founders made not only a surprising discovery when they observed that occupation influenced recovery from illness, but they also translated that discovery into action by forming the National Society for the Promotion of Occupational Therapy.

At this point an interesting turn occurred. Once occupational therapy was identified, the demand for services quickly followed. The literature that I reviewed became silent about the scientific aspects of this great "discovery."

World War I was followed by legislation mandating occupational therapy services in rehabilitation. The depression brought with it demands for retraining the unemployed. World War II, followed by the Korean War, the Vietnam War, and the "wars" on poverty, stroke, heart disease, cancer, and other disabling conditions, created a great demand for occupational therapists (9). We responded.

Our tools, techniques, and values were quickly adapted to new categories of clients. We moved into many new environments to provide services: hospitals, rehabilitation centers, community mental health centers, private practice, community treatment centers, physicians' of-

Perspectives on Purposeful Activity: Foundation and Future of Occupational Therapy

fices, nursing homes, home health, well baby clinics, and school systems. We managed by training aides and volunteers or by becoming consultants and by supervising others.

Not only did we move into new environments, but we also adapted our repertoire of tools. We used arts and crafts, splinting and orthotics, therapeutic use of self, pre-vocational exploration, neurodevelopmental and kinesiological theories and techniques, activities of daily living, and more recently, exercise routines previously used in physical therapy.

Sensory-integrative therapy emerged, but it came primarily from a research base. Its adherents used a test (the Southern California Sensory Integrative Test) designed to diagnose and treat certain deficits. Treatment programs oriented to specific problems were planned and an attempt was made to formulate and organize both diagnosis and treatment into a theoretical framework.

Change, "meeting needs," and adaptation have been a way of life for us. We have been responsive to society's demands and to the needs of our clients. Indeed, those needs and demands have had priority over the needs of the profession and of its members.

We met the everchanging challenges for delivery of services and created many jobs. This ensured the survival of our profession, the importance of which cannot be minimized. We adapted well and our efforts have without question produced a significant result: a greater demand for occupational therapists than we have ever been able to supply.

This growth was not accomplished without a price, however, and today we are beginning to pay that price.

The conditions under which our profession rapidly developed were such that demand for services quickly increased and has continued unabated. There was little time for our founders' visions to be nurtured, expanded, or understood intellectually or conceptually—rather, there was demand that the ideas, the convictions, the values be put into action immediately.

Part of the price we now pay is that our directions frequently seem to be predicated not upon the observations and concepts of our founders but upon external sources and influences: the influence of medicine, the perceived power of the Federal government, sources of reimbursement for treatment, and limited vision and lack of confidence in our potential, as reflected in a narrow concept of practice and cluttered professional education programs specifying breadth rather than depth. Argyris and Schon, in *Theory and Practice: Increasing Professional Effectiveness*, state that factors such as these reflect the demands or expectations of special interest groups but that they are external to the nature of professional practice and education (6).

With each new direction we have taken, the shortage of qualified personnel has increased. To respond to the problem of personnel shortages, we have experimented

and continue to experiment with a variety of ways to recruit, certify, and retread personnel for entry into our profession. Some plans have been creative and innovative; others were taken in anticipation of government action (if we fail to act, the government will). Attempts to "fill the gap" have been an obsession with us.

Abraham Maslow is reported to have once said that "If the only tool you have is a hammer you tend to see every problem as a nail" (10). We seem to have taken this approach, believing that if we can just recruit enough students, provide amnesty for enough persons who have "dropped out," or promote enough COTAs to OTRs, our problems will be solved.

Dubos proposes an interesting perspective that seems applicable to our situation. As a proponent of adaptation, he warns that, if adaptation is carried too far, without awareness of the consequences, the desired change may be harmful rather than helpful. He illustrates this point by describing how the body adapts to air pollution on a short-term basis, but develops chronic bronchitis or emphysema if the stress of short-term adaptive processes must continue indefinitely. In crowded social environments, individuals put on blinders and no longer perceive the crowd; in so doing, however, they sacrifice a certain quality of interpersonal life (7).

Dubos provided this additional description. He related that Pasteur once taught the physiology of architecture at the Ecole des Beaux Arts in Paris. To demonstrate the importance of good ventilation, he conducted the following experiment. He placed a bird in a bell jar in which the oxygen was not renewed so that it gradually diminished. The bird adapted by decreasing its activity and remaining almost immobile. Pasteur then removed the bird and replaced it with a new one, abruptly introducing it to an atmosphere low in oxygen. The new bird began to move about and promptly died. Not only did this demonstration illustrate the importance of good ventilation, but it also demonstrated that we unconsciously adapt to unfavorable circumstances, but only if they occur slowly (7).

The principles of human adaptation presented by Dubos can be applied to professions as well as to people. We have adapted over time to medical and social need and demand but without recognizing the consequences of our adaptive behavior. Some of these consequences as they now confront us are listed below.

First, we have not considered the impact of introducing new therapists, who are still maturing and are educated only at the baccalaureate level, into the stress-producing environments that exist today. We have had time to acclimate ourselves and have acquired some of the requisite knowledge, skills, and tools through experience, but new therapists are often introduced to the environment abruptly.

Second, our sole focus on meeting needs of the disabled and of society has led to the neglect of the importance of fostering, nurturing, and supporting people who move into more demanding, challenging, and often lonely positions as administrators, clinical specialists, researchers, and curriculum directors. One has only to see the number of vacancies for curriculum directors or researchers to understand the nature of the problem. When therapists move into these positions, almost every segment of our profession wants and needs something from them: participation in a task force, continuing education opportunities, membership on or chairing a committee. Yet, as a profession, we offer little support to people in these positions.

Clinical or entry-level therapists sell a commodity that is primarily patient oriented: skill in diagnosing certain kinds of problems relating to performance; a treatment procedure, methodology, or technique; a splint or an adaptive device. The commodity that a researcher, a faculty member, or an administrator sells is an idea, a concept. Regardless of the commodity that we offer, however, we need documentation of its worth, its value, its potential dangers, and the conditions under which it is most effective. We have been so busy selling the commodity that we have neglected the work that must be done to substantiate the value of that commodity. The more we move up and extend our contacts, the more documentation for support is required.

My personal experience and explorations lead me to suggest that people in general, people as professionals, and professions composed of people, all need to be nurtured. Many forms of sustenance are required to strengthen and prepare or to renew and revitalize us, especially in times of rapidly changing conditions and high stress, both of which are found in abundance today.

Finally, the third consequence of our overadaptation to society's needs and demands is reflected in the fact that we have defined our problem as one of insufficient human resources at the entry level—or lack of nails—rather than defining conceptual problems and perplexing questions. A theoretical framework cannot emerge from the problem of insufficient personnel. Nor does the availability of jobs attract thoughtful persons who want to commit themselves, their energies, and their resources to a career.

The absence of well-defined theories limits our scope, our focus, and our research. It puts us in the position of relying on such things as role-delineation studies—studies of past performance and activity to support our endeavors. These studies do not provide a base of knowledge to support us. The absence of a solid theoretical foundation also causes us to overemphasize old values and their "rightness." It leads, I believe, to our condemnation of medicine for its lack of humanitarianism, its dehumanizing approach, its reductionism—since this further justifies our position.

So, as our evolution has brought us face-to-face with society's expectations for research and of the need for scientific support (or at least examination of) our therapeutic rationale and procedures, *we* fall back on old values and seek to defend our positions.

We face a painful conflict, and we are ill prepared for the new directions with their implications for change in our lives. The tragedy is that we are also ill prepared to defend our services and our education.

How, then, has our conceptual development progressed, and what hope is there for us?

A review of our literature suggests that conceptual development was initiated by our founders. It then was generally dormant until Dr. Reilly, in 1961 (see Chapter 6), translated the vision and "discovery" of our founders into an hypothesis:

That man, through the use of his hands as they are energized by mind and will, can influence the state of his own health.

She attributed this hypothesis to our founders and said of it:

"The splendor of its vision goes far beyond rating it as an idea conceived once in a lifetime or even once in a century. Rather, it falls in the class of one of those great beliefs which has advanced civilization. Its magnificence lies in the optimistic vote of confidence it gives to human nature. It implies that there is a reservoir of sensitivity and skill in the hands of man which can be tapped for his health. It implies the rich adaptability and durability of the central nervous system which can be influenced by experiences. And more than all this, it implies that man, through the use of his hands, can creatively deploy his thinking, feelings and purposes to make himself at home in the world and to make the world his home."

Dr. Reilly continues: "For a profession organized around this hypothesis it sets few limits to its growth. It merely endows a group with the obligation to acquire reliable knowledge leading to a competency to serve the belief. Because this is an hypothesis about health, it requires that this knowledge be made available for the guidance of physicians and that it be made applicable to a wide range of medical problems."

Reilly concluded her lecture with a suggestion that the hypothesis would begin its proof when we identified the drive in Man for occupation and would continue as we shaped our services to fill that need. ". . . we belong," she said, "to a profession that requires the mind to look at the history of man's achievements throughout civilization. It requires the spirit to respond to the wonders of what man has accomplished with his hands." (11)

Consider for a moment the beauty and power of Reilly's statement—and the potential that it offers to each of us as we join with our clients to assist them in fulfilling this potential in their lives. This is our heritage, our legacy, our challenge. It gives us a direction that can be sought regardless of the environment in which we work. It offers tremendous potential for channeling our values into productive outcomes. It requires no distinction of age or category of disease. It is universal.

This hypothesis, too, lay dormant for a period of time, although work in related areas was progressing.

Most recently, in the fall of 1980, Kielhofner *et al.* published a series of four articles in which a model of human occupation emanating from Reilly's hypothesis was proposed (12). It is suggested in this model that occupation, or function, is central to human life and that the occupational therapist is uniquely qualified to address deficits or problems causing dysfunction. The purpose of occupational therapy is to facilitate the transition of persons with illnesses or disabilities from a state of dependency and dysfunction to or toward a state of full participation and meaningful function in the environments in which they live. Consequently, we address the problems or deficits unique to each individual as well as the social system in which he or she functions and lives.

We have targeted for ourselves a level of performance that is high indeed: an approach to holistic treatment that requires consideration of many complex factors, frequently crossing interdisciplinary lines to understand and grasp the principles of:

1. normal development in all spheres throughout the life span;
2. pathology and its relation to function and dysfunction;
3. adaptation and change;
4. learning and acquisition of competence;
5. integrative processes; and
6. human interaction within the context of the environment.

We now add to this list of requirements an understanding of the principles of occupational behavior and general systems theory. And, as if this is not enough, we must also understand research—because it is by and through research that we determine whether or not our theoretical constructs have substance and produce the results that we claim. The knowledge acquired from research and its findings may enable us to explain, with some degree of assurance, how, under what conditions, and when therapeutic intervention is effective. It makes possible prediction, with some degree of certainty, to say when and with whom our methods of intervention will be beneficial. It may even lead to some degree of control over factors that produce or aggravate disability and dysfunction.

Research can be viewed as a form or system of communication, for it is the language of scientists and of critical thinkers. When persons from other disciplines examine and understand the methods by which we have critically evaluated and analyzed what we do, they can have confidence in what we say we produce or accomplish.

I believe that the works of Reilly and Kielhofner *et al.* (as well as that of Ayres, although in a slightly different context) are significant contributions to the conceptual development needed by our profession. This work is very rudimentary, but it begins to formulate the conceptual questions to be addressed, uniquely, by our profession. It also offers potential for drawing the separate and disparate parts of our profession together under one conceptual umbrella and for connecting these parts not only to each other but to the whole.

We have identified for ourselves a goal that is extremely complex and of enormous magnitude for we must have knowledge to understand the cause of dysfunction, to diagnose dysfunction as it affects performance and occupation, to identify and establish the appropriate program and process for specific individuals that will result in adaptation and ultimately integration, to bring about change in society and in technology so that both share responsibility for adapting to the needs of humans—and all living things on this earth.

Without question, this goal, this sense of direction, offers a service needed by society now and one that will be needed in ever increasing ways as technology expands. As Dubos said, the most tragic problem confronting industrialized nations is that society is increasingly unable to provide people with a function that has a profound meaning for their lives.

How, then, can we pursue this goal—and make it a reality rather than a vision or a set of values for people who want to do good things?

Thoughts for the Future

I have no certain answers for us, but I can share with you some of my thoughts, my tentative suggestions. I, like you, have intuitive feelings, beliefs, and some empirical evidence from my observations and practice that suggest we have the potential to offer "A sufficiently vital and unique service for medicine to support and society to reward." (11) Ideally, this will be a stimulus for our most creative thinking so that, together, we can find appropriate answers for us and for our profession.

First, it is important to recognize the conflict that confronts us: our desire to retain values that have been an integral part of our profession and, on the other hand, our recognition of the importance of science and research—accompanied by our fears about the directions in which science and research may take us. The potential changes have frightening implications for us—professionally and personally. None of us can help but wonder, "What will happen to me in this process of change?" Will there be a place for me to continue working, and how will I fit? What will happen to my program, my patients, my students, my job?" These questions must be addressed.

Second, I believe that we must redefine the problems that our profession is to address. We must have a sense of direction, a series of perplexing questions to which we, as a profession, commit ourselves. The problem is not one of a shortage of people; it is a shortage of ideas, of concepts, of critically defined questions and problems that attract people, that captivate their imaginations and tap their creativity, that use their intellectual capacity, that say to them, "Here is a problem, a perplexing question of great social value and individual meaning. Join us. Become an occupational therapist and help us find answers." Saving lives is important—but what is the redeeming value of saving lives if they cannot be lived with dignity and meaning?

This has been brought home to me through two recent experiences. In the first instance, I was driving home one day and, as I turned a corner near my house, I saw an older woman sitting on the ground, near the corner. She waved, and I waved back. A moment later it occurred to me to stop and walk back to see about her. She greeted me with obvious relief and said, "I thought no one would ever stop." She had stumbled and fallen and could not get up by herself. After asking about injuries, I helped her get to her feet, and we talked a bit. As I started to leave, she asked if I knew how old she was. "Oh, perhaps 60," I replied. "No," she laughed, "I'm 96." Then she stood tall and straight, looked down at me, and said, "I take a walk everyday—but today I stumbled on something I didn't see and fell." Being a bit shaken at her age, my fear of potential injury to her, and not knowing quite what to do, I asked if she would like me to walk home with her.

"Oh, no," she replied, with tears welling in her eyes and a look of terror crossing her face, "I live with my daughter, and if I can't walk by myself, she'll put me in a nursing home—I don't want to be put away." How tragic that people must devote their energies and spend their last years struggling to avoid being put away.

In the second experience, I have, with my family, watched helplessly as a rapidly progressive nervous system degeneration has deprived my mother of her ability to use her body, to communicate, to function.

Medical science and humanistic, caring physicians have literally saved her life but neither the art nor the science of medicine has freed her of the indignity of her illness: incontinence; total loss of speech and ability to form words with her lips; contractures, rigidity, and spasticity in her hands, arms, trunk, and body that prohibit other forms of communication except through limited signs and signals; difficulties with eating, chewing, swallowing, and even keeping the food in her mouth. She is totally dependent on the sensitivity, awareness, and understanding of others to comprehend and respond to every need that she has; her sharp, alert, functioning mind is locked inside a useless body. She knows all that goes on; she hears, sees, cries, laughs, thinks, and feels—but our ability to comprehend is so limited.

I have watched as caring family and friends come to visit. Interaction is so limited and so uncomfortable that sometimes we come in twos or threes and end up talking to each other as though mother is not there. Or we are afraid, perhaps of tiring her or perhaps of our own discomfort and helplessness—and so we move into another room to sit and talk.

I, too, share this sense of helplessness and know how difficult it is to "treat" the members of one's family. I recognize the limitations of my own knowledge of the art and science of our practice. Still, this experience has given me a new appreciation for the potential of our profession as well as a greater realization of the complexity of the issues that we seek to address.

In addition to identifying the problems, the perplexing questions, to which we address ourselves, we must develop plans and strategies, or "road maps," to guide us as we commit ourselves and our resources to the process of seeking answers. It is necessary to recognize that each set of questions may produce some answers, but answers will also create new questions. Our search may be unending.

Third, we should set aside our condemnations of medicine and science, our contempt for basic research and reductionism. Instead, we should focus our energies and resources on those things *we* need to do. As I have learned to recognize and read the messages my own body sends to my unaware mind, I increasingly recognize that my anger is not usually about something "out there," but is a result of my frustration, pain, or anxiety about my own feelings of inadequacy, or impotence, my inability to accomplish or fulfill personal needs or certain expectations. We can learn, wisely, from the experiences of others, and avoid their pitfalls, but let us use our energies creatively and constructively to fulfill our purposes.

Fourth, I believe that we need to recognize and acknowledge the power of knowledge. We work in environments where one is measured against standards of knowledge and where power, emanating from knowledge, resides with those who have knowledge. Our own professional goals, as they are implicitly reflected in our values, require a high level of achievement, knowledge, and experience. We need to recognize the value that knowledge, of itself, has, how it can support *all* of us, and how it can nurture and open doors for us.

It is easy to be frightened by knowledge—by those who are perceived as being knowledgeable. My graduate students are frightened of my knowledge and of the control over their lives that it may give me. I, in turn, am frightened at their knowledge of clinical practice—and fearful of exposing my ignorance. It is only when we both acknowledge our fears and know that we can each make a unique contribution to strengthen the totality of our mutual experience that we move forward together.

Fifth, we need to acknowledge the validity of our professional value system. These values are expressed in the total context of our lives: How we care for ourselves and each other, how we treat our environment, and how we behave toward our colleagues, our friends, our families, and all the other creatures and living things that inhabit this earth we call home. We value freedom to make choices; independence to exercise those decisions; physical ability to come and go as we please; health; the warmth and meaning of home, friends, and privacy; the opportunity to engage intellect and creativity in meaningful activity; and the inherent spirituality and dignity that enables us to appreciate love and beauty—in all its forms.

Each of us, as professionals and as individual members of society, must retain and support our values. We value people, and their right to dignity. We value their desire to integrate themselves into life to the extent possible for them—and we seek to help them enter the mainstream of life: to shop in markets, to attend movies, to listen to the music of great symphonies; to see and feel the beauty of ballet, to work, to play, to watch, to feel. Government should not have to be responsible for bringing about such attitudes; we should accept that responsibility because it is just and right for us to do so, because we believe that every human being has the right and the responsibility to participate in life to the extent he or she is capable and desires to do so.

Still, we must also recognize some of the limitations inherent in acting on values alone or without the requisite knowledge base. A healthy respect for knowledge enables us to translate values into action effectively, thereby increasing our chances of producing lasting results.

Finally, we need to put our fears of specialization to rest. Dubos says that most of the great discoveries have been intuitive and have come from phenomenologists: people who see a problem as a whole without looking at its inner mechanisms or detailed parts (7). The discovery itself usually comes in the form of a surprise, an unexpected outcome of an event, observation, or experiment. As I said earlier, occupational therapy was just such a discovery—the observation that patients and clients who engaged in activity or occupation seemed to recover.

However, Dubos states that the great discovery alone may not be sufficient. There must also be people who are logicians and analysts, people who are committed to understanding and explaining how, when, and under what conditions the unexpected outcome, the surprise occurs. This process has two parts at work in occupational therapy. One is that of looking at the whole organism in relation to its environment. This is a complicated relationship, according to Dubos, that requires a complex response by the organism. The complexity of this problem (which Dubos calls adaptation, and we call occupational therapy) "may well require development of a new scientific approach because existing scientific methodologies may not be applicable to its resolution.... This new science would have to learn to predict the total organism's response to very complex situations." (7)

The second part of this process is an examination of the individual and of his or her deficits and assets, followed by a plan that promotes improved function through reduction of deficits and strengthening of assets. In this and other instances, Dubos stresses the importance of the reductionist approach to provide explanations. Further, both Dubos and general systems theorists emphasize the relevance, and indeed critical importance, of bringing specialists from many areas together to solve problems. The science of adaptation, says Dubos, "must be viewed from the perspectives of medicine, technology, architecture, and social life because not only must humans adapt to new conditions, but technology and environments must also be adapted to human needs."(7)

The discovery of our founders and the work of Reilly; Kielhofner *et al.*; and of Ayres and others provide the sketchy outlines of a model that may ultimately provide a unifying theoretical or conceptual force in our profession, integrating under one umbrella our concepts and treatment approaches in areas as diverse as pediatrics and gerontology, as disparate as physical dysfunction, sensory integration, and psychiatry; and even providing a coherent, logical place for hand specialists, feeding specialists, and activity specialists. We need generalists *and* specialists, for each has a contribution to make. The potential contribution of each increases the value of the whole if appropriate connections and linkages can be established through research and theory development.

Our traditional values, when supplemented and supported by knowledge, offer us the potential to become a powerful presence in our society—powerful in that we provide a resource that enables individuals to live their lives as they want, to become what they want to be.

I believe that we do not have to sacrifice our old values for new ones but that we can merge the old and the new, thereby strengthening each. Our old values, when combined with the new, emphasizing science and knowledge, can forge powerful new directions for our profession. In so doing, we will acquire new competence. The process of adaptation will bring about change, but integration can provide us with a unity and wholeness that we have not yet achieved.

Perhaps, as we think of old values and new directions, of the concepts and meaning of competence, adaptation, and integration, we should heed the advice of Pericles when he spoke to the Athenians:

> Fix your eyes on the greatness of your profession as you have it before you day by day; fall in love with her, and when you feel her great, remember that her greatness was won by people with courage, with knowledge of their duty, and with a vision that all things are possible.(13)

Acknowledgments

The author gratefully acknowledges the guidance and direction given by Fanny B. Vanderkooi and Florence M. Stattel as she entered the occupational therapy profession, as well as the contributions of Ann P. Grady, Gail

---

Fidler, Donna King, Elizabeth J. Yerxa, the faculty and students at Washington University, and other friends and colleagues for their intellectual stimulation and challenge, friendship, and support of her personal, conceptual, and professional development.

References

1. Yerxa EJ: Authentic occupational therapy. *Am J Occup Ther* 21: 6, 1967.

2. Ayres AJ: Occupational therapy for motor disorders resulting from impairment of the central nervous system. *Rehab Lit* October 1960.

3. Wiest A: *Activity Book for the Ill, Convalescent, and Disabled of All Kinds as Well as the Hand of the Physician*, Stuttgart: Ferdnand Emke, Anje Ruil, *Am J Occup Ther* 21: 280–324, 1967.

4. Tracy S: *Studies in Invalid Occupations*, Boston: Whitcomb and Burrows, 1910.

5. Yerxa EJ: *The Present and Future Audacity of Occupational Therapy*, unpublished paper presented at Washington University, St. Louis, MO, October 1980.

6. Argyris C, Schon D: *Theory in Practice: Increasing Professional Effectiveness*, San Francisco: Jossey Books, Pub., 1980.

7. Dubos R, Escandi JP: *Quest: Reflections on Medicine, Science, and Humanity*, New York: Harcourt, Brace, Jovanovich, 1979.

8. Merton RK: On the shoulders of giants, quoted in Gould SJ: *The Panda's Thumb*, New York: W.N. Norton & Co., 1980.

9. Johnson JA: Commitment to action. *Am J Occup Ther 30:* 135–148, 1976.

10. Maslow A: *Quest*, May–June, 1977.

11. Reilly M: Occupational therapy can be one of the great ideas of 20th century medicine. *Am J Occup Ther 16:* 1–9, 1962 (Reprinted as Chapter 6).

12. Kielhofner G, et al.: A model of human occupation, Parts 1–4, *Am J Occup Ther 34:* 572–581; 34: 657–670; 34: 731–737; 34: 777–788, 1980.

13. Quotation from Hislop H: The not-so-impossible dream, *Phys Ther 55:* 1069–1080, 1975.

Chapter 64

How High Do We Jump? The Effect of Reimbursement on Occupational Therapy

Brenda S. Howard, OTR

To what extent does reimbursement influence the practice of occupational therapy? Many occupational therapists agree that reimbursement affects clinical practice. Documentation, length and frequency of treatment, use of treatment modalities, and the need for regulation are all cited in the everyday conversation of clinicians as being related to reimbursement, at least in part. Less visible, and sometimes less comfortable, influences of reimbursement may be clinicians' ability to treat some diagnoses and not others, the development of specialty areas of treatment as new avenues of reimbursement open up, and the lack of development of some specialties because of limited reimbursement. However, the influences behind the initiation and continuance of third-party dictation of clinical practice and the question of how far dictation of practice really goes are rarely explored.

An understanding of the history and directions of reimbursement in the United States and of the depth of influence these reimbursement trends have on the development of occupational therapy will help occupational therapists put the influence of reimbursement into perspective.

History of Occupational Therapy in Relation to Reimbursement

"Historically, the reimbursement method for occupational therapy has driven its delivery system" (Foto, 1988a, p. 564). The history of occupational therapy reimbursement may be divided into three eras of change: the institution of modern health insurance, beginning in the 1920s and ending in the 1950s; the events leading up to and following the initiation of Medicare and Medicaid in the 1960s; and the control of costs that has begun in the current era of prospective payment (Baum, 1985).

The occupational therapy profession was born out of the Moral Treatment movement in the second half of the

19th century. Moral Treatment signified a change from custodial care of mentally ill people to care based on the "law of love" (Bockoven, 1971, p. 223). Adolph Meyer, whose work preceded the profession, linked occupational therapy to Moral Treatment by describing diseases as problems of adaptation, appropriate use of time as the remedy for habit deterioration, and occupational therapy as the means of teaching the structuring of time (Meyer, 1922/1977 [see Chapter 2]). In fact, the first definition of the profession, written in 1918, was "a means of instruction and employment in productive occupation" (Hopkins & Smith, 1978, p. 10). Meyer's philosophy of occupation in mental health strongly influenced the philosophy and history of occupational therapy as a whole (Hopkins & Smith, 1978).

In the decades following the Civil War, although occupational therapy was still in its infancy, the philosophy of Moral Treatment, as used in mental health, was already declining. This decline was largely due to a shift in popular thought from a moral–emotional model to a technological–pathological approach in which the scientific method was embraced (Bockoven, 1971). This happened in spite of the established efficacy of Moral Treatment (Bockoven, 1971; Peloquin, 1989 [see Chapter 4]). Mental health also shifted to an organic, pathology-based frame of reference in the early 1900s (Bockoven, 1971).

The shift in popular philosophy affected not only mental health practice but the entire medical community (Bockoven, 1971). The Flexner Report, published in 1906 (see Feldstein, 1987), marked a change in the philosophy underlying medical treatment. Generated by the American Medical Association in an effort to upgrade the quality of medical schools (Feldstein, 1987), the Flexner Report emphasized a unifactorial, biomedical, scientific model of disease. As a result of the report, medicine shifted to more scientific, laboratory-based concepts (Waitzkin, 1978).

During the formative years of the profession, occupational therapy persisted in its view that adaptation to and engagement in the environment were strong components of health, in spite of differing popular philosophy (Bockoven, 1971). However, the financial constraints of the depression years precipitated a significant turning point in the profession's development. In the middle of the 1930s, the American Occupational Therapy Association (AOTA) asked the American Medical Association to establish standards for training institutions and take over accreditation of occupational therapy schools. It was this decisive step that formally placed occupational therapy in the position of a medical ancillary (Rerek, 1971). This action, although it achieved its purpose of survival, limited nonmedical practice opportunities for the future in that occupational therapy was now tied to the health care industry by educational standards and financial concerns. Thus, the profession's struggle between its roots in Moral Treatment and the medical model/scientific method began.

From the 1940s to the 1960s, occupational therapy was involved in the rehabilitation movement, which began with the return of World War II disabled veterans. New antibiotic medications and advanced methods in surgery helped injured soldiers survive their wounds, and rehabilitation helped them to be independent with the resulting disabilities. Rehabilitation was also economically advantageous. During this time, association with the rehabilitation movement (and possibly with the medical community) made occupational therapists "uncomfortable with their simple operating principle that it was good for disabled people to keep active" (Mosey, 1971, p. 235). New treatment methods (e.g., orthotics, vocational evaluation, neuromuscular facilitation), borrowed from other professions, were added to the occupational therapists' repertoire at a pace so rapid that it was impossible to assimilate these changes into the profession's theoretical base (Mosey, 1971).

The rehabilitation movement was accompanied by changes in payment for health care services. Before this, health insurance had been based in local, private systems. Increases in the cost of medical care exceeded the limitations of this system. National health insurance was debated, but instead payment for health care was installed as an employee benefit controlled by private industry. The American Medical Association successfully campaigned against national health insurance, in conjunction with organized labor, which wanted to retain health insurance as a bargaining tool (Somers & Somers, 1961). The medical profession fought national health care coverage because it viewed "involvement of the federal government as a fatal intrusion in the hallowed doctor–patient relationship and believed that it would lead to the increasing bureaucratization of medicine" (Luft, 1978, p. 3). By the middle of the 1960s, physicians no longer had enough political power to stop government-supported health insurance (Luft, 1978), in part due to the increased political power of consumer groups (Freidson, 1975). With more support for government involvement in health care, Medicare and Medicaid were born in 1966. With their advent, the established traditions of payment and organization in health care were permanently altered (Freidson, 1975).

Few changes in the provision of services were anticipated with the start of Medicare. Diasio (1971) recognized that Medicare and Medicaid would allow the development of occupational therapy in community health care for the elderly and the poor. Reilly (1966) feared that an increased use of paramedical staff, including therapists, would cause funds for their wages to be spread thin, causing salary stagnation and the dreaded threat of symbiosis with physical therapy. As occupational therapists clarified their role, however, and as the use of more paramedical staff (therapists included) resulted in a shortage of therapists, Reilly's fears did not come true (Baum, 1985).

From the 1960s to the early 1980s, occupational therapy continued to enjoy a political climate favorable to health care, and its services grew (Davy, 1984a). However, costs began to escalate as health care facilities took advantage of available capital. Consequently, Congress set limits on Medicare reimbursement as part of the Tax Equity and Fiscal Responsibility Act of 1982 (Public Law 97–248). In the following year the Social Security Amendments of 1983 (Public Law 98–21) were enacted, which set the stage for the phasing in of the prospective payment and diagnosis-related group (DRG) forms of reimbursement (Russell, 1989).

With the cost constraints of the late 1970s and 1980s and the inception of prospective payment, occupational therapists found that accurate documentation was crucial to reimbursement (AOTA, 1989). In addition, demand for inpatient occupational therapy services decreased, and demand for outpatient services increased (Foto, 1988a). Shorter hospital stays have resulted in higher volumes of patients for occupational therapy services; further, the new payment system encourages provision of "the fewest number of services possible" (Baum, 1985, p. 779) to meet goals. All of this has led to concern over how to maintain service quality (Baum, 1985). For example, occupational therapists have found that their poorer clients receive limited support from government programs for therapy services. Thus, clinicians must struggle to provide helpful services during limited contact with these patients (Foto, 1988a).

In 1986, Congress passed the Occupational Therapy Medicare Amendments (Section 9337 of Public Law 99–509) in response to the need for more community-based treatment. These amendments extended full coverage to occupational therapy services under Medicare Part B. Payment was authorized for patients in skilled nursing facilities, rehabilitation agencies, home health care, and private practice (AOTA, 1989). Medicare Part B coverage has provided financial support for the expansion of private practice and contractual occupational therapy services in the past few years.

The Effect of Changes in Reimbursement on the Profession

The current environment of cost containment leaves occupational therapists "caught between the pressures of patients' demands for quality care and the drive to contain costs," which "creates professional and emotional conflict" (Foto, 1988a, p. 564). The effect of reimbursement on the definition of occupational therapy and on practice, management, professional ethics, and the profession's response will be discussed in the following paragraphs.

The Definition of Occupational Therapy

The definition of occupational therapy has been shaped by changing reimbursement patterns. In a special issue of the *American Journal of Occupational Therapy* (Davy, 1984c), detailed articles supplied information on coverage available for various practice areas of occupational therapy. This implied that what occupational therapists can do, and therefore what they are, is defined at least in part by what is reimbursed. In addition, what is not covered is outlined so that therapists do not perform noncovered services, or at least do not define what they do in a noncovered manner. In the same issue, Davy (1984b) described the great lengths to which the profession has gone to get itself defined by insurance companies in order to ensure coverage.

Further substantiation of this point is found in *Medicare Outpatient Physical Therapy and Comprehensive Outpatient Rehabilitation Facility Manual* (Department of Health and Human Services, 1989). Section 503 of this document, entitled "Guidelines for Submitting Claims for Outpatient Occupational Therapy Services," defines the services that are covered under Medicare Part B. One important feature of this document is its definition of what is not occupational therapy. If it is not in the guidelines, it is not paid for. Therefore, clinicians cannot perform or document services that are not in the guidelines if they wish to obtain reimbursement under Medicare Part B. Because this document is becoming a standard used by most insurance companies, its significance in defining occupational therapy is substantial. Fortunately for the profession, occupational therapists assisted in its development at the government's request (AOTA, 1989).

Practice

Because the descriptions of the coverage available in various practice areas are used by occupational therapists in documenting their services, occupational therapists must now treat within the boundaries of these descriptions. Clinicians may therefore find themselves changing or limiting their modes of treatment to comply with reimbursement restrictions. For example, the occupational therapy guidelines for Medicare Part B specifically state that daily feeding programs are not considered skilled occupational therapy once the adapted procedures have been implemented (AOTA, 1989). Therefore, an occupational therapist may design a feeding program for a patient in a skilled nursing facility with Medicare Part B coverage but may have limited financial support for continued intervention. Patients with Medicare coverage are not the only ones affected. Outpatient care is another clinical area in which limitations in various forms of reimbursement dictate occupational therapy service provision: "Many times, because of a patient's lack of health insurance, we must turn even the most appropriate treatment candidates away from our

|outpatient| departments" (Burke & Cassidy, 1991, p. 174 |see Chapter 65|). Not only the frequency but also the nature of treatment has changed. Clinicians are now asked to provide diagnosis-based treatment protocols that will guarantee coverage for services. These protocols may or may not fit in with individual patient needs (Burke & Cassidy, 1991 |see Chapter 65|).

At a deeper and more disturbing level, changing reimbursement patterns have caused shifts in the definition of occupational therapy that have led, in turn, to changes in professional roles (e.g., occupational therapists' role with the chronically ill). Reilly (1971) explained the disparity that led to this change:

> There is an enormous obstruction outside the control of the profession that seriously impairs the delivery of service. It is the absence of economic support to chronic medicine. The commitment and hence the capitalization in medicine is directed toward the reduction and prevention of pathology and the treatment of acute phases of illness. Occupational therapy makes its investments in the health residual which follows pathology and hence focuses on the chronic aspect of the illness and is concerned with health rather than pathology. (p. 245)

Indeed, program design and treatment of acute phases of chronic illness are currently among the few occupational therapy services for persons with chronic illness that are supported by Medicare (AOTA, 1989).

New directions in reimbursement provide the capital for the development of new and existing clinical areas. Foto (1988a) gave examples of occupational therapy's ability to provide what insurance companies now want (e.g., wellness programs, reduced hospital stays, treatment at a lower level of care |therapist rather than physician| where appropriate, the return of patients to the highest possible functional level). She wrote, "Since occupational therapists offer these services, we should be in demand. But we must educate the industry . . ." (Foto, 1988a, p. 564). Her statements suggest that shifts in reimbursement will shape occupational therapy by the profession's need or desire to be where the reimbursement is. For example, records of facilities developed recently indicate that they include skilled nursing homes, outpatient services, and home health care (Russell, 1989). Could it be that, with the 1986 change in Medicare Part B reimbursement, these areas are once again profitable for occupational therapy? One could argue that the recent surge in the number of contracting agencies providing therapies for these clinical areas is another direct result of improved reimbursement. The type and quality of therapy services also appears to have changed with this resurgence: Agencies are reimbursed on a treatment unit basis, so therapists must account for their time by units of productivity. This means that little time is left to develop programs for services to chronically ill people or nonreimbursable nursing home residents.

The current climate of cost containment may have an effect on available treatment technology. This trend is hard to predict due to the varied nature of regulation and the effects of national values and lobbying groups on federal legislation. Aaron and Schwartz (1984) speculated that in the case of high-technology equipment, "the demand will be fully met in some cases; in others, constraints on expenditures will reduce either quality or quantity" (p. 115). What will this mean for occupational therapy? It may mean that patients will have to be prioritized for available equipment and that treatments that rely on high-technology equipment will go up in cost because of lower supply and higher demand. This could lead to greater access to technology for those who can pay and less access for the poor.

Management

Changes in reimbursement have also meant changes in management style for occupational therapy departments. Productivity and efficiency are becoming high-priority goals, because departments must handle more patients with fewer staff. Changes to increase productivity may include attempting to meet treatment goals in fewer treatment sessions; performing evaluations and treatments that focus on decreasing lengths of stay by addressing primarily the problems that are keeping patients in hospitals; and use of occupational therapy assistants, aides, volunteers, and part-time staff to meet treatment goals at the lowest cost possible. An emphasis on efficiency could require computer documentation for faster charting and evening and weekend treatment to speed recovery (Scott, 1984). Such programs for increased productivity need to be studied to determine their efficacy and to determine whether they allow patients sufficient time for the rest needed to recover.

In addition to changes in program design, productivity concerns cause managers to justify staff positions based on reimbursement data. Foto (1988b) suggested the use of the Medicare cost report to justify hiring more staff. This report covers not the number of treatments given, but the number of treatments reimbursed. Foto's suggestion highlights the fiscal constraints under which managers are operating and the extent to which reimbursement issues are linked to clinical issues.

Ethics

Reimbursement constraints can influence changes in professional ethics. The Occupational Therapy Code of Ethics, Principle 1, Item H, states: "The individual shall establish fees, based on cost analysis, that are commensurate with services rendered" (AOTA, 1988, p. 795). In light of cost constraints and the need to justify staff, there is a risk that this principle may be interpreted loosely, resulting in ethical abuses. Possible abuses include overbilling for services (e.g., rounding up times), providing services that are not necessary for functional goals, overpricing of services, overworking employees to maintain revenues, and focusing efforts on those programs that bring in revenue but are not clinically effective (Mullins, 1989).

Reimbursement concerns raise new ethical questions: Is it ethical to make changes in the provision of services based on the patient's method of payment, or on the basis of reimbursability rather than diagnosis? Discrimination in providing health services may work both ways: The nonreimbursable patient may receive subminimal care, which compromises quality, and the patient with ample reimbursement may be treated beyond the limit of goals for cost containment. The free market medical system provides few checks and balances:

> The market is the provider's best friend. It gives providers license to supply inaccurate information, to limit service only to those patients with an ability to pay, to charge whatever they wish, and to reduce quality of care to achieve greater profitability. (Sloan, Blumstein, & Perrin, 1988, p. 237)

The Profession's Response

The responses of occupational therapy as a profession to changes in reimbursement fall into three categories: regulation, public relations, and political action. Although the justification for regulation (licensure) of health care professionals has been consumer protection (Sloan et al., 1988), an equally important consequence for occupational therapy is improved reimbursement (see Moyers, 1988). Licensure of occupational therapists exists in 46 states (Javernick, 1991).

Increased dialogue and public relations efforts with third-party payers will distribute control of the health care industry more equally between providers and payers (Hertenstein, 1989). Occupational therapists who enter into dialogue with insurance companies must be prepared to address the insurance industry's needs (Foto, 1988a) and use the industry's language of functional independence and patient dignity to discuss occupational therapy services (Foto, 1988b). By addressing insurance industry concerns, occupational therapists may find it necessary to compromise on clinical issues. Other responses to reimbursement concerns include mobilizing to accommodate managed care, breaking through coverage barriers of health maintenance organizations (Foto, 1988b), and recruiting new occupational therapists so that services will continue to be available at a lower cost level (Baum, 1985).

Political action within the profession consists of lobbying for a better understanding of occupational therapy issues among legislators (Baum, 1985; Foto, 1988b). Being politically active is crucial to taking a proactive stance in managing change in health care (Foto, 1988b).

Discussion

Occupational therapy does not exist in a vacuum; societal influences are a dominant factor in precipitating change. Neither research nor pure theory appears to have the impact on occupational therapy practice that society does. The societal influence of reimbursement for health care has substantially affected occupational therapy in definition, practice, management, ethics, and the profession's response. Reimbursement has altered occupational therapy by at least four means: control, understanding (e.g., of disease), language, and values.

Control

It is a Marxist premise that increased concentration of capital in the hands of the few leaves others unempowered (Waitzkin, 1978). With capital for health care centralized in insurance companies and government programs, it is to be expected that these third-party payers exert great control over the health care system. Control in occupational therapy has been altered by placing the definition of the profession, in part, in the hands of those who hold the capital. In other words, occupational therapy is being controlled to some extent by payers who participate in defining it. Examples, mentioned earlier, include the proliferation or demise of specialty areas according to reimbursability (as with the increase in hand therapy and work hardening and the decrease in inpatient care and contact with pediatric clients); changes in service provision according to coverage (e.g., limited provision of services to patients with limited reimbursement); and the need to justify the number of staff members in occupational therapy departments by the number of treatments reimbursed.

Understanding

Virchow, who studied social epidemiology and social medicine, focused on two major themes regarding the understanding of disease. He believed that the origin of disease is multifactorial (not just physical) and that successful improvements in health care must be the result of concurrent improvements in economic, political, and social reforms (as cited by Waitzkin, 1978). One can extrapolate from Virchow that it is necessary to maintain a consistent understanding of the whole health care system, the ways it seeks to remediate disease, and the economic and political changes that affect the system.

Shifts in popular ideology have caused occupational therapy to change its understanding of itself. For example, the modern urgency for research attempts to establish occupational therapy within the biomedical/scientific model, indicating how far occupational therapy understanding has shifted from its connection to Moral Treatment philosophy. Research, therefore, becomes not just a measure of efficacy, but a method to justify occupational therapy according to the dominant model in health care practice. Because reimbursement rewards the unifactorial medical model, it becomes difficult to survive economically while clinging to a philosophy based on multifactorial causes of disease. Compromise—by assimilating aspects of the medical model—allows for survival, but limits options for social effectiveness.

Language

Sapir and Whorf (Sapir, 1929) developed a hypothesis of linguistic relativity that held that the way things are talked about affects understanding of them. When this hypothesis is applied to occupational therapy, the way the profession is discussed changes how it is perceived. Subtle changes in occupational therapy philosophy have occurred simply through changes in the language with which thoughts are framed. By using the language of insurance companies (e.g., *skilled occupational therapy*) in documentation and definition, occupational therapy shifts into new clinical dimensions (e.g., use of objective tests and measurements) and discards old practices (e.g., use of activity for its intrinsic qualities). Framing occupational therapy in the appropriate language makes it acceptable and reimbursable to third-party payers. Language has affected management in particular; the words *cost containment*, *productivity*, and *efficacy* now occupy and shape the department manager's thoughts (Gray, 1983; Mullins, 1989).

Values

In our society, individualism and private enterprise are valued. With cost containment, the prevailing values in health care become clearer: Technology and the scientific method are valued more than the holistic use of a variety of treatment methods; the young and productive are valued more than the old and frail; and acute treatment is valued more than chronic care (Waitzkin, 1987). Reimbursement within a system that embraces these values shapes the practice of occupational therapy. What our profession valued at its inception contrasts with the values of the current health care system; the tension between societal values and the values of the profession continues to be a source of conflict for many clinicians.

Implications

How high do we jump? Should reimbursement dictate clinical practice? No one sector of society should control the health care field or any aspect of it. Accountability is a necessary part of participation in health care to ensure a broader distribution of power so that all interested parties may be assured of representation. The fact remains, however, that third-party payers have exerted substantial control over the profession, with an unclear understanding of how occupational therapy has influenced trends in reimbursement. It is also unclear how much say patients have in occupational therapy practice.

Occupational therapists occasionally need to step outside of the health care arena and view the interplay between the various sources of control in health care, so that reasons for actions and reactions will become clearer. For example, when clinicians understand the financial pressures that their health care institutions face, it is easier to view frustrations with service provision to individual patients as symptoms of a larger problem. It is also imperative to view the profession from the point of view of the other players—the patient, the insurance carrier, and other disciplines—so that cooperation and dialogue are welcomed when occupational therapy's role in the health care system is negotiated.

Occupational therapists also need to understand who they are as occupational therapists. Proactive, systematic vocational planning is then possible (Howard, 1990). Vocational planning includes defining ethical practice, framing the definition in language that is not easily bent, and lobbying for it through public relations activities and political action. It also includes examining the conflicting goals of quality service and cost containment and setting guidelines by which to practice within the boundaries of both.

The occupational therapist may use other means to maintain a fair distribution of power. Baum (1985) recommended looking to payment sources other than third-party payment to free occupational therapists to be self-directive. She mentioned workers' compensation, liability insurance, corporate funds, public health funds, and Social Security as a few examples. Another option is to practice in nontraditional (i.e., nonmedical) settings that allow greater impact on patient populations without reimbursement constraints. Occupational therapists working as employee health directors in industry are an example of nontraditional practitioners with an impact on prevention. A third means of vocational planning is volunteerism. If higher salaries and staff shortages are contributing to escalating costs and limited access for poor and rural patients, then volunteering is one option. Although most occupational therapists do not have the opportunity for full-time volunteer work, some are able to donate an hour a week to a free clinic. Others are able to offer a week or two a year of consultation services to programs for needy people. Still others participate in local and national advocacy groups for persons with disabilities.

We as occupational therapists must be aware that social factors influence the direction of the profession. Reimbursement issues not only frustrate clinical practice but participate in shaping occupational therapy. We must be aware of the causes of constraints on practice in order to be proactive in issues of health care policy.

References

Aaron, J., & Schwartz, W. B. (1984). *The painful prescription: Rationing hospital care.* Washington, DC: Brookings Institution.

American Occupational Therapy Association. (1988). Occupational therapy code of ethics. *American Journal of Occupational Therapy, 42,* 795–796.

American Occupational Therapy Association. (1989, September 16). *Insuring payment through documentation: A common sense approach* [American Occupational Therapy Association workshop presented in Indianapolis].

Baum, C. M. (1985). Growth, renewal, and challenge: An important era for occupational therapy. *American Journal of Occupational Therapy, 39,* 778–784.

Bockoven, J. S. (1971). Legacy of Moral Treatment—1800's to 1910. *American Journal of Occupational Therapy, 25,* 223–225.

Burke, J. P., & Cassidy, J. C. (1991). The Issue Is—Disparity between reimbursement-driven practice and humanistic values of occupational therapy. *American Journal of Occupational Therapy, 45,* 173–176. (Reprinted as Chapter 65).

Davy, J. D. (1984a). Nationally Speaking—Status report on reimbursement for occupational therapy services. *American Journal of Occupational Therapy, 38,* 295–298.

Davy, J. D. (1984b). Preferred provider organizations. *American Journal of Occupational Therapy, 38,* 327–329.

Davy, J. D. (Guest Ed.). (1984c). Reimbursement [Special issue]. *American Journal of Occupational Therapy, 38* (5).

Department of Health and Human Services. (1989, May). *Medicare outpatient physical therapy and comprehensive outpatient rehabilitation facility manual* (DHHS Publication No. 9, Transmittal No. 87). Washington, DC: Health Care Financing Administration.

Diasio, K. (1971). The modern era—1960 to 1970. *American Journal of Occupational Therapy, 25,* 237–242.

Feldstein, P. J. (1987). Policies of the American Medical Association: Self-interest or public-interest? In H. D. Schwartz (Ed.), *Dominant issues in medical sociology* (pp. 549–558). New York: Newbery Award Records.

Foto, M. (1988a). Nationally Speaking—Managing changes in reimbursement patterns, Part 1. *American Journal of Occupational Therapy, 42,* 563–565.

Foto, M. (1988b). Nationally Speaking—Managing changes in reimbursement patterns, Part 2. *American Journal of Occupational Therapy, 42,* 629–631.

Freidson, E. (1975). *Doctoring together: A study of professional social control.* Chicago: University of Chicago Press.

Gray, B. (1983). *The new health care for profit: Doctors and hospitals in a competitive environment.* Washington, DC: Brookings Institution.

Hertenstein, R. D. (1989). Third party concerns. *Cancer, 64* (July Suppl.), 319.

Hopkins, H. L., & Smith, H. D. (Eds.). (1978). *Willard and Spackman's occupational therapy* (5th ed.). Philadelphia: Lippincott.

Howard, B. S. (1990, December 3). Systematic vocation for OTs. *OT Forum,* pp. 8–12.

Javernick, J. A. (1991, March 28). Wyoming therapists gain licensure. *OT Week,* pp. 2, 16.

Luft, H. S. (1978). *Poverty and health.* Cambridge, MA: Ballinger Publishing.

Meyer, A. (1977). The philosophy of occupation therapy. *American Journal of Occupational Therapy, 31,* 639–642. (Original work published 1922). (Reprinted in Chapter 2).

Mosey, A. C. (1971). Involvement in the rehabilitation movement—1942–1960. *American Journal of Occupational Therapy, 25,* 234–236.

Moyers, P. (1988, June) *Licensure fund raising campaign.* Open form letter distributed at the June 1988 Indiana Occupational Therapy Conference, Mitchell, IN.

Mullins, L. L. (1989). Hate revisited: Power, envy, and greed in the rehabilitation setting. *Archives of Physical Medicine and Rehabilitation, 70,* 740–744.

Occupational Therapy Medicare Amendments (Public Law 99–507), § 9337.

Peloquin, S. M. (1989). Looking Back—Moral Treatment: Contexts considered. *American Journal of Occupational Therapy, 43,* 537–544. (Reprinted in Chapter 4).

Reilly, M. (1966). The challenge of the future to an occupational therapist. *American Journal of Occupational Therapy, 20,* 221–225.

Reilly, M. (1971). The modernization of occupational therapy. *American Journal of Occupational Therapy, 25,* 243–246.

Rerek, M. D. (1971). The depression years—1929 to 1941. *American Journal of Occupational Therapy, 25,* 231–233.

Russell, L. B. (1989). *Medicare's new hospital payment system: Is it working?* Washington, DC: Brookings Institution.

Sapir, E. (1929). The status of linguistics as a science. *Language, 5,* 207–214.

Scott, S. J. (1984). The Medicare prospective payment system. *American Journal of Occupational Therapy, 38,* 330–334.

Sloan, F. A., Blumstein, J. F., & Perrin, J. M. (Eds.). (1988). *Cost, quality, and access in health care.* San Francisco: Jossey-Bass.

Social Security Amendments of 1983 (Public Law 98–21).

Somers, H. M., & Somers, A. R. (1961). *Doctors, patients, and health insurance.* Washington, DC: Brookings Institution.

Tax Equity and Fiscal Responsibility Act of 1982 (Public Law 97–248).

Waitzkin, H. (1978). A Marxist view of medical care. *Annals of Internal Medicine, 89,* 264–278.

Waitzkin, H. (1987). A Marxian interpretation of the growth and development of coronary care technology. In H. D. Schwartz (Ed.), *Dominant issues in medical sociology* (2nd ed., pp. 613–624). New York: Newbery Award Records.

Chapter 65

Disparity between Reimbursement-Driven Practice and Humanistic Values of Occupational Therapy

Janice Posatery Burke, MA, OTR/L, FAOTA

Joanne C. Cassidy, MEd, OTR/L

In January 1990, clinicians, educators, and researchers met at the Directions for the Future Symposium in San Diego to delineate, discuss, and debate a wide range of economic, political, and social issues that are influencing the evolution of occupational therapy practice and education. By examining these factors in an open and thorough way, therapists believe they will be able to develop proactive positions that will ensure the continued well-being of the field.

In this paper, we will consider two distinctly opposing forces that dramatically affect and present considerable obstacles to occupational therapists. On the one hand, occupational therapists are taught to embrace a fundamental, humanistically based philosophy of practice that emphasizes the importance of the individual. On the other hand, they are expected to practice in an economically defined health care environment, where issues of reimbursement for service are highly valued and are among the key factors to be considered when making evaluation and treatment decisions.

Humanistic-Valued Practice

Adolf Meyer is among the early leaders of the field credited with advocating treatment that centers on a "profound respect for the patient and his efforts to get through this life with a maximum of gratification and a minimum of discomfort" (Muncie, 1959, p. 1322). During the early years of the profession's development, this notion formed the keystone of professional practice. This approach directed therapists to emphasize work, play, and social activities and placed with therapists a moral obligation and responsibility as agents of society to any person whose future as a member of that society was jeopardized (Bockoven, 1971). With this perspective, occupational therapists placed the utmost respect on "human individuality and on a fundamental perception of the individual's need to engage in creative activity in relation to his fellow man" (Bockoven, 1971, p. 223). This initial orientation is still very much a part of current practice, as evidenced by the preamble to the *Occupational Therapy Code of Ethics* (American Occupational Therapy Association [AOTA], 1988), which states that therapists "are committed to furthering people's ability to function fully within their total environment" (p. 795).

Additional concepts and concerns such as habit training were added to our repertoire of characteristically humanistic-based practice and directed us toward an involved role with our patients. As a primary aspect of treatment, habit training was used to enlist patients' interests as they established a sense of personal usefulness. To do so, therapists were taught to consider the person as well as the environment and the effect each had on the other (Ryon, 1925; Slagle, 1934).

Throughout its professional development, occupational therapy has continued to remain strongly oriented to the individual. Information was accumulated that would allow therapists to administer evaluation and treatment that would be highly sensitive to and inclusive of an individual's culture, values, and beliefs. Therapists found that involvement of the patient in his or her own treatment was the most natural way to ensure behavioral change. The patient's goals were used to form the basis of the treatment session, and the patient's active involvement was enlisted to ensure a successful outcome. It followed that if therapists were to create individually designed, personally meaningful treatment programs then they must spend considerable time and energy getting to know each patient as a person. In this way, the therapist could determine what was needed.

Our conflict in the 1990s lies in how these individually oriented, humanistic values can survive within the current climate of health care. What economic, political, and social factors are impinging on our deeply ingrained humanistic philosophy of care, and how shall we act in relation to those forces?

Shifting Our Allegiance

In the current practice of occupational therapy, we have been forced to shift our allegiance from focusing solely on the patient to a more expanded concern that incorporates the needs of our employers to remain financially solvent. This shift has increased our attention to efficient discharges, shortened lengths of stay, maintenance of high census, development of referral networks, and provision of care in the least costly way. Like physicians, we have had to amend our traditional allegiance to the patient due to increased fiscal restraint, which requires that we now consider the economic realities of the hospitals in which we work. We must interweave the moral commitment we have to the individual with the economic responsibilities we have to our employer (Cassidy, 1988). This dilemma surfaces daily in outpatient care, where patterns for reimbursement for services are typically narrowly defined and limited in scope. This has resulted in an environment in which conflicting forces are at work: People have a need for the service, and therapists are trained to provide the needed service, but there is no viable mechanism available to pay for the service. Many times, because of a patient's lack of health insurance, we must turn even the most

appropriate treatment candidates away from our departments. In present-day practice, "the economics of the system rather than the need or condition of the patient dictates the amount and level of occupational therapy service" (Perinchief, 1988, p. 166).

Another effect of this economically driven situation is that we are faced with the pressure of providing a certain treatment protocol that is based on diagnosis. The frequency of treatment is dictated not by the patients' needs but rather by administrative directive. To follow this directive guarantees a charge for the cost of rehabilitation while that patient is eligible for such charges based on third-party reimbursement criteria (Neuhaus, 1988).

In reimbursement-driven practice, many decisions are predicated on factors outside of the therapist. Indeed, changing reimbursement patterns have demanded new service provision models. We must therefore ask ourselves whether we as occupational therapists will be able to create new treatment models that meet reimbursement guidelines and still maintain our strong commitment to individuals, holistic care, and occupational role performance.

More and more it appears that we must use a technical, protocol-driven approach to treatment. This mechanistic approach clashes with our preferred approach to the person as an individual, because, according to Neuhaus (1988), we must practice "in a climate where technology and cost containment may overshadow the needs of the individual patient" (p. 288). The conflict is further complicated, because "it is difficult to set realistic priorities that have some meaning for the patient when the patient's length of hospital stay has been determined on the basis of a diagnostic category that denies the individuality of the patient in general as well as the specific needs of that particular person" (Neuhaus, 1988, p. 291).

These obvious practice dilemmas raise key questions, such as (a) Does providing cost-effective care mean giving up quality of care and a commitment to quality-of-life issues? (b) Do we have enough time to get to know the person, develop individually valued goals, elicit motivation and participation, and provide opportunities for individually meaningful successes? and (c) Are we uncomfortable with providing what we may consider to be less than quality care and compensating in other ways, such as prescribing additional or special adaptive devices and equipment?

Identifying the Consumer

The term *consumer* is no longer reserved for the patient alone; it now extends to the government (policy makers, legislators, health care systems), health maintenance organizations, third-party payers, for-profit hospital corporations, and school administrators. With this expanded roster of agents to whom the therapist is held accountable comes the pressure of a complex of concerns and vested interests that increase the likelihood of ethical conflicts (Hansen, 1990).

Demonstrating our effectiveness to third-party reimbursers requires that we be able to explain and justify treatment to a variety of administrators and health and education officials. Again, the nature of our practice conflicts with how outsiders view efficacy. Occupational therapy goals are oriented to the individual, and the outcomes of treatment are individually significant; by their nature, these outcomes are not statistically significant. Conversely, in economics, belief systems are built when proof is generated in large numbers that can be generalized to the population.

Where reimbursement issues are concerned, other persons, including families who may be paying a significant portion of the bill, will also need to understand and have trust in the rationale behind our treatment methods if they are going to invest their money in such treatment. In addition to paying for our services, families will have to invest their interest and time by actively participating in treatment with their family member. This unusual demand on our part contrasts with the more traditional and authoritarian position taken by other health care practitioners. Rather than being asked to stand aside and relinquish control, families are required to actively participate in the problem solving, decision making, and implementation of treatment. Surprised by this demand for involvement, families may grapple with the perceived value of such therapy. Their confusion is typified by their repeated inquiries for an explanation of our service, especially in terms of the outcomes they can expect for their family member. Many therapists find these inquiries difficult to handle. Their reluctance to promise outcomes stems from their respect for the individual and their knowledge of the complex factors that influence behavior and skill development.

The need to influence public policy makers, legislators, and insurance regulatory bodies to ensure our inclusion in standards and regulations for health care and associated policy decisions (e.g., education, home care, employment) requires us to move in many other unfamiliar ways. Will we be able to convince them that occupational therapy is a primary and essential service (Cassidy, 1988)? Our ability to do this may be influenced by how different and almost simplistic our practice looks, with its focus on daily living skills, as compared with the high-tech professions and environments in which we practice (Burke, 1984).

The subtle complexity of everyday activities (Fleming, 1990) may appear to be less important or to require less professional skill when compared with the operating suite, a physical therapy hydrotherapy unit, or a dialysis unit. Our practice, which uses common sense objects in everyday ways, may cause others to diminish our importance and our skill as part of a modern health care team (Fleming, 1990).

Our role in home care exemplifies this dilemma. In home care reimbursement regulations, occupational therapy is considered a secondary service. This means that an occupational therapist is unable to open a case and provide intervention to the increasing number of homebound patients who are leaving acute care settings before they have been able to fully benefit from occupational therapy. Because therapists are working under the restricted timetables of acute care, they will frequently sketch out a brief plan to justify further occupational therapy for a given patient who is homebound. When the patient is discharged and assigned to a home health agency the occupational therapy plan is reviewed by a primary service provider, typically a nurse or a physical therapist. Upon reading the plan to provide training for daily living skills, a nurse or physical therapist will often ignore the unstated expertise that is required to teach daily living skills and instead assume by the very commonness of the goals and activities that his or her own treatment plan will suffice toward the accomplishment of these goals.

Summary

The humanistic-driven versus reimbursement-driven issues that we have outlined present complex ethical dilemmas to occupational therapists concerned with "assuring the best quality of life possible for their patients" (Hansen, 1990, p. 4). As we approach the 21st century, we find ourselves increasingly involved in a careful examination of the "ethical parameters of our practice" (Hansen, 1990, p. 7). As called for by AOTA's Directions for the Future plan (Fleming, Johnson, Marina, Spergel, & Townsend, 1987), we must make some decisions and act in ways that will lead to our appropriate inclusion in the health care marketplace. Some of those ways are outlined in the directives below.

Establish mechanisms to ensure that patients receive occupational therapy. Ideally, the acute care role for which we are best suited is triage. In triage, we would assess the person's level of need and his or her readiness to engage in rehabilitation. On the basis of assessment findings, a patient would be assigned to a rehabilitation setting, nursing home, outpatient care setting, or home health care agency. This would depend on our ability to secure our role as essential service providers.

Resolve personnel issues, especially in the areas of retention and recruitment. Therapists may not be attracted to or be able to stick with positions in acute and rehabilitation care centers because of their frustration with the medical model; the associated lack of support for the kind of service we want to give; and the burnout we experience from the high-paced, mechanically and technically centered care. Implementation of strategies such as the triage system outlined above may help us to mitigate our personnel shortages.

Increase the social commitment to the value of health. Current societal values associated with health care provision are reflected in an unequal provision of service based on economic and social class, including racial and ethnic distinctions. Why are some people turned away from health and rehabilitation programs while others are allowed to receive care for varying periods of time and in a variety of settings? Once we affirm that all people have an equal right to equal health care, we will be able to provide occupational therapy in a way that is consistent with our humanistic philosophy.

Develop an acute awareness of and knowledge about health care reimbursement. Information on "the limitation of that coverage and of the alternatives for coverage" (Perinchief, 1988, p. 166) is critical in planning and implementing optimum treatment programs. Such information can help therapists succeed in their "unspoken contract with the patient to provide optimum care, which includes ensuring that the service provided is reimbursable" (Moyers, 1990, p. 15). Additionally, a thorough investigation of alternative and less costly service provision models, such as consultation, and the effect of these models on patient care status must be acted on.

Educate Consumers. As consumers assume the responsibilities of their role, they will harness their power and position with reimbursement sources. Educated consumers will be able to turn their anger and frustration at being denied rehabilitation or occupational therapy for home health care into efforts to call, write, lobby, and otherwise influence their lawmakers and their insurance agencies. By doing so, consumers ensure that the health policies and procedures reflecting their true preferences for care are appropriately developed and included in laws and regulations governing health care.

References

American Occupational Therapy Association. (1988). Occupational therapy code of ethics. *American Journal of Occupational Therapy, 12,* 795–796.

Bockoven, J. S. (1971). Occupational therapy—A historical perspective. Legacy of Moral Treatment—1800's to 1910. *American Journal of Occupational Therapy, 25,* 223–225.

Burke, J. P. (1984). Occupational therapy: A focus for roles in practice. *American Journal of Occupational Therapy, 38,* 24–28.

Cassidy, J. C. (1988). Access to health care: A clinician's opinion about an ethical issue. *American Journal of Occupational Therapy, 42,* 295–299.

Fleming, M. (1990). *A common sense practice in an uncommon world.* Paper presented at the institute on Clinical Reasoning, Tufts University–Boston School of Occupational Therapy, Medford, MA.

Fleming, M. H., Johnson, J. A., Marina, M., Spergel, E. L., & Townsend, B. (Eds.). (1987). *Occupational therapy: Directions for the future.* Rockville, MD: American Occupational Therapy Association.

Hansen, R. (1990). Ethical considerations. In C. B. Royeen (Ed.), *AOTA self study series: Assessing function* (No. 10). Rockville, MD: American Occupational Therapy Association.

Moyers, P. (1990). Reimbursement for functions assessment. In C. B. Royeen (Ed.), *AOTA self study series: Assessing function* (No. 8). Rockville, MD: American Occupational Therapy Association.

Muncie, W. (1959). The psychobiological approach. In S. Arieti (Ed.), *American handbook of psychiatry* (Vol. 11, pp. 1317–1335). New York: Basic.

Neuhaus, B. E. (1988). Ethical considerations in clinical reasoning: The impact of technology and cost containment. *American Journal Of Occupational Therapy, 42,* 288–294.

Perinchief, J. (1988). Influences of the health care system on occupational therapy practice. In H. Hopkins & H. Smith (Eds.), *Willard and Spackman's occupational therapy* (7th ed.) (pp. 165–167). Philadelphia: Lippincott.

Ryon, W. G. (1925). Habit training for mental patients. *Occupational Therapy and Rehabilitation, 4,* 235–239.

Slagle, E. (1934). Occupational therapy: Recent methods and advances in the United States. *Occupational Therapy and Rehabilitation, 13,* 289–298.

Chapter 66

Creating Excellence in Patient Care

Kathleen Barker Schwartz, EdD, OTR, FAOTA

Occupational therapists today are working in health care organizations that operate from an efficiency perspective. That is, administration's goals are concerned with increasing efficiency in order to succeed financially. Experts argue that this approach can put quality at risk (Snoke, 1987; Starr, 1988). This paper proposes an alternative approach—the excellence perspective—as a way to address quality and at the same time sustain productivity.

The chapter traces the evolution of the efficiency perspective and provides a critique of this approach as applied to health care organizations. It examines the historical origins of the excellence perspective and describes its use in business and its potential for health care. To illustrate how the excellence perspective can be successfully applied to health, a case study of an inpatient unit in a large teaching hospital in northern California is presented.

The Efficiency Perspective and Health Care Management

The efficiency perspective originated in industry with principles introduced by Frederick Winslow Taylor in the early 1900s (Copley, 1923). Taylor declared that "scientific management" would enhance productivity by increasing worker performance and increase profitability by reducing labor costs (Taylor, 1919). A critical feature of scientific management was the creation of a class of managers who were guided primarily by concerns for efficiency and profit (Hoxie, 1916). In response to Taylor's ideas, labor unions argued that if scientific management took hold, the craftsman would lose his autonomy and become little more than an animated tool of management (Montgomery, 1984).

Taylor's ideas did take hold. Indeed, scientific management ideology provides the foundation for the efficiency perspective in management today (Drucker, 1954). A basic assumption of this perspective is that resources are finite and must be carefully controlled in order to achieve productivity. Control of scarce resources such as time, money, and staff is accomplished through a hierarchical organizational structure in which formal authority is delegated to managers who are responsible for monitoring efficiency and profitability (Perrow, 1970).

Although the efficiency perspective has exerted considerable influence in industry and business since 1920, the perspective has taken much longer to permeate health care management. Although there is evidence to show that the doctrine of scientific management was preached to doctors as well as to businessmen (Haber, 1964), there is little data to show that the efficiency perspective was influential in the formative years of American hospitals.

Health care institutions were not identified with the business concern of profitability in the early years of the 20th century. The health care system at that time consisted of either charity or voluntary hospitals whose goals were humanitarian in nature (Starr, 1982). In many instances, doctors had authority over both the administrative and the clinical aspects of hospital care and thus fulfilled the roles of technical expert and manager. This was in contrast to industry where the skilled worker, or "doer," became separated from the manager, or "thinker" (Reich, 1983). One prominent Chicago physician evidently was mindful of events in industry when he warned his colleagues, "If we wish to escape the thralldom of commercialism, if we wish to avoid the fate of the toolless workers, we must control the hospital" (Holmes, 1906, p. 320).

Indeed it was a shift in control and purpose that brought the efficiency perspective to health care organizations. By 1970, the humanitarian emphasis had shifted to a concern for the best way to run hospitals as businesses (Drucker, 1973). The health care industry expanded from hospitals into rehabilitation centers, outpatient services, nursing homes, and community programs. Accompanying this expansion was growth in the private insurance industry and in federal insurance programs through Medicare and Medicaid. The physician–manager role eroded and governance became separated from clinical management. Hospital administrators with master's degrees in business administration took over the business functions of hospitals, guided by the efficiency perspective.

The efficiency perspective has been justified on the grounds that health care in the United States is big business, and therefore health care organizations should be run according to a business model, which emphasizes efficiency. Given modern concerns about rising costs in health care, the need for the efficiency perspective was deemed obvious: This approach enables management to focus on the goals of productivity and cost control.

Differences between business and health care, however, raise questions as to the goodness of fit with the efficiency perspective. One important difference lies in the mission of the organization. In business, profits are the top priority. In health care, quality patient care is the predominant goal. Some for-profit health care facilities do exist, but a large proportion of health care institutions remain nonprofit. Even the nonprofit facilities, however, have begun to shift their emphasis away from quality and toward cost reduction as a result of the cost-containment movement.

This shift in focus has highlighted a growing conflict between practitioner and administrator. Differing professional orientations place the administrator trained from a business perspective on the side of efficiency and the practitioner trained from a humanistic perspective on the side of quality. Whereas the administrator focuses on the efficient use of funds and increased productivity, the health care practitioner desires freedom to act in the full interests of the patient and resources to provide the most advanced treatment ("Balancing Health Care Costs," 1988).

One way to address this dilemma of efficiency versus quality is to reframe the question: Can all organizations achieve quality as well as efficiency? Some management theorists argue that this is possible, if organizations use the excellence perspective.

The Excellence Perspective and Health Care Management

The origins of the excellence perspective can be traced to the work of Mary Parker Follett (Follett, 1924; Fox & Urwick, 1973). Follett articulated her management philosophy in the first part of the 20th century, at the same time that scientific management was gaining popularity. She proposed that businesses would be effective only when they created an environment that stimulated each member to make his or her fullest contribution. Indeed, she argued that the strength of an organization depended on its ability to create a "working unit," in which shared values and common interests could evolve (Follett, 1987). Follett proposed that the best way to create organizational environments that fostered such working units was through shared decision making and participative governance, a position in direct opposition to the authoritarian approach advocated by Taylor.

Follett's interest in creating an environment in which people could contribute fully was probably due in part to her own experience as a woman. She was also influenced by the idealistic leanings of several of her instructors at Harvard and by her professional experience as the founder of a group of community centers called the Roxbury League (Cabot, 1934; Crawford, 1971). The prescience of Follett's vision has recently been acknowledged (Mullins, 1979; Parker, 1984). March (1965) claimed Follett was ahead of her time: Her ideas did not fit in with the management wisdom of her age, an age dominated by the efficiency perspective.

Contemporary management theorists challenge the efficiency perspective. They argue that it has not helped American business, which is suffering from declines in product quality and in productivity (Reich, 1983). They urge that we move away from the concern of efficiency and toward a focus on excellence (Peters & Austin, 1985;

Peters & Waterman, 1982). They claim that if one emphasizes excellence as the primary goal, then productivity is not sacrificed but, rather, is enhanced (Walton, 1985).

Studies of successful businesses that exemplify the excellence perspective show several common elements. (Deal & Kennedy, 1982; Waterman, 1987). A key element is the definition of a vision that can guide the direction and activities of an organization. This vision should be shared, that is, the organization's members must value its mission. Leadership is a critical factor (Kouzes & Posner, 1989). It is the leader with a vision who helps shape the organization. Leaders create an environment that fosters collaboration, one that encourages and recognizes the contributions of all members. Case studies show that organizations committed to a shared goal, with leaders who direct the organization's resources toward that goal, create an environment that achieves quality and productivity (Posner, Kouzes, & Schmidt, 1985).

Since the first writings on this management perspective were published, much interest has been expressed, as has some criticism. Questions arise as to how an organization creates a vision, which is a vague concept at best. How does an organization convince its members to work toward a shared goal? How does one become the kind of leader who can shape an environment that enables members to achieve excellence and productivity? Recent writings by organizational theorists who support this perspective have attempted to answer these questions (Bradford & Cohen, 1984).

For example, Kouzes and Posner (1989) used data from their research based on 1,372 questionnaires and interviews to describe how leaders bring forth the best in themselves and others. The authors discussed the concept of vision, which they said is not mysterious and which can be defined as mission, goal, purpose, or simply the desire to make something happen that will contribute to quality. Kouzes and Posner described the ways that effective leaders create an environment in which members want to achieve excellence: (a) they enable others to see the possibilities a vision holds; (b) they are willing to take risks and experiment with new ideas; (c) they enable others to act and therefore to feel strong, capable, and committed; (d) they lead by example, through actions that support their words; and (e) they encourage others through genuine acts of caring. The authors' book is replete with descriptions of acts of leadership that contributed to excellence in performance. Examples are cited from both the public sector and private industry.

Deal, Kennedy, and Spiegel (1983) addressed the specific application of the excellence perspective to health care institutions. They asserted that although this perspective is not abundant in health care, some organizations do exemplify excellence. As examples, they described a prestigious urban teaching hospital and a community rehabilitation facility. Although these organizations differ in size (large versus small), mission (acute care versus long-term care), and financial status (nonprofit versus for profit), they share certain elements. Deal et al. found each organization was committed to being the best. For one, this meant the best teaching hospital; for the other, the best rehabilitation facility. This vision was shared by all members and shaped by leaders who committed the necessary resources to achieve this goal. Individual contributions were encouraged and recognized. Within the rehabilitation facility, the occupational therapy department was well respected for its contribution to excellence. Its members were encouraged to contribute and, in fact, developed several patient care programs. The director of occupational therapy had recently been promoted to vice president; at that level she anticipated having a greater opportunity to further her vision of excellence in patient care (D. Robinson, personal communication, October 30, 1982).

Case Study

The Asian and Pacific American Psychiatric Inpatient Program at San Francisco General Hospital in San Francisco, California, opened in 1980. It later served as the model for the development of four other inpatient programs to serve Latinos, Blacks, women, and patients with AIDS-related psychiatric illnesses. These five programs, designed to provide culturally sensitive psychiatric care to minority and ethnic patients, were recently awarded a certificate of significant achievement by the American Psychiatric Association (American Psychiatric Association, 1987).

It all began when Francis Lu, MD, participated in a 1979 National Institute for Mental Health conference on ethnic and minority curriculum development. Out of that conference grew his idea about how to provide the best culturally sensitive care to ethnic and minority patients. Lu envisioned an Asian-focus unit in which patients of that ethnic background would come together with professionals of the same background. He believed that acutely disturbed patients could benefit from services provided by professionals who spoke the same language and understood cultural values and beliefs. This view is supported by experts who argue that successful treatment can only occur when the professional comes to understand the patient's story, that is, the way a person views himself or herself in the world (Coles, 1989; Taylor, 1989).

Dr. Lu laid the groundwork for this idea through discussions with the hospital's administration. The department of psychiatry at San Francisco General Hospital is a joint undertaking of the city and county of San Francisco and the University of California, San Francisco. Lu persuaded the administration that his idea would assist the hospital to better address the needs of San Francisco's diverse population. He proposed that a core group of mental health professionals who shared a similar vision could provide more effective diagnosis and treatment. He argued that for the same cost as traditional treatment, higher quality care would be achieved. No special grants or funding were requested; however, Lu did gain administrative support for the concept of a focus unit as well as a commitment to provide funds for recruitment. Leaders in the Asian community were approached, and they expressed their support for the idea. According to the 1980 census, 21.3 percent of San Francisco's residents are Asian American.

The unit began with two professionals of Asian origin, Lu and one nurse. The staff grew to consist of a program director, a senior attending physician, nurses, social workers, and an occupational therapist—all of Asian descent. Those who came to work on the unit did so because they shared the vision of an Asian-focus patient care unit. The unit offered professionals the opportunity to contribute their knowledge of Asian languages and culture. Once the vision was established, the professionals shaped the unit's direction and goals. The goals were (a) to provide culturally sensitive psychiatric care, (b) to provide multi-disciplinary training opportunities, and (c) to develop a body of research to improve both patient care and education.

The way patient treatment was conducted was determined by the developing unit's vision and goals. The staff employed treatment approaches most likely to provide excellent patient care that was culturally sensitive. An ethnomedical approach to diagnosis and treatment was viewed as more consistent with the unit's goal than the traditional biomedical model. This ethnomedical approach not only focuses on diagnosis and precipitating incident but explores information regarding previous life and stresses in the home country; the escape experience and refugee events; and language, cultural, financial, and racial problems encountered in the United States. The staff also explores beliefs the patient might hold about illness, for example, the belief that disease is caused by an excess or deficiency of yin and yang. This approach provides treatment based on an understanding of the patient's perceived symptoms and difficulties (Lee, 1985).

The milieu is designed to make patients comfortable. Rice and tea are routinely served with meals. Ethnic newspapers, books, and music tapes are available. Family members are allowed to bring home cooked food during their visits. Great importance is placed on family involvement and linkages with the community once the person is discharged. Evelyn Lee, EdD, became program director in 1982. Lu described Dr. Lee as a charismatic and caring leader who has energetically directed the unit toward its mission to provide psychotic and severely depressed Asian American patients with an environment that understands their pain and their cultural background (F. Lu, personal communication, November 30, 1989).

Lisa Lai, OTR, was hired in 1982 as the unit's occupational therapist. Lai has relied on general principles of occupational therapy coupled with creativity and her knowledge of Asian language and culture. Occupational therapy treatment uses occupation that is both meaningful and purposeful; Lai uses an approach to treatment that takes into account both patients' functional needs and their values and beliefs. For example, the cooking group features recipes from various Asian and Pacific countries. Support for treatment that addresses both the meaning and the purpose of occupation has been a growing theme in the professional literature (Yoder, Nelson, & Smith, 1989). Lai asserts that treatment that combines professional expertise with a sensitivity to the language and values of patients can result in major changes in patients status and responsiveness to treatment (L. Lai, personal communication, November 30, 1989).

In summary, the Asian-focus unit exemplifies many of the characteristics of the excellence perspective. It began with an idea, a vision, that would join others in the pursuit of excellence in patient care. This vision represents the shared values and beliefs of the professionals within the unit. Its leaders epitomize the leadership qualities of the excellence perspective: They have enabled others to see the possibilities of their vision, they have experimented with new ideas, and they have encouraged professionals within the unit to make individual contributions. They lead through example and encourage through caring. Development of the Asian-focus unit was hard work; it took several years to achieve the cohesion it has now. Its evolution required patience, a commitment of resources from the administration, and energy and understanding from the professionals within the unit. Recruitment has been and remains an issue. The unit must attract and retain competent professionals with an Asian background and language capability who share the same sense of mission. Although the program has gained national recognition for its innovative approach, there is a feeling expressed by some within the facility that the program promotes a segregated approach to treatment, one that separates patients as well as staff. This belief assumes that the focus units maintain a separate mission from the rest of the organization. Another viewpoint, however, is that the focus units simply offer one way to achieve the overall mission of the hospital, which is to provide quality patient care for the residents of San Francisco. Further research is planned to document the effectiveness of the focus unit in patient treatment (Lee & Lu, 1989).

Discussion

One might ask, if the excellence approach leads to higher quality patient care, why is it not used by more health care organizations? The answer, in part, is that people act in ways that are most comfortable. As this paper has shown, the efficiency perspective is pre-dominant in health care. Efficiency has become the primary goal; quality patient care is a secondary goal. Common wisdom dictates that if one focuses on efficiency, one gets productivity and reasonable patient care. Excellence in patient care has been presumed to be something that could only be achieved at a financial risk. Research has contributed to disproving this assumption, but common wisdom dies hard. We must also examine the nature of leadership in health care organizations. Administrators tend to be conservative, particularly in a climate that is so heavily focused on cost containment and short-term financial performance. The majority of leaders using the excellence perspective are from organizational cultures noted for being more innovative, such as high technology. Finally, there can be little energy for innovation in an environment where the vision is survival. Only when one replaces that vision with one of excellence can energy be freed for making changes that can contribute to quality patient care as well as to productivity.

Implications for Occupational Therapy

As this case study has shown, health care professionals were the leaders in developing a program to achieve quality patient care. Because many administrators are preoccupied with finances, it will probably fall to health professionals to continue to lead the focus on excellence. Occupational therapists can contribute to this effort by developing ideas to increase the quality services within our domain.

As the profession of occupational therapy plans for its future, one vision that emerges is that of the multifaceted occupational therapist, a person who is a competent clinician, a supporter of and contributor to research, and a strong manager–leader (Directions for the Future, 1990). This vision says we can no longer afford to have occupational therapists who are knowledgeable only about patient evaluation and treatment. Instead, we need people who are able to articulate the profession's contribution and introduce new ideas that can lead practice. This requires leadership ability and management knowledge. Occupational therapists can use the excellence perspective as a guide to program innovation. It is a perspective that fits with the occupational therapist's concern for quality patient care and the administration's concern for productivity.

Acknowledgments

I express my appreciation to the staff and patients of the Asian and Pacific American Psychiatric Inpatient Program at San Francisco General Hospital, San Francisco, California. In particular I would like to cite the assistance of Francis Lu, MD Assistant Clinical Professor of Psychiatry, University of California, San Francisco;

Evelyn Lee, EdD, Assistant Clinical Professor of Psychiatry, University of California, San Francisco; Lisa Lai, OTR, Staff Occupational Therapist, San Francisco General Hospital; and Judy Levin, OTR Senior Occupational Therapist, San Francisco General Hospital.

References

American Psychiatric Association, (1987, Oct 16). *Six exceptional programs for the mentally ill share hospital and community awards.* News release.

Balancing health care costs and quality. (1988, June). *Occupational Therapy News*, p. 3.

Bradford, D. L., & Cohen, A. R.(1984). *Managing for excellence.* New York: Wiley.

Cabot, R. (1934). Mary Parker Follett: An appreciation. *Radcliffe Quarterly, 18*, 81.

Coles, R. (1989). *The call of stories.* Boston: Houghton Mifflin.

Copley, F. B. (1923). *Frederick W Taylor: Father of scientific management.* New York: Harper & Brothers.

Crawford, D. (1971). Mary Parker Follett. In D. Crawford (Ed.), *Notable American women 1607–1950* (pp. 639–641). Cambridge, MA: Belknap Press.

Deal, T. E., & Kennedy, A. A. (1982). *Corporate cultures.* Reading, MA: Addison–Wesley.

Deal, T. E., Kennedy, A. A., & Spiegel, A. H. (1983). How to create an outstanding hospital culture. *Forum. 26*, 21–34.

Directions for the Future. (1990, January). Meeting of the American Occupational Therapy Association, San Diego, CA.

Drucker, P. F. (1954). *The practice of management.* New York: Harper & Row.

Drucker, P. F. (1973). *Management: Tasks, responsibilities, practices.* New York: Harper & Row.

Follett, M. P. (1924). *Creative experience.* New York: Longmans, Green.

Follett, M. P. (1987). Freedom and coordination. Lectures in business organization. In A. Brief (Ed.), *Ancestral Books in the Management of Organizations.* New York: Garland.

Fox, M., & Urwick, L. (Eds). (1973). *Dynamic administration: The collected papers of Mary Parker Follett.* London: Pitman.

Haber, S. (1964). *Efficiency and uplift.* Chicago: University of Chicago Press.

Holmes, B. (1906). The hospital problem. *Journal of the American Medical Association, 38*, 320.

Hoxie, R. F. (1916). *Scientific management and labor.* New York: D. Appleton.

Kouzes, J., & Posner, B. (1989). *The leadership challenge.* San Francisco: Jossey–Bass.

Lee, E. (1985). Inpatient psychiatric services for Southeast Asian refugees. *Southeast Asian Mental Health.* Washington, DC: National Institute for Mental health.

Lee, F., & Lu, F. (1989). Assessment and treatment of Asian American survivors of mass violence. *Journal of Traumatic Stress, 2,* 93–120.

March, J. (Ed.). (1965). *Handbook of organizations.* Chicago: Rand McNally.

Montgomery, D. (1984). *Worker's control in America.* London: Cambridge University Press.

Mullins, L. (1979). Approaches to management. *Management Accounting, 57,* 15–18.

Parker, L. D. (1984). Control in organizational life: The contribution of Mary Parker Follett, *Academy of Management Review, 9,* 736–745.

Perrow, C. (1970). *Organizational analysis.* Monterey, CA: Brooks/ Cole.

Peters, T., & Austin, N. (1985). *A passion for excellence: The leadership difference.* New York: Random House.

Peters, T., & Waterman, R. (1982). *In search of excellence: Lessons from America's best-run companies.* New York: Harper & Row.

Posner, B. Z., Kouzes, J. M., & Schmidt, W. H. (1985). Shared values make a difference. *Human Resource Management, 24,* 293–309.

Reich, R. B. (1983). *The next American frontier.* New York: Times Books.

Snoke, A. W. (1987). The hospital administrator. *Hospital Topics, 65,* 23–29.

Starr, P. (1982). *The social transformation of American medicine.* New York: Basic.

Starr, P. (1988, March 20). Increasingly, life and death issues become money matters. *New York Times,* p. E1.

Taylor, F. W. (1919). *The principles of scientific management.* New York: Harper & Brothers.

Taylor, S. E. (1989). *Positive illusions.* New York: Basic.

Walton, R. E. (1985). From control to commitment in the workplace. *Harvard Business Review, 63,* 77–84.

Waterman, R. H. (1987). *The renewal factor.* New York: Bantam.

Yoder, R. M., Nelson, D. L., & Smith, D. A. (1989). Added-purpose versus rote exercise in female nursing home residents. *American Journal of Occupational Therapy, 43,* 581–586.

Chapter 67

Sustaining the Art of Practice in Occupational Therapy

Suzanne M. Peloquin, PhD, OTR

Occupational therapists have seen an effort within their profession to unearth historical roots, to articulate a philosophical base, to elucidate models for practice, and to validate theoretical concepts through research. The search for a professional identity and for professional credibility is essential; it has also been intense. The purpose of this article is to explore a concept that has been under-represented in occupational therapy literature over the last decade: the art of the practice of occupational therapy.

The art of occupational therapy is the soul of its practice. Therapy as an art is an old theme; literature as a nurturer of the soul is an older theme still. The occupational therapy literature with its many references to paradigms, constructs and variables reflects a considerable effort to articulate the profession's scientific basis. A profession committed to balance can perhaps sustain its art by reflecting on the images of caring and helpful occupation seen in fictional literature.

The Art of Occupational Therapy

In 1972, the American Occupational Therapy Association (AOTA) Council on Standards defined occupational therapy as "the art and science of directing man's participation in selected tasks to restore, reinforce and enhance performance, facilitate learning of those skills and functions essential for adaptation and productivity, diminish or correct pathology, and to promote and maintain health" (p. 204). Years later, AOTA's Representative Assembly accepted a more comprehensive definition that begins as follows:

> Occupational therapy is the use of purposeful activity with individuals who are limited by physical injury or illness, psychosocial dysfunction, developmental or learning disabilities, poverty and cultural differences or aging process in order to maximize independence, prevent disability and maintain health. (1981, p. 798)

Definitions evolve over time to reflect changes in priorities and orientations. It is not surprising that the descriptive phrase "art and science," which validates a blend of practice components, was deleted between 1972 and 1981 as the profession's emphasis turned toward scientific research and accountability.

In spite of this deletion from the profession's official definition, the practice of occupational therapy remains a blend of art and science. There is an art to the practice of any therapeutic endeavor. Mosey (1981) discussed art relative to the practice of occupational therapy. She first defined the art of practice negatively, stating that the art of practice is not (a) a desire to help others, (b) the skilled application of scientific knowledge, or (c) simply being a systematic or sympathetic practitioner. Mosey wrote, "The capacity to establish rapport, to empathize, and to guide others to know and make use of their potential as participants in a community of others illustrates the art of occupational therapy" (p. 4). Without art, she claimed, occupational therapy would become the application of scientific knowledge in a sterile vacuum.

Mosey (1981) elaborated those characteristics commonly held by practitioners she called "masters in the art of practice" (p. 23). The artful practitioner perceives the individual as indivisible into various parts or subsystems. Although practitioners reduce the human organism into subsystems in order to understand the patient more clearly, the art of practice reintegrates those subsystems to see a whole person. Meeting the patient as an individual enables the practitioner to empathize with the patient and to accept his or her feelings, ideas, and values. The meaning that the patient places on his or her life, relationships, and environment guides the therapist–patient collaboration toward growth, independence, and the use of potential.

The science of practice, Mosey (1981) said, is a phenomenon fundamental to all professions. In occupational therapy practice, science is the gathering of data through systematic clinical observations or through more formalized research projects to help develop new theories or to verify, refine, or refute existing theories relevant to the practice. The art and the science of occupational therapy together constitute its practice.

Devereaux (1984) (see Chapter 33) identified the caring relationship as the art rather than the science of health care. She wrote, "Occupational therapists are specialists in making care happen. We know how to enrich all the transactions in the relationship with the patient. These become caring gestures" (p. 794) (in Chapter 33). Devereaux characterized the particular caring of occupational therapists as singular among professionals: helping the patient reconnect to those occupations that are meaningful to him or her. She said, "Occupational therapists care by helping people disengage from despair and dysfunction and by helping them look forward, to see their loss as being able to be ameliorated through adaptation and occupation" (p. 794) (in Chapter 33).

Within the context of her definition of caring, Devereaux (1984) (see Chapter 33) highlighted a major assumption that informs the theory and the practice of occupational therapy: that adaptation occurs through the use of occupation. According to Reed and Sanderson (1983), occupational therapy theory and practice build on several assumptions. Although it is difficult to summarize these assumptions, Reed and Sanderson demonstrated that it is possible. They categorized a long list that included assumptions about: (a) human beings; (b) occupational performance; (c) health, wellness, and illness; (d) the receipt of health care services; (e) the provision of health care; (f) occupational therapy; and (g) the therapeutic use of occupations. In the art of practice, as occupational therapists engage meaningfully with patients, they discuss assumptions. They formulate treatment plans based on mutual assumptions chosen from among several possible categories. A cluster of assumptions gleaned from Reed and Sanderson's comprehensive list seems central to the caring connection described by Devereaux. These assumptions relate to occupation and figure prominently in any dialogue with patients about their connection with meaningfulness:

Each individual must perform some occupation or have the occupations performed for the person to survive.

A person adapts or adjusts (grows and develops) through the use of and participation in various occupations.

Occupations may be divided into three major areas: self-maintenance, productivity and leisure.

A balance of occupations is facilitatory to the maintenance of a satisfying life.

Occupations permit a person to fulfill individual and group needs.

Occupations must be relevant and useful to the individual in relating to the environment. (p. 70)

The art of practice supports the entire structure of occupational therapy. Caring, informed by assumptions about occupation, constitutes the base for those elements Devereaux (1984) (see Chapter 33) considered essential to an effective relationship in occupational therapy: (a) competence, (b) belief in the dignity and worth of the person, (c) belief that each person has the potential for change and growth, (d) communication, (e) values, (f) touch, and (g) sense of humor. Caring transforms a science of occupation into a therapeutic practice.

Mastery of the art of practice in the fullness described by Mosey (1981) and Devereaux (1984) (see Chapter 33) is a challenge. One need only reflect on the current demands faced by practitioners to acknowledge the difficulty. The brief length of patients' stays, the demands for productivity, the documentation criteria for third-party reimbursers and accrediting agencies, and the requirements for research and quality assurance all demand the time and energy required for caring. Occupational therapy practitioners need affirmation that the art of practice is valued and that those assumptions about occupation that are communicated through caring are relevant to patients. Today's health care system does not tend to nurture the art; it does not encourage consistent patient–therapist dialogue about assumptions.

Associates of occupational therapy in medicine have been vocal in their articulation of the struggle to retain the humane side of practice. Engel (1977) wrote of physicians' disenchantment with an approach to disease that neglects the patient, with a dominance of procedures over patient sensitivities, and with a biomedical emphasis that disregards human meaning. Pellegrino (1979) claimed that the concepts of discreteness of disease processes and specificity of therapeutic agents have transformed the ethos of medicine. Therapeutics as we know it today, a little more than a century old, has been beneficial for humankind on the whole. But the impact of scientific advances and technological successes has profoundly compromised the relationship between patient and physician.

Patients resent the fragmentation of their care. Public distress has resulted in a series of measures to acknowledge the patient, the person, and his or her rights: quality assurance, the patient's bill of rights, legal concern with informed consent, and the regulation of experimentation on human beings. These measures systematize a defense against a powerful medical system that tends to forget or ignore the individual patient. The health care system demands scientific competence; the legal system demands acknowledgment of individual rights. There is no escaping the reality: Practitioners must engage in the science of practice in order to function in the health care system. And yet, patients and professionals alike recognize the sterility of a human service practice devoid of its art, its caring. Rights can be legislated, but caring cannot. The art of practice, not so valued or nurtured by the health care system, requires sustenance from other sources.

Literature: Toward an Affirmation of the Art of Practice

A new field, literature and medicine, suggests a source of sustenance for the art of occupational therapy practice. Jones (1987) characterized literature and medicine as a recent phase in the medical humanities experiment in medical education. She identified two approaches to literature that justify its incorporation into medical education: the aesthetic and the moral. Trautmann (1978) described the aesthetic approach: "to teach a student to read, in the fullest sense" (p. 36). The fictional world, she said, reveals "relationships between people and within a single personality" (p. 33). In reading fiction, one "must look at words in their personal and social contexts" (p. 36). Trautmann said that through literature one can make the leap to empathy, to compassion. Through literature, one can achieve affirmation of personal dignity—affirmation of a personhood threatened by the health care system.

Coles (1979), a physician, described the second approach to literature, the moral approach. He wrote that "the point of a medical humanities course devoted to literature is ethical reflection" (p. 445). Coles believed that novelists and clinicians alike focus on the everyday life and on the unique nature of the human being. He said that there is a continuing tension between one's idealism and life's demands. Novelists, he said, can move one to scrutinize assumptions, expectations, and values, to reflect on a life either as it is being lived or as one hopes to live it.

Images from fictional literature viewed within the context of either the aesthetic or the moral approach can nurture the art of occupational therapy practice. The art of practice, is, after all, intrinsically centered on images—images of relationships, of qualities that make relationships meaningful, of occupation's meaning in a life.

The aesthetic approach to literature can help, in its scrutiny of relationships, to validate the meaningfulness of "the capacity to establish rapport, to empathize, and to guide others to know and make use of their potential as participants in a community of others" (Mosey, 1981, p. 4). The moral approach can prompt reflection about practice elements and about assumptions that inform practice. Both approaches can validate the practitioner's commitment to the art, to caring, and to caring connections.

Yerxa and Sharrott (1986), in their endorsement of a liberal arts education for occupational therapists, wrote

> Occupational therapy's knowledge base requires an understanding of medical conditions, but it is not the medical condition per se that is of the greatest significance; rather, it is the occupational nature of the human being. Thus, although our knowledge, in practice, is primarily applied to people who are ill and disabled, the science of occupation and its concern with the play–work continuum, adaptation, and competence development applies to all people, disabled or not. (p. 158)

Literature, read in its fullest sense and reflected upon, can contribute to an understanding of the human condition.

Mosey (1981) described the process of learning the art of practice: "The individual who strives to bring art to practice must be able to engage in the often uncomfortable process of learning more about one's self, changing one's self, and gaining knowledge about how one's values and expectations may differ from those of others" (p. 25). In the world of fiction one can find a mirror reflecting back, for recognition and appraisal, one's self, one's values, and one's expectations. One can also find in the world of fiction a window opening onto a world of others, their values, and their expectations. Literature can facilitate learning the art of practice.

Fiction: A Reflection of the Art of Practice

The concept of reading fiction to enhance the art of practice will no doubt elicit varied responses from widely diverse occupational therapy practitioners. Avid, discriminating readers use the process already, but nonreaders may not be intrinsically motivated to turn to fiction without a clear indication that the process can enhance their skill in the art of practice. Although the process seems particularly suited to the educational system, it is equally adaptable to any continued learning endeavor.

The fictional world is populated by occupational therapists and patients. Some images from that world reflect practitioners inept in the art of practice and patients vocal about that ineptitude. Fiction also contains images that seriously challenge assumptions about occupation. If one expects sustenance from the literature, one needs to know how to handle the negative images.

Reading in a fuller sense can be affirming, even if the fictionalized occupational therapist happens to be a rogue or a villain. If one can agree that the character's interpersonal style lacks care, that agreement affirms one's endorsement of a different style: "I'll be (or I am) a different kind of occupational therapist." This can be affirming. Reading in the fuller sense, one can find other characters whose interactional styles are favorably represented. To reflect on characteristics worth emulating is to once again affirm one's belief in caring and in the art of practice.

An encounter in the fictional world with a blatant repudiation of an assumption about occupational therapy may be disturbing. By reading in the moral sense, that is, reading to examine human values, one can step out of one's own world of assumptions to consider those of others. This experience can enrich later dialogues with patients. The exploration of another world through fiction can enable one to better understand real patients whose values differ from one's own. The reflection and the broadening of view made possible through fiction can facilitate the meeting of each patient as an individual.

In *The Cracker Factory* (Rebeta-Burditt, 1977), an occupational therapist working in a private psychiatric hospital is characterized in a most unflattering manner. The protagonist in this story is Cassie, a young woman admitted to the hospital because she is depressed and abusing alcohol. Cassie does not single the occupational therapist out for criticism; the therapist is one of several characters seen as oppressive. Cassie describes her hospital experiences satirically. She depicts the occupational therapist in an interactionally challenging scene: attempting to motivate patients to come to a therapy group. Cassie names the therapist "Brunhilde, the misplaced Viking Lady" and "the Dictator of OT" (p.

114). Both names suggest an abuse of power. One expects ferocious and bloody battle with a Viking and arbitrary orders from a dictator. The names, unfortunately, seem apt. The therapist "marches around the seventh floor telling all the patients that their doctor has 'ordered' Occupational Therapy" (p. 114). Rather than discussing with individual patients the merits of therapy or its relevance to them personally, she invokes the power of the doctor's order. She "herds them out in the hall" and "goosesteps them out the door" (p. 114). There is no evidence of rapport here, no humor, no recognition of patients as individuals. Harshness dominates the scene.

The occupational therapist insists that the patients "must come IMMEDIATELY" (p. 114). When patients try to hide from her by taking a shower, "She doesn't care. Wet or screaming, it makes no difference. She drags them along anyway" (pp. 114–115). A caring touch is replaced by dragging and goose-stepping. Notably absent are a respect for patients' dignity and an acknowledgment of patients' rights. There is clearly no empathy. Instead, there are threats: "If you don't go to OT, it will be written down on your chart and you won't get out of here" (p. 114). Cassie's perception of the motivational attempt is one of intimidation. The reader is forced to agree.

Practitioners may recognize in this portrayal the familiar struggle inherent in the motivational process. Ultimately, the patient has the right to refuse all treatment, for whatever reason. Furthermore, the patient has every right to dispute or to reject any and all assumptions about the therapeutic process. Meanwhile, the concerned practitioner, invested in the patient as a person, tries to communicate possible benefits, to convey a deep personal interest, to attempt to collaborate, and to walk away from the motivational effort only when convinced that the patient has sufficient information to have made a real choice.

Powerful images from *The Cracker Factory* stimulate reflection about the motivational attempt. Does even the best attempt feel, to the patient, like a battle? If so, what interpersonal elements might signal a truce? Cassie's view clearly reminds therapists that a patient who has little control over an environment perceives those in control as dictators. What therapist characteristics might impress a patient differently? *The Cracker Factory* provides a clue to anyone reading in the fuller sense.

One favorite nurse escapes Cassie's sharp criticism: the nurse she calls Tinkerbell. Tink does not invoke rules or orders. She makes exceptions to the rules when possible. Cassie comes in from the cold, after a late-night Alcoholics Anonymous meeting, and Tink tosses her a set of keys saying, "The kitchen is officially closed but you may go in if you like" (p. 221). Cassie is "delighted, feeling like a friend" (p. 221). Tink takes time to establish rapport, to be with Cassie, to talk with her. She asks personal questions, and she encourages Cassie to share. When Cassie says of herself, "I doubt I'll ever have the ability to be that open," Tink says, "Give it time. . . . When you're more comfortable, you'll loosen up" (p. 222). When Cassie asks Tink a personal question, Tink agrees to answer, saying, "Okay, Cassie, I'll play fair" (p. 223). She shares a personally painful situation. Unlike Brunhilde, whom Cassie describes as not caring, Cassie tells Tink, "You care," to which Tink nods and replies, "I care" (p. 227). But Tink admits personal shortcomings. She says, "I have limitations like everyone else" (p. 227). She tells Cassie, "I prefer involvement on a limited basis, caring on my terms, the way I handle it best, the way I'm most effective" (p. 227). Tink's disclosure of personal weaknesses has therapeutic value. She can say, "Cassie . . . from where I'm standing, I have a clear view of *your* strengths" (p. 227). Tink's display of humanity reinforces Cassie's humanity. In Cassie's worldview, Tink is a caring person; the occupational therapist is not. The art in Tink's practice of nursing contrasts harshly with the absence of art in the occupational therapist's practice.

Interactional characteristics make a difference to patients in fiction and in reality. The exaggeration and striking contrast between one occupational therapist and one nurse used in *The Cracker Factory* can generate powerful responses and productive thinking. The kind of reflection that is prompted by an encounter with forceful fictional characters can nurture the art of practice.

Images of Occupation and Caring Connections

In addition to specific images of occupational therapists in literature, there are images of occupation and of caring people associated with occupation. Two literary pieces, Kesey's *One Flew Over the Cuckoo's Nest* (1962) and Shem's *The House of God* (1978), have achieved a measure of notoriety for their portrayals of health care environments in which professional caring is painfully compromised.

Kesey's novel depicts a state mental institution. The story is told from the point of view of the Chief, an electively mute, chronically ill American Indian patient. The Chief's delusional system and active visual and auditory hallucinations contribute to the image that patients are caught in a gigantic unyielding machine designed to socialize them into conformity. The typical hospital day is monotonous: Acutes and Chronics alike submit to the order imposed by the Big Nurse, The Chief describes the atmosphere: "There's something strange about a place where the men won't let themselves loose and laugh, something strange about the way they all knuckle under to that smiling flour-faced old mother [Big Nurse]" (p. 48). He describes group discussion among the patients as "telling things that wouldn't ever let them look one another in the eye again" (p. 49). He characterizes the therapies offered as being all the same and unable to engage the patient: "Ten-forty, -forty five, -fifty,

patients shuttle in and out to appointments in ET or OT or PT" (p. 38). The environment is devoid of meaningful occupation and meaningful interpersonal exchange; the result is dehumanizing.

Shem describes an equally maladaptive environment in *The House of God*. Roy Basch is an intern at the House of God, a hospital where the "emphasis was on doing everything always for everyone forever to keep the patient alive" (pp. 25–26). The House of God is filled with gomers, "human beings who have lost what goes into being human beings" (p. 38). Within this environment, interns and residents lack support from their supervisors, struggle against exhaustion, and grapple with life, death, and ethical issues. Tired interns focus on getting sleep: "I wish she would die so I could just go to sleep" (p. 135). They try to learn "enough medicine to worry less about saving patients and more about saving themselves" (p. 150). They always seem on the edge of sanity and control. Roy says, "I'm scared that one of these nights, with nobody else around, when someone starts to abuse me, I'm going to lose control and beat the shit out of some poor bastard" (pp. 232–233). There is no balance of occupations, no rest, and no leisure. Roy describes his inner state at his worst point: "I had been as far from the world of humans as I could get. . . . I had been sarcastic. I'd avoided feeling everything, as if feelings were little grenades" (p. 361). Roy Basch, denied a balance of occupations and cut off from meaningful human exchange by the demands and stresses of work, lives in an environment as dehumanized as that portrayed by the Chief.

Kesey and Shem provide hope for both the Chief and Roy Basch: there is a way out of these maladaptive environments and these dehumanizing worlds. Other people lead the way out, people who can laugh, who can relate, who can touch. People help the Chief and Roy to make connections with helpful occupations.

In *One Flew Over the Cuckoo's Nest*, McMurphy enters the Chief's world: "He sounds big. I hear him coming down the hall, and he sounds big in the way he walks.... He talks a little the way Papa used to, voice loud and full of hell" (p. 16). McMurphy laughs. The Chief says, "I realize all of a sudden it's the first laugh I've heard in years" (p. 16). McMurphy's activity level is contagious. He plays cards and Monopoly, he pitches pennies, he commandeers a tub room for a game room, he socializes and gambles incessantly, he struggles with Big Nurse over the use of the TV. The longer McMurphy stays, the more in touch with reality the Chief becomes. McMurphy organizes two activities (or occupations) in particular that seem to make meaningful connections for others: a basketball game on the ward and a fishing trip.

McMurphy "talk[s] the doctor into letting him bring a ball back from the gym" (p. 174). In response to the nurse's objections, the doctor observes: "A number of the players, Miss Ratched, have shown marked progress since that basketball team was organized; I think it has proven its therapeutic value" (p. 175). The team increases a feeling of solidarity among the patients. The Chief, though not on the team, says, "We got to go to the gym and watch our basketball team" (p. 176). The game "let most of (them) come away feeling there'd been a kind of victory" (p. 176) despite their 20-point loss. The image of this patients' team is familiar to most occupational therapists: "Our team was too short and too slow, and Martini kept throwing passes to men that nobody but him could see" (p. 176). The adaptive effects represented in this image of the game validate a major occupational therapy assumption about the human condition.

When basketball season is over, McMurphy plans a fishing trip. He deceives authorities into thinking that two maiden aunts will sponsor the expedition. Instead, he engages the help of a prostitute. The Chief focuses his attention increasingly on McMurphy's energy and strength. When he speaks for the first time in years, he speaks to McMurphy. After having been withdrawn for years, the Chief yearns to reach out. He thinks, "I just want to touch him because he's who he is" (p. 188). McMurphy signs the Chief up for the fishing trip. The Chief reflects: "I was actually going out of the hospital with two whores on a fishing boat; I had to keep saying it over and over to myself to believe it" (p. 191).

Images of the fishing trip powerfully present the competence, mastery, and connectedness with others possible through occupation. The activity meets both group and individual needs. The trip is an occupation enjoyable to these men both in the doing and in the end product: the successful catch. Fiction here validates on a dramatic level what a formal analysis might predict about this particular activity for a group of institutionalized patients. Each person on the expedition benefits in some way from the activity. The Chief's experience is representative of that of the others. On the ride he says, "I could feel a great calmness creep over me, a calmness that increased the farther we left land behind us" (p. 208). He recalls that he "was as excited as the rest" (p. 209). He fishes independently: "I was too busy cranking at my fish to ask him [McMurphy] for help" (p. 210). The clearest representation of the healing effect of the experience is the spread of McMurphy's laughter. The Chief says, "I notice Harding is collapsed beside McMurphy and is laughing too. And Scanlon from the bottom of the boat .... It started slow and pumped itself full, swelling the men bigger and bigger. I watched, part of them, laughing with them" (p. 212). The Chief explains that McMurphy knows about laughter: "He knows you have to laugh at the things that hurt you just to keep yourself in balance, just to keep the world from running you plumb crazy" (p. 212). From within the context of a dehumanizing state institution, a real person, capable of relating and capable of touching lives, makes connections for these men using occupations that help them heal. This image can nurture the art of occupational therapy practice.

In *The House of God*, Roy Basch's experience cuts him off from a number of caring peers. Two people manage to help Roy reconnect through occupations. Roy's girlfriend, Berry, quietly reflects back to him the changes she sees. Toward the end of the novel she says, "Roy, I'm worried. . . . You're isolated. . . . You're hypomanic. . . . For me, tonight, you're a dead man. There's no spark of life" (p. 349). She organizes a trip to see a performance of the mime Marcel Marceau. Roy tries to get out of going at the last minute, so Berry has four of Roy's friends literally carry him out of the hospital to the performance. Seeing the mime perform, Roy reflects, "All of a sudden I felt as if a hearing aid for all my senses had been turned on. I was flooded with feeling" (p. 359). Later he says, "Berry welcomed me back to her, and I felt her caring arms around me for the first time. Awakening, I began to thaw" (p. 360). The performance, in its dramatic portrayal of the human struggle, touches Roy and reconnects him with his innermost self. He says, "I realized that what had been missing [from the House of God experience] was all that I loved. I would be transformed. I'd not leave that country of love again" (p. 363). Soon after the performance, Roy describes his internship: "I hated this. The whole year sucked" (p. 374). Berry asks him, "Why not become a psychiatrist? . . . Being with people was all that kept you going this year, Roy. And 'being with' is the essence of psychiatry" (p. 374). Berry, having connected Roy to a powerful experience that enabled him to feel again, suggests an occupation in which his need to feel and care might be allowed to grow. This healing image is also one that validates the art of occupational therapy practice.

The Fat Man is a caring resident in *The House of God*. In some ways a renegade like Kesey's McMurphy, the Fat Man shares survival skills in an insane world. He teaches interns to "buff" charts and to "turf" hopeless cases elsewhere (p. 61). He models caring behaviors among patients who can comprehend the care. He invokes 13 laws of the House of God, all raucous and outrageous, but aimed to counterbalance the senseless thrust of an institution to apply technological procedures regardless of human cost. One law reads: "The only good admission is a dead admission" (p. 420). Patients love Fats, and Roy asks, "As crass and as cynical as you are?" (p. 213). Fats answers, "That's why: I'm straight with 'em and I make 'em laugh at themselves. . . . I make them feel like they're still part of life, part of some grand nutty scheme instead of alone with their diseases" (pp. 213–214). Roy reflects on this: "I was touched. Here was what medicine could be: human to human. Like all our battered dreams" (pp. 215–216).

The Fat Man sees his residency as only a part of the nutty scheme of things. He attends to other satisfying occupations. He dabbles with inventions such as his "anal mirror" (p. 107). Fats expounds on his invention: "The anus is a great curiosity to almost all mankind" (p. 107). Roy is never quite sure how tongue-in-cheek this invention idea really is. But the idea reflects a comic relief, a reprieve from the daily grind. Fats models a life outside the House of God. He manages a private practice out of his home, saying, "What's the sense of being a licensed doc if you don't use it 'to relieve pain and suffering'? This GP work is terrific—these are my neighbors, my people" (p. 372). His life connects beyond his occupation at the dehumanizing House of God. Fats touches others; he can also be touched. When an intern commits suicide, Roy recalls that "the Fat Man was crying. Quiet tears filled his eyes, fat wet tears of desperation and loss" (p. 313). Fats can touch Roy: When he comes to apologize for the recent distance between them, he links pinkies with Roy. Roy remembers, "It was perfect, a magical moment. . . . He'd sensed my emptiness, and he'd responded. His touch meant I wasn't alone. He and I were connected" (p. 373).

Fats also helps the interns consider meaningful occupational connections. Toward the end of their rotation, he works with the interns to select specialty areas. Using chalk and a blackboard, he lists the advantages and disadvantages that the interns see in each specialty. The exercise, one largely of values clarification, helps Roy. He says, "By the end of the Fat Man's colloquium, the remarkable had happened: on paper, Psychiatry was the clear winner" (p. 381). Fats is able to touch the lives of the interns. Through caring gestures he helps connect them with meaningful occupations.

Conclusion

Reflection about the art of occupational therapy is less widespread in the professional literature than is reflection about the science of occupational therapy. This is a matter of concern in that occupational therapy is a blend of art and science. The art of practice includes the ability to establish rapport, to empathize, and to facilitate choices about occupational and human potential within a community of others. Engaging in the art of practice commits the therapist to an encounter with an individual who is a collaborator in his or her plan for treatment. Collaboration includes a discussion of each patient's personal goals and of professional and personal assumptions about both the human condition and the meaning of occupation in a life. Without the caring elements that ground the therapist–patient relationship and the dialogue that grounds collaborative treatment planning, occupational therapy would be reduced to a sterile science of occupation.

The current health care system does not encourage the art of practice. Medical practitioners, propelled by the scientific model, have recently returned to a consideration of their lost art. Systematized patient defenses against the depersonalization and fragmentation of their care have affirmed the popular need for care in addition to cure. Practitioners looking to sustain their art have had to turn to sources other than the health care system. The new discipline of literature and medicine attempts to support a humane medical practice through the insightful reading of fiction, and it has the potential to sustain the art of occupational therapy practice as well. By reading fictional literature in its fullest, aesthetic sense, one can reflect on and affirm the importance of relationships and caring in practice by comparing and contrasting those various personal characteristics most conducive to helping. Reading fictional literature in its moral sense can enable practitioners to explore values and assumptions about the human condition and, more specifically, about the importance and meaning of occupation in a life. This reading process is adaptable to the educational system as well as to any other continued education format.

Examples from three fictional works illustrate that both positive and negative images of occupational therapy and occupation can affirm commitment to artful practice. Reading fiction can validate the competence, mastery, and human connectedness with others possible through occupation. Reading fictionalized stories of occupational therapists and other caregivers can affirm those personal qualities of warmth, genuineness, humor, and empathy that are essential in the establishment of a helpful bond.

The art of occupational therapy practice requires validation, though perhaps not in the same manner as does its science. The reading of fictional literature can provide occupational therapists with sustaining images: images of relationships, images of qualities that make relationships meaningful, and images of the meaning of occupation in a life. Reflection on these images can reaffirm one's commitment to the art of providing occupation as therapy.

Acknowledgments

I extend special thanks to Dr. Anne Hudson Jones, Institute for the Medical Humanities, The University of Texas Medical Branch, whose flexibility and encouragement made it possible to integrate course material with occupational therapy issues. I also thank Doreen S. McCarty for typing the manuscript.

References

American Occupational Therapy Association Council on Standards. (1972). Occupational therapy: Its definition and functions. *American Journal of Occupational Therapy, 26*, 204–205.

American Occupational Therapy Association Representative Assembly minutes—1981. (1981). *American Journal of Occupational Therapy 35*, 792–802.

Coles, R. (1979). Medical ethics and living a life. *New England Journal of Medicine, 301,* 444–446.

Devereaux, E. B. (1984). Occupational therapy's challenge: The caring relationship. *American Journal of Occupational Therapy, 38,* 791–798. (Reprinted in Chapter 33.)

Engel, G. L. (1977). The need for a new medical model: A challenge for biomedicine. *Science, 196,* 129–135.

Jones, A. H. (1987). Reflections, projections, and the future of literature-and-medicine. In D. Wear, M. Kohn, & S. Stocker (Eds.), *Literature and medicine: A claim for a discipline* (pp. 29–40). McLean, VA: Society for Health and Human Values.

Kesey, K. (1962). *One flew over the cuckoo's nest.* New York: New American Library, Signet Books.

Mosey, A. C. (1981). *Occupational therapy: Configuration of a profession.* New York: Raven Press.

Pellegrino, E. D. (1979). In M. J. Vogel, & C. E. Rosenberg (Eds.), *The therapeutic revolution: Essays in the social history of American medicine* (pp. 245–266). Philadelphia: University of Pennsylvania Press.

Rebeta-Burditt, J. (1977). *The cracker factory.* New York: Bantam Books.

Reed, K. L., & Sanderson, S. R. (1983). *Concepts of occupational therapy.* Baltimore: Williams & Wilkins.

Shem, S. (1978). *The House of God.* New York: Dell Publishing.

Trautmann, J. (1978). The wonders of literature in medical education. In D. Self (Ed.), *The role of the humanities in medical education* (pp. 32–44). Norfolk, VA: Teagle & Little.

Yerxa, E., & Sharrott, G. (1986). Liberal arts: The foundation for occupational therapy education. *American Journal of Occupational Therapy, 40,* 153–159.

Chapter 68

Dreams, Dilemmas and Decisions for Occupational Therapy Practice in a New Millennium: An American Perspective

Elizabeth J. Yerxa, EdD, OTR, FAOTA

Humankind is poised to take a giant step into the 21st century. Will the year 2000 bring a great leap forward into a more humane, healthy, enlightened global community, or will it begin a downward spiral, toward an irretrievable loss of the dream for a good life? Scientists, philosophers, public policy makers, optimists, and pessimists are debating their visions of the future, looking into crystal balls filled with light or darkness.

Assumptions

As I enter this debate I bring a set of assumptions. The 21st century will possess characteristics that are of great importance to occupational therapists and the persons we serve.

First, the next century will begin an *era of chronicity* beyond that which the world has ever known. The population of persons with impairments will increase markedly, as will the number of persons at risk. This era of chronicity will result from the successes of medical technology, the aging of the populace, and the preservation of biological life on an unprecedented scale (Robinson, 1988).

Second, *new knowledge* emanating from the sciences, philosophy, literature, and the arts will affirm the significance of the uniqueness, individuality and wholeness of each person (Edelman, 1992; Thelen, 1990). This new knowledge will enlighten scientists about life span development and the evolution of our species. Research, at last, will emphasize human purpose, action, goal-directedness, interests, curiosity, and consciousness, as well as the joy, despair, or boredom that persons experience when they engage in their daily rounds of activity (Csikszentmihalyi, 1975).

Third, daily life will increase in *complexity* (Toffler, 1981). Successful accomplishment of the activities of daily living will be much more challenging because of increased urbanization, the diversity of cultures interacting, the multiplicity of social role expectations, high technology, and the difficulty of educating children for competency in an instantaneously changing environment.

Fourth, the future will bring an *increased emphasis on personal power, autonomy, self-direction, and self-responsibility*, with a decrease in the influence of traditional paternalistic political and social systems. Persons will demand to control their own destinies and to participate in the decisions that affect them.

Fifth, the 21st century will see a *new conceptualization of health*, a shift away from the old idea that health means the absence of disease, pathology, or impairments. The new idea of health is reflected, for example, in Pörn's (in press) philosophy. He defined health as persons' capacities to achieve their goals and purposes through possession of a repertoire of skills.

Sixth, the new era will bring an *increased awareness of attending to the demands of the environments in which persons actually live and work*. Persons will learn such skills as mathematical computation, not by classroom drills and tests divorced from the pulsating rhythms of life, but in the real world of the supermarket, office, and shopping mall.

Research has demonstrated not only that transferring skills from the academic environment to the real world is difficult but that the skills learned are different (Lave, 1988). Thus learning a skill in a classroom might develop competency for schoolwork but not for the challenges of daily life.

Dreams

Within this context of the future, being an optimist and an occupational therapist (and the two characteristics usually do go together), I have a dream. My most audacious dream is that the 21st century will begin the millennium of occupation. Occupation, as engagement in self-initiated, self-directed, adaptive, purposeful, culturally relevant, organized activity, speaks to my assumptions about the future in compelling ways. The era of chronicity requires that some profession recognize and reclaim the potential of persons with chronic conditions or at risk of developing them, so that these persons can achieve their purposes and so that social barriers to their self-definition will be removed. I nominate occupational therapy as that profession.

The new understanding emanating from the sciences about individuality and wholeness needs to be synthesized with the 70 years of knowledge about human activity, development, learning, and evolution that are embedded in the rich history of occupational therapy. We knew it all the time! For example, we knew that infants are driven by their unique curiosity to explore the world, learn from their experiences, and thus shape their nervous systems (Reilly, 1974). Engagement in occupation cannot be divorced from the meaning it possesses for the person.

The increased complexity of daily life for all persons demands a profession that knows a great deal about daily routines and how persons manage and thrive in their environments. My global travels have shown that occupational therapists everywhere focus on engagement in daily life, regardless of other differences in practice. Alvin Toffler (1981), the futurologist, proposed that all persons, not just those with impairments, will need "life organizers" (p. 377) to help them deal with the complexity of daily life in the 21st century. I nominate occupational therapists to be tomorrow's life organizers, using our knowledge of activities of daily living to help persons get their lives together in a complex world.

As for the increased emphasis on autonomy and personal responsibility, occupational therapists have always involved patients or other participants in formulating and carrying out their programs. In fact, authentic occupational therapy cannot take place unless the patient becomes his or her own agent of competency via occupation. Many other health care professionals do not know how to help the patient do this because they are trained in an old paternalistic model of acute care. In his book, *Medicine at the Crossroads*, Konner recommended that physicians adopt a "new model" of the physician–patient bond called the "patient as colleague" (1993, p. 14) model, in which the physician and patient exchange views and plan treatment or prevention together. Occupational therapists who have used a similar approach for decades can catalyze change in the entire health care system through their skill and example. In this way more persons will take responsibility for their own health.

A vision of health as the possession of a repertoire of skills to achieve one's own purposes fits with occupational therapy's traditional emphasis on skill, mastery, and competence that can be attained regardless of pathology or impairment. It also suggests that occupation that develops skills can prevent illness and influence health by developing competency and making life worth living. This view of health is compatible with Reilly's (1962) (see Chapter 6) great hypothesis that human beings, through the use of their hands as energized by mind and will, can influence the state of their own health. Such a perspective on health implies that every human being has resources that can be reclaimed through occupational therapy (Montgomery, 1984).

Research demonstrating that persons need to learn skills in the environments in which their skills will be used supports occupational therapists who create a "just right challenge" (p. 251) from the environment so that the person can make an adaptive response (Robinson, 1977). It also supports the importance of providing occupational therapy in the home, community, supermarket, shopping mall, workplace, or school, not in artificial environments such as clinics or hospitals. I opened my eyes to the importance of the real life environment when I provided occupational therapy to children with cerebral palsy in a home program after 2 years of similar work in a hospital. Not only was it easier for children to learn skills when the skills did not have to be transferred to a different environment (as was necessary in the hospital), but as an occupational therapist, I could experience the challenges of their daily lives and employ them in increments that assured both a just-right challenge and a high probability of success (Burke, 1977).

Biological evolution, in all creatures, advances in relation to real environmental challenges, not *before* such challenges occur (Jordan, 1991). Nature does not plan ahead; only when an organism is faced with a real environmental challenge can it adapt. Occupational therapists who provide service in real life environments are not only practical but are employing the most sophisticated form of intervention supported by neurobiology, evolutionary biology and anthropology.

Decisions and Dilemmas

What implications do these perspectives of the future hold for occupational therapy practice? Arnold Beisser (1988), a physician who became almost totally paralyzed as a result of poliomyelitis, described his experience as follows:

> More important [than the physical helplessness] was being *separated from so many of the elemental routines that occupied people*. . . . I no longer felt connected with the familiar roles I had known in family, work, sports. My *place in the culture was gone*. (pp. 166–167) [Italics added]

Occupational therapists will need to establish their priorities for practice in the millennium of occupation. I recommend a decision in favor of the vital, fundamental issues that are most important to the person and society: survival, work, contribution, participation, delight in one's own actions. Focus on these will influence health through development of a repertoire of skills that reconnects persons to the elemental routines of their culture, restoring their place in the world. The dilemma is that the organization of the U.S. health care system provides most of its resources for acute care, modalities, and techniques in an artificial environment that values short-term, measurable, physical changes and is not prepared to address these fundamental issues. As a result, the experiences recorded by articulate persons with disabilities—Lewis Puller (1991), Robert Murphy (1990), Arnold Beisser (1988), and Andre Dubus (1991) — as well as our research on persons with disabilities living in the community (Burnett & Yerxa, 1980) show major unmet needs for help in dealing with such elemental issues as skills for living in the community, being part of one's culture, and having something satisfying to do. These authors and our research subjects did not mention occupational therapy in connection with their difficulties in daily living or their need to develop a new repertoire of skills at home or at work. If occupational therapy was mentioned at all it was as a minor aspect of acute care in the hospital.

The era of chronicity cries out for practice founded on an optimistic view of persons, their resources and potential; one that emphasizes what is right, such as intrinsic motivation, rather than what is wrong, such as organ impairment. In spite of the Americans With Disabilities Act of 1990 (Public Law 101–336), persons with disabilities are too often stigmatized as second class citizens or disposable persons. Unfortunately, this social attitude is so pervasive that persons with disabilities may be denied many social opportunities or internalize the stigma themselves, leading to depression and denial. This is a major dilemma. In the future world of genetic engineering and probable euthanasia, persons with disabilities are at risk of being eliminated as they were in Nazi Germany. Through new knowledge of occupation practiced by occupational therapists, these persons will be able to achieve their own purposes and to contribute to the variety and richness of society. Occupational therapists who are allies and advocates for persons with disabilities will help change society's attitudes from "those people are inferior" to "these people are fundamentally human, just like the rest of us." Through occupation this profession will reaffirm its commitment to persons with chronic conditions, a commitment initially made by Adolph Meyer (1922) (see Chapter 2) and Eleanor Clarke Slagle (1922).

A final implication is that occupational therapy practice will be enriched and broadened by new interdisciplinary knowledge of occupation, which some of us have named *occupational science*. Tomorrow's world needs a profession that views persons as both unique and whole, who create themselves through engagement in activity as driven by their interests and curiosity. Thus occupation, rather than being trivial, will be seen as the essential connector between the developing human organism and its environment, a creator of unique neural networks, motor patterns, and life-affirming mastery.

Science and philosophy's new interest in the wholeness of human beings belies the specialism that has permeated society and medicine. Persons have been divided into minds and bodies to fit into specialists' categories of mental health and physical disabilities. One of the greatest strengths of occupational therapy education has been its insistence on preparing students to look at persons as having not only muscles and joints but feelings, perceptions, families, communities, and unique patterns of daily activity. Ours is one of the few health professions that is educated to think this way, whose practitioners can serve anyone who needs to develop skills in the presence of a challenge labeled physical, psychiatric, developmental, or environmental. Our science and clinical experiences will help reconnect the human mind and body. Strengthening our generalist outlook with new knowledge will make our profession much more adaptable to the changing conditions of tomorrow's world environment. Evolutionary biology has taught us that specialists such as dinosaurs perish when their environment changes, whereas generalists such as cockroaches and human beings survive and prosper (Jordan, 1991).

A dilemma is created by the U.S. health care system's low priority on providing resources for those labeled mentally ill and the resulting attrition in the numbers of occupational therapists adopting such practice. New knowledge of occupation that relates to skill, adaptation to changing circumstances, temporality, management and organization of the environment, and obtaining satisfaction through one's own action has a great deal to offer persons who are given psychiatric diagnostic labels. The millennium of occupation will reaffirm the commitment to improving the life opportunities of all persons regardless of diagnostic labels, because it is the right thing to do in a compassionate society and because occupational therapists have the knowledge and skill to make it happen. In the millennium of occupation, occupational therapists will enable human beings as whole persons to be reconnected with their culture through skills. Persons with disabilities will no longer be endangered or be isolated on islands of abnormality, but will perceive themselves as skilled, competent, and capable of mastery. The era of chronicity will be answered by the millennium of occupation. Health will ultimately be perceived not as the absence of impairment but as possession of a repertoire of skills to achieve one's own purposes. Robert Murphy (1990), an anthropologist paralyzed by a spinal cord tumor, at the end of his, "journey into the world of the disabled," said that

> the essence of the well-lived life is the defiance of negativity, inertia and death. Life has a liturgy that must be continually celebrated and renewed; it is a feast whose sacrament is consummated in the paralytic's breaking out from his prison of flesh and bone, and in his quest for autonomy. (p. 230)

Occupational therapists, in the new millennium of occupation, can provide a key to the prison and tools for the quest for autonomy.

References

Americans With Disabilities Act of 1990 (Public Law 101–336). 42 U. S. C., § 12101.

Beisser, A. (1988). *Flying without wings: Personal reflections on being disabled.* New York: Doubleday.

Burke, J. P. (1977). A clinical perspective on motivation: Pawn versus origin. *American Journal of Occupational Therapy, 31,* 254–258.

Burnett, S., & Yerxa, E. J. (1980). Community-based and college-based needs assessment of physically disabled persons. *American Journal of Occupational Therapy, 34,* 201–207.

Csikszentmihalyi, M. (1975). *Beyond boredom and anxiety: The experience of play in work and games.* San Francisco: Jossey-Bass.

Dubus, A. (1991). *Broken vessels. Essays by Andre Dubus.* Boston: David R. Godine.

Edelman, G. (1992). *Bright air, brilliant fire. On the matter of mind.* New York: Basic.

Jordan, W. (1991). *Divorce among the gulls: An uncommon look at human nature.* San Francisco: North Point.

Konner, M. (1993). *Medicine at the crossroads.* New York: Pantheon.

Lave, J. (1988). *Cognition in practice.* New York: Cambridge University Press.

Meyer, A. (1922). The philosophy of occupational therapy. *Archives of Occupational Therapy, 1,* 1–10. (Reprinted as Chapter 2).

Montgomery, M. A. (1984). Resources of adaptation for daily living: A classification with therapeutic implications for occupational therapy. *Occupational Therapy in Health Care. 1,* 9–33.

Murphy, R. F. (1990). *The body silent.* New York: Norton.

Pörn, I. (In press). Health and adaptedness. *Theoretical Medicine.*

Puller, L. B. (1991). *Fortunate son. The autobiography of Lewis B. Puller, Jr.* New York: Grove Weidenfeld.

Reilly, M. (1962). Occupational therapy can be one of the great ideas of 20th century medicine. *American Journal of Occupational Therapy, 16,* 1–9. (Reprinted as Chapter 6).

Reilly M. (1974). *Play as exploratory learning.* Beverly Hills, CA: Sage.

Robinson, A. (1977). Play: The arena for acquisition of rules for competent behavior. *American Journal of Occupational Therapy, 31,* 248–253.

Robinson, I. (1988). The rehabilitation of patients with long term physical impairments: The social context of professional roles. *Clinical Rehabilitation, 2,* 339–347.

Slagle, E. C. (1922). Training aids for mental patients. *Occupational Therapy and Rehabilitation, 1,* 11–14.

Thelen, E. (1990). Dynamical systems and the generation of individual differences. In J. Colombo & J. W. Fagan (Eds.), *Individual differences in infancy: Rehability, stability, and prediction.* Hillsdale, NJ: Erlbaum.

Toffler, A. (1981). *The third wave.* New York: Bantam.

Chapter 69

Dreams, Dilemmas, and Decisions for Occupational Therapy Practice in a New Millennium: A Canadian Perspective

Helene J. Polatajko, PhD, OT(C)

My dreams for occupational therapy in the new millennium are predicated on what I imagine the world will be like in that millennium. Although I would like to believe that the world will be free of war, disease, illness, indeed all sources of human misery, I do not believe that to be the destiny of humanity. Rather, I believe that there will always be some phenomena that will result in less-than-ideal situations for humankind. Whether these phenomena will result in disability or handicap, however, is another issue.

I Dream of a World Free of Handicap

In my dream, the world will be free of handicap in the new millennium. Free not because we have learned to rehabilitate those with disabilities but because we have learned to create an environment that allows those with different abilities to live with dignity. Free not because we have allowed those with disabilities to end their lives but because we have enabled those with different abilities to have meaningful lives. Free not because we have learned to prevent disability but because we have learned to eliminate handicap. In other words, I dream of a world that honors, respects, and values differences, a world that enables living with different abilities.

Before I go on describing my dream and its implications for occupational therapy, let me clarify how I am using the terms *disability* and *handicap* and how they relate to each other. In attempting to establish an international classification for the long-term functional and social consequences of disease, the World Health Organization (WHO) identified three distinct and independent classifications: impairment, disability, and handicap. *Impairment* is defined as "any loss of psychological, physiological, or anatomical structure or function resulting from any cause" (1980, p. 27). *Disability* is defined as "any restriction or lack (resulting from an impairment) of ability to perform an activity in the manner or within the range considered normal for a human being" (p. 28). *Handicap* is "a disadvantage for a given individual, resulting from an impairment or disability, that limits or prevents the fulfillment of a role that is normal (depending on age, sex, and social and cultural factors) for that individual" (p. 29). In the vernacular of occupational therapy, handicap is a disadvantage that limits or prevents occupational role performance. Although WHO considers these classifications to be independent, there is, as apparent from the WHO definitions, a causal relationship between them (see Figure 1). It should be noted, however, that not all impairment leads to disability, nor does all disability lead to handicap. Indeed, because handicap is viewed as a disadvantage, and disadvantage is a social construct, disability must be seen as neither a necessary nor a sufficient condition for the creation of a handicap. In my dream the world will be free of handicaps because of occupational therapy—not the occupational therapy we know now, but the occupational therapy that surely must evolve because *occupation* is a powerful idea. To quote Thomas Jefferson, "It is neither wealth nor splendour, but tranquility and occupation, which give happiness" (cited in Foley, 1967, p. 399).

The great psychologist Hebb (1966) noted long ago that "living things must be active" (p. 248); that the need for activity and the avoidance of boredom, the result of inactivity, are important determinants of human behavior. Recently, two courageous young persons, one Canadian and one American, provided dramatic personal testimony of the vital importance that activity or the lack of it, has in determining human behavior.

In Canada, a 25-year-old woman caught national media attention when she fought the legal system for the right to refuse life-sustaining treatment. Having spent 2½ years in a hospital bed because of a disease that resulted in the permanent loss of all her independent function, including respiration, Nancy B. pleaded for the right to die. She told the judge that a life without the ability to do is not worth living ("Woman makes plea," 1991). She won her case. On February 13, 1992, Nancy B. died.

In the United States, 29-year-old Larry McAfee had a motorcycle accident that left him unable to walk, eat, or even breathe independently. After a year of intensive rehabilitation, out of finances, Larry was also doomed to a life in a hospital bed where, he said, "I used to just lie there on my back, being just so bored" (Schindehette & Wescott, 1993, p. 85). Two years later, "broken in spirit after being warehoused in a series of institutions, McAfee fought for the legal right to shut off his life-sustaining respirator" (Schindehette & Wescott, 1993, p. 85). Larry McAfee won his case. However, he is alive and well and living in the first independent-care home in the state of Georgia. While engaged in his fight to die, he discovered that he had options other than boredom, that in an environment that enabled occupation he could have an active, meaningful life. But Larry McAfee warned, "if ever I have to return to an institution, then I prefer death" (Schindeherte & Wescott, p. 86).

I Dream of a World Where Occupation Is a Powerful Idea

My dream for occupational therapy in the 21st century is that we will not only know unequivocally that occupation is a powerful idea but also choose to act on that idea, for "any powerful idea is absolutely fascinating and absolutely useless until we choose to use it" (Bach, 1988, p. 119).

Occupational therapy is in an exciting, transitional phase—a paradigm shift, as Kielhofner has described it (1992). If we make the right decisions now, if we frame the emerging paradigm well, I believe that the occupational therapy of the future will be quite different from the one we know today.

The occupational therapy we know now fails to realize the full potential of occupation. As Kielhofner (1992) and numerous others have pointed out, practice today is heavily influenced by the medical model. Practice is focused, primarily, on reducing impairment through the therapeutic use of purposeful activity. To quote Henderson et al. (1991), "the use of purposeful activity is the core of occupational therapy" (p. 370). In Canada, a similar emphasis on the therapeutic use of activity prevails. The definition of occupational therapy adopted by our national association begins with "Occupational therapy is the art and science which utilizes the analysis and application of activities" (Canadian Association of Occupational Therapists [CAOT], 1991, p. 140).

I Dream of a Discipline Focused on Occupation

In my dream, the occupational therapy of the future will realize the full potential of occupation. Practice will be grounded firmly in an occupational model. The focus of practice will shift from reducing impairment through purposeful activity to preventing handicap through occupational enablement.

My dream is predicated on two developments in our discipline, both called for by Ann Grady in her presidential address at the 72nd Annual Conference of the American Occupational Therapy Association. Grady asked occupational therapists to revisit and reaffirm the concepts and visions held by the founders of the discipline, to "reaffirm the idea that being meaningfully occupied provides direction for individuals and that successful engagement in the activity leads to individual satisfaction and promotes health and well-being (1992, p. 1062), and to "provide the leadership needed to continue developing knowledge based on our founders' vision and to find a myriad of ways to apply that knowledge to the challenges of practice in the 21st century" (p. 1065).

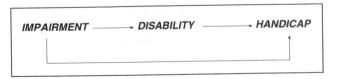

Figure 1. World Health Organization disablement model.

For my dream to come true, we, as occupational therapists must

- affirm that occupation is a powerful idea
- adopt occupation as *the* core concept
- entrench occupation in our value system
- become experts in enabling occupation.

My dream is that our continued study of occupation will make it possible, in the new millennium, for us to move beyond the rhetoric of the day and translate our values into action.

In my 1992 Muriel Driver Lecture, I articulated what I and a group of colleagues believe to be the core values of occupational therapy (see Appendix D). I elaborate on these briefly below and describe what I think it means to translate these into action as we embrace occupation as the core concept of our discipline. (For a more extensive discussion, see Polatajko, 1992.)

The values statement concerns itself with the core elements of this discipline. The first two, the individual and human life, are shared with all health care disciplines. The third, occupation, distinguishes occupational therapy from the rest. Occupational therapists view humans as occupational beings with a basic need to do.

Translating the Rhetoric into Action

Translating these values into action means, first of all, acknowledging some basic assumptions about occupation.

Occupation is a basic survival need. Occupation is essential to the well-being of every person much in the same way that sleep and food are; occupational deprivation, like sleep deprivation or food deprivation, results in serious mental and physical deterioration of the person and may even result in death—often at the individual's own hand.

Occupation is an extremely complex, multilevel, multifaceted construct. Occupation has cognitive, affective, physical, and environmental attributes and is individually determined; therefore, the study of occupation requires the investigation of the occupation, the person performing that occupation, the environmental context, and their interaction.

Occupational competence is the result of a goodness of fit between the person, the occupation, and the environment. Competence is defined as adequacy or sufficiency, answering all the requirements of an environment (Pridham & Schutz, 1985). That is, the occupational competence of any given person is determined by the interaction between the skills necessary to perform the occupation, the abilities of the person, and the demands of the environment in which the occupation is to be performed (see Figure 2).

Translating these values into action also means that:

Practice is client driven. The client's right to autonomy is taken seriously, and the client is understood to be a *prosumer* (defined by Toffler [1981, p. 11] as a fusion of producer and consumer) of occupational therapy services, keenly interested in exercising choice over the services that she or he accepts and accepting only those services that can be tailored to meet his or her needs.

Practice is founded on an ideology of empowerment (as defined by Rappaport, 1981). The role of occupational therapist is understood to be one of enhancing possibilities for persons to control their own lives at both a personal and a social level.

The ultimate goal of practice is wholly and solely the enablement of occupational competence. The purpose of practice is to alter the person's ability, the occupation, or the environment so that the person can achieve the necessary balance between ability and the environmental demands to enable occupational competence (see Figure 3).

Practice is context focused. Given the ideology of empowerment and the nature of occupation, services must be oriented toward, if not provided in, the person's context, that is, his or her physical, social, and cultural environment.

Practitioners take on many roles in enabling occupational competence. The traditional roles of hands-on clinician, administrator, researcher, and educator are not always adequate to enable occupational competence. Often, particularly when competence requires environment changes, new forms of practice are necessary, such as program designer, consultant, public educator, lobbyist, policy maker, and social critic.

Practitioners use many and any tools. Activity is only one of many tools used to enhance occupational competence. Practitioners use a variety of tools to enable clients; these may include technology, assistive devices, environmental adaptation, attitudinal shift, family education, social education, and policy change.

The domain of concern of the discipline is occupation. The body of knowledge of the discipline is centered on occupation. Scholarly inquiry is focused on understanding the phenomenon of occupation and the determinants of occupational competence. Given the complex nature of occupation, the study of occupation is multidisciplinary and multimethodological.

Occupational therapists are experts in occupation. As my dream comes true there will be a great deal of change for occupational therapy (see Figure 4). These changes will present all occupational therapists—present practitioners, administrators, researchers and educators alike—with dilemmas that each of us will have to resolve for ourselves and that the profession will have to resolve as a whole.

As my dream comes true there will be a great deal of change that will create dilemmas, not only for occupational therapists, but for the world in general. Once the central importance and power of occupation is realized, it will necessitate a shift in such basic notions as quality of life and human rights. This shift has already begun, as shown by the cases of Nancy B. and Larry McAfee.

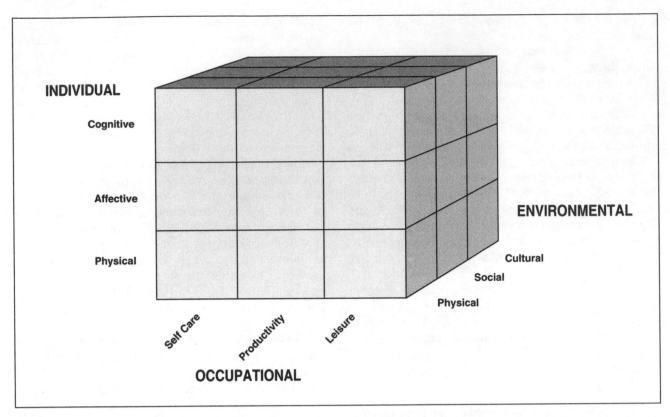

Figure 2. Occupational competence model. Reprinted with permission from Polatajko, H. J. (1992). Naming and framing occupational therapy: A lecture dedicated to the life of Nancy B. *Canadian Journal of Occupational Therapy, 59*, 189–200. Reprinted with permission of CAOT Publications.

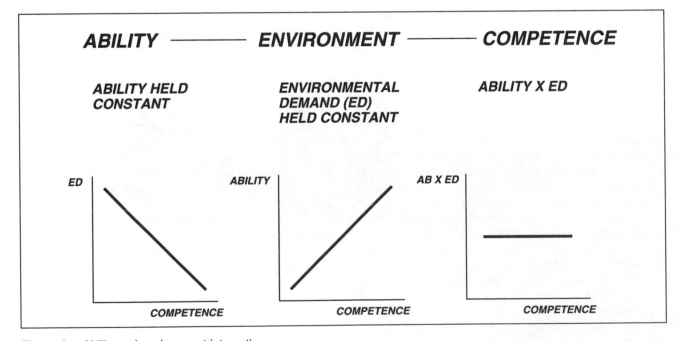

Figure 3. Ability and environment interaction.

OT...	Will no longer be...	But...
Ideology	Treatment	Empowerment
Model	Medical	Enabling
Goal	Impairment Reduction	Occupational Competence
Function	To Cure	To Enable
Role	Clinician	Multifaceted
Setting	Institution	Occupational Context
Hallmark	Activity	Occupational Perspective
Activity	**THE Means**	**THE End**

Figure 4. Changes for occupational therapy in the coming millennium.

I believe that mine is not an impossible dream. Rather, I believe that we, as a discipline, are uniquely poised to make this dream come true—to lead the way in health care. Steven Lewis, former Ambassador of Canada to the United Nations, speaking at the CAOT conference in June 1991, said:

> There is no other discipline that is so eclectic, so far ranging and whose core principles are at the very heart of where the health care system is going .... You are the only health profession that has fully embraced the concepts of health promotion, prevention, community-based care and the individual as centre to the process. ("Perspectives '91." 1991, p. 11)

As with all change, this change will be experienced with some hesitation, discomfort, and, I hope, excitement. But when my dream comes true, I believe that occupational therapists will be instrumental in helping the world to enable all to achieve occupational competence and therefore eliminate handicap.

Appendix

Occupational Therapy Values Statement

Occupational Therapy Values
As Occupational Therapists,
We value
- the individual
- human life
- occupation

About the individual,
We believe that humans are occupational beings, that:
- every individual has intrinsic dignity and worth
- every individual has the right to autonomy
- each individual is a unique whole
- each individual has abilities and competencies
- each individual has the capacity for change

- individuals are social beings
- individuals shape and are shaped by their environment

About human life,
We believe that all human life has value, that:
- the value of human life is based on meaning, not perfection
- quality of life is as valued as quantity

About occupation,
We believe that occupation is a basic human need, that:
- occupation is an essential component of life
- occupation gives meaning to life
- occupation organizes behavior
- occupation has developmental and contextual dimensions
- occupation is socioculturally determined

(Conceptual Framework Think Tank, 1992)
University of Western Ontario-Occupational Therapy
Adapted from H.J. Polatajko (1992). Naming and framing occupational therapy: A lecture dedicated to the life of Nancy B. *Canadian Journal of Occupational Therapy, 59,* 193. Adapted with permission of CAOT Publications.

References

Bach, R. (1988). *One.* New York: Dell.

Canadian Association of Occupational Therapists. (1991) *Canadian occupational therapy guidelines for client-centered practice.* Toronto: Author.

Foley, J.P. (1967). *The Jeffersonian cyclopedic comprehensive collection of the views of Thomas Jefferson.* New York: Russel & Russel.

Grady, A.P. (1992). Nationally Speaking—Occupation as vision. *American Journal of Occupational Therapy, 46,* 1062–1065.

Hebb, D.O. (1966). *A textbook of psychology.* Philadelphia: Saunders.

Henderson, A., Cermak, S., Coster, W., Murray, E., Trombly, C., & Tickle-Degnen, L. (1991). Occupational science is multidimensional. *American Journal of Occupational Therapy, 45,* 370–372.

Kielhofner, G. (1992). *Conceptual foundations of occupational therapy.* Philadelphia: Davis.

Perspectives '91—Taking the initiative. (1991). *National, 8* (5), 11.

Polatajko, H.J. (1992). Naming and framing occupational therapy: A lecture dedicated to the life of Nancy B. *Canadian Journal of Occupational Therapy, 59,* 189–200.

Pridham, K.R., & Schutz, M.E. (1985). Rationale for a language for naming problems from a nursing perspective. *Image: The Journal of Nursing Scholarship, XVII* (4), 122–127.

Rappaport, J. (1981). In praise of paradox: A social policy of empowerment over prevention. *American Journal of Community Psychology, 9* (1), 1–25.

Schindehette, S., & Wescott, G. (1993, January 18). Deciding not to die. *People,* pp. 85–86.

Toffler, A. (1981). *The third wave.* Toronto: Bantam.

Woman makes plea to end life. (1991, November 29). *The Globe and Mail,* Section A, p. 4.

World Health Organization. (1980). *International classification of impairments, disabilities and handicaps (ICIDH).* Geneva, Switzerland: Author.

Appendices
Introduction

This text concludes with thirteen appendices which supplement a number of the text's chapters and/or areas of focus to serve as an additional resource for the reader.

The first appendix contains the official AOTA **Definition of OT Practice for State Regulation**. This clear, succinct overview of the field of Occupational Therapy emphasizes the use of purposeful activity in OT practice and provides the reader with a useful, holistic definition of our profession. The inherent worth and vital importance of purposeful activity to Occupational Therapy is reinforced in the next two appendices which present the **Philosophical Base of Occupational Therapy**, and AOTA's **Position Paper on Purposeful Activity**. The latter appendix also provides the reader with key concepts, definitions and principles regarding the use of purposeful activity in evaluation and intervention.

The ethical and humane use of purposeful activity requires a recognition of and a commitment to professional values and attitudes. Appendix D presents AOTA's official statement defining the **Seven Core Values and Attitudes of Occupational Therapy Practice**; providing a strong affirmation of our profession's philosophical base. The following appendix also affirms OT's philosophical base, but in addition it provides the reader with a rare look at our profession's historical roots. This appendix contains an **Address in Honor of Eleanor Clarke Slagle** which was delivered by Adolf Meyer at a testimonial banquet on September 14, 1937, in Atlantic City, New Jersey. This event, on the eve of Slagle's retirement from professional life, also featured a speech by the First Lady, of the time, Eleanor Roosevelt (Quiroga, 1985). Regrettably, Mrs. Roosevelt's complete testimony to Slagle is not available, but fortunately Meyer's is. His intimate knowledge of Mrs. Slagle's significant contributions to our profession and to the clients she worked with led to this stirring tribute to the woman who "personified" Occupational Therapy.

The next six appendices provide the reader with information that will facilitate the practical application of key OT concepts and principles. Appendix F includes the **Life Style Performance Profile** which outlines key areas for assessment according to the practice model presented in Chapter 11 by Gail Fidler. Evaluation and intervention guidelines relevant to Section II—The Environmental Contexts of Purposeful Activity—are presented in the next appendix which includes AOTA's **Position Paper on Occupational Therapy and the Americans with Disabilities Act (ADA)**. Knowledge of ADA is critical to ensure OT practitioners work collaboratively and effectively with consumers to empower them in their work environments (as described in Chapter 22 by Crist and Stoffel) and in their communities of choice (as presented by Grady in Chapter 23). The next appendix supplements Chapter 45 that explored the use of adjunctive modalities in Occupational Therapy. It includes AOTA's **Position Paper on Physical Agent Modalities (PAMs),** providing important information on the use of PAMs as an adjunct to or in preparation for purposeful activity. Ethical considerations necessary for the appropriate use of PAMs in OT practice are justifiably emphasized.

The third Edition of AOTA's **Uniform Terminology for OT Practice**, an **Activity Analysis Form** and an **Activity Analysis Sample** based upon this uniform terminology are provided in the next three appendices. While it may be human nature, (or at least student nature) to go straight to the definitions of terms, I urge the reader to take the time to carefully consider the highly relevant clinical examples which highlight the interrelationships between the performance components, performance areas and performance contexts and which translates these into realistic practice situations. In addition, reflect on the discussion of the "person-activity-environment fit" and the application to practice guidelines. Thoughtful consideration of these issues will ensure that uniform terminology is used as an integrative holistic tool, rather than a reductionist one.

Activity analysis also risks being approached in a reductionistic manner; therefore, the activity analysis form and sample included here strive to present a comprehensive and integrative approach to activity analysis, adaptation, gradation, and synthesis. Uniform terminology was selected as a framework for this activity analysis because it provides comprehensive definitions of terms to assist the neophyte in analyzing all aspects of an activity. Sections on activity adaptation, gradation and synthesis are included to facilitate a thorough exploration of the therapeutic potential of selected activities. The application of this complete framework will assist the reader in designing meaningful purposeful activities for evaluation and intervention in all areas of OT practice.

To effectively use purposeful activity in a diversity of practice situations requires the development and maintenance of a solid theoretical base along with a broad network of resources; therefore, the last two appendices provide listings of activity resources and references pertinent to the major topics covered in this text. These listings are not intended to be all inclusive, as an exhaustive bibliography and resource guide are in themselves books. However, I have carefully selected literature and resources that I have found to be relevant and applicable to current OT education and practice. Resources listed include professional and consumer organizations, educational, vocational, and recreational services, environmental and home modification companies and suppliers of play/leisure equipment and craft activities. The reference lists at the end of each chapter also provide a wealth of well researched resources. Readers who actively use these references and resources will strengthen their philosophical foundation, develop their clinical expertise, and enhance the quality of their collaboration with the consumers of OT services.

Reference

Quiroga, V.A. (1995). *Occupational Therapy: The First 30 Years—1900 to 1930*. Bethesda, MD: American Occupational Therapy Association.

Appendix A

Definition of Occupational Therapy Practice for State Regulation

"Occupational therapy" is the use of purposeful activity or interventions designed to achieve functional outcomes which promote health, prevent injury or disability and which develop, improve, sustain, or restore the highest possible level of independence of any individual who has an injury, illness, cognitive impairment, psychosocial dysfunction, mental illness, developmental or learning disability, physical disability, or other disorder or condition. It includes assessment by means of skilled observation or evaluation through the administration and interpretation of standardized tests and measurements.

Occupational therapy services include but are not limited to:

1. The assessment and provision of treatment in consultation with the individual, family, or other appropriate persons; and

2. interventions directed toward developing, improving, sustaining or restoring daily living skills, including self-care, skills and activities that involve interactions with others and the environment, work readiness or work performance, play skills or leisure capacities, or enhancing educational performance skills; and

3. developing, improving, sustaining or restoring sensory-motor, perceptual or neuromuscular functioning; or range of motion; or emotional, motivational, cognitive, or psychosocial components of performance; and

4. education of the individual, family or other appropriate persons in carrying out appropriate interventions.

These services may encompass assessment of need and the design, development, adaptation, application or training in the use of assistive technology devices; the design, fabrication or application of rehabilitative technology such as selected orthotic devices; training in the use of orthotic or prosthetic devices; the application of physical agent modalities as an adjunct to or in preparation for purposeful activity; the application of ergonomic principles; the adaptation of environments and processes to enhance functional performance; or the promotion of health and wellness.

This definition was originally published in the *American Journal of Occupational Therapy, 48*, 1072–1073. Copyright © 1994, American Occupational Therapy Association.

Appendix B

The Philosophical Base of Occupational Therapy

Man is an active being whose development is influenced by the use of purposeful activity. Using their capacity for intrinsic motivation, human beings are able to influence their physical and mental health and their social and physical environment through purposeful activity. Human life includes a process of continuous adaptation. Adaptation is a change in function that promotes survival and self-actualization. Biological, psychological, and environmental factors may interrupt the adaptation process at any time throughout the life cycle. Dysfunction may occur when adaptation is impaired. Purposeful activity facilitates the adaptive process.

Occupational therapy is based on the belief that purposeful activity (occupation), is including its interpersonal and environmental components, may be used to prevent and mediate dysfunction, and to elicit maximum adaptation. Activity as used by the occupational therapist includes both an intrinsic and a therapeutic purpose.

This statement was adopted by the April 1979 Representative Assembly of The American Occupational Therapy Association, Inc. as Resolution C #531–79. The text can be noted below:
American Occupational Therapy association (1979). The philosophical base of occupational therapy. *American Journal of Occupational Therapy, 33,* 785.
American Occupational Therapy Association (1979). Policy 1.11. The philosophical base of occupational therapy. In *Policy Manual of The American Occupational Therapy Association. Inc.* Rockville, MD: Author.

Appendix C

Position Paper: Purposeful Activity

The American Occupational Therapy Association (AOTA) submits this paper to clarify the use of the term *purposeful activity*, a central focus of occupational therapy throughout its history. People engage in purposeful activity as part of their daily life routines, in the context of occupational performance (AOTA, 1979 [see Appendix B]). Occupation refers to active participation in self-maintenance, work, leisure, and play. Purposeful activity refers to goal-directed behaviors or tasks that comprise occupations. An activity is purposeful if the individual is an active, voluntary participant and if the activity is directed toward a goal that the individual considers meaningful (Evans, 1987; Gilfoyle, 1984; Mosey 1986; Nelson, 1988 [reprinted as Chapter 41]). The purposefulness of an activity lies with the individual performing the activity and with the context in which it is done (Henderson et al., 1991). The meaning of an activity is unique to each person, influenced by his or her life experiences (Mosey 1986; Pedretti, 1982), life roles, interests, age, and cultural background, as well as the situational context in which the activity occurs. Occupational therapy practitioners (i.e., registered occupational therapists and certified occupational therapy assistants) are committed to the use of purposeful activity to evaluate, facilitate, restore, or maintain individuals' abilities to function in their daily occupations.

Occupational therapists use activities to evaluate an individual's capacities to meet the functional demands of his or her environment and daily life. On the basis of an evaluation, the occupational therapy practitioner, in collaboration with the individual, designs activity experiences that offer the individual opportunities for effective action. Purposeful activities assist and build upon the individual's abilities and lead to achievement of personal functional goals.

Purposeful activity provides opportunities for persons to achieve mastery of their environment, and successful performance promotes feelings of personal competence (Fidler & Fidler, 1978 [reprinted as Chapter 7]). A person who is involved in purposeful activity directs attention to the goal rather than to the processes required for achievement of the goal. Engagement in purposeful activity within the context of interpersonal, cultural, physical, and other environmental conditions requires and elicits coordination among the individual's sensory motor, cognitive, and psychosocial systems. Purposeful activity may involve the independent use of complex cognitive processes, such as premeditation, reflection, planning, and use of symbolic cues. Conversely, it may involve less complex processes and take place in an environment of external structure, support, and supervision (Allen, 1987; Henderson et al., 1991). Engagement in purposeful activity provides direct and objective feedback of performance both to the occupational therapy practitioner and the individual.

The therapeutic purposes for which purposeful activity is used include mastery of a new skill, restoration of a deficient ability, compensation for functional disability, health maintenance, or prevention of dysfunction. To use purposeful activity therapeutically, an occupational therapy practitioner analyzes the activity from several perspectives. First, the activity is examined to identify its component parts to determine which skills and abilities are necessary to complete the task. Second, it is examined in terms of the context in which it will be performed. Third, the practitioner considers the person's age, occupational roles, cultural background, gender, interests, and preferences that may influence the meaningfulness of the activity for the individual. All this information is considered together to assist the occupational therapy practitioner in synthesizing (i.e., adapting, grading, and combining) activities for therapeutic purposes for a particular individual.

Purposeful activities cannot be prescribed on the basis of analysis of their inherent characteristics alone; rather, by definition, prescription of purposeful activity is individual-specific. An occupational therapy practitioner grades or adapts a chosen activity for an individual to promote successful performance or elicit a particular response. Grading activities challenges the patient's abilities by progressively changing the process, tools, materials, or environment of a given activity to gradually increase or decrease performance demands. These incremental modifications are made in response to the individual's dynamic changes and provide opportunities for gradual development of skill and related therapeutic benefits. The grading of activities is accomplished by modifying the sequence, duration, or procedures of the task; the individual's position; the position of the tools and materials; the size, shape, weight, or texture of the materials; the nature and degree of interpersonal contact; the extent of physical handling by the occupational therapy practitioner during performance; or the environment in which the activity is attempted. Supportive or assistive devices or techniques may be used to enhance the effectiveness of an activity or to facilitate performance (Henderson et al., 1991; Pedretti & Pasquinelli, 1990). Such techniques or devices are considered facilitative or preparatory to performance of purposeful activity and engagement in occupations.

If the therapy goal is to enhance a performance component so that an individual can engage in an occupational performance area, the selected activity and environmental conditions are manipulated to present graded challenges to the specific skills required. When an individual's successful completion of a task is a priority, occupational therapy practitioners adapt the task and the environment to facilitate performance. Adaptation is a process that changes an aspect of the activity or the environment to enable successful performance and accomplish a particular therapeutic goal. Adaptation of a task may require the use of assistive devices and techniques or grading strategies.

Occupational therapy education provides the necessary background for using activities as therapeutic modalities by instructing the student about behavioral and biological sciences related to the use and meaning of activity, about the nature of purposeful activity, about the process of activity analysis and synthesis, and about the application of activity to therapeutic problems within occupational therapy frames of reference.

In summary, purposeful activity occurs within the context of work, self-care, play, and leisure activities and is used therapeutically to evaluate, facilitate, restore, or maintain individuals' abilities to function competently within their daily occupations. The occupational therapy practitioner's commitment to those whom he or she serves is to guide them in the use of purposeful activities so as to empower them to enhance the quality of their being in the daily reality where they live as parents, children, students, homemakers, workers, or retirees (Reilly, 1966).

Prepared by Jim Hinojosa, PhD, OTR, FAOTA, Joyce Sabari, PhD, OTR, and Lorraine Pedretti, MS, OTR, with contributions from Mark S. Rosenfeld, PhD, OTR, and Catherine Trombly, ScD, OTR/L FAOTA, for The Commission on Practice (Jim Hinojosa, PhD, OTR, FAOTA, Chairperson).
Approved by the Representative Assembly April 1983. Revised and approved by the Representative Assembly June 1993.

References

Allen, C. K. (1987). 1987 Eleanor Clarke Slagle Lecture—Activity: Occupational therapy's treatment method. *American Journal of Occupational Therapy, 41,* 563–575.

American Occupational Therapy Association. (1979). Resolution C, 531–79: The philosophical base of occupational therapy. *American Journal of Occupational Therapy, 33,* 785. Reprinted as Appendix B.

Evans, K. A. (1987). Nationally Speaking—Definition of occupation as the core concept of occupational therapy. *American Journal of Occupational Therapy, 41,* 627–628.

Fidler, G. S., & Fidler, J. W. (1978). Doing and becoming: Purposeful action and self-actualization. *American Journal of Occupational Therapy, 32,* 305–310. (Reprinted as Chapter 7).

Gilfoyle, E. M. (1984). Eleanor Clarke Slagle Lectureship 1984: Transformation of a profession. *American Journal of Occupational Therapy, 38,* 575–584.

Henderson, A., Cermak, S., Coster, W., Murray, E., Trombly, C., & Tickle-Degnen, L. (1991). The Issue Is—Occupational science is multidimensional. *American Journal of Occupational Therapy, 45,* 370–372.

Mosey, A. C. (1986). *Psychosocial components of occupational therapy.* New York: Raven.

Nelson, D. L. (1988). Occupation: Form and performance. *American Journal of Occupational Therapy, 42,* 633–641. (Reprinted as Chapter 41).

Pedretti, L. W. (1982, May). *The compatibility of current treatment methods in physical disabilities with the philosophical base of occupational therapy.* Paper presented at the 62nd Annual Conference of the American Occupational Therapy Association, Philadelphia, PA.

Pedretti, L. W., & Pasquinelli, S. (1990). A frame of reference for occupational therapy in physical dysfunction. In L. W. Pedretti & B. Zoltan (Eds.), *Occupational therapy practice skills for physical dysfunction* (pp. 1–17). St. Louis: Mosby.

Reilly, M. (1966). The challenge of the future to an occupational therapist. *American Journal of Occupational Therapy, 20,* 221–225.

Appendix D

Core Values and Attitudes of Occupational Therapy Practice

Introduction

In 1985, the American Occupational Therapy Association (AOTA) funded the Professional and Technical Role Analysis Study (PATRA). This study had two purposes: to delineate the entry-level practice of OTRs and COTAs through a role analysis and to conduct a task inventory of what practitioners actually do. Knowledge, skills, and attitude statements were to be developed to provide a basis for the role analysis. The PATRA study completed the knowledge and skills statements. The Executive Board subsequently charged the Standards and Ethics Commission (SEC) to develop a statement that would describe the attitudes and values that undergird the profession of occupational therapy. The SEC wrote this document for use by AOTA members.

The list of terms used in this statement was originally constructed by the American Association of Colleges of Nursing (AACN) (1986). The PATRA committee analyzed the knowledge statements that the committee had written and selected those terms from the AACN list that best identified the values and attitudes of our profession. This list of terms was then forwarded to SEC by the PATRA Committee to use as the basis for the Core Values and Attitudes paper.

The development of this document is predicated on the assumption that the values of occupational therapy are evident in the official documents of the American Occupational Therapy Association. The official documents that were examined are: (a) *Dictionary Definition of Occupational Therapy* (AOTA, 1986), (b) *The Philosophical Base of Occupational Therapy* (AOTA, 1979) (reprinted as Appendix B), (c) *Essentials and Guidelines for an Accredited Educational Program for the Occu-*

pational Therapist (AOTA, 1991a), (d) *Essentials and Guidelines for an Accredited Educational Program for the Occupational Therapy Assistant* (AOTA, 1991b), and (e) *Occupational Therapy Code of Ethics* (AOTA, 1988). It is further assumed that these documents are representative of the values and beliefs reflected in other occupational therapy literature.

A *value* is defined as a belief or an ideal to which an individual is committed. Values are an important part of the base or foundation of a profession. Ideally, these values are embraced by all members of the profession and are reflected in the members' interactions with those persons receiving services, colleagues, and the society at large. Values have a central role in a profession and are developed and reinforced throughout an individual's life as a student and as a professional.

Actions and attitudes reflect the values of the individual. An attitude is the disposition to respond positively or negatively toward an object, person, concept, or situation. Thus, there is an assumption that all professional actions and interactions are rooted in certain core values and beliefs.

Seven Core Concepts

In this document, the *core values and attitudes* of occupational therapy are organized around seven basic concepts—altruism, equality, freedom, justice, dignity, truth, and prudence. How these core values and attitudes are expressed and implemented by occupational therapy practitioners may vary depending upon the environments and situations in which professional activity occurs.

Altruism is the unselfish concern for the welfare of others. This concept is reflected in actions and attitudes of commitment, caring, dedication, responsiveness, and understanding.

This appendix was previously published in the *American Journal of Occupational Therapy, 47*, 1085–1086.

Equality requires that all individuals be perceived as having the same fundamental human rights and opportunities. This value is demonstrated by an attitude of fairness and impartiality. We believe that we should respect all individuals, keeping in mind that they may have values, beliefs, or life-styles that are different from our own. Equality is practiced in the broad professional arena, but is particularly important in day-to-day interactions with those individuals receiving occupational therapy services.

Freedom allows the individual to exercise choice and to demonstrate independence, initiative, and self-direction. There is a need for all individuals to find a balance between autonomy and societal membership that is reflected in the choice of various patterns of interdependence with the human and nonhuman environment. We believe that individuals are internally and externally motivated toward action in a continuous process of adaptation throughout the life span. Purposeful activity plays a major role in developing and exercising self-direction, initiative, interdependence, and relatedness to the world. Activities verify the individual's ability to adapt, and they establish a satisfying balance between autonomy and societal membership. As professionals, we affirm the freedom of choice for each individual to pursue goals that have personal and social meaning.

Justice places value on the upholding of such moral and legal principles as fairness, equity, truthfulness, and objectivity. This means we aspire to provide occupational therapy services for all individuals who are in need of these services and that we will maintain a goal-directed and objective relationship with all those served. Practitioners must be knowledgeable about and have respect for the legal rights of individuals receiving occupational therapy services. In addition, the occupational therapy practitioner must understand and abide by the local, state, and federal laws governing professional practice.

Dignity emphasizes the importance of valuing the inherent worth and uniqueness of each person. This value is demonstrated by an attitude of empathy and respect for self and others. We believe that each individual is a unique combination of biologic endowment, sociocultural heritage, and life experiences. We view human beings holistically, respecting the unique interaction of the mind, body, and physical and social environment. We believe that dignity is nurtured and grows from the sense of competence and self-worth that is integrally linked to the person's ability to perform valued and relevant activities. In occupational therapy we emphasize the importance of dignity by helping the individual build on his or her unique attributes and resources.

Truth requires that we be faithful to facts and reality. Truthfulness or veracity is demonstrated by being accountable, honest, forthright, accurate, and authentic in our attitudes and actions. There is an obligation to be truthful with ourselves, those who receive services, colleagues, and society. One way that this is exhibited is through maintaining and upgrading professional competence. This happens, in part, through an unfaltering commitment to inquiry and learning, to self-understanding, and to the development of an interpersonal competence.

Prudence is the ability to govern and discipline oneself through the use of reason. To be prudent is to value judiciousness, discretion, vigilance, moderation, care, and circumspection in the management of one's affairs, to temper extremes, make judgments, and respond on the basis of intelligent reflection and rational thought.

Summary

Beliefs and values are those intrinsic concepts that underlie the core of the profession and the professional interactions of each practitioner. These values describe the profession's philosophy and provide the basis for defining purpose. The emphasis or priority that is given to each value may change as one's professional career evolves and as the unique characteristics of a situation unfold. This evolution of values is developmental in nature. Although we have basic values that cannot be violated, the degree to which certain values will take priority at a given time is influenced by the specifics of a situation and the environment in which it occurs. In one instance dignity may be a higher priority than truth; in another prudence may be chosen over freedom. As we process information and make decisions, the weight of the values that we hold may change. The practitioner faces dilemmas because of conflicting values and is required to engage in thoughtful deliberation to determine where the priority lies in a given situation.

The challenge for us all is to know our values, be able to make reasoned choices in situations of conflict, and be able to clearly articulate and defend our choices. At the same time, it is important that all members of the profession be committed to a set of common values. This mutual commitment to a set of beliefs and principles that govern our practice can provide a basis for clarifying expectations between the recipient and the provider of services. Shared values empowers the profession and, in addition, builds trust among ourselves and with others.

References

American Association of Colleges of Nursing. (1986). *Essentials of College and University Education for Professional Nursing. Final report.* Washington, DC: Author.

Prepared by Elizabeth Kanny, MA, OTR, for the Standards and Ethics Commission (Ruth A. Hansen, PhD, OTR, FAOTA, Chairperson). Approved by the Representative Assembly June 1993.

American Occupational Therapy Association. (1986, April). *Dictionary definition of occupational therapy.* Adopted and approved by the Representative Assembly to fulfill Resolution #596-83. (Available from AOTA, 1383 Piccard Drive, PO Box 1725, Rockville, MD 20849–1725).

American Occupational Therapy Association. (1988). Occupational therapy code of ethics. *American Journal of Occupational Therapy, 42,* 795–796.

American Occupational Therapy Association. (1991a). Essentials and guidelines for an accredited educational program for the occupational therapist. *American Journal of Occupational Therapy, 45,* 1077–1084.

American Occupational Therapy Association. (1991b). Essentials and guidelines for an accredited educational program for the occupational therapy assistant. *American Journal of Occupational Therapy, 45,* 1085–1092.

American Occupational Therapy Association. (1979). The philosophical base of occupational therapy. *American Journal of Occupational Therapy, 33,* 785. (Reprinted as Appendix B).

Appendix E

Address in Honor of Eleanor Clarke Slagle

Adolf Meyer

.

It is a great privilege to have an opportunity to speak on this occasion which honors a friend and long-time coworker, our Mrs. Eleanor Clarke Slagle, as a person and as the personification of occupational therapy. Presidents and officers have come and gone but for 20 years Mrs. Slagle has brought into the field just that kind of personality which proved highly fruitful and auspicious: she has been, not a dictator, not a boss, but a leader by example, a human being and human factor among human beings, a cultivator of human relationships, in gathering around herself coworkers and in making coworkers of the patients. Such is the human being Mrs. Slagle and what she means to us and to the thousands of patients who have been and are still reached by her and her pupils. And inseparable from this personal human side, there stands before us the nature and character of the product of her work and the spirit and philosophy her life and life-work exemplify, that which brings us together in this assembly and in this large and impressive organization.

This gathering and the work achieved by this body with Mrs. Slagle as the head worker are enough of a testimonial for a cause and its leading and stabilizing captain. Obviously Mrs. Slagle has had her ideal not only in perpetuating herself in a special role but in training a rank and file ever able to furnish timber for leadership from the ranks and in the ranks, and growth from the ranks.

For 20 years, from the beginning of our organization, Mrs. Slagle has, as treasurer and secretary, done that work of continuity which with changing presidents and changing topics represents the very constitution of this growing

This chapter was previously published in *Occupational Therapy in Mental Health, 5,* (3), 109–113.

force in the ranks of dealing with those who, for a time and sometimes for good, are forced into that army that needs shelter and protection and among whom the work of restoring health and better ways of prevention and achievement of the handicapped brings care and cure.

In these days in which we are perhaps too much inclined to look upon leadership as a profession, and upon professional agitators as the reapers of honor and power, it is a tremendous satisfaction to see one of the chief workers completing 20 years in that office which personifies the very constitution of this body. Mrs. Slagle and Dr. Dunton have been the spirits in the ranks and from the ranks and for the ranks, not imposed managers, but the souls of the essence of the work, giving freely of their time and experience while carrying on the work itself.

In the great division of labor we need continuity and examples that survive the changes and are embodiments of the very essentials which only the best workers can perpetuate in steady growth, in stability of motion and promotion, those who see that ever new deals are fair deals, deals embodying the wisdom of those who do and actually work and never cease to grow and to create.

Growth and work and achievement and attainment are all a function of that one virtual commodity time, that steady rhythm of day and night, of seasons and years, not a mere eternal return but eternal progression. No two days can be quite the same, and no two years; but there has to be an element of continuity and cohesion; and for this it takes those starting with enough personality, capable of maintaining themselves and of remaining forces and centers of growth. And as in the nature of humanity, generation follows generation, the young work beside the old and the old work beside the young, those capable of being the bearers of continuity are few and rare and, we are glad to see, honored and sought as the very essence of progress.

Mrs. Slagle comes from the same source and soil that gave me my first opportunities and encouragement: the opportunity to realize the need for more, the need for growth, the opportunity to find similarly minded forces and the spirit of action that has to go with knowledge and vision to make it both fertile and practical: Illinois, large needs and large enterprises, a whole group of aspiring forces and engaging problems, needs in practice and needs in hospitals, close to Missouri, wanting to be shown and shown by actual work and performances. The educator, the social worker and the physician were bound to get together. Miss Lathrop was one of the great links. As the great gardener Froebel in education and his pupil Grossman in the therapeutic training of psychopaths by work recognized the need of a setting for work and for therapy in sound use of time, so there was the shaping of an atmosphere of work and action at Kankakee, encouraged by the social spirit about Hull House, all working for the training by action and not only by word. The old ideal of the Middle Ages, pray and work, took real form in the union of one's best thought and work, and when we opened the Phipps Clinic for action, Miss Lathrop was able to lend us Mrs. Slagle as the model and instigator of workmanship in the service of therapy. That the greatest benefit for the sufferer was to come from the philosophy of time and its use and from the right person to exemplify it was natural in the pragmatic atmosphere of the middle west and Mrs. Slagle brought the fruit of experience to our new center. She started us and, like all good workers, inspired others, so that, when she was needed for more and more training of new forces, she left with us the workers who carried on while she was drawn into that field of training and teaching and organizing, that did so much in the emergencies of that international madness called war and again for the needs arising from the madness and the immaturity and blunderings even in peace. As a contributor to the philosophy of time and life, as a cultivator of life and health in activity, Mrs. Slagle has become a guide, philosopher and friend of hundreds and hundreds, and as I said, the embodiment of example and principle. What she has added in the nearly twenty-five years since she came to help us is a proud record, a rare fulfillment of a life still growing and still progressing.

The demands of actual life and work where it is most needed have wrought a wonderful change in turning psychology from esoteric contemplation into the service of actual life. Real needs and real opportunities have led us into modern psychobiology and a science of human nature and behavior. And the basis of this modern psychobiology is not mere analysis and preaching of

license, but a study and cultivation of the person and action. This is how the old principle of engaging patients in activity has become the basic setting of all modern therapy. Pathology is no longer a kind of gloating over what can be found at autopsy. It is the study of the mistakes and maladjustments, the failures of man to use his best sense and opportunities. Mistakes become damage and damage becomes disease and disease in turn has to be brought back to where it is treated as "poor work" to be replaced by good and helpful work. This is the role of occupational therapy, not merely making a lot of stereotyped articles but releasing or implanting and fostering action with the reward and joy of achievement. I have heard Mrs. Slagle quote from a passage in the first paper I ever wrote on the treatment of nervous and mental disorders, addressed to the Chicago Pathological Society in February, 1893, nearly forty-five years ago, in which I asked my colleagues for the discussion of the kind of work which could be expected from and recommended to American ladies. I do not know why I picked on the ladies; I suppose because the doctors present were all men and I felt I knew them. I said: 'Experience alone can give suggestions in this line.' I called it mental hygiene, foreshadowing what I now mean by "mind," the person in action, good or bad, helpful and effective or mere restlessness, often overactive only as the result of fatigue and mismanagement.

I should like to be able to voice adequately what so many of my patients have gained through Mrs. Slagle and her pupils and what it all means not only for the sufferer but also for the healthy of our time. When the development of machinery supersedes the driving power of necessity in the development of habits and possibilities of work, we turn to the ingenuity of those who know the creative possibilities available not only for the sick but for the rank and file of those with "time on their hands."

From reveling in thoughts of eternity, we now have the great task to inject again the joys of activity of the day so that we may make a return of the pleasure of the day's work an efficient competitor with the mere pleasure and glamor of night life. We are grateful to Mrs. Slagle and her pupils and coworkers for their devotion and skill and creative zeal and achievements in the furtherance of the joy and rewards of work and creation.

It must be a great satisfaction to Mrs. Slagle to see the onward march of what had but slender beginnings. There is a need of leisure for the spreading of the wisdom that has come from the wide experience under difficult conditions. As wisdom grows there comes the demand for a spreading into wider usefulness. Today we have come into a period of prostitution of the capacity and love for work to the service of the something and the somebody else of mere wages. We have more and more cause to search for the natural inducements to work and the opportunities for new creative principles. We have to study work for its own rewards and to honor and cherish it and to cultivate it so as to make it deserve the honor and joy. Working under the difficulties met by the psychiatric occupational worker should and will give us much material for a usable knowledge of the relation of person and work, worker and work, and worker and leadership.

What is the work one can love and live with and live on? What are the conditions of work that are needed if the worker is to love the work and to live on and through it?

I shall never forget the deplorable words of a Secretary of Labor in a discussion of immigration. He told us we needed some immigration to get labor to do the dirty work which no American parent would want his children to do.

We occupational workers know that there is no work that cannot be shaped so as to find its worker able to get satisfaction from the doing and the result.

In these days in which continuity of purpose seems overshadowed by doctrines of change and where leadership in a democratic sense threatens to be belittled and to degenerate in other lands into highpower dictatorships, it is a matter of great joy and cheer to see respect and honor brought to a leader of unusual modesty and gentleness.

In the midst of talk and reality of change we see careers of continuity of progress, of action and creativeness in the ranks, and as part of the ranks.

We see those natural and inspiring instances in which a rare individual becomes a live and effective example of ideas and ideals as the living and active person, and persons expressive of ideals.

And we are glad to see those persons who become living symbols of great movements and realizations, in the midst of the younger and the budding generations, sharing with them the experience of a lifetime and the spirit of everbudding youth.

It is the pride of democracy to cherish its leaders as parts of the ranks, as influence by example, and as recipients of recognition and of fellowship in the rank and file.

We like to see it brought home that a lifetime of work and service and devotion and leadership in a cause also finds its recognition, and recognition and esteem its expression.

Appendix F

The Life-style Performance Profile

The Life-style Performance Profile presents a structure for organizing and identifying performance skills and deficits within the context of an individual's sociocultural norms and characteristic patterns of responding to and managing life tasks. It offers a focus for describing sociocultural and environmental factors that can be tapped as resources to support the development of skills. It helps to delineate external forces that interfere with learning and require intervention. Since impaired performance is related to neuropsychological factors and interpersonal components as well as sociocultural ones, the assessment process must include the evaluation of these components. Specific concerns addressed in the Life-style Performance frame of reference are:

This appendix was originally published in S.C. Robertson, (Ed), (1988). *FOCUS: Skills for assessment and treatment*, p. 3–38.

Skill and skill level, "appropriate" balance determined by: age, culture, and biology

Self-care and Maintenance	Self-needs/Intrinsic Gratification	Service to Others
Self-care: Washing Dressing Eating Toileting	Acknowledgment of own personal needs and interests	Role identity and responsibilities: Household and financial management Job market role Support/care of dependents Student role Family member role
	Interests manifested	
Self maintenance: Food preparation Shopping Money management Transportation Daily schedule—time Care of: Living area Personal belongings	Interests actually pursued Abilities and skills being used Skill deficits Intrinsic gratification values and attitudes	Role/job demands and pressures Skills required Existing skills Skill deficits
Self support	External resources/barriers: Family/social Culture Economics Environment	Appropriateness of role identity/responsibilities
Existing skills		Service values and attitudes
Skill deficits		External resources/barriers: Family/social Culture Economics Environment
Self care values and attitudes		
External resources/barriers: Family/social Culture Economics Environment		

Reciprocal Relationships

Patterns of relating
Friends
Peers
Family
Groups
Intimacy

Interpersonal
Values
Expectation of self/others
Roles and responsibilities

Skills required
Existing skills/assets
Skill deficits

External resources
Family
Culture
Economics
Environment

Appendix G

Position Paper: Occupational Therapy and the Americans With Disabilities Act (ADA)

The American Occupational Therapy Association (AOTA) applauds the Americans With Disabilities Act (ADA) (Public Law 101–336) as landmark legislation passed by Congress to promote the integration of individuals with disabilities into the mainstream of society. Since its inception, the profession of occupational therapy has worked to foster independence in individuals with disabilities through the teaching and modification of independent living skills, work behaviors and skills, and compensatory strategies to minimize the limiting effect physical or mental impairments may have on the life of an individual.

The ADA prevents discrimination against individuals with disabilities by extending to them the same civil rights protection guaranteed under the law to individuals on the basis of race, creed, sex, national origin, and religion. Furthermore, the ADA provides comprehensive civil rights protection for individuals with disabilities in the areas of employment, public accommodations, transportation, state and local government services, and telecommunications, and the power to enforce these rights. The AOTA supports these mandates and urges all occupational therapy practitioners to embrace opportunities to empower individuals with disabilities in the following five areas specified by the ADA.

1. Employment
2. Public accommodations
3. State and local government
4. Public transportation
5. Telecommunications

This appendix was previously published in the *American Journal of Occupational Therapy, 47*, 1082-1083. Copyright © 1993, American Occupational Therapy Association.

Employment

Historically, occupational therapy practitioners have played a significant role in assisting individuals with disabilities to enter into or return to the work force. Under the employment provisions of the ADA, the occupational therapy practitioner continues to maintain a significant role in this area. Occupational therapy practitioners' understanding of everyday functional abilities and the demands that work places on individuals with disabilities enables them to assist consumers, employers, human resource professionals, risk and safety managers, occupational health personnel, and supervisors in developing reasonable accommodations to allow a person with a physical or mental disability access to the work force.

Occupational therapy practitioners' training and expertise in the areas of job-site analysis, combined with their knowledge of work, human performance, and function, places them in a unique position to assist employers in implementing the ADA. The occupational therapist performs a job-site analysis to identify the essential and marginal functions of a job, and the job's environmental, cognitive, and psychological considerations. The job-site analysis provides a basis for the development of job descriptions written in specific functional terms. These job descriptions, based on the job-site analysis, become a working document that allows employers to provide accurate, job-specific information to job applicants and the human resources staff.

The occupational therapist may work as a consultant to teach human resources professionals how to use the functional job description as a tool during the interview process. Occupational therapy practitioners' education and understanding of sensorimotor, cognitive, psychosocial, and motor dysfunction, and how these affect the individual, place them in an excellent position to sensitize coworkers and supervisors to use proper disability etiquette to interact with, supervise, and work effectively with persons with disabilities. As consultants, occupational therapy practitioners may play a key role in dispelling the myths, misconceptions, stereotypes, and fears about disabilities found in the workplace.

To meet the new challenges presented to individuals with disabilities by the ADA's employment provisions, occupational therapists can work with employers to assess the occupational performance of individuals to determine their ability to perform the essential functions of a given job, with or without reasonable accommodations. Where accommodations are required to facilitate job performance, occupational therapists may recommend appropriate adaptive equipment, auxiliary aids, job restructuring, task adaptation, schedule changes, or work site or workstation modifications to enable these prospective or returning employees to perform the essential functions of their jobs.

Occupational therapy practitioners can play a key role in the employer's determination of whether an individual poses a direct threat to himself or herself or others in the workplace. Where a direct threat is found, occupational therapy practitioners can suggest reasonable accommodations to reduce the risk of harm. Employers, risk and safety managers, and human resources directors who wish to develop injury prevention programs that comply with the ADA will also benefit from the occupational therapist's consultation. This may include developing post-offer, job-related employee screenings and evaluations for high-risk injury positions.

Working in concert with individuals with disabilities, including work-related injuries, occupational therapy practitioners develop strategies to prepare the individual for employment. Through job-seeking skills training, clients are taught what to expect during the interview process, which reasonable accommodations to suggest and how to suggest them, and what their rights are during the application and interview process.

Public Accommodations

The occupational therapy practitioner facilitates compliance with the ADA's public accommodations provisions by working with architects, engineers, businesses, other professionals, and the consumer to determine the accessibility of places frequented by the general public and specified in the ADA, such as stores, theaters, health clubs, restaurants, hotels, office buildings, physicians' offices, and hospitals. Where inaccessible facilities, programs, goods, or services are identified, occupational therapy practitioners, on the basis of their knowledge of

the functional abilities of individuals with disabilities, suggest adaptive equipment, auxiliary aids, policy changes, alternative methods of service provision, and environmental adaptations to make the facilities, programs, goods, or services accessible and usable. By promoting compliance with the ADA, the occupational therapy practitioner expands the individual's access to public accommodations in the mainstream of independent living.

State and Local Government Services

In the area of state and local services, the occupational therapy practitioner can consult with program staff from local governments to assist in integrating individuals with disabilities into the various services provided by the government agencies. For example, if a county provides a summer day camp for children through its parks department, an occupational therapy practitioner can develop a program to allow children with disabilities an equal opportunity to participate in the same camp program. Occupational therapy practitioners can also assist local governments to acquire auxiliary aids or adaptations needed to make other programs and services accessible to individuals with disabilities. Occupational therapy practitioners can serve as a resource for government task forces and departments providing consultation for ADA compliance in the areas of employment, accessibility, and communication.

Public Transportation

The ADA requires public transportation systems to provide more access to individuals with disabilities on the basis of their knowledge of accessibility requirements, auxiliary aides, and functional mobility limitations of individuals, occupational therapy practitioners can assist public and private transportation system planners with providing access to buses, taxicabs, trains, airplanes, and subway systems. For example, occupational therapy practitioners can assist with making terminals accessible and suggesting that schedules be made available in alternative formats.

Telecommunications

The ADA's telecommunications provision requires the establishment of interstate and intrastate telecommunications relay services for individuals with hearing and speech impairments. Occupational therapy practitioners can assist telecommunications companies in assessing the need for information relay systems and can provide information about assistive device acquisition and training issues related to individuals with disabilities.

In summary, occupational therapy practitioners play a key role in educating the public as well as individuals with disabilities about their rights and responsibilities under the ADA. The occupational therapy practitioner's understanding of work and task analysis, knowledge of the functional limitations of disability, and experience with adaptive equipment provision and environmental adaptation places the practitioner in a unique position to serve as a resource in ADA-related matters. The AOTA supports the fundamental purposes of the ADA and encourages its members to assist the public in complying with its mandates to promote the entry of individuals with disabilities into the mainstream of independent living.

Reference

Americans With Disabilities Act of 1990 (Public Law 101-336), 42 U.S.C. § 12101.

Prepared by Barbara L. Kornblau, JD, OTR, DAAPM for The Commission on Practice (Jim Hinojosa, PhD, OTR, FAOTA, Chairperson).

Approved by the Representative Assembly June 1993.

This document was originally prepared as a White Paper (October 1991 to June 1993) for the American Occupational Therapy Association and was revised as a Position Paper for the Commission on Practice.

Appendix H

Position Paper: Physical Agent Modalities

The American Occupational Therapy Association, Inc. (AOTA), asserts that "physical agent modalities may be used by occupational therapy practitioners when used as an adjunct to or in preparation for purposeful activity to enhance occupational performance and when applied by a practitioner who has documented evidence of possessing the theoretical background and technical skills for safe and competent integration of the modality into an occupational therapy intervention plan" (AOTA, 1991a, p. 1075). The purpose of this paper is to clarify the parameters for the appropriate use of physical agent modalities in occupational therapy. Physical agent modalities are defined as those modalities that produce a response in soft tissue through the use of light, water, temperature, sound, or electricity. Physical agent modalities include, but are not limited to, paraffin baths, hot packs, cold packs, Fluidotherapy, contrast baths, ultrasound, whirlpool, and electrical stimulation units (e.g., functional electrical stimulation [FES]/neuromuscular electrical stimulation [NMES] devices, and transcutaneous electrical nerve stimulator [TENS]) (AOTA, 1991b).

Physical agent modalities can be categorized as "adjunctive methods" (Pedretti & Pasquinelli, 1990, pp. 3–4). An adjunctive method is one that is used in conjunction with or in preparation for patient involvement in purposeful activity. Adjunctive methods support and promote the acquisition of the performance components necessary to enable an individual to resume or assume the skills that are a part of his or her daily routine. As such, the exclusive use of physical agent

This appendix was previously published in the *American Journal of Occupational Therapy, 16*, 1090-1091.

modalities as a treatment method during a treatment session without application to a functional outcome is not considered occupational therapy. Physical agent modalities can be appropriately integrated into an occupational therapy program only when they are used to prepare the patient for better performance and prevention of disability through self-participation in work, self-care, and play and leisure activities (AOTA, 1979).

The safe selection, application, and adjustment of physical agent modalities, however, is not considered entry-level practice. The specialized learning necessary for proper use of these modalities typically requires appropriate postprofessional education, such as continuing education, in-service training, or graduate education. Documentation of the theoretical and technical education necessary for safe and appropriate use of any physical agent modalities should include, but not be limited to: course(s) in human anatomy; principles of chemistry and physics related to specific properties of light, water, temperature, sound, or electricity, as indicated by the selected modality; physiological, neurophysiological, and electrophysiological changes that occur as a result of the application of the selected modality; the response of normal and abnormal tissue to the application of the modality; indications and contraindications related to the selection and application of the modality; guidelines for treatment and administration of the modality; guidelines for preparation of the patient, including education about the process and possible outcomes of treatment (i.e., risks and benefits); and safety rules and precautions related to the selected modality. Education should also include methods for documenting the effectiveness of immediate and long-term effects of treatment and characteristics of the equipment, including safe operation, adjustment, indications of malfunction, and care. Supervised use of the physical agent modality should continue until service competency and professional judgment in selection, modification, and integration into an occupational therapy program are assured (AOTA, 1991b). As with all media, when a registered occupational therapist delegates the use of a physical agent modality to a certified occupational therapy assistant, both shall comply with appropriate supervision requirements and ensure that their use is based on service competency (AOTA, 1991c).

The Occupational Therapy Code of Ethics (AOTA, 1988) supports safe and competent practice in the profession and provides principles that can be applied to physical agent modality use. Principle 2 (Competence) states that "occupational therapy personnel shall actively maintain high standards of professional competence" (p. 795) and places expectations on practitioners to demonstrate competency by meeting competency-based standards. Principle 2B states that "the individual shall recognize the need for competence and shall participate in continuing professional development" (p. 795), which obliges practitioners to maintain competency by involvement in continuing education. In particular, therapists who choose to use physical agent modalities must stay abreast of current research findings regarding the efficacy of physical agent modality use. In addition, Principle 3A states that "the individual shall be acquainted with applicable local, state, federal, and institutional rules and Association policies and shall function accordingly" (p. 795) and requires practitioners to comply with all rules, regulations, and laws. All state laws and regulations related to physical agent modality use have precedence over AOTA policies and positions.

References

American Occupational Therapy Association. (1979). Policy 1.12. Occupation as the common core of occupational therapy. In *Policy manual of the American Occupational Therapy Association, Inc.* Rockville, MD: Author.

American Occupational Therapy Association. (1988). Occupational therapy code of ethics. *American Journal of Occupational Therapy, 42,* 795–796.

American Occupational Therapy Association. (1991a). Official: AOTA statement on physical agent modalities. *American Journal of Occupational Therapy, 45,* 1075.

American Occupational Therapy Association. (1991b). *Physical Agent Modality Task Force report.* Rockville, MD: Author.

American Occupational Therapy Association. (1991c). Registered occupational therapists and certified occupational therapy assistants and modalities [Policy 1.25]. *American Journal of Occupational Therapy, 45,* 1112–1113.

Pedretti, L. W., & Pasquinelli, S. (1990). A frame of reference for occupational therapy in physical dysfunction. In L. W. Pedretti & B. Zoltan (Eds.), *Occupational therapy practice skills for physical dysfunction* (3rd ed., pp. 1–17). St. Louis: Mosby.

Prepared by Mary Jo McGuire, MS, OTR, for the Commission on Practice (Jim Hinojosa, PhD, OTR, FAOTA, Chair).

Approved by the Representative Assembly March 1992.

Appendix I

Uniform Terminology for Occupational Therapy—Third Edition

This is an official document of The American Occupational Therapy Association. This document is intended to provide a generic outline of the domain of concern of occupational therapy and is designed to create common terminology for the profession and to capture the essence of occupational therapy succinctly for others.

It is recognized that the phenomena that constitute the profession's domain of concern can be categorized, and labeled, in a number of different ways. This document is not meant to limit those in the field, formulating theories or frames of reference, who may wish to combine or refine particular constructs. It is also not meant to limit those who would like to conceptualize the profession's domain of concern in a different manner.

Introduction

The first edition of Uniform Terminology was approved and published in 1979 (AOTA, 1979). In 1989, the *Uniform Terminology for Occupational Therapy—Second Edition* (AOTA, 1989) was approved and published. The second document presented an organized structure for understanding the areas of practice for the profession of occupational therapy. The document outlined two domains. PERFORMANCE AREAS (activities of daily living |ADL|, work and productive activities, and play or leisure) include activities that the occupational therapy practitioner[1] emphasizes when determining functional abilities. PERFORMANCE COMPONENTS (sensorimotor, cognitive, psychosocial, and psychological aspects) are the elements of performance that occupational ther-

[1] "Occupational therapy practitioner" refers to both registered occupational therapists and certified occupational therapy assistants.

apists assess and, when needed, in which they intervene for improved performance.

This third edition has been further expanded to reflect current practice and to incorporate contextual aspects of performance. *Performance Areas, Performance Components, and Performance Contexts* are the parameters of occupational therapy's domain of concern. *Performance areas* are broad categories of human activity that are typically part of daily life. They are activities of daily living, work and productive activities, and play or leisure activities. *Performance components* are fundamental human abilities that—to varying degrees and in differing combinations—are required for successful engagement in performance areas.

These components are sensorimotor, cognitive, and psychosocial and psychological. *Performance contexts* are situations or factors that influence an individual's engagement in desired and/or required performance areas. Performance contexts consist of *temporal* aspects (chronological, developmental, life cycle, and disability status); and *environmental* aspects (physical, social, and cultural). There is an interactive relationship among performance areas, performance components considered as they relate to participation in performance areas. Performance areas and performance contexts are taken into consideration when determining function and dysfunction relative to performance areas and performance components, and in planning intervention. For example, the occupational therapist does not evaluate strength (a Performance component) in isolation. Strength is considered as it affects necessary or desired tasks (performance areas). If the individual is interested in homemaking, the occupational therapy practitioner would consider the interaction of strength with homemaking tasks. Strengthening could be addressed through kitchen activities, such as cooking and putting groceries away. In some cases, the practitioner would employ an adaptive approach and recommend that the family switch from heavy stoneware to lighter-weight dishes, or use lighter-weight pots on the stove to enable the individual to make dinner safely without becoming fatigued or compromising safety.

Occupational therapy assessment involves examining performance areas, performance components, and performance contexts. Intervention may be directed toward elements of performance areas (e.g., dressing, vocational exploration), performance components (e.g., endurance, problem solving), or the environmental aspects of performance contexts. In the latter case, the physical and/or social environment may be altered or augmented to improve and/or maintain function. After identifying the performance areas the individual wishes or needs to address, the occupational therapist assesses the features of the environments in which the tasks will be performed. If an individual's job requires cooking in a restaurant as opposed to leisure cooking at home, the occupational therapy practitioner faces several challenges to enable the individual's success in different environments. Therefore, the third critical aspect of performance is the performance context, the features of the environment that affect the person's ability to engage in functional activities.

This document categorizes specific activities in each of the performance areas (ADL, work and productive activities, play or leisure). This categorization is based on what is considered "typical," and is not meant to imply that a particular individual characterizes personal activities in the same manner as someone else. Occupational therapy practitioners embrace individual differences, and so would document the unique pattern of the individual being served, rather than forcing the "typical" pattern on him or her and family. For example, because of experience or culture, a particular individual might think of home management as an ADL task rather than "work and productive activities" (current listing). Socialization might be considered part of a play or leisure activity instead of its current listing as part of "activities of daily living," because of life experience or cultural heritage.

Examples of Use in Practice

Uniform Terminology—Third Edition defines occupational therapy's domain of concern, which includes performance areas, performance components, and performance contexts. While this document may be used by occupational therapy practitioners in a number of different areas (e.g., practice, documentation, charge systems, education, program development, marketing, research, disability classifications, and regulations), it focuses on the use of uniform terminology in practice. This docu-

ment is not intended to define specific occupational therapy programs or specific occupational therapy interventions. Examples of how performance areas, performance components, and performance contexts translate into practice are provided below.

- An individual who is injured on the job may have the potential to return to work and productive activities, which is a performance area. In order to achieve the outcome of returning to work and productive activities, the individual may need to address specific performance components, such as strength, endurance, soft tissue integrity, time management, and the physical features of performance contexts, like structures and objects in his or her environment. The occupational therapy practitioner, in collaboration with the individual and other members of the vocational team, uses planned interventions to achieve the desired outcome. These interventions may include activities such as an exercise program, body mechanics instruction, and job site modifications, all of which may be provided in a work hardening program.

- An elderly individual recovering from a cerebral vascular accident may wish to live in a community setting, which combines the performance areas of ADL with work and productive activities. In order to achieve the outcome of community living, the individual may need to address specific performance components, such as muscle tone, gross motor coordination, postural control, and self-management. It is also necessary to consider the sociocultural and physical features of performance contexts, such as support available from other persons, and adaptations of structures and objects within the environment. The occupational therapy practitioner, in cooperation with the team, utilizes planned interventions to achieve the desired outcome. Interventions may include neuromuscular facilitation, practice of object manipulation, and instruction in the use of adaptive equipment and home safety equipment. The practitioner and individual also pursue the selection and training of a personal assistant to ensure the completion of ADL tasks. These interventions may be provided in a comprehensive inpatient rehabilitation unit.

- A child with learning disabilities is required to perform educational activities within a public school setting. Engaging in educational activities is considered the performance area of work and productive activities for this child. To achieve the educational outcome of efficient and effective completion of written classroom work, the child may need to address specific performance components. These include sensory processing, perceptual skills, postural control, motor skill, and the physical features of performance contexts, such as objects (e.g., desk, chair) in the environment. In cooperation with the team, occupational therapy interventions may include activities like adapting the student's seating in the classroom to improve postural control and stability, and practicing motor control and coordination. This program could be developed by an occupational therapist and supported by school district personnel.

- The parents of an infant with cerebral palsy may ask to facilitate the child's involvement in the performance areas of activities of daily living and play. Subsequent to assessment, the therapist identifies specific performance components, such as sensory awareness and neuromuscular control. The practitioner also addresses the physical and cultural features of performance contexts. In collaboration with the parents occupational therapy interventions may include activities such as seating and positioning for play, neuromuscular facilitation techniques to enable eating, facilitating parent skills in caring for and playing with their infant, and modifying the play space for accessibility. These interventions may be provided in a home-based occupational therapy program.

- An adult with schizophrenia may need and want to live independently in the community, which represents the performance areas of activities of daily living, work and productive activities, and leisure activities. The specific performance categories may be medication routine, functional mobility, home management, vocational exploration, play or leisure performance, and social interaction. In order to achieve the outcome of living independently, the individual may need to address specific performance components, such as topographical orientation; memory; categorization; problem solving; interests; social conduct; time management; and sociocultural features of performance contexts, such as social factors (e.g., influence of family and friends) and roles. The occupational thera-

py practitioner, in cooperation with the team, utilizes planned interventions to achieve the desired outcome. Interventions may include activities such as training in the use of public transportation, instruction in budgeting skills, selection and participation in social activities, instruction in social conduct, and participation in community reintegration activities. These interventions may be provided in a community-based mental health program.

- An individual with a history of substance abuse may need to reestablish family roles and responsibilities, which represent the performance areas of activities of daily living, work and productive activities, and leisure activities. In order to achieve the outcome of family participation, the individual may need to address the performance components of roles; values; social conduct; self-expression; coping skills; self-control; and the sociocultural features of performance contexts, such as custom, behavior, rules, and rituals. The occupational therapy practitioner, in cooperation with the team, utilizes planned interventions to achieve the desired outcomes. Interventions may include roles and values exercises, instruction in stress management techniques, identification of family roles and activities, and support to develop family leisure routines. These interventions may be provided in an inpatient acute care unit.

Person-Activity-Environment Fit

Person-activity-environment fit refers to the match among the skills and abilities of the individual; the demands of the activity; and the characteristics of the physical, social, and cultural environments. It is the interaction among the performance areas, performance components, and performance contexts that is important and determines the success of the performance. When occupational therapy practitioners provide services, they attend to all of these aspects of performance and the interaction among them. They also attend to each individual's unique personal history. The personal history includes one's skills and abilities (performance components), the past performance of specific life tasks (performance areas), and experience within particular environments (performance contexts). In addition to personal history, anticipated life tasks and role demands influence performance.

When considering the person-activity-environment fit, variables such as novelty, importance, motivation, activity tolerance, and quality are salient. Situations range from those that are completely familiar, to those that are novel and have never been experienced. Both the novelty and familiarity within a situation contribute to the overall task performance. In each situation, there is an optimal level of novelty that engages the individual sufficiently and provides enough information to perform the task. When too little novelty is present, the individual may miss cues and opportunities to perform. When too much novelty is present, the individual may become confused and distracted, inhibiting effective task performance.

Humans determine that some stimuli and situations are more meaningful than others. Individuals perform tasks they deem important. It is critical to identify what the individual wants or needs to do when planning interventions.

The level of motivation an individual demonstrates to perform a particular task is determined by both internal and external factors. An individual's biobehavioral state (e.g., amount of rest, arousal, tension) contributes to the potential to be responsive. The features of the social and physical environments (e.g., persons in the room, noise level) provide information that is either adequate or inadequate to produce a motivated state.

Activity tolerance is the individual's ability to sustain a purposeful activity over time. Individuals must not only select, initiate, and terminate activities, but they must also attend to a task for the needed length of time to complete the task and accomplish their goals.

The quality of performance is measured by standards generated by both the individual and others in the social and cultural environments in which the performance occurs. Quality is a continuum of expectations set within particular activities and contexts.

Uniform Terminology for Occupational Therapy—Third Edition

Occupational Therapy is the use of purposeful activity or interventions to promote health and achieve functional outcomes. *Achieving functional outcomes* means to develop, improve, or restore the highest possible level of independence of any individual who is limited by a physical injury or illness, a dysfunctional condition, a cognitive impairment, a psychosocial dysfunction, a mental illness, a developmental or learning disability, or an adverse environmental condition. Assessment means the use of skilled observation or evaluation by the administration and interpretation of standardized or nonstandardized tests and measurements to identify areas for occupational therapy services.

Occupational therapy services include, but are not limited to:

1. the assessment, treatment, and education of or consultation with the individual, family, or other persons; or

2. interventions directed toward developing, improving, or restoring daily living skills, work readiness or work performance, play skills, or leisure capacities, or enhancing educational performances skills; or

3. providing for the development, improvement, or restoration of sensorimotor, oral-motor, perceptual or neuromuscular functioning; or emotional, motivational, cognitive, or psychosocial components of performance.

These services may require assessment of the need for and use of interventions such as the design, development, adaptation, application, or training in the use of assistive technology devices; the design, fabrication, or application of rehabilitative technology such as selected orthotic devices; training in the use of assistive technology, orthotic or prosthetic devices; the application of physical agent modalities as an adjunct to or in preparation for purposeful activity; the use of ergonomic principles; the adaptation of environments and processes to enhance functional performance; or the promotion of health and wellness (AOTA, 1993, p 1117).

I. PERFORMANCE AREAS

Throughout this document, activities have been described as if individuals performed the tasks themselves. Occupational therapy also recognizes that individuals arrange for tasks to be done through others. The profession views independence as the ability to self-determine activity performance, regardless of who actually performs the activity.

A. *Activities of Daily Living*—Self-maintenance tasks.

1. *Grooming*—Obtaining and using supplies; removing body hair (use of razors, tweezers, lotions, etc.); applying and removing cosmetics; washing, drying, combing, styling, and brushing hair; caring for nails (hands and feet), caring for skin, ears, and eyes; and applying deodorant.

2. *Oral Hygiene*—Obtaining and using supplies; cleaning mouth; brushing and flossing teeth; or removing, cleaning, and reinserting dental orthotics and prosthetics.

3. *Bathing/Showering*—Obtaining and using supplies; soaping, rinsing, and drying body parts; maintaining bathing position; and transferring to and from bathing positions.

4. *Toilet Hygiene*—Obtaining and using supplies; clothing management; maintaining toileting position; transferring to and from toileting position; cleaning body; and caring for menstrual and continence needs (including catheters, colostomies, and suppository management).

5. *Personal Device Care*—Cleaning and maintaining personal care items, such as hearing aids, con-

tact lenses, glasses, orthotics, prosthetics, adaptive equipment, and contraceptive and sexual devices.

6. *Dressing*—Selecting clothing and accessories appropriate to time of day, weather, and occasion; obtaining clothing from storage area; dressing and undressing in a sequential fashion; fastening and adjusting clothing and shoes; and applying and removing personal devices, prostheses, or orthoses.

7. *Feeding and Eating*—Setting up food; selecting and using appropriate utensils and tableware; bringing food or drink to mouth; cleaning face, hands, and clothing; sucking, masticating, coughing, and swallowing; and management of alternative methods of nourishment.

8. *Medication Routine*—Obtaining medication, opening and closing containers, following prescribed schedules, taking correct quantities, reporting problems and adverse effects, and administering correct quantities using prescribed methods.

9. *Health Maintenance*—Developing and maintaining routines for illness prevention and wellness promotion, such as physical fitness, nutrition, and decreasing health risk behaviors.

10. *Socialization*—Accessing opportunities and interacting with other people in appropriate contextual and cultural ways to meet emotional and physical needs.

11. *Functional Communication*—Using equipment or systems to send and receive information, such as writing equipment, telephones, typewriters, computers, communication boards, call lights, emergency systems, Braille writers, telecommunication devices for the deaf, and augmentative communication systems.

12. *Functional Mobility*—Moving from one position or place to another, such as in-bed mobility, wheelchair mobility, transfers (wheelchair, bed, car, tub, toilet, tub/shower, chair, floor). Performing functional ambulation and transporting objects.

13. *Community Mobility*—Moving self in the community and using public or private transportation, such as driving, or accessing buses, taxi cabs, or other public transportation systems.

14. *Emergency Response*—Recognizing sudden, unexpected hazardous situations, and initiating action to reduce the threat to health and safety.

15. *Sexual Expression*—Engaging in desired sexual and intimate activities.

B. Work and Productive Activities—Purposeful activities for self-development, social contribution, and livelihood.

1. *Home Management*— Obtaining and maintaining personal and household possessions and environment.

   a. *Clothing Care*—Obtaining and using supplies; sorting, laundering (hand, machine, and dry clean); folding; ironing; storing; and mending.

   b. *Cleaning*—Obtaining and using supplies; picking up; putting away; vacuuming; sweeping and mopping floors; dusting; polishing; scrubbing; washing windows; cleaning mirrors; making beds; and removing trash and recyclables.

   c. *Meal Preparation and Cleanup*—Planning nutritious meals; preparing and serving food; opening and closing containers, cabinets and drawers; using kitchen utensils and appliances; cleaning up and storing food safely.

   d. *Shopping*—Preparing shopping lists (grocery and other); selecting and purchasing items; selecting method of payment; and completing money transactions.

   e. *Money Management*—Budgeting, paying bills, and using bank systems.

   f. *Household Maintenance*—Maintaining home, yard, garden, appliances, vehicles, and household items.

   g. *Safety Procedures*—Knowing and performing preventive and emergency procedures to maintain a safe environment and to prevent injuries.

2. *Care of Others*—Providing for children, spouse, parents, pets, or others, such as giving physical care, nurturing, communicating, and using age-appropriate activities.

3. *Educational Activities*—Participating in a learning environment through school, community, or work-sponsored activities, such as exploring educational interests, attending to instruction, managing assignments, and contributing to group experiences.

4. *Vocational Activities*—Participating in work-related activities.

   a. *Vocational Exploration*—Determining aptitudes; developing interests and skills, and selecting appropriate vocational pursuits.

   b. *Job Acquisition*—Identifying and selecting work opportunities, and completing application and interview processes.

   c. *Work or Job Performance*—Performing job tasks in a timely and effective manner; incorporating necessary work behaviors.

d. *Retirement Planning*—Determining aptitudes; developing interests and skills; and selecting appropriate avocational pursuits.

e. *Volunteer Participation*—Performing unpaid activities for the benefit of selected individuals, groups, or causes.

C. *Play or Leisure Activities*—Intrinsically motivating activities for amusement, relaxation, spontaneous enjoyment, or self-expression.

1. *Play or Leisure Exploration*—Identifying interests, skills, opportunities, and appropriate play or leisure activities.

2. *Play or Leisure Performance*—Planning and participating in play or leisure activities. Maintaining a balance of play or leisure activities with work and productive activities, and activities of daily living. Obtaining, utilizing, and maintaining equipment and supplies.

II. PERFORMANCE COMPONENTS

A. *Sensorimotor Component*—The ability to receive input, process information, and produce output.

1. *Sensory*

   a. *Sensory Awareness*—Receiving and differentiating sensory stimuli.

   b. *Sensory Processing*—Interpreting sensory stimuli.

      (1) *Tactile*—Interpreting light touch, pressure, temperature, pain, and vibration through skin contact/receptors.

      (2) *Proprioceptive*—Interpreting stimuli originating in muscles, joints, and other internal tissues that give information about the position of one body part in relation to another.

      (3) *Vestibular*—Interpreting stimuli from the inner ear receptors regarding head position and movement.

      (4) *Visual*—Interpreting stimuli through the eyes, including peripheral vision and acuity, and awareness of color and pattern.

      (5) *Auditory*—Interpreting and localizing sounds, and discriminating background sounds.

      (6) *Gustatory*—Interpreting tastes.

      (7) *Olfactory*—Interpreting odors.

   c. *Perceptual Processing*—Organizing sensory input into meaningful patterns.

      (1) *Stereognosis*—Identifying objects through proprioception, cognition, and the sense of touch.

      (2) *Kinesthesia*—Identifying the excursion and direction of joint movement.

      (3) *Pain Response*—Interpreting noxious stimuli.

      (4) *Body Scheme*—Acquiring an internal awareness of the body and the relationship of body parts to each other.

      (5) *Right-Left Discrimination*—Differentiating one side from the other.

      (6) *Form Constancy*—Recognizing forms and objects as the same in various environments, positions, and sizes.

      (7) *Position in Space*—Determining the spatial relationship of figures and objects to self or other forms and objects.

      (8) *Visual-Closure*—Identifying forms or objects from incomplete presentations.

      (9) *Figure Ground*—Differentiating between foreground and background forms and objects.

      (10) *Depth Perception*—Determining the relative distance between objects, figures, or landmarks and the observer, and changes in planes of surfaces.

      (11) *Spatial Relations*—Determining the position of objects relative to each other.

      (12) *Topographical Orientation*—Determining the location of objects and settings and the route to the location.

2. *Neuromusculoskeletal*

   a. *Reflex*—Eliciting an involuntary muscle response by sensory input.

   b. *Range of Motion*—Moving body parts through an arc.

   c. *Muscle Tone*—Demonstrating a degree of tension or resistance in a muscle at rest and in response to stretch.

   d. *Strength*—Demonstrating a degree of muscle power when movement is resisted, as with objects or gravity.

   e. *Endurance*—Sustaining cardiac, pulmonary, and musculoskeletal exertion over time.

   f. *Postural Control*—Using righting and equilibrium adjustments to maintain balance during functional movements.

   g. *Postural Alignment*—Maintaining biomechanical integrity among body parts.

   h. *Soft Tissue Integrity*—Maintaining anatomical and physiological condition of interstitial tissue and skin.

3. *Motor*

   a. *Gross Coordination*—Using large muscle groups for controlled, goal-directed movements.

b. *Crossing the Midline*—Moving limbs and eyes across the midsagittal plane of body.

c. *Laterality*—Using a preferred unilateral body part for activities requiring a high level of skill.

d. *Bilateral Integration*—Coordinating both body sides during activity.

e. *Motor Control*—Using the body in functional and versatile movement patterns.

f. *Praxis*—Conceiving and planning a new motor act in response to an environmental demand.

g. *Fine Coordination/Dexterity*—Using small muscle groups for controlled movements, particularly in object manipulation.

h. *Visual-Motor Integration*—Coordinating the interaction of information from the eyes with body movement during activity.

i. *Oral-Motor Control*—Coordinating oropharyngeal musculature for controlled movements.

B. *Cognitive Integration and Cognitive Components*—The ability to use higher brain functions.

1. *Level of Arousal*—Demonstrating alertness and responsiveness to environmental stimuli.

2. *Orientation*—Identifying person, place, time, and situation.

3. *Recognition*—Identifying familiar faces, objects, and other previously presented materials.

4. *Attention Span*—Focusing on a task over time.

5. *Initiation of Activity*—Starting a physical or mental activity.

6. *Termination of Activity*—Stopping an activity at an appropriate time.

7. *Memory*—Recalling information after brief or long periods of time.

8. *Sequencing*—Placing information, concepts, and actions in order.

9. *Categorization*—Identifying similarities of and differences among pieces of environmental information.

10. *Concept Formation*—Organizing a variety of information to form thoughts and ideas.

11. *Spatial Operations*—Mentally manipulating the position of objects in various relationships.

12. *Problem Solving*—Recognizing a problem, defining a problem, identifying alternative plans, selecting a plan, organizing steps in a plan, implementing a plan, and evaluating the outcome.

13. *Learning*—Acquiring new concepts and behaviors.

14. *Generalization*—Applying previously learned concepts and behaviors to a variety of new situations.

C. *Psychosocial Skills and Psychological Components*—The ability to interact in society and to process emotions.

1. *Psychological*

a. *Values*—Identifying ideas or beliefs that are important to self and others.

b. *Interests*—Identifying mental or physical activities that create pleasure and maintain attention.

c. *Self-Concept*—Developing the value of the physical, emotional, and sexual self.

2. *Social*

a. *Role Performance*—Identifying, maintaining, and balancing functions one assumes or acquires in society (e.g., worker, student, parent, friend, religious participant).

b. *Social Conduct*—Interacting by using manners, personal space, eye contact, gestures, active listening, and self-expression appropriate to one's environment.

c. *Interpersonal Skills*—Using verbal and non-verbal communication to interact in a variety of settings.

d. *Self-Expression*—Using a variety of styles and skills to express thoughts, feelings, and needs.

3. *Self-Management*

a. *Coping Skills*—Identifying and managing stress and related factors.

b. *Time Management*—Planning and participating in a balance of self-care, work, leisure, and rest activities to promote satisfaction and health.

c. *Self-Control*—Modifying one's own behavior in response to environmental needs, demands, constraints, personal aspirations, and feedback from others.

III. PERFORMANCE CONTEXTS

Assessment of function in performance areas is greatly influenced by the contexts in which the individual must perform. Occupational therapy practitioners consider performance contexts when determining feasibility and appropriateness of interventions. Occupational therapy practitioners may choose interventions based on an understanding of contexts, or may choose interventions directly aimed at altering the contexts to improve performance.

A. *Temporal Aspects*
1. *Chronological*—Individual's age.
2. *Developmental*—Stage or phase of maturation.
3. *Life Cycle*—Place in important life phases, such as career cycle, parenting cycle, or educational process.
4. *Disability Status*—Place in continuum of disability, such as acuteness of injury, chronicity of disability, or terminal nature of illness.
B. *Environment*
1. *Physical*—Nonhuman aspects of contexts. Includes the accessibility to and performance within environments having natural terrain, plants, animals, buildings, furniture, objects, tools, or devices.
2. *Social*—Availability and expectations of significant individuals, such as spouse, friends, and caregivers. Also includes larger social groups which are influential in establishing norms, role expectations, and social routines.
3. *Cultural*—Customs, beliefs, activity patterns, behavior standards, and expectations accepted by the society of which the individual is a member. Includes political aspects, such as laws that affect access to resources and affirm personal rights. Also includes opportunities for education, employment, and economic support.

References

American Occupational Therapy Association. (1979). Occupational therapy product output reporting system and uniform terminology for reporting occupational therapy services. Rockville, MD: Author.

American Occupational Therapy Association. (1989). Uniform terminology for occupational therapy—Second edition. *American Journal of Occupational Therapy, 43*, 808–815.

American Occupational Therapy Association. (1993). Definition of occupational therapy practice for state regulation (Policy 5.3.1). *American Journal of Occupational Therapy, 47*, 1117-1121.

Authors

The Terminology Task Force:
Winifred Dunn, PhD, OTR, FAOTA, Chairperson
Mary Foto, OTR, FAOTA,
Jim Hinojosa, PhD, OTR, FAOTA
Barbara Schell, PhD, OTR/L, FAOTA
Linda Kohlman Thomson, MOT, OTR, FAOTA
Sarah D. Hertfelder, MEd, MOT, OTR/L, Staff Liaison
for
The Commission on Practice
Jim Hinojosa, PhD, OTR, FAOTA, Chairperson
Adopted by the Representative Assembly 7/94

NOTE: This document replaces the following documents, all of which were rescinded by the 1994 Representative Assembly:
Occupational Therapy Product Output Reporting System (1979)
Uniform Terminology for Reporting Occupational Therapy Services—First Edition (1979)
Uniform Occupational Therapy Evaluation Checklist (1981)
Uniform Terminology for Occupational Therapy—Second Edition (1989)

Uniform Terminology, Third Edition: Application To Practice

Introduction

This document was developed to help occupational therapists apply *Uniform Terminology—Third Edition* to practice. The original grid format (Dunn, 1988) enabled occupational therapy practitioners to systematically identify deficit and strength areas of an individual and to select appropriate activities to address these areas in occupational therapy intervention (Dunn & McGourty, 1990). For the third edition, the profession is highlighting "Contexts" as another critical aspect of performance. A second grid provides therapy practitioners with a mechanism to consider the contextual features of performance in activities of daily living (ADL), work and productive activity, and play/leisure. "Performance Areas" and "Performance Components" (Figure A) focus on the individual. These features are imbedded in the "Performance Contexts" (Figure B).

On the original grid (Dunn, 1988), the horizontal axis contains the Performance Areas of Activities of Daily Living, Work and Productive Activities, and Play or Leisure Activities (see Figure A). These Performance Areas are the functional outcomes occupational therapy addresses. The vertical axis contains the Performance Components, including Sensorimotor Components, Cognitive Components, and Psychosocial Components. The Performance Components are the skills and abilities that an individual uses to engage in the Performance Areas. During an occupational therapy assessment the occupational therapy practitioner determines an individual's abilities and limitations in the Performance Components and how they affect the individual's functional outcomes in the Performance Areas.

The grid in Figure B can be used to analyze the contexts of performance for a particular individual. For example, when working with a toddler with a developmental disability who needs to learn to eat, the occupational therapy practitioner would consider all the Performance Contexts features as they might impact on this toddler's ability to master eating. Unlike the grid in Figure A, in which the occupational therapy practitioner selects *both* Performance Areas (i.e., what the individual wants or needs to do) and the Performance Component (i.e., a person's strengths and needs), in this grid (Figure B) the occupational therapy practitioner only selects the Performance Area. After the Performance Area is identified through collaboration with the individual and significant others, the occupational therapy practitioner considers ALL Performance Contexts features as they might impact on performance of the selected task.

Intervention Planning

Intervention planning occurs both within the general domain of concern of occupational therapy (i.e., uniform terminology) and by considering the profession's theoretical frames of reference that offer insights about how

---

to approach the problem. In Figure A, the occupational therapy practitioner considers the Performance Areas that are of interest to the individual and the individual's strengths and concerns within the Performance Components. The intervention strategies would emerge from the cells on the grid that are placed at the intersection of the Performance Areas and the targeted Performance Components (strength and/or concern). For example, if a child needed to improve sensory processing and fine coordination for oral hygiene and grooming, an occupational therapy practitioner might select a sensory integrative frame of reference to create intervention strategies, such as adding textures to handles and teaching the child sand and bean digging games. Dunn and McGourty (1989) discuss this in more detail.

When using Figure B, the occupational therapy practitioner considers the Performance Contexts features in relation to the desired Performance Area. The occupational therapy practitioner would analyze the individual's temporal, physical, social, and cultural contexts to determine the relevance of particular interventions. For example, if the child mentioned above was a member of a family in which having messy hands from sand play was unacceptable, the occupational therapy practitioner would consider alternate strategies that are more compatible with their lifestyle. For example, perhaps the family would be more interested in developing puppet play. This would still provide the child with opportunities to experience the textures of various puppets and the hand movements required to manipulate the puppets in play context, without adding the messiness of sand. When occupational therapy practitioners consider contexts, interventions become more relevant and applicable to individuals' lives.

Case Example 1

Sophie is a 75-year-old lady, who was widowed three years ago, is recovering from a cerebral vascular accident and has been transferred from an acute care unit to an inpatient medical rehabilitation unit. Prior to her admission, she was living in a small house in an isolated location and has no family living nearby. She was driving independently and frequently ran errands for her friends. She is adamant in her goal to return to her home after discharge. All of her friends are quite elderly and are not able to provide many resources for support.

Sophie and the team collaborated to identify her goals. Sophie decided that she wanted to be able to meet her daily needs with little or no assistance. Almost all of the Performance Areas are critical in order to achieve the outcome of community living in her own home. Being able to cook all of her meals, bathe independently, and

have alternative transportation available is necessary. Because of their significant impact on the patient's function in the Performance Areas, some of the Performance Components that may need to be addressed are figure ground, muscle tone, postural control, fine coordination, memory, and self-management.

In the selection of occupation therapy interventions, it is critical to analyze the elements of Performance Contexts for the individual. The physical and social elements of her home environment do not support returning home without modifications to her home and additional social supports being established. Railings must be added to the front steps, provision of and instruction in the use of a tub seat, and instruction in the use of specialized transportation may need to occur. If this same individual had been living in an apartment in a retirement community prior to her CVA, the contexts of performance would support a return home with fewer environmental modifications being needed. Being independent in cooking might not be necessary due to meals being provided, and the bathroom might already be accessible and safe. If the individual had friends and family available, the social support network might already be established to assist with shopping and transportation needs. The occupational therapy interventions would be different due to the contexts in which the individual will be performing. Interventions must be selected with the impact of the Performance contexts as an essential element.

Case Example 2

Malcolm is a 9-year-old boy who has a learning disability which causes him to have a variety of problems in the school. His teachers complain that he is difficult to manage in the classroom. Some of the Performance Components that may need to be addressed are his self control such as interrupting, difficulty sitting during instruction, and difficulty with peer relations. Other children avoid him on the playground, because he doesn't follow rules, doesn't play fair, and tends to anger quickly when confronted. The performance component impairment with concept formation is reflected in his sloppy and disorganized classroom assignments.

The critical elements of the Performance Contexts are the temporal aspect of age-appropriateness of his behavior and the social environmental aspect of his immature socialization. The significant cultural and temporal aspects of his family are that they place a high premium on athletic prowess.

The occupational therapy practitioner intervenes in several ways to address his behavior in the school environment. The occupational therapy practitioner focuses on structuring the classroom environment and facilitating consistent behavioral expectations for Malcolm by educational personnel. She also consults with the teachers to develop ways to structure activities which will support his ability to relate to other children in a positive way.

In contrast, another child with similar learning disabilities, but who is 12 years old and in the 7th grade might have different concerns. Elements of the Performance Contexts are the temporal aspect of the age-appropriateness of his behavior; and the social environmental context of school where "bullying" behavior is unacceptable and in which completing assignments is expected. In addressing the cultural Performance Contexts the occupational therapy practitioner recognizes from meeting with parents that they have only average expectation for academic performance but value athletic accomplishments.

Since teachers at his school consider completion of home assignments to be part of average performance, the occupational therapy practitioner works with the child and parents on time management and reinforcement strategies to meet this expectation. After consultation with the coach, she works with the father to create activities to improve his athletic abilities. When occupational therapy practitioners consider family values as part of the contexts of performance, different intervention priorities may emerge.

Authors

The Terminology Task Force:
Winnie Dunn, PhD, OTR, FAOTA, - Chairperson
Mary Foto, OTR, FAOTA
Jim Hinojosa, PhD, OTR, FAOTA
Barbara A. Boyt Schell, PhD, OTR, FAOTA
Linda Kohlman Thomson, MOT, OTR, OT(C), FAOTA
Sarah D. Hertfelder, MEd, MOT, OTR - Staff Liaison
     for
The Commission on Practice - 1994
Jim Hinojosa, PhD, OTR, FAOTA, Chairperson

This document replaces the 1989 *Application of Uniform Terminology to Practice* that accompanied the *Uniform Terminology for Occupational Therapy—Second Edition.*

I. PERFORMANCE AREAS	II. PERFORMANCE COMPONENTS	III. PERFORMANCE CONTEXTS

A. Activities of Daily Living
  1. Grooming
  2. Oral Hygiene
  3. Bathing/Showering
  4. Toilet Hygiene
  5. Personal Device Care
  6. Dressing
  7. Feeding and Eating
  8. Medication Routine
  9. Health Maintenance
  10. Socialization
  11. Functional Communication
  12. Functional Mobility
  13. Community Mobility
  14. Emergency Response
  15. Sexual Expression
 	
B. Work and Productive Activities
  1. Home Management
    a. Clothing Care
    b. Cleaning
    c. Meal Preparation/Cleanup
    d. Shopping
    e. Money Management
    f. Household Maintenance
    g. Safety Procedures
  2. Care of Others
  3. Educational Activities
  4. Vocational Activities
    a. Vocational Exploration
    b. Job Acquisition
    c. Work or job Performance
    d. Retirement Planning
    e. Volunteer Participation
 	
C. Play or Leisure Activities
  1. Play or Leisure Exploration
  2. Play or Leisure Performance
	A. Sensorimotor Component
	  1. Sensory
	    a. Sensory Awareness
	    b. Sensory Processing
	    (1) Tactile
	    (2) Proprioceptive
	    (3) Vestibular
	    (4) Visual
	    (5) Auditory
	    (6) Gustatory
	    (7) Olfactory
	    c. Perceptual Processing
	    (1) Stereognosis
	    (2) Kinesthesia
	    (3) Pain Response
	    (4) Body Scheme
	    (5) Right-Left Discrimination
	    (6) Form Constancy
	    (7) Position in Space
	    (8) Visual-Closure
	    (9) Figure Ground
	    (10) Depth Perception
	    (11) Spatial Relations
	    (12) Topographical Orientation
	  2. Neuromusculoskeletal
	    a. Reflex
	    b. Range of Motion
	    c. Muscle Tone
	    d. Strength
	    e. Endurance
	    f. Postural Control
	    g. Postural Alignment
	    h. Soft Tissue Integrity
	  3. Motor
	    a. Gross Coordination
	    b. Crossing the Midline
	    c. Laterality
	    d. Bilateral Integration
	    e. Motor Control
	    f. Praxis
	    g. Fine Coordination/Dexterity
	    h. Visual-Motor Integration
	    i. Oral-Motor Control
	
	B. Cognitive Integration and Cognitive Components
	  1. Level of Arousal
	  2. Orientation
	  3. Recognition
	  4. Attention Span
	  5. Initiation of Activity
	  6. Termination of Activity
	  7. Memory
	  8. Sequencing
	  9. Categorization
	  10. Concept Formation
	  11. Spatial Operations
	  12. Problem Solving
	  13. Learning
	  14. Generalization
	
	C. Psychosocial Skills and Psychological Components
	  1. Psychological
	    a. Values
	    b. Interests
	    c. Self-concept
	  2. Social
	    a. Role Performance
	    b. Social Conduct
	    c. Interpersonal Skills
	    d. Self-Expression
	  3. Self-Management
	    a. Coping Skills
	    b. Time Management
	    c. Self-Control
		A. Temporal Aspects
		  1. Chronological
		  2. Developmental
		  3. Life Cycle
		  4. Disability Status
		
		B. Environment Aspects
		  1. Physical
		  2. Social

Figure A. Uniform Terminology Grid (Perfomance Areas and Performance Components)

PERFORMANCE AREAS

Column headers (left to right):
Activities of Daily Living · Grooming · Oral Hygiene · Bathing/Showering · Toilet Hygiene · Personal Device Care · Dressing · Feeding and Eating · Medication Routine · Health Maintenance · Socialization · Functional Communication · Functional Mobility · Community Mobility · Emergency Response · Sexual Expression · Work and Productive Activities · Home Management · Care of Others · Educational Activities · Vocational Activities · Play or Leisure Activities · Play/Leisure Exploration · Play/Leisure Performance

PERFORMANCE COMPONENTS

A. Sensorimotor Component

Sensory
- Sensory Awareness
- Sensory Processing
  - (1) Tactile
  - (2) Proprioceptive
  - (3) Vestibular
  - (4) Visual
  - (5) Auditory
  - (6) Gustatory
  - (7) Olfactory
- Perceptual Processing
  - (1) Stereognosis
  - (2) Kinesthesia
  - (3) Pain Response
  - (4) Body Scheme
  - (5) Right-Left Discrimination
  - (6) Form Constancy
  - (7) Position in Space
  - (8) Visual-Closure
  - (9) Figure Ground
  - (10) Depth Perception
  - (11) Spatial Relations
  - (12) Topographical Orientation

Neuromusculoskeletal
- Reflex
- Range of Motion
- Muscle Tone
- Strength
- Endurance
- Postural Control
- Postural Alignment
- Soft Tissue Integrity

Motor
- Gross Coordination
- Crossing the Midline
- Laterality
- Bilateral Integration
- Motor Control
- Praxis
- Fine Coordination/Dexterity
- Visual-Motor Integration
- Oral-Motor Control

	PERFORMANCE AREAS																								
PERFORMANCE COMPONENTS	Activities of Daily Living	Grooming	Oral Hygiene	Bathing/Showering	Toilet Hygiene	Personal Device Care	Dressing	Feeding and Eating	Medication Routine	Health Maintenance	Socialization	Functional Communication	Functional Mobility	Community Mobility	Emergency Response	Sexual Expression	Work and Productive Activities	Home Management	Care of Others	Educational Activities	Vocational Activities	Play or Leisure Activities	Play/Leisure Exploration	Play/Leisure Performance
B. Cognitive Integration and Cognitive Components																								
1. Level of Arousal																								
2. Orientation																								
3. Recognition																								
4. Attention Span																								
5. Initiation of Activity																								
6. Termination of Activity																								
7. Memory																								
8. Sequencing																								
9. Categorization																								
10. Concept Formation																								
11. Spatial Operations																								
12. Problem Solving																								
13. Learning																								
14. Generalization																								
C. Psychosocial Skills and Psychological Components																								
1. Psychological																								
a. Values																								
b. Interests																								
c. Self-Concept																								
2. Social																								
a. Role Performance																								
b. Social Conduct																								
c. Interpersonal Skills																								
d. Self-Expression																								
3. Self-Management																								
a. Coping Skills																								
b. Time Management																								
c. Self-Control																								

Figure B. Uniform Terminology Grid (Perfomance Areas and Performance Contexts)

PERFORMANCE AREAS

PERFORMANCE CONTEXTS

A. Temporal Aspects

Chronological
Developmental
Life Cycle
Disability Status

B. Environment

Physical
Social
Cultural

Performance Areas columns:
Activities of Daily Living, Grooming, Oral Hygiene, Bathing/Showering, Toilet Hygiene, Personal Device Care, Dressing, Feeding and Eating, Medication Routine, Health Maintenance, Socialization, Functional Communication, Functional Mobility, Community Mobility, Emergency Response, Sexual Expression, Work and Productive Activities, Home Management, Care of Others, Educational Activities, Vocational Activities, Play or Leisure Activities, Play/Leisure Exploration, Play/Leisure Performance

Appendix J

Activity Analysis Form: Based on Uniform Terminology for Occupational Therapy – Third Edition (American Occupational Therapy Association, 1994)

Be certain to refer to this publication for definitions of all terms and guidelines for application of Uniform Terminology to practice.

I. ACTIVITY DESCRIPTION

Directions: Fill in the blank spaces with information about your selected activity. Be clear and specific.

A.   Activity: _____

B.   Description of activity as *normally* performed. Briefly describe your selected activity and then identify the sequential steps and time required to successfully complete this activity.

C.   Considerations for activity use in treatment. Describe any special issues one would need to consider if this activity was used in a clinical setting. Be certain to address safety precautions and possible contraindications for activity performance. Specify the equipment, materials, and space needed to perform the activity. Identify the cost of the activity's equipment and materials and the cost of therapist's time for activity preparation, supervision, and cleanup.

II. PERFORMANCE AREAS

Directions: Identify the relevance of your selected activity to each occupational performance area listed. Your selected activity may be an inherent and required component of an occupational performance area or it may enhance a performance area (for example: brushing one's teeth is an inherent part of oral hygiene and it can enhance socialization). In addition, skill in an occupational performance area may be needed as a precursor for performance of your selected activity or your activity may require subsequent engagement in a performance area (for example: diapering a baby requires one to first budget money to purchase the diapers and then the subsequent activities of safely disposing of the diaper and washing one's hands). Provide a clear rationale as to how and why your activity relates or does not relate to each of the performance areas.

A.   Activities of Daily Living

   1.   Grooming

   2.   Oral Hygiene

   3.   Bathing/Showering

   4.   Toilet Hygiene

   5.   Personal Device Care

6. Dressing

7. Feeding and Eating

8. Medication Routine

9. Health Maintenance

10. Socialization

11. Functional Communication

12. Functional Mobility

13. Community Mobility

14. Emergency Response

15. Sexual Expression

B. Work and Productive Activities

1. Home Management

a. Clothing Care

b. Cleaning

c. Meal Preparation/Cleanup

d. Shopping

e. Money Management

f. Household Maintenance

g. Safety Procedures

2. Care of Others

3. Educational Activities

4. Vocational Activities
a. Vocational Exploration

b. Job Acquisition

c. Work or Job Performance

d. Retirement Planning

e. Volunteer Participation

C. Play or Leisure Activities

1. Play or Leisure Exploration

2. Play or Leisure Performance

III. PERFORMANCE COMPONENTS

Directions: Indicate the performance components required to complete your selected activity. Explain how this performance component is used during this activity. If a performance component is not required to do the activity, write N/A beside it and explain why this performance component is not required to do this activity.

A. Sensorimotor Component

1. Sensory

a. Sensory Awareness

b. Sensory Processing

(1) Tactile

(2) Proprioceptive

(3) Vestibular

(4) Visual

(5) Auditory

(6) Gustatory

(7) Olfactory

c. Perceptual Processing

(1) Stereognosis

(2) Kinesthesia

(3) Pain Response

(4) Body Scheme

(5) Right-Left Discrimination

(6) Form Constancy

(7) Position in Space

(8) Visual-Closure

(9) Figure Ground

(10) Depth Perception

(11) Spatial Relations

(12) Topographical Orientation

2. Neuromusculoskeletal

   a. Reflex

   b. Range of Motion

   c. Muscle Tone

   d. Strength

   e. Endurance

   f. Postural Control

   g. Postural Alignment

   h. Soft Tissue Integrity

3. Motor

   a. Gross Coordination

   b. Crossing the Midline

   c. Laterality

   d. Bilateral Integration

   e. Motor Control

   f. Praxis

   g. Fine Coordination/Dexterity

   h. Visual-Motor Integration

   i. Oral-Motor Control

B. Cognitive Integration and Cognitive Components

  1. Level of Arousal

2. Orientation

3. Recognition

4. Attention Span

5. Initiation of Activity

6. Termination of Activity

7. Memory

8. Sequencing

9. Categorization

10. Concept Formation

11. Spatial Operations

12. Problem Solving

13. Learning

14. Generalization

C. Psychosocial Skills and Psychological Components

  1. Psychological

    a. Values

    b. Interests

    c. Self-Concept

  2. Social

    a. Role Performance

    b. Social Conduct

    c. Interpersonal Skills

    d. Self-Expression

  3. Self-Management

    a. Coping Skills

    b. Time Management

    c. Self-Control

IV. PERFORMANCE CONTEXTS

Directions: Indicate and describe the temporal and environmental relevance and requirements of your selected activity.

A. Temporal Aspects

1. Chronological

2. Developmental

3. Life Cycle

4. Disability Status

B. Environment

1. Physical

2. Social

3. Cultural

V. ACTIVITY ADAPTATION, GRADATION, AND SYNTHESIS

Directions: Describe how your selected activity can be adapted and graded to be used in OT intervention. Interventions may be directed towards components of the performance areas (e.g. money management, retirement planning), the performance components (e.g. dexterity, social role performance) or the environmental aspects of performance contexts (e.g. modifying or structuring the environment to improve or maintain function). Be certain your adaptations and gradations address both psychosocial and physical aspects of performance.

A. Activity Adaptations: Identify elements of the activity that can be changed or altered so that a client can perform the activity.

B. Activity Gradation: Identify elements of the activity that can be graded and the degree of gradability possible.

C. Activity Synthesis: Describe and explain how your activity can be designed to meet the following goals of intervention for a client and/or patient population. For background information on these 5 types of intervention, please refer to Mosey, A. C. (1986). *Psychosocial Components of Occupational Therapy*, (pp. 335–358). New York: Raven Press.

1. For the purpose of meeting health needs.

2. For the purpose of prevention.

3. For the purpose of maintenance.

4. For the purpose of management.

5. For the purpose of change.

Appendix K

Activity Analysis Sample

1. ACTIVITY DESCRIPTION

Directions: Fill in the blank spaces with information about your selected activity. Be clear and specific.

A. Activity: Jumping Rope

B. Description of activity as *normally* performed. Briefly describe your selected activity and then identify the sequential steps and time required to successfully complete this activity.

—Hold jump rope by handles (one in each hand). Arms parallel to side, using wrist rotation swing the rope over head and towards the front. Jump over rope when rope reaches floor. Repeat.

Sequence of major steps, time required for each step-

   1-Obtain rope 1–2 min.
   2-Clear space 1 min.
   3-Get in position. Stand straight, arms at side with handle in each hand and rope is to back, resting on achilles tendon. 10 sec.
   4-Swing rope above head by moving arms backwards and rotating wrist. As rope approaches front, jump off the floor with both feet so that rope may pass underneath feet. 5 sec.
   5-Continue rotating rope so that rope arcs overhead and underneath feet in a continuous motion until fatigued (depends on the physical condition of the individual and on their interest level) 1–10 min or more.

C. Conditions for activity use in therapy. Describe any special issues one would need to consider if this activity was used in a clinical setting. Be certain to address safety precautions and possible contraindications for activity performance. Specify the equipment, materials, and space needed to perform the activity. Identify the cost of the activity's equipment and materials and the cost of therapist's time for activity preparation, supervision, and cleanup.

Precautions—It is important to allow room to prevent a passerby from getting hit with rope. Also, comfortable, non-binding clothing should be worn as well as supportive flat-heeled footwear such as sneakers. It is not advisable to wear loose chains or jewelry as these may "catch" on the rope.

Contraindications—Caution must be considered when providing this activity for a suicidal person; rope can be used to hang him or herself. This is not an appropriate activity for people with bad knees, bad backs or wrist fractures. Jumping rope may aggravate the condition. Individuals who do not have basic equilibrium, sensorimotor and cognitive skills may not be able to safely complete this task.

Equipment needed and cost:

1-jump rope, $2.00–$12.00, prices vary depending on the quality of the jump rope.

²-Cost in therapist time: No additional time needed for preparation and cleanup. Time for supervision of activity is equal to duration of activity (see IB above). If jumping rope is used as a group activity, time will be needed to gather group and instruct members on group goals. If therapist needs to teach activity, 5–30 minutes will be needed depending upon client's learning abilities and gross motor skills.

II. PERFORMANCE AREAS

Directions: Identify the relevance of your selected activity to each occupational performance area listed. Your selected activity may be an inherent and required component of an occupational performance area or it may enhance a performance area (for example: brushing one's teeth is an inherent part of oral hygiene and it can enhance socialization). In addition, skill in an occupational performance area may be needed as a precursor for performance of your selected activity or your activity may require subsequent engagement in a performance area (for example: diapering a baby requires one to first budget money to purchase the diapers and then the subsequent activities of safely disposing the diaper and washing one's hands). Provide a clear rationale as to how and why your activity relates or does not relate to each of the performance areas.

A. Activities of Daily Living

1. Grooming—This is not important for jumping rope alone, but could influence the interactions of others. The decision to participate in group jumping or instruction can be affected by how attractive an individual feels or how attractive others appear. Also, if a person jumps rope vigorously, they may need to groom themselves prior to engaging in other activities.
2. Oral Hygiene—Generally, not applicable, may be a factor if in a group, as noted above.
3. Bathing/Showering—After jumping rope vigorously, an individual may want to bathe or shower prior to engaging in other activities.
4. Toilet Hygiene—Not applicable (N/A). However, a person may toilet as a precursor to jumping rope to increase their comfort level.
5. Personal Device Care—A person who wears eye glasses may want to remove them or attach a safety band to the glasses prior to jumping rope.

6. Dressing—Appropriate dressing skills are needed. Person needs to know which clothing is best suited to wear for exercise. For example: sneakers, loose fitting or stretching clothing.
7. Feeding and Eating—Proper nourishment can influence the level of stamina required to jump rope. Jumping rope may increase one's thirst and/or appetite.
8. Medication Routine—If a person is on medication, they will need to be aware of potential side effects their medication may have on their ability to exercise. Some side effects of medications (eg: dizziness, postural hypotension, akathesia, tremors, etc.) may contraindicate jumping rope. Safety and ability to maintain balance are potential concerns.
9. Health Maintenance—Jumping rope is definitely related to the maintenance of health as it is an exercise which can develop and maintain physical fitness.
10. Socialization—Not applicable if jumping rope alone. May be needed if jumping rope in a group situation (ie: playground, gym)
11. Functional Communication—Not applicable, unless a person uses a voicebox for oral communications with others.
12. Functional Mobility—Functional ambulation is a precursor to the ability to jump.
13. Community Mobility—Jumping rope can be done in one's home environment. If a person wants to travel to a gym or playground in their community, they will need community mobility skills.
14. Emergency Response—Required if and when a person loses his or her balance, experiences angina or has an asthma attack due to exercise.
15. Sexual Expression—Not directly applicable. Feeling fit may contribute to one's sexual identity.

B. Work and Productive Activities

1. Home Management
   a. Clothing Care—Not directly applicable. One may need to launder sweaty clothes after jumping rope vigorously or mend clothes damaged in a fall.
   b. Cleaning—N/A.
   c. Meal Preparation/Cleanup—Not directly applicable. One may want to prepare food if jumping rope facilitated an increased appetite.
   d. Shopping—A person may need to shop for a jump rope and/or exercise clothing if these items are not available to them.

e. Money Management—N/A.

f. Household Maintenance—A person would need to maintain outside of home for a clear jumping space (eg: cut lawn, sweep driveway).

g. Safety Procedures—A person jumping rope will need to recognize potential hazards, such as, wet or uneven surface. If a person falls when jumping rope, he or she will need to know how to take care of any incurred injury (ie: cuts, sprains).

2. Care of Others—Not directly applicable. However, a parent or caregiver can teach a child to jump rope and engage in this activity together.

3. Educational Activities—N/A.

4. Vocational Activities (Generally not applicable. This activity may influence vocational activities if work interests or pursuits were in the fields of fitness or child care [ie: working or volunteering at the YMCA or community center])—

a. Vocational Exploration

b. Job Acquisition

c. Work or Job Performance

d. Retirement Planning

e. Volunteer Participation

C. Play or Leisure Activities

1. Play or Leisure Exploration—Jumping rope can help someone explore their interests in physical activities. It can help develop fitness skills and create a number of opportunities to engage in an enjoyable leisure activity.

2. Play or Leisure Performance—Once a jump rope is obtained, it can be used often to maintain a balance of leisure with in one's life. Jumping rope requires a moderate amount of space and only one piece of very portable equipment, therefore, preparation and planning time is minimal.

III. PERFORMANCE COMPONENTS

Directions: Indicate the performance components required to complete your selected activity. Explain how this performance component is used during this activity. If a performance component is not required to do the activity, write N/A beside it and explain why this

performance component is not required to do this activity.

A. Sensorimotor Component

1. Sensory

a. Sensory Awareness—The ability to receive and differentiate many senses, as noted below, is required to jump rope.

b. Sensory Processing

(1) Tactile—Utilized to feel grip on jump rope handles.

(2) Proprioceptive—Used to know upper and lower extremity joint positions in relation to each other as one jumps.

(3) Vestibular—This is essential to maintain balance while jumping.

(4) Visual—Used to see position of rope while jumping. Vision can also help scan jumping area and surface to ensure safety. However, one can jump rope without vision if vestibular and proprioceptive senses are intact.

(5) Auditory—This is not necessary to jump rope but it can be helpful for counting repetitions (hearing rope hit floor). Audition can also enhance quality of the jumping rope experience if one jumps to music or rhymes.

(6) Gustatory—N/A.

(7) Olfactory—N/A.

c. Perceptual Processing

(1) Stereognosis—May be used to distinguish handles from rope without looking.

(2) Kinesthesia—This is essential to know the excursion and direction of arm and leg movement while jumping.

(3) Pain Response—N/A. (only used if one falls and injures self)

(4) Body Scheme—Used throughout the activity for many body parts are employed in jumping rope.

(5) Right-Left Discrimination—Not required in regular jump rope because both sides of the body move simultaneously. However, this may be required when learning and performing more

complex jump rope routines (ie: double dutch, crossovers).

  (6) Form Constancy—Used to recognize jump rope in different forms (ie: coiled, knotted, elongated)

  (7) Position in Space—This is essential in order to jump within the confines of jumping rope's arc and to not trip over the rope.

  (8) Visual-Closure—May be used to identify rope even when entire rope is not in sight (i.e.: if it is behind back, over head).

  (9) Figure Ground—This may be used to find the jump rope within a crowded closet, toy chest, or gym bag.

  (10) Depth Perception—Used to judge the distance needed between self and objects, buildings or people to ensure rope does not hit anything.

  (11) Spatial Relations—Used to know the position of the jump rope in relation to other items in the environment (eg: playground equipment).

  (12) Topographical Orientation—Used to determine the appropriate setting to engage in jumping rope and used to get to that desired location.

2. Neuromusculoskeletal

  a. Reflex—Intact reflexes (i.e.: righting reflexes) are required to perform voluntary coordinated movements. Also, lower level reflexes (eg: ATNR, STNR) must be integrated.

  b. Range of Motion—Active ROM of upper extremities is required to turn rope and active ROM is required in lower extremities to jump. Trunk flexion, extension and rotation are also used when picking up rope and jumping.

  c. Muscle Tone—Good muscle tone is required throughout activity.

  d. Strength—Minimal strength needed to pick up rope and turn it.

  e. Endurance—This is essential for jumping rope requires cardiac, pulmonary, and musculoskeletal exertion over time. The amount of endurance needed depends on the length of time one jumps.

  f. Postural Control—This is essential to maintain balance as one jumps.

  g. Postural Alignment—This is used as one jumps and body parts move; particularly used to maintain proper body mechanics (ie: back and trunk).

  h. Soft Tissue Integrity—This would become a factor if a person jumped in bare feet on a rough surface or gripped handles of rope too tightly for an extended period of time resulting in skin breakdown.

3. Motor

  a. Gross Coordination—This is essential for coordinating arms and legs while jumping.

  b. Crossing the Midline—In regular jump rope this is not required. This is required in more complex jump rope moves (ie: crossovers, double dutch).

  c. Laterality—N/A. Jumping rope requires use of both sides of the body.

  d. Bilateral Integration—This is essential as both sides of the body are used simultaneously to swing rope and jump.

  e. Motor Control—Jumping rope requires a number of movement patterns. The need for motor control will increase as complexity of jumping routine increases.

  f. Praxis—This is essential when learning the activity of jumping rope.

  g. Fine Coordination/Dexterity—A minimal amount is needed to manipulate handles of jump rope. Increased dexterity may be needed to take out a knot if rope becomes tangled.

  h. Visual-Motor Integration—This is essential to see the arc of the rope as it moves and then to coordinate jumping with the rope's movement.

  i. Oral-Motor Control—Not required, unless one pauses during jumping rope to drink or eat.

B. Cognitive Integration and Cognitive Components

1. Level of Arousal—One must be alert and respond to environmental stimuli to be able to jump rope safely.

2. Orientation—Orientation to situation and place is necessary to understand the appropriate environment in which to engage in this activity, so as not to disturb or endanger other people. Example: A crowded room, a designated quiet area, a stair well. Orientation to time is used to know when to jump rope and for how long. Orientation to person is not required to jump rope, unless one is jumping rope with others.

3. Recognition—The ability to recognize a jump rope is required. Recognition of persons can be helpful if jumping in a social setting.

4. Attention Span—This is needed to follow directions, practice the various components of jump roping and repeat sequence over a period of time. A minimum of 5 minutes is needed. Maximum attention span needed will depend upon how long person jumps.

5. Initiation of Activity—Required to begin jumping rope.

6. Termination of Activity—Required to stop jumping rope prior to the initiation of excessive fatigue or muscle pain.

7. Memory—This is necessary to remember directions and to consciously recall the steps of jumping rope until it becomes automatic. Memory can also be used when recalling more complex jump rope routines or songs and rhymes used when jumping rope.

8. Sequencing—Required if doing a complex double dutch routine to be certain motor actions are in order.

9. Categorization—N/A.

10. Concept Formation—Not generally applicable. May be used if designing a new jump rope routine.

11. Spatial Operations—Used to mentally manipulate the position of the rope in relationship to self and objects in environment.

12. Problem Solving—Used if person has difficulty with the task (eg: rope is tangled, rope too long or too short)

13. Learning—Required to acquire the skill of jumping rope.

14. Generalization—Gross motor skills and behaviors to maintain balance and safety can be generalized to jumping rope.

C. Psychosocial Skills and Psychological Components

1. Psychological

   a. Values—Jumping rope can be reflective of a belief in developing and maintaining physical fitness. There is a value to exercise for many people.

   b. Interests—Jumping rope can be a physical activity that is pleasurable. It can develop interest in physical fitness.

   c. Self-Concept—Jumping rope successfully can give one a sense of pride, control, and physical power. It can facilitate a positive body image. Difficulties encountered while jumping rope can teach one to accept one's limitations and learn to form realistic expectations and self-appraisal (ie: I'm clumsy and it's ok).

2. Social

   a. Role Performance—Jumping rope can be related to one's role as a parent, child care worker, playground attendant. School age children often jump rope during recess. If one is involved in competitive double dutch team competition, the role of player and/or team leader will be relevant.

   b. Social Conduct—Not utilized if jumping alone. If jumping in social setting (ie: gym, playground) the ability to use manners, and express self appropriately is critical. Being aware of one's personal space using eye contact, gestures and active listening can enhance the quality of this activity. (ie: Knowing when to "jump in" during a complex routine).

   c. Interpersonal Skills—Not required if jumping alone. If jumping in a social setting, interpersonal skills are essential. Verbal and nonverbal communication can be used when learning to jump rope and when jumping in a group (ie: double dutch).

   d. Self-Expression—Used when expressing pride, enjoyment and/or frustration with task.

3. Self-Management

   a. Coping Skills—Used if a difficulty arises (eg: falling, rope tangled). If waiting one's "turn" to jump one must be patient. Generally, jumping rope is not highly stressful and it can even be used as a physical release of tension.

   b. Time Management—Jumping rope can be planned and used as a routine leisure and/or health maintenance activity.

   c. Self-Control—N/A if jumping alone. Used if in a group situation (ie: need to wait turn, part of a double dutch group).

IV. PERFORMANCE CONTEXTS

Directions: Indicate and describe the temporal and environmental relevance and requirements of your selected activity.

A. Temporal Aspects

1. Chronological: Participants in this activity can range in age from approximately 5 years old to 65 years of age or older (depending upon one's physical status).
2. Developmental: To engage in this activity one must have complete reflex development and moderate coordination.
3. Life Cycle: People in all stages of life (child, adolescent, adult and elder) can all engage in this activity if physically able.
4. Disability Status: Jumping rope would generally be contraindicated in the acute stages of an illness or disability. It can be a useful activity for the rehabilitation stage of disability or in helping someone cope with the limitations of a chronic illness or disability. It can be helpful for health maintenance and prevention of further disability.

B. Environment

1. Physical: A flat, clear, non-skid surface free of obstacles is required (a minimum space of 5' x 8' is desirable). Jump rope may be done inside (ie: in a gym) or outside (ie: driveway, playground).
2. Social: Jump rope is a recreational activity which can involve family and friends. If one jumps rope in a community setting or as a member of a team, one's social network would be expanded and the social norms, routines and role expectations of this network will influence the individual.
3. Cultural: A wide variety of cultures engage in this activity, however activity variations may be culturally defined (ie: double dutch competitions are more common in American inner cities than in European farm communities). Some cultures may define this activity according to gender (ie: only girls jump rope in a school playground but boys can jump rope in a gym to train to be a boxer).

V. ACTIVITY ADAPTATION, GRADUATION, AND SYNTHESIS

Directions: Describe how your selected activity can be adapted and graded to be used in OT intervention. Interventions may be directed towards components of the performance areas (e.g. money management, retirement planning), the performance components (e.g. dexterity, social role performance) or the environmental aspects of performance contexts (e.g. modifying or structuring the environment to improve or maintain function). Be certain your adaptations and gradations address both psychosocial and physical aspects of performance.

A. Activity Adaptations: Identify elements of the activity that can be changed or altered so that a client can perform the activity.

There are several adaptations which can be made to enable a client to perform the activity. Built up handles can be added to the jump rope for persons who do not have a tight cylindrical grasp. Handles can be inserted into "universal cuffs" or specially constructed gloves to hold the jump rope ends if a person does not have any functional grasp. One end of a jump rope can be attached to a rotating hook on a wall to enable a person to turn the rope with only one hand. A brightly colored rope can help someone with visual impairments see the rope as it turns. Verbal or auditory cues (eg: encouragement, music) can be added to the activity to help a person with cognitive deficits attend to the activity and to provide needed psychosocial support.

B. Activity Gradation: Identify elements of the activity that can be graded and the degree of gradability possible.

The activity can be graded according to:

a) Duration: Jumping rope can begin with just a few repetitions and can work up to many minutes. An increase in duration would be particularly beneficial to cardiac patients who need to increase their aerobic activities and overall cardiac-pulmonary function. Children who are hyperactive or have attention deficits could benefit by sustaining and controlling their focus on jumping rope.
b) Range of motion: When grading the activity for ROM of the upper extremities, an individual jumping alone uses predominantly UE flexion and extension, while turning the rope for another jumper uses more abduction, adduction, pronation, and supination. Swinging the rope for others in double-dutch jumping entails bilateral crossing over the midline. All forms of jumping rope use LE flexion and extension.
c) Resistance: The jump rope can initially be made of lightweight rope. Weighted handles would

increase resistance when jumping. Adding ankle and wrist weights would allow for greater resistance. Grading the activity in this way would help increase strength for those with upper extremity weakness and increase cardiopulmonary endurance in general.

d) Complexity: Visual cue cards and demonstration can be used for those with perceptual or cognitive problems, apraxia or aphasia. Verbal instruction and cuing can decrease complexity while the addition of rhymes, songs, rhythms and additional steps and routines can increase complexity.

e) Socialization: This activity can begin as a solitary or 1:1 activity. It can then progress to a parallel activity. Double dutch or Chinese jump rope requires increased cooperation. Songs, music or games can be used in group jump roping activities to increase socialization. Team competitions require the highest level of social skills. Jumping rope can encourage increased attendance at a gym, fitness class, school or playground.

f) Independence: Grading can begin with 1:1 instruction and support. Decreasing this guidance will increase independence. Becoming a leader of a double dutch team requires the highest level of independence.

C. Activity Synthesis: Describe and explain how your activity can be designed to meet the following goals of intervention for a client and/or patient population. For background information on these 5 types of intervention, please refer to Mosey, A. C. (1986). *Psychosocial Components of Occupational Therapy.* (pp. 335–358). New York: Raven Press.

1. For the purpose of meeting health needs.

    The activity of jumping rope can meet basic psychophysical needs by providing sensory stimulation and gross motor activity. This can be appropriate for persons with chronic mental and/or physical illness who may lack independent sensorimotor activities.

    Jumping rope can be incorporated into a daily routine ensuring an adequate temporal balance between work, rest and play. It is a fun activity which can meet a person's need for pleasure and serve as a tension releaser. This can be helpful for a person lacking leisure skills and exhibiting temporal dysfunction. Jumping rope can be a social activity and if done in a group, it

can meet an individual's need for group association and/or psychosocial deficits.

2. For the purpose of prevention.

    As a physical activity, jumping rope can aid in the primary prevention of obesity and cardiovascular disease. When this activity is performed in a group or community setting isolation and depression can be prevented through peer socializations and the receiving of encouragement from others.

3. For the purpose of maintenance.

    Jumping rope regularly can maintain a person's physical health, especially their cardiovascular fitness, muscle tone and gross motor coordination. This can be very beneficial for the elderly. Being able to jump rope independently can contribute to the maintenance of self-esteem, especially if one had viewed themselves as clumsy and uncoordinated (eg: an adolescent with a developmental disability). Regular participation in a leisure activity can maintain a person's ability to balance their work, play, and rest. Jumping rope to music can be relaxing and help maintain a sense of well being. Jumping rope as a family can help maintain positive parent-child and/or sibling relationships. This activity can also contribute to the maintenance of social interaction skills if done in a group or community setting.

4. For the purpose of management.

    This activity can be used to manage undesirable or disruptive behaviors as it can allow for a socially acceptable release of physical and emotional energy. A person may be able to vent their anger and/or frustrations by jumping vigorously. Using music or song to accompany the rope jumping can also provide an emotional release. The routine, repetitive and rhythmic nature of this activity can also help manage anxiety or confusion in persons with psychosocial and/or cognitive deficits. Clients may also become motivated to manage their hygiene needs and/or socially inappropriate behaviors in response to group norms and their desire to be accepted by their peers.

5. For the purpose of change.

    Jumping rope can be used to increase coordination, strength and endurance in persons with physical and/or developmental disabilities. These improved abilities can then be generalized to other functional activities. Jumping rope can also increase an individual's situational coping skills as he or she learns to deal with feelings associated with learning a new physical activity (ie: clumsiness). Coping skills can be increased as person deals with learning more complex routines in a group setting. Mastering the activity of jumping rope can also increase one's self esteem and sense of pride in one's physical abilities. Jumping rope in a group or as a member of a team can increase one's socialization skills especially the ability to attend to others, wait one's turn, cooperate and compete in a socially acceptable manner. This can be beneficial to individuals with psychosocial deficits of all ages.

Adolescents with physical, psychosocial and/or developmental disabilities may need to develop a common identity with their peer group. This can be facilitated through the use of popular music (ie: rap, hip hop) and the wearing of stylish fashions during jump rope routines and/or double dutch team competitions.

Appendix L

Supplemental Reference Lists

Developmental Aspects of Purposeful Activity

Aitken, M.J. (1982). Self-concept and functional independence in the hospitalized elderly. *American Journal of Occupational Therapy, 36*, 243-250.

Anderson, J., & Hinojosa, J. (1984). Parents and therapists in a professional partnership. *American Journal of Occupational Therapy, 38*, 452-461.

Arnetz, B. (1985). Gerontonic occupational therapy-Psychology and social predictiors of praticipation and therapeutic benefits. *American Journal of Occupational Therapy, 39*, 460-465.

Ayres, A.J. (1980). *Sensory Integration and the Child.* Los Angeles, CA: Western Psychological Services.

Ayres, A.J. (1986). *Developmental Dyspraxia and Adult Onset Apraxia.* Torrance, CA: Sensory Integration Interantional.

Bailey, D. (1971). Vocational theories and work habits related to childhood development. *American Journal of Occupational Therapy, 25*, 298.

Baker, B.L., & Bughtman, A.J. (1989). *Steps to Independence: A Skills Training Guide for Parents and Teachers of Children with Special Needs (2nd ed).* Baltimore, MD: Paul H. Brooks Publishing Company.

Baker, C., & Long, T. (1994). *Tips from Tots.* Palo Alto, CA: VORT Corporation.

Becker, G. (1980). *Growing Old in Silence: Deaf People in Old Age.* Berkeley, CA: University of California Press.

Branholm, I.B., & Fugl-Meyer, A.R. (1992). Occupational role preferences and life satisfaction. *Occupational Therapy Journal of Research, 12 (3)*, 159-171.

Bowe, R. (1980). *Rehabilitating America: Toward Independence for Disabled and Elderly People.* New York, NY: Harper & Row.

Bricker, D. (1993). *An Activity-Based Approach to Early Intervention.* Palo Alto, CA: VORT Corporation.

Brofenbrenner, U. (1979). *The Ecology of Human Development: Experiments by Human Development: Experiments by Nature and Design.* Cambridge, MA: Harvard University Press.

Brunner, J., Jolly, A. & Silava, K. (Eds) (1976). *Play its Role in Development and Evolution.* New York, NY: Basic Books.

Cermak, S. A., Stein, F. & Abelson, C. (1973). Hyperactive children and activity group therapy model. *American Journal of Occupational Therapy, 26 (6)*, 311-315.

Clancy, H. & Clark, M.J. (1990). *Occupational Therapy with Children.* New York, NY: Churchill Livingston.

Clark, P. (1979a). Human development through occupation: theoretical framework in contemporary occupational therapy practice. Part 1. *American Journal of Occupational Therapy, 33*, 505-541.

Clark, P. (1979b). Human development through occupation: A philosophy and conceptual model for practice. Part 2. *American Journal of Occupational Therapy, 33*, 577-585.

Csikszentmihalyi, M. & Larson, R. (1976). What play says about behavior. *Ontario Psychologist, 8*, 5-11.

Csikszentmihalyi, M. & Larson, R. (1984). *Being Adolescent.* New York, NY: Basic Books.

Cynkin, S. (1979). *Occupational Therapy: Toward Health through Activities.* Boston, MA: Little, Brown and Co.

Davis, L.J. & Kirkland, M. (Eds) (1986). *Role of Occupational Therapy with the Elderly.* Rockville, MD: American Occupational Therapy Association.

DePoy, E., Werrbach, G. & Archer, L. (1992). Retirement adjustment: a rehabilitation dilemma. *American Journal of Occupational Therapy, 7 (4)*, 55-63.

Dunn, W. (Ed.) (1991). *Pediatric Occupational Therapy: Facilitating Effective Service Provision.* Thorofare, NJ: Slack Inc.

Eisenberg, M.G., Sutkin, L.C. & Jansen, M.A. (1984). *Chronic Illness and Disability Through the Life Span: Effects on Self and Family.* New York, NY: Springer.

Erickson, E. (1971). *Toys and Reason: Stages in the Ritualization of Experience.* New York, NY: W. W. Norton.

Feil, N. (1982). *Validation-The Feil Method: How to Help the Disoriented Old-Old.* Cleveland, OH: Feil Productions.

Florey, L. (1971). An approach to play and play development. *American Journal of Occupational Therapy, 25,* 275

Gailey, R. (1992). Recreational pursuits for elders with amputation. *Topics in Geriatric Rehabilitation, 8 (1),* 39-58.

Gilfoyle, E.M., Grady, A.P. & Moore, J.C. (1981). *Children Adapt.* Thorofare, NJ: Charles B. Slack.

Gralewicz, A. (1973). Play deprivation in multihandicapped children. *American Journal of Occupational Therapy, 27,* 70-72.

Gregory, M.D. (1983). Occupational behavior and life satisfaction among retirees. *American Journal of Occupational Therapy, 37,* 548-553.

Hamill, C.M. & Oliver, R.C. (1980). *Therapeutic Activities for the Handicapped Elderly.* Rockville, MD: Aspen Systems Corporation.

Hasselkus, B.R. (1992). The meaning of activity: Day care for persons with Alzheimer's disease. *American Journal of Occupational Therapy, 46,* 199-206.

Hasselkus, B. (1978). Relocation stress and the elderly. *American Journal of Occupational Therapy, 32,* 631-636.

Hatter, J.K. & Nelson, D.L. (1987). Altruism and task participation in the elderly. *American Journal of Occupational Therapy, 41,* 379-381.

Heard, C. (1977). Occupational role acquisition: A perspective on the chronically disabled. *American Journal of Occupational Therapy, 31,* 243-247.

Helm, M. (Ed) (1987). *Occupational Therapy with the Elderly.* New York, NY: Churchill Livingstone.

Herrmann, C. (1990). A descriptive study of daily activities and role conflict in single adolescent mothers. *Occupational Therapy in Health Care, 6,* 53-68.

Hinojosa, J., Anderson, J. & Strauch, C. (1988). Pediatric occupational therapy in the home. *American Journal of Occupational Therapy, 42,* 17-22.

Janicki, M. & Wisniewski, H. (Eds) (1985). *Aging and Developmental Disabilities-Issues and Approaches.* Baltimore, MD: Paul H. Brookes.

Kautzman, L. (1991). Facilitating adult learning in occupational therapy patient education programs. *Occupational Therapy Practice, 2,* 1-11.

Keilhofner, G. (1981). An ethnographic study of deinstitutionalized adults: Their community setting and daily experiences. *Occupational Therapy Journal of Research, 1,* 125-142.

Kielhofner, G. & Barris, R. (1984). Collecting data on play: A critique of available methods. *Occupational Therapy Journal of Research, 4,* 150-181.

Kielhofner, G., Barris, R., Bauer, D., Shoestock, B. & Walker, L. (1983). A comparison of play behavior in nonhospitalized and hospitalized children. *American Journal of Occupational Therapy, 37,* 305-312.

Kiernat, J.M. (1991). *Occupational Therapy and the Older Adult: A Clinical Manual.* Rockville, MD: Aspen Publishers.

Kolman, C. (1987). Changing life roles after physical injury. *Occupational Therapy Forum. Atlantic Edition, 11 (43),* 12-13, 17.

Kramer, P. & Hinojosa, J. (1995). Epiphany of human occupation. In C.B. Royeen (Ed). *The Practice of the Future: Putting Occupation Back into Therapy* (Lesson 8, p.5-17). Bethesda, MD: American Occupational Therapy Association.

Kultgen, P. & Habenstein, R. (1984). Processes and goals in aftercare programs for deinstitutionalized elderly mental patients. *Gerontologist, 24,* 167-173.

Kubler-Ross, E. (1969). *On Death & Dying.* New York, NY: MacMill.

Kubler-Ross, E. (1978). *To Live Until We Say Good-bye.* New Jersey: Prentice Hall.

Lane, S.J. (1995). Use it or lose it. In C.B. Royeen (Ed). *The Practice of the Future: Putting Occupational Back into Therapy.* (Lesson 9, pp 19-21). Bethesda, MD: American Occupational Therapy Association.

Lawritten, M.P., Wendley, P.G. & Byerts, T.O. (1982). *Aging and the Environment: Theoretical Approaches.* New York, NY: Springer.

Lawton, M.P. (1980). *Environment and Aging.* Monterey, CA: Brooks-Cole.

Lawton, M.P. & Brody, E. (1969). Assessment of older people: Self-maintaining and instrumental activities of daily living. *Gerontologist, 9,* 179-186.

Lewis, S.C. (1979). *The Mature Years: A Geriatric Occupational Therapy Text.* Thorofare, NJ: Slack.

Lewis, S.C. (1988). *Providing for the Older Adult-A Gerontological Handbook.* New Jersey: Slack.

Lewis, S.C. (1989). *Elder Care in Occupational Therapy.* Thorofare, NJ: Slack.

Llorens, L.A. (1970). Facilitating Growth and Development: The Promise of Occupational Therapy. *American Journal of Occupational Therapy, 24,* 93-101.

Llorens, L.A. (1976). *Application of a Developmental Theory for Health and Rehabilitation.* Rockville, MD: American Occupational Therapy Association.

Llorens, L. & Rubin, E. (1987). *Developing Ego Functions in Disturbed Children.* Detroit, MI:

Mace, N.L. (1987). Principles of activities for persons with dementia. *Physical and Occupational Therapy in Geriatrics, 5 (3),* 13-27.

Marino-Shorn, J.A. (1985). Morale, work and leisure in retirement. *Physical and Occupational Therapy in Geriatrics, 4 (2),* 49-59.

Matsutsuyu, J. (1971). Occupational behavior-A perspective on work and play. *American Journal of Occupational Therapy, 25,* 291-293.

Maurer, P.A. (1971). Antecedents of work behavior. *American Journal of Occupational Therapy, 25,* 295.

McKinney, Vreeberg & West (1985). *Extending Horizons: A Resource for Assisting Handicapped Youth in their Transition from Vocational Education to Employment.* Columbus, OH: National Center for Research in Vocational Education.

Michelman, S. (1971). The importance of creative play. *American Journal of Occupational Therapy, 25,* 285-290.

Mobily, K.E. (1982). Motivational aspects of exercise for the elderly: Barriers and solutions. *Physical and Occupational Therapy in Geriatrics, 1,* 43-53.

Mullins, C.S., Melson, D.L. & Smith, D.A. (1987). Exercise through dual-purpose activity in the institutional elderly. *Physical and Occupational Therapy in Geriatrics, 5*, 29-39.

Neistadt, M.E. (1986). Occupational therapy treatment goals for adults with developmental disabilities. *American Journal of Occupational Therapy, 40*, 672-678.

Neistadt, M.E. (1988). Occupational therapy for adults with perceptual deficits. *American Journal of Occupational Therapy, 42*, 434-440.

Nelson, D.L. (1984). *Children with autism and other Pervasive Disorders of Developmental and Behavior: Therapy through Activities.* Thorofare, NJ: Slack, Inc.

Nelson, D.L. & Stucky, C. (1992). The roles of occupational therapy in preventing futher disability of elderly persons in long-term care facilities. In J. Rothman & R. Levine (Eds), *Prevention Practice: Strategies for Physical and Occupational Therapy*, (pp19-35). Philadelphia, PA: Saunders.

New York City Alzheimer's Resource Center (1985). *Caring-A Guide to Managing the Alzheimer's Patient at Home.* New York, NY: Author.

Norman, A.N. & Crosby, P.M. (1990). Meeting the challenge: Role of occupational therapy in a geriatric day hospital. *Occupational Therapy in Mental Health, 10 (3)*, 65-78.

Nystrom, E.P. (1974). Activity patterns and leisure concepts among the elderly. *American Journal of Occupational Therapy, 28*, 337-345.

Palmer, F. & Barrows, C. (1985, December). Vocational activities for adolescents: A program description. *Mental Health Special Interest Section Newsletter*, pp. 1-2.

Pratt, P.N. & Allen, A.S., (Eds) (1995). *Occupational Therapy for Children*, 3rd ed., St. Louis, MO: C.V. Mosby Co. 1989.

Provost, J. (1990). *Work, Play and Type: Achieving Balance in your Life.* Palo Alto Psychologists' Press.

Redman-Bentley, D. (1982). Parent expectations for professionals providing services to their handicapped children. *Physical and Occupational Therapy in Pediatrics, 2*, 13-26.

Reilly, M. (Ed). *Play as Exploratory Learning* (pp. 247-266). Beverly Hills, CA: Sage Publications.

Robinson, A. (1977). Play: The arena for the acquisition of rules of competent behavior. *American Journal of Occupational Therapy, 31*, 248.

Royeen, C.B. (1994). The human life cycle: Paradigmatic shifts in occupation. In C.B. Royeen (Ed). *The Practice of the Future: Putting Occupation back into Therapy*, (Lesson 11, pp. 5-22). Rockville, MD: American Occupational Therapy Association.

Searle, M.S. (1991). Leisure, aging and mental health: A review of the clinical evidence. *Topics in Geriatric Rehabilitation, 7 (2)*, 1-12.

Shannon, P. (1970). The work model: A basis for occupational therapy programming. *American Journal of Occupational Therapy, 24*, 215.

Sherman, E. & Newman, E.S. (1977). The meaning of cherished personal possessions for the elderly. *Journal of Aging and Human Development, 8*, 181-192.

Singleton, J.S., Forbes, W.F & Agwani, N. (1993). Stability of activity across lifespan. *Activities, Adaptation and Aging, 18 (1)*, 19-28. New York, NY: Haworth Press.

Smelser, N. & Erikson, E. (1980). *Work and Love in Adulthood.* Cambridge, MA: Harvard University Press.

Synder, S. (1985). Comprehensive inpatient treatment for the young adult patient. *Occupational Therapy in Mental Health, 5 (4)*, 47-58.

Sparling, J.W. (1982). Bridging the generation gap through occupation. *Occupational Therapy News, 36 (10)*, 7.

Takata, N. (1969). The play history. *American Journal of Occupational Therapy, 23*, 314-318.

Tickle, L. & Yerxa, E. (1981). Need satisfaction of older persons living in the community and in institutions, part 2: Role of activity. *American Journal of Occupational Therapy, 35*, 650-655.

Tyler, B. & Kogan, K.L. (1977). Reduction of stress between mothers and their handicapped children. *American Journal of Occupational Therapy, 31*, 151-155.

Vandenburg, B. & Keilhofner, G. (1982). Play in evolution, culture, and individual adaptation: Implications for therapy. *American Journal of Occupational Therapy, 36*, 20.

Wilson, D.S., Allen, C.K., McCormick, G. & Burton, G. (1989). Cognitive disability and routine task behaviors in a community-based population with senile dementia. *Occupational Therapy Practice, 1 (1)*, 58-66.

Wood, W. (1993). Occupation and the relevance of primatology to occupational therapy. *American Journal of Occupational Therapy, 47*, 515-522.

Yerxa, E.J. & Baum, S. (1986). Engagement in daily occupations and life satisfaction among people with spinal cord injuries. *Occupational Therapy Journal of Research, 6*, 271-283.

Zager, R.P. & Marquette, C.H. (1981). Developmental considerations in children and early adolescents with spinal cord injury. *Archives of Physical Medicine and Rehabilitation, 62*, 427-431.

Environmental Contexts: Physical, Sociocultural, and Temporal Influences on Activity

Adams, R. (1993). The role of occupational therapist in community mental health. In R.P. Cottrell (Ed). *Psychosocial Occupational Therapy: Proactive Approaches*, (pp165-168). Bethesda, MD: American Occupational Therapy Association.

Alton, I. & Chelmers, M. (1980). *Culture and Environment.* Monterey, CA: Brooks/Cole.

American Occupational Therapy Association (1993). *Design for Aging: Strategies for Collaboration Between Architechts and Occupational Therapists.* Rockville, MD: American Occupational Therapy Association.

Anderson, P.P. & Fenichel, E.S. (1989). *Serving culturally Diverse Families of Infants and Toddlers with Disabilities.* Washington, DC: National Center for Clinical Infant Programs.

Barnes, K. (1991). Modification of the physical environment. In C. Baum, & C. Christiansen (Eds). *Occupational Therapy-Overcoming Human Performance Deficits.* Thorofare, NJ: Slack.

Barney, K. (1989). Cultural awareness perspectives. *Introduction, Gerontology Special Interest Section Newsletter, 12 (2)*, 1-2. Rockville, MD: American Occupation Therapy Association.

Barris, R. (1987). Activity: The interface between person and environment. *Physical and Occupational Therapy in Geriantrics, 5 (2)*, 39-49.

Baum, C. (1991). Identification and use of environmental resources. In C. Baum and C. Christiansen (Eds). *Occupational Therapy Overcoming Human Performance Deficits*, (pp. 789-802). Thorofare, NJ: Slack, Inc.

Baum, C.M. & Luebben, A.J. (1985). Assessing community resources to support independent living, in *Pivot: Planning and Implementing Vocational Readiness in Occupational Therapy*. Rockville, MD: The American Occupational Therapy Association, 95-98.

Beck, M.A. & Callahan, D.K. (1980). Impact of institutionalization on the posture of chronic schizophrenic patients. *American Journal of Occupational Therapy, 74*, 332-335.

Benzig, P. & Strickland, R. (1983). Occupational therapy in a community based prevention program. *Occupational Therapy in Mental Health, 3 (1)*, 15-30.

Blakeney, A.B. (1987). Appalachian values: Implications for occupational therapists. *Occupational Therapy in Health Care, 4*, 57-72.

Bowen, R., Jones, R. & Shriver, D. (1993). Statement: The role of occupational therapy in the independent living movement. *American Journal of Occupational Therapy, 47*, 1079-1080.

Bowker, I.H. (1982). *Humanizing Institutions for the Aged*. Lexington, MA: D.C. Heath and Company.

Brockett, M. (1987). Cultural variations in Bay Area Functional Performance Evaluation scores-Considerations for occupational therapy. *Canadian Journal of Occupational Therapy, 54*, 195-199.

Brofenbrenner, U. (1979). *The Ecology of Human Development: Experiments by Human Development: Experiments by Nature and Design*. Cambridge, MA: Harvard University Press.

Cranbury, J.G., Barnett, J. & Goldman, N. (1993). *Readily Achievable Checklist: a Survey for Accessibility*. Rockville, MD: American Occupational Therapy Association.

Crist, P.H. (1993). Community living skills: A psychoeducational community based program. In R.P. Cottrell (Ed). *Psychosocial Occupational Therapy: Proactive Approaches*, (pp. 169-176). Rockville, MD: American Occupational Therapy Association.

Csikzentmikhalyi, M. (1990). *Flow. The Psychology of Optimal Experience*. New York, NY: Harper Perennial.

Csikzentmikhalyi, M. & Rochberg-Halton, E. (1981). *The Meaning of Things, Domestic Symbols and the Self*. New York, NY: Camridge University Press.

Dasler, P.J. (1993). Deinstitutionalizing the occupational therapist. In R.P. Cottrell (Ed). *Psychosocial Occupational Therapy: Proactive Approaches*, (pp. 25-29). Rockville, MD: American Occupational Therapy Association.

Davidson, H. (1991). Assessing environmental factors. In C. Christiansen (Eds). *Occupational Therapy-Overcoming Human Deficits*. Thorofare, NJ: Slack.

DiJoseph, L. M. (1982). Independence through activity: Mind, body, and environment interaction in therapy. *American Journal of Occupational Therapy, 36*, 740-744.

Dillard, M., Adenian, L., Flores, O., Lai, L., McRae & Shapir, M. (1992). Culturally competent occupational therapy in a diversely populated mental health center. *American Journal of Occupational Therapy, 46*, 721-725.

Dunn, W., Brown, C., McClain, L.H., & Westman, K. (1994). The ecology of human performance: A contextual perspective on human occupation. In C.B. Royeen (Ed). *The Practice of the Future: Putting Occupation back into Therapy. (1)*, 12-51. Rockville, MD: American Occupational Therapy Association.

Dunning, H. (1972). Environmental occupational therapy. *American Journal of Occupational Therapy, 26*, 292-298.

Ellmer, R. & Olbrisch, M.E. (1983). The contribution of a cultural perspective in understanding and evaluating client satisfaction. *Evaluation and Program Planning, 6*, 275-281.

Friedlob, S.A., Janis, G.A. & Deets, Aron, C. (1993). A hospital connected halfway house program for individuals with long-term neuropsychiatric disabilities. In R.P. Cottrell (Ed). *Psychosocial Occupational Therapy: Proactive Approaches*, (pp. 139-146). Bethesda, MD: American Occupational Therapy Association.

Gallardo, G. & Kirchman, M.M. (1987). Age Integrated or Age Segregated Living for Semi-Independent Elderly People. *Physical and Occupational Therapy in Geriatrics*.

Goldenberg, K. (1993). Toronto's home-based aftercare program: An exciting model. In R.P. Cottrell (Ed). *Psychosocial Occupational Therapy: Proactive Approaches*, (pp. 187-190). Bethesda, MD: American Occupational Therapy Association.

Goldman, N. (Ed) (1987). *Achieving Physical and Communication Accessibility*. Rockville, MD: American Occupational Therapy Association.

Gray, M. (1972). Effects of hospitalization on work-play behavior. *American Journal of Occupational Therapy, 26*, 180-185.

Grossman, J. (1977). Nationally speaking: Preventive health care and community programming. *American Journal of Occupational Therapy, 31*, 351-354.

Gutheil (1985). The therapeutic milieu: Changing times and theories. *Hospital and Community Psychiatry, 36*, 1279-1285.

Haarmann, A. (1990). *Lanuage in its Cultural Embedding*. New York, NY: Mouton de Gruyter.

Haggard, L. & Williams, D. (1992). Identify affiramation through leisure activities: Leisure symbols of the self. *Journal of Leisure Research, 24 (19)*, 1-18.

Hasslekus, D.R. & Brown, M. (1983). Respite care for community elderly. *American Journal of Occupational Therapy, 37*, 83-88.

Helman, C. (1984). *Culture, Health and Illness*. Bristol, England: John Wright and Sons.

Hemphill, B.J. & Werner, P.C. (1993). Deinstitutionalization: A role for Occupational therapy in the state hospital. In R.P. Cottrell (Ed). *Psycchosocial Occupational Therapy Proactive Approaches*, (pp. 31-37). Bethesda, MD: American Occupational Therapy Association.

Howe, M.C. & Briggs, A.K. (1982). Ecological systems model for occupational therapy. *American Journal of Occupational Therapy, 36*, 322-327.

Jackson, G.A. (1993). Short-term psychiatric treatment: How will occupational therapy adapt? In R.P. Cottrell (Ed). *Psychosocial Occupational Therapy Proactive Approaches*, (pp. 21-24). Bethesda, MD: American Occupational Therapy Association.

Jaffe, E. (1982). Role of occupational therapy as a community consultant: Primary preventiona mental health programming. *Occupational Therapy in Mental Health, 1 (2)*, 47-62.

Jamison, M. (1985). The interaction of culture and learning: Implications for occupational therapy. *Canadian Journal of Occupational Therapy, 52*, 5-8.

Jung, C. (1964). *Man and his Symbols*. New York, NY: Doubleday.

Kavanagh, M. (1990 March). Way station: A model community support program for persons with severe mental illness. *Mental Health Interest Section Newsletter*, (pp. 6-8).

Kielhofner, G. (1981). An ethnographic study of deinstitutionalized adults: Their community settings and daily life experiences. *Occupational Therapy Journal of Research, 1*, 125-142.

Klapp, O.E. (1991). *Inflation of Symbols*. New Brunswick, NJ: Transaction.

Kleinman, A., Eisenberg, L. & Good, B. (1978). Culture, illness, and care: Clinical lessons from anthropologic and cross-cultural research. *Annals of Internal Medicine, 88*, 251-258.

Knadson, D., Cable, T. & Beck, L. (1995). *Interpretation of Cultural and Natural Resources*. State College, PA: Venture Publishing.

Krofting, L.H., Krefting, D.V. (1991). Cultural influences on performance. In C. Chritiansen and C. Baum (Eds). *Occupational Therapy-Overcoming Human Performance Deficits*. Thorofare, NJ: Slack.

Krespy, M., Maeda, E. & Rothwell, N. (1976). The apartment program: Community living option for halfway house residents. *Hospital and Community Psychiatry, 27*, 153-154, 159.

Law, M. (1991). The environment: A focus for occupational therapy. *Canadian Journal of Occupational Therapy*, 171-179.

Lawritten, M.P., Wendley, P.G. & Byerts, T.O. (1982). Aging and the environment: *Theoretical Approaches*. New York, NY: Springer.

Lawton, M.P. (1982). Competence, environmental press, and the adaption of older people. In M.P. Lawton, P.G. Windley & T.O. byerts (Eds). *Aging and the Environment: Theoretical Approaches*. New York, NY: Springer.

Lawton, M.P. (1986). *Environment and Aging*. Albany, NY: Conter for the Study of Aging.

Levine, R.E. (1984). The cultural aspects of home care delivery. *American Journal of Occupational Therapy, 38*, 734-738.

Lewis, I. M. (Ed) (1977). *Symbols and Sentiments: Cross-Cultural Studies in Symbolism*. New York, NY: Academic Press.

Lindsay, J. (1971). The injured workman-Do cultural influences affect his rehabilitation? *Canadian Journal of Occupational Therapy, 38*, 15-19.

Litterst, T.A.E. (1985). A reappraisal of anthropological fieldwork methods and the concept of culture in occupational therapy research, *American Journal of Occupational Therapy 39*, 602-604.

Llorens, L.A. (1984). Changing balance: Environment and individuals. *American Journal of Occupational Therapy, 38*, 575-584.

Mach, A. (1993). *Symbols, Conflicts and Identity*. Albany, NY: State University of New York Press.

Maguire, G.A. (1979). Volunteer program to assist the elderly to remain in home settings. *American Journal of Occupational Therapy, 33*, 98-101.

Maslen, D. (1982). Rehabilitation training for community living skills: Concept and techniques. *Occupational Therapy in Mental Health, 2 (1)*, 33-49,

Mauras-Corsino, E., Daniewicz, C.V. & Swan, L.C. (1985). The use of community networks for chronic psychiatric patients. *American Journal of Occupational Therapy, 39*, 374-378.

Mechanic, D. (1986). The concept of illness behavior: Culture, situation, and personal predisposition. *Psychological Medicine, 16*, 1-7.

Morse, A. (1987). A cultural intervention model for developmentally disabled adults: An expanded role for occupational therapy. *Occupational Therapy in Health Care, 4*, 103-113.

Neistadt, L. (1993). Adult day care: A model for changing times. In R.P. Cottrell (Ed). *Psychosocial Occupational Therapy Proactive Approaches*, (pp. 465-472). Bethesda, MD: American Occupational Therapy Association.

Nesbit, J. & Johnson, C. (1993). Facilitating transition from hospital inpatient to community resident for mental health clients: A consultative model. *Occupational Therapy Practice, 4*, 54-59.

Paschke, M.J. (1984). Day care within a community mental health center. *Physical and Occupational Therapy in Geriatrics, 3 (4)*, 67-70.

Peterson, R. (1990). Symposium: The many facts of culture. *Contemporary Sociology, 19*, 498-499.

Pierce, C.M. & Dickson, R. (1962). The occupational therapy shop as a culture. *American Journal of Occupational Therapy, 16*, 231-235.

Radonsky, V.E., Jackson, H., Barton, S., Fedak, K. & Marim, M. (1986). Step ahead-Occupational therapy in the community. *Occupational Therapy in Mental Health, 6 (2)*, 79-87.

Randall, D. (1989). *Strategies for Working with Culturally Diverse Communities and Clients*. Ravensdale, WA: Idyll Arbor, Inc.

Robinson, L. (1987). Patient compliance in occupational therapy home health programs: Sociocultural considerations. *Occupational Therapy in Health Care, 4*, 127-137.

Rogers, J. (1989). The occupational therapy home assessment: the home as a therapeutic environment. *Journal of Home Health Care Practitioners, 2 (1)*, 73-81.

Rogers, J.C., Marcus, C.L. & Snow, T.L. (1987). Maude: A case of sensory deprivation. *American Journal of Occupational Therapy, 41*, 673-676.

Rosenthal, L.A. & Howe, M.C. (1984). Temporal adaptation among day versus night shift workers. *Occupational Therapy in Mental Health, 4 (2)*, 59-78.

Searles, H. (1960). *The Nonhuman Environment*. New York, NY: International Universities.

Shawski, K.A. (1987). Ethnic/racial considerations in occupational therapy. *Occupational Therapy in Health Care, 4*, 37-49.

Sorenson, J. (1994, June 6). Symbolism: The missing link in OT today. *Advance*, (p. 5).

Spechler, J.W. (1995). *Reasonable Accommodation: Profitable Commpliance with the Americans with Disabilities Act.* Delray Beach, FL: St. Lucie Press.

Spencer, J. (1987). Environmental assesment strategies. *Topice in Geriatric Rehabilitation, 3 (1)*, 35-41.

Szekais, B. (1985). Risk factors for institutionalization in a community elderly population. *Physical and Occupational Therapy in Geriatric, 4 (1)*, 33-43.

Taria, E. (1984). An occupational therapist's perspecitive on environmental adaptations for the disabled elderly. *Occupational Therapy in Health Care, 1 (4)*, 25-33.

Takata, N. (1971). The play milieu: A preliminary appraisal. *American Journal of Occupational Therapy, 35*, 644-649.

Tully, K. (1986). *Improving Residential Life for Disabled People.* New York, NY: Churchill Livingstone.

Turner, V. (1974). *Dramas, Fields, and Metaphors: Symbolic Action in Human Society.* Itaca, NY: Cornell University Press.

Turner, V. (1986). *The Anthropology of Performance.* New York, NY: PAJ.

Turner, V.W. (1967). *The Forest of Symbols.* Ithaca, NY: Cornell University Press.

U.S. Consumer Product Safety Commission (1986). *Safety for Older Consumers: Home Safety Checklist.* Washington, DC.

Wells, S.A. (1994). *A Multicultural Education and Resource Guide for Occupational Therapy Educators and Practitioners.* Bethesda, MD: American Occupational Therapy Association.

Westland, G. (1985). Dipping into community mental health: An aspect of the occupational therapist's role. *British Journal of Occupational Therapy, 48 (9)*, 260-262.

Weimer, R.B. & West, W.L. (1970). Occupational therapy in community health care. *American Journal of Occupational Therapy, 24 (5)*, 323-328.

Wilberding, D. (1993). The quarterway house: More than an alternative of care. In R.P. Cottrell (Ed). *Psychosocial Occupational Therapy Proactive Approaches*, (pp. 127-135). Bethesda, MD: American Occupational Therapy Association.

Wilcock, A.A. (1993). Keynote paper: Biological and sociocultural aspects of occupation, health and health promotion. *British Journal of Occupational Therapy, 56*, 200-203.

Williams, G. (1987). Disablement and social contest of daily activity. *International Disability Studies, 9*, 97-102.

Woodside, H. (1993). The day center and its role as a social network. In R.P. Cottrell (Ed). *Psychosocial Occupational Therapy Proactive Approaches*, (pp. 329-332). Bethesda, MD: American Occupational Therapy Association.

Yasuda, L. & Royeen, C.B. (1994). Considering environmental contexts: Thinking about functional outcomes. In C.B. Royeen (Ed). *The Practice of the Future: Putting Occupation back into Therapy*, (Lesson 1), (pp. 9-11). Rockville, MD: American Occupational Therapy Association.

Yelton, D. & Nielson, C. (1991). Understanding Applachian values: Implications for occupational therapists. *Occupational Therapy in Mental Health, 11*, 173-195.

Zisserman, L. (1981). The modern family and rehabilitation of the handicapped: A macrosociological view. *American Journal of Occupational Therapy, 35*, 13-20.

Evaluations

Allen, C.K. (1985). *Occupational Therapy for Psychiatric Diseases: Measurement and Management of Cognitive Disabilities.* Boston, MA: Little, Brown and Co.

American Occupational Therapy Association (1984). Hierarchy of competencies relating to the use of standardized instruments and evaluation techniques by occupational therapists. *American Journal of Occupational Therapy, 38*, 803-804.

Anderson, A.P. (1985). Work potential evaluation in mental health. *American Journal of Occupational Therapy, 39*, 695-663.

Asher, I.E. (1989). *An Annotated Index of Occupational Therapy Evaluation Tools.* Rockville, MD: American Occupational Therapy Association.

Backman, C. (1994). Assessment of self-care skills. In C.Christiansen (Ed). *Ways of Living: Self-care Strategies for Special Needs.* Bethesda, MD: American Occupational Therapy Association.

Barris, R., Oakley, F. & Kielhofner, G. (1987). The role checklist. In Hemphill, B.J. (1987). *Mental Health Assesment in Occupation Therapy.* Thorofare, NJ: Slack.

Benson, J. & Clark, F. (1982). A guide for insturment development and validation. *American Journal of Occupational Therapy, 36*, 783-788.

Bledsoe, N. & Shepard, J. (1982). Reliability and validity of a preschool play scale. *American Journal of Occupational Therapy, 36*, 783-788.

Bloomer, J.S. & Williams, S.K. (1987). *The Bay Area Functional Performance Evaluation, (Research Ed.).* Palo Alto, CA: Consulting Psychologists Press.

Bolton, B. (1987). *Handbook of Measurement and Evaluation in Rehabilitation.* Baltimore, MD: Paul H. Brookes.

Brayman, S. & Kirby, T. (1982). The comprehensive occupational therapy evaluation. In Hemphill, B. (Ed) (1982). *The Evaluation Process in Psychiatric Occupational Therapy.* Thorofare, NJ: Slack, Inc.

Brockett, M.M. (1987). Cultural varitations in Bay Area Functional Performance Evaluation Scores-Considerations for Occupational Therapy. *Canadian Journal of Occupational Therapy, 54 (4)*, 195-199.

Casanova, J.S. & Ferber, J. (1976). Comprehensive evaluation of basic living skills. *American Journal of Occupational Therapy, 30 (2)*, 101-105.

Christiansen, C. (1991). Occupational performance assessment. In C. Christiansen & C. Baum (Eds). *Occupational Therapy-Overcoming Human Performance Deficits.* Thorofare, NJ: Slack.

Clarke, E.N. & Peters, M. (1984). *Scorable Self-Care Evaluation.* Tucson, AZ: Therapy Skill Builders.

Denton, P. (1988). Assessing the patient's functional performance. *Hospital and Community Psychiatry, 39 (9)*, 935-936.

Dombrowski, L.B. (1990). *Functional Needs Assessment Program for Chronic Psychiatric Patients.* Tucson, AZ: Therapy Skill Builders.

Dunn, W. (1980). Evaluation of pre-schoolers. *Sensory Integration, Special Interest Section Newsletter, 3 (3)*.

Dunn, W. (1981). *A Guide to Testing Clinical Observations in Kindergartners*. Rockville, MD: The Occupational Therapy Association.

Farrell-Holtan, J. (1990). The occupational therapist's role in interdisciplinary team assessment of the cognitively impaired elderly. *Occupational Therapy in Mental Health, 10 (3)*, 53-63.

Fidler, G.S. (1982). The activity laboratory: A structure for observing and assessing perceptual, integrative and behavioral strategies. In Hemphill, B. *The Evaluation Process in Psychiatric Occupational Therapy*, (pp195-207). Thorofare, NJ: Slack Inc.

Fidler, G. (1988). The life style performance profile. In Robertson, S. (Ed) *Mental Health Focus: Skills for Assessment and Treatment*. Rockville, MD: American Occupational Therapy Association.

Fisher, A.G. (1992). Functional measures, part I: What is function, what should we measure, and how should we measure it? *American Journal of Occupational Therapy, 46 (2)*, 183-185.

Florey, L.L. & Michelman, S.M. (1982). Occupational role history: A screening tool for psychiatric occupational therapy. *The American Journal of Occupational Therapy, 36*, 301-308.

Gallo, J.J., Reichel, W. & Anderson, L. (1995). *Handbook of Geriatric Assessment*. Gaithersberg, MD: Aspen Publisher.

Good-Ellis, M.A., Fine, S.B., Spencer, J.H. & DiVittis, A. (1987). Developing a role activity performance scale. *American Journal of Occupational Therapy, 41 (4)*, 232-241.

Halpern, A.S. & Fuhrer, M.D. (Eds). *Functional Assessment in Rehaiblitation*. Baltimore, MD: Paul H. Brookes.

Hemphill, B.J. (Ed) (1982). *The Evaluation Process in Pshychiatric Occupational Therapy*. Thorofare, NJ: Slack Inc.

Hemphill, B.J. (Ed) (1988). *Mental Health Assessment in Occupational Therapy*. Thorofare, NJ: Slack Inc.

Houston, D., Williams, S.L., Bloomer, J. & Mann, W.C. (1989). The Bay Area Functional Performance Evaluation: Development and standardization. *American Journal of Occupationnal Therapy, 43 (3)*, 170-183.

Intagliata, S. & Sullivan, B. (1991). Development and implementation of the Rehabilitation Institute of Chicago Functional Assessment Scale. *Occupational Therapy Practice, 2*, 26-37.

Jacobs, K. (1985). *Occupational Therapy: Work Related Programs and Assessments*. Boston, MA: Little, Brown, and Co.

Jackoway, I., Rogers, J. & Snow, T. (1987). The role change assessment: An interview tool for evaluating older adults. *Occupational Therapy in Mental Health, 7 (1)*, 17-38.

Johnson, T.P., Vinnecombe, B.T. & Merrill, G.W. (1980). The independent living skills evaluation. *Occupational Therapy in Mental Health, 1 (2)*, 5-18.

Kaplan, K. & Kielhofner, G. (1989). *Occupational Analysis Interview and Rating Scale*. Thorofare, NJ: Slack.

Katz, N., Itzkovich, M., Auerbach, S. & Elazar, B. (1989). Lowenstein Occupational Therapy Cognitive Assessment (LOTCA). Battery for brain-injured patients: Reliability and valididty. *American Journal of Occupational Therapy, 43*, 184-191.

Kielhofner, G. & Henry, A.D. (1988). Development and investigation of the occupational performance history interview. *American Journal of Occupational Therapy, 42 (8)*, 489-498.

Kielhofner, G., Henry, A. & Walens, D. (1989). *A User's Guide to the Occupational Therapy Performance History Interview*. Rockville, MD: American Occupational Therapy Association.

King, L.J. (1982). The person symbol as an assessment tool. In Hemphill, B.J. (Ed). *The Evaluation Process in Psychiatric Occupational Therapy*, (pp.169-194). Thorofare, NJ: Slack.

King-Thomas, L. & Hacker, B.J. (1987). *A Therapist's Guide to Pediatric Assessment*. Boston, MA: Little, Brown and Co.

Kohlman-Thomas, L. (1992). *KELS: The Kolman Evaluation of Living Skills*. Rockville, MD: American Occupational Therapy Association.

Law, M. & Letts, L. (1989). A critical review of the scales of activities of daily living. *American Journal of Occupational Therapy, 43*, 522-528.

Lawton, M.P. & Brody, E. (1969). Assessment of older people: Self maintaining and instrumental activities of daily living. *Gerontologist, 9*, 179-186.

Leonardelli, C.A. (1988a). The Milwaukee evaluation of daily living skills (MEDLS). In B. Hemphill (Ed). *Mental Health Assessment in Occupational Therapy*, (pp.151-162). Thorofare, NJ: Slack.

Leonardelli, C.A. (1988b). *The Milwaukee Evaluation of Daily Living Skills: Evaluation in Long-term Psychiatric Care*. Thorofare, NJ: Slack.

Lerner, C. (1979). The magazine picture collage: Its clinical use and validity as an assessment device. *American Journal of Occupational Therapy, 33 (8)*, 500-504.

Lerner, C. & Ross, G. (1977). The magazine picture collage: Development of an objective scoring system.), 156-161. *American Journal of Occupational Therapy, 31 (3)*, 156-161.

Linder, T.W. (1994). *Transdisciplinary Play Assessment*. Palo Alto, CA: VORT Corporation.

Mann, W.C., Huselid, R. (1993). An abbreviated task-oriented assessment (Bay Area Funcctional Performance Evaluation). *American Journal of Occupational Therapy, 47*, 111-118.

Matheson, L. (1984). *Work Capacity Evaluation: Interdisciplinary Approach to Industrial Rehabilitation*. Trabuco Canyon, CA: Eric.

Matheson, L. & Ogden, L.D. (1983). *Work Tolerance Screening*. Trabuco Canyon, CA: Rehabilltation Institute of Southern California.

Mathews, R.M., Whang, P.L. & Fawcett, S.B. (1982). Behavioral assessment of occupational skills in learning disabled adolescents. *Journal of Learning Disabilities, 15*, 38-41.

Matsutsuyu, J. (1967). The interest checklist. *American Journal of Occupational Therapy, 32*, 628-630.

McGourty, L.K. (1988). Kohlman evaluation of living ckills. In B. Hemphill, (Ed). *Mental Health Assessment in Occupational Therapy*, (pp. 133-146). Thorofare, NJ: Slack.

Moorhead, L. (1969). The occupational history. *American Journal of Occupational Therapy, 23 (4)*, 329-334.

Oakley, F., Kielhofner, G., Barris, R. & Reichler, R. (1986). The role checklist: Development and empirical assessment of reliability. *Occupational Therapy Journal of Research, 6 (3)*, 157-170.

Peloquin, S. (1983). The development of an occupational therapy interview/therapy set procedure. *American Journal of Occupational Therapy, 37 (7)*, 457-461.

Pollock, N. (1993). Client centered assessment. *American Journal of Occupational Therapy 42*, 298-301.

Robertson, S. (Ed). *Mental Health Focus: Skills for Assessment and Treatment.* Rockville, MD: American Occupational Therapy Association.

Rogers, J.C., Holm, M.B., Goldstein, G., McCue, M. & Nussbaum, P.D. (1994). Stability and change in functional assessment of patients with geropsychiatric disorders. *American Journal of Occupational Therapy, 48*, 914-918.

Rogers, J.C. & Masagatani, G. (1982). Clinical reasoning of occupational therapists during the initial assessment of physically disabled patients. *Occupational Therapy Journal of Research, 2*, 195-219.

Scholle-Maritn, S. (1987). Application of the model of human occupation: Assessment in child and adolescent psychiatry. *Occupational Therapy in Mental Health, 7 (2)*, 3-22.

Shaw, C. (1982). The interview process. In Hemphill, B.J. (Ed). *The Evaluation Process in Psychiatric Occupational Therapy*, (pp.15-42). Thorofare, NJ: Slack Inc.

Sheer, S.J. (1990). *Multidisciplinary Perspectives in Vocational Assessment of Impaired Workers.* Rockville, MD: Aspen Publishers.

Smith, R.O. (1990). Administration and Scoring Manuel. *OT Fact (Occupational Therapy Functional Assessment Compilation Tool).* Rockville, MD: The American Occupational Therapy Association, Inc.

Spencer, J.C. (1987). Environmental assessment strategies. *Topics in Geriatric Rehabilitation, 3 (1)*, 35-41.

Takata, N. (1969). The play history. *American Journal of Occupational Therapy, 23*, 314-318.

VORT Corporation. (1995). *HELP: The Hawaii Early Learning Profile.* Palo Alto, CA: Author.

Watts, J.H., Kielhofner, G., Bauer, D.F., Gregory, M.D. & Valentine, D.B. (1986). The assessment of occupational functioning: A screening tool for use in long-term care. *American Journal of Occupational Therapy, 14*, 65-69, 79.

Weggs, L.S. (1960). Eleanor Clarke Slagle lecture: The essentials of work evaluation. *American Journal of Occupational Therapy, 40 (4)*, 231-240.

Whagner, A.D., Myers, A.C., Blazer, D.G., & Matteson, M.A. (1984). *Mental Health Assessment and Therapeutic Intervention with Older Adults.* Rockville, MD: Aspen Publishers.

Williams, S.L. & Bloomer, J. (1987). *Bay Area Functional Performance Evaluation Administration and Scoring Manuel. (2nd ed).* Palo Alto: Consulting Psychologists Press.

Witt, P. & Ellis, G. (1985). *The Leisure Diagnostic Battery: Users Manuel and Sample Forms.* State College, PA: Venture Publishing Inc.

Yerxa, E.J., Burnett-Bualieu, S., Stocking, J.S. & Azen, S.P. (1988). Development of the satisfaction with performance scaled questionaire. *American Journal of Occupational Therapy, 42 (4)*, 215-221.

Historical and Philosophical Foundations of Occupational Therapy

Allen, C.K. (1987). Activity: Occupational therapy's treatment method. American *Journal of Occupational Therapy, 41 (9)*, 563-575.

American Occupational Therapy Association (1987). *Occupational Therapy: Directions for the Future.* Rockville, MD: American Occupational Therapy Association.

American Occupational Therapy Association (1979). Resolution D, # 532-79, Occupation as the common core of occupational therapy. *American Journal of Occupational Therapy, 33*, 785.

Azima, H. & Azima, F. (1959). Outline of a dynamic theory of occupational therapy. *American Journal of Occupational Therapy, 8 (5)*, 215.

Barris, R., Kielhofner, G. & Watts, J. (1988). *Bodies of Knowledge in Psychosocial Practice.* Thorofare, NJ: Slack.

Bing, R.K. (1967). William Rush Dunton, Jr.: American psychiatrist and occupational therapist, 1986-1966. *American Journal of Occupational Therapy, 21 (3)*, 172-175.

Bockhoven, J.S. (1971). Legacy of moral treatment-1800s to 1910. *American Journal of Occupational Therapy, 25*, 223-225.

Bowman, I. (1985). *Guide of the Archives of the American Occupational Therapy Association.* Rockville, MD: American Occupational Therapy Association.

Brienes, E.B. (1995). Evaluation, adaptation and culture. In C.B. Royeen (Ed). *The Practice of the Future: Putting Occupation Back into Therapy, (Lesson 9)* (pp. 5-27). Bethesda, MD: American Occupational Therapy Association.

Bienes, E.B. (1995). *Occupational Therapy Activities from Clay to Computers: Theory and Practice.* Philadelphia, PA: F.A. Davis.

Brienes, E.B. (1986). *Origins and Adaptations: A Philosophy of Practice.* Lebanon, NJ: Seri-Rehab.

Brienes, E.B. (1990). Genesis of occupations: A philosophical model for therapy. *Australian Occupational Therapy Journal, 37*, 45-49.

Brown, M. & Ellis, R.K. (1986). Purposeful activities: Yesterday, today and tomorrow. *Physical Disabilities Special Interest Section Newsletter, 9 (4)*, 4-5. Rockville, MD: American Occupational Therapy Association.

Bruce, M. & Borg, B. (1987). *Frames of Reference in Psychosocial Occupational Therapy.* Thorofare, NJ: Slack.

Burke, J.P. (1983). Defining occupation: Importing and organizing interdisciplinary knowledge. In G. Kiehofner (Ed). *Health Through Occupation: Theory and Practice in Occupational Therapy,* (pp.125-138). Philadelphia, PA: F.A. Davis.

Charmaz, K. (1991). *Good Days, Bad Days: The Self in Chronic Illness and Time.* New Brunswick, NJ: Rutgers University.

Christiansen, C. (1994). *Ways of Living: Self-care Strategies for Special Needs.* Rockville, MD: American Occupational Therapy Association.

Christiansen, C.H. & Bauman, C.M. (Eds) (1991). *Occupational Therapy: Overcoming Human Performance Deficits.* Thorofare, NJ: Slack.

Clark, F. (1993). Occupational embedded in a real life: Interweaving occupational science and occupational therapy: 1993 Eleanor Clark Slagle Lecture. *American Journal of Occupational Therapy, 57*, 1067-1078.

Clark, F., Parham, D., Carlson, M., Frank, G., Jackson, J., Pierce, D., Wolfe, R. & Zemke, R. (1991). Occupational Science: Academic innovation in the service of occupational therapy's future. *American Journal of Occupational Therapy, 45*, 300-310.

Cracknell, E. (1993). To do is to be. *British Journal of Occupational Therapy, 56*, 391.

Csikzentmihalyi, M. (1990). *Flow.* New York, NY: Harper and Row.

Diasio-Serett, K. (1985). Another look at occupational therapy's history: Paradigm of pair-of-hands? *Occupational Therapy in Mental Health, 5,* 1-31.

Driver, M.F. (1968). A philosophic view of the history of occupational therapy in Canada. *Canadian Journal of Occupational Therapy, 35*, 53-60.

Dunton, W.R. (1918). The principles of occupational therapy. *Public Health Nursing, 10,* 316-321.

Dunton, W.R. (1926). An historical note. *Occupational Therapy and Rehabilitation, 5 (6)*, 427-439.

Dunton, W.R. (1928). *Prescribing Occupational Therapy for Nurses.* Springfield, IL: Charles C. Thomas.

Dunton, W.R. (1931). Occupational therapy. *Occupational Therapy and Rehabilitation, 10 (2)*, 113-121.

Early, M.B. (1987). *Mental Health Concepts and Techniques for the Occupational Therapy Assistant.* New York, NY: Raven Press.

Englehardt, H.T. (1977). Defining occupational therapy: The meaning of therapy and the virtues of occupation. *American Journal of Occupational Therapy 31 (10)*, 675-690.

Fidler, G. & Fidler, J. (1963). *Occupational Therapy: A Communication Process in Psychiatry.* New York, NY: Macmillan Co.

Fike, M.L. (1984). The role of occupational therapy in psychological rehabilitation of the physically disabled. In *Rehabilitation Psychology*, (pp. 221-223). Rockville, MD: Aspen Systems Corporation.

Haas, L.J. (1924). One hundred years of occupational therapy, a local history. *Archives of Occupational Therapy 3*, 83-100.

Hagedorn, R. (1992). *Occupational Therapy: Foundations for Practice: Models, Frames of Reference and Core Skills.* New York, NY: Churchill.

Hall, H.J. (1923). *O.T. a New Profession.* Concord: Rumford Press.

Henderson, A. (1988). Occupational therapy knowledge: From practice to theory. *American Journal of Occupational Therapy, 42 (9)*, 567-576.

Jung, C. (1964). *Man and His Symbols.* New York, NY: Doubleday.

Kielhofner, G. (1978). General system theory: Implications for the theory and action in occupational therapy. American Journal of Occupational Therapy, 32, 637-645.

Kielhofner, G. (1982). A heritage of activity: Development of theory. *American Journal of Occupational Therapy, 36 (11)*, 723-730.

Kielhofner, G. (Ed) (1983). *Health Through Occupation: Theory and Practice in Occupational Therapy.* Philadelphia, PA: F.A. Davis.

Kielhofner, G. (1985). *A Model of Human Occupation: Theory and Application.* Baltimore, MD: Williams and Wilkins.

Kielhofner, G. (1988). Occupational therapy-base in occupation (pp.84-92). In Hopkins, H. & Smith, H. (Eds). *Willard & Spackman's Occupational Therapy.* Philadelphia, PA: J.B. Lippincott.

Kielhofner, G. & Burke, J.P. (1977). Occupational therapy after 60 years: An account of changing identity and knowledge. *American Journal of Occupational Therapy, 31*, 675-689.

Kielhofner, G. (1978). General system theory: Implications for the theory and action in occupational therapy. *American Journal of Occupational Therapy, 32*, 637-645.

Jackson, M. (1993). From work to therapy: The changing politics of occupation in the twentieth century. *British Journal of Occupational Therapy, 56*, 360-364.

Kleinman, B.L. & Bulkley, B.L. (1982). Some implications of a science of adaptive responses. *American Journal of Occupational Therapy, 36 (1)*, 15-19.

Levine, R. & Bravyley, C.R. (1991). Occupation as a therapeutic medium. In C. Christiansen & C. Baum (Eds). *Occupational Therapy: Overcoming Human Performance Deficits*, (pp. 592-631). Thorofare, NJ: Slack.

Licht, S. (1947a). William Rush Dunton, Jr. *Occupational Therapy and Rehabilitation, 26 (2)*, 47-52.

Licht, S. (1947b). The objectives of occupational therapy. *Occupational Therapy and Rehabilitation, 26 (1)*, 17-22.

Llorens, L. (1984). Theoretical conceptualizations of occupational therapy: 1960-1982. *Occupational Therapy in Mental Health, 4*, 1-14.

Lyons, B.G. (1983). Purposeful versus human activity. *American Journal of Occupational Therapy, 37 (7)*, 493-498.

McColl, M.A., Law, M. & Stewart, D. (). *Theoretical Basis of Occupational Therapy: An Annotated Bibliography of Applied Theory in the Professional Literature.* Thorofare, NJ: Slack, Inc.

Marshall, E.M. (1985). Looking back. *American Journal of Occupational Therapy, 39*, 297-300.

Mayer, M.A. (1988). Analysis of information processing and cognitive disability theory. *American Journal of Occupational Therapy, 42*, 176-183.

Mosey, A. (1970). *Three Frames of Reference for Mental Health.* Thorofare, NJ: Slack.

Mosey, A.C. (1974). An alternative: The biopsychosocial model. *American Journal of Occupational Therapy, 28 (3)*, 137-140.

Mosey, A.C. (1981). *Occupational Therapy: Configuration of a Profession.* New York, NY: Raven Press.

Mosey, A.C. (1985). A monistic of pluralistic approach to professional identity. *Amercian Journal of Occupational Therapy, 39 (8)*, 504-509.

Mosey, A. (1986). *Psychosocial Components of Occupational Therapy.* New York, NY: Raven Press.

Reed, K.L. (1993). The beginnings of occupational therapy. In H.L. Hopkins & H.D. Smith (Eds). *Willard and Spackman's Occupa-*

tional Therapy, (8th Edition), (pp.26-43). Philadelphia, PA: Lippincott.

Reed, K.L. (1984). *Models of Practice in Occupational Therapy.* Baltimore, MD: Williams & Wilkins.

Reed, K. & Sanderson, S.R. (1980). *Concepts of Occupational Therapy.* Baltimore, MD: Williams & Wilkins.

Reilly, M. (1977). A response to: Defining occupational therapy: The meaning of therapy and the virtues of occupation. *American Journal of Occupational Therapy, 31,* 673-674.

Reilly, M. (1971). The modernization of occupational therapy. *American Journal of Occupational Therapy, 25,* 243-246.

Reilly, M. (1966). The challenge of the future to an occupational therapist. *American Journal of Occupational Therapy, 20,* 221-225.

Rogers, J.C. (1982a). Order and disorder in medicine and occupational therapy. *American Journal of Occupational Therapy, 36,* 29-35.

Rogers, J.C. (1982b). The spirit of independence: The evolution of a philosophy. *American Journal of Occupational Therapy, 36,* 709-715.

Sands, I. (1928). When is occupation curative? *Occupational Therapy and Rehabilitation, 7,* 115-122.

Schultz, S. & Schakade, J.K. (1992). Occupational adaptation: Toward a holistic approach for contemporary practice, part 2. *American Journal of Occupational Therapy, 46,* 917-925.

Shannon, P.D. (1986). Philosophical considerations for the practice of occupational therapy. In Ryan, S.E. (Ed). *The Certified Occupational Therapy Assistant: Roles and Responsibilities,* (pp. 38-44). Thorofare, NJ: Slack.

Shannon, P.D. (1977). The derailment of occupational therapy. *American Journal of Occupational Therapy, 31 (4),* 229-234.

Slagle, E.C. (1914). History of the development of occupation for the insane. *Maryland Psychiatric Quarterly, 4 (1),* 14-20.

Slagle, E.C. (1917). The Department of Occupational Therapy. *Institutional Quarterly, 10,* 29-32.

Slagle, E.C. (1922). Training aides for mental patients. *Archives of Occupational Therapy, 1 (1),* 11-18.

Slagle, E.C. (1931). The training of occupational therapists. *Psychiatric Quarterly, 31 (5),* 12-20.

Slagle, E.C. (1934). The occupational therapy programme in the state of New York. *Journal of Mental Science, 80,* 639-649.

Slagle, E.C. (1936). Editorial: From the heart. *Occupational Therapy and Rehabilitation, 16 (6),* 343-345.

Slagle, E.C. (1938). Occupational therapy. *Trained Nurse and Hospital Review, 100,* 375-382.

Smith, M.B. (1974). Competence and adaptation: A perspecitve on therapeutic ends and means. *American Journal of Occupational Therapy, 28 (1),* 11-15.

Spackman, C.S. (1967). The World Federation of Occupational Therapists. *American Journal of Occupational Therapy 21,* 301-309.

Tracy, S.E. (1912). *Studies in Invalid Occupation: A Manual for Nurses and Attendants.* Boston, MA: Whitcomb and Burrows.

West, W.L. (1984). A reaffirmed philosophy and practice of occupational therapy for the 1980s. *Amercian Journal of Occupational Therapy, 38,* 15-23.

White, R.W. (1959). Motivation reconsidered: The concept of competence. *Psychological Review, 66,* 297-233.

White, R.W. (1971). The urge toward competence. *American Journal of Occupational Therapy, 25,* 271-274.

Wish-Baratz, S. (1989). Looking back: Bird T. Baldwin: A holistic scientist in occupational therapy's history. *American Journal of Occupational Therapy, 43,* 257-260.

Woodside, H. (1976). Dimensions of the occupational behavior model. *Canadian Journal of Occupational Therapy 43,* 11.

Woodside, H.H. (1971). Occupational therapy: A historical perspective: The development of occupational therapy-1910-1929. *American Journal of Occupational Therapy, 25,* 226-230.

Yerxa, E.J. (1967). Authentic occupational therapy. *American Journal of Occupational Therapy 21,* 1-9.

Yerxa, E. (1978). The philosophical base of occupational therapy. *In Occupational therapy: 2001 A.D.* Rockville, MD: American Occupational Therapy Association.

Yerxa, E. (1988). Oversimplification: The hobgoblin of theory and practice in occupational therapy. *Canadian Journal of Occupational Therapy, 55 (1),* 5-6.

Yerxa, E.J. (1992). Some implications of occupational therapy's history for epistemology, values and relation to medicine. *American Journal of Occupational Therapy, 46,* 79-83.

Young, M.E. & Quinn. (1992). *Theories and Principles of Occupational Therapy.* New York, NY: Chruchill Livingston.

Rehabilitative Equipment, Technological Aids and Environmental Modifications

Adaptive Environments Center (1981). *Environments for All Children.* Washington, DC: National Center for a Barrier Free Environment.

American Association of Retired Persons (1985). *Your Home, Your Choice: A Workbook for Older People and Their Families.* Washington, DC: Author.

American Insititute of Architects Foundation (1985). *Design For Aging: An Architect's Guide.* Washington, DC: The AIA Press.

American National Standards Institute, Inc (1986). *American National Standard for Buildings and Facilities Providing Accessiblity and Usability for Physically Handicapped People.* New York, NY: American National Standards Institute.

American Occupational Therapy Association (1989). *Technology Review '89: Perspecitves on Occupational Therapy Practice.* Rockville, MD: Author.

Anderson, H. (1981). *The Disabled Homemaker.* Springfield, Il: Charles C. Thomas.

Angelo, J. & Smith, R.O. (1989). The critical role of occupational therapy in augmentative communication services. In American Occupational Therapy Association, *Technology Review '89: Perspectives on Occupational Therapy Practice,* (pp. 49-54). Rockville, MD: AOTA.

Architecture and Transportation Barriers Compliance Board (1985). *Uniform Federal Accessibility Standards.* Washington, DC.

Bailey, R.W. (1989). *Human Performance Engineering, 2nd Edition.* Englewood Cliffs, NJ: Prentice Hall.

Bain, B.K. (1989). Assessment of clients for technological assistive devices. In American Occupational Therapy Association, *Technology Review '89: Perspectives on Occupational Therapy Practice,* (pp. 55-59). Rockville, MD: AOTA.

Barnes, M.R. & Crutchfield, C.A. (1994). *Patient at Home: A Manual for Exercise Programs, Self-help Devices, and Home Care Products, 2nd Edition.* Thorofare, NJ: Slack, Inc.

Batt, R.C. & Lounsbury, P.A. (1990). Teaching the patient with cognitive deficits to use a computer. *American Journal of Occupational Therapy, 44,* 364-367.

Batavia, A., DeJong, C., Eckenhoff, E. & Materson, R. (1990). After the Americans with Disabilities Act: The role of the rehabilitation community. *Archives of Physical Medicine and Rehabilitation, 71,* 1014-1015.

Bednar, M.J. (1982). *Barrier-free Environments.* New York, NY: Van Nostrand Rheinhold.

Blackman, J.A. (Ed) (1995). *Technology in Early Intervention.* Frederick, MD: Acpen

Blackstone, S.W. (1986). *Augmentative Communication. An Introduction.* Rockville, MD: American Speech Language-Hearing Association.

Borden, P.A. & Vanderheiden, G.C. (Eds) (1988). *Rehab/education Resourcebook Series Update.* Madison, WI: University of Wisconsin, Trace R & D Center Reprint Service.

Brandenburg, S.A. & Vanderheinden, G.C. (Eds) (1987a). *Rehab/education Resourcebook Series: Resource Book 1 Communication Aids.* Boston, MA: Little, Brown, and Company.

Brandenburg, S.A. & Vanderheinden, G.C. (Eds) (1987b). *Rehab/education resourcebook series: Resource Book 2 Switches, Training, and Environmental Control.* Boston, MA: Little, Brown, and Company.

Brandenburg, S.A. & Vanderheinden, G.C. (Eds) (1987c). *Rehab/education Resourcebook Series: Resource Book 3 Software and Hardware.* Boston, MA: Little, Brown, and Company.

Browkaw, E.H. (1984). Adaptation of media. *The American Journal of Occupational Therapy, 2 (2),* 77.

Burges, J.H. (1986). *Designing for Humans: The Human Actor in Engineering.* Princeton, NJ: Petrocelli Books.

Campbell, C.L. (1986). Introduction: Robotics and the disabled. In F.L. Cromwell (Ed). *Computer Applications in Occupational Therapy,* (pp. 93-98). New York, NY: The Haworth Press.

Cary, J.R. (1978). *How to Create Interiors for the Disabled.* New York, NY: Pantheon Books.

Church, G. and Glennen, S. (1992). *The Handbook of Assistive Technology.* San Diego, CA: Singular Publishing Company.

Clark, E.N. (Ed) (1986). *Microcomputers: Clinical Applications.* Thorofare, NJ: Slack.

Cochran, W. (1981). Restrooms. *Access Information Bulletin.* Washington, DC: National Center for a Barrier Free Environment.

Cohen, U. & Weissman, G.D. (1991). *Holding on to Home: Designing Environments for People with Dementia.* Baltimore, MD: John Hopkins Press.

Cohen, U. & Day, K. (1993). *Contemporary Environments for People with Dementia.* Baltimore, MD: John Hopkins Press.

Coleman, C.L. (Ed) (1988). *Action Augmentative Communicatioon Training Modules.* Sacramento, CA: Assistive Device Center.

Colvin, M. & Korn, T. (1984). Eliminating barriers to the disabled. *American Journal of Occupational Therapy, 38 (11),* 748-753.

Cook, A.M. & Hussey, S.M. (1995). *Assistive Technologies: Principles and Practice.* St. Louis, MO: Mosby.

Cromwell, F.S. (Ed) (1986). *Computer Applications in Occupational Therapy.* New York, NY: The Haworth Press.

Dickey, R. & Shealey, S.H. (1987). Using technology to control the environment. *The American Journal of Occupational Therapy, 41 (11),* 722-725.

Dickman, I.R. (1983). *Making Life more Livable: Simple Adaptaions for th Homes of Blind and Visually Impaired Older People.* New York, NY: American Foundation for the Blind.

Eastman Kodak Company (1983). *Ergonomic Design for People at Work, Vol. 1.* New York, NY: Van Nostrand Reinhold Company.

Ellek, D. (1991). The Americans with Disabilities Act of 1990. *American Journal of Occupational Therapy, 45 (2),* 177-179.

Enders, A. (1989). *Assistive Technology Sourcebook.* Bothesda, MD: RESNA Press.

Federal Register (1988). *Technology Related Assistance for Individuals with Disabilities Act of 1988,* PL 100-407.

Finkley, E. (1988). Occupational therapy in augmentative communication. *Occupational Therapy News, 42 (5),* 14-15.

Fishman, I. (1987). *Electronic Communication Aids.* Boston, MA: College-Hill Press.

Garee, B.E. (1979). *Ideas for Making Your Home Accessible.* Bloomington, IL: Cheever Publishing.

Gay, K. (1986). *Ergonomics: Making Products and Places fit People.* Hillside, NJ: Enslow Publishers.

Gilfoyle, M. Elnora, D/Sc, OTR, FAOTR, Grady, Ann P., MA, OTR, FAOTR, & Moore, Josephine, C., PhD, OTR, FATR. (1993). *Children Adapt a Theory of Sensorimotor-Sensory Development, Second Edition.* Thorofare, NJ: Slack, Inc.

Gilkeson, G.E. & Krouskop, T.A. (1987). A Master's degree program in occupational therapy with a rehabilitation technology focus. *The American Journal of Occupational Therapy, 41 (11),* 22.

Glass, K. & Hall, K. (1987). Occupational therapists' views about th use of robotic aids for people with disabilities. *The American Journal of Occupational Therapy 41 (11),* 745-747.

Goldenberg, E.P. (1979). *Special Technology for Special Children.* Baltimore, MD: University Park Press.

Goldsmith, S. (1976). *Designing for the Disabled, (3rd ed).* London: RIBA Publications Limited.

Grandjean, E. (1971). *Fitting the Task to the Man- An Ergonomic Approach.* London: RIBA Publications Limited.

Hale, G. (Ed) (1979). *The Source Book for the Disabled.* London: Imprint Books, Ltd.

Hall, M. (1987). Unlocking information technology. *The American Journal of Occupational Therapy, 41 (11),* 722-725.

Hayden, M.J. (1992). Disability awareness workshop: Helping businesses comply with the Americans with Disabilities Act of 1990. *American Journal of Occupational Therapy, 46*, 461-465.

Hopf, P. & Raeber, J. (1984). *Access for the Handicapped: The Barrier-free Regulations for Design and Construction in all 50 States*. New York, NY: Van Nostrand Reinhold Company.

Hussey, S.M. (Ed) (1991). Developmental Disabilities. *Special Interest Section Newsletter Special Issue on Assistive Technology*. Rockville, MD: American Occupational Therapy Association.

Kailes, J.I. & Jones, D. (1993). *A Guide to Planning Accessible Meetings*. Houston, TX: ILRU Research and Training Center on Independent Living.

Kiewel, H. (1986). Ramps, Stairs, and Floor Treatments. *Access Informantion Bulletin*. Washington, DC: Paralyzed Vetrans of America.

Lebonvich, W.L. (1993). *Design for Dignity: Studies in Accessibility*. Sommerset, NJ: John Wiley and Sons.

Lee, K.S. & Thomas, D.J. (1990). *Control of Computer Based Technology for People with Disabilities*. Toronto, Canada: University of Toronto Press.

Meredith Corp. (1981). *The Accessible Home: Remodeling Concerns for the Disabled*. Better Homes and Gardens Remodeling Ideas, July, 65-79.

Mancuso, L.L. (1990). Reasonable accomodations for workers with psychiatric disabilities. *Prosocial Rehabilitation Journal, 14*, 3-19.

Mayall, J. & Desharnais, G. (1994). *Positioning in an Wheelchair: A Guide for Professional Caregivers of the Disabled Adults, 2nd Edition*. Thorofare, NJ: Slack, Inc.

Parker, M.G., Thorslund, M. (1991). The use of technical aids among community based elderly. *American Journal of Occupational Therapy, 45 (8)*, 712-718.

Raschko, B. (1982). *Housing Interiors for the Disabled and Elderly*. New York, NY: Van Nostrand Reinhold Company.

Reichle, J., York, J. & Sigafoos, J. (1991). *Implementing Augmentative and Alternative Communication: Strategies for Learners with Severe Disabilities*. Baltimore, MD: Paul H. Brookes Publishing Company.

Sandler, A., Thruman, S., Meddock, T. & DuCette, J. (1985). Effects of environmental modifications on the behavior of persons with severe handicaps. *Journal of the Association for Persons with Severe Handicaps, 10 (3)*, 157-163.

Skolaski-Pellitteri, T. (1983). Environmental adapations which compensate for dementia. *Physical and Occupational Therapy in Geriatrics, 3*, 25-32.

Skolaski-Pellitteri, T. (1984). Environmental intervention for the demented person. *Physical and Occupational Therapy in Geriatrics, 3*, 25-32.

Smith, R.O. (1991). Technological approaches to performance enhancement. In C. Christiansen and C. Baum (Eds). *Occupational Therapy, Overcoming Human Performance Deficits*. Thorofare, NJ: Slack.

Sorensen, R. (1979). *Design for Accessibility*. New York, NY: McGraw-Hill Book Company.

Stockdell, S.M. & Crawfork, M.S. (1992). An industrial model for assisting enployers to comply with the Americans with Disabilities Act of 1990. *American Journal of Occupational Therapy 46*, 427-433.

Technology-Related Assistance for Individuals with Disabilities (ACT) (1988). (Public Law 100-407), 29 USC 2202.

U.S. Consumer Product Safety Commission (1986). *Safety for Older Consumers*. Washington, DC: U.S. Consumer Product Safety Commission.

U.S. Departments of Education (1987, October). *Access to Information by Users with Disabilities: Initial Guide*. Washington, DC: Author.

Vanderheiden, G.C. (1987). Service delivery mechanisms in rehabilitation technology. *American Journal of Occupational Therapy, 41*, 703-710.

Verville, R. (1990). The Americans with Disabilities Act: An analysis. Archives of *Physical Medicine and Rehabilitation, 71*, 1010-1013.

Webster, J.B. & Cook, A.M. (Eds) (1979). *Clinical Engineering: Principles and Practices*. Englewood Cliffs, NJ: Prentice Hall.

Webster, J.G., Cook, A.M., Tompkins, W.J. & Vanderheiden, G.C. (Ed) (1985). *Electronic Devices for Rehabilitation*. New York, NY: John Wiley & Sons.

Wittmeyer, M. & Barrett, J.E. (1980). *Housing Accessibility Checklist*. Seattle, WA: University of Washington Press.

Wittmeyer, M.B. & Stolov, W.C. (1978). Educating wheelchair patients on home architectural barriers. *American Journal of Occupational Therapy, 32*, 557.

Wylde, M., Baron-Robbins, A. & Clark, S. (1994). *Building for a Lifetime: The Design and Construction of Fully Accessible Homes*. Newton, CT: Taunton Press.

Young, H. & Tornyay, R. (1995). *Choices Making a Good Move to a Retirement Community*. Thorofare, NJ: Slack, Inc.

Research: Applied Scientific Inquiry in Purposeful Activity

Adelstein, L.A. & Nelson, D.L. (1985). Effects of sharing versus non-sharing on affective meaning in collage activities. *Occupational Therapy in Mental Health, 5*, 29-45.

Bakaski, R., Bhambhani, Y. & Madill, H. (1991). The effects of task preference on performance during purposeful and nonpurposeful activities. *American Journal of Occupational Therapy, 45*, 912-916.

Banning, M.R. & Nelson, D.L. (1987). The effects of activity-elicited humor and group structure on group cohesion and affective responses. *American Journal of Occupational Therapy, 41*, 510-514.

Barlow, D.H., Hayes, S.C. & Nelson, R.O. (1984). *The Scientist-Practitioner: Research and Accountability in Clinical Settings*. New York, NY: Pergamon.

Block, M.W., Smith, D.A. & Nelson, D.L. (1989). Heart rate, activity, duration and affect in added purpose versus single purpose jumping activities. *American Journal of Occupational Therapy, 43*, 25-30.

Boyer, J., Colman, N., Levy, L. & Manoly, B. (1989). Affective responses to activities: A comparative study. *American Journal of Occupational Therapy, 43*, 81-88.

Bundy, A.C., Pendergast, N., Steffan, J.A. & Thorn, D. (1990). *Reviews of Selected Literature on Occupation and Health.* Rockville, MD: American Occupational Therapy Association.

Carter, B.A., Nelson, D.L. & Duncombe, L.W. (1983). The effect of psychological type on the mood and meaning of two collage activities. *American Journal of Occupational Therapy, 39*, 688-693.

Christiansen, C.H. (1981). Toward resolution of crisis: Research requisites in occupational therapy. *Occupational Therapy Journal of Research, 1 (2)*, 115-124.

Christiansen, C.H. (1986). Research: An economic imperative. *Occupational Therapy Journal of Research, 3*, 195-198.

Christiansen, C.H. (1986). Research as reclamation. *Occupational Therapy Journal of Research, 6*, 323-326.

Clark, F. (1993). Occupation embedded in real life: Interweaving occupational science and occupational therapy: 1993 Eleanor Clark Slagle lecture. *American Journal of Occupational Therapy, 47*, 1067-1078.

Creighton, C. (1988, April 28). Therapeutic activities study shows free time unfulfilling for many. *OT Week, 2*, 16.

DeCarlo, J.J. & Mann, W.C. (1985). The effectiveness of verbal versus groups in improving self perceptions of interpersonal communication skills. *American Journal of Occupational Therapy, 39*, 20-27.

DeKuiper, W.P., Nelson, D.L. & White, B.E. (1993). Materials-based occupation vs. Imagery vs. rote exercise: A replication and extension. *Occupational Therapy Journal of Research, 13*, 183-197.

Dunton, W.R. (1934). The need and value of research in occupational therapy. *Archives of Occupational Therapy, 13 (6)*, 325.

Fahl, M.A. (1970). Emotionally disturbed children: Effects of cooperative and competitive activity on peer interaction. *American Journal of Occupational Therapy, 24*, 31-33.

Gilfoyle, E.M. & Christiansen, C.H. (1987). Research: The quest for truth and the key to excellence. *American Journal of Occupational Therapy, 41*, 7-9.

Gillette, N. (1979). Practice, education and research. In American Occupational Therapy Association. *Occupational Therapy: 2001 A.D.* (pp.18-25). Rockville, MD: Author.

Grady, A.P. (1987). Naturally speaking-Research: Its role in enforcing the professional image. *American Journal of Occupational Therapy, 41*, 415-420.

Hasselkus, B.R. (1991). Qualitative research: Not another orthodoxy. *Occupational Therapy Journal of Research, 11 (1)*, 3-7.

Heck, S.A. (1988). The effect of purposeful activity on pain tolerance. *American Journal of Occupational Therapy, 42*, 577-581.

Jacobshagen, I. (1990). The effect of interruption of activity on affect. *Occupational Therapy in Mental Health, 10 (2)*, 35-46.

Johnson, E. (Ed) (1990). *Readings in Occupational Therapy Research.* Rockville, MD: American Occupational Therapy Association.

Katz, N. & Cohen, E. (1991). Meaning ascribed to four craft activities before and after extensive learning. *Occupational Therapy Journal of Research, 11*, 24-39.

Kazdin, A.E. (Ed) (1992). *Methodological Issues and Strategies in Clinical Research.* Washington, DC: American Psychological Association.

Kielhofner, G. & Takata, N. (1980). A study of mentally retarded person: Applied research in occupational therapy. *American Journal of Occupational Therapy, 34*, 252-258.

Kircher, M.A. (1984). Motivation as a factor of perceived exertion in purposeful versus nonpurposeful activity. *American Journal of Occupational Therapy, 38*, 165-170.

Kleinman, B.L. & Stalcup, A. (1991). The effect of a graded craft activities on visual motor integration in an inpatient child psychiatry population. *American Journal of Occupational Therapy, 45*, 324-330.

Kremer, E.R.H., Nelson, D.L. & Duncombe, L.W. (1984). Effects of selected activities on affective meaning in psychiatric clients. *American Journal of Occupational Therapy, 38*, 522-528.

LaMore, K.L. & Nelson, D.L. (1993). The effects of options on performance of an art project in adults with mentla disabilities. *American Journal of Occupational Therapy, 47*, 397-401.

Lang, E.M., Nelson, D.L. & Bush, M.A. (1992). Comparison of performance in materials-based occupation, imagery-based occupation, and rote exercise in nursing home residents. *American Journal of Occupational Therapy, 46*, 607-611.

Licht, B.C. & Nelson, D.L. (1990). Adding meaning to a design copy task through representational stimuli. *American Journal of Occupational Therapy, 44*, 408-413.

Line, J. (1969). Case method as a scientific form of clinical thinking. *American Journal of Occupational Therapy, 23*, 308-313.

Llorens, L.A. (1993). Activity analysis: Agreement between participants and observers on perceived factor in occupational components. *Occupational Therapy Journal of Research, 13 (3)*, 198-211.

MacRae, A. (1993). An overview of theory and research on hallucinations: Implications for occupational therapy. In R.P. Cottrell (Ed). *Psychosocial Occupational Therapy: Proactive Approaches*, (pp. 401-409). Rockville, MD: American Occupational Therapy Association.

Malkin, M. & Hons, C.Z. (1993). *Research in Therapeutic Recreation: Concepts and Methods.* State College, PA: Venture Publishing.

Marks, R.G. (1987). Statistical design considerations to incorporate into published research articles. *Occupational Therapy in Mental Health, 7 (3)*, 37-53.

Maurer, T.L., Smith, D.A. & Armetta, C.L. (1989). Single purpose vs. added purpose activity: Performance comparisons with chronic schizophrenics. *Occupational Therapy in Mental Health, 9 (3)*, 9-20.

Miller, L. & Nelson, D.L. (1987). Dual-purpose activity versus single-purpose activity in terms of duration on task, exertion level, and affect. *Occupational Therapy in Mental Health, 7*, 55-67.

Mitcham, M.D. (1985). *Integrating research into Occupational Therapy.* Rockville, MD: American Occupational Therapy Foundation.

Morton, S.G., Barnett, D.W. & Hale, L.S. (1992). Comparison of performance measuure of an added-purpose task versus a single-purpose task for upper extremities. *American Journal of Occupational Therapy, 46,* 128-133.

Mosey, A.C. (1989). The proper focus of scientific inquiry in occupational therapy: Frames of reference (Editorial). *Occupational Therapy Journal of Research, 9 (4),* 195-201.

Mosey, A.C. (1992). *Applied Scientific Inquiry in the Health Professions: An Epistemological Orientation.* Bethesda, MD: American Occupational Therapy Association.

Mullins, C.S., Nelson, D.L. & Smith, D.A. (1987). Exercise through dual-purpose activity in the institutionalized elderly. *Physical and Occupational Therapy in Geriatrics, 5,* 29-39.

Mumford, M. (1974). A comparison of interpersonal skills in verbal and activity groups. *American Journal of Occupational Therapy, 28,* 281-283.

Neistadt, M.E. (1994). The effects of different treatment activities on functional fine motor coordination in adults with brain injury. *American Journal of Occupational Therapy, 48,* 877-883.

Nelson, D.L. (1993, June). The experimental analysis of occupation. *Developmental Disabilities Special Interest Section Newsletter, 16,* 7-8.

Nelson, D., Thompson, G. & Moore, J. (1982). Identification of factors affective meaning in four selected activities. *American Journal of Occupational Therapy, 36,* 505-509.

Ostrow, P.C. & Kaplan, K.L. (Eds) (1987). *Occupational Therapy in Mental Health: A Guide to Outcomes Research.* Rockville, MD: American Occupational Therapy Association.

Ostrow, P.C., Spencer, F.M. & Johnson, M. (1987). *The cost-effectiveness of Rehabilitation: A Guide to Research Relevant to Occupational Therapy.* Rockville, MD: American Occupational Therapy Association. *OT Week (1987 January) 1 (1).*

Reed, K.L. (1984). Understanding theory: The first step in learning about research. *American Journal of Occupational Therapy, 38,* 677-682.

Reilly, M. (1974). *Play as Exploratory Learning: Studies in Curiosity Behavior.* Beverly Hills, CA: Sage.

Reisman, J.E. & Blakeney, A.B. (1993). Exploring sensory integrative treatment in chronic schizophrenia. In R.P. Cottrell (Ed). *Psychosocial Occupational Therapy: Proactive Approaches,* (pp.411-419). Rockville, MD: American Occupational Therapy Association.

Rogers, J.C. & Holm, M.B. (1994). Accepting the challenge of outcome research: Examining the effectiveness of occupational therapy practice. *American Journal of Occupational Therapy, 48,* 871-876.

Royeen, C.B. (1988). *Philosophy and Methodologies of Research Tradition in Occupational Therapy: Process, Philosophy and Status.* Thorofare, NJ: Slack.

Royeen, C.B. (1989). *Clinical Research Handbook: An Analysis for the Service Professions.* Thorofare, NJ: Slack.

Schwartzberg, S.L., Howe, M.C. & McDermott (1982). A comparison of three treatment group formats for facilitating social interaction. *Occupational Therapy in Mental Health, 2,* 1-16.

Sefton, J. & Mummery, W.K. (1995). *Benefits of Recreation Research.* State College, PA: Venture Publishing.

Slade, S., Falkowski, W., A.K. & Slade, P. (1975). Immediate psychological effects of various occupational therapy activities on psychiatric patients: a pilot study. *The British Journal of Occupational Therapy, 38,* 172-173.

Steffan, J.A. & Nelson, D.L. (1987). The effects of tool scarcity on group climate and affective meaning within context of a stenciling activity. *American Journal of Occupational Therapy, 41 (7),* 449-453.

Stein, F. (1989). *Anatomy of Clinical Research: An Introduction to Scientific Inquiry in Medicine, Rehabilitation, and Related Health Professions.* Thorofare, NJ: Slack.

Taber, F., Baron, S. & Blackwell, A. (1953). A study of a task-directed and free choice group. *American Journal of Occupational Therapy, 7,* 118-124.

Taylor, E. & Manguno, J. (1991). Use of treatment activities in occupational therapy. *American Journal of Occupational Therapy, 45,* 317-322.

Thibodeaux, C.S. & Ludwig, F.M. (1988). Intrinsic motivation in product-oriented and non-product-oriented activities. *American Journal of Occupational Therapy, 42,* 169-175.

VanDeusen, J. & Harlowe, D. (1987). The efficacy of the ROM dance program for adults with rheumatoid arthritis. *American Journal of Occupational Therapy, 41,* 90-95.

Yerxa, E. (1983). Research priorities. *American Journal of Occupational Therapy, 37 (10),* 699.

Yerxa, E. (1987). Research: The key to the development of occupational therapy as an academic discipline? *American Journal of Occupational Therapy, 41,* 415-419.

Yoder, R.M., Nelson, D.L. & Smith, D.A. (1989). Added purpose versus rote exercise in female nursing home residents. *American Journal of Occupation Therapy, 43 (9),* 581-595.

Zimmer-Branum, S. & Nelson, D.L. (1995). Occupationally embedded exercise versus rote exercise: A choice between occupational forms by elderly nursing home residents. *American Journal of Occupational Therapy, 49,* 397-402.

Therapeutic Activities: Principles and Methods

Agacinski, K. & Stern, D. (1984). A two track program enhances therapeutic gains for chronically ill in a day hospital population. *Occupational Therapy in Mental Health, 4,* 15-22.

Ager, C. (1986). Therapeutic aspects of volunteer and advocacy activities. *Physical and Occupational Therapy in Geriatrics, 5 (2),* 3-11.

Allen, C.K. (1985). *Occupational Therapy for Psychiatric Diseases: Measurement and Management of Cognitive Disabilities.* Boston, MA: Little, Brown.

Allen-Burket, A. (1988). *Time Well-spent: A Manual for Visiting Older Adults.* Ravensdale, WA: Idyll Arbor Inc.

Allen, C.K. & Earhart, C.A. (1992). *Occupational Therapy Treatment Goals for the Physically and Cognitively Disabled.* Rockville, MD: American Occupational Therapy Association.

Allen, G. & Peppers, S. (1988, March). Use of a therapeutic choir as an agent of change in patients. *Mental Health Special Interest Section Newsletter,* (pp. 2-3).

American Occupational Therapy Association (1985). *PIVOT: Planning and Implementing Vocational Readiness in OT*. Rockville, MD: Author.

Angle, D.K. & Buxton, J.M. (1991). *Community Living Skills for Workbook for the Brain Injured Adult*. Frederick, MD: Aspen Publishers.

Ascher-Svanum, H. & Krause, A.A. (1991). *Psychoeducational Groups for Patients with Schizophrenia: A Guide for Practitioners*. Rockville, MD: Aspen Publishers.

Barris, R., Cordero, J. & Christiaansen, R. (1986). Occupational therapists' use of media. *American Journal of Occupational Therapy, 40*, 679-684.

Barter, J.T., Qerirol, J.F. & Ekstrom, S.P. (1984). A psychoeducational approach to educating chronic mental patients about community living. *Hospital and Community Psychiatry, 35*, 793-797.

Bernard, A. (1992). The use of music as a purposeful activity: A preliminary investigation. *Physical and Occupational Therapy in Geriatrics, 10 (3)*, 35-45.

Berry, B.L. & Lukens, H.C. (1975). Integrating occupational therapy into other activities in a day treatment program. *Hospital and Community Psychiatry, 26*, 569-574.

Bissell, J.C. & Mailloux, Z. (1981). The use of crafts in occupational therapy for the physically disabled. *American Journal of Occupational Therapy 35*, 369-374.

Blose, D.A. & Smith, L.L. (1995). *Thrifty Nifty Stuff for Little Kids*. Tucson, AZ: Therapy Skill Builders.

Borg, B. & Bruce, M.A. (1991). *The Group System: The Therapeutic Activity Group in Occupational Therapy*. Thorofare, NJ: Slack.

Bowlby, C. (1993). *Therapeutic Activities with Persons Disabled by Alzheimers Disease and Related Disorders*. Frederick, MD: Aspen Publishers.

Breines, E.B. (1995). *Occupational Therapy Activities: From Clay to Computers: Theory and Practice*. Philadelphia, PA: FA Davis.

Bricker, D. (1994). *An Activity-based Approach to Early Intervention*. Palo Alto, CA: VORT Corporation.

Brockema, M.C., Danz, K.H. & Schloemer, C.V. (1975). Occupational therapy in a community after care program. *American Journal of Occupational Therapy, 29*, 22-27.

Brown, T., Harwood, K., Heckman, J., & Short, I. (Eds) (1989). *Mental Health Protocols for Occupational Therapy*. Baltimore, MD: Chess Publishers.

Bruce, M.A. (1988). Occupational therapy in group treatment. In D.W. Scott & N. Katz (Eds), *Occupational Therapy in Mental Health: Principles in Practice*. Philadelphia, PA: Taylor and Francis.

Buettner, L. & Martin, S. (1995). *Therapeutic Recreation in the Nursing Home*. State College, PA: Venture Publishing.

Burnside, I.M. (Ed) (1986). *Working with the Elderly: Group Process and Techniques (2nd Ed)*. Boston, MA: Jones and Bartlett Publications.

Caplaw-Lindler, E., Harpaz, L. & Samberg, S. (1979). *Therapeutic Dance/Movement-Expressive Activities for Older Adults*. New York, NY: Human Sciences Press.

Chandani, A. (1990). What really is therapeutic activity? *British Journal of Occupational Therapy, 53*, 15-18.

Charlesworth, E.A. & Nathan, R.G. (1984). *Stress Management: A Comprehensive Guide to Wellness*. New York, NY: Antheneum.

Cole, M. (1993). *Group Dynamics in Occupational Therapy*. Thorofare, NJ: Slack.

Coling, M.C. & Garrett, J.N. (1995). *Activity-based Intervention Guide with more than 250 Multi-sensory Play Ideas*. Tucson, AZ: Therapy Skill Builders.

Copley, J. (1986). Development of a psychosocial group for the chronic physically disabled adult. *Advance, 2 (4)*, 1, 2, 7.

Cotton, D.H. (1990). *Stress Management: An Integrated Approach to Therapy*. New York, NY: Brunner/Mazel.

Conviensky, M. (1986, June). Addressing performance components in day treatment: A program description. *Mental Health Special Interest Newsletter*, (pp. 3-4).

Crist, P.A.H., Thomas, P.P. & Stone, B.L. (1984). Prevocational and sensorimotor training in chronic schizophrenia. *Occupational Therapy in Mental Health, 4 (2)*, 23-27.

Cromwell, F.S. (1985). *Work-related programs in Occupational Therapy*. New York, NY: Haworth Press.

Cromwell, F.S. (Ed) (1984). *Occupational Therapy Strategies and Adaptations for Independent Daily Living*. New York, NY: Haworth Press.

Cynkin, S. (1979). *Occupational Therapy: Toward Health Through Activities*. Boston, MA: Little, Brown.

Cynkin, S. & Robinson, A.M. (1990). *Occupational Therapy and Activities Health: Toward Heath through Activities*. Boston, MA: Little, Brown.

Dattilo, J. (1994). *Inclusive Leisure Services: Responding to the Rights of People with Disabilities*. State College, PA: Venture Publishing.

Davis, C.M. (1995). *Alternative Therapies: An Introduction*. Thorofare, NJ: Slack, Inc.

Davis, M., McKay, M. & Eskelman, R. (1982). *The Relaxation and Stress Reduction Workbook (2nd Ed)*. Oakland, CA: New Harbinger.

Davis-Koska, A., Kraml, D., Miyake, S. & Rochford, C (1986). Using purpose to engage the patient with depression. *Occupational Therapy in Health Care, 3 (1)*, 41-53.

Demers, L.M. (1992). *Work Hardening: A Practical Guide*. Stoneham, MA: Andover, Medical Publishers.

Denton, P. (1986). *Psychiatric Occupational Therapy: A Workbook of Practical Skills*. Boston, MA: Little, Brown.

Department of Army. (1971). *Craft Techniques in Occupational Therapy: Technical Manual*. Washington, DC: Department of Army.

Dowling, J.R. (1985). *Keeping Busy: A Handbook of Activities for Persons with Dementia*. Baltimore, MD: John Hopkins Press.

Drake, M. (1992). *Crafts in Therapy and Rehabilitation*. Thorofare, NJ: Slack, Inc.

Dumcombe, L.W. & Howe, M.C. (1985). Group work in occupational therapy: A survery of practice. *American Journal of Occupational Therapy, 39 (3)*, 163-170.

Egan, M. (1992). Focus: Physical agent modalities: Useful tools for requiring function. *OT Week, 6 (18),* 14-15.

Falk-Kessler, J., Momich, C. & Perel, S. (1991). Therapeutic factors in occupational therapy groups. *American Journal of Occupational Therapy, 45 (1),* 59-66.

Fidler, G.S. (1969). The task-oriented group as a context for treatment. *American Journal of Occupational Therapy, 23 (1),* 43-48.

Fidler, G.S. (1984). *Design of Rehabilitation Services in Psychiatric Hospital Settings.* Rockville, MD: American Occupational Therapy Association.

Fine, S. (1983). *Occupational Therapy: The Role of Rehabilitation and Purposeful Activity in Mental Health Practice.* Rockville, MD: American Occupational Therapy Association.

Finn, G.L. (1972). The occupational therapist in prevention programs. *American Journal of Occupational Therapy, 26,* 59-66.

Frye, B. (1990). Art and multiple personality disorder: An expressive framework for occupational therapy. *American Journal of Occupational Therapy, 44,* 1013-1022.

Gauthier, L. & Dalziel, S. (1987). The benefits of group occupational therapy for patients with Parkinson's disease. *American Journal of Occupational Therapy 41 (6),* 360-365.

Gibson, D. (Ed) (1988). Group process and structure in psychosocial occupational therapy [Special Issue]. *Occupational Therapy in Mental Health, 8 (3).*

Glickstein, J.K. (1988). *Therapeutic Interventions in Alzheimer's Disease-A program of Functional Communication Skills for Activities of Daily Living.* Rockville, MD: Aspen Publishers.

Gliner, J.A. (1985). Purposeful activity in motor learning: An event approach to motor skill acquisition. *American Journal of Occupational Therapy, 39,* 28-34.

Hamill, C.M. & Oliver, R.C. (1980). *Therapeutic Activities for the Handicapped Elderly.* Rockville, MD: Aspen Publishers.

Hansen, M., Ritter, G., Gutmann, M. & Christiansen, B. (1990). *Understanding Stress: Strategies for a Healthier Mind and Body.* Rockville, MD: American Occupational Therapy Association.

Harwood, K.J. & Wenzl, D. (1990). Admissions to discharge: A psychogeriatric transitional program. *Occupational Therapy in Mental Health, 10 (3),* 79-100.

Hellen, C.R. (1992). *Alzheimer's disease: Activity-forced Care.* Stoneham, MA: Andover Medical Publishers.

Hemphill, B.J., Peterson, C.Q. & Werner, P.C. (1991). *Rehabilitation in Mental Health: Goals and Objectives for Independent Living.* Thorofare, NJ: Slack, Inc.

Henry, A.D., Delson, D. & Duncombe, L.W. (1984). Choice making in group and individual activity. *American Journal of Occupational Therapy, 38 (4),* 245-251.

Herring, K.L. & Wilkinson, S. (1995). *Action Alphabet: Snesorimotor activities for Groups.* Tucson, AZ: Therapy Skill Builders.

Hibbard, T., Camitelli, J. & Lieberman, H.J. (1989). Off-unit activites programming for long-stay psychiatric inpatients: Clinical and administrative effects. *Occupational Therapy in Mental Health, 9 (1),* 49-61.

Hickerson-Crist, P.A., Thomas, P.P. & Stone, B.L. (1984). Prevocational and sensorimotor training in chronic schizophrenia. *Occupational Therapy in Mental Health, 4 (2),* 23-37.

Higden, J.F. (1990). Expressive therapy in conjuction with psychotherapy in the treatment of persons with multiple personality disorder. *American Journal of Occupational Therapy, 44,* 991-993.

Hirama, H. (1992). *Activity Analysis: A primer.* Baltimore, MD: Chess Publications.

Hollis, L.I. (1986). Identifying occupational therapy: the use of purposeful activities. *Physical Disabilities Special Interest Section Newsletter, 9 (4), 2-3.* Rockville, MD: American Occupational Therapy Association.

Howe, M.C. & Schwartzbrg, S.L. (1988). Structure and process in designing a functional group. *Occupational Therapy in Mental Health, 8 (3),* 1-8.

Howe, M.C., Weaver, C.T. & Dulay, J. (1981). The development of a work-oriented day center program. *American Journal of Occupational Therapy, 35,* 711-718.

Kaminsky, J. (1988, July 28). Group therapy provides extra push for motivating rehabilitation clients. *OT Week,* (pp. 4-5).

Kanellos, M. (1985). Enhancing vocational outcomes of spinal cord-injured persons: The occupational therapist's role. *American Journal of Occupational Therapy, 39,* 726-733.

Kaplan, K.L. (1988). *Directive Group Therapy: Innovative Mental Health Treatment.* Thorofare, NJ: Slack.

Kemp, B. & Kelinplatz, F. (1985). Vocational rehabilitation of the older worker. *American Journal of Occupational Therapy, 39,* 322-326.

Kerstien, M.E. (1993, June 10). Reach up and tie something: Simple macrame draws out patients' skills. *OT Week, 7 (23),* 16-17.

Kling, T.I. (1993). Brief or new: Hand strengthening with a computer for purposeful activity. *American Journal of Occupational Therapy, 47,* 635-637.

Klimowicz, R. (1987). Sensorimotor activities on a short-term inpatient unit. *Occupational Therapy Forum, 4 (2),* 1, 3-6.

Korb, K.L., Azok, S.K. & Leutenberg, E.A. (1989). *Life Management Skills.* Beechwood, OH: Wellness Reproductions.

Korb, K.L., Azok, S.K. & Leutenberg, E.A. (1991). *Life Management Skills II.* Beechwood, OH: Wellness Reproduction.

Jacobs, K. (Ed) (1990). Work: Occupational therapy interventions. *Occupational Therapy Practice, 1,* 1-87.

Johnson, D.W. & Johnson, F.P. (1982). *Joining Together: Group Theory and Group Skills.* Englewood Cliffs, NJ: Prentice Hall.

Johnson, J. (1986). *Wellness: A Context for Living.* Thorofare, NJ: Slack.

Lamport, N., Coffey, M. & Hersch, G. (1993). *Activity Analysis Handbook, 2nd Edition.* Thorofare, NJ: Slack, Inc.

Llorens, L.A. (1973). Activity analysis for cognitive-perceptual-motor dysfunction. *American Journal of Occupational Therapy, 27,* 453-456.

Llorens, L. (1986). Activity analysis: Agreement among factors in a sensory processing model. *American Journal of Occupational Therapy, 40 (2),* 103-110.

Lewin, J.V. & Lewin, R.A. (1987). On treatment integration: Psychotherapy and work therapy. *Occupational Therapy in Mental Health, 7 (3),* 21-36.

Levy, L.L. (1987a). Psychosocial intervention and dementia, Part 1: State of the art, future directions. *Occupational Therapy in Mental Heath, 7 (1),* 69-107.

Levy, L.L. (1987b). Psychosocial intervention and dementia, part II: The cognitive disability perspecitive. *Occupational Therapy in Mental Health, 7 (4),* 13-36.

Linder, T.W. (1995). *Transdisciplinary Play-based Intervention.* Palo Alto, CA: VORT Corporation.

Lobdell, K., Johnson, C., Nesbitt, J. & Clave, M. (1986). *Therapeutic Crafts: A Practical Approach.* Thorofare, NJ: Slack, Inc.

Mace, N. (1987). Principles of activities for persons with dementia. *Physical and Occupational Therapy in Geriatrics, 5 (3),* 13-27.

Marcus, E. & Granovetter, R. (1994). *Making It Easy-Crafts and Cooking Activities for Handicapped Learners.* Palo Alto, CA: VORT Corporation.

Matheson, L., Ogden, L., Violette, K. & Schultz, K. (1985). Work hardening: Occupational therapy in industrial rehabilitation. *American Journal of Occupational Therapy, 39,* 314-321.

McCram Griffith, R. (1990). *Protocols for Adapting Activities to the Changing Needs of People with Dementia.* Baltimore, MD: Chess Publications.

McDermott, A.A. (1988). The effect of three group formats on group interaction patterns. *Occupational Therapy in Mental Health, 8 (3),* 69-89.

McPhee. (1992). The use of physical agent modalities: A result of an identity crisis or an extension of the profession. *Physical Disabilities Special Interest Section Newsletter, 15 (3),* 6-7.

McSurp, E., Howard, L. & Schlitt, D. (1990). The planning group: An example of learning through doing. *Occupational Therapy Forum, 5 (1),* 1, 3-5.

Mosey, A.C. (1970). The concept and use of developmental groups. *American Journal of Occupational Therapy, 24 (4),* 272-275.

Mosey, A. (1973). *Activities Therapy.* New York, NY: Raven Press.

Mumford, M.S. (1974). A comparison of interpersonal skills in verbal and activity groups. *American Journal of Occupational Therapy, 28,* 281-283.

Muslin, D. (1982). Rehabilitation training for community living skills. *Occupational Therapy in Mental Health, 2 (1).*

Napier, R.N. & Gershenfeld, M.K. (1983). *Making Groups Work: A Guide for Group Leaders.* Boston, MA: Houghton Mifflin.

Neidstadt, M.E. & Marques, K. (1984). An independent living skills training program. *American Journal of Occupational Therapy, 38,* 671-676.

Neidstadt, M.E., McAuley, D., Zecha, D. & Shannon, R. (1993). An analysis of a board game as a treatment activity. *American Journal of Occupational Therapy, 47,* 154-160.

Nelson, D.L. (1984). *Childern with Autism and other Pervasive Disorders of Development and Behavior: Therapy through Activities.* Thorofare, NJ: Slack.

Ogden, L.D. (1979). Activity guidelines dor subacute and high-risk cardiac patients. *American Journal of Occupational Therapy, 33,* 291-298.

Paire, J.A. & Karney, R.J. (1984). The effectiveness of sensory stimulation for geropsychiatric inpatients. *American Journal of Occupational Therapy, 38,* 505-509.

Powers, P. (1991). *The Activity Gourmet.* State College, PA: Venture Publishing.

Rabinowitz, E. (1986). Day care and Alzheimer's disease: A weekend program in New York City. *Physical and Occupational Therapy in Geriatrics, 4 (3),* 95-103.

Radonsky, V.E., Haffenbreidel, J., Harper, C., Kilgman, K. & Timms, C. (1987). Occupational therapy in vocational readiness. *Occupational Therapy in Mental Health, 7 (3),* 83-92.

Ramsbey, N. (1993). Is purposeful activity effective in remediating physical impairments and restoring functions? *Journal of Occupational Therapy Students, 7 (2),* 7-14.

Remocker, A.J. & Storch, E. (1987). *Action Speaks Louder: A Handbook of Structured Group Techniques.* New York, NY: Chruchill Livingstone.

Richert, G.Z. & Meryyman, M.B. (1987). The vocational continuum: A model for providing vocational services in a partial hospitalization program. *Occupational Therapy in Mental Health, 7 (3),* 1-20.

Robertson, S.C. (Ed) (1989). *Mental Health Focus: Skills for Assessment and Treatment.* Rockville, MD: American Occupational THerapy Association.

Rogers, J.C. (1989). Therapeutic activity and health status. *Topics in Geriatric Rehabilitation, 4 (4),* 1-11.

Ross, M. (1991). *Integrative Group Therapy: The Structured Five-stage approach (2nd ed).* Thorofare, NJ: Slack.

Ross, M. & Burdick, D. (1981). *Sensory Integration: A Training Manual for Therapists and Teachers for Regressed, Psychiatic and Geriatric Patient Groups.* Thorofare, NJ: Slack.

Sampson, E.E. & Marthas, M. (1981). *Group Process for the Health Professions (2nd ed).* New York, NY: John Wiley & Sons.

Saxon, S.V. & Etten, M.J. (1984). *Psychosocial Rehabilitative Programs for Older Adults.* Springfield, IL: Charles C. Thomas.

Scott, D.W. & Katz, N. (1988). *Occupational Therapy in Mental Health: Principles in Practice.* New York, NY: Taylor and Francis.

Sheridan, C. (1987). *Failure-free Activities for the Alzheimer's Patient: A Guidebook for Caregivers.* San Francisco, CA: Cottage Books.

Simmons, P.L. & Mullins, L. (1992). *Acute Psychiatric Care: An Occupational Therapy Guide to Exercises in Daily Living.* Thorofare, NJ: Slack, Inc.

Smith, P.A., Burrow, H.S. & Whitney, J.N. (1959). Psychological attributes of occupational therapy crafts. *American Journal of Occupational Therapy, 13,* 25-26.

Stein, F. & Tallant, B. (1988). Applying the group process to psychiatric occupational therapy, part 2: A model for a therapeutic group in psychiatric occupational therapy. *Occupational Therapy in Mental Health, 8 (3),* 29-52.

Taira, E.D. (Ed) (1986). Therapeutic interventions for the person with dementia [Special Issue]. *Physical and Occupational Therapy in Geriatrics, 4 (3).*

Tedrick, T. & Green, E. (1995). *Activity Experiences and Programming within Long-term Care.* State College, PA: Venture Publishing.

Thibodeux, C.D. & Ludwig, F.M. (1988). Intrinsic motivation in product-oriented activities. *American Journal of Occupational Therapy, 42,* 169-175.

Tigges, K.N. & Marcil, W.M. (1986, January/February). Maximizing quaity of life for the homebound patient. *The American Journal of Hospice Care,* (pp. 21-23).

Trombly, C. (1982). Include exercise in purposeful activity [Letter to the editor]. *American Journal of Occupational Therapy, 36,* 467-468.

Tubesing, N. & Tubesing, D. (1983). *Structured Exercises in Stress Management.* Buluth, MN: Whole Person Press.

Van Deusen, J. & Harlowe, D. (1987). Te efficacy of the ROM dance program for adults with rheumatoid arthritis. *American Journal of Occupational Therapy, 41 (2),* 90-95.

VanderRoest, L.L. & Clments, S.T. (1983). *Sensory Integration: Rationale and Treatment Activities for Groups.* Grand Rapids, MI: South Kent Health Services, Inc.

Weston, D.L. (1961). The dimensions of crafts. *American Journal of Occupational Therapy, 15,* 1-5.

Weston, D.L. (1960). Therapeutic crafts. *American Journal of Occupational Theray, 14,* 121-122, 133.

Widerstrom, A.H. (1995). *Achieving Learning Goals through Play.* Tucson, AZ: Therapy Skill Builders.

Wilberding, D. (1987). Rehabilitation through activities for the chronic schizophrenic patient. In AOTA (Ed). *The Chronically Mentally Ill: Issues in Intervention Proceedings,* (pp. 34-47). Rockville, MD: Editor.

Webb, L.J. (1973). The therapeutic social club. *American Journal of Occupational Therapy, 27,* 81-83.

Webster, D. & Schwartzberg, S.L. (1992). Patient's perception of curative factors in occupational therapy groups. *Occupational Therapy in Mental Health: A Journal of Psychosocial Practice and Research, 12 (1).*

White, B. & Keller, M.J. (1992). *Therapeutic Recreation: Cases and Exercises.* State College, PA: Venture Publishing.

Woolfolk, R.L. & Lehrer, P.M. (Eds) (1984). *Principles and Practice of Stress Management.* New York, NY: Guilford.

Yalom, I. (1975). *The Theory and Practice of Group Psychotherapy.* New York, NY: Basic Books.

Yalom, I.D. (1983). *Inpatient Group Psychotherapy.* New York, NY: Basic Books.

Zander, A. (1971). *Motives and Goals in Groups.* New York, NY: Academic Press.

Zogola, J.M. (Ed) (1987). *Doing Things: A Guide to Programming Activities for Persons with Alzheimer's Disease and Related Disorders.* Baltimore, MD: John Hopkins University Press.

The Therapeutic Relationship

Able, E. & Nelson, M. (Eds). *Circle of Caring.* New York, NY: State University of New York Press.

Arnstein, S.M. (1990). Intrinsic motivation. *American Journal of Occupational Therapy, 44,* 462-463.

Bandura, A. (1977). Self-efficacy: Toward a unifying theory of behavioral change. *Psychological Review, 84,* 191-215.

Bandura, A. (1982). Self-efficacy mechanisms in human agency. *American Psychologist, 37,* 122-147.

Baum, C.M. (1980). Occupational therapists put care into health system. *American Journal of Occupational Therapy, 34,* 505-517.

Benham, P.K. (1988). Attitudes of occupational therapy personnel toward persons with disabilities. *American Journal of Occupational Therapy, 42,* 305-311.

Benjamin, A. (1974). *The Helping Interview (2nd ed).* Boston, MA: Houghton Mifflin.

Benner, P. (1984). *From Novice to Expert: Excellence and Power in Clinical Nursing Practice.* Reading, MA: Addison-Wesley.

Bernheim, K.F. (1993). Principles of professional and family collaboration in R.P. Cottrell (Ed). *Psychosocial Occupational Therapy: Proactive Approaches,* (pp. 297-299). Bethesda, MD: American Occupational Therapy Association.

Blackman, J.A. (1995). *Working with Families in Early Intervention.* Frederick, MD: Aspen.

Bond, J.E. (1986). Increasing motivation in the practice of occupational therapy. *Occupational Therapy Forum. II (32),* 22-24.

Branner, L.M. (1985). *The Helping Relationship: Process and Skills (3rd ed).* Englewood Cliffs, NJ: Prentice Hall.

Burke, J.P. (1977). A clinical perspective on motivation: Pawn vs. origin. *American Journal of Occupational Therapy, 31,* 254-258.

Burke, J.P., Miyake, S., Keilhofner, G. & Barris, R. (1983). The demystification of health care and demise of the sick role: Implications for occupational therapy. In G. Kielhofner (Ed), *Health Through Occupation,* (pp. 197-210). Philadelphia, PA: F.A. Davis.

Brunfield, A. (1985). *Multiple Sclerosis: A Personal Exploration.* New York, NY: Demos Publications.

Carberry, H. (1983). Psychological mothods for helping the angry, resistant and negative patient. *Cognitive Rehabilitation, 1 (4),* 4-5.

Charash, L., Lovelace, R., Wolf, S., Sutscher, A., Roye, D.P., & Leach, C. (Eds) (1987). *Realities in Coping with Progressive Neuromuscular Disorders.* Philadelphia, PA: Charles Press.

Corbin, J.M. & Strauss, A. (1988). *Unending Work and Care: Managing Chronic Illness at Home.* San Francisco, CA: Jossey-Bass.

Davis, C.M. (1994). *Patient-practitioner Interaction: An Experimental Manual for Developing the Art of Health Care.* Thorofare, NJ: Slack, Inc.

Deci, E.L. & Ryan, P.M. (1985). *Intrinsic Motivation and Self Determination in Human Behavior.* New York, NY: Plenum Press.

De Loach, C. & Greer, B.J. (1981). *Adjustment to Severe Disability.* New York, NY: McGraw Hill.

Dwoney, J., Reidel, G. & Kitischer, A. (Eds) (1981). *Bereavement of Physical Disability: Recommitment to Life, Health, and Function.* New York, NY: Arno Press.

Egan, G. (1986). *The Skilled Helper: A Systematic Approach to Effective Helping (3rd Ed).* Monterey, CA: Brooks/Cole.

Falvo, D.R. (1991). *Medical and Psychosocial Aspcets of chronic Illness and Disability.* Rockville, MD: Aspen Publishers.

Finch, J. & Groves, D. (Eds). *A Laborer of Love: Women, Work and Caring.* Boston, MA: Routledge and Kegan Paul.

Fleming, M. (Ed) (1990). *Preceedings of the Clinical Reasoning Institute for Occupational Therapy Educators.* Medford, MA: Tufts University.

Florey, L.L. (1969). Intrinsic Motivation: The dynamics of occupational therapy theory. *American Journal of Occupational Therapy, 23,* 319-322.

Fondiller, E.D., R., L.J. & Neuhaus, B.F. (1990). Values influencing clinicla reasoning in occupational therapy. *Occupational Therapy Journal of Research, 10 (1),* 41-55.

Frank, A.W. (1991). *At the Will of the Body: Reflections of Illness.* Boston, MA: Houghton Mifflin.

Frank, G. (1994). The personal meaning of self-care occupations. In C.Christiansen (Ed) *Ways of Living: Self-Care Strategies for Special Needs,* (pp. 27-49). Rockville, MD: American Occupational Therapy Association.

Freda, M. (1993). Sexuality and disability-Treating the whole person in R.P. Cottrell (Ed), *Psychosocial Occupational Therapy: Proactive Approaches,* (pp. 449-550). Bethesda, MD: Aerican Occupational Therapy Association.

Gage, M. (1992). The appraisal model of coping: An assessment and intervention model for occupational therapy. *American Journal of Occupational Therapy, 46,* 353-362.

Geskie, M.A. & Salasek, J.L. (1988). Attitudes of health care personnel towards persons with disabilities. In H.E. Yuker (Ed), *Attitudes Toward Persons with Disabilities,* (pp. 187-200). New York, NY: Springer Publishing Company.

Gilfoyle, E.M. (1980). Caring: A philosophy for practice. *American Journal of Occupational Therapy.*

Goffman, E. (1963). *Stigma: Notes on the Management of a Spoiled Identity.* Englewood Cliffs, NJ: Prentice Hall.

Grogan, G. (1991a). Anger management: A perspecitve for occupational therapy, part 1. *Occupational Therapy in Mental Health, 11 (2/3),* 149-171.

Groves, J.F. (1978). Taking care of the hateful patient. *New England Journal of Medicine, 298,* 883-887.

Harvey, L. (1984). Advocacy and the aged: A case for the therapist advocate. *Physical and Occupational Therapy in Geriatrics, (3/2),* 5-15.

Henderson, G. & Bryan, W.V. (1984). *Psychosocial Aspects of Disability.* Springfield, IL: Charles C. Thomas.

Hubbard, S. (1991). Toward a truly holistic approach to occupational therapy. *British Journal of Occupational Therapy, 54,* 415-418.

Huss, A.J. (1977). Touch with care or a caring touch. *American Journal of Therapy, 31,* 17-18.

Hutchins, D.E. & Cole, C.S. (1986). *Helping Relationships and Strategies.* Pacific Grove, CA: Brooks/Cole.

Kasch, M.C. (1985). Motivation and activity. (Letter to the editor), *American Journal of Occupational Therapy, 34,* 114-115.

King, L.J. (1980). Creative caring. *American Journal of Occupational Therapy, 34,* 529-534.

Kircher, M.A. (1984). Motivation as a factor in purposeful vs nonpurposeful activity. *American Journal of Occupational Therapy, 38,* 165-170.

Kelinman, A. (1980). *Patients and Healers in the Context of Culture.* Los Angeles, CA: University of California Press.

Kubler-Ross, E. (1978). *To Live Until We Say Good-bye.* Englewood Cliffs, NJ: Prentice Hall.

Kubler-Ross, E. (1981). *Living with Death and Dying.* New York, NY: Macmillan.

Leete, F. (1993). Patient's accounts of stress and coping in schizophrenia in R.P. Cottrell (Ed), *Psychosocial Occupational Therapy: Proactive Approaches,* (pp. 283-288). Bethesda, MD: American Occupational Therapy Association

Marinelli, R.P. & Dell Orto, A.E. (1984). *The Psychological and Social Impact of Physical Disability (2nd ed).* New York, NY: Springer.

Mattingly, C. (1989). *Thinking with Stories: Story and Experience in Clinical Practice. Unpublished Doctrinal Dissertation.* Massachusetts Institute of Technology. Cambridge, MA.

Mattingly, C. (1991). What is clinical reasoning? *American Journal of Occupational Therapy, 45,* 979-986.

Mattingly, C. & Fleming, M. (1994). *Clinical Reasoning, Forms of Inquiry in a Therapeutic Practice.* Philadelphia, PA: F.A. Davis.

McConchie, S.D. (1993). Establishing support and advocacy groups in R.P. Cottrell (Ed), *Psychosocial Occupational Therapy: Proactive Approaches,* (pp. 315-318). Behtesda, MD: American Occupational Therapy Association.

Miller, J.F. (1983). *Coping with Chronic Illness, Overcoming Powerlessness.* Philadelphia, PA: F.A. Davis.

Moos, R.H. (Ed) (1977). *Coping with Physical Illness.* New York, NY: Plenum Press.

Mosey, A. (1986). *Psychosocial Components of Occupational Therapy.* New York, NY: Raven Press.

Mueller, S. and Suto, M. (1993). Starting a stress management program. In R.P. Cottrell (Ed), *Psychosocial Occupational Therapy: Proactive Approaches,* (pp. 319-322). Bethesda, MD: American Occupational Therapy Association.

Murphy, R.F. (1987). *The Body Silent.* New York, NY: Henry Holt.

Nager, M. (1990). *Perspectives on Disabilities.* Palo Alto, CA: Health Markets Research.

Navarra, T. (1995). *A Word to the Wise: Wisdom for Caregivers.* Thorofare, NJ: Slack, Inc.

Navarra, T., Lipkowitz, M.A. & Navarra, J.G. (1990). *Therapeutic Communication: A Guide to Effective Interpersonal Skills for Health Care Professionals.* Thorofare, NJ: Slack.

Nelson, C.E. & Payton, D.D. (1991). The issue is—a system for involving patients in program planning. *American Journal of Occupational Therapy, 45 (8),* 753-755.

O'Hara, C.C. & Harren, M. (1987). *Rehabilitation with Brain Injured Survivors: An Empowerment Approach.* Rockville, MD: Aspen Publishers.

Parham, D. (1987). Nationally speaking—Toward professionalism: The reflective therapist. *American Journal of Occupational Therapy, 41,* 555-561.

Parsons, T. (1975). The sick role and the role of the physician reconsidered. *Health and Society.* 257-278.

Payton, O.D. (Ed) (1986). *Psychosocial Aspects of Clinical Practice.* New York, NY: Chruchill Livingston.

Payton, O.D., Nelson, C. & Ozer, M. (1990). *Patient Participation in Program Planning: A Manual for Therapists.* Philadelphia, PA: F.A. Davis.

Peloquin, S.M. (1993). The depersonalization of patients: A profile gleaned form narratives. *American Journal of Occupational Therapy, 47,* 830-837.

Peloquin, S.M. (1990). The patient-therapist relationship in occupational therapy: Understanding visions and images. *American Journal of Occupational Therapy, 44 (1),* 13-21.

Peloquin, S.M. (1990). The patient-therapist relationship in occupational therapy: Understanding visions and images. In R.P. Cottrell (Ed), *Psychosocial Occupational Therapy: Proactive Approaches,* (pp. 267-275). Bethesda, MD: American Occupational Therapy Association.

Purtilo, R.B. (1990). *Health Professional and Patient Interaction, 4th edition.* Philadelphia, PA: W.B. Saunders.

Register, C. (1988). *Living with Chronic Illness: Days of Patience and Passion.* New York, NY: Macmillan.

Reily, M. (1984). The importance of the client versus patient issue for occupational therapy. *American Journal of Occupational Therapy, 38 (6),* 404-406.

Robinson, V.M. (Ed) (1991). *Human and the Health Professions: The Therapeutic Use of Humor in Health Care, 2nd Edition.* Thorofare, NJ: Slack, Inc.

Robinson, V. (1977). *Humor and the Health Professions.* Thorofare, NJ: Slack, Inc.

Rogers, C. (1961). *On Becoming a Person.* Boston, MA: Houghton Mifflin.

Rogers, J.C. & Figone, J.J. (1979). Psychosocial parameters in treating the person with quadriplegia. *American Journal of Occupational Therapy, 33,* 432-439.

Rousso, M., O'Malley, S.G. & Severance, M. (1988). *Disabled, Female and Proud: Stories of Ten Women with Disabilities.* Boston, MA: Exceptional Parent Press.

Sabari, J.S. (1985). Professional socialization: Implications for occupational therapy. *American Journal of Occupational Therapy, 39,* 96-102.

Sachs, D. & Labovitz, D.R. (1994). The caring occupational therapist within the scope of professional roles and boundaries. *American Journal of Occupational Therapy, 48,* 997-1005.

Schon, D. (1983). *The Reflective Practitioner: How Professionals Think in Action.* New York, NY: Basic.

Schontz, F.C. (1975). *The Psychological Aspects of Physical Illness and Disability.* New York, NY: Macmillan.

Shapiro, D. (1982). *Loss, Motivation and Activity in Bereavement of the Physically Disabled.* New York, NY: Arno Press.

Sharrott, G.W. & Cooper-Forops, C. (1986). Theories of motivation in occupational therapy: An overview. *American Journal of Occupational Therapy, 40,* 249-257.

Sharrott, G.W. & Yerxa, E.J. (1985). Promises to keep: Implications of the referent "patient" versus "client" for those served by occupational therapy. *American Journal of Occupational Therapy, 39 (6),* 401-406.

Shulman, L. (1984). *The Skills of Helping Individuals and Groups, 2nd Edition.* Itasca, IL: F.E. Peacock.

Teitelman, J.L. (1982). Eliminating learned helplessness in older rehabilitation patients. *Physical and Occupational Therapy in Geriatrics, 1 (4),* 3-10.

Teusink, J.P. & Mahler, S. (1993). Helping families cope with Alzheimer's disease. In R.P. Cottrell (Ed), *Psychosocial Occupational Therapy: Proactive Approaches,* (pp. 333-337). Bethesda, MD: American Occupational Therapy Association.

Tigges, K.N. & Marcil, W.M. (1988). *Terminal and Life-threatening Illness: An Occupational Behavior Perspective.* Thorofare, NJ: Slack.

Turner, I.M. (1993). The healing power of repect-A personal journey. In R.P. Cottrell (Ed) *Psychosocial Occupational Therapy: Proactive Approaches,* (pp. 259-265). Bethesda, MD: American Occupational Therapy Association.

Vargo, J.W. (1993). Some psychological effects of physical disabilities. In R.P. Cottrell (Ed), *Psychosocial Occupational Therapy: Proactive Approaches,* (pp. 433-436). Bethesda, MD: American Occupational Therapy Association.

Yerxa, E.J. (1980). Occupational Therapy's role in creating a future climate of caring. *American Journal of Occupational Therapy, 34,* 529-534.

Appendix M

Supplemental Resource Lists

Environment and Home Modification

Access Board, Department of Justice
1331 F Street, Northwest
Suite 1000
Washington, DC 20004
202-272-5434
Issues standards in accordance with the Architectural Barriers Act, responds to complaints of violations against this act, and enforces compliance of the Act.

Accessibility Equipment Manufacturers Association
4001 East 138th Street
Grand View, MO 64030
816-763-3100
Provides information on products on the market.

Adaptive Environments Center
374 Congress Street
Suite 301
Boston, MA 02210
617-695-1225
Provides design consultation and publications.

AM-ABLE
(All Modifications for a Barrier-Free Life and Environment)
8240 Parkway Drive
Suite 107
La Mesa, CA 91942
619-262-2532
Provides design consultation, general construction, and an extensive library.

American Institute of Architects (AIA)
202-626-7492
800-365-2724
AIA offers a variety of publications on designing for the elderly and people with disabilities. The AIA library will do bibliographic searches on specific architecturally related questions for a fee.

American Association of Retired Persons (AARP)
AARP Fulfillment Department
601 E Street, NW
Washington, DC 20049
202-434-2277
AARP publishes and distributes a free guide to home modifications entitled *The DoAble Renewable Home: Making Your Home Fit Your Needs*.

Architecture and Barrier-Free Design Program
Paralyzed Veterans of America
801 18th Street, NW
Washington, DC 20006
202-416-7642
Publisher/distributor of a free publication *Making your Home Accessible*.

Center for Accessible Housing
North Carolina State University
Box 8613
Raleigh, NC 27695-8613
919-515-3082
919-515-3023 (Fax)
This center provides assistance and resources to improve the quality and availability of housing for people with disabilities to individuals and industry through research, collaborative efforts with manufacturers, training, and information services. Resources include an information and referral service, a technical design assistance service, and publications. Training is provided directly to people with disabilities, disability advocates, designers, professionals in the building industry, housing providers, and

---

design students at the post-secondary level. All materials and solutions provided by the center are based on the principles of universal design.

Century 21 Real Estate Corporation
P.O. Box 19564
Irvine, CA 92713-9564
714-553-2100

Century 21 distributes a free brochure entitled *Easy Access Housing for Easier Living* that includes a checklist to assist home buyers in evaluating accessibility.

Disabled Opportunities Center
7323 Engineer Road
San Diego, CA
619-573-0800

A model home that displays the latest in assistive devices and environmental design. An occupational therapist, architect, and contractor are available for advice, and items can be ordered through the center.

Eastern Paralyzed Veterans Association
75-20 Astoria Boulevard
Jackson Heights, NY 11370-1178
718-803-EPVA
800-444-0120

Distributors of a free 43 page booklet entitled *Wheelchair House Designs* and a free pamphlet *Wheeling to Fire Safety*. Both publications provide information relevant to all persons with disabilities, not just for those who use wheelchairs.

Easy Street Environments
6031 South Maple Avenue
Tempe, AZ 85283
602-345-8442

Easy Street Environments® provide life-size props for persons with disabilities in rehabilitation centers, allowing them to practice common tasks so that living independently outside the rehabilitation center is less daunting. Among Easy Street's stations are a bank, office, clothing store, grocery store, pharmacy, car, and a fast food restaurant. There's also a work unit complete with a ladder, conveyor belt, and other equipment. A variety of surfaces, including vinyl tile, undulating deep pile "turf," parquet wood, brick sidewalk, concrete street, curb and curb cut, and crosswalk ramp are provided. Lifesize murals add depth and realism.

Independent Living Research Utilization Program (ILRU)
ILRU Research and Training Center
2223 South Sheppard
Suite 1000
Houston, TX 77019
713-520-0232
713-520-5136 (TDD)

ILRU provides information, technical assistance and training, and conducts research on independent living. A bimonthly publication, numerous reports, and a directory of independent living centers in US are available.

Independent Production Fund
45 West 45th Street, 15th Floor
New York, NY 10036
212-221-6310

This audiovisual company has produced a video library entitled *Everyone Wins!*, which features creative ways to eliminate the use of restraints and provide quality care to nursing home residents. Eight videos are supplemented with training manuals and handouts suitable for designing and marketing programs to management, staff in service training, and/or family education.

National Council on Independent Living (NCIL)
211 Wilson Boulevard
Suite 405
Arlington, VA 22201
703-525-3406
703-525-3407 (TDD)

NCIL is a membership organization of independent living centers in the United States. Independent living skills training, technical assistance, information referrals, peer counseling, and a quarterly newsletter are available.

National Kitchen and Bath Association
687 Willow Grove Street
Hackettstown, NJ 07840
800-843-6522

This member association provides lists of accessible kitchen and bath designs and information on products for enhancing accessibility.

Universal Designers and Consultants Inc.
1700 Rockville Pike
Suite 110
Rockville, MD 20852
301-770-7890

UD&C specializes in assisting clients in making facilities accessible to persons with disabilities in compliance with the ADA. Services include facility surveys, strategic planning, product identification, site and facility designs, telephone consulting, and attitudinal training. Publications, software, and videos are available.

Shared Housing Resource Center, Inc.
431 Pine Street
Burlington, VT 05401
802-862-2727

A national clearinghouse for more than 400 shared housing programs throughout the country. This center promotes shared housing, answers consumer inquiries, and assists professionals in the development and implementation of shared housing programs.

Universal Design Initiative of the Assistive Technology Program
National Rehabilitation Hospital
P.O. Box 222514
Chantilly, VA
703-378-5079

Producer and distributor of videos and resources on universal design.

Untie the Elderly
> The Kendel Corporation
> P.O. Box 100
> Kenrett Square, PA 19348
> 610-388-5500

An interdisciplinary program to eliminate physical and chemical restraints in health care settings. Informative publications, newsletters, audiovisuals, inservices, and workshops provide practical, ethical alternatives to the use of restraints. Many suggestions emphasize the use of purposeful activity as an effective method to manage behavior.

US Access Board (formerly known as the Architectural and Transportation Compliance Board)
> 1331 F Street, NW
> Suite 1000
> Washington, DC 20004-1111
> 202-272-5434
> 202-272-5449 (TDD)

The Board is an independent federal regulatory agency charged with issuing standards and regulations regarding the accessibility of public and private facilities. It publishes pamphlets, brochures, and articles about architectural accessibility; federal buildings; airports; federal law; and design. It also processes complaints about accessibility, often recommending adaptations to achieve compliance with federal standards. It enforces the Architectural Barrier Act and develops guidelines for ADA compliance. In addition, its Office of Technical services provides technical assistance and training on the removal of barriers in areas of architecture, transportation, communication, and attitudes.

Leisure, Recreation, and Play

Also see Professional Organizations, Family and Social Supports; Therapeutic Activities and Equipment Suppliers, as many of these professional and consumer resources provide a diversity of information and services relevant to leisure pursuits and recreational activities (e.g., books, videos, games, exercise groups, swimming programs, field trips, discount tickets, and transportation).

Ability Journal
> C2 Publishing
> 1682 Langley Avenue
> Irvine, CA 92714-5633
> 714-854-8700

A bimonthly magazine that emphasizes entertainment, and technology of interest to the general public and the personal achievements of persons with disabilities.

ABLED! Active, Beautiful, Loving, Exquisite Disabled Woman
> 12211 Fondren, Suite 703
> Houston, TX 77035
> 713-726-1132

A non-profit organization that publishes a free quarterly newsletter in print and audio cassette format, focused on women with disabilities. Thematic articles and regular columns focus on health, beauty, careers, leisure, legal concerns, and other issues related to being a woman with a disability.

Accent on Living
> P.O. Box 700
> Bloomington, IL 61701
> 309-378-2961

A quarterly magazine focusing on the needs and concerns of persons with disabilities. Articles cover organizations, products, and ideas for daily living, recreation, and humor. A *Buyer's Guide*, a sourcebook on products and services, is also available.

Access to Recreation, Inc.
> 2509 E. Thousand Oaks Blvd.
> Suite 430
> Thousand Oaks, CA 91362
> 805-498-7535
> 800-634-4351

Access to Recreation is a catalog featuring adaptive recreation equipment for persons with physical disabilities. It offers many items, including camera mounts, adapted golf clubs, fishing reels, exercisers, bowling ball ramps, games, and knitting aids.

American Automobile Association (AAA)
> 1000 AAA Drive
> Heathrow, FL 32746-5063
> 407-444-7961

In addition to their traditional services for motorists (i.e., trip planning and roadside services), the AAA publishes an extensive, geographically arranged directory of organizations and companies that provide driving evaluations, specialized driver training, vehicle modifications, and other services to drivers with disabilities.

American Athletic Association of the Deaf (AAAD)
> 3607 Washington Boulevard
> Suite 4
> Ogden, UT 84403
> 801-393-8710
> 801-393-7916 (TTD)

A membership organization providing yearround sports and recreation opportunities for people who are deaf. A quarterly newsletter, AAAD *Bulletin*, and a quarterly magazine, *Deaf Sports Review* are also provided to members.

Choice Magazine Listening
> 85 Channel Drive
> Port Washington, NY 11050
> 516-586-8280

A free bimonthly recorded service for persons unable to use regular print because of visual or physical disabilities. Choice Magazine Listening provides, on 4-track cassette tapes, eight hours of unabridged articles, fiction and poetry form such publications as *Smithsonian*, *The New Yorker*, *Foreign Affairs*, *The New York Times Magazine*, *The Atlantic*, *Esquire*, *Sports Illustrated*, *Audubon*, and *The Wall Street Journal*. Talking book 4-track cassette tape players are available free from the Library of Congress, National Library Service for the Blind and Physically Handicapped, Washington, DC.

Compeer, Inc.

Monroe Square, Suite B-1
259 Monroe Avenue
Rochester, NY 14607
800-836-0475

Compeer is a program that trains volunteers to serve as a caring friend to a person with mental illness. Volunteers are asked to make a minimum commitment of one hour per week for a year to meet at mutually convenient times with their friend to share activities like walking, shopping, going to the movies, or just chatting at a coffee shop. Compeer also provides a telephone calling service to support individuals awaiting a oneto-one match and special services for men, women, and children who are homeless. Volunteers receive 5 hours of training, and ongoing education and support from Compeer staff.

Descriptive Video Service (DVS)

WGBH-TV
125 Western Avenue
Boston, MA 02134
617-492-2777, ext. 5400
800-736-3099
800-333-1203

DVS is a national service of WGBH-TV that provides audio description for a wide variety of public television (PBS) programs. DVS also produces and distributes dozens of home videos with audio description, including popular Hollywood dramas, comedies, family programs, action/ adventure, sci fi movies, mysteries, documentaries, and educational programs.

Disabilities Digest

P.O. Box 44275
Cincinnati, OH 45244-0275
513-528-0404

A bimonthly subscription magazine which aims to provide a central source of information and a forum for disability for all people. Each issue has an editorial theme (e.g., ADA, sexuality, education). Regular departments include Arts and Leisure, Business, Family and Health, Science and Medicine, and Communication.

Disability Today

627 Lyons Lane
Suite 203
Oakville, ON, Canada L6J527
905-338-6894

A quarterly Canadian subscription magazine which emphasizes advancing equity and opportunity for persons with disabilities. Feature articles focus on legal issues, environmental access, rehabilitation sports, education, and leisure. Regular departments include news, computers, prevention, marketplace, and resources.

Disabled Sports USA

451 Hungerford Drive, Suite 100
Rockville, MD 20850
301-217-0960

Disabled Sports USA's nationwide network of nearly 70 community-based chapters and affiliates offers a wide variety of activities, including camping, hiking, biking, horseback riding, 10K runs, water skiing, white water rafting, rope courses, mountain climbing, sailing, yachting, canoeing, kayaking, aerobic fitness, and snow skiing. Special youth programs are also available.

Handicap Introductions (HI)

35 Wisconsin Circle
Suite 205
Chevy Chase, MD 20815
301-656-8723

A network for persons with disabilities and non-disabled people who do not view disabilities as barriers to an active social life. HI operates as an international dating service with most "matches" occurring across the United States via phone calls and mailed correspondence. Successful "matches" have resulted in strong friendships, social dates, interstate visits and over 100 marriages.

Handicapped Scuba Association

116 W. El Portal, Suite 104
San Clemente, CA 92672
610-692-7824

A non-profit organization providing diver education programs for persons with disabilities. A dive club, refresher courses, diving excursions, listings of accessible hotels/ resorts, videos, and lecture presentations are available. Instructor training courses, diver certification, and dive buddy programs are also available.

International Bible Society

1820 Jet Stream Drive
Colorado Spring, CO 80921-3696

The International Bible Society publishes a Bible designed specifically for the reading convenience of people with physical disability, "New International Version New Testament and Psalms for the Physically Disabled." Features include: large, 13 point type, special spiral binding to enable the book to be easily opened and remain open, and special coated paper that makes pages easy to turn by hand or with a mouth stick.

Kaleidoscope: International Magazine of Literature, Fine Arts, and Disability

United Disability Services
326 Locust Street
Akron, OH 44302
216-762-9755

A semi-annual subscription literary magazine. Each issue addresses a theme through fiction, poetry, personal essays, and photography. Information about current literature, films, research treatment programs, and health care trends is also included.

Mainstream—Magazine of the Abled-Disabled

P.O. Box 370598
San Diego, CA 92137-0598

A subscription magazine featuring articles, editorials, and commentaries on education, employment, recreation, technology, healthcare, advocacy, and politics.

Matilda Ziegler Magazine for the Blind
80 Eighth Avenue
Room 1304
New York, NY 10011
212-242-0263
212-633-1601 (Fax)

The *Matilda Ziegler Magazine for the Blind* is a monthly that reprints articles covering a wide range of subjects taken from some of the nation's foremost newspapers and periodicals; it also gives news of particular interest to persons who are blind and visually impaired. The magazine, published in Grade 2 braille and on four-track, half-speed cassette, was founded in 1907 by E. Matilda Ziegler, whose endowment covers the cost of free distribution of the magazine to any person who is blind who requests it.

Mouth: The Voice of Disability Rights
61 Brighton Street
Rochester, NY 14607
716-442-2916 (Fax only)

A bimonthly subscription magazine available in standard print, large print, and audio cassette format (hardship subscriptions of $1 or $2 are available). Mouth emphasizes activism and methods to revolutionize the way society, organizations, and sociopolitical systems view and treat persons with disabilities.

Moving Forward
P.O. Box 3553
Torrance, CA 90510-3553
310-320-8793

A national newspaper for people with disabilities. Regular features include national and international news relevant to persons with disabilities, legal and ADA information, research reports, sports, travel, and opinion columns.

National Library Service for the Blind and Physically Handicapped
The Library of Congress
1291 Taylor Street, NW
Washington, DC 20542
202-707-5100

A free national library for individuals who cannot use standard printed materials due to visual or physical limitations (e.g., low vision, paralysis, weakness, incoordination). Talking books, large print and braille books, magazines, and musical scores are available. Special cassette players, phonographs, amplifiers, and remote controls are also loaned for free. A diversity of topics ranging from adventures, mysteries, classics, cookbooks, drama, fine arts, history, humor, music, science and nature, science fiction, westerns, travel, and best sellers are offered for all age ranges.

National Arts and Disability Center (NADC)
300 UCLA Medical Plaza
Room 3330
Los Angeles, CA 90095
310-794-1141

NADC provides technical assistance and information on art schools and organizations, assistive technology, and related topics.

National Foundation of Wheelchair Tennis (NFWT)
940 Calle Amanecer, Suite B
San Clemente, CA 92672
714-361-3663

An organization promoting recreational and competitive wheelchair tennis through instructional clinics, camp programs and competitive tournaments. Publications and videos are available.

National Wheelchair Basketball Association (NWBA)
P.O. Box 6001
2850 North Garey Avenue
Pomona, CA 91769-6001
909-596-7733 x2212 or x2210

A national organization to promote wheelchair basketball. NWBA has 175 teams competing in 25 conferences annually. A wheelchair basketball training camp is also provided.

National Wheelchair Softball Association (NWSA)
1616 Todd Court
Hastings, MN 55033
612-437-1792

NWSA is the national governing body for wheelchair softball in the US. Local league play and tournaments are available.

National Amputee Golf Association
11 Walnut Hill Road
P.O. Box 1228
Amherst, NH 03031
800-633-6242

A membership organization open to anyone who has an upper or lower extremity amputation and who enjoys golfing. Learn-to-Golf clinics for the physically disabled and modified golf equipment are available.

New Mobility
Miramar Communications Inc.
23815 Stuart Ranch Road
P.O. Box 8987
Malibu, CA 90265
800-543-4116
310-317-4522

A monthly subscription magazine focusing on disability lifestyle, culture, and resources.

North American Riding for the Handicapped Association (NARHA)
P.O. Box 33150
Denver, CO 80233
800-369-RIDE

A non-profit organization dedicated to promoting equine activities for persons with disabilities. Publications and videos that provide information on therapeutic riding and riding programs are available. A "start-up packet" is available to assist with the development of new programs. NARHA is also the parent organization of the American Hippotherapy Association (AHA) which promote research, education, and communication among occupational and physical therapists and others using horses as a treatment approach with persons with disabilities.

PN / Paraplegia News
Paralyzed Veterans of America Inc.
2111 East Highland Avenue
Suite 180
Phoenix, AZ 85016-4702
602-224-0500

A monthly publication providing information for wheelchair user. Legislative updates, computer columns, and articles on adaptive equipment, wheelchairs, and accessibility are included.

SABAH, Inc.
(Skating Association for the Blind and Handicapped, Inc.)
548 Elmwood Avenue
Buffalo, NY 14222
716-883-9728

SABAH teaches ice skating to people of all ages and abilities at their own pace. SABAH has developed special equipment for persons with mental, physical, or emotional disabilities, enabling them to learn to ice skate. SABAH also offers training seminars for therapists.

Sports and Spokes
2111 East Highland Avenue
Suite 180
Phoenix, AZ 85016
602-224-0500

A bimonthly journal on competitive sports and recreation for persons with disabilities. Junior, adult, and wheelchair sports are featured.

The Disability Rag and Resource
P.O. Box 145
Louisville, KY 40201
502-452-5343

A bimonthly subscription magazine available in a multitude of formats; standard print, large print, cassette, braille, and diskette. Its' focus is on disability rights, and each issue addresses a theme not often addressed in other disability press publications. Regular columns include book and film reviews, fiction, poetry, editorials, and media watch.

Theater Access Project (TAP)
Theater Development Fund
1501 Broadway
New York, NY 10036
212-221-0885

TAP's aim is to increase the access of New York's theater to the physical disabled. Services include sign-interpreted performances, preferential seating, ticket ordering by mail and discounted tickets to plays, musicals, concerts, and dance recitals. While TAP only serves the New York theater, many major cities provide similar accessibility services. For information contact each city's office for the disabled.

Toys R' Us Toy Guide for Differently-Abled Kids
This shopping guide contains toys that are educational, entertaining, and meet the standards set by the U.S. Consumer Products Safety Commission. They have been professionally tested by children with disabilities. Copies of this free guide are available at any Toys R' Us store.

Twin Peaks Press
P.O. Box 129
Vancouver, WA 98666-0129
206-694-2462
800-637-2256

A publisher and distributor of directories and books for persons with disabilities. Its free Disability Bookshop Catalog lists more than 400 books of interest for persons with disabilities, which are available for mail-order purchase.

Very Special Arts (VSA)
The John F. Kennedy Center for the Performing Arts
Washington, DC 20566
800-933-VSA1

A non-profit organization dedicated to enriching the lives of the individuals with physical and/or mental disabilities through participation in the arts. VSA coordinates programs in music, dance, creative dramatics, and the visual arts. Publications, videos, technical assistance, demonstrations, conferences, seminars, workshops, and arts festivals are offered throughout the country for all age groups.

Voyager Outward Bound School
111 3rd Avenue South
Suite 120
Minneapolis, MN 55401

Voyager Outward Bound's mission is to conduct adventure-based educational courses structured to inspire self esteem, self reliance, concern for others and care for the environment. A "Mixed Ability" course designed for both physically challenged and able-bodied participants is offered to enable persons with physical disabilities to participate in the Outward Bound experience.

Wheelchair Archery Sports Section
3595 E. Fountain Blvd., Suite L-1
Colorado Springs, CO 80910
719-574-1150

An organization promoting recreational and competitive archery for person with disabilities. Adaptive equipment is available to enable persons with upper extremity weakness to participate in archery events.

Wheelchair Athletics of the USA/NWAA
3595 E. Fountain Blvd., Suite L-1
Colorado Springs, CO 80910
719-574-1150

An organization which promotes a number of recreational and competitive wheelchair sports including track, field, and road racing.

Wilderness on Wheels Foundation (WOW)
7125 W. Jefferson Avenue - No. 155
Lakewood, CO 80235
303-988-2212

This non-profit foundation has constructed a mile-long accessible boardwalk through the Rockies, 60 miles southwest of Denver. People with disabilities can hike, fish, cookout, and camp along the trail. There is no charge.

World At Large
Dept. M
P.O. Box 190330
Brooklyn, NY 11219
800-285-2743
800-AT-LARGE

A weekly tabloid-sized large type subscription news magazine the presents stories selected from and published simultaneously by US News and World Report, Time, and other magazines. World and national news, education, health, the arts, sports, and crossword puzzles are among its featured articles.

Therapeutic Activities and Equipment Suppliers

Attainment Company
504 Commerce Parkway
Verona, WI 53593
800-327-4269

Distributor of Life Skill Programs for people with developmental or acquired disabilities. Products include step-by-step illustrated materials for shopping, cooking, community activities, grooming, and housekeeping.

BiFolkal Productions Inc.
809 Williamson Street
Madison, WI 53703
608-251-2818

A non-profit corporation producing materials for use in activities with older adults. Multisensory kits are designed to encourage reminiscence and the inter-generational sharing of memories. A comprehensive catalog and a free quarterly newsletter of program ideas are available. Many public libraries loan BiFolkal Kits for free.

Books on Special Children
P.O. Box 305
Congers, NY 10920-0305
914-638-1236

A distributor of books on children with special needs: for parents, caregivers, and professionals.

Childswork/Childsplay
Center for Applied Psychology, Inc.
P.O. Box 1586
King of Prussia, PA 19406

A distributor of therapeutic games, self-help books and reference materials which focus on addressing the mental health needs of children and their families. Many of their self-awareness and esteem-building products are suitable for all ages.

Clinician's View
6007 Osuna Road, NE
Albuquerque, NM 87109
505-880-0058
505-880-0059 (Fax)

Producers and distributors of therapeutic and clinical videos, continuing education seminars, and publications form infant and pediatric treatment to adult rehabilitation, home health, and ADA.

Craft Resources
P.O. Box 828
Fairfield, CT 06430
800-243-2874

A distributor of needlecraft, arts and crafts, and supplies.

Creative Crafts International
16 Plains Road
P.O Box 819
Essex, CT 06426
800-666-0767

A distributor of arts and crafts equipment and supplies.

Crestwood Company
6625 N. Sidney Place
Milwaukee, WI 53209-3259
414-352-5678

Distributor of communications aids for children and adults and adapted toys for children with special needs.

Cross Creek Recreational Products
P.O. Box 409A
Amenia, NY 12501
212-685-3672

A distributor of therapeutic activities developed for people with Alzheimer's disease and related dementia diseases, multi-infarct stroke patients, the developmentally disabled, mentally retarded adults, and the psychiatrically impaired.

Dick Blick Company
P.O. Box 1267
Galesburg, IL 61401
309-343-6181 x235
800-933-2542

A distributor of arts and crafts materials including kits and open stock materials.

Electronic Industries Foundation (EIF)
919 18th Street NW
Suite 900
Washington, DC 20006
202-955-5814

EIF provides general information on assistive devices and their applications, as well as alternative devices for persons with disabilities.

Geriatric Resources Inc.
931 South Semoran Boulevard
Suite 200
Winter Park, FL 32792
800-359-0390
407-678-1616

Producers and distributors of products to help improve the quality of life and manage potentially problematic behaviors for persons with dementia. Products are grouped functionally according to cognitive abilities and level of cognitive decline. Products include memory aids, reminiscent games, puzzles, sensory stimulation products, audio cassettes and educational texts.

Glanz-Richman Rehabilitation Associates, LTD
1560 Indian Trail
Riverwoods, IL 60015
708-945-1917

Publisher and distributor of evaluation, treatment, and activity manuals for the psychogeriatric patient population. Publication emphasis is on meeting the needs of clients residing in nursing homes and complying with OBRA regulations.

Gold Timers
(A Division of Incentives for Learning, Inc.)
111 Center Avenue, Suite I
Pacheco, CA 94553
510-682-2428

Publishers and distributors of games, activities, textbooks, books on tape, videos, and adult appropriate coloring books. Most items focus on language development, behavior management, reminiscence, and/or the needs of persons with Alzheimer's.

Imaginart Therapy Materials
307 Arizona Street
Bisbee, AZ 85603
800-828-1376

Distributor of publications on therapeutic activities, puzzles, games, communication programs, and activity kits.

Knight's Woodcraft for Therapeutic Activities
P.O. Box 900888
San Diego, CA 92190-9988
619-265-1668

A distributor of woodcrafts kits, tools, and supplies.

Nasco
901 Janesville Avenue
Fort Atkinson, WI 52538-0901
800-558-9595

A distributor of arts and crafts, teaching aids, supplies, and equipment.

National Mobility Equipment Dealers Association (NMEDA)
909-East Skagway Avenue
Tampa, FL 33604
800-833-0427
813-932-8566

This member association provides information and referrals on equipment funding, safety, legislation, driver evaluation, adaptive vehicle modification and related areas of concern regarding mobility for persons with disabilities.

National Rehabilitation Information Center (NARIC)
8455 Colesville Road, Suite 935
Silver Spring, MD 20910-3319
800-346-2742
301-588-9284

MARIC is a library and information center, housing more than 40,000 documents in all aspects of disability and rehabilitation. Services include ABLEDATA; a national computerized data bank giving information about commercially-available rehabilitation aids and equipment, and REHABDATA; a database providing a descriptive listing of all NARIC documents on a particular topic or combination of topics. All products and services are available in a multitude of formats to ensure accessibility to all persons with disabilities. NARIC is staffed by specialists trained to provide individualized assistance to meet the unique needs of the user. Publications addressing consumer and practitioner needs are available.

Psychological Corp.
Communications/Therapy Skill Builders
P.O. Box 839954
San Antonio, TX 78283-3954
602-232-7500
800-866-4446

A publisher and distributor of texts, videos, patient education manuals, activity materials, games, and equipment suitable for a variety of patient populations. *Cognitive Rehabilitation: Group Games and Activities* is particularly relevant to many practice settings.

Rifton for People with Disabilities
P.O. Box 901
Rifton, NY 12471-0901
800-336-5948
914-658-8065

Manufacturers of adaptive devices, chairs, tables, positioning equipment, hand-driven tricycles, community playthings, and wooden day care equipment.

S&S Arts and Crafts
P.O. Box 513
Department 2082
Colchester, CT 06415
800-243-9232

A distributor of arts and crafts supplies and equipment.

Sammons Preston Inc.
P.O. Box 5071
Bolingbrook, IL 60440-5071
800-323-5547

A distributor of evaluation, treatment, and rehabilitation supplies and equipment.

Society for the Advancement of Rehabilitation and Assistive Technology (RESNA)
1101 Connecticut Avenue, NW

Suite 700
Washington, DC 20036
202-857-1199

A membership organization which addresses research, development, dissemination, and utilization of knowledge in rehabilitative and assistive technology. A journal, Assistive Technology, a newsletter, numerous publications, and an annual conference are provided.

Tandy Leather Company
1400 Everman Parkway
Ft. Worth, TX 76113
817-551-9778

A distributor of leather craft projects, kits, tools, and books.

The ROM Institute
3601 Memorial Drive
Madison, WI 53704
608-243-2451

Producer of the ROM Dance Instructional Media kit, which is a tool for teaching range of motion exercise, relaxation, and pain management to elderly, arthritis, or Parkinson patients.

The Leather Factory
P.O. Box 50429
Ft. Worth, TX 76105
817-496-4414

A distributor of leather, leathercraft tools, and supplies.

The Lighthouse Inc.
Low Vision Products
36-02 Northern Boulevard
Long Island City, NY 11101
800-453-4923

A non-profit vision rehabilitation agency providing a diversity of consumer services. Their products catalog offers a number of assistive devices, games, and hobbies for the visually impaired. Many items are also appropriate for persons with physical and/or cognitive disabilities.

Therapro, Inc.
225 Arlington Street
Framingham, MA 01701
508-872-9494

Producer and distributor of therapeutic activities to stimulate sensation, perception, and cognition. Adaptive equipment, developmental learning material, books, and assessments are also sold.

Therapy Skill Builders
3830 E. Bellevue
P.O. Box 42050-H92
Tucson, AZ 85733
602-323-7500

A publisher and distributor of texts, videos, patient education manuals, games, and equipment suitable for a variety of patient populations across the life span.

Tools of the Trade
13005 8th Avenue NW
Seattle, WA 98177
206-363-8104

Manufacturer and distributor of toys that can be used for therapy for the very young to the very old. Each toy lists age ranges and specific purposes the toys can be used for.

"2 to 6" The Early Childhood Report
Biddle Publishing Co.
P.O. Box 1305
Brunswick, ME 04011
207-833-5016

This publication is a multidisciplinary digest of current information, reviews, and activities to enhance the learning and development of children aged 2 to 6. Contents include an activities page, children's book and toy review, medical column, and literature reviews in the areas of early childhood education, socialemotional development, sensory-motor development, speech and language, and more—all presented in terms of developmental age versus grade level or chronological age.

Vanguard Crafts
1081 East 48th Street
Brooklyn, NY 11234
718-377-5188

An arts and crafts supplier and distributor. Project packs and individual materials are available.

Veteran Leather Company, Inc.
204 25th Street
Brooklyn, NY 11232
718-768-0300

A manufacturer and distributor of leather, tools, kits, and other leathercraft supplies.

Wellness Reproductions, Inc.
23945 Mercantile Road
Beachwood, OH 44122-5924
216-831-9209
800-669-9208

Producers and distributors of therapeutic products and psychoeducational materials. Their publications, *Life Management Skills I, II, III, and IV*, each contain 50 reproducible activity handouts covering a wealth of functional skills, (e.g., stress management, assertiveness, goal setting, discharge planning, leisure, and community integration). Posters, games, and videos are also available. All products can be easily graded and utilized with a diversity of patient populations.

Whole Persons Associates
1702 E. Jefferson
Duluth, MN 55812
800-247-6789

A distributor of print and audiovisual publications that address the areas of stress management and wellness promotion. Complete course packages are available.

World Wide Games
P.O. Box 517
Department 2082
Colchester, CT 06415
800-243-9232

A distributor of games to generate social integration and improve coordination and concentration. Many are suitable for one hand, wheelchair use, or for the vision impaired.

Educational and Vocational Rehabilitation

American Printing House for the Blind (APH)
1839 Frankfort Avenue
P.O. Box 6085
Louisville, KY 40206-0085
502-895-2405

APH is the official source of educational texts for visually handicapped students (primary through secondary level) throughout the United States and its possessions. It maintains the Central Catalog, which is a listing of textbooks available in large type, braille, and recorded format that are produced by APH and by commercial companies. It also engages in research; manufactures and sells assistive devices and produces recreational and religious literature in special format.

Association for Education and Rehabilitation of the Blind and Visually Impaired
206 North Washington Street, Suite 320
Alexandria, VA 22314
703-548-1884

This organization promotes the advancement of education, guidance, and vocational rehabilitation of blind and visually impaired children and adults. It maintains job exchange services and a speaker's bureau, offers continuing-education seminars and publishes several journals and newsletters.

Association on Higher Education and Disability (AHEAD)
P.O. Box 21192
Columbus, OH 43221
614-488-4972

AHEAD is a membership organization for individuals involved in the development of policy and in the provision of quality support services to serve the needs of persons with disabilities involved in all areas of higher education. It publishes the quarterly magazine, *Journal of Postsecondary Education and Disability*, a newsletter, the Alert, and numerous consumer, educational, and training booklets, texts, and videos.

Association on Handicapped Student Service Programs in Postsecondary Education (AHSSPPE)
P.O. Box 21192
Columbus, OH 43221-0192
614-488-4972

AHSSPPE is a membership organization for individuals involved in the provision of quality support services to disabled students in higher education. A quarterly publication Journal of *Postsecondary Education and Disability*, a newsletter: *the Alert*, several special interest groups, numerous informational publications, training workshops, and conferences are provided to members.

Breaking New Ground Resource Center
Agricultural Engineering Dept.
Purdue University
West Lafayette, IN 47907
317-494-5088
800-825-4264

The Breaking New Ground Resource Center assists farmers and ranchers who are physically disabled. Publications include newsletters, technical articles, resource manuals, and video tapes/slide set. Major areas of focus include technical devices, prosthetics, worksite modifications, and hand controls to enable farmers and ranchers to continue their work.

CAREERS and the DISABLED
Equal Opportunity Publications, Inc.
150 Motor Parkway, Suite 420
Hauppauge, NY 11788
516-273-0066

A career magazine for people with disabilities, published three times per year. A nominal subscription fee is charged.

Center on Education and Training for Employment (CETE)
The Ohio State University
1900 Kenny Road
Columbus, OH 43210
614-292-4353
800-848-4815

CETE is a non-profit organization which provides access to current research, curricular resources, and other products pertaining to vocational education and training.

Closing The Gap (CTG)
P.O. Box 68
Henderson, MN 56044
612-248-3294

CTG disseminates information on up-to-date computer technologies and commercially available hardware and software that enables persons with disabilities to utilize computers for education, work, and independent living. A bimonthly newspaper, workshops, and an annual international conference are provided.

Coalition for Disabled Musicians
P.O. Box 1002M
Bay Shore, NY 11706
516-586-0366

A self-help non-profit organization which gives persons with disabilities the opportunity to pursue their musical dreams. Accessible rehearsal and studio space, music workshops, seminars, and lessons are provided. Amateurs and professionals can join a diversity of studio and stage bands.

Consumer Information Center
P.O. Box 100
Pueblo, CO 81002
719-948-3334

A publisher and distributor of consumer education information sheets and booklets. Topics include health, education, federal benefit programs, the Americans with Disabilities Act (ADA), mental illness, AIDS, cancer, and Alzheimer's disease. Most publications are free. Others have a nominal charge. Many are excellent for use as consumer education tools in psychoeducational groups.

Council for Exception Children (CEC)
1920 Association Drive
Reston, VA 22091-1589
703-620-3660
800-328-0272

CEC is a non-profit organization dedicated to quality education for all exceptional children; preschool, gifted, culturally and linguistically diverse, physically disabled, learning disabled and youth in transition from school to work. CEC has 17 specialized divisions and over 1,000 chapters in the US and Canada. CEC publishes the journals *Teaching Exceptional Children* and *Exceptional Children*. Each specialized division publishes journals, newsletters, books and monographs, and sponsors conferences and other professional development programs. CEC's Center for Special Education Technology distributes information on assistive technology, funding, and training.

Educational Resources Information Center (ERIC)
ERIC is a federally funded information system on schooling, education, and related topics, and a bibliographic database with more than 850,000 articles and documents on all aspects of education. ERIC is composed of 16 clearinghouses, each focusing on a different aspect of education. Each clearinghouse offer free information packets on selected topics. ERIC *Digests* (brief overviews of current topics), books, reports, directories, minibibliographies, references and referrals, customized searches, and prepackaged computer searches on selected topics. Clearinghouses relevant to OT include, but are not limited to:
Adult, Career, and Vocational Education (CE)
Ohio State University
Center on Education and Training for Employment
1900 Kenny Road
Columbus, OH 43210-1090
614-292-4353
800-848-4815
614-292-1260 (Fax)
Disabilities and Gifted Education (EC)
The Council for Exceptional Children
1920 Association Drive
Reston, VA 22091-1589
703-264-9474
800-328-0272

Information and Technology
Syracuse University
4-194 Center for Science and Technology
Syracuse, NY 13244-4100
315-443-3640
800-464-9107
315-443-5448 (Fax)
You can contact any ERIC clearinghouse for a complete listing of ERIC programs and services.

Freedom's Wings International
1832 Lake Avenue
Scotch Plains, NJ 07076
908-232-6354

A membership organization providing flight training with FAA-certified instructors, handcontrolled equipped aircraft, and support equipment for persons with disabilities who wish to become pilots.

HEATH Resource Center
(Higher Education And The Handicapped)
One Dupont Circle
Suite 800
Washington, DC 20036-1193
202-939-9320
800-544-3284

HEATH gathers and disseminates information about educational support services, policies, procedures, adaptations, and opportunities at American campuses, vocational-technical schools, and other post-secondary training entities for persons with disabilities to enable them to develop to their fullest potential through postsecondary education and training. HEATH participates in national conferences, training sessions, and workshops; prepares policy background information for the Department of Education; publishes resource papers, pamphlets, directories, and newsletters; and identifies people who are knowledgeable about disability issues for administrators, counselors, and others at the state or local level.

Job Accommodation Network (JAN)
918 Chestnut Ridge Road
Suite 1
Morgantown, WV 26506

JAN is an information and consulting services providing individualized accommodation solutions to enable persons with disabilities to work It is a free service provided by the President's Committee on Employment of People with Disabilities.

Job Opportunities for the Blind (JOB)
1800 Johnson Street
Baltimore, MD 21230
800-638-7518
410-659-9314

A nation-wide employment listing referral and resource service for persons who are blind. Publications include a bi-monthly job magazine, proceedings of JOB seminars, and informational booklets on job seeking employment skills and ADA. All publications are available in multi-formats, including audio cassette and Braille.

Lift Inc.
P.O. Box 1072
Mountside, NJ 07092
908-789-2443
800-552-5438

Lift is a non-profit organization which recruits, trains, and hires individuals with disabilities as computer professional for corporate clients throughout the country. A comprehensive 6 month at home training program and advanced technological aids are provided so that persons with severe disabilities can succeed. Job placements at corporate sites and/or at home using telecommunications are available.

Mobility International USA (MIUSA)
P.O. Box 10767
Eugene, OR 97403
503-343-1284

A national non-profit organization that helps integrate people with disabilities into international educational exchange programs and travel. It offers educational exchange programs, international workcamps, and travel information and referral services for individual or group travel. A quarterly newsletter, resource texts, travel guides, and videotapes are available.

Modern Talking Picture Service
Captioned Films/Videos Program
4707 140th Avenue North
Clearwater, FL 34622
813-532-0706

A free-loan service of educational and theatrical captioned films/videos to assist deaf/hearing impaired persons in their educational and recreational pursuits. Classic features, the latest Hollywood releases, short subjects, continuing educational titles, afterschool specials, and school subjects from preschool through college are available.

National Industries for the Severely Handicapped (NISH)
2235 Cedar Lane
Vienna, VA 22182
703-560-6800
703-560-6512 (TDD)

A federally funded agency which seeks to provide employment to persons with severe disabilities through Federal contracts. A monthly publication, NISH News is available.

National Theater Workshop of the Handicapped (NTWH)
354 Broome Street
Suite 5-1
New York, NY 10013
212-941-9511

NTWH is a training production and advocacy organization serving adults with disabilities. NTWH offers professional instruction in acting, oral interpretation, music, movement and dance, playwriting, theater management and technical theater. The Theater Workshop maintains a professional repertory theater company which showcases the talents of its students in every form of theater.

President's Committee on Employment of People with Disabilities
1331 F Street, NW
Washington, DC 20004-1107
202-376-6200

The President's Committee on Employment of People with Disabilities publishes and distributes free pamphlets, newsletters, publications, and posters covering such topics as education, employment, accessibility, and adapting the work site. Additional publications and videos are available for purchase. Collaboration with employers is emphasized and all disabilities (physical, psychological, and/or learning) are considered.

Prevention Plus, Inc.
5775 Wayzata Boulevard
Suite 700
Minneapolis, MN 55416

A consulting company specializing in the prevention and management of work injuries through the production and distribution of publications and audiovisuals on ergonomics, safety, back injury, and cumulative trauma.

Recording for the Blind and Dyslexic (RFB&D)
20 Roszel Road
Princeton, NJ 08540
609-452-0606

RFB&D is a non-profit service organization that provides recorded educational books and related library services to people with print disabilities (i.e., blindness, low vision, learning disabilities, or other physical impairments that effect reading). RFB&D has an extensive lending library of books (over 80,000) already recorded, including educational texts, fiction, drama, and poetry in a number of languages and a recording service for additional titles.

Stout Vocational Rehabilitation Institute (SVRI)
School of Education and Human Service
University of Wisconsin-Stout
Menomenee, WI 54741-0790
715-232-2475

SVRI provides vocational rehabilitation services, conducts research, provides training, and produces and disseminates information to further the potential of persons with disabilities. SVRI is comprised of 4 centers to effectively meet the needs of persons with disabilities and their service providers. These centers are the Projects with Industry Center, Center for Rehabilitation Technology, Research and Training Center, and Vocational Center.

The Dole Foundation
> 1819 H Street NW, Suite 340
> Washington, DC 20006-3603
> 202-457-0318

A non-profit organization dedicated to expanding employment opportunities for persons with disabilities. It disseminates information, provides grants, and distributes numerous publications to educate consumers, employers, and the public about the employment of working-aged people with disabilities, and to assist employers in making accommodations for workers with disabilities

Trace Research and Development Center
> University of Wisconsin-Madison
> S-151 Waisman Center
> 1500 Highland Avenue
> Madison, WI 53705-2280
> 608-262-6966

The Trace Center is a leading research and development site focusing in the areas of disability access to computers and information systems. Trace produces the Co-Net CD-ROM, containing the Cooperative Electronic Library on Disability. This is an integrated collection of information resources in an easy-to-use computer database form, and includes ABLEDATA and REHABDATA. Trace also publishes a Resource book containing a comprehensive listing of assistive technologies for communication, control, and computer.

University of Illinois Film Center
> 1325 S. Oak Street
> Champaign, IL 61820
> 800-FOR-FILM

A distributor of thousands of educational and health-related videos. Videos are available for sale or short-term and long-term rentals. Many are relevant to patient education and/or staff training programs.

Vocational Studies Center
> University of Wisconsin-Madison
> 964 Educational Sciences Building
> 1025 West Johnson Street
> Madison, WI 53706
> 608-263-2929

The Vocational Studies Center is a research, development, and service center which provides technical assistance and products to assist vocational educators and rehabilitation therapists. Resources available include curriculum development aids, audiovisual materials, and textbooks. Many products are specific to persons with disabilities and are suitable for diverse educational levels and age groups.

Professional Organizations, Family and Social Supports

Also see Leisure, Recreation, and Play resources, for this list includes a number of publications, magazines and newsletters which often provide a great deal of supportive information for consumers and their families.

Alexander Graham Bell Association for the Deaf
> 3417 Volta Place, N.W.
> Washington, DC 20007
> 202-337-5520

A non-profit organization providing advocacy services and financial assistance to children and adults with hearing impairments. Financial aid for newborns and school-aged children, and college scholarships for young adults and adults are provide. General information and a catalog of educational publications are available.

Alzheimer's Disease and Related Disorders Association (ADRDA)
> 919 North Michigan Avenue
> Suite 1000
> Chicago, IL 60611
> 800-621-0379

A national, non-profit organization serving individuals with Alzheimer's disease or related dementias, and their families. Diagnostic and treatment referrals, information packets and fact sheets, local support groups and respite care, legal and financial assistance, an autopsy assistance network, educational seminars and research abstracts, and a print and video library are available to member.

American Parkinson's Disease Association (APDA)
> Suite 401
> 60 Bay Street
> Staten Island, NY 10301
> 718-981-8001
> 800-223-2732

A non-profit organization dedicated to finding a cure and easing the burden of Parkinson's disease. APDA funds research to increase knowledge and improve the treatment of Parkinson's disease. Local support groups for patients and their families, and educational publications are available.

American Paralysis Association
> 500 Morris Avenue
> Springfield, NJ 07081
> 201-379-2690
> 800-526-3456

A non-profit organization providing a toll-free spinal cord injury (SCI) Hotline. The hotline provides information and referrals to individuals who have sustained an SCI, and their families. Referrals include resources for peer support, rehabilitation facilities, professional experts, and local SCI organizations.

American Amputee Foundation (AAF)
P.O. Box 250218
Hillcrest Station
Little Rock, AR 72225
501-666-2523

AAF provides information and referrals for amputees and their families. A semi-annual newsletter, self-help guides, peer counseling, and low cost loans for purchase of prostheses. Assistance with insurance claims, justification letters to payers, testimony and life planning, home modifications and technical assistance are also provided.

American Heart Association
7320 Greenville Avenue
Dallas, TX 75231
800-242-8721
214-373-6300

A national, non-profit organization serving individuals with heart disease, and their families. Educational information, treatment referrals, prevention programs, patient and family support groups, and research funding are provided.

American Association of People with Disabilities (AAPD)
4401 Connecticut Avenue, NW
Suite 223
Washington, DC 20008

A private non-profit organization which aims to provide a unified voice for persons with disabilities, support full implementation and enforcement of ADA, enhance the productivity, independence and full integration of persons with disabilities, and educate and influence government policy makers and the public on the rights and issues of persons with disabilities.

American Association of Retired Persons (AARP)
1909 K Street
Washington, DC 20049
202-434-2277

A membership organization for persons over 50 providing a diversity of educational and service programs. Health care referrals and consumer advocacy, pre-retirement planning, a Volunteer Talent bank, tax assistance and financial counseling, criminal justice assistance, widow-persons services, audiovisual and print publications, and the bi-monthly journal *Modern Maturity*, are provided to members. ASRP is a member of the Long-term Care Campaign and has special initiatives focusing on minority affairs, women, and worker equity.

American Foundation for the Blind (AFB)
1615 M Street, N.W.
Suite 250
Washington, DC 20036
202-457-1487
800-232-5463

AFB is a non-profit organization whose mission is to enable people who are blind or visually impaired to achieve equality of access and opportunity to ensure freedom of choice in their lives. AFB operates the National Technology Center, which serves as a resource for research and development, evaluations, and information services on technology for blind and visually impaired people and their families, professionals in blindness and low vision fields, employers, educators, researchers, and private industry. AFB also operates an American with Disabilities Act (ADA) Consulting Group, the Careers and Technology information Bank, and a Talking Book program. Regional support centers are available nationwide. Publications, adaptive equipment, health care information, and leisure activities are available from AFB's product catalog. AFB also publishes the *Guide to Toys for Children Who are Blind or Visually Impaired*.

American Cancer Society
1599 Clifton Road, N.E.
Atlanta, GA 30329
800-ACS-2345
404-320-3333

A national, non-profit organization dedicated to serving the needs of individuals with cancer, and their families. Public education, consumer information, treatment referrals, advocacy, and research are national priorities. State and local chapters provide a diversity of direct services, including patient and family support groups, peer counseling, rehabilitation programs, home care equipment and supplies, and transportation to and from treatment appointments. Audiovisual, publications, newsletters, research briefs, workshops, and a national conference are available.

American Diabetes Association
National Service Center
P.O. Box 25757
1660 Duke Street
Alexandria, VA 22314
703-549-1500
800-ADA-DISC

A private, non-profit, membership organization concerned with the diagnosis, treatment, and research for a cure of diabetes. Public, patient, family, and professional educational services and literature are available. A monthly periodical and an annual conference are provided to members.

American Council of the Blind
1155 15th Street, N.W.
Washington, DC 20005
202-467-5081
800-424-8666

A national membership organization concerned with improving the quality of life for blind and visually impaired people. Services include toll-free information and referrals, scholarship assistance to postsecondary students, public education and awareness training, legal assistance, and consumer advocacy. The *Braille Forum*, a free bimonthly magazine, and an annual national convention are available to members.

American Epilepsy Society

638 Prospect Avenue
Hartford, CT 06105-4298
203-232-4825

A professional membership organization promoting interdisciplinary communication and exchange of clinical information about epilepsy Peer review research and a quarterly publication, *Epilepsia*, are provided.

Amyotrophic Lateral Sclerosis (ALS) Association

15300 Ventura Boulevard
Sherman Oaks, CA 91403
818-990-2151

A non-profit organization devoted to research on ALS and to the provision of information and supportive services to persons with ALS, and their families.

Andrus Gerontology Center

University of Southern California
University Park MC-0191
Los Angeles, CA 90089-0191
213-740-6060

The Andrus Gerontology Center has a phone network program for caregivers who are unable to leave their homes to attend caregiver support groups. The center has developed a series of audiotapes entitled "Care-line" that can be used by phone network members to develop social support, increase coping skills, provide information on practical concerns, and develop strategies to manage their caregiving tasks and responsibilities. The Care-line audiotapes (with a program guide) are available for purchase from the Andrus Gerontology Center.

Arthritis Foundation

1314 Spring Street, N.W.
Atlanta, GA 30309
404-872-7100
800-283-7800

A non-profit organization serving the needs of individuals with rheumatoid arthritis, osteoarthritis, ankylosing spondylitis, scleroderma, systemic lupus erythematosus, juvenile arthritis, or fibrositis. Educational packets, treatment information, research findings, and support groups are available for consumers, their families, and the professionals who work with them. The arthritis Health Professions Association (AHPA), a section of the Arthritis Foundation, serves as a professional membership organization, publishes professional literature, and conducts continuing education programs annually.

Association for Children and Adults with Learning Disabilities

4156 Library Road
Pittsburgh, PA 15234
412-881-2253

A private, non-profit, membership organization devoted to learning disabilities. A national center, regional offices, and local chapters provide educational information, diagnostic testing, treatment referrals, remedial centers' newsletters, and publications to consumers, their families, and health care professionals.

Association for Retarded Citizens (ARC)

National Headquarters
500 East Border Street
Suite 300
P.O. Box 300649
Arlington, TX 76010
817-261-6003

ARC is a non-profit national association devoted to improving the welfare of all children and adults with mental retardation, and their families. ARC provides services to parents and other individuals, organizations, and communities for jointly meeting the needs of people with mental retardation. Fact sheets, informational booklets, a bimonthly newsletter, and an electronic mail and information services are available.

Autism Society of America

8601 Georgia Avenue
Suite 503
Silver Spring, MD 20910
301-565-0433

A national agency dedicated to the education and welfare of people with autism. Priorities are research and education. An information and referral service, publications, reading lists, and a quarterly newsletter are provided.

Canine Companions for Independence

P.O. Box 446
1221 Sebastapol Road
Santa Rosa, CA 95402
707-528-0830

A non-profit organization that trains dogs to help persons with disabilities perform activities of daily living and maintain their independence. A promotional and educational video. "What a difference a dog makes," is available.

Center for Consumer Healthcare Information

4000 Birch Street
Suite 112
Newport Beach, CA 92660
800-627-2244

Publisher of the *Case Management Resource Guide*, an annually updated reference book that covers more than 50 categories of health care resources, including home care, rehabilitation, psychiatric and addiction treatment, and long-term care services. Entries contain detailed information on services, credentials, staffing, admission restrictions, special programs, contact names, phone numbers, and addresses.

Children of Aging Parents (CAP)
1609 Woodbourne Road
Woodbourne Office Campus
Suite 302-A
Levittown, PA 19067
215-945-6900

A national organization providing education, information, and referrals on elder care. Peer counseling and support groups are available to assist family caregivers.

Children's Hospice International
901 North Washington Street
Alexandria, VA 22314
703-684-0330

A non-profit organization that provides medical and technical assistance, treatment referrals, education, and research on hospice care for children.

Disabilities Resources, Inc. (DRI)
Four Glatter Lane
Centerreach, NY 11720-1032

A non-profit organization established to promote and improve awareness, availability, and accessibility of information to persons with disabilities to help them "live, learn, love, work, and play independently". DRI publishes the *Disability Resource Monthly*, a subscription newsletter that monitors, previews, and reports on resources for independent living.

Disability Connection
Apple Worldwide Disability Solutions Group
20525 Mariani Avenue
Cupertino, CA 95014

An on-line source of information and forum for networking for people with disabilities. The Disability Connection is available as part of e-World, Apple's global on-line information and electronic mail service. It features resources from some of the world's leading disabilities and rehabilitation organizations. Features of the electronic forum include: Exceptional Parent Forum, Assistive Technology Center, The Trace R&D Center Forum, Meeting Centers, and Face to Face, a forum to connect users with disability vendors, organizations, and advocacy groups.

Disability, Pregnancy, and Parenthood International
Auburn Press Inc.
9954 South Walnut Terrace, # 201
Palos Hills, IL 60465
515-276-1233

This quarterly publication focuses on the interests and needs of parents and prospective parents with disabilities. Included are personal accounts, conference reports, book reviews, and articles.

Epilepsy Foundation of America (EFA)
4351 Garden City Drive
Landover, MD 20785
301-459-3700
800-332-1000

EFA is a national, non-profit organization for persons with epilepsy, their families, and the professionals who work with them. Public education, consumer advocacy, treatment referrals, phone counseling, and support groups are provided. Educational publications, information packets, and newsletters are available.

Family Survival Project
425 Bush Street
Suite 500
San Francisco, CA 94108
415-434-3388
800-445-8106

A resource center for families, friends, and professionals who are caregivers for adults with brain injuries. Fact sheets and consultations on legal, financial, and respite care concerns are available.

Gay Men's Health Crisis, Inc. (GMHC)
129 West 20th Street
New York, NY 10011
212-807-6655

GMHC is a comprehensive, non-profit, educational and health care organization serving persons with AIDS of all ages, regardless of sexual orientation. GMHC develops and distributes material that address the various aspects of AIDS (general information, risk reduction, medical and psychological issues, testing, health insurance, legal concerns, etc.) to fulfill the needs of different audiences. It conducts public forums, seminars for health care professionals, workshops for people at risk, and educational research programs. GMHC also provides support services for all people with AIDS, which includes crisis intervention counseling; a "buddy" program (helping with daily living tasks); recreational programs; pediatrics programs; support and therapy groups (for people with AIDS and their care partners); and legal, financial, and health care advocacy.

Handykapppers, Inc.
P.O. Box 4294
Naperville, IL 60567-42
708-350-5263

A consumer-owned company specializing in educational seminars and videotapes designed to help persons utilizing wheelchairs adjust to their physical challenges.

Helen Keller National Center for Deaf-Blind Youths and Adults (HKNC)
111 Middle Neck Road
Sands Point, NY 11050-1299
516-944-8900 (Voice)
516-944-8637 (TTY)

HKNC provides diagnostic evaluation, shortterm comprehensive rehabilitation and personal adjustment training, work experience, and placement. Services in the field include 10 regional offices, some 40 affiliated agencies, a National Training Team, Services for Older Adults Who Are DeafBlind, and a Technical Assistance Center. The Center maintains a national register of deafblind persons, conducts research to develop and/or modify aids and devices for the deafblind population, provides community education, publishes a national magazine, and provides publications on curriculum and services. HKNC's role is to ensure that people who are deaf-blind receive the skills training and supports necessary to enable them to live and work in the community of their choice.

Help for Incontinent People, Inc. (HIP)
P.O. Box 544
Union, SC 29739
803-579-7900
800-BLADDER

A not-for-profit organization dedicated to improving the quality of life for people with incontinence. HIP functions as a clearinghouse of information and services on incontinence for consumers, their families, and health care professionals. It provides education, advocacy, and support about the causes, prevention, diagnoses, treatment, and management alternatives for incontinence. The *Resource Guide of Incontinent Products and Services*, a newsletter, audio/visual programs, and educational leaflets are available.

Helping Hands: Simian Aides for the Disabled, Inc.
1505 Commonwealth Avenue
Boston, MA 02135
617-787-4419

A non-profit organization that trains capuchin monkeys to provide skilled assistance to quadriplegics, enabling them to perform numerous activities of daily living independently.

Huntington's Disease Society of America
Dept. P
140 W. 22nd Street
New York, NY 10011
800-345-4372

A non-profit organization devoted to research education and the provision of services to persons with Huntington disease, and their families.

International Hearing Dog, Inc.
5901 East 89th Avenue
Henderson, CO 80640
303-287-3277

A non-profit organization that trains dogs to respond to sounds in the home. The "hearing ear" dogs are placed free with individuals who are deaf or hearing impaired, increasing their safety and independence.

Learning Disabilities Association (LDA)
4156 Library Road
Pittsburgh, PA 15234
412-341-1515

LDA is a private, non-profit organization devoted to providing support and advocacy services for children and adults with learning disabilities. Informational and referral services are provide to consumers, families, and professionals. State and local chapters, a national legislative committee, bimonthly newsbriefs, and an annual conference are available.

Let's Face It
P.O. Box 711
Concord, MA 01742
508-371-3186

An international mutual self-help organization dedicated to helping people with facial difference, their families, and the professionals who work with them to understand and solve the problems of living with facial disfigurement.

Life Services for the Handicapped, Inc.
352 Park Avenue South
Suite 703
New York, NY 10010-1709
212-532-6740

A non-profit organization that has set up a discretionary trust fund and life service program to enable families to leave resources to their children with disabilities without their children losing public entitlements. Assistance to help families plan for the longterm, life-care needs of their family members with disabilities is available. A quarterly newsletter, Life Lines, provides current information on long-term care issues, trends, benefits, and programs.

Lighthouse National Programs
Lighthouse National Center for Vision and Aging
Lighthouse National Center for Vision and Child
 Development
800 Second Avenue
New York, NY 10017
212-808-0077
212-808-5544 (TDD)
800-334-5497

A non-profit rehabilitation organization that provides information and resources for care across the United States for persons with visual impairments. Patient clinics, technical assistance, consultation, professional training, and professional and public education through print and audiovisual publications are provided.

Lupus Foundation of America
1717 Massachusetts Avenue, N.W.
Washington, DC 20036
800-558-0121

A non-profit organization providing funds for research, education, and patient and family information. Support groups are available for persons with systemic lupus erythematsus and related disorders.

Muscular Dystrophy Association (MDA)

3300 East Sunrise Drive
Tucson, AZ 85718
602-529-2000

A non-profit organization funding research to find potential cures and effective treatments for 40 neuromuscular disorders. Local chapters provide a diversity of services to patients and their families. Services include diagnostic clinics; occupational, physical, and speech therapy; genetic counseling; equipment supplies and repairs; support groups for patients and their families; and summer camp programs for persons aged 6 to 21. Information packets on many neuromuscular disorders, MDA research, and services are available.

National Organization for Rare Disorders (NORD)

P.O. Box 8923
New Fairfield, CT 06812-1783
203-746-6518

NORD is a private, non-profit, health-care service that serves as an information clearinghouse on rare disorders. (Rare disorders are defined as those affecting 200,000 people or fewer). Individualized information packets on symptoms, treatment, research, support groups, and self-help organizations are provided for a multitude of rare disorders. NORD will research consumer requests and help members and/or their families network with persons who are affected with the same or similar rare disorder.

National Information Center on Deafness

Gallaudet University
800 Florida Avenue, N.E.
Washington, DC 20002
202-651-5051

A private information and referral service for persons who are deaf or hearing impaired. Resource listings and fact sheets are available.

National Organization on Disability (NOD)

910 16th Street, N.W.
Suite 600
Washington, DC 20006
202-293-5960
800-248-ABLE

A private, non-profit organization that aims to increase acceptance of all men, women, and children with physical or mental disabilities and to increase their participation in every aspect of life. Educational publications, training manuals, technical assistance, and a computerized database are available. Special emphasis is placed on local community integration for persons with disabilities through a national network of Community Partnership Programs.

National Rehabilitation Association (NRA)

1910 Association Drive
Suite 205
Reston, VA 22091-1502
703-715-9090

A national membership organization of consumers, family members, and professionals interested in the advocacy of programs and services for people with disabilities. Special divisions include the National Association for Independent Living, the Job Placement Division, the National Association of Rehabilitation Instructors, the National Association of Service Providers in Private Rehabilitation, and the Vocational Evaluation and Work Adjustment Association. State, regional, and national conferences, educational seminars, and numerous publications, including the Journal of Rehabilitation, Rehab USA, and NRA Newsletter, are available to members.

National Stroke Association

300 East Hampden Avenue
Englewood, CO 80110-2622
303-762-9922

A non-profit organization whose aim is to reduce the incidence and severity of stroke through prevention, treatment, rehabilitation, and research. Professional and consumer education, print, and audiovisual publications, family, and self-help groups, and a quarterly newsletter are provided.

National Self-Help Clearinghouse

25 West 43rd Street
New York, NY 10036
212-642-2944

A national clearinghouse providing information and referrals on self-help groups and organizations. Publications and resource lists are available.

National Osteogenesis Imperfecta Foundation, Inc. (OIF)

P.O. Box 14807
Clearwater, FL 34629-4087
813-855-7077

A national voluntary organization dedicated to serving the needs of individuals with Osteogenesis Imperfecta (OI) or Brittle Bone Disorder. Services include a quarterly newsletter, extensive literature, educational videos, a nationwide parent contact network, and national conferences.

National Multiple Sclerosis Society

733 3rd Avenue
New York, NY 10017
800-624-8236
212-986-3240

A non-profit organization dedicated to serving persons with Multiple Sclerosis (MS) and their families, while supporting research to find the cure for and cause of MS. National, regional, and local chapters provide a wide range of direct services to clients and their families, including medical clinics, support groups, individual counseling, career development services, water therapy, occupational therapy, home health aide assistance, recreational programs, transportation assistance, equipment loan programs, a mail-order prescription plan, and advocacy services. Print and video publications, professional education and training programs, a newsletter, and a journal are available to members.

National Alliance for the Mentally Ill

2101 Wilson Boulevard
Suite 302
Arlington, VA 22201
800-950-NAMI

NAMI is a self-help, support, and advocacy organization for persons with mental illnesses, their families and friends, and concerned professionals. NAMI provides educational publications, informational packets, audiovisuals, and research support on a multitude of topics. Its goals are to enable members to share concerns, learn about mental illnesses, and receive practical advice on treatment and community resources. Special interest networks offer additional support regarding children and adolescents, consumers (patients), culture and language concerns, curriculum and training (for professionals), forensic issues, guardianships and trusts, the homeless and missing, religious outreach, siblings and adult children, and veterans. NAMI is a strong advocate for improved services for persons with severe mental illnesses and for increased research into the causes and treatments of mental illnesses.

National Information Center for Children and Youth with Disabilities (NICHCY)

(Acronym refers to previous name)
P.O. Box 1492
Washington, DC 20013
800-999-5599
703-893-6061

NICHCY provides free information to assist parents, educators, care-givers, advocates, and others in helping children and youth with disabilities become participating members of the community. As a national information clearinghouse, NICHCY maintains databases with current information on disability topics; provides information on local , state, and/or national disability groups for parents and professionals; distributes information packets on a multitude of disabilities; and provides technical assistance to parent and professional groups NICHCY publishes *News Digest*, an issue paper that compiles articles on current research and relevant program information, and *Transition Summary*, which reports on current effective practices that assist persons with disabilities in the transition from school to work, other postsecondary programs, and to independent living in the community.

National Association for Visually Handicapped (NAVH)

22 West 21st Street
New York, NY 10010
212-889-3141

NAVH is a non-profit organization that serves as a national information and referral agency for all partially sighted (not totally blind) persons. It offers large-print textbooks, testing materials, visual aids, leisure reading, largeprint periodic newsletters for adults and children, and informational literature for the partially sighted and their families, and the professionals and paraprofessionals working with them.

National Aphasia Association

Murray Hill Station
P.O. Box 1807
New York, NY 10156-0611
800-922-4622

A non-profit organization devoted to increasing the public's awareness of aphasia and providing information and service referrals to persons with aphasia, and their families. Information packets, reading lists, communication hints, newsletters, and local support groups are available.

National Association for the Dually Diagnosed (NADD)

110 Prince Street
Kingston, NY 12401
800-331-5362

A multidisciplinary membership association devoted to serving those who have both mental illness and mental retardation. Newsletters, regional and local workshops, a national conference, and information dissemination are provided.

National Ataxia Foundation (NAF)

750 Twelve Oaks Center
15500 Wayzata Boulevard
Wayzata, MN 55391
612-473-7666

A non-profit organization serving individuals with hereditary ataxia, and their families. NAF provides educational publications and referral services to patients, families, and health care professionals. Genetic counseling and research are strongly supported, as there is no screening test, cure, or effective treatment for the hereditary ataxias.

National Association for Parents of the Visually Impaired

P.O. Box 317
Watertown, MA 02272-0317
800-562-6265

A self-help organization that addresses the needs of parents and families of visually impaired children and promotes public understanding of the needs and rights of the child with a visual impairment. Six regional support networks are available.

National Head Injury Foundation
1140 Connecticut Avenue, N.W.
Suite 812
Washington, DC 20036
202-296-6443
800-444-6443

A national, non-profit organization devoted to issues affecting persons with brain injuries, and their families. The dissemination of information, educational resources, publications, and referrals are provided.

National Easter Seal Society
70 East Lake Street
Chicago, IL 60601
312-726-6200
800-221-6827

A national, non-profit organization dedicated to helping people with disabilities achieve maximum independence. Prevention programs, rehabilitation services, technological assistance, public education, and advocacy services are provided through a nationwide network of affiliates and chapters. An extensive library, including print and audiovisual publications on diagnostic and clinical topics, caregiving, and the Americans with Disabilities (ADA) may be accessed.

National Diabetes Information Clearinghouse
P.O. Box NDIC
9000 Rockville Pike
Bethesda, MD 20892
301-468-2162

A national informational and referral service on diabetes and its complications for consumers, their families, professionals, and the general public. Topical bibliographies, educational publications, conference proceedings, and monographs are available.

National Depressive and Manic-Depressive Association
(NDMDA)
730 North Franklin
Suite 501
Chicago, IL 60610
312-642-0049

A non-profit organization dedicated to improving the availability and quality of health care, eliminating discrimination and stigma, and developing and maintaining support groups for persons with depressive and/or manic-depressive illnesses. Research and partnerships with professionals are also emphasized. Informational literature, a newsletter, audiovisuals, service referrals, research support, a national clearinghouse, and an annual conference are available.

National Down Syndrome Congress
1800 Dempster Street
Park Ridge, IL 60068-1146
800-232-NDSC

A private, non-profit, national organization serving individuals of all ages who have Down syndrome, and their families. Educational information and a referral service are available.

Orton Dyslexia Society
Chester Building
Suite 382
8600 La Salle Road
Baltimore, MD 21284
410-296-0232

A membership organization that provides information on dyslexia to the general public, consumers, families, and professionals. Regional and national conferences, a quarterly newsletter, and an annual scholarly journal are available to members.

Paralyzed Veterans of America
801 18th Street, N.W.
Washington, DC 20006
202-USA-1300
800-424-8200

A national organization dedicated to ensuring that veterans with paralysis receive all the benefits and services they are entitled to. Patient education, medical research, consumer advocacy, accessibility, legal assistance, and sports programs are emphasized. The monthly journal *Paraplegia News*, the bimonthly *Sports and Spokes*, and many educational publications are available to members.

Recovery, Inc.
802 North Dearborn Street
Chicago, IL 60610
312-337-5661

An international self-help organization for former patients and other persons with mental health problems. Recovery stresses cooperation and education with professionals. Its purpose is to prevent relapses and to forestall chronicity in former and current patients. Literature, weekly meetings, and panel demonstrations are available.

Self-Help for Hard-of-Hearing People
7800 Wisconsin Avenue
Bethesda, MD 20814
301-657-2248
301-657-2249 (TDD)

A non-profit, consumer organization dedicated to serving the needs of people with hearing loss, their families, and their friends. Public education, advocacy, treatment referrals, support groups, and research funding into the causes and potential cures for hearing loss are provided.

Siblings for Significant Change
105 East 22nd Street
New York, NY 10010
212-420-0776

Siblings for Significant Change is a non-profit organization designed to unite siblings of individuals with disabilities, to advocate for services, and to improve conditions for their families. The dissemination of information, a speaker's bureau, conferences, and workshops are provided to promote greater public awareness of the needs of the disabled and their families.

Support Dogs for the Handicapped, Inc.

301 Sovereign
Suite 113
St. Louis, MO 63011
314-394-6163

An organization that trains dogs to help persons with disabilities perform activities of daily living and maintain functional independence.

Support Source

420 Rutgers Avenue
Swarthmore, PA 19081
215-544-3605

Publisher of caregiver education manuals and caregiver seminar workbooks.

The Association for Persons with Severe Handicaps (TASH)

11201 Greenwood Avenue North
Seattle, WA 98133
206-361-8870

TASH is an international non-profit membership organization dedicated to improving the quality of life and providing education and advocacy for persons with severe cognitive disabilities. A monthly newsletter, the quarterly *Journal for Persons with Severe Handicaps*, numerous print and audiovisual publications, and an annual conference are provided to members.

The Long-Term Care Campaign

P.O. Box 27394
Washington, DC 20038
202-393-2092

The Long-Term Care Campaign is a coalition of 140 national organizations, including AOTA, dedicated to enacting comprehensive legislation to protect American families against the devastating costs of long-term care. Professional and consumer information, and print and audiovisual publications are available.

The Sibling Information Network

The A.J. Pappanikou Center
991 Main Street
East Hartford, CT 06108
203-282-7050

The Network serves as a clearinghouse of information, ideas, projects, literature, and research regarding siblings and other issues related to the needs of families with members who have disabilities. A newsletter containing program descriptions, requests for assistance, conference announcements, reviews of research, literature summaries, discussion articles, and research reports is published quarterly. A newsletter insert specifically for children ages 5 through 15, called "SIBPAGE" is also available.

The National Council on the Aging, Inc. (NCOA)

409 Third Street, S.W.
Washington, DC 20024
202-479-1200

A private, non-profit, membership organization committed to improving the lives of older persons, NCOA serves as a national source of information, training, technical assistance, advocacy, and research on virtually every aspect of aging. Specialized units focus on the areas of adult day care, community-based long-term care, seniors centers, senior housing, health promotion, rural aging, older worker employment, spirituality and aging, and financial services for elders. A bimonthly magazine, *Perspective on Aging*, the quarterly *Abstracts in Social Gerontology: Current Literature on Aging*, the bimonthly NCOA Networks, and numerous publications, workshops, and conferences are available to members.

United Cerebral Palsy, Inc. (UCP)

1522 K Street, N.W.
Suite 1112
Washington, DC 20005
202-371-0622

A private, non-profit, national organization serving adults and children with cerebral palsy, their families, and the professionals who work with them. Educational information, treatment referrals, and advocacy services are available. Services provided by local chapters include early intervention programs, summer camps, assisted living programs, family support groups, and peer counseling. Emphasis is placed on community integration, competitive employment opportunities, and the utilization of environmental control units and assistive technologies to maximize the independence and quality of life for persons with cerebral palsy.

Video Press

University of Maryland
School of Medicine
Suite 133
100 Penn Street
Baltimore, MD 21201-1082
800-328-7450
410-706-5497

This service offers sales and rentals of award winning videocassettes for health professionals and educators. An extensive collection is available with an emphasis on gerontology, long-term care, mental health, terminal illness, and pediatrics. Many focus on quality of life issues; providing case studies and documentaries of clients and caregivers.

Well Spouse Foundation (WSF)
P.O. Box 28876
San Diego, CA 92198-0876
619-673-9043

WSF is a non-profit, national organization with more than 50 regional support groups, devoted to meeting the needs of the 7 to 9 million individuals who care for spouses with chronic illness or disability. Support groups, networking contacts, monthly bulletins, and a quarterly newsletter are available to give emotional support, and to raise consciousness about and advocate for the spouses and children of the chronically ill.

Index

Humanistic values, reimbursement, disparity, 595–598

Humanistic-valued practice, 595–596

Humor, 489–492

  elements, 490–491

  seminar and workshop presentations, 491–492

  state of the art, 490–491

  therapeutic relationship, 323

I

Identification group, 289–292

  defined, 290

  development theory, 290

  occupational therapy method, 296

  social activity club, 202

  sociological framework, 296

  theoretical basis, 289–292

  theoretical model, 290

Identity, adolescent, 266

Illness experience, disease, contrasted, 353

Imagery

  elderly, 519–524

  purpose, 519–524

  repetitive exercise, 519–524

Immigrant, culture, 165–166

Inclusion, 229

  communication, 236

  interactive strategies, 236–238

  nature, 232–234

Inclusion movement, 233

Inclusive community, 229–239

  historical aspects, 230

  importance, 230

  value-based practices, 234

Individualizing treatment, 344

Individuals with Disabilities Education Act, 233

Industrial Rehabilitation Act, 20

Insanity

  moral treatment, 40

    new therapeutic environments, 41–42

  philosophy, 40

Institutionalization, elderly, effects, 210

Integration, defined, 578

Intention, automation interaction, 246

Interaction planning

  terminology, 659–660

  Uniform Terminology for Occupational Therapy, 659–660

Interactive reasoning, 344–346

  interpersonal intelligence, 345

  perspectives, 344

  values, 345

Interest

  defined, 300

  determinants, 300

  elderly, 300

Interpersonal intelligence, interactive reasoning, 345

Interpersonal relatedness domain, Life Style Performance Model, 119

Intrapersonal communication, 237

Intrinsic gratification domain, Life Style Performance Model, 118

J

Johnson, Susan Cox, 19–20

Justice, 636

K

Kidner, Thomas Bessell, 20–21

Kinetic analysis, 401

Knowing, 201

  philosophy, 202

Knowledge, clinical reasoning, 329, 332–333

L

Language, 592

Lathrop, Julia, 32

Lazarus Project, 209–215

  community model, 212–213

    building, 214

    concept development, 213–214

    implementation, 213–214